COMPLETE GUIDE TO
SYMPTOMS, ILLNESS & SURGERY

D0574967

COMPLETE GUIDE TO
SYMPTOMS, ILLNESS & SURGERY

Where does it hurt? What does it mean?
A doctor answers your questions.

H. Winter Griffith, M.D.

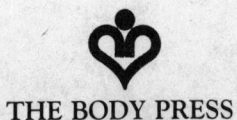

THE BODY PRESS

Cover Photo: Balfour Walker

Published by The Body Press, a division of Price Stern Sloan, Inc.
360 North La Cienega Boulevard
Los Angeles, California 90048

ISBN: 0-89586-334-0
Library of Congress Catalog Card Number: 85-80120
©1985 HPBooks, Inc.
Printed in U.S.A.

Notice: The information in this book is true and complete to the best of our knowledge. The book is intended only as a supplementary guide to medical treatment. It is not intended as a replacement for sound medical advice from a doctor. Only a doctor can include the variables of an individual's age, sex and past medical history needed for proper medical care. This book does not contain every possible factor relating to medical symptoms, illnesses or surgeries. Important decisions about treating an ill person must be made by the individual and his doctor. All recommendations herein are made without guarantees on the part of the author, the technical consultants or Price Stern Sloan. The author and publisher disclaim all liability with the use of this information.

15 14 13 12 11

Contents

About the Author

H. Winter Griffith, M.D., a Fellow of the American Academy of Family Practice, has authored several medical books, including the best-selling *Complete Guide to Prescription & Non-Prescription Drugs,* published by HPBooks, Inc. He also wrote three editions of *Instructions for Patients, Drug Information for Patients, Instructions for Dental Patients, Information and Instructions for Pediatric Patients* and *Pediatrics for Parents.* Dr. Griffith received his medical degree from Emory University in 1953. After 20 years in private practice, he established a basic medical-science program at Florida State University. He then became an Associate Professor of Family and Community Medicine at the University of Arizona College of Medicine.

Technical Consultants

Daniel Levinson, M.D.
Associate Professor of Family and Community Medicine, University of Arizona College of Medicine.
Fellow of the American Board of Family Practice.

Evan W. Kligman, M.D.
Medical Director, Geriatrics Primary Care Centers, Department of Family and Community Medicine, University of Arizona College of Medicine.
Diplomate of the American Board of Family Practice.

Donald J. McFarlane, M.D.
Clinical Professor, University of Arizona College of Medicine.
Fellow of the American College of Surgeons.

Sally Watkins, R.N.
Head Nurse, Family Practice Residency Program, University of Arizona College of Medicine.
Member of the Health Education Committee, Family Practice Office, University of Arizona College of Medicine.

Preface

I first came across Winter Griffith's name when asked to take over the U.S. Food and Drug Administration's patient information program. When reviewing correspondence from the 1960s, I found a letter from a Florida doctor asking if there was any problem in distributing written drug information to patients.

As far as I know, no one had previously thought of providing specific written information to patients. This was Dr. Griffith's idea and goal, and it has become his lifelong mission.

Until the 1970s, patient education consisted of doctors patting patients on their heads and telling them to call if they had problems. Doctors did not discuss risks and side effects of drugs for fear of how patients would react.

Some doctors still have this attitude. But most doctors and patients recognize that information about risks and benefits of drug treatment is not only a patient's right, it is a *patient's responsibility*. Taking care of oneself means active participation in treatment decisions. Promoting participation between doctor and patient is the purpose of this book.

Winter Griffith is the godfather of patient education. His first books were compilations of simple instruction sheets that doctors could hand out to patients. The sheets contained information the doctor wanted patients to know about illness and treatment. These instruction sheets are still copied an average of 16 million times a year and distributed to patients.

Dr. Griffith's later books have evolved to contain information the patient wants to know! Over the years, Dr. Griffith has come to understand people's needs for accurate, understandable information.

Some doctors think patients want to make their own decisions about health care, so they try to control the amount of information patients receive. Dr. Griffith understands that people want to decide *with* their doctors about treatment and other decisions affecting their health.

This book is a patient-advocate bible. It provides the information people want about symptoms, illnesses and surgeries.

The beauty of this book is that it explains what happens to the patient, why it happens, what risks are involved, what to expect in diagnosis and treatment, and how to monitor treatment.

The book is chock-full of usable information. Dr. Griffith has mastered the art of transmitting technical information. There is no medical jargon—just solid, helpful facts.

I could not end this preface without a personal note about the author. I tend to distrust most people in the patient education field. "Do-gooders" sometimes have hidden agendas. After more than a decade of working closely with Dr. Griffith as colleague and friend, I haven't discovered his hidden agenda. I have come to believe that he is what he says he is. Dr. Griffith sees his role as a medical missionary, translating sound medical advice into useful information. I hope everyone who uses this book feels the author's genuine warmth and concern that radiate from its pages.

Louis A. Morris, Ph.D.
Head, Patient Education, Research, and Labeling Branch
U.S. Food and Drug Administration

Take Care of Yourself

As a patient, you can and should share responsibility with your doctor for your medical care. Knowing the "what," "why," and "how" of an illness enables you to get maximum benefit from your medical treatment.

Several years ago, I set a personal goal to translate complicated, technical medical information into up-to-date, easily understood information that any interested layman could use. *Complete Guide to Prescription and Non-Prescription Drugs,* published by HPBooks in 1983, was a major step toward that goal. The public's response to that effort has been overwhelmingly positive.

This book is another major step. It has evolved out of more than 25 years as a family doctor and teacher, answering questions of patients and medical students.

CHANGING TIMES

Early in my practice, patients would come to me for help with the attitude, "Do something to make me better." At that time, my attitude—and that of most colleagues—was, "Do what I tell you and things will get better—but don't ask too many questions. A little knowledge is a dangerous thing." We had been trained to be authoritarian in our dealings with patients.

These attitudes are self-defeating. Fortunately, they are changing, and enlightened medical professionals welcome this change as an important way to improve health care.

Many thoughtful and assertive patients have taught us they wish to be more involved. They don't want to be passive and powerless in matters that affect their own bodies. They don't want instructions or advice that is incomplete or lacking in credibility. They seek—and sometimes demand—enough information so they can think for themselves and participate in important medical decisions affecting them.

I wrote this book—with the help of many friends—for those persons who want additional responsibility for their own health and that of their families.

THE INFORMATION GAP

The information in this book barely scratches the surface of all information in medical literature. It is a scant amount of the knowledge doctors have acquired. In addition to a medical education, most doctors have extensive clinical experience—and ideally, a great deal of wisdom and compassion.

But somehow, and sometimes for justifiable reason, a doctor's medical information does not get translated and transmitted into usable form for the most important member of the health-care team—the patient.

Even when information *is* competently conveyed to the patient by a doctor, nurse or other health professional, the patient has no follow-up written checklist to remind and reinforce what he or she has learned. This book is intended to provide you with the missing checklist and to supplement information you have received from your doctor.

SIMPLE, CONCISE INFORMATION

Condensing the available mass of medical and surgical knowledge into one volume has required much simplification. I have tried not to omit major facts and concepts, but of necessity, many details have been left out.

It is impossible to include all the factors and circumstances that affect each individual's health. Thus, your doctor may take into account other factors not included here when he or she makes a precise diagnosis and recommends treatment for you.

WHAT YOU CAN FIND IN THIS BOOK

This book contains three major sections: Symptoms, Illnesses and Disorders, and Surgeries. Information for each is organized in chart form. The three chart formats vary somewhat, and each format is explained in detail in the following pages.

The book contains an appendix section to supplement information in the charts. General instructions that apply to many illnesses or disorders need not be repeated on each chart, so they are included in the general appendix section.

The 21 appendix entries include: a number of special diets; suggestions to reduce stress and maximize longevity; instructions for breast self-exam, back care and exercise programs; an immunization schedule; directions for reducing fever, preparing hot and cold soaks and taking care of casts; and guidelines for safe drug use.

A special feature of the book is a list of resources for additional information. If you want more, in-depth information about symptoms, illnesses, surgeries or other medical problems discussed in this book, the list provides a starting place to find more information.

The resource list contains names and addresses of volunteer and government health agencies devoted to specific disorders. It also contains a list of recent medical books available in most public libraries.

WHAT YOU CAN'T FIND IN THIS BOOK

This book will not help you diagnose or treat your own illnesses very often. Printed words cannot replace the knowledge and expertise that your doctor provides.

A book is no substitute for communication between you and your doctor. Only your doctor knows your medical history and special circumstances. Only you know the intensity and exact quality of your symptoms. The printed page cannot capture or convey the *feelings* that accompany illness.

HOW YOU WILL BENEFIT

Yet, armed with introductory knowledge about diseases and surgical procedures discussed in this book, you are in a strong position in the following ways:

• You can better understand the nature of your illness.
• You can more easily recognize circumstances when a doctor's help is necessary.
• You can learn useful facts about how to prevent disease and injury.
• You can confirm and refresh your memory about facts regarding your illness.
• You can review a checklist of ways to make yourself better if you are ill.
• You can discuss issues with your doctor when treatment outlined in the book differs from what your doctor advises. Doctors do not always agree on the best course of treatment for a particular illness. When information from different medical sources has varied, I have tried to provide the general, up-to-date medical consensus.

If your doctor's recommendations differ, they may be very valid. However, you should feel free to explore the options with your doctor. He or she should welcome and answer your questions. If not, consider consulting another doctor.

I believe your best chance to achieve and maintain optimal health is to participate fully in taking care of yourself. I hope this book provides a tool to help you reach that goal.

Guide to Symptom Charts

The symptom charts are designed to suggest one or more illnesses and disorders that a specific symptom might indicate. Each chart focuses on one common symptom. For example, the chart for *excessive sweating* appears on the facing page.

These charts do not include every possible sign or symptom the human body can exhibit, but they represent the most familiar and easily recognizable ones.

The charts provide a guide for how serious symptoms are. They give you clues as to what symptoms can mean. They refer you to other sections of the book for further information. *However, they are not intended as self-diagnosis charts.* No book should replace a competent doctor's diagnosis! The charts are only to help you decide how to proceed when you or someone else develops symptoms.

Refer to the numbers on the sample chart for an explanation of each heading described below.

1—SYMPTOM NAME

Charts are titled and arranged alphabetically by the name that is most common or that best describes the symptom (**SWEATING, EXCESSIVE**).

In cases where the symptom name is ambiguous, or the symptom can apply to several parts of the body, the body part is part of the title. For example, **SWELLING** (a symptom) appears as separate charts titled: **ABDOMINAL SWELLING; ANKLES, SWOLLEN; SWELLING OR LUMP;** and **TESTICLES, PAINFUL OR SWOLLEN.** One chart is alphabetized by the symptom name, **SWELLING.** The rest are alphabetized by the body part the swelling affects.

If you can't find your symptom under its own name, refer to the index or check alphabetically for the main part of the body it affects.

2—SYMPTOMS & FACTORS

The main symptom is grouped in the first column with other symptoms or factors that frequently accompany it. Each group represents a separate illness or disorder that the symptom can indicate.

For instance, excessive sweating can mean many things, depending on what other symptoms appear with it. When accompanied by chest pain, excessive sweating can be a sign of heart attack, the first entry. When accompanied instead by weight loss, coughing with blood, fever and fatigue, the second entry, it can be a strong indication of serious lung disorders. The third entry relating to a disorder of the thyroid gland presents yet another possibility.

The symptom groups are arranged in order from the most serious possible illness to the least serious. This is merely an approximation, as it varies with individuals.

For example, heart attack is listed first on the sample chart as the gravest emergency. Symptoms of tuberculosis,

SWEATING, EXCESSIVE

SYMPTOMS & FACTORS	POSSIBLE PROBLEM	WHAT TO DO*
• Excessive sweating. • Chest pain.	Heart attack.	• Call doctor now! • See Heart Attack. • See Coronary-Artery Disease.
• Excessive sweating at night. • Weight loss. • Persistent cough with blood in sputum. • Fever. • Fatigue.	• Lung inflammation or infection. • Cancer.	• See Tuberculosis. • See Hodgkin's Disease. • See Lung Cancer.
• Excessive sweating, plus 2 or more of following: • Weight loss. • Increased appetite. • Anxiety. • Sleeping problems.	Overactive thyroid gland.	See Hyperthyroidism.
• Excessive sweating. • Use of prescription, non-prescription or illegal drug.	Adverse reaction or side effect of drug.	• Consult doctor about prescription drug. • Discontinue use of non-prescription or illegal drug.
• Excessive sweating. • Fever.	Normal occurrence with fever.	See Fever charts (in Symptoms section).
• Excessive sweating. • Anxiety or excitement.	Normal occurrence with stress.	See Anxiety.
• Excessive sweating. • Overweight.	Effect of excess weight.	See Obesity.
• Excessive sweating in woman older than 38. • Irregular menstrual periods.	Hormone changes; end of menstrual cycles approaching.	See Menopause.
Excessive sweating in woman during menstrual period.	No underlying disorder.	Nothing.
• Excessive sweating. • Use of synthetic material, such as nylon, for clothing or blankets.	Increased skin heat.	Wear natural fibers. such as cotton.
Excessive sweating in teenager.	Normal occurrence during adolescence.	Nothing.

*All references are to Illness section unless noted otherwise.

SYMPTOMS 99

Hodgkin's disease and lung cancer, the second entry, can also be life-threatening. However, these conditions usually deteriorate slowly and don't pose immediate danger. Therefore, they appear below heart attack. Obviously, this judgment can vary between individuals. When in doubt, consult your doctor.

Often, none of the symptom groups will match your present problem. Your doctor knows your medical history and can perform a physical examination and use laboratory tests to diagnose your condition.

3—POSSIBLE PROBLEM

The center column provides a short description of what a symptom group can indicate and what major body parts it affects. This column also briefly defines the illness or disorder to which you are referred in the third column.

In some cases, a group of symptoms can indicate more than one illness—sometimes they are totally unrelated. In that event, each description is listed next to an editor's bullet. For instance, the second group of symptoms that we have discussed can indicate lung inflammation or infection, or cancer.

No attempt has been made to include every possible illness or disorder signaled by a symptom group. The identifications are based on illnesses that are *most obvious, most common or most serious*. For similar reasons, many rare illnesses described on illness charts in this book have not been referred to on symptom charts.

4—WHAT TO DO

The most serious medical problems that require immediate help are listed first in the third column. They usually are preceded by directions to call your doctor *now*. Below that, you will often be directed to the illness chart in this book that explains the problem. For instance, the first entry has the instructions:

- Call doctor now!
- See Heart Attack.
- See Coronary-Artery Disease.

All "See . . ." instructions refer to illness charts. Exceptions to this rule will be noted on the symptom chart.

If the chart says "Call doctor now," don't waste precious time looking up the illness in this book. Wait to read more about it when the crisis has passed. Call your doctor immediately!

If anyone develops dramatic symptoms that you think represent life-threatening danger, call for *emergency help*. Dial 0 or 911 and report your address or location (with directions).

In extreme situations, render what first aid you can, such as giving cardiopulmonary resuscitation (CPR). Yell for help from anyone within range.

Additional emergency information appears on pages 893 to 896.

Guide to Illness & Disorder Charts

The information about illnesses and disorders is organized in condensed, easy-to-read charts.

Each one is described in a one-page format shown in the sample chart, **HYPERTHYROIDISM,** on page 15.

Major sections of the chart format are numbered and explained in the next few pages.

Most of the charts in this section refer to an illness. In some cases, however, charts refer to disorders or problems that are not really illnesses. The chart, **TEETHING,** is not about a disease—or even a disorder. It deals with a normal process that all people experience. It would be a disorder only if it did *not* occur.

But teething can be a medical problem. It often affects an infant's sense of well-being, and it may require treatment. Because teething is so common, and because some treatments for it are appropriate and others are not, it is included with illness charts.

1—CHART NAME

Charts are arranged alphabetically by the most-common name for the illness, disorder or medical problem. Other names for these appear in parentheses below the main heading. Hyperthyroidism does not have another name, so it appears alone. However, a disease such as German measles is also known as rubella, and its chart lists both: **GERMAN MEASLES (Rubella).**

Sometimes names for various medical problems vary in different geographic regions. All names in this book, including alternate names, are cross-referenced in the index.

To find information about a medical problem, check the index. You may also look up its major symptom in the symptom charts. If you can't find the illness chart you want, ask your doctor or nurse for alternate names by which the disorder is known.

2—GENERAL INFORMATION

This section includes seven topics: *Definition; Body Parts Involved; Sex or Age Most Affected; Signs and Symptoms; Causes; Risk Increases With;* and *How to Prevent.* Each is discussed separately.

3—DEFINITION

A short definition of the problem or disease is provided. Sometimes the definition must include information from other categories, such as causes, body parts involved and others. The definition may also include information of general interest, such as how common a disease is, or whether it is contagious, cancerous or inherited.

4—BODY PARTS INVOLVED

This is usually a list of specific body parts or organs, such as bones, skin or liver. Sometimes general body systems, such as central nervous system, genitourinary system or gastrointestinal system, will be listed. The list usually includes body parts affected at the beginning of the disease, as many diseases spread to other body parts as they progress.

Of course, some illnesses involve all body cells—even from the beginning. Then the words "Total body" appear.

5—SEX OR AGE MOST AFFECTED

Some medical problems affect specific population groups only. Others affect all ages and both sexes indiscriminately. This section explains whether the medical problem occurs more often in males or females, or whether the incidence is about equal in either sex. It also lists the age group usually affected. These are generalizations, and variations can occur with specific individuals.

Sometimes labels, such as "newborns" or "adolescents," are used to describe age ranges. These labels are arbitrary names for specific ages, but they are commonly used in medical texts. Following are the age classifications:
• Newborns (0 to 2 weeks)
• Infants (2 weeks to 1 year)
• Young children (1 to 5 years)
• Older children (5 to 12 years)
• Adolescents (12 to 20 years)
• Young adults (20 to 40 years)
• Middle-aged adults (40 to 60 years)
• Older adults (over 60 years).

6—SIGNS AND SYMPTOMS

Signs are observed. *Symptoms* are felt or experienced.

A sign may be observed by the patient or by someone else, or it may represent physical findings determined by laboratory tests, X-rays and other diagnostic measures. Symptoms are feelings only the patient can describe.

Refer to the chart. The first item under this heading—hyperactivity— is a sign. It can be observed by the patient and others around him or her.

The next three items—feeling warm or hot all the time, tremors, and sweating—are signs *and* symptoms. They can be observed by others and they can be felt by the patient. The fifth—itching skin—is a symptom that only the patient can feel and describe.

Signs and symptoms are listed together in this book; no attempt is made to separate the two. On most charts, a wide range of possible signs and symptoms are listed. *It is unlikely that any patient will have all, or even most, of the possible signs and symptoms.* The presence or absence of signs and symptoms may vary according to:
• The age and sex of the patient.
• Extent of the illness.
• The stage of the illness.
• Medical and family history.
• Current state of health.

7—CAUSES

Many times the cause of a disorder is unknown. Causes for most medical problems include the following:
• Inherited (congenital) defects.
• Infections from bacteria, viruses, parasites, yeasts or fungi. All of these are sometimes referred to as "germs," but most people associate "germs" with bacteria only.
• Physical injury.
• Toxins (poisons) from a wide range of sources, such as contaminated food, environmental pollution and bites from poisonous snakes or insects.
• Allergies.
• Tumors. These may be benign or malignant. Benign tumors do not spread to adjacent or distant organs and threaten life. Malignant (cancerous) tumors can.

HYPERTHYROIDISM

GENERAL INFORMATION

DEFINITION—Overactivity of the thyroid, an endocrine gland that regulates all body functions.

BODY PARTS INVOLVED—Thyroid gland and most other body organs, especially the endocrine system, which includes the pituitary gland, parathyroid glands, pancreas, adrenal glands, and ovaries or testicles.

SEX OR AGE MOST AFFECTED—Adults between ages 20 and 50, mostly women.

SIGNS & SYMPTOMS
- Hyperactivity.
- Feeling warm or hot all the time.
- Tremors.
- Sweating.
- Itching skin.
- Pounding, rapid, irregular heartbeat.
- Weight loss, despite overeating. Older persons may gain weight.
- Marked anxiety and restlessness.
- Sleeplessness.
- Fatigue and weakness.
- Protruding eyes (exophthalmos) and double vision (sometimes).
- Diarrhea (sometimes).
- Hair loss (sometimes).
- Goiter (sometimes).

CAUSES
- Thyroid nodules or tumors.
- Pituitary disorders.
- Ovarian disorders.

RISK INCREASES WITH
- Family history of hyperthyroidism.
- Stress.

HOW TO PREVENT—No specific preventive measures.

WHAT TO EXPECT

APPROPRIATE HEALTH CARE
- Self-care after diagnosis.
- Doctor's treatment.
- Surgery to remove part of the thyroid, if medication does not control the disorder.

DIAGNOSTIC MEASURES
- Your own observation of symptoms.
- Medical history and physical exam by a doctor.
- Laboratory blood studies.
- EKG (see Glossary).
- Radioactive studies such as I131 uptake (see Glossary).

POSSIBLE COMPLICATIONS
- Congestive heart failure.
- "Thyroid storm"—a sudden worsening of all symptoms. This is a life-threatening emergency.
- Misdiagnosis as a psychiatric anxiety reaction.

PROBABLE OUTCOME—Usually curable with medication or surgery. Allow 6 months of treatment for the condition to stabilize.

HOW TO TREAT

NOTE—Follow your doctor's instructions. These instructions are supplemental.

GENERAL MEASURES—Since this condition develops gradually, symptoms may be difficult to recognize. If family and friends mention changes in your behavior or appearance, consult your doctor.

MEDICATION—Your doctor may prescribe:
- Antithyroid drugs to depress thyroid activity.
- Beta-adrenergic blockers to decrease a rapid heartbeat.
- Radioactive iodine, which selectively destroys thyroid cells.

ACTIVITY—Rest in bed as much as possible until the disorder is cured.

DIET—Eat a diet high in protein to replace tissue lost from thyroid overactivity.

CALL YOUR DOCTOR IF

- You have symptoms of hyperthyroidism.
- Symptoms worsen suddenly, especially after surgery.
- New, unexplained symptoms develop. Drugs used in treatment may produce side effects.

13

14

15

16

17

18

19

20

ILLNESSES & DISORDERS 359

- Endocrine disorders. This means too many or too few hormones are produced from the pituitary gland, thyroid gland, parathyroid gland, pancreas, adrenal glands, ovaries, testicles or thymus gland.
- Mental or emotional disorders, such as anxiety, depression or schizophrenia.
- Diseases caused by defects in the body's immune system. These include disorders of hypersensitivity, such as rheumatic fever, rheumatoid arthritis, systemic lupus erythematosus and many others.

8—RISK INCREASES WITH
Many disorders have known risk factors that can trigger the problem, make it more likely to occur or increase its duration and intensity. The most common risk factors include:
- Age, especially older persons or newborns and infants.
- Stress—either physical or emotional.
- Anxiety, depression and other mental or emotional problems.
- Fatigue or overwork.
- Poor nutrition due to improper diet or disease.
- Obesity.
- Recent or chronic illness that can lower resistance to other diseases.
- Recent surgery or injury.
- Genetic factors, such as family or ethnic tendency toward a disease.
- Use of drugs, such as alcohol, tobacco, caffeine, narcotics, psychedelics, hallucinogens, marijuana, sedatives, hypnotics or cocaine.
- Use of medications, whether prescription or non-prescription. Even necessary drugs cause adverse reactions and side effects that can complicate treatment and outcome of medical problems.
- Exposure to allergens, environmental pollutants or poisons.
- Geographic areas.
- Crowded or unsanitary living conditions.
- Socioeconomic factors.

9—HOW TO PREVENT
Prevention can be of two types—prevention of the initial disease or prevention of a relapse or recurrence after recovery.

Prevention of any medical problem is the *best treatment*. Researchers continue to discover ways to prevent, delay or diminish some illness, pain, disability and untimely deaths. These are included whenever available.

The causes and risk factors for a disease often provide the best clues for prevention. Many diseases, however, cannot be prevented at present.

10—WHAT TO EXPECT
This section includes four topics: *Appropriate Health Care; Diagnostic Measures; Possible Complications;* and *Probable Outcome.* Each is discussed separately below.

11—APPROPRIATE HEALTH CARE
Self-care or home care is often listed as the first form of appropriate health care. It is an important part of care for almost all disorders. Sometimes total self-care suffices if you have previous experience with a medical problem and

a source to review important points in treatment.

Usually, however, a medical problem should be diagnosed by a doctor before you attempt self-care. Once your doctor diagnoses an illness and outlines a treatment program, self-care or home care is often important. Treatment measures outlined in this book are designed to guide you, whether you are caring for yourself or taking care of someone else.

Effective self-care includes maintaining a positive attitude about yourself and being determined to improve or heal. During illness, a sense of humor and a positive outlook are just as helpful as medication or other treatment measures.

A doctor's care is often necessary, not only to diagnose and prescribe treatment for a medical problem, but to supervise self-care (or hospitalization, when necessary) and to provide additional medical treatment such as surgery.

In addition, even the simplest medical problems sometimes develop complications and require a doctor's care. In those cases, a doctor's treatment can be appropriate even though it applies to a small fraction of cases.

Find a competent personal physician who communicates well with you and with whom you can establish mutual respect.

Psychotherapy, counseling or biofeedback training may be the only useful health care for a medical problem caused mainly by stress or emotional problems.

Counseling and therapy are also helpful in providing personal and family support, especially with illnesses that are terminal or represent major lifestyle adjustments.

Rehabilitation is often helpful for illnesses or injuries that cause temporary or permanent disability. Rehabilitation may be provided by trained physical therapists or physiatrists (medical doctors who specialize in physical therapy). If rehabilitation is mentioned as appropriate health care, ask your doctor for information specific to your disability.

12—DIAGNOSTIC MEASURES

Your own observation of symptoms is usually the first—and often, most important—diagnostic measure. It is the first step toward medical treatment. For that reason, it is listed under this heading on almost all illness charts. Exceptions are made for a few medical problems, such as those that are signaled by unconsciousness, in which case self-observation is impossible.

A medical history and physical exam by a doctor are also almost universal requirements before treatment for any disorder can begin. Even if a medical problem is usually treated at home, a history and exam will be necessary if complications develop that require medical treatment.

Additional diagnostic measures include laboratory studies and other medical tests. The most-common include:
• Studies of body fluids, such as blood, serum, plasma or spinal fluid.

• Microscopic and chemical examination of excreted material, such as urine or stools.
• CAT (computerized axial tomography) scans or X-rays of the affected body part.
• EKG (electrocardiogram), EEG (electroencephalogram) and EMG (electromyogram).
• Therapeutic trial of medication. This is used sometimes for a critically ill patient without a specific diagnosis while awaiting laboratory results.

You may not undergo every diagnostic test listed on the chart, and conversely, you may undergo tests *not* listed. Some tests are performed only if previous tests have not provided enough information. Others are performed only when complications develop. All medical diagnostic tests mentioned in this book are defined in the Glossary.

13—POSSIBLE COMPLICATIONS

Complications are additional medical problems triggered by or as a result of the original illness. Complications sometimes occur, despite accurate diagnosis and competent treatment. Some are preventable, a few are inevitable—but most are rare.

14—PROBABLE OUTCOME

A very important concern in any illness is the patient's question, "What is going to happen to me? How will this disease or injury affect my life?"

No one can completely predict the outcome of an accident or illness. The predictions in this section are guesses based on averages.

Patients and doctors work toward

optimal results, but medicine is an inexact science. Response to treatment depends on many variables, and there are many unanswered questions about health and disease.

Some illnesses are considered incurable at present. The term "incurable" is a general one that includes everything from insignificant conditions that are mere annoyances to fatal diseases that bring certain death in a short time. For that reason, additional information about life expectancy is usually included for incurable illnesses. Again, individual variations are common, but the predictions are an attempt to answer a patient's most important questions. They help you adopt optimistic but realistic expectations.

In almost all cases—no matter how serious the illness—symptoms can be relieved or controlled to minimize pain and discomfort.

15—HOW TO TREAT

This section provides the checklist mentioned earlier that reminds you of instructions your doctor has given you. The information should not replace your doctor's instructions, because treatments vary a great deal between individuals.

If the instructions don't seem to fit your problem, ask your doctor or nurse for answers that apply uniquely to you.

The four major headings include: *General Measures; Medication; Activity;* and *Diet.*

16—GENERAL MEASURES

The instructions under this heading apply to home treatment. They cover common matters, such as soaks for skin problems, use of crutches, appropriate clothing, bandages or bathing.

They are not complete and may not apply to everybody, but they provide a good review of general measures helpful for most patients.

17—MEDICATION

Information under this heading is generally of two types—drugs your doctor may prescribe, and non-prescription drugs you can take safely.

Prescription drugs are named by generic name or drug class. A brief description of a drug's purpose and effect is given. For more information about a specific drug, see the Glossary. It contains entries for generic drugs and drug classes mentioned in this book.

Additionally, you may refer to my book, *Complete Guide to Prescription and Non-Prescription Drugs*, published by HPBooks.

For general instructions about safe use of medicine, see Appendix 21.

18—ACTIVITY

Patients are often confused about whether they must stay in bed during an illness. They are often concerned with returning to work or school, and whether activity will be restricted after recovery. These questions are answered under this heading.

Additionally, guidelines are given for resuming sexual relations—an important area that patients are sometimes reluctant to mention. If the illness has been life-threatening, as with a heart attack, or if it involves abdominal or genital organs, this is particularly pertinent information.

Exercise references are often included, and when not specified otherwise, references to regular physical exercise mean *aerobic* exercise (see Appendix 20).

19—DIET

Diet information can vary from "no special diet" to references to the following diets included in the Appendix section:
- Regular, well-balanced diet that is high in fiber.
- Recommended diet for persons over 50.
- Pregnancy and lactation (breast-feeding) diet.
- Milk-restricted diet.
- Gluten-restricted diet.
- Allergy diet.
- Liquid diet.
- Low-fat diet.
- Low-salt diet.
- Weight-loss diet.
- Soft diet.

For additional specialized diets, consult your doctor or a dietitian.

20—CALL YOUR DOCTOR IF

For most medical problems, a phone call or visit to your doctor is recommended to establish a diagnosis.

After diagnosis, when the course of an illness differs from what is expected, your doctor wants to know. Many developing complications can be averted with prompt medical treatment. Specific symptoms are usually listed that indicate complications.

Of course, if any other symptoms begin that you believe are related to your illness or the drugs you take, call your doctor about them, too.

Guide to Surgery Charts

The information about common surgeries is organized in charts with a format similar to that for illness and disorder charts (see sample chart on facing page).

Generally, surgeries discussed in this section are those commonly performed as treatment for a disorder, such as thyroid-gland removal, or as a diagnostic procedure, such as dilatation and curettage. The surgery topics may be about such minor procedures as a toenail removal, or such major lifesaving procedures as a heart transplant.

Sometimes a surgery is mentioned on an illness chart as part of treatment for that disorder. For instance, thyroid-gland removal is mentioned on the chart for hyperthyroidism (the previous sample chart) as a treatment for patients whose disorder does not respond to other treatment.

Each major heading on the surgery charts is numbered in the sample chart, and the numbered sections are explained in the next few pages.

1—NAME OF SURGERY

Charts are arranged alphabetically by the name that most simply describes the surgical procedure. In some cases, medical professionals refer to the surgery by a more technical name. The technical name appears in parentheses below the main title.

Thyroid-gland removal is clearly understood by everyone, but your surgeon may refer to it as *thyroidectomy*. Both names are included on the chart, and the surgery appears in the index under both names.

2—GENERAL INFORMATION

This section contains four topics: *Definition; Body Parts Involved: Reasons for Surgery* and *Surgical Risk Increases With.* Each topic is discussed separately.

3—DEFINITION

A short definition of the surgery may include information about how common the procedure is and whether or not the medical problem requiring surgery is caused by congenital defects or is the result of disease or injury.

4—BODY PARTS INVOLVED

As discussed with illness charts, body parts can refer to specific organs, such as the brain, or to body systems, such as the central nervous system.

Body parts are often defined in the text, if space permits. If you are not familiar with the body parts involved in a procedure, and the parts are not defined in text, refer to the Glossary for information.

5—REASONS FOR SURGERY

This section lists the most common reasons for a surgical procedure. (Of course, it cannot include *all* possible reasons).

If the medical problems listed are unfamiliar to you, refer to the index. Some have separate illness charts, and the rest are explained in the Glossary.

6—SURGICAL RISK INCREASES WITH

Risk factors make a surgery more complicated or delay healing. Following are common risk factors for most surgeries:

THYROID-GLAND REMOVAL
(Thyroidectomy)

 GENERAL INFORMATION

DEFINITION—Removal of part or all of the thyroid gland.

BODY PARTS INVOLVED—Thyroid gland, the organ in the neck below the Adam's apple that controls the body's metabolism.

REASONS FOR SURGERY
- Hyperthyroidism in pregnant women and children.
- Benign or cancerous tumors of the thyroid.
- Thyroglossal cysts (see Glossary).

SURGICAL RISK INCREASES WITH
- Adults over 60.
- Obesity.
- Smoking.
- Poor nutrition.
- Untreated hyperthyroidism.
- Use of antithyroid medication and iodides before surgery decreases risk. Ask your doctor.

 WHAT TO EXPECT

WHO OPERATES—General surgeon.

WHERE PERFORMED—Hospital.

DIAGNOSTIC TESTS
- Before surgery: Blood studies; sonograms; CAT scan; needle biopsy; or radioactive-iodine uptake and scan (see Glossary).
- After surgery: Blood studies.

ANESTHESIA—General anesthesia by inhalation and injection, with an airway tube placed in the windpipe.

DESCRIPTION OF OPERATION
- An incision is made in the neck following natural skin lines.
- Blood supply to the thyroid gland is clamped.
- All or part of the thyroid gland is cut free and removed, and a drain is left in place. In certain cases, some normal thyroid gland tissue is left intact.
- The skin is closed with sutures or clips, which can usually be removed in 2 to 10 days after surgery.

POSSIBLE COMPLICATIONS
- Hoarseness, if vocal-cord nerves are damaged during surgery.
- Hypothyroidism.
- Hypoparathyroidism.
- Excessive bleeding.
- Surgical-wound infection.

AVERAGE HOSPITAL STAY—3 to 7 days.

PROBABLE OUTCOME—Underlying problem cured in most patients. Cancer that is present but has not spread may require radiation treatment. Allow about 6 weeks for recovery from surgery.

 POSTOPERATIVE CARE

NOTE—This information is supplemental and should not replace your doctor's instructions.

GENERAL MEASURES
- A hard ridge should form along the incision. As it heals, the ridge will recede gradually.
- Use an electric heating pad, a heat lamp or a warm compress to relieve incisional pain.
- Bathe and shower as usual. You may wash the incision gently with mild unscented soap.

MEDICATION—Your doctor may prescribe:
- Pain relievers. Don't take prescription pain medication longer than 4 to 7 days. Use *only* as much as you need.
- Thyroid hormones.

ACTIVITY
- Return to work and normal activity as soon as possible. This reduces postoperative depression and irritability, which are common.
- Resume driving 2 weeks after you return home.
- Resume sexual relations when able.

DIET—No special diet.

 CALL YOUR DOCTOR IF

- Pain, swelling, redness, drainage or bleeding increases in the surgical area.
- You develop signs of infection: headache, muscle aches, dizziness or a general ill feeling and fever.
- You develop symptoms of hypothyroidism: excessive weakness, fatigue, intolerance to cold, menstrual irregularities, constipation, or dry and coarse skin and hair.

SURGERIES 785

- Stress, anxiety, depression or other emotional problems.
- Poor nutrition from any cause.
- Chronic illness.
- Recent illness, surgery or injury.
- Genetic factors.
- Obesity.
- Smoking.
- Alcoholism.
- Age, especially newborns and infants or older adults.
- Use of drugs of abuse, such as narcotics, psychedelics, hallucinogens, marijuana, sedatives, hypnotics or cocaine.
- Use of some drugs or medications, whether prescription or non-prescription. Medicines most likely to increase surgical risk include antihypertensives, muscle relaxants, tranquilizers, sleep inducers, insulin, sedatives, cortisone, beta-adrenergic blockers, calcium-channel blockers and antibiotics.

These same drugs, of course, are lifesaving for some serious illnesses, but they can complicate treatment and outcome of other medical or surgical problems.

7—WHAT TO EXPECT

This section includes eight topics: *Who Operates; Where Performed; Diagnostic Tests; Anesthesia; Description of Operation; Possible Complications; Average Hospital Stay;* and *Probable Outcome.* Each topic is discussed separately.

8—WHO OPERATES

A routine surgery is often performed by a general surgeon or by a doctor who specializes in the body system involved. For instance, either a general surgeon or an obstetrician-gynecologist might remove an ovarian cyst.

Highly complicated surgeries, such as a heart transplant, are usually done by surgeons with additional specialized training.

We have included the type of surgeon most likely to perform the procedure, but variations can occur. In many communities general surgeons perform operations that are customarily performed elsewhere by a surgical subspecialist.

Your surgeon should not be uneasy about discussing with you before surgery his previous experience and education. Most competent surgeons welcome and sometimes recommend a second opinion, when the surgery to be performed is elective rather than an emergency.

9—WHERE PERFORMED

A surgical procedure may be performed in any of the following places:
- A doctor's office.
- An independent, outpatient surgical facility.
- A hospital outpatient surgical facility.
- The operating room of a hospital.
- An emergency room.

10—DIAGNOSTIC TESTS

Diagnostic tests related to surgery can occur before, during or after the surgical procedure.

Laboratory studies are helpful in diagnosis and in providing necessary anatomical information prior to surgery. Many tests are the same as those discussed earlier in diagnosis of illnesses.

Some tests are especially useful in

surgery. Examples include:
● Special X-ray studies of the gastrointestinal tract (upper GI series or lower GI series).
● Intravenous studies of the kidney and urinary tract (intravenous pyelogram and retrograde pyelogram).
● Coronary angiography (X-ray studies of the coronary arteries performed during a cardiac catheterization procedure).
● Biopsy (microscopic study of tissue) before surgery to establish a diagnosis prior to extensive surgery (usually for cancer), and biopsy afterward of tissue removed during the surgical procedure.

11—ANESTHESIA

Anesthesia makes surgery possible without pain. Prior to giving anesthesia, most surgeons prescribe preoperative medications. These generally consist of:
● Tranquilizers or sedatives to help reduce apprehension.
● Pain relievers (frequently a narcotic drug such as morphine). This medication also reduces apprehension and decreases the amount of anesthesia needed.
● An anticholinergic drug, such as scopolamine or atropine, to decrease secretions from the nose, throat and lungs during the operation.

The type of anesthesia used depends on the surgical problem, the age and general condition of the patient, and sometimes on the availability of personnel to administer the anesthesia.

If an operation can be performed with any of several types of anesthesia, you have a right to know the advantages and disadvantages of each. If you wish, you have the right to

participate in the selection. Don't hesitate to ask questions.

If a chart lists several anesthesia options for a surgery, you will have one of them, but not all.

The various types of anesthesia include:

Local Anesthesia—This is usually an injectable form of a drug ending in "caine," such as novocaine or xylocaine.

Local anesthesia is frequently injected into an injury site, such as a fracture, and bleeding from the injury disperses the anesthetic to all pain-sensitive parts of the injury. Local anesthesia may also be used to block a specific nerve bundle, allowing a pain-free procedure such as a tooth extraction.

Local anesthetics are sometimes combined with epinephrine to reduce bleeding in certain procedures, such as dental surgery or removal of superficial skin lesions.

Before you have an injection of local anesthesia, tell your doctor or dentist about any allergic responses you have had to local anesthesia in the past. Also inform him or her about any prescription or non-prescription drugs you take, and about any cardiovascular disease, heartbeat irregularities or peripheral vascular disease you have. The use of local anesthetics with epinephrine under these circumstances can sometimes complicate the disorder.

Spinal Anesthesia—An injection of local anesthetic into the spinal canal, above the level of the surgery site, is known as spinal anesthesia. It relieves pain satisfactorily for many procedures below the waist, such as surgery of the rectum, genitourinary tract or lower extremities.

A special type of low-spinal anesthesia is called caudal anesthesia or "saddle block" (it affects the body area that comes into contact with a horse saddle).

General Anesthesia—This form of anesthesia is generally administered by inhalation, injection and an airway tube.

A short-acting hypnotic or sedative is injected into a vein. It quickly produces light sleep and allows placement of an airway tube (endotracheal tube) without discomfort. The tube is connected to hoses that lead to gas machines.

The anesthesiologist controls the flow of anesthesia gases and monitors many body functions, such as blood pressure, breathing rate, pulse and EKG, while the patient sleeps.

When you awaken, the endotracheal tube may still be in place or may have been removed. Unless respiration needs continued machine support, the endotracheal tube is usually removed in the recovery room.

The tube will make your throat sore for about 24 hours. This is normal and requires no treatment.

12—DESCRIPTION OF OPERATION

The surgical procedure is described in brief, non-technical terms. Individual surgeons may use slightly varying techniques, but the basic steps are included and only details vary.

If you want additional information, your surgeon can give more details or a librarian can suggest resource materials with fuller descriptions and explanations.

During some surgeries of the gastrointestinal tract, a hollow tube (Levin tube) is passed through your nose into your stomach after you are asleep. The tube will probably be in place when you awaken in the recovery room. The purpose of the tube is to keep the stomach empty to prevent vomiting or aspiration of material while you are asleep. It also keeps the stomach decompressed until normal muscular movement of the gastrointestinal tract can resume after surgery. An empty stomach is more comfortable and helps prevent complications that may arise if the stomach becomes distended with air or gas.

The average time in surgery and in the recovery room are left out because variations are too great. Factors that affect the time limits depend upon:
- The exact techniques chosen.
- The experience and preference of the surgeon.
- The availability and experience of assistants and operating room personnel.
- The presence or absence of complications during surgery.
- The age and condition of the patient prior to surgery.

Don't hesitate to ask your surgeon to estimate the time your operation will require.

13—POSSIBLE COMPLICATIONS

Complications are additional medical problems related to the surgery that occur during or after the procedure. They sometimes happen despite accurate diagnosis, skillful surgery, competent assistance and well-equipped operating rooms. Some complications are preventable, and some occur frequently—but most are rare.

14—AVERAGE HOSPITAL STAY

This estimate is based on an average. It varies according to how healing and recuperation progress and whether complications develop before, during or after surgery. It is also influenced by the amount insurance companies will allow as reimbursement of specific procedures.

15—PROBABLE OUTCOME

This heading relates to the surgery's effect on the underlying disorder and the average length of time required to recover from surgery. Estimates are based on the assumption that complications do not occur and healing proceeds normally. Complications can alter the course of healing dramatically. A positive outlook following surgery is an important factor in good outcome and rapid healing.

16—POSTOPERATIVE CARE

This section generally provides instructions for self-care during recuperation after hospitalization. It should serve as a reminder for instructions given you by your surgeon. It should not replace your doctor's instructions.

The section has four major topics: *General Measures; Medication; Activity;* and *Diet.*

17—GENERAL MEASURES

Some questions are almost universal following surgery. Most patients are unsure how to care for a surgical wound. They have questions about pain, bathing, stitches, clothing and other matters. These questions are answered in this section.

18—MEDICATION

Drugs usually prescribed after surgery are described, along with brief instructions for their use.

See Appendix 21, Safe Use of Medicine, for general instructions.

19—ACTIVITY

Resumption of activity is a strong area of concern for post-surgical patients. Guidelines are provided for when to return to school or work, when to resume driving, when to resume sexual relations and what types of exercise are appropriate.

20—DIET

During surgery with general anesthesia, the gastrointestinal tract is kept empty. After the patient awakens, clear liquids are usually provided until the gastrointestinal tract begins to function again. When appropriate, this information is included in the surgery charts. Additional diet instructions usually refer to special diets in the Appendix section, as described earlier.

21—CALL YOUR DOCTOR IF

Call your doctor if healing and recuperation after surgery don't follow the usual course of events. Excessive bleeding and general or surgical-wound infection are common dangers after most surgical procedures, and these are always mentioned on surgery charts when appropriate.

Other reasons listed can serve as reminders of possible complications. If you develop symptoms you believe are related to your illness—even if they don't appear on the chart—call your doctor about them.

ABDOMINAL PAIN, RECURRENT ATTACKS

SYMPTOMS & FACTORS	POSSIBLE PROBLEM	WHAT TO DO*
• Recurrent pain in upper abdomen. • Poor appetite. • Unexplained weight loss.	• Tumor. • Disorder of pancreas.	• See Stomach Cancer. • See Pancreatitis. • See Pancreas Cancer.
• Recurrent pain in lower abdomen. • Recurrent diarrhea, usually without blood. • No fever.	• Inflammation of large intestine. • Tumor.	• See Diverticular Disease. • See Large-Intestine Cancer.
• Recurrent pain in lower abdomen. • Nausea. • Recurrent diarrhea. • General ill feeling. • Fever during attacks. • Blood or mucus in stool.	Inflammatory disease of large intestine.	See Ulcerative Colitis.
• Recurrent pain in lower abdomen. • Recurrent diarrhea, usually without blood or mucus in stool. • General ill feeling. • Fever during attacks.	Inflammation of small intestine.	See Crohn's Disease.
• Recurrent pain in upper right abdomen that may spread to chest, back or shoulders. • No fever.	Gallbladder disorder.	See Gallstones.
• Recurrent pain in upper right abdomen. • Vomiting. • Fever during attacks.	Gallbladder inflammation.	See Acute Cholecystitis or Cholangitis.
Recurrent pain in upper abdomen that is usually relieved by milk, bland food or antacid medicine.	• Stomach inflammation. • Peptic-ulcer disease.	• See Gastritis. • See Duodenal Ulcer. • See Stomach Ulcer.
• Recurrent pain in lower abdomen. • Alternating diarrhea and constipation. • Recurrent, burning pain in upper abdomen, especially when bending forward or lying down.	• Disorder of muscle contractions in colon. • Stomach acid in esophagus.	• See Spastic Colitis. • See Heartburn.

*All references are to Illness section unless noted otherwise.

ABDOMINAL PAIN, SUDDEN ATTACK

SYMPTOMS & FACTORS	POSSIBLE PROBLEM	WHAT TO DO*
• Severe abdominal pain, plus any of following: • Temperature of 100F (37.8C) or higher. • Constipation. • Abdominal swelling. • Vomiting.	Serious abdominal disorder.	• Call doctor now. • See Intestinal Obstruction. • See Appendicitis. • See Aneurysm. • See Peritonitis.
• Severe abdominal pain. • Menstrual period late 4 or more weeks. • Shoulder pain. • Abdominal pain that began in small of back, spreading to genital area. • No fever at onset of pain. • Smoky or bloody urine.	• Pregnancy developing outside uterus. • Kidney colic.	• See Ectopic Pregnancy. • See Kidney Stones.
• Abdominal pain. • Diarrhea. • Vomiting.	• Food poisoning. • Infection of digestive tract.	• See Salmonella Infections. • See Gastroenteritis.
• Pain in lower abdomen in woman. • Green-yellow, heavy or bad-smelling vaginal discharge.	Infection of reproductive organs.	• See Pelvic Inflammatory Disease. • See Ovarian Cyst.
• Abdominal pain that began in small of back, spreading to genital area. • Fever. • Frequent, painful, occasionally bloody urination.	Infection in urinary tract.	• See Bladder Infection. • See Acute Kidney Infection.
• Burning pain of abdominal skin with tenderness along pain route. • Skin blisters.	Virus infection of sensory nerves.	See Shingles.
• Pain in upper right abdomen that may spread to chest, back or shoulders. • Nausea or vomiting.	Gallbladder disorder.	• See Gallstones. • See Pancreatitis. • See Heart Attack.
• Mild pain in lower abdomen. • Constipation or gas. • Recent diet change, such as adding more fiber.	Intestinal disturbance caused by diet change.	Consult doctor if discomfort persists longer than 3 hours.
• Pain in lower abdomen in females. • Unexplained vaginal bleeding.	Several disorders.	See Unexpected Vaginal Bleeding (in Symptoms section).
Abdominal pain following excessive consumption of alcohol or food.	Stomach inflammation.	• See Gastritis. • See Indigestion.
Recurrent abdominal pain for 1 week or more.	Several disorders.	See Recurrent Abdominal Pain (in Symptoms section).

*All references are to Illness section unless noted otherwise.

ABDOMINAL SWELLING

SYMPTOMS & FACTORS	POSSIBLE PROBLEM	WHAT TO DO*
● Abdominal swelling in last 24 hours. ● Severe abdominal pain, plus any of following: ● Fever. ● Diarrhea or constipation. ● Vomiting.	Serious abdominal disorder.	● Call doctor now. ● See Intestinal Obstruction.
● Abdominal swelling. ● Swollen ankles. ● Breathing difficulty, especially at night.	Fluid in abdomen and other body parts caused by heart condition.	● Consult doctor. ● See Congestive Heart Failure.
● Abdominal swelling. ● Puffy ankles that hold a dent when pressed with finger. ● Decreased urination.	Kidney disorder.	● Consult doctor. ● See Glomerulo-nephritis. ● See Wilm's Tumor (children only).
● Abdominal swelling. ● Yellow skin and eyes.	Liver disorder.	● Consult doctor. ● See Cirrhosis of the Liver.
● Lower abdominal swelling that is slowly increasing. ● No signs of pregnancy. ● Persistent constipation.	● Tumor. ● Intestinal disorder.	● See Ovarian Cyst. ● See Constipation.
Abdominal swelling in woman 1 to 5 days before or during menstrual period.	Fluid retention caused by hormone changes.	See Premenstrual Syndrome.
● Abdominal swelling. ● Overweight.	Effect of excess weight.	See Obesity.
● Abdominal swelling in woman of childbearing age. ● Tender, enlarged breasts. ● Morning nausea. ● No menstrual period for 2 months or longer.	Pregnancy.	Consult doctor to confirm pregnancy.

*All references are to Illness section unless noted otherwise.

ANKLE PAIN

SYMPTOMS & FACTORS	POSSIBLE PROBLEM	WHAT TO DO*
• Pain in ankle. • Ankle swollen, red and hot. • Fever. • Recent infection, such as gonorrhea.	Joint infection.	See Infectious Arthritis.
• Pain in ankles or other joints. • Affected joints red, warm, swollen. • Fever. • General ill feeling. • Recent illness, such as sore throat or skin infection.	Complication of prior streptococcal infection.	• Consult doctor. • See Rheumatic Fever.
• Severe pain in ankle following injury. • Ankle can't move or bear weight. • Ankle swells rapidly and turns blue.	• Severe injury. • Broken bone.	• See Sprains & Strains. • See Bone Fracture.
• Pain in ankles or other joints, such as knees or fingers. • Affected joints red, warm, swollen. • No fever.	• Joint inflammation. • Degenerative condition of joints.	• See Rheumatoid Arthritis. • See Juvenile Rheumatoid Arthritis (children only). • See Gout. • See Osteoarthritis.
• Moderate pain in ankle following injury. • Ankle can move and bear weight.	Mild ligament injury.	See Sprains & Strains.

*All references are to Illness section unless noted otherwise.

ANKLES, SWOLLEN

SYMPTOMS & FACTORS	POSSIBLE PROBLEM	WHAT TO DO*
• Swollen ankle. • Calf of swollen leg tender. • Pain when flexing ankle.	Blood clot in deep vein.	• Call doctor now. • See Deep-Vein Thrombosis.
• Swollen ankles. • Chronic breathing difficulty that is worsening. • Cough that is worse when lying down.	Fluid in lungs and other body parts caused by heart condition.	• See Congestive Heart Failure. • See Glomerulo-nephritis.
• Swollen ankles. • Pregnancy.	Common occurrence during pregnancy, but may be sign of high blood pressure.	See Toxemia of Pregnancy.
Swollen, painful ankle.	Several disorders.	See Ankle Pain (in Symptoms section).
• Swollen ankle. • Injury to ankle in last 4 months.	Normal swelling following injury.	If ankle becomes painful, consult doctor.
• Swollen ankles. • Recent confinement for several hours, such as car, bus, train, airplane. • No pain.	Normal occurrence.	• Elevate legs. When possible, avoid prolonged sitting or standing—move around frequently. • If swelling persists more than 48 hours, consult doctor.
• Swollen ankles. • Use of oral contraceptives, cortisone drugs or non-steroidal anti-inflammatory drugs.	• Adverse reaction or side effect of drug. • Blood clot in deep vein.	• Consult doctor. • See Deep-Vein Thrombosis.
• Swollen ankles. • Menstrual period due in a few days.	Fluid retention caused by hormone changes or excess salt intake.	See Premenstrual Syndrome.

*All references are to Illness section unless noted otherwise.

ANXIETY

SYMPTOMS & FACTORS	POSSIBLE PROBLEM	WHAT TO DO*
• Anxiety, plus any of following: • Inability to listen attentively and remember. • Clinging dependency. • Cold or hot flashes. • Cool, sweaty hands. • Abdominal cramps. • Diarrhea or constipation. • Dizziness. • Dry mouth. • Lack of concentration. • Faintness. • Rapid heartbeat. • Impotence in men. • Low frustration level. • Muscle tension and pain (backache, neckache, headache). • Painful menstruation. • Painful sexual intercourse. • Pale or flushed skin. • Restlessness. • Tightness in chest. • Frequent urination.	Effect of stress or unrecognized fear.	See Anxiety (in Illness section).
Anxiety about any of following: enclosed spaces; airplanes; crowds; heights; "going crazy"; infection; or death.	Psychological disorder.	Consult doctor.
• Anxiety, plus 2 or more of following: • Weight loss. • Bulging eyes. • Excessive sweating. • Fatigue. • Rapid or irregular heartbeat.	Overactive thyroid gland.	See Hyperthyroidism.
Persistent anxiety without other symptoms.	Effect of stress.	See Anxiety (in Illness section).
• Anxiety. • Dizziness or lightheadedness. • Rapid breathing. • Frequent sighing.	Decreased carbon dioxide in blood.	See Hyperventilation Syndrome.
• Anxiety. • Use of prescription or non-prescription drug.	Adverse reaction or side effect of drug.	• Consult doctor about prescription drug. • Discontinue use of non-prescription drug.
• Anxiety. • Recent withdrawal from tobacco, alcohol or drug, such as sleeping pills.	Withdrawal symptom.	• Consult doctor about drug withdrawal. • See Drug Abuse & Addiction. • See Alcoholism.

*All references are to Illness section unless noted otherwise.

APPETITE LOSS

SYMPTOMS & FACTORS	POSSIBLE PROBLEM	WHAT TO DO*
• Appetite loss. • Use of vitamins or prescription or non-prescription drugs, especially: anticancer drugs; digitalis; aminophylline; narcotics; antihistamines; ephedrine; methylphenidate; diphenylhydantoin; or amphetamines.	Adverse reaction or side effect of drug.	• Consult doctor about prescription drug. • Discontinue use of non-prescription drug.
• Appetite loss (sudden). • Headache. • Nausea or vomiting. • Bloody urine. • Decreased urination. • Puffy face.	Kidney disorder.	See Glomerulonephritis.
• Appetite loss. • Nausea at sight of food, plus 2 or more of following: • Jaundice (yellow skin and eyes). • Vomiting. • Tenderness over liver area. • Fever. • Weakness and fatigue.	Liver disorder.	• See Acute Viral Hepatitis. • See Hepatitis in Children. • See Cirrhosis of the Liver.
• Appetite loss. • Weight loss. • Vague feeling of illness or fatigue.	Cancer.	Consult doctor.
• Appetite loss, plus 2 or more of following: • Fever. • Sore throat. • Headache. • Painful swelling in neck, armpit or groin. • Fatigue. • Jaundice (yellow skin and eyes). • Pain in upper right abdomen.	Virus infection.	See Infectious Mononucleosis.
• Appetite loss. • Fatigue. • Weight loss. • Hair loss. • Craving for salt. • Skin that darkens. • Dizziness on standing.	Inadequate cortisone hormone.	See Addison's Disease.

*All references are to Illness section unless noted otherwise.

APPETITE LOSS (continued)

SYMPTOMS & FACTORS	POSSIBLE PROBLEM	WHAT TO DO*
• Appetite loss with weight gain. • Loss of energy, fatigue. • Puffy face. • Decreased sex drive. • Dry skin and hair. • Constipation. • Low voice.	Underactive thyroid gland.	See Hypothyroidism.
• Appetite loss. • Excessive alcohol consumption.	Vitamin deficiency caused by alcohol.	See Alcoholism.
• Appetite loss. • Weight loss, plus 2 or more of following: • Paleness. • Sore, red, smooth, burning tongue. • Yellowish skin.	Vitamin B-12 and folic-acid deficiency.	See Pernicious Anemia.
• Gradual appetite loss in woman 45 or older. • Fatigue. • Menstrual changes.	Normal occurrence with decreasing estrogen level of menopause.	Consult doctor.
• Appetite loss. • Pain or pressure in stomach. • Excessive consumption of alcohol or food.	Stomach inflammation caused by alcohol or spices.	See Gastritis.
• Appetite loss. • Nausea and vomiting. • Fever.	Irritation or infection of digestive tract.	See Gastroenteritis.
• Appetite loss in child. • Irritability. • Paleness.	Disorder of red-blood cells.	See Iron-Deficiency Anemia.
• Appetite loss. • Depression or anxiety.	Effect of stress.	• See Depression. • See Anxiety. • See Anorexia Nervosa.
• Appetite loss. • Nausea. • Pregnancy or possible pregnancy.	Effect of hormone change during pregnancy.	Eat small, frequent meals.
Appetite loss in child around age 2.	Normal occurrence caused by slowed growth rate.	Nothing. Appetite will return when growth accelerates.

*All references are to Illness section unless noted otherwise.

ARM OR HAND PAIN

SYMPTOMS & FACTORS	POSSIBLE PROBLEM	WHAT TO DO*
• Pain in arm during exercise. • Feeling of pressure in chest.	Temporary lack of oxygen to heart.	• Call doctor if pain lasts longer than 5 minutes. • See Angina Pectoris. • See Coronary-Artery Disease.
• Pain in elbow, wrist or finger joint. • Affected joint red and swollen. • Fever. • General ill feeling.	Bone or joint infection.	• Consult doctor. • See Osteomyelitis. • See Infectious Arthritis.
• Severe pain in arm following injury. • Arm misshapen.	Broken bone.	• Call doctor now. • See Bone Fracture.
• Pain in elbow, wrist or finger joints. • Affected joints red, warm, swollen. • Fever. • Recent illness, such as sore throat, gonorrhea or skin infection.	Complication of prior streptococcal infection.	See Rheumatic Fever.
• Pain in elbow, wrist or finger joint. • Affected joint red, warm, swollen.	Joint inflammation.	• See Osteoarthritis. • See Rheumatoid Arthritis. • See Juvenile Rheumatoid Arthritis (children only). • See Bursitis. • See Gout.
• Pain in arm or hand. • Numbness or tingling in arm or hand. • Stiff neck and cracking sound with neck movement.	Pressure on nerves in neck.	See Cervical Spondylosis.
• Pain in arm or hand. • Numbness or tingling in arm or hand, especially at night. • No recent injury.	Pressure on nerves in wrist.	See Carpal-Tunnel Syndrome.
• Pain in elbow, wrist or finger joint when bending arm or hand. • No redness or swelling.	Tendon inflammation.	See Tendinitis.
• Severe pain in arm following injury. • Arm not misshapen.	Muscle or ligament injury.	• See Pulled or Torn Muscle. • See Sprains & Strains.

*All references are to Illness section unless noted otherwise.

BACKACHE

SYMPTOMS & FACTORS	POSSIBLE PROBLEM	WHAT TO DO*
• Sudden backache. • Recent fall or injury to back, plus any of following: • Difficulty moving arm or leg. • Loss of bladder or bowel control. • Numbness or tingling in extremities.	Damaged spinal cord.	• Call doctor now. • Don't move injured person.
• Sudden sharp pain down back of leg. • Recent heavy lifting or strenuous exercise.	Pressure on large nerve in leg.	See Ruptured Disk.
• Chronic backache. • Numbness or tingling in extremities that is worsening.	Pressure on spinal cord.	See Spinal-Cord Tumor.
• Sudden backache in person over age 60. • Sharp pain in one place over the spine. OR • Recent confinement to bed or wheelchair.	Bone damage caused by softening of bones.	• Consult doctor. • See Osteoporosis.
• Backache. • Fever. • Painful urination.	• Kidney infection. • Virus infection.	• See Acute Kidney Infection. • See Influenza.
• Sudden backache. • Recent fall or injury to back. • Pain only at injury site.	Muscle injury.	See Pulled or Torn Muscle.
• Backache in person older than 60. • Pain in other joints.	Degenerative condition of joints.	See Osteoarthritis.
• Backache. • Overweight. OR • Use of chair too high or too low for desk. OR • Recent heavy lifting or strenuous exercise. OR • Recent use of jackhammer or other heavy equipment.	Strain of back muscle or ligament.	• See Appendix 15 for suggestions for back care. • See Obesity.
Backache that is worse in morning.	• Lack of adequate back support during sleep. • Chronic inflammation.	See Ankylosing Spondylitis.

*All references are to Illness section unless noted otherwise.

BOWEL, LACK OF CONTROL

SYMPTOMS & FACTORS	POSSIBLE PROBLEM	WHAT TO DO*
• Lack of bowel control. • Convulsions or unconsciousness.	Brain abnormality, such as tumor or stroke.	Call doctor now.
• Lack of bowel control. • Lump just inside anus.	Rectal tumor.	See Large-Intestine Cancer.
• Lack of bowel control, plus any of following: • Slurred speech. • Weakness or paralysis of any part of body. • Unconsciousness. • Blurred vision.	• Decreased blood supply to brain. • Pressure on spinal cord.	• See Stroke. • See Spinal-Cord Tumor.
• Lack of bowel control. • Acute diarrhea.	Powerful, uncontrollable bowel function.	See Acute Diarrhea.
• Frequent leakage of small amounts of stool. • Chronic constipation. especially in child or person over 65.	Stretched anus caused by constipation.	See Fecal Impaction.
• Lack of bowel control, plus any of following: • Recent childbirth with episiotomy. • Recent surgery of vagina. • History of rectal surgery. • Anal fissure or fistula. • Hemorrhoids.	Rectal or anal abnormalities caused by any of several factors.	Consult doctor.
Lack of bowel control in a young child who once was toilet-trained.	• Regressive behavior. • Emotional disturbance caused by factors such as: new siblings; change in home or school; divorce of parents; parental withdrawal, neglect or abuse.	See Encopresis.
• Lack of bowel control. • Mental retardation.	Failure to achieve control due to intellectual deficit.	Continue attempts to toilet train. Place person on toilet at regular times. Provide rewards for success.

*All references are to Illness section unless noted otherwise.

BREAST PAIN OR LUMPS

SYMPTOMS & FACTORS	POSSIBLE PROBLEM	WHAT TO DO*
Breast pain or lump that can be felt or seen.	• Cyst. • Tumor.	• See Fibrocystic Breast Disease. • See Breast Cancer.
• Pain or tenderness in breasts before menstrual periods. • Irregular periods. • Woman over age 38.	Thickening of gland tissue in breasts caused by hormonal changes.	See Menopause.
• Throbbing pain in breast of new mother. • Hard, tender, red lump on breast, or inflamed nipple. • Fever.	Breast infection.	See Breast Abscess.
• Pain, swelling and tenderness in new mother. • Fever.	Breast inflammation.	See Mastitis.
• Pain or tenderness in breasts. • Possible pregnancy.	Common sensitivity as breasts enlarge during pregnancy.	Wear a support bra.
Swollen, tender, hard breasts within 4 days of delivering baby.	Engorgement of breast tissue with milk.	Consult doctor.
• Sore nipples in woman who is breast-feeding. OR • Sharp pain in nipple of nursing mother when breast-feeding baby. • No fever. • No other symptoms related to breast.	Cracked or sore nipples. Common occurrence during first weeks of breast-feeding.	Wash nipples and apply lanolin cream after breast-feeding. Consult doctor if fever develops.
• Pain or tenderness in breasts. • Menstrual period due in a few days.	Discomfort caused by hormone changes.	See Premenstrual Syndrome.

*All references are to Illness section unless noted otherwise.

BREATH, BAD

SYMPTOMS & FACTORS	POSSIBLE PROBLEM	WHAT TO DO*
• Bad breath. • Persistent cough with bad-smelling sputum.	Chronic lung infection.	• See Bronchiectasis. • See Lung Abscess.
• Bad breath. • Fever.	Common occurrence with fever and illness.	See Fever charts (in Symptoms section).
Bad breath that smells like oranges.	Sugar in the urine.	See Diabetes Mellitus.
• Bad breath that smells like ammonia. • Kidney disease.	Kidney failure.	See Chronic Kidney Failure.
• Bad breath. • Bleeding gums. OR • Aching teeth and gums when eating hot, cold or sweet foods.	Gum inflammation.	• See Gingivitis. • See Periodontitis.
• Bad breath. • Sore mouth or tongue.	Infection or sores in mouth or tongue.	See Sore Mouth (in Symptoms section).
• Bad breath. • Dentures.	Food particles trapped in dentures.	See Denture Problems.
• Bad breath. • No visit to dentist in last 6 months.	Tooth decay or plaque deposits.	• Consult dentist. • See Tooth Decay.
• Bad breath. • Poor dental hygiene.	Food particles trapped in teeth.	See Tooth Decay.
• Bad breath. • Recent consumption of garlic, onions or alcohol.	Metabolism of these substances.	Nothing. Breath will return to normal.

*All references are to Illness section unless noted otherwise.

BREATHING DIFFICULTY

SYMPTOMS & FACTORS	POSSIBLE PROBLEM	WHAT TO DO*
• Sudden breathing difficulty. • Severe chest pain spreading to jaw, neck or arms.	Life-threatening heart attack.	• Call doctor now! • See Heart Attack. • See Coronary-Artery Disease.
• Sudden breathing difficulty. • Sharp chest pain that worsens with inhalation.	• Blood clot in lung. • Collapsed lung.	• Call doctor now. • See Pulmonary Embolism. • See Pneumothorax.
• Sudden breathing difficulty. • Chest pain.	Temporary lack of oxygen to heart.	See Angina Pectoris.
• Chronic breathing difficulty that is worsening. • Swollen ankles.	Fluid in lungs and other body parts caused by heart condition.	See Congestive Heart Failure.
• Breathing difficulty. • Fever. • Cough with green-yellow or brownish sputum.	Infection of breathing passages.	• See Pneumonia (all charts). • See Acute Bronchitis.
• Mild breathing difficulty. • Noisy breathing.	Spasm of bronchial tubes.	See Wheezing (in Symptoms section).
• Chronic breathing difficulty that is worsening. • Persistent cough with thick gray or green-yellow sputum. • Dusty working conditions.	Lung inflammation.	• See Pneumoconiosis. • See Silicosis. • See Asbestosis.
• Chronic breathing difficulty that is worsening. • Persistent cough with gray or green-yellow sputum. • No dusty working conditions.	Chronic inflammation or infection of breathing passages.	• See Chronic Bronchitis. • See Emphysema. • See Bronchiectasis.
• Breathing difficulty. • Lightheadedness. • Numbness or tingling in hands and feet.	Decreased carbon dioxide in blood.	• See Hyperventilation Syndrome. • See Anxiety.

*All references are to Illness section unless noted otherwise.

BRUISING OR BLOOD SPOTS UNDER THE SKIN, UNEXPLAINED

SYMPTOMS & FACTORS	POSSIBLE PROBLEM	WHAT TO DO*
• Unexplained bruising or blood spots under skin. • Kidney or liver disorder.	Abnormal platelet function.	See Chronic Kidney Failure.
• Unexplained blood spots under skin. • Fever. • Pain in affected area. • Headache. • Weakness. • General ill feeling.	Bacterial, viral or parasitic infection.	Consult doctor.
• Unexplained bruising or blood spots under skin. • Use of prescription or non-prescription drug, such as: anticoagulants; aspirin; sulfa drugs; digitoxin; quinine; quinidine; antihistamines; phenothiazines; antidepressants; local anesthetics; ionidec; penicillin; mercury; bismuth; cortisone drugs; or anticonvulsants.	Adverse reaction or side effect of drug.	Consult doctor.
Unexplained bruising in healthy child.	Child abuse.	Notify authorities.
• Unexplained bruising or blood spots under skin. • Swollen gums that bleed occasionally. • Pain in arms or legs.	Poor nutrition.	• Consult doctor. • Take vitamin-C supplements.
Unexplained blood spots under skin following violent coughing, vomiting or choking.	Raised pressure in blood vessels of head and neck.	Consult doctor.
• Unexplained bruising in newborn. • Jaundice (yellow skin and eyes).	Blood disorder.	See Rh Incompatibility.
• Unexplained bruising or blood spots under skin. • Recent virus infection.	Blood disorder.	• Call doctor now. • See Thrombo-cytopenia.
• Unexplained bruising on lower extremities. • Abdominal pain. • Red, swollen and tender joints.	Allergic disorder.	See Allergic Purpura.

*All references are to Illness section unless noted otherwise.

BUMPS ON SKIN

SYMPTOMS & FACTORS	POSSIBLE PROBLEM	WHAT TO DO*
• Dark, slow-growing lump. OR • Change in mole size or color. • Borders of mole become irregular. • Bleeding or pain in mole.	Skin cancer.	See Malignant Melanoma.
Single lump that grows.	• Skin growth caused by virus. • Skin cancer, especially if center is an open sore. • Spread of cancer from other body parts.	• Consult doctor. • See Basal-Cell Skin Cancer. • See Squamous-Cell Skin Cancer.
• Bumps or rash. • Fever.	Several disorders.	See Rash with Fever (in Symptoms section).
Rough, small bumps on skin of anus, vagina or penis.	Skin growth caused by virus.	See Venereal Warts.
• Light-red bumps with raised edges. • Severe itching.	Allergic reaction.	See Hives.
Painful, red bump with white or yellow center in part of body with hair.	Infected hair follicle.	See Boils.
Thickened bump on toe.	Skin thickening caused by pressure.	See Corn or Callus.
Rough, hard bump on hand or foot with tiny black dots in bump.	Skin growth caused by virus.	See Warts.
Red bumps on cheeks, on either side of nose and on scalp (sometimes).	Autoimmune disorder.	See Discoid Lupus Erythematosus.

*All references are to Illness section unless noted otherwise.

BURPING OR GAS

SYMPTOMS & FACTORS	POSSIBLE PROBLEM	WHAT TO DO*
• Burping that worsens after eating fatty foods. • Pain in upper right abdomen that may spread to back.	Gallbladder disorder.	See Gallstones.
• Gas. • Pale, bad-smelling stool. • Unexplained weight loss.	Poor digestion.	See Malabsorption.
Burping that worsens when bending or lying down.	Stomach acid in esophagus.	See Heartburn.
• Gas. • Alternating constipation and diarrhea. • Lower abdominal pain that is relieved by passing gas or bowel movements.	Disorder of muscle contractions in colon.	See Spastic Colitis.
• Burping. • Discomfort and fullness after eating.	• Air swallowed while eating. • Tumor.	• See Indigestion. • See Stomach Cancer.
• Gas. • High-fiber diet.	Effect of high-fiber foods.	Nothing. Improves eventually without diet change.

*All references are to Illness section unless noted otherwise.

CHEST PAIN

SYMPTOMS & FACTORS	POSSIBLE PROBLEM	WHAT TO DO*
• Severe chest pain beneath breastbone, spreading to jaw, neck or arms. • Sweating. • Anxious feeling. • Sudden breathing difficulty. • Nausea, vomiting.	Life-threatening heart attack.	• Call doctor now! • See Heart Attack. • See Rapid Heartbeat. • See Coronary-Artery Disease.
• Chest pain. • Sudden breathing difficulty. • Recent surgery. OR • Recent injury or illness requiring bed confinement.	Blood clot from leg or pelvis that has lodged in lung.	• Call doctor now. • See Pulmonary Embolism. • See Atelectasis.
• Severe chest pain, spreading to jaw, neck or arms. • No other symptoms.	• Temporary lack of oxygen to heart. • Life-threatening heart damage.	• Call doctor now. • See Angina Pectoris. • See Coronary-Artery Disease.
• Sharp chest pain that worsens with inhalation. • Sudden breathing difficulty. • No other factors.	Collapsed lung.	• Call doctor now. • See Pneumothorax.
• Chest pain. • Shortness of breath. • Cough. • Fever.	• Lung infection. • Inflammation of membranes around lungs.	• See Pneumonia (all charts). • See Pleurisy.
Chest pain without symptoms or factors listed on this chart.	Many disorders, including stress and anxiety.	Consult doctor.
• Chest pain on one side. • Burning feeling at pain site. • Pain unaffected by breathing. • Skin rash at pain site.	Virus infection of sensory nerves.	See Shingles.
• Chest pain. • Cough with green or gray-yellow sputum.	Infection of bronchial tubes.	See Acute Bronchitis.
• Chest pain on one side. • Recent chest injury, chest surgery or severe cough.	Pulled muscle or broken rib.	• See Pulled or Torn Muscle. • See Bone Fracture.
Chest pain that worsens when bending or lying down.	Stomach acid in esophagus.	See Heartburn.
Chest pain that worsens when swallowing.	Several disorders.	See Swallowing Difficulty (in Symptoms section).

*All references are to Illness section unless noted otherwise.

CONFUSION (PERSON OVER AGE 65)

SYMPTOMS & FACTORS	POSSIBLE PROBLEM	WHAT TO DO*
• Confusion. • Slurred speech. • Weakness in extremities.	Decreased blood supply to brain.	• Call doctor now. • See Stroke. • See Transient Ischemic Attack (T.I.A.).
• Sudden confusion. • Unusually long time since eating. OR • Use of insulin or oral hypoglycemic drug.	Low blood sugar.	Drink sweet drink or eat sweet snack. If confusion lasts longer than 10 minutes, call doctor.
• Confusion appearing over several weeks. • Fall or head injury in last 2 months.	Effect of injury.	• Call doctor now. • See Subdural Hemorrhage & Hematoma.
• Sudden confusion. • Signs of physical illness, such as fever, cough or loss of bladder control.	Effect of illness.	Call doctor now.
• Sudden confusion • Cold abdomen. • Recent chill.	Drop in body temperature.	See Hypothermia.
• Sudden confusion. • Change in prescription. OR • Use of mind-altering drugs, such as marijuana or cocaine.	Adverse reaction or side effect of drug.	Consult doctor.
• Confusion appearing over several weeks, plus 2 or more of following: • Inability to remember recent events. • Decline in attention to personal appearance or cleanliness. • Personality change.	• Poor nutrition. • Mental deterioration.	• See Vitamin-C Deficiency. • See Vitamin-B Deficiencies. • See Dementia.

*All references are to Illness section unless noted otherwise.

CONFUSION (PERSON UNDER AGE 65)

SYMPTOMS & FACTORS	POSSIBLE PROBLEM	WHAT TO DO*
• Confusion, plus any of following: • Blurred vision. • Dizziness. • Numbness or tingling in any part of body. • Speaking difficulty. • Weakness in extremities.	Decreased blood supply to brain.	• Call doctor now. • See Stroke. • See Transient Ischemic Attack (T.I.A.).
• Sudden confusion. • Recent head injury.	Brain injury.	• Call doctor now. • See Head Injury.
• Confusion in a woman of childbearing age. • Sudden fever of 101F (38.3C) or higher. • Vomiting. • Skin rash.	Infection.	• Call doctor now. • See Toxic Shock Syndrome.
• Confusion. • Fever of 103F (39.4C) or higher.	Effect of fever.	• Call doctor now. • See Fever.
• Confusion, plus any of following: • Heart disease. • Lung disease. • Diabetes.	Complication of underlying disorder.	Call doctor now.
• Confusion, plus any of following: • Agitation. • Delirium. • Disorientation. • Hallucinations. • Inability to recognize others.	• Mental illness. • Sugar in the urine. • Bleeding inside skull. • Tumor.	• Call doctor now. • See Diabetes Mellitus. • See Subdural Hemorrhage & Hematoma. • See Brain Tumor.
• Confusion. • Use of drugs, including: antihistamines; appetite suppressants; muscle relaxants; pain killers; sedatives; tranquilizers; or mind-altering drugs, such as marijuana, cocaine, L.S.D. and heroin.	• Adverse reaction or side effect of drug. • Drug interaction.	Consult doctor.
• Confusion. • Alcohol consumption, either alone or with drug.	• Adverse reaction or side effect of alcohol. • Drug interaction.	• Consult doctor. • Stop drinking alcohol.

*All references are to Illness section unless noted otherwise.

CONSTIPATION

SYMPTOMS & FACTORS	POSSIBLE PROBLEM	WHAT TO DO*
• Constipation. • Pain in lower abdomen within last week.	Inflammation of large intestine.	• See Diverticular Disease. • See Large-Intestine Cancer.
• Chronic constipation. • Recurrent pain in lower abdomen.	Disorder of muscle contractions in colon.	See Spastic Colitis.
• Constipation, plus 2 or more of following: • Fatigue. • Unexplained weight gain. • Dry skin or hair. • Decreased tolerance to cold.	Underactive thyroid gland.	See Hypothyroidism.
• Constipation. • Pain with bowel movements. • Occasional blood in stool.	• Varicose veins in anus. • Split in skin around anus.	• See Hemorrhoids. • See Constipation (in Illness section).
• Chronic tendency toward constipation. • Frequent suppression of urge for bowel movement. OR • Regular laxative use.	Poor bowel reflexes.	See Constipation (in Illness section).
• Constipation. • Use of prescription or non-prescription drug.	Adverse reaction or side effect of drug.	• Consult doctor about prescription drug. • Discontinue use of non-prescription drug.
Constipation while dieting.	Lack of adequate water or fiber in diet.	Include more fiber in your diet. For a balanced diet, see Appendix 1.
• Chronic tendency toward constipation. • No other symptoms.	Lack of adequate water or fiber in diet.	See Constipation (in Illness section).

*All references are to Illness section unless noted otherwise.

COUGH

SYMPTOMS & FACTORS	POSSIBLE PROBLEM	WHAT TO DO*
• Sudden violent cough. • Inhalation of foreign object.	Normal coughing to expel object from lungs.	Consult doctor if cough lasts longer than 1 hour.
Persistent cough without sputum.	• Tumor. • Heart disorder. • Spasm of bronchial tubes. • Irritation of bronchial tubes from smoking.	• Request chest X-ray. • See Lung Cancer. • See Congestive Heart Failure. • See Asthma.
• Cough. • Shortness of breath.	Several disorders.	See Breathing Difficulty (in Symptoms section).
• Recent cough with green-yellow or rusty sputum. • Fever. • Breathing difficulty.	Lung infection.	• See Pneumonia (all charts). • See Histoplasmosis. • See Valley Fever. • See Psittacosis.
• Persistent cough with sputum that is worsening. • Fever. • Unexplained weight loss. • Fatigue. • Excessive sweating at night.	Lung infection or inflammation.	• See Tuberculosis. • See Bronchiectasis. • See Lung Abscess.
• Sudden cough without sputum. • Inhalation of irritating substance or fumes.	Irritation of breathing passages.	Avoid exposure to chemicals, dust and cigarettes.
• Recent cough without sputum. • Hoarseness or voice loss.	Inflammation of vocal cords.	See Voice Loss or Hoarseness (in Symptoms section).
• Recent cough. • Fever.	Inflammation or infection of breathing passages.	• See Acute Bronchitis. • See Influenza.
• Persistent cough following cold or flu. • History of persistent cough during previous cold or flu seasons.	Chronic inflammation or infection of bronchial tubes.	See Chronic Bronchitis.
• Recent cough. • Stuffy or runny nose. • Sore throat.	Virus infection.	See Common Cold.

*All references are to Illness section unless noted otherwise.

COUGH WITH BLOOD

SYMPTOMS & FACTORS	POSSIBLE PROBLEM	WHAT TO DO*
• Cough with blood. • Recent surgery. OR • Recent bed confinement because of illness or injury.	Blood clot in lung.	• Call doctor now. • See Pulmonary Embolism.
• Cough with blood. • Persistent cough following recent cold or flu.	Bleeding in breathing passages.	Call doctor now.
• Persistent cough with blood for several weeks. • Fever of 100F (37.8C) or higher. • Unexplained weight loss. • Fatigue. • Excessive sweating at night.	• Bacterial inflammation or infection of lung. • Tumor.	• See Tuberculosis. • See Lung Cancer. • See Lung Abscess.
• Cough with blood or frothy pink or brownish sputum. • Breathing difficulty. • History of high blood pressure or heart disorder.	Fluid in lungs.	• Consult doctor. • See Pulmonary Edema.
• Cough with blood or brownish sputum. • Fever of 102F (38.9C) or higher.	Lung infection.	See Pneumonia (all charts).

*All references are to Illness section unless noted otherwise.

COUGHING IN CHILDREN

SYMPTOMS & FACTORS	POSSIBLE PROBLEM	WHAT TO DO*
• Cough. • Severe breathing difficulty. • Wheezing. OR • Bluish face or fingertips.	• Spasm of bronchial tubes. • Swelling in vocal cords.	• Call doctor now. • See Asthma. • See Croup.
• Cough. • Fever. • Rapid or difficult breathing.	Infection of breathing passages.	• Call doctor now. • See Acute Bronchitis. • See Bronchiolitis. • See Pneumonia (all charts).
• Severe uncontrollable cough. • Noisy "whooping" gasps for air following cough.	Bacterial lung infection.	See Whooping Cough.
• Cough. • Noisy breathing with wheezing. • Possible inhalation of small foreign object, such as peanut.	Normal coughing to expel object from lung.	Consult doctor if coughing lasts longer than 1 hour.
• Persistent cough in an infant. • Abdominal swelling. • Frequent, bad-smelling stools.	Inherited disorder.	See Cystic Fibrosis.
• Cough. • Fever. • No other symptoms.	Virus infection.	• See Common Cold. • See Influenza.
• Cough. • Chronic runny or stuffy nose.	Enlarged adenoids.	Consult doctor.
• Cough. • Adult smokers in house or child may have smoked.	Irritation caused by tobacco smoke.	• Adult smokers should smoke outside. • Talk to child about hazards of smoking.

*All references are to Illness section unless noted otherwise.

CRYING, EXCESSIVE
(INFANT 0 TO 6 MONTHS)

SYMPTOMS & FACTORS	POSSIBLE PROBLEM	WHAT TO DO*
• Excessive crying. • Irritability. • Lethargy. • Poor appetite. • Fever.	Infection.	• Consult doctor. • See Fever (Child 0 to 2 Years) in Symptoms section.
• Excessive crying. • Irritability. • Lethargy. • Poor appetite.	Minor illness.	Consult doctor if symptoms persist longer than 1 day.
Excessive crying in infant younger than 3 months, usually after feeding.	Irritation of digestive tract.	See Colic in Infants.
• Excessive crying. • Crying stops after feeding. • Crying resumes less than 2 hours after feeding.	• Inadequate nourishment. • Thirst.	• If breast-feeding. feed on demand and increase sucking time. • If bottle-feeding, increase amount offered. • Offer water between feedings. • See Colic in Infants.
• Excessive crying. • Rash in diaper area.	Chemical skin irritation.	See Diaper Rash.
Crying until picked up.	Boredom or loneliness.	• Touch and talk to infant more. • Place infant within sight of you.
• Crying. • Cool or chilly environment.	Cold.	• Dress infant warmly. • Move infant into warm room.
Crying in infant younger than 3 months before falling asleep.	Muscle jerks and twitches when falling asleep.	Wrap infant firmly in blanket before putting to bed.

*All references are to Illness section unless noted otherwise.

DEPRESSION

SYMPTOMS & FACTORS	POSSIBLE PROBLEM	WHAT TO DO*
• Depression, plus 3 or more of following: • Loss of energy, fatigue. • Difficulty sleeping, waking up or daytime sleepiness. • Reduced sex drive. • Loss of pleasure in usual activities. • Poor appetite or unexplained weight loss. • Overeating and weight gain. • Feelings of excessive guilt, worthlessness, self-reproach. • Decreased ability to think, concentrate or make decisions. • Recurrent thoughts of death, suicide or suicide attempt. • Crying, tearfulness. • Decline in social activity or talkativeness. • Hallucinations.	• Psychological disorder. • Sugar in the urine. • Underactive or overactive thyroid gland. • Cancer.	• Consult doctor. • See Depression (in Illness section). • See Diabetes Mellitus. • See Hyperthyroidism. • See Pancreas Cancer. • See Anorexia Nervosa. • See Bulimia. • See Hypothyroidism.
Depression in a woman following childbirth.	Common occurrence for several weeks after delivery.	See Postpartum Depression.
• Depression. • Use of prescription or non-prescription drug. OR • Excessive alcohol consumption.	Adverse reaction or side effect of drug or alcohol.	• Consult doctor. • See Alcoholism.
• Depression. • Recent virus infection with fever such as flu, infectious mononucleosis or hepatitis.	Common occurrence for 3 to 6 months following infection.	Consult doctor if depression worsens or lasts longer than 2 weeks.
Depression following traumatic or sad event, such as death in family.	Normal occurrence for 3 to 6 months following such experiences.	See Depression (in Illness section).

*All references are to Illness section unless noted otherwise.

DIARRHEA
(INFANT 0 TO 6 MONTHS)

SYMPTOMS & FACTORS	POSSIBLE PROBLEM	WHAT TO DO*
• Diarrhea. • Fever. • Vomiting.	• Infection of digestive tract. • Ear infection.	• See Gastroenteritis in Infants & Children. • See Middle-Ear Infection.
• Diarrhea. • Baby content, alert and feeding well. • Baby taking non-prescription drug.	Adverse reaction or side effect of drug.	• Consult doctor. • Discontinue use of drug unless recommended by doctor.
• Diarrhea. • Baby taking prescription drug for some other disorder.	Adverse reaction or side effect of drug.	Consult doctor. Dose may need adjustment, substitution or discontinuation.
• Diarrhea. • Itching at night. OR • Worms in stool.	Parasites.	• See Pinworms. • See Roundworms.
• Diarrhea. • Recent addition of solids to diet.	Baby too young to digest solid food.	• Consult doctor. • Wait until age 4 months before trying solids.
• Diarrhea. • Baby seems content, alert and feeds well on bottle feedings. • Sugar added to any formula or water. OR • Less than recommended amount of water added to baby's orange juice. OR • Fruit juice sweetened with sugar.	Upset digestion due to excess sugar.	• Consult doctor. • Don't add sugar to baby's food. • Use recommended amounts of water to dilute juice.

*All references are to Illness section unless noted otherwise.

DIARRHEA
(PERSON OVER 6 MONTHS)

SYMPTOMS & FACTORS	POSSIBLE PROBLEM	WHAT TO DO*
• Diarrhea. • Blood in stool.	Inflammation of large intestine.	• See Ulcerative Colitis. • See Bacillary Dysentery.
• Diarrhea for 24 hours or longer. • Vomiting • Abdominal pain. • Consumption of spoiled or contaminated food.	Effect of toxins in food.	See Salmonella Infections.
• Diarrhea. • Use of prescription or non-prescription drug.	Adverse reaction or side effect of drug.	• Consult doctor about prescription drug. • Discontinue use of non-prescription drug.
• Diarrhea. • Nausea or vomiting.	Bacterial or parasitic infection of digestive tract.	• See Gastroenteritis. • See Giardiasis.
Recurrent attacks of diarrhea during periods of stress.	Effect of stress.	• See Anxiety. • See Spastic Colitis.
• Recurrent attacks of diarrhea. • Pain in lower abdomen.	Several disorders.	See Recurrent Abdominal Pain (in Symptoms section).

*All references are to Illness section unless noted otherwise.

DIZZINESS

SYMPTOMS & FACTORS	POSSIBLE PROBLEM	WHAT TO DO*
● Dizziness, plus any of following: ● Speaking difficulty. ● Blurred vision. ● Numbness or tingling in any part of body. ● Weakness or paralysis in extremities.	Decreased blood supply to brain.	● Call doctor now. ● See Stroke. ● See Transient Ischemic Attack, (T.I.A.). ● See Subarachnoid Hemorrhage.
● Dizziness. ● Recurrent morning headache. ● Nausea or vomiting.	● Bleeding inside skull. ● Tumor.	● Call doctor now. ● See Subdural Hemorrhage & Hematoma. ● See Brain Tumor.
● Dizziness. ● Irregular heartbeat.	Heart-rhythm disorder.	● See Atrial Fibrillation. ● See Heart-Rhythm Irregularity. ● See Heart Block.
● Dizziness. ● Use of prescription or non-prescription drug.	Adverse reaction or side effect of drug.	● Consult doctor about prescription drug. ● Discontinue use of non-prescription drug.
● Dizziness. ● Decreased hearing. ● Noises in ear.	Infection or disorder of inner ear.	● See Labyrinthitis. ● See Meniere's Disease.
Dizziness when turning head in person over age 50.	Pressure on nerves in neck.	See Cervical Spondylosis.
Dizziness when standing suddenly.	● Temporary drop in blood pressure. ● Disorder of red blood cells.	● Avoid rising suddenly. ● See Iron-Deficiency Anemia.

*All references are to Illness section unless noted otherwise.

EAR, RINGING OR BUZZING SOUNDS

SYMPTOMS & FACTORS	POSSIBLE PROBLEM	WHAT TO DO*
• Ear noises. • Use of prescription or non-prescription drug.	Adverse reaction or side effect of drug.	• Consult doctor about prescription drug. • Discontinue use of non-prescription drug.
• Ear noises. • Hearing loss.	Damaged auditory nerve.	See Hearing Impairment or Loss.
• Strange, loud ear noises. • Severe, uncomfortable tickling in ear.	Insect in outer-ear canal.	Consult doctor.
Ear noises after airplane flight.	Middle-ear damage caused by change in air pressure.	See Barotitis Media.

*All references are to Illness section unless noted otherwise.

EARACHE

SYMPTOMS & FACTORS	POSSIBLE PROBLEM	WHAT TO DO*
• Earache. • Sticky, green-yellow discharge from ear.	Infection of outer-ear canal or middle ear.	• See Outer-Ear Infection. • See Middle-Ear Infection. • See Ruptured Eardrum.
• Earache. • Fever.	Infection of middle ear.	See Middle-Ear Infection.
• Earache. • Stuffy nose.	Common occurrence with cold or allergy.	See Middle-Ear Infection.
Earache that worsens when earlobe is pulled.	Infection of outer-ear canal.	See Outer-Ear Infection.
• Earache. • Pain in tooth or jaw.	• Tooth or gum infection. • Inflammation of joint in jaw.	• Consult dentist. • See Tooth Abscess. • See Temporo-Mandibular Joint Syndrome.
• Earache. • Blocked feeling in ear that cannot be cleared by swallowing. • Diminished hearing.	Wax in ear canal.	See Earwax Blockage.
• Earache that began during airplane flight. • Blocked feeling in ear that cannot be cleared by swallowing.	Middle-ear damage caused by change in air pressure.	See Barotitis Media.

*All references are to Illness section unless noted otherwise.

EYE PAIN

SYMPTOMS & FACTORS	POSSIBLE PROBLEM	WHAT TO DO*
• Severe eye pain. • Recent eye injury with visible damage. • Loss of vision.	Serious injury.	Call doctor now.
• Pain behind eye, plus any of following: • Eyes sensitive to light. • Lethargy. • Confusion. • Pain that worsens when bending head forward. • Severe headache.	• Inflammation of membranes around brain. • Bleeding in membrane around brain.	• Call doctor now. • See Aseptic Meningitis. • See Bacterial Meningitis. • See Subarachnoid Hemorrhage.
• Eye pain in one eye. • Blurred vision. • Eye sensitive to light.	• Excess pressure in eye. • Inflammation of iris.	• See Acute Glaucoma. • See Iritis.
• Eye pain. • Eye injury without visible damage.	Minor injury.	See Eye Contusion or Laceration.
• Pain behind eye. • Area of tenderness over nose or cheekbones. • Pain that worsens when bending forward. • Recent cold or nasal allergies.	Sinus infection.	See Sinus Infection.
• Pain behind eye. • Tenderness in temple on affected side.	Inflammation of arteries in temples.	• Call doctor now. • See Polymyalgia Rheumatica or Temporal Arteritis.
• Eye pain. • Watery, red eye.	Foreign object in eye.	See Foreign Body in Eye.
• Eye pain. • Red, swollen eyelid. • Red eye.	Infection of hair follicle on eyelid.	See Sty.
• Eye pain. • Red eye. • Gritty feeling in eye. • Stickiness around eye.	Infection of eye membrane.	See Conjunctivitis.
• Eye pain. • Red eye. • Gritty feeling in eye.	Inadequate tear production.	Use non-prescription artificial tears. Consult doctor if discomfort lasts longer than 2 days.
• Eye pain. • Eyelid curls inward. • Red eyelid and eye.	Disorder of eyelid.	See Entropion.

*All references are to Illness section unless noted otherwise.

FACE PAIN

SYMPTOMS & FACTORS	POSSIBLE PROBLEM	WHAT TO DO*
• Face pain, plus any of following: • Chest pain. • Neck pain. • Shoulder pain. • Arm pain.	Heart attack.	• Call doctor now! • See Heart Attack. • See Coronary-Artery Disease. • See Atherosclerosis.
• Severe pain on one side of face over eye. • Redness of white of eye. • Blurred vision.	Excess pressure in eye.	See Acute Glaucoma.
Sharp pain on one side of face when face is touched or when chewing.	Damaged nerve.	See Tic Douloureux.
• Sudden, throbbing pain in temple. • General ill feeling. • Tender scalp.	Inflammation of arteries in temples.	See Polymyalgia Rheumatica or Temporal Arteritis.
• Pain on one side of face between eye and nose. • Runny nose and eye.	Vascular headache.	• See Migraine Headache. • See Tension or Vascular Headache.
• Face pain. • Recent rash at site of pain.	Virus infection of sensory nerves.	See Shingles.
• Pain or tenderness around eyes and cheekbones that worsens when bending head forward. • Recent cold or nasal allergies.	Sinus infection.	See Sinus Infection.
Throbbing pain on one side of face that worsens at night, when eating or when touching a particular tooth.	Infection around tooth.	• Consult doctor or dentist. • See Tooth Abscess.
• Aching pain over or around jaw joint. • Jaw that sometimes clicks when opening. • Frequent headaches.	Inflammation of joint in jaw.	See Temporo-Mandibular Joint Syndrome.

*All references are to Illness section unless noted otherwise.

FACIAL SKIN PROBLEMS

SYMPTOMS & FACTORS	POSSIBLE PROBLEM	WHAT TO DO*
• Change in face mole's size, color or sensitivity. OR • A new mole or lump on face.	Skin cancer.	See Malignant Melanoma.
Sore on face or lip that doesn't heal in 3 weeks.	Skin cancer.	• See Basal-Cell Skin Cancer. • See Squamous-Cell Skin Cancer.
• Blistery rash on one side of face. • Painful, burning sensation at site 1 or 2 days before rash appears.	Virus infection of sensory nerves.	See Shingles.
Blisters that burst and become crusty.	Skin infection.	See Impetigo.
Red, itching, scaling rash on face.	Allergic reaction.	See Eczema.
Any of following conditions on face: • Painful, red bumps. • Bumps with white or yellow centers. • Blackheads.	Skin disorder beginning after puberty.	See Acne.
• Flushed face, plus one of following: • Stress. • Consumption of alcohol or spicy food. • Adult over 40.	Disorder of tiny blood vessels.	See Acne Rosacea.
Blister or red, rough or painful area around mouth.	Virus infection.	See Cold Sores.
• Rough, red patch on cheek, nose or forehead. • Person over age 35.	Skin damage caused by sun exposure.	• See Sunburn. • See Actinic Keratosis.
Patch of skin on face that is lighter or darker than surrounding skin.	Disorder of skin pigment.	See Vitiligo.

*All references are to Illness section unless noted otherwise.

FAINTNESS OR FAINTING

SYMPTOMS & FACTORS	POSSIBLE PROBLEM	WHAT TO DO*
• Faintness or fainting. • Feeling that heart speeds or slows before faintness. • Known heart disease.	Heart-rhythm disorder.	• Call doctor now. • See Heart Block. • See Heart-Rhythm Irregularity. • See Atrial Fibrillation.
• Faintness, plus any of following: • Blurred vision. • Speaking difficulty. • Confusion. • Numbness or tingling in any part of body. • Weakness or paralysis in extremities.	Decreased blood supply to brain.	• Call doctor now. • See Transient Ischemic Attack. • See Stroke.
Faintness after several hours in strong sunshine or hot environment.	Heat exhaustion.	• Call doctor now. • See Heatstroke or Heat Exhaustion.
• Faintness. • Unusually long time since eating . OR • Diabetes.	Low blood sugar.	• Drink sweetened juice or beverage or eat something sugary or starchy. • See Functional Hypoglycemia. • See Hypoglycemia of Diabetes.
• Faintness. • Fatigue. • Shortness of breath. • Person older than 50.	• Heart disease. • Disorder of red blood cells.	• See Congestive Heart Failure. • See Pernicious Anemia.
• Faintness. • Use of drug for high blood pressure.	Adverse reaction or side effect of drug.	Consult doctor.
• Faintness. • Dizziness.	Several disorders.	See Dizziness (in Symptoms section).
• Faintness when standing suddenly. OR • Faintness following bed confinement.	Temporary drop in blood pressure.	Avoid rising suddenly.
• Faintness. • Breathing deeply, rapidly or sighing before faintness.	Effect of stress. No underlying disorder.	• See Hyperventilation Syndrome. • See Anxiety. • Consult doctor if happens repeatedly.
Faintness when turning head in person older than 50.	Pressure on nerves in neck.	See Cervical Spondylosis.
• Fainting. • Shortness of breath before faintness. • Recent strenuous exercise.	Temporary change in blood chemistry.	Consult doctor if happens repeatedly.

*All references are to Illness section unless noted otherwise.

FATIGUE (continued on next page)

SYMPTOMS & FACTORS	POSSIBLE PROBLEM	WHAT TO DO*
• Fatigue. • Chest discomfort with exertion that is relieved by rest.	Narrowing of coronary arteries.	• Consult doctor. • See Atherosclerosis. • See Coronary-Artery Disease. • See Heart-Valve Disease.
• Fatigue. • Appetite loss. • Weight loss.	• Cancer. • Disorder of red blood cells.	• Consult doctor. • See Anemia (all charts).
• Fatigue in a child who fails to grow normally. • Shortness of breath. • Blueness under fingernails.	Congenital heart disease.	Consult doctor.
• Fatigue. • Appetite loss. • Nausea at sight of food, plus 2 or more of following: • Jaundice (yellow skin and eyes). • Vomiting. • Tenderness over liver. • Fever. • Weakness.	Liver disorder.	• See Acute Hepatitis. • See Hepatitis in Children. • See Cirrhosis of the Liver.
• Fatigue, plus 2 or more of following: • Appetite loss. • Fever. • Headache. • Painful swelling in neck, armpit or groin. • Jaundice (yellow skin and eyes). • Sore throat.	Virus infection.	See Infectious Mononucleosis.
• Fatigue. • Use of prescription or non-prescription drug.	Adverse reaction or side effect of drug.	• Consult doctor about prescription drug. • Discontinue use of non-prescription drug.
• Fatigue. • Cough. • Fever. • Weight loss. • Shortness of breath.	• Lung infection. • Tumor.	• See Tuberculosis. • See Bronchiectasis. • See Pneumonia (all charts). • See Influenza. • See Lung Cancer.

*All references are to Illness section unless noted otherwise.

FATIGUE (continued)

SYMPTOMS & FACTORS	POSSIBLE PROBLEM	WHAT TO DO*
• Fatigue. • Coarse skin and hair. • Low voice. • Loss of sex drive. • Puffy face.	Underactive thyroid gland.	See Hypothyroidism.
• Fatigue. • Fever. • Headache, plus any of following: • Nausea, vomiting or diarrhea. • Drowsiness. • Cough. • Sore throat. • Pain in neck. • Aches in bones or joints. • Skin rash. • Pain in back. • Painful urination.	Bacterial or viral infection.	Consult doctor.
• Fatigue. • Appetite loss. • Weight loss. • Hair loss. • Craving for salt. • Skin that darkens.	Inadequate cortisone hormone.	See Addison's Disease.
• Fatigue in woman at menopause. • Appetite loss.	Normal occurrence with decreasing estrogen level of menopause.	Consult doctor.
• Fatigue. • Pregnancy. • Shortness of breath.	Dietary deficiency of pregnancy, particularly of protein, calcium, vitamins or iron.	• Consult doctor. • Eat more meat, fish. poultry, eggs or dried beans. • Drink 2 extra glasses of skim milk daily. • Take iron supplement and prenatal vitamin supplement.
• Fatigue. • Depression or anxiety.	Effect of stress.	• See Depression. • See Anxiety.

*All references are to Illness section unless noted otherwise.

FEVER
(CHILD 0 TO 2 YEARS)

SYMPTOMS & FACTORS	POSSIBLE PROBLEM	WHAT TO DO*
• Fever. • Convulsions.	Effect of high fever.	• Call doctor now. • See Febrile Convulsion.
• Fever. • Infant of 3 months or younger.	Many possibilities.	Consult doctor. Signs of illness at this age require prompt medical evaluation.
• Fever. • Rash.	Several disorders.	See Rash with Fever (in Symptoms section).
• Fever. • Noisy breathing.	Swelling in vocal cords.	• Consult doctor. • See Croup.
• Fever. • Rapid or difficult breathing.	Infection of breathing passages.	• Call doctor now. • See Acute Bronchitis. • See Bronchiolitis. • See Pneumonia (all charts).
• Fever. • Runny nose. • Recent exposure to contagious disease, such as measles, mumps or chickenpox.	Early stage of contagious illness.	Consult doctor.
• Fever. • Crying as if in pain. • Pulling at ear.	Infection of middle ear.	• Consult doctor. • See Middle-Ear Infection.
• Fever. • Diarrhea.	Infection of digestive tract.	• Consult doctor. • See Gastroenteritis in Infants & Children.
• Fever. • Runny nose.	Virus infection.	• See Common Cold. • Consult doctor if temperature rises.
• Fever. • Hot weather or environment. • Infant overdressed.	Overheating.	• Remove some of infant's clothing. • Offer water to drink. • Give cool bath.

*All references are to Illness section unless noted otherwise.

FEVER
(CHILD OVER 2 YEARS)

SYMPTOMS & FACTORS	POSSIBLE PROBLEM	WHAT TO DO*
• Fever. • Child seems very ill, plus any of following: • Stiff neck. • Pain when bending head forward. • Eyes sensitive to light. • Headache. • Vomiting.	Infection of membranes around brain.	• Call doctor now. • See Aseptic Meningitis.
• Fever. • Convulsions.	Several disorders.	• Call doctor now. • See Febrile Convulsions.
• Fever. • Earache. • Child pulls at ear.	Infection of middle ear.	See Middle-Ear Infection.
• Fever of 102F (38.9C) or higher. • No other symptoms.	Infection.	Consult doctor.
• Fever. • Cough. • Rapid or difficult breathing.	Infection of breathing passages.	See Pneumonia (all charts).
• Fever. • Rash.	Several disorders.	See Rash with Fever (in Symptoms section).
• Fever. • Abdominal pain.	Several disorders.	See Sudden Attack of Abdominal Pain (in Symptoms section).
• Fever. • Diarrhea.	Infection of digestive tract.	See Gastroenteritis.
• Fever. • Swelling between ear and jaw.	Virus infection.	See Mumps.
• Fever. • Sore throat or hoarseness.	Infection of upper respiratory tract.	• See Tonsillitis. • See Pharyngitis. • See Laryngitis.
• Fever. • Cough. • Runny nose.	Virus infection.	• See Common Cold. • See Influenza. • Consult doctor if temperature rises.
• Fever. • Runny nose. • Recent exposure to contagious disease, such as measles, mumps or chickenpox.	Early stage of contagious illness.	Consult doctor.

*All references are to Illness section unless noted otherwise.

FEVER
(PERSON OVER AGE 12)

SYMPTOMS & FACTORS	POSSIBLE PROBLEM	WHAT TO DO*
• Fever. • Headache, plus any of following: • Pain bending forward. • Lethargy. • Confusion. • Nausea or vomiting.	Infection of membranes around brain.	• Call doctor now. • See Aseptic Meningitis.
• Fever. • Pain in back below last rib.	Infection of urinary tract.	See Acute Kidney Infection.
Fever after several hours in strong sunshine or hot environment.	Heat exhaustion.	See Heatstroke or Heat Exhaustion.
• Fever. • Cough. • Shortness of breath. even when resting.	Lung infection.	See Pneumonia (all charts).
• Fever for 24 hours without other symptoms. OR • Recurrent fever, or higher, with normal temperature between fevers.	Several disorders.	• Consult doctor. • See Fever of Undetermined Origin (in Illness section).
• Fever. • Cough with gray-yellow sputum. OR • Wheezing.	Infection of bronchial tubes.	See Acute Bronchitis.
• Fever. • Cough. • Headache. • Aches in bones or joints. • Stuffy or runny nose.	Virus infection.	• See Common Cold. • See Influenza.
• Fever. • Use of prescription or non-prescription drug.	Adverse reaction or side effect of drug.	• Consult doctor for prescription drug. • Discontinue use of non-prescription drug.
• Fever. • Painful urination. • Frequent urination.	Urinary-tract infection.	• See Bladder Infection. • See Acute Kidney Infection.
• Fever. • Sore throat.	Throat infection.	• See Tonsillitis. • See Pharyngitis.
• Fever. • Rash.	Several disorders.	See Rash with Fever (in Symptoms section).
• Fever. • Nausea or vomiting. • Diarrhea.	Infection of digestive tract.	See Gastroenteritis.

*All references are to Illness section unless noted otherwise.

FOOT PROBLEMS

SYMPTOMS & FACTORS	POSSIBLE PROBLEM	WHAT TO DO*
• Pain in toe joints. • Affected joints red, warm, swollen. • Fever. • Recent illness, such as sore throat or skin infection.	Complication of prior streptococcal infection.	See Rheumatic Fever.
Pain in foot following injury.	• Broken bone. • Ligament injury.	• See Bone Fracture. • See Sprains & Strains.
• Pain in foot joint, especially big toe. • Affected joint red, warm, swollen.	Joint inflammation.	See Gout.
Pain in foot after walking or running.	• Circulatory disorder. • Bone injury.	• See Atherosclerosis. • See Buerger's Disease.
• Pain on bottom on foot. • Red, swollen area on sole.	Infection caused by a penetrating wound or splinter.	Consult doctor. You may need tetanus protection.
• Pain on bottom of foot. • Small growth or area on sole that hurts when walking.	Skin growth caused by virus.	See Plantar Warts.
• Itching foot. • Skin between toes red, soft and peeling.	Fungus infection.	See Athlete's Foot.
• Pain in toe joints. • Affected joints red, warm, swollen.	Inflammatory disease of joints.	See Rheumatoid Arthritis.
• Pain or tenderness in foot joint, especially big toe. • Affected joint red, warm, swollen. • Use of prescription drug to prevent fluid retention (diuretic).	Adverse reaction or side effect of diuretic drug.	• Consult doctor. • See Gout.
• Aching feet. • Recent walking or prolonged standing.	• Fracture. • Ligament strain caused by fallen arches.	• See March Fracture. • Consult doctor if pain persists.
• Aching feet. • Significant overweight.	Effect of excess weight.	See Obesity.
• Pain in toe joints, ankles, knees or hips. • Person over age 50.	Degenerative condition of joints.	See Osteoarthritis.
Excessively sweaty feet.	No underlying disorder.	• Wash and dry feet twice a day. Apply talcum powder. • Wear cotton socks.

*All references are to Illness section unless noted otherwise.

HAIR GROWTH IN WOMEN, EXCESSIVE

SYMPTOMS & FACTORS	POSSIBLE PROBLEM	WHAT TO DO*
• Excessive hair growth over 4 or 5 months. • Unexplained weight gain. • Menstrual changes or absent periods. • Deep voice.	Disorder or tumor of ovaries or adrenal gland.	• See Benign Ovarian Tumor. • See Ovarian Cyst. • See Ovarian Cancer. • See Cushing's Syndrome. • See Stein-Leventhal Syndrome.
• Excessive hair growth over 2 months or less. • Use of prescription drug, such as hormones, cortisone drugs or anticonvulsants.	Adverse reaction or side effect of drug.	Consult doctor.
• Excessive hair on face or body that developed before age 20. • Similar hairiness in other female family members.	Genetic causes; no underlying disorder.	Consult cosmetologist for removal of unwanted hair.
Excessive hair growth, especially on face, in woman who has had ovaries removed or is over age 40.	Normal occurrence with decreasing estrogen level of menopause.	• Consult doctor. • Consult cosmetologist for removal of unwanted hair.
Excessive hair growth during pregnancy.	Hormone changes of pregnancy.	Nothing. Hair growth decreases after delivery.

*All references are to Illness section unless noted otherwise.

HAIR LOSS

SYMPTOMS & FACTORS	POSSIBLE PROBLEM	WHAT TO DO*
• Hair loss. • Use of prescription drug, especially for cancer or circulatory disorders.	Adverse reaction or side effect of drug.	Consult doctor.
Sudden hair loss in patches on head.	Skin disorder.	• See Lichen Planus. • See Alopecia Areata. • See Ringworm. • See Telogen Effluvium.
Hair thinning in a woman within 2 to 3 months following childbirth.	Effect of hormonal changes.	Nothing. Hair growth will return to normal.
Gradual hair loss in women, especially thinning of hair on top of head.	Normal occurrence with aging.	See Pattern Baldness (Male & Female).
Receding front hairline or thinning of hair on top of head in men.	Hereditary baldness occurring in men at any age.	See Pattern Baldness (Male & Female).
• Hair loss. • Frequent use of any of following hair-care products or styles: permanent waves; dyes; bleaches; curling irons or hot rollers; straighteners; tight braids; ponytails; or cornrows.	Hair damage.	• Change hair style; avoid damaging products or styles. • Consult doctor if hair loss persists.
• Hair loss. • Unconscious pulling on hair.	Effect of stress.	See Anxiety.
Hair loss in 2 to 3 months following serious illness and high fever.	Temporary effect of illness.	Nothing. Hair should return to normal within few months.

*All references are to Illness section unless noted otherwise.

HALLUCINATIONS

SYMPTOMS & FACTORS	POSSIBLE PROBLEM	WHAT TO DO*
• Hallucinations, plus any of following: • Agitation. • Confusion. • Inability to recognize other people. • Signs of physical illness, such as fever.	Delirium.	Call doctor now.
• Hallucinations. • Use of prescription drug.	Adverse reaction or side effect of drug.	Consult doctor.
• Hallucinations. • Excessive alcohol consumption. OR • Use of mind-altering drugs, such as LSD.	Adverse reaction of alcohol or drug.	• Discontinue use of alcohol or drug. • Consult doctor if hallucinations last longer than 4 hours. • See Drug Abuse & Addiction. • See Alcoholism.
• Hallucination of hearing voices that accuse one of real or imagined misdeeds. • Feelings of guilt.	Psychiatric disorder.	Consult doctor.
Hallucination of seeing or hearing close relative or friend who has recently died.	Common experience following such events.	Hallucinations should cease eventually. Consult doctor if hallucinations last longer than 6 weeks.
Hallucinations when falling asleep or on waking.	Common occurrence at these times.	Nothing.

*All references are to Illness section unless noted otherwise.

HEADACHE

SYMPTOMS & FACTORS	POSSIBLE PROBLEM	WHAT TO DO*
• Severe headache that worsens when bending head forward. • Eyes sensitive to light. • Lethargy. • Confusion. • No recent head injury.	Bleeding in membrane around brain.	• Call doctor now. • See Subarachnoid Hemorrhage & Hematoma. • See Brain or Epidural Abscess.
• Headache. • Lethargy. • Nausea or vomiting. • Recent head injury.	Bleeding inside skull.	• Call doctor now. • See Extradural Hemorrhage.
• Headache that worsens when bending head forward. • Fever. • Eyes sensitive to light.	Infection of membranes around brain.	• Call doctor now. • See Aseptic Meningitis. • See Bacterial Meningitis.
• Headache. • Eye pain. • Blurred vision. • Nausea or vomiting. • No injury to eye.	Excess pressure in eye.	• Call doctor now. • See Acute Glaucoma.
• Habitual headache on waking; no excessive alcohol consumption. • Double vision. • Nausea or vomiting.	• High blood pressure. • Brain tumor.	• See Hypertension. • See Brain Tumor.
• Headache. • Use of prescription or non-prescription drug.	Adverse reaction or side effect of drug.	• Consult doctor about prescription drug. • Discontinue use of non-prescription drug.
• Severe headache. • Fever.	Common occurrence with infection.	See Fever charts (in Symptoms section).
• Headache. • Recent head injury. • No other symptoms.	Common occurrence after head injury.	See Head Injury.
• Headache. • Vision disturbance before headache. • Nausea or vomiting.	Severe vascular headache.	See Migraine Headache.

*All references are to Illness section unless noted otherwise.

HEADACHE (continued)

SYMPTOMS & FACTORS	POSSIBLE PROBLEM	WHAT TO DO*
• Headache in forehead or back of head. • Tense, stressed feeling. • Sleeping difficulty.	Effect of stress.	• See Anxiety. • See Tension or Vascular Headache. • See Depression.
• Headache. • Decreased consumption of caffeine-containing beverages (coffee, colas, cocoa, tea).	Caffeine withdrawal.	• Reduce consumption of caffeine gradually. • Use a non-prescription pain reliever, such as acetaminophen.
• Headache, plus any of following: • Unusually long time since eating. • Excessive alcohol consumption. • Stuffy, smoky or noisy room. • Exposure to strong sunlight.	Circumstantial headache. No underlying disorder.	Use a non-prescription pain reliever, such as acetaminophen.
• Pain or tenderness around eyes and cheekbones that worsens when bending head forward. • Recent cold or nasal allergies.	Sinus infection.	See Sinus Infection.
• Headache without pain around eyes and cheekbones. • Runny or stuffy nose.	Virus infection.	See Common Cold.
Headache after reading or straining to see.	Strain on neck muscles (not strain on eyes.)	See Tension or Vascular Headache.
• Headache after excessive alcohol consumption. • Nausea or vomiting.	"Hangover."	Use a non-prescription pain reliever, such as acetaminophen.

*All references are to Illness section unless noted otherwise.

HEARING LOSS

SYMPTOMS & FACTORS	POSSIBLE PROBLEM	WHAT TO DO*
• Hearing loss. • Use of prescription or non-prescription drug.	Adverse reaction or side effect of drug.	• Consult doctor about prescription drug. • Discontinue use of non-prescription drug.
• Hearing loss. • Sticky, green-yellow discharge from ear.	• Infection of outer-ear canal or middle ear. • Injury to eardrum.	• See Outer-Ear Infection. • See Middle-Ear Infection. • See Ruptured Eardrum.
• Hearing loss. • Dizziness.	Disorder or infection of inner ear.	• See Labyrinthitis. • See Meniere's Disease.
• Hearing loss, especially of high-pitched sounds. • Exposure to excessive noise, such as a jackhammer.	Damage caused by exposure to harmful noise levels.	See Hearing Impairment or Loss.
• Hearing loss. • Earache.	Infection or blockage.	See Earache (in Symptoms section).
Gradual hearing loss in person over age 60.	Common occurrence with aging.	Consult doctor.
• Gradual hearing loss over several weeks or months. • Similar hearing loss in other family members.	Poor function of middle-ear bones.	See Otosclerosis.
• Hearing loss. • Recent cold or sore throat.	Blockage of canal between middle ear and back of throat (eustachian tube).	• See Common Cold. • Consult doctor if hearing loss lasts longer than 3 days.
Gradual hearing loss over several weeks or months without other symptoms.	Earwax blockage.	See Earwax Blockage.

*All references are to Illness section unless noted otherwise.

HEARTBEAT IRREGULARITY

SYMPTOMS & FACTORS	POSSIBLE PROBLEM	WHAT TO DO*
• Irregular heartbeat. • General ill feeling. • History of heart disease.	Disorder of heart rate or rhythm.	• Call doctor now. • See Atrial Fibrillation. • See Heart-Rhythm Irregularity. • See Heart Block. • See Rapid Heartbeat. • See Potassium Imbalance. • See Aneurysm. • See Heart-Valve Disease. • See Calcium Imbalance. • See Idiopathic Hypertrophic Subaortic Stenosis.
• Irregular heartbeat. • Use of prescription or non-prescription drugs, such as: thyroid medication; digitalis preparations; diuretics; diet pills; stimulants; caffeine; decongestants; cold remedies, including nasal sprays; illegal drugs, including marijuana, cocaine, psychedelics, amphetamines.	Adverse reaction or side effect of drug.	• Consult doctor about prescription drug. • Discontinue use of non-prescription or illegal drug.
• Irregular heartbeat. • Unexplained weight loss. • Anxiety. • Excessive sweating. • Fatigue.	Overactive thyroid gland.	See Hyperthyroidism.
• Rapid or irregular heartbeat. • Recent tension or worry.	Effect of stress.	See Anxiety.
• Irregular heartbeat. • Excessive smoking. • Excessive consumption of caffeine-containing beverages such as coffee, cola, tea or cocoa.	Effect of nicotine or caffeine.	Decrease nicotine or caffeine use.
• Rapid or irregular heartbeat. • Fever.	Infection.	See Fever charts (in Symptoms section).

*All references are to Illness section unless noted otherwise.

IMPOTENCE, SEXUAL

SYMPTOMS & FACTORS	POSSIBLE PROBLEM	WHAT TO DO*
• Sexual impotence. • Use of prescription or non-prescription or mood-altering drugs, such as: antihypertensives; amphetamines; narcotics; cocaine; antidepressants; antihistamines; antiulcer medicines; diuretics; hormones including birth-control pills; beta-adrenergic blockers; tranquilizers; reserpine; marijuana; digitalis; skeletal-muscle relaxants; sedatives; hypnotics; or phenothiazines.	Adverse reaction or side effect of drug.	• Consult doctor about prescription drug. • Discontinue use of non-prescription drug.
• Sexual impotence. • Chronic illness.	• Low level of testosterone (male sex hormone). • Diminished blood circulation to genitals.	• Consult doctor. • See Atherosclerosis. • See Diabetes Mellitus. • See Cirrhosis of the Liver. • See Hypothyroidism. • See Multiple Sclerosis. • See Enlarged Prostate. • See Underactive Pituitary Gland.
• Sexual impotence. • Excessive alcohol consumption.	Effect of alcohol.	See Alcoholism.
• Sexual impotence. • Anxiety or depression.	Effect of stress.	• See Anxiety. • See Depression.
• Sexual impotence. • History of sexually transmitted disease.	Scarring or other effect of infection.	• See Syphilis. • See Gonorrhea. • See Urethritis.
• Sexual impotence. • History of premature ejaculation or other sexual dysfunction.	Psychosexual problem.	See Male Sexual Impotence.
• Sexual impotence. • Acute illness with fever.	Temporary effect of illness.	Nothing. Sexual function will return when illness subsides.

*All references are to Illness section unless noted otherwise.

ITCHING

SYMPTOMS & FACTORS	POSSIBLE PROBLEM	WHAT TO DO*
• Itching. • Yellow skin and eyes.	• Blood disorder. • Liver disorder.	Call doctor now.
• Itching. • General ill feeling.	• Blood disorder. • Kidney disorder. • Overactive thyroid gland. • Adverse reaction or side effect of drug. • Cancer.	• Consult doctor. • See Polycythemia. • See Acute Kidney Failure. • See Hyperthyroidism. • See Drug Hypersensitivity.
• Itching. • Rash. • No fever.	Several skin disorders.	See Rash without Fever (in Symptoms section).
Itching in genital area in females.	Irritation or infection.	See Vaginal Itching (in Symptoms section).
• Itching or bleeding around anus. • Painful bowel movements.	• Varicose veins in anus. • Split in skin around anus.	• See Hemorrhoids. • See Anal Fissure.
• Itching head. • Tiny white spots on hair that won't come off.	Parasites.	See Lice.
• Itching head. • Small bald patches on scalp.	Fungus infection.	See Ringworm.
Itching around anus, especially at night.	Parasites.	See Pinworms.
• Itching hands. • Hands are frequently wet or exposed to chemicals.	Effect of chemicals or moisture.	See Contact Dermatitis.
• Itching. • New clothing.	Allergic reaction.	• Wash new clothing before wearing. • Avoid irritating fabrics.
Itching around anus following severe diarrhea.	Normal response to irritation.	Apply ointment containing zinc oxide.

*All references are to Illness section unless noted otherwise.

KNEE PAIN

SYMPTOMS & FACTORS	POSSIBLE PROBLEM	WHAT TO DO*
• Pain in knee following injury. • Knee won't bear weight. • Knee misshapen.	Broken bone or dislocation.	• Call doctor now. • See Bone Fracture. • See Dislocation or Subluxation.
• Pain in knee. • Knee red, warm, swollen. • Fever. • General ill feeling.	Bone or joint infection.	See Osteomyelitis.
• Pain in knee and other joints. • Affected joints red, warm, swollen. • Fever. • Recent illness. such as sore throat, gonorrhea or skin infection.	Complication of prior infection.	• See Rheumatic Fever. • See Infectious Arthritis.
• Pain in knee. • Knee "catches" or won't bear weight.	Injured knee cartilage.	See Sprains & Strains.
• Pain in knee or other joints. • Affected joints red, warm, swollen. • No fever.	Joint inflammation.	• See Bursitis. • See Gout. • See Rheumatoid Arthritis. • See Juvenile Rheumatoid Arthritis (children only). • See Osgood-Schlatter Disease (older children and adolescents only).
• Chronic pain in knee. • Knee sometimes "catches" or won't support weight. OR • Persistent discomfort in knee, fingers or other joints without other symptoms.	Degenerative joint disease.	See Osteoarthritis.
• Pain in knee in child under 12. • Hip pain. • Limp.	Degenerative condition of hip joint in children.	See Legg-Perthes Disease.

*All references are to Illness section unless noted otherwise.

LEG PAIN

SYMPTOMS & FACTORS	POSSIBLE PROBLEM	WHAT TO DO*
• Pain in calf when flexing ankle. • Swollen, tender calf.	Blood clot in deep vein.	• Call doctor now. • See Deep-Vein Thrombosis.
• Leg pain following injury. • Leg won't bear weight.	Broken bone.	• Call doctor now. • See Bone Fracture.
• Pain in calf. • One vein red, hot and hard.	Blood clot in superficial vein.	See Superficial Thrombophlebitis.
• Persistent pain in one part of leg. • Fever. • General ill feeling.	• Bone infection. • Cancer.	• See Osteomyelitis. • See Multiple Myeloma.
Sharp pain down back of leg, especially when coughing, sneezing or laughing hard.	Pressure on large nerve in leg.	• See Ruptured Disk. • See Backache (in Symptoms section).
• Pain in calf after walking 100 yards or more. • Pain disappears with rest.	Circulatory disorder.	• See Atherosclerosis. • See Buerger's Disease. • See Arterial Thrombosis & Embolus.
• Leg pain. • Painful or stiff hip on same side as leg pain.	Degenerative condition of joints.	See Osteoarthritis.
• Leg pain. • Muscles tighten briefly— usually while asleep—then return to normal.	Several disorders.	See Muscle Cramp (in Symptoms section).
• Leg ache, especially after standing a long time. • Prominent veins in legs.	Disorder of veins.	See Varicose Veins.
• Leg pain following strenuous exercise or following injury. • Leg can bear weight.	Muscle injury.	See Pulled or Torn Muscle.

*All references are to Illness section unless noted otherwise.

MEMORY PROBLEMS

SYMPTOMS & FACTORS	POSSIBLE PROBLEM	WHAT TO DO*
• Inability to remember a period of time. • Recent head injury.	Brain injury.	• Call doctor now. • See Head Injury.
Inability to remember episodes of excessive alcohol consumption.	Effect of alcohol.	• Consult doctor. • See Alcoholism.
• Inability to remember *recent* events while remembering *long-ago* events. plus 2 or more of following: • Poor attention span in conversations or with instructions. • Decline in attention to personal appearance or cleanliness. • Personality change. • Decline in ability to cope with everyday matters.	Mental deterioration.	• See Dementia. • See Vitamin-B Deficiencies. • See Alzheimer's Disease.
• Inability to remember a period of time. • Use of prescription or non-prescription drug, especially for sleeping difficulty.	Adverse reaction or side effect of drug.	Consult doctor.
Total memory loss.	Psychological disorder.	Consult doctor.
• Inability to remember everyday things, such as location of keys, pens, glasses, or forgetting items on shopping list. • Depression or tension.	Effect of stress.	• See Depression. • See Anxiety.
Gradual decline over past 10 years in ability to remember everyday things in person over age 50.	Common occurrence with aging; no underlying disorder.	• Consult doctor at next appointment. • Write lists to help your memory. This is not the beginning of serious mental decline.
• Inability to remember a period of time, plus events surrounding any of the following: • Epileptic seizure. • Diabetic coma. • Period before and after surgery. • Severe, feverish illness such as meningitis or pneumonia.	Common occurrence following these situations.	Nothing.

*All references are to Illness section unless noted otherwise.

MENSTRUAL PERIODS, LATE OR ABSENT

SYMPTOMS & FACTORS	POSSIBLE PROBLEM	WHAT TO DO*
• Menstrual periods absent, plus 2 or more of following: • Unexplained weight gain. • Masculine voice. • Abnormal hairiness.	Hormone imbalance.	Consult doctor.
• Menstrual periods absent. • Recent quick weight loss from drastic dieting. OR • Current participation in strenuous exercise program.	Hormone changes.	See Secondary Amenorrhea.
• Menstrual periods absent, plus: • Recent illness. OR • Tension or worry. OR • Change in lifestyle. such as new job or new home.	Effect of stress.	See Secondary Amenorrhea.
Menstrual periods absent since discontinuing use of oral contraceptives.	Hormone changes caused by discontinuing pill.	See Secondary Amenorrhea.
• Menstrual period late by 2 or more weeks. • Sexual intercourse within last month.	Pregnancy.	Consult doctor to confirm pregnancy.
Menstrual periods absent in woman over age 38.	Normal menstrual irregularities at this age.	See Menopause.
• Menstrual periods absent. • Use of prescription drug.	Adverse reaction or side effect of drug.	Consult doctor.
Menstrual periods absent since delivery of baby.	Normal occurrence caused by hormone changes following childbirth.	• If bottle-feeding. consult doctor if periods do not resume within 8 weeks after delivery. • If breast-feeding. consult doctor if periods do not resume within 4 weeks after weaning.
Menstrual periods have never started.	Hormone changes of puberty have not occurred.	• Consult doctor if older than 16. • See Primary Amenorrhea.

*All references are to Illness section unless noted otherwise.

MENSTRUAL PERIODS, PAINFUL OR HEAVY

SYMPTOMS & FACTORS	POSSIBLE PROBLEM	WHAT TO DO*
• Menstrual periods more painful or heavier than usual. • Bad-smelling vaginal discharge. • Fever.	Infection of reproductive organs.	• Call doctor now. • See Pelvic Inflammatory Disease.
• Current menstrual period more painful or heavier than usual. • Period arrived 1 week or more late.	• Early pregnancy and miscarriage. • Pregnancy outside uterus.	• Consult doctor. • See Miscarriage. • See Ectopic Pregnancy.
Menstrual period more painful or heavier than usual, especially during last days of period.	Disorder of lining of pelvic organs.	• See Endometriosis. • See Dysmenorrhea.
Menstrual periods more painful or heavier since receiving intrauterine contraceptive device (IUD).	Common side effect of using IUD.	Consult doctor.
• Menstrual periods more painful or heavier than usual. • No other pelvic or genital symptoms.	Benign growth in uterus.	See Fibroid Tumors of the Uterus.
Menstrual periods painful or heavy since discontinuing use of oral contraceptives.	Hormone changes caused by discontinuing pill.	Consult doctor.
• Menstrual periods painful. • Periods began within last 3 years. • Healthy otherwise.	No disease.	See Dysmenorrhea.
Menstrual period heavy in woman who has recently delivered a baby.	Normal occurrence during first 2 menstrual periods following childbirth.	Consult doctor if heavy periods persist.
Menstrual flow always heavy.	No underlying disorder.	Consult doctor for blood test for anemia.

*All references are to Illness section unless noted otherwise.

MOUTH, SORE

SYMPTOMS & FACTORS	POSSIBLE PROBLEM	WHAT TO DO*
• Sore mouth. • Fever. • Sores in mouth. • Use of prescription or non-prescription drugs.	Adverse reaction or side effect of drug.	Call doctor now.
• Sore mouth. • Fever. • Red, painful gums that bleed easily. • Bad breath.	• Bacterial infection. • Cancer.	• See Trench Mouth. • See Leukemia.
• Sore mouth. • Painful ulcers with red edges, white centers.	Infection or inflammation.	See Canker Sores.
• Sore mouth. • Blisters or red, rough or painful areas on lips or in mouth.	Virus infection.	• See Cold Sores. • See Hand, Foot & Mouth Disease.
• Sore mouth. • Creamy-white patches in mouth or tongue.	Fungus infection.	See Thrush.
• Sore mouth. • Rough or split corners of mouth.	Vitamin or mineral deficiency.	• See Vitamin-B Deficiencies. • See Folic-Acid-Deficiency Anemia. • See Aplastic Anemia.
• Sore mouth. • Use of new cosmetics.	Allergic reaction caused by chemical.	Discontinue use of new cosmetic.

*All references are to Illness section unless noted otherwise.

MUSCLE CRAMP

SYMPTOMS & FACTORS	POSSIBLE PROBLEM	WHAT TO DO*
Recurrent leg cramps when walking.	Circulatory disorder.	• See Atherosclerosis. • See Buerger's Disease. • See Arterial Thrombosis & Embolus.
Muscle cramp following exposure to heat.	Heat exhaustion.	See Heatstroke or Heat Exhaustion.
• Recurrent muscle cramps. • Tender nodules on skin. • Stiffness and weakness.	Infammation of connective tissue.	See Fibrositis.
• Muscle cramp. • Use of diuretic drug for high blood pressure or heart disorder.	Adverse reaction or side effect of drug.	Consult doctor.
• Muscle cramp while relaxed or resting in bed. OR • Muscle cramp in arm or leg during or after exercise. OR • Muscle cramp after sitting in awkward position.	Common occurrence; usually no underlying disorder.	Massage muscle and use heat to relieve pain.

*All references are to Illness section unless noted otherwise.

NECK PAIN

SYMPTOMS & FACTORS	POSSIBLE PROBLEM	WHAT TO DO*
• Sudden neck pain, especially when bending head forward, plus any of following: • Lethargy. • Confusion. • Eyes sensitive to light. • Nausea or vomiting. • Severe headache.	Infection or bleeding in membrane around brain.	• Call doctor now. • See Aseptic Meningitis. • See Subarachnoid Hemorrhage.
• Sudden, severe neck pain. • Recent strong jolt. • Difficulty controlling arms or legs. • Loss of bowel or bladder control.	Damaged spinal cord.	Call doctor now.
• Severe neck pain. • Sharp pain in shoulders or arms when moving head.	• Slipped disk in neck. • Neck-muscle injury.	• See Ruptured Disk. • See Whiplash. • See Torticollis.
• Severe neck pain. • Swelling in side or back of neck.	Infection.	See Swelling or Lump (in Symptoms section).
• Stiffness or severe neck pain on waking. • No pain before going to bed.	Uncomfortable sleeping position.	Consult doctor if neck pain lasts longer than 24 hours.
• Chronic neck pain that is worsening. • Numbness or tingling in arm or hand. • Person over age 50.	Pressure on nerves in neck.	See Cervical Spondylosis.
• Sudden, severe neck pain. • Injury to neck.	Muscle injury.	See Pulled or Torn Muscle.

*All references are to Illness section unless noted otherwise.

NIGHTMARES

SYMPTOMS & FACTORS	POSSIBLE PROBLEM	WHAT TO DO*
• Recurrent nightmares. • Excessive alcohol consumption.	Effect of alcohol.	See Alcoholism.
• Nightmares. • Use of prescription drug.	Adverse reaction or side effect of drug.	Consult doctor.
• Nightmares. • Tension or worry.	Effect of stress.	See Anxiety.
Nightmares following traumatic or sad experience, such as an accident or death of loved one.	Common occurrence following such experiences.	Consult doctor if nightmares persist longer than 6 weeks.
• Nightmares. • Recent alcohol withdrawal.	Withdrawal symptom.	See Alcoholism.
• Nightmares. • Physical illness. • Fever.	Common occurrence during feverish illness.	Nothing.
• Nightmares. • Recent withdrawal of drug, such as sleeping pills.	Common occurrence under circumstances.	Nothing. Dreams should return to normal in several days.
Occasional nightmares without other symptoms or factors.	Common occurrence.	Nothing.

*All references are to Illness section unless noted otherwise.

NOSE, STUFFY OR RUNNY

SYMPTOMS & FACTORS	POSSIBLE PROBLEM	WHAT TO DO*
• Stuffy or runny nose (thick, cloudy, yellow-green discharge). • Pain or tenderness around eyes and cheekbones that worsens when bending head forward.	Sinus infection.	See Sinus Infection.
• Stuffy or runny nose (clear, watery discharge), plus any of following: • Fever. • Cough. • Headache. • Aches in bones or joints. • Sore throat.	Virus infection.	• See Common Cold. • See Influenza.
• Stuffy or runny nose (clear, watery discharge). • Itching eyes. • Sneezing.	Nasal allergy.	See Hay Fever.

*All references are to Illness section unless noted otherwise.

NUMBNESS, TINGLING OR PRICKLING

SYMPTOMS & FACTORS	POSSIBLE PROBLEM	WHAT TO DO*
● Numbness or tingling on one side of body, plus any of following: ● Weakness in extremities. ● Dizziness. ● Confusion. ● Blurred vision. ● Speaking difficulty.	Decreased blood supply to brain.	● Call doctor now. ● See Stroke. ● See Transient Ischemic Attack (T.I.A.).
● Numbness or tingling in an arm or leg. ● Weakness in the affected side. ● Recent heavy lifting or strenuous exercise.	Pressure on nerves.	See Ruptured Disk.
● Numbness or tingling in any part of body. ● Use of prescription drug.	Adverse reaction or side effect of drug.	Consult doctor.
● Numbness or tingling in fingers or toes. ● Blue fingers or toes in cold weather. ● Redness and pain when numbness subsides and feeling returns.	Disorder of blood circulation in fingers and toes.	See Raynaud's Disease.
● Numbness or tingling in hands. ● Stiff neck. ● Person over age 35.	Pressure on nerves in neck.	● See Cervical Spondylosis. ● See Thoracic-Outlet-Obstruction Syndrome.
● Numbness or tingling in hands and fingers, especially at night. ● Sharp pain in hand or arm. especially at night. ● Weak grip.	Pressure on nerves in wrist.	See Carpal-Tunnel Syndrome.
● Numbness or tingling in hands and face, especially around lips. ● Dizziness. ● Fever (occasionally).	Decreased carbon dioxide in blood.	● See Hyperventilation Syndrome. ● Consult doctor if fever is present.
Numbness or tingling in feet or hands after sitting in one position a long time or waking from deep sleep.	● Stretching of or pressure on a nerve. ● Temporary decrease in blood supply to a nerve. ● No underlying disorder.	Nothing. Feeling returns in a few minutes.

*All references are to Illness section unless noted otherwise.

PUPILS OF DIFFERENT SIZE

SYMPTOMS & FACTORS	POSSIBLE PROBLEM	WHAT TO DO*
• Pupils of different size. • Recent injury to head or eye.	Bleeding inside skull.	• See Head Injury. • See Subdural Hemorrhage & Hematoma. • See Extradural Hemorrhage.
• Pupils of different size. • Headache. • Nausea or vomiting without nausea. • Blurred or double vision.	• Tumor. • Expanding brain lesion.	• Call doctor now. • See Brain Tumor. • See Brain Abscess. • See Head Injury. • See Aneurysm.
• Pupils of different size. • Fever. • Headache that worsens when bending forward. • Lethargy. • Stiff neck. • Eyes sensitive to light.	Infection of membranes around brain.	• Call doctor now. • See Aseptic Meningitis. • See Bacterial Meningitis. • See Viral or Aseptic Encephalitis.
• Pupils of different size. • Pain in eye. • Nausea.	Excess pressure in eye.	See Acute Glaucoma.
• Pupils of different size. • Decreased sweating on side with dilated pupil. • Drooping eyelid on affected side.	• Birth injury. • Tumor in chest. • Lymph-node pressure.	Consult doctor.
• Pupils of different size (occasionally). • No other symptoms or factors.	Unknown.	Nothing as long as pupils return to normal.
• Pupils of different size. • No recent injury. • Similar unequal pupils in other family members.	Genetic causes. No underlying disorder.	Nothing.

*All references are to Illness section unless noted otherwise.

RASH WITH FEVER

SYMPTOMS & FACTORS	POSSIBLE PROBLEM	WHAT TO DO*
• Purple spots, plus 2 or more of following: • Fever. • Headache. • Pain when bending head forward. • Eyes sensitive to light. • Vomiting.	Infection of membranes around brain.	• Call doctor now. • See Bacterial Meningitis.
• Red rash in woman of childbearing age. • Fever of 101F (38.3C) or higher. • Rapid heartbeat. • Fatigue and weakness. • Excessive thirst.	Bacterial infection.	• Call doctor now. • See Toxic Shock Syndrome.
• Purple rash. • Fever.	Allergic disorder.	• Call doctor now. • See Allergic Purpura.
• Red rash. • Paleness around mouth. • Fever of 102F (38.9C) or higher. • Bright red, sore throat. • Swollen tonsils. • Enlarged glands in neck.	Complication of preceding streptococcal infection.	• Call doctor now. • See Scarlet Fever.
• Red spots or blotches on face or trunk. • Fever, plus 2 or more of following: • Dry cough. • Sore, red eyes. • Runny nose. • Sore Throat. • Headache.	• Virus infection. • Rickettsia infection.	• See Measles. • See Hand, Foot & Mouth Disease. • See Rocky Mountain Spotted Fever.
• Raised, red, itching bumps that become blisters on face, trunk and genitals. • Fever.	Virus infection.	See Chickenpox.
• Red rash. • Fever. • Swelling on both sides of neck or at base of skull.	Virus infection.	See German Measles.

*All references are to Illness section unless noted otherwise.

RASH WITHOUT FEVER

SYMPTOMS & FACTORS	POSSIBLE PROBLEM	WHAT TO DO*
• Light-red bumps with raised edges. • Severe itching.	Allergic reaction.	See Hives.
• Itching rash. • Use of prescription or non-prescription drug.	Adverse reaction or side effect of drug.	• Call doctor now. • See Drug Hypersensitivity.
• Itching rash around genitals or anus. • No other symptoms or factors.	• Sugar in urine. • Vaginal infection.	• See Diabetes Mellitus. • See Monilial Vaginitis.
Red bumps in a small area without other symptoms.	Insect bites.	See Insect Bites & Stings.
• Red rash scattered over body. • Severe itching at night. • Gray lines or red, sore spots between fingers or on wrists.	Parasites.	See Scabies.
Red, scaling patch that spreads into a ring.	Fungus infection.	See Ringworm.
Itching, red, scaling or moist rash under cosmetics, jewelry or new clothing.	Allergic reaction.	See Contact Dermatitis.
• Itching, red, scaling or moist rash, plus: • Recent contact with plant. such as poison ivy, poison oak, poison sumac, primrose or mango. OR • Recent contact with irritating detergents or other chemicals.	Allergic reaction.	See Contact Dermatitis.
Itching, red, scaling or moist rash, especially on hands.	Skin disorder aggravated by stress.	See Atopic Dermatitis.
Rash without fever in child under 2.	Several disorders.	See Skin Problems (Child Under Age 2) in Symptoms section.

*All references are to Illness section unless noted otherwise.

SEXUAL INTERCOURSE, PAINFUL FOR MAN

SYMPTOMS & FACTORS	POSSIBLE PROBLEM	WHAT TO DO*
• Pain during ejaculation. • Burning when urinating. • Discharge from penis.	Infection of urethra or prostate gland.	• See Urethritis. • See Prostatitis. • See Gonorrhea.
• Pain in penis during intercourse. • Red, swollen, tender bumps or sores on skin or tip of penis.	Skin inflammation or infection.	• See Genital Herpes. • See Balanitis.
• Pain in penis during intercourse. • Partner tense, difficult to arouse or uncomfortable during intercourse.	Lack of lubrication in partner's vagina.	• See Dyspareunia. • See Vaginismus.
• Pain in tip of penis after intercourse. • Use of rubber condom. OR • Partner uses contraceptive cream or douching solution.	Allergic reaction to cream, solution or condom.	See Dyspareunia.
• Pain in penis before, during or after intercourse. • No other symptoms or factors.	Psychosexual problem.	• See Dyspareunia. • See Male Sexual Impotence.

*All references are to Illness section unless noted otherwise.

SEXUAL INTERCOURSE, PAINFUL FOR WOMAN

SYMPTOMS & FACTORS	POSSIBLE PROBLEM	WHAT TO DO*
• Painful intercourse only when partner penetrates vagina deeply. • Heavy, painful periods.	Disorder of lining of pelvic organs.	See Endometriosis.
• Painful intercourse. • Abnormal vaginal discharge.	Several disorders.	See Abnormal Vaginal Discharge (in Symptoms section).
• Painful intercourse. • Tenderness over bladder. • Frequent, painful urination.	Bladder inflammation.	See Bladder Infection.
Painful intercourse in woman past menopause or over age 45.	Normal occurrence caused by decreased vaginal secretions.	• See Vaginismus. • See Dyspareunia. • See Menopause.
• Painful intercourse. • Recent childbirth.	Inflammation or scarring caused by a stretched or torn vagina or episiotomy repair.	• Wait at least 3 weeks before resuming sexual relations after childbirth. • Consult doctor if pain lasts longer than 8 weeks.
• Painful intercourse. • Vaginal itching.	Several disorders.	See Vaginal Itching (in Symptoms section).
• Painful intercourse. • Vagina seems too tight.	Muscle spasm.	• See Vaginismus. • See Dyspareunia.
• Painful intercourse. • Recent start or increase in sexual activity.	No underlying disorder.	• Wait 2 to 3 days for symptoms to disappear before resuming sex. • See Vaginismus. • See Dyspareunia.

*All references are to Illness section unless noted otherwise.

SHOULDER PAIN

SYMPTOMS & FACTORS	POSSIBLE PROBLEM	WHAT TO DO*
• Pain in shoulder following injury. • Inability to move shoulder. • Shoulder misshapen. • Bruising in affected area.	Broken bone or dislocation.	• Call doctor now. • See Bone Fracture. • See Dislocation or Subluxation.
• Sudden pain in shoulder in woman of childbearing age. • Menstrual period late 4 weeks or more. • Sudden pain in lower abdomen.	Pregnancy developing outside uterus.	• Call doctor now. • See Ectopic Pregnancy.
• Sudden pain in shoulder or other joint. • Affected joint red, warm, swollen. • Fever. • Recent illness, such as sore throat or skin infection.	Complication of prior streptococcal infection.	See Rheumatic Fever.
• Pain in shoulder and other joints. • Affected joints red, warm, swollen.	Inflammatory disease of joints.	See Rheumatoid Arthritis.
• Sudden pain in shoulder. • No fever.	Shoulder inflammation.	See Gout.
• Pain in shoulder, especially when moving arm. • No other symptoms.	Shoulder inflammation.	See Bursitis.
• Pain in shoulder when moving arm. • Stiffness and severity of pain increasing.	Severe shoulder inflammation.	See Frozen Shoulder.
• Pain in shoulder following injury. • Shoulder appearance normal • Shoulder movement uncomfortable.	Injury to shoulder-cuff muscle or ligament.	• See Pulled or Torn Muscle. • See Sprains & Strains.

*All references are to Illness section unless noted otherwise.

SKIN PROBLEMS
(CHILD UNDER AGE 2)

SYMPTOMS & FACTORS	POSSIBLE PROBLEM	WHAT TO DO*
• Rash. • Fever.	Several disorders.	See Rash with Fever (in Symptoms section).
Dark red or purple spots that don't fade when skin is pressed or stretched.	Allergic disorder.	• Call doctor now. • See Allergic Purpura.
Rash, spots, blisters or discoloration in infant 3 months or younger.	Several disorders.	Consult doctor.
Inflamed skin with itching, flaking patches.	Allergic skin disorder.	See Eczema.
Blisters on face that burst and become crusty.	Skin infection.	See Impetigo.
Rash in diaper area.	Chemical skin irritation.	See Diaper Rash.
• Rash or blotches. • Hot weather or environment.	Sweat retention.	• Remove excess clothing. • Consult doctor if rash lasts longer than 24 hours or child seems ill. • See Prickly Heat.
Greasy, scaling, crusty patches on scalp.	Cradle cap.	Use half-strength coal-tar cream on affected areas. Your pharmacist can provide this. Cradle cap usually disappears when hair grows.
Patch of skin that is lighter or darker than surrounding skin.	• Disorder of skin pigment. • Inherited skin lesion.	• See Pityriasis Alba. • See Benign Skin Lesions.

*All references are to Illness section unless noted otherwise.

SKIN PROBLEMS
(PERSON OVER AGE 2)

SYMPTOMS & FACTORS	POSSIBLE PROBLEM	WHAT TO DO*
• A new mole or dark lump. OR • Change in a mole that has been present since childhood in person over age 12.	Skin cancer.	See Malignant Melanoma.
• Rash. • Use of prescription or non-prescription drug.	Adverse reaction or side effect of drug.	Call doctor now.
• Rash. • Fever.	Several disorders.	See Rash with Fever (in Symptoms section).
Skin problems in child under 2.	Several disorders.	See Skin Problems (Child Under Age 2) in Symptoms section.
• Blistery rash. • Burning sensation at site 1 or 2 days before rash appears.	Virus infection of sensory nerves.	See Shingles.
Red skin areas covered with silvery scales.	Chronic skin disorder.	See Psoriasis.
Skin problem on feet.	Several disorders.	See Foot Problems (in Symptoms section).
Skin problem on face.	Several disorders.	See Facial Skin Problems (in Symptoms section).
Bumps on skin.	Several disorders.	See Bumps on Skin (in Symptoms section).
Patch of skin that is lighter or darker than surrounding skin.	Disorder of skin pigment.	• See Vitiligo. • See Pityriasis Alba.
Reddish, scaly, oval patches on chest, back or abdomen without fever or other symptoms.	Inflammatory skin disorder.	See Pityriasis Rosea.
Itching rash without fever.	Several disorders.	See Rash Without Fever (in Symptoms section).
Itching without change in skin appearance.	Several disorders.	See Itching (in Symptoms section).

*All references are to Illness section unless noted otherwise.

SLEEPING PROBLEMS

SYMPTOMS & FACTORS	POSSIBLE PROBLEM	WHAT TO DO*
• Fitful sleep. • Shortness of breath when awake.	Fluid in lungs caused by heart condition.	See Congestive Heart Failure.
• Sleeping problems. • Use of prescription or non-prescription drug, such as appetite suppressants. decongestants or diuretics.	Adverse reaction or side effect of drug.	Consult doctor.
• Inability to fall asleep. • Daytime tension.	Effect of stress.	See Anxiety.
• Wakefulness during night, plus 2 or more of following: • Reduced sex drive. • Inability to concentrate. • Lowered self-esteem. • Feelings of guilt, worthlessness, self-reproach. • Fatigue. • Loss of pleasure in usual activities. • Poor appetite or overeating.	Depression.	See Depression.
• Sleeping problems. • Recent withdrawal from narcotics, tranquilizers, sleeping pills or alcohol.	Withdrawal symptom.	Nothing. Normal sleep pattern should return within several weeks.
• Sleeping problems. • Use of illegal drug.	Adverse reaction or side effect of drug.	• Discontinue use of drug. • See Drug Abuse & Addiction.
• Sleeping problems, plus 2 or more of following: • Excessive sweating. • Unexplained weight loss. • Increased appetite. • Anxiety. • Rapid or irregular heartbeat.	Overactive thyroid gland.	See Hyperthyroidism.
Sleeping problems following late, heavy dinner or consumption of 3 or more alcoholic beverages at night.	Common occurrence.	• Eat lighter or earlier dinner. • Decrease alcohol consumption.
• Sleeping problems. • Use of caffeine-containing beverage or drug.	Stimulant effect of caffeine.	Decrease use of caffeine, especially during late afternoon or evening.
• Sleeping problems. • Sedentary lifestyle.	Common occurrence.	See Appendix 20. for exercise recommendations.
Change in sleep pattern in person over age 60.	Normal occurrence; less sleep needed with aging.	Nothing.

*All references are to Illness section unless noted otherwise.

SPEAKING DIFFICULTY

SYMPTOMS & FACTORS	POSSIBLE PROBLEM	WHAT TO DO
• Speaking difficulty, plus any of following: • Blurred vision. • Numbness or tingling in any part of body. • Weakness in extremities. • Dizziness.	Decreased blood supply to brain.	• Call doctor now. • See Stroke. • See Transient Ischemic Attack (T.I.A.). • See Aneurysm. • See Arterial Thrombosis & Embolism.
• Speaking difficulty. • Use of prescription or non-prescription drug.	Adverse reaction or side effect of drug.	Consult doctor.
• Expressionless speech with abnormal tone and phrasing. • Trembling that is worst at rest. • Shuffling walk.	Disorder of central nervous system.	See Parkinson's Disease.
• Inability to complete words without repeating first consonants. OR • Inability to speak when ready to say something.	Stammering or stuttering in children, and stress in adults.	Consult doctor.
Normal pronunciation, but confused words or ideas in person under age 45.	Psychiatric disorder.	Consult doctor.
• Normal pronunciation but confused words or ideas, plus 2 or more of following: • Poor attention span with conversations or instructions. • Decline in attention to personal appearance or cleanliness. • Personality changes.	Mental deterioration.	See Alzheimer's Disease.
Speaking difficulty because of inability to move muscles on one side of face.	Disorder of facial nerves.	See Bell's Palsy.
Speaking difficulty because of pain in mouth or tongue.	Infection or sores in mouth or tongue.	See Sore Mouth (in Symptoms section).

*All references are to Illness section unless noted otherwise.

STOOL, ABNORMAL APPEARANCE

SYMPTOMS & FACTORS	POSSIBLE PROBLEM	WHAT TO DO*
• Very dark or black stool. • Pain or discomfort in abdomen.	Bleeding in digestive tract.	• Call doctor now. • See Stomach Ulcer. • See Duodenal Ulcer. • See Stomach Cancer. • See Large-Intestine Cancer. • See Diverticular Disease.
• Blood in stool. • No fever or illness.	• Varicose veins or break around anus. • Tumor.	• Consult doctor. • See Hemorrhoids. • See Anal Fissure.
• Blood in stool. • General ill feeling. • Fever.	Inflammatory disease of intestinal tract.	• See Ulcerative Colitis. • See Bacillary Dysentery.
• Pale stool. • Yellow skin and eyes.	Gallbladder or liver disorder.	• Call doctor now. • See Acute Cholecystitis or Cholangitis. • See Acute Viral Hepatitis.
• Pale, foamy, bulky, bad-smelling stool. • No jaundice.	Poor digestion.	See Malabsorption.
• Stool that is very dark, black or contains black material, plus any of following: • Recent consumption of green, leafy vegetables. • Current use of iron-supplement tablets. • Recent use of Pepto-Bismol.	No underlying disorder.	Nothing.

*All references are to Illness section unless noted otherwise.

SWALLOWING DIFFICULTY

SYMPTOMS & FACTORS	POSSIBLE PROBLEM	WHAT TO DO*
• Swallowing difficulty. • Muscle weakness of neck, chest and extremities. • Drooping eyelids. • Double vision. • No fever.	Toxin from contaminated food.	• Call doctor now. • See Botulism.
• Swallowing difficulty. • Sore throat. • Recent swallowing of foreign object, such as fish bone.	Object stuck in throat.	Call doctor now.
• Swallowing difficulty that is worsening. • Sensation that food is stuck high in chest. • Unexplained weight loss.	• Disorder of nerves that control esophagus muscles. • Tumor.	• See Esophagus Cancer. • See Hiatal Hernia. • See Esophageal Stricture or Corrosive Esophagitis.
• Swallowing difficulty. • Sore throat. • Fever.	Throat infection.	• Request throat culture. • See Strep Throat. • See Tonsillitis. • See Pharyngitis. • See Diphtheria.
• Swallowing difficulty. • Drooping eyelids. • Arm and leg weakness.	Autoimmune disorder.	See Myasthenia Gravis.
• Swallowing difficulty. • Sensation that food is stuck high in chest. • Occasional chest pain, especially when bending forward or lying down.	Discomfort in upper digestive tract.	See Heartburn.
Normal swallowing with sensation that food is stuck.	Effect of stress.	• Increase fluid intake when eating. • See Anxiety.

*All references are to Illness section unless noted otherwise.

SWEATING, EXCESSIVE

SYMPTOMS & FACTORS	POSSIBLE PROBLEM	WHAT TO DO*
• Excessive sweating. • Chest pain.	Heart attack.	• Call doctor now! • See Heart Attack. • See Coronary-Artery Disease.
• Excessive sweating at night. • Weight loss. • Persistent cough with blood in sputum. • Fever. • Fatigue.	• Lung inflammation or infection. • Cancer.	• See Tuberculosis. • See Hodgkin's Disease. • See Lung Cancer.
• Excessive sweating, plus 2 or more of following: • Weight loss. • Increased appetite. • Anxiety. • Sleeping problems.	Overactive thyroid gland.	See Hyperthyroidism.
• Excessive sweating. • Use of prescription, non-prescription or illegal drug.	Adverse reaction or side effect of drug.	• Consult doctor about prescription drug. • Discontinue use of non-prescription or illegal drug.
• Excessive sweating. • Fever.	Normal occurrence with fever.	See Fever charts (in Symptoms section).
• Excessive sweating. • Anxiety or excitement.	Normal occurrence with stress.	See Anxiety.
• Excessive sweating. • Overweight.	Effect of excess weight.	See Obesity.
• Excessive sweating in woman older than 38. • Irregular menstrual periods.	Hormone changes; end of menstrual cycles approaching.	See Menopause.
Excessive sweating in woman during menstrual period.	No underlying disorder.	Nothing.
• Excessive sweating. • Use of synthetic material, such as nylon, for clothing or blankets.	Increased skin heat.	Wear natural fibers, such as cotton.
Excessive sweating in teenager.	Normal occurrence during adolescence.	Nothing.

*All references are to Illness section unless noted otherwise.

SWELLING OR LUMP

SYMPTOMS & FACTORS	POSSIBLE PROBLEM	WHAT TO DO*
Lump in breast.	• Cyst. • Cancer.	• Consult doctor. • See Fibrocystic Breast Disease. • See Breast Cancer.
Swelling in armpit.	• Infection in arm. • Cancer.	• Consult doctor. • See Breast Cancer.
Lump or swelling in neck, armpit or groin without other symptoms or factors.	• Infection. • Tumor.	• See Hodgkins Disease. • See Lymphoma.
• Lump or swelling in neck, armpit or groin. • Use of prescription drug, especially for epilepsy or thyroid disorder.	Adverse reaction or side effect of drug.	Consult doctor.
Soft lump or swelling in groin or near navel that disappears when pressed or enlarges with cough.	Protruding intestinal tissue.	See Hernia.
Swelling between ear and jaw.	• Virus infection of glands. • Infection around tooth. • Disorder or tumor of salivary gland.	• See Mumps. • See Tooth Abscess. • See Salivary-Duct Stones. • See Salivary-Gland Tumor.
• Lump or swelling in neck, armpit or groin. • Fever.	Virus infection.	See Infectious Mononucleosis.
Swelling or lump in child 3 months or younger.	Several disorders.	Consult doctor.
• Swelling on both sides of neck, toward front. • Sore throat.	Bacterial or viral infection.	• See Tonsillitis. • See Pharyngitis. • See Infectious Mononucleosis.
• Swelling at both sides of back of neck. • Pink rash. • Fever.	Virus infection.	See German Measles.

*All references are to Illness section unless noted otherwise.

SWELLING OR LUMP (continued)

SYMPTOMS & FACTORS	POSSIBLE PROBLEM	WHAT TO DO*
Tender or hard lump in neck just below Adam's apple.	Inflammation or tumor of thyroid.	● See Thyroiditis. ● See Thyroid Tumor.
● Tender lump on elbow or in armpit. ● Fever. ● Exposure to cats.	Virus infection.	See Cat-Scratch Fever.
Firm swelling in groin that does not disappear when pressed.	● Infection in leg or genitals. ● Protruding intestinal tissue.	● Consult doctor. ● See Hernia.
● Swelling on sides of neck. ● Sore, cut or insect bite on head or neck.	Infected bite or wound.	● Consult doctor. ● See Insect Bites & Stings.
● Tender swelling in armpit, groin, elbow or base of neck. ● Sore, cut or insect bite on hand, arm, leg or shoulder on same side as swelling.	Infected bite or wound.	● Consult doctor. ● See Insect Bites & Stings.
● Painful, red lump or swelling. ● Recent injury to area.	Bleeding under skin.	● See Pulled or Torn Muscle. ● See Sprains & Strains.
Painful, red bump with white or yellow center in part of body with hair.	Infected hair follicle.	See Boils.
Swelling in front of neck with movement when swallowing.	Thyroid goiter.	Consult doctor.
● Swelling in neck, armpit or groin. ● Recent vaccination, such as tetanus or typhoid.	Swelling caused by vaccination.	Consult doctor.
Painless swelling near joint that is overused.	Ganglion cyst.	Consult doctor.

*All references are to Illness section unless noted otherwise.

TESTICLES, PAINFUL OR SWOLLEN

SYMPTOMS & FACTORS	POSSIBLE PROBLEM	WHAT TO DO*
• Sudden, painful swelling in testicle. • No injury to genital area.	• Twisted testicle. • Infection of glands in testicle.	• Call doctor now. • See Testicle Torsion. • See Epididymitis.
• Sudden, painful swelling in testicle. • Recent injury to genital area.	Internal injury.	Call doctor now.
Swelling of one testicle.	Cyst or tumor.	• Consult doctor. • See Cancer of the Testicle.
• Pain in testicles. • Painless, rubbery strands extending up scrotum. • No injury to testicles.	Enlarged veins in testicle.	Consult doctor.
• Pain in testicles. • Swelling between ear and jaw. • Fever.	Virus infection of glands.	• Consult doctor. • See Mumps.
Painless swelling of testicles.	• Fluid accumulation. • Enlarged veins in testicle. • Protruding intestinal tissue.	• Consult doctor. • See Hernia.

*All references are to Illness section unless noted otherwise.

THROAT, SORE

SYMPTOMS & FACTORS	POSSIBLE PROBLEM	WHAT TO DO*
● Sore throat. ● Fever. ● Swelling on both sides of neck toward front. ● Red, swollen tonsils with specks of pus on surface.	Bacterial or viral infection.	● Request throat culture. ● See Tonsillitis. ● See Strep Throat. ● See Infectious Mononucleosis. ● See APC Disease. ● See Diphtheria.
● Sore throat. ● Excessive smoking or alcohol consumption. OR ● Smoke-filled environment.	Throat irritation or inflammation.	See Pharyngitis.
● Sore throat. ● Dripping nose. ● Itching eyes.	Allergic reaction.	See Hay Fever.
● Sore throat. ● Hoarseness or voice loss.	Several disorders.	See Voice Loss or Hoarseness (in Symptoms section).
● Sore throat. ● Fever, plus any of following: ● Aches in bones or joints. ● Cough. ● Headache. ● Stuffy or runny nose.	Virus infection.	● See Common Cold. ● See Influenza.
● Sore throat. ● Fever. ● Swelling or tenderness between ear and jaw.	Virus infection of glands.	See Mumps.

*All references are to Illness section unless noted otherwise.

TONGUE, SORE

SYMPTOMS & FACTORS	POSSIBLE PROBLEM	WHAT TO DO*
• Sore tongue. • Use of prescription or non-prescription drugs.	Adverse reaction or side effect of drug.	Consult doctor.
• Sore tongue. • Pain one one side of face.	Nerve inflammation or damage.	See Tic Douloureux.
• Sore tongue. • Hard lump on tongue or in mouth.	• Infection. • Tumor.	• Call doctor now. • See Benign Mouth or Tongue Tumor. • See Oral Cancer.
• Sore tongue. • Diarrhea with loose, bulky, bad-smelling stool. • Retarded growth.	Poor digestion.	See Malabsorption.
• Sore tongue. • Discomfort involves whole tongue.	• Inflammation or infection. • Allergy. • Anemia.	• See Pernicious Anemia. • See Iron-Deficiency Anemia. • See Anemia during Pregnancy. • See Tongue Inflammation.
• Sore tongue. • Discomfort confined to one spot.	Abrasion from denture or irregular tooth.	Consult dentist.
• Sore tongue. • Cracked, fissured, red, tongue. • Mouth ulcers.	Poor nutrition.	• Consult doctor. • See Vitamin-B Deficiencies.

*All references are to Illness section unless noted otherwise.

TOOTHACHE

SYMPTOMS & FACTORS	POSSIBLE PROBLEM	WHAT TO DO*
• Gnawing pain in lower teeth and neck. • Chest discomfort beneath beastbone. • Shoulder or arm pain. • Sweating.	Insufficient oxygen to heart.	• Call doctor now. • See Angina Pectoris. • See Coronary-Artery Disease.
• Toothache, plus any of following: • Fever. • Swollen face or gums. • Continual pain that interferes with sleep.	• Advanced tooth decay. • Infection around tooth.	• Call dentist now. • See Tooth Abscess. • See Tooth Decay.
• Toothache over several teeth. • Red, swollen, bleeding gums.	Gum infection.	See Periodontitis.
• Toothache during or just after eating. • No recent dental work.	Tooth cavity.	See Tooth Decay.
• Recurrent toothache. • No other symptoms.	Tooth decay.	• Consult dentist. • See Tooth Decay.
• Toothache when biting food. • Recent tooth filling.	• Common occurrence following a filling. • Filling not level.	Consult dentist if pain lasts longer than 1 week.

*All references are to Illness section unless noted otherwise.

TREMBLING OR TWITCHING

SYMPTOMS & FACTORS	POSSIBLE PROBLEM	WHAT TO DO*
• Trembling or twitching, especially of tongue and face muscles. • Use of prescription or non-prescription drug, especially phenothiazine.	Adverse reaction or side effect of drug.	• Consult doctor about prescription drug. • Discontinue use of non-prescription drug.
Trembling in one part of body, especially when affected part is at rest.	Disorder of central nervous system.	See Parkinson's Disease.
• Trembling. • Alcohol withdrawal.	Withdrawal symptom.	See Alcoholism.
• Trembling. • Excessive consumption of coffee or tea. OR • Use of non-prescription drug containing caffeine.	Adverse effect of caffeine.	Decrease use of caffeine.
• Trembling, plus 2 or more of following: • Weight loss. • Fatigue. • Excessive sweating.	Overactive thyroid gland.	See Hyperthyroidism.
Twitching in one small part of body, such as eyelid.	Fatigue or tension. Usually no underlying disorder.	• See Anxiety. • Consult doctor if you feel ill or if muscles seem weak.
Trembling in any part of body without other symptoms or factors.	Inherited tendency to tremble from anxiety or stress.	Consult doctor to confirm diagnosis.
Unexpected body jerks when falling asleep.	Involuntary muscle spasms. No underlying disorder.	Nothing.

*All references are to Illness section unless noted otherwise.

URINATION, FREQUENT

SYMPTOMS & FACTORS	POSSIBLE PROBLEM	WHAT TO DO*
• Frequent urination. • Pain with urination.	Several disorders.	See Painful Urination (in Symptoms section).
• Frequent urination, especially at night. • Increased urine production, plus 2 or more of following: • Increased hunger and thirst. • Itching around genitals or anus. • Fatigue. • Weight loss.	Sugar in urine.	See Diabetes Mellitus.
• Frequent urination in man older than 50, plus 2 or more of following: • Involuntary urine leak after urination. • Weak urinary stream. • Difficulty starting urination. • Increased waking at night to urinate.	Disorder of prostate gland.	• See Enlarged Prostate. • See Prostatitis.
• Frequent urination in a woman. • Intense urge to urinate, followed quickly by uncontrollable urine leak.	Urge incontinence.	See Stress Incontinence.
• Frequent urination, especially at night. • Increased urine production. • Excessive consumption of tea, coffee, cola or alcohol.	Effect of caffeine or alcohol.	Decrease consumption of caffeine or alcohol.
• Frequent urination. • Difficulty controlling bladder.	Several disorders.	See Urination, Lack of Control (in Symptoms section).
• Frequent urination, especially at night. • Increased urine production. • Use of diuretic drug for heart disease or high blood pressure.	Effect of diuretic drug.	Consult doctor if uneasy.
• Frequent urination. • Anxiety or excitement. OR • Cold weather.	Normal occurrence.	Nothing.
• Frequent urination. • Possible pregnancy.	Normal occurrence during first 3 months and last 3 months of pregnancy.	Consult doctor to confirm pregnancy.

*All references are to Illness section unless noted otherwise.

URINATION, LACK OF CONTROL

SYMPTOMS & FACTORS	POSSIBLE PROBLEM	WHAT TO DO*
• Lack of urinary control. • Lack of bowel control.	• Irritation or infection of digestive tract. • Decreased blood supply to brain.	• See Gastroenteritis. • See Stroke.
• Lack of urinary control. • Use of prescription drug.	Adverse reaction or side effect of drug.	Consult doctor.
• Lack of urinary control. • Constipation for longer than 1 week.	Pressure on bladder from fecal impaction.	See Fecal Impaction.
• Lack of urinary control. • Cloudy, bad-smelling urine.	Infection of urinary tract.	• See Bladder Infection. • See Urethritis.
Dribbling of urine after urination in male over age 50.	• Disorder of prostate gland. • Inflammation of urethra.	• See Enlarged Prostate • See Urethritis.
• Lack of urinary control in person over age 60, plus 2 or more of following: • Inability to remember recent events. • Decline in attention to personal appearance or cleanliness. • Personality change.	• Poor nutrition. • Mental deterioration.	• See Vitamin-B Deficiencies. • See Alzheimer's Disease. • See Dementia.
Small urine leak in female following intense urge to urinate.	Urge incontinence.	See Stress Incontinence.
Small urine leak in female when coughing, sneezing, laughing or running.	Abnormalities in reproductive system.	See Stress Incontinence.
Lack of urinary control in child over age 3-1/2.	Several causes.	See Bed-Wetting.
• Lack of urinary control. • Chronic illness.	Several disorders.	• Call doctor now. • See Multiple Sclerosis. • See Syphilis. • See Ruptured Disk.

*All references are to Illness section unless noted otherwise.

URINATION, PAINFUL

SYMPTOMS & FACTORS	POSSIBLE PROBLEM	WHAT TO DO*
• Painful urination in man. • Thick, yellow-green discharge from penis.	Sexually-transmitted infection.	• See Gonorrhea. • See Urethritis.
• Painful urination in woman. • Bad-smelling vaginal discharge. • Pain or tenderness in lower abdomen. • Fever.	Sexually-transmitted infection.	• See Gonorrhea. • See Urethritis.
• Painful urination in man. • Heavy feeling or dull pain between scrotum and anus. • Fever.	Infection of prostate gland.	See Prostatitis.
• Painful urination. • Pain in one side of back, between waist and last rib. • Fever.	Kidney infection.	See Acute Kidney Infection.
• Painful urination. • Frequent urination.	Bladder inflammation.	See Bladder Infection.
• Painful urination. • Painful blisters on genitals. • Fever.	Sexually-transmitted virus infection.	See Genital Herpes.
• Painful urination in female. • Green-yellow or white discharge from vagina. • Itching around genitals.	Vaginal infection.	• See Monilial Vaginitis. • See Trichomonal Vaginitis.

*All references are to Illness section unless noted otherwise.

URINE, ABNORMAL COLOR

SYMPTOMS & FACTORS	POSSIBLE PROBLEM	WHAT TO DO*
• Clear, dark-brown urine. • Pale stool. • Yellow skin and eyes.	Liver disorder.	• Call doctor now. • See Acute Viral Hepatitis.
Pink, red or smoky-brown urine.	Disorder of urinary tract.	• Consult doctor. • See Cystitis. • See Enlarged Prostate. • See Kidney Cancer. • See Bladder Tumor. • See Tuberculosis. • See Bladder Stones. • See Chronic Kidney Infection. • See Wilm's Tumor (children only). • See Hypernephroma.
• Dark yellow or orange urine. • Fever. OR • Very hot weather. OR • Decreased fluid intake.	Concentrated urine.	• See Fever charts (in Symptoms section). • See Heatstroke or Heat Exhaustion. • Increase fluid intake.
• Dark yellow or orange urine. • Vomiting. • Diarrhea.	Concentrated urine.	• See Recurrent Attacks of Vomiting (in Symptoms section). • See Diarrhea (in Symptoms section).
• Pink, red or smoky-brown urine. • Use of new prescription drug in last 24 hours.	Side effect of drug.	Consult doctor if color change not expected.
• Dark yellow or orange urine. • Recent use of laxatives containing senna. OR • Recent consumption of rhubarb.	Effect of chemicals in these substances.	Nothing.
• Pink, red or smoky-brown urine. • Recent consumption of beets, blackberries or other red food.	Effect of natural or artificial color.	Nothing.
Green or blue urine.	Effect of artificial color in food or drug.	Nothing.

*All references are to Illness section unless noted otherwise.

VAGINAL BLEEDING, UNEXPECTED

SYMPTOMS & FACTORS	POSSIBLE PROBLEM	WHAT TO DO*
Vaginal bleeding during first 3 months of pregnancy.	Spontaneous abortion.	• Call doctor now. • See Miscarriage.
Vaginal bleeding during 4th to 9th month of pregnancy.	Abnormal location of of placenta.	• Call doctor now. • See Placenta Previa. • See Abruptio Placenta.
• Unexpected vaginal bleeding. • Severe abdominal pain. • Pregnancy possible.	Pregnancy developing outside uterus.	See Ectopic Pregnancy.
• Unexpected vaginal bleeding. • Severe abdominal pain. • Current use of intrauterine contraceptive device (IUD).	Pregnancy developing outside uterus.	See Ectopic Pregnancy.
• Unexpected vaginal bleeding in woman over age 45. • Last menstrual period more than 6 months ago.	• Hormone changes. • Tumor, especially if over age 45.	• See Menopause. • See Uterine Cancer. • See Cancer of Cervix. • See Post-Menopausal Uterine Bleeding.
• Unexpected vaginal bleeding. • Heavy, watery vaginal discharge or bleeding immediately after sexual intercourse.	Tumor.	• See Cervical Erosion. • See Cancer of Cervix. • See Uterine Cancer.
Unexpected vaginal bleeding between menstrual period.	Uterine bleeding.	• See Dysfunctional Uterine Bleeding. • See Fibroid Tumors of the Uterus.
• Unexpected vaginal bleeding. • Recent insertion of intrauterine contraceptive device (IUD).	Complications caused by IUD.	Consult doctor.
• Unexpected vaginal bleeding. • Use of oral contraceptives.	Breakthrough bleeding; common occurrence in women taking pill.	Consult doctor.
• Unexpected vaginal bleeding in puberty. • Menstrual periods began recently. OR • More frequent menstrual periods than usual. • Unexpected vaginal bleeding after skipping periods. • Woman over age 38.	Hormone changes that accompany beginning and ending of menstrual cycles.	See Menopause.

*All references are to Illness section unless noted otherwise.

VAGINAL DISCHARGE, ABNORMAL

SYMPTOMS & FACTORS	POSSIBLE PROBLEM	WHAT TO DO*
• Green-yellow, bad-smelling vaginal discharge. • Pain in lower abdomen. • Frequent or painful urination.	Infection of reproductive organs.	• See Pelvic Inflammatory Disease. • See Gonorrhea.
• Heavy, bad-smelling vaginal discharge 2 or more days after childbirth. • Fever. • Abdominal pain.	Infection of uterus.	See Puerperal Infection.
• Heavy vaginal discharge. • Vaginal pain.	Irritation or infection of cervix.	See Cervicitis.
• Green-yellow, bad-smelling vaginal discharge. • No other symptoms.	Vaginal infection.	See Trichomonal Vaginitis.
• Heavy vaginal discharge that is normal in color and consistency. • Vaginal itching or soreness.	Irritation or infection.	See Vaginal Itching (in Symptoms section).
White, curd-like vaginal discharge.	Vaginal fungus infection.	See Monilial Vaginitis.
• Green-yellow, bad-smelling vaginal discharge. • Tampon, diaphragm or cervical cup left in vagina.	Vaginal infection.	• Remove tampon. diaphragm or cup if you can. • If not, consult doctor.
• Heavy vaginal discharge that is normal in color and consistency. • Use of oral contraceptives. OR • Possible pregnancy.	Normal occurrence caused by hormone changes.	Consult doctor to confirm pregnancy.
• Red or brown vaginal discharge. • Occasional spotting of blood between menstrual periods.	Several disorders.	• See Cervical Polyps. • See Unexpected Vaginal Bleeding. (in Symptoms section).
Heavy vaginal discharge that is normal in color and consistency occurring during middle days between periods.	Normal occurrence during ovulation.	Nothing.

*All references are to Illness section unless noted otherwise.

VAGINAL ITCHING

SYMPTOMS & FACTORS	POSSIBLE PROBLEM	WHAT TO DO*
• Vaginal itching, plus 2 or more of following: • Unexplained weight loss. • Increased hunger and thirst. • Frequent urination. • Fatigue.	Sugar in urine.	• See Diabetes Mellitus. • See Monilial Vaginitis.
• Vaginal itching. • Unusual vaginal discharge.	Several disorders.	• See Vulvovaginitis before Puberty (children only). • See Abnormal Vaginal Discharge (in Symptoms section).
• Vaginal itching. • Use of antibiotics.	Vaginal infection.	• Consult doctor. • See Monilial Vaginitis.
• Vaginal itching. • Use of chemical spray, ointment, cream, douche or contraceptive foam.	Irritation caused by chemical or drug.	• Consult doctor. • Discontinue use of possible irritant.
Vaginal itching in woman over age 38.	Decreasing level of estrogens at menopause.	• See Menopause. • See Pruritis Vulvae.

*All references are to Illness section unless noted otherwise.

VISION DISTURBANCE OR LOSS

SYMPTOMS & FACTORS	POSSIBLE PROBLEM	WHAT TO DO*
• Vision disturbance. • Recent head injury.	Bleeding inside skull.	• Call doctor now. • See Subdural Hemorrhage & Hematoma.
Sudden, partial or total loss of vision in one or both eyes.	• Decreased blood supply to back of eye or brain. • Disorder of central nervous system.	• Call doctor now. • See Stroke. • See Transient Ischemic Attack. • See Brain Tumor. • See Multiple Sclerosis.
• Blurred vision in one eye. • Eye pain.	Excess pressure in eye.	See Acute Glaucoma.
• Blurred vision in one eye. • Flashing lights. • Floating spots. • No pain.	Disorder of blood vessels and structures in back of eye.	See Retinal Detachment.
• Double vision. • Bulging eyes.	• Overactive thyroid gland. • Tumor. • Inflammation of tissue behind eye.	• Consult doctor. • See Hyperthyroidism. • See Exophthalmos. • See Eye Tumor.
• Blurred vision. • Person over age 50.	• Clouding of eye lens. • Decreased blood supply to back of eye.	See Cataract.
• Blurred vision in past 2 days. • Eye pain.	Inflammation of iris.	See Iritis.
• Blurred vision. • Use of prescription drug.	Adverse reaction or side effect of drug.	Consult doctor.
• Blurred vision. • Diabetes.	Diabetic retinopathy (retina injury).	Consult doctor.
• Flashes of light or wavy spots in vision. • Severe headache. • Nausea and vomiting.	Severe vascular headache.	See Migraine Headache.

*All references are to Illness section unless noted otherwise.

VOICE LOSS OR HOARSENESS

SYMPTOMS & FACTORS	POSSIBLE PROBLEM	WHAT TO DO*
• Voice loss or hoarseness for longer than 1 week. OR • Recurrent attacks of hoarseness or voice loss in last 6 months.	• Inflammation of vocal cords. • Tumor.	• See Laryngitis. • See Larynx Cancer. • See Vocal-Cord Nodules.
• Voice loss or hoarseness. • Tender or hard lump in neck just below Adam's apple.	Tumor of thyroid.	See Thyroid Tumor.
• Hoarseness, plus 2 or more of following: • Dry skin or hair. • Decreased tolerance for cold. • Fatigue. • Unexplained weight gain.	Underactive thyroid gland.	See Hypothyroidism.
Hoarseness following excessive smoking or alcohol consumption.	Inflammation of vocal cords caused by alcohol or tobacco.	See Laryngitis.
Hoarseness following cold, cough or sore throat.	Inflammation of vocal cords caused by nasal drainage.	See Laryngitis.
Hoarseness following excessive use of voice.	Inflammation of vocal cords caused by overuse.	See Laryngitis.
• Hoarseness. • Recent tension or depression.	Effect of stress.	See Anxiety.

*All references are to Illness section unless noted otherwise.

VOMITING (INFANT 0 TO 6 MONTHS)

SYMPTOMS & FACTORS	POSSIBLE PROBLEM	WHAT TO DO*
• Forceful vomiting. • Possible accidental ingestion of drug or poison.	Chemical irritation of stomach and toxic effect of chemical on brain.	Call doctor now or go to emergency room.
• Vomiting. • Fever of 101F (38.3C) rectally or higher, plus any of following: • Lethargy. • Eyes sensitive to light. • General ill appearance. • Crying with urination.	• Infection in membranes around brain. • Urinary-tract infection.	Call doctor now.
• Vomiting. • Recurrent attacks of screaming or crying, as if in great pain.	Blockage in intestines.	• See Intussusception. • See Intestinal Obstruction.
• Vomiting. • Fever.	Infection.	See Fever in Infants (in Symptoms section).
• Vomiting. • Failure to gain weight. • Withdrawn affect.	Emotional deprivation from lack of touching or attention.	See Failure to Thrive.
• Vomiting. • Cough or runny nose.	Virus infection.	Consult doctor if vomiting lasts longer than 6 hours.
• Vomiting. • Swelling or lump in groin or testicle.	Protruding intestinal tissue.	See Hernia.
• Vomiting. • Diarrhea.	Infection of digestive tract.	See Gastroenteritis in Infants & Children.
• Infant vomits forcefully after each feeding. • Infant appears healthy. • Infant is male and younger than 4 months.	Constriction in outlet to stomach.	See Congenital Pyloric Stenosis.
• Vomiting. • Infant appears healthy. • No other symptoms.	• Single episode—no underlying disorder. • More than one episode— several disorders, such as food allergies or milk intolerance.	• Consult doctor if vomiting lasts longer than 6 hours. • Consult doctor for repeated vomiting.
• Infant spits up small amount of milk during or just after bottle-feeding. • Infant appears healthy. • New bottle nipple.	Hole in nipple may be wrong size.	Adjust hole size in nipple.
• Vomiting. • Recent playful bouncing.	Disturbed equilibrium.	Don't bounce after feedings.

*All references are to Illness section unless noted otherwise.

VOMITING, RECURRENT ATTACKS

SYMPTOMS & FACTORS	POSSIBLE PROBLEM	WHAT TO DO*
• Recurrent vomiting. • Poor appetite. • Constant pain in upper abdomen.	Tumor.	See Stomach Cancer.
• Recurrent vomiting without nausea. • Recurrent headaches, especially in morning.	• Bleeding inside skull. • Tumor.	• Consult doctor. • See Subdural Hemorrhage & Hematoma. • See Brain Tumor.
• Recurrent vomiting. • Use of prescription or non-prescription drug.	Adverse reaction or side effect of drug.	Consult doctor.
• Recurrent vomiting. • Occasional pain or tenderness in upper right abdomen. • Fever.	Gallbladder inflammation.	See Acute Cholecystitis or Cholangitis.
• Recurrent vomiting. • Occasional pain or tenderness in upper right abdomen. • No fever.	Gallbladder disorder.	See Gallstones.
• Recurrent vomiting. • Poor appetite. • Jaundice (yellow skin and eyes).	Gallbladder or liver disorder.	• See Gallstones. • See Acute Viral Hepatitis.
• Recurrent vomiting. • Pain or tenderness in center of upper abdomen. • Discomfort relieved by vomiting.	Peptic-ulcer disease.	• See Duodenal Ulcer. • See Stomach Ulcer.
Vomiting within hours after drinking alcohol.	Stomach inflammation.	See Gastritis.
• Recurrent vomiting. • Burning sensation in chest or upper abdomen, especially when bending forward or lying down.	Stomach acid in esophagus.	See Heartburn.
• Recurrent vomiting at approximately same time each day. • Possible pregnancy.	Vomiting of early pregnancy.	See Morning Sickness During Pregnancy.
Recurrent, self-induced vomiting.	Psychological disorder.	See Bulimia.

*All references are to Illness section unless noted otherwise.

VOMITING, SUDDEN ATTACK

SYMPTOMS & FACTORS	POSSIBLE PROBLEM	WHAT TO DO*
● Vomiting. ● Headache, plus any of following: ● Eyes sensitive to light. ● Drowsiness or confusion. ● Pain when bending head forward.	Infection or bleeding in membranes around brain.	● Call doctor now. ● See Aseptic Meningitis. ● See Bacterial Meningitis. ● See Subarachnoid Hemorrhage.
● Vomiting. ● Headache. ● Head injury in last 24 hours.	Brain injury.	● Call doctor now. ● See Head Injury.
Vomiting of blood or dark "coffee ground" material.	Bleeding in stomach.	● Call doctor now. ● See Stomach Ulcer.
● Vomiting. ● Abdominal pain or swelling. ● Inability to have bowel movement.	Blockage in intestines.	● Call doctor now. ● See Intestinal Obstruction.
● Vomiting. ● Eye pain. ● Blurred vision.	Excess pressure inside eye.	● Call doctor now. ● See Acute Glaucoma.
● Vomiting. ● Severe abdominal pain. ● No pain relief from vomiting.	Several disorders.	● Call doctor now. ● See Appendicitis.
● Vomiting. ● Use of prescription or non-prescription drug.	Adverse reaction or side effect of drug.	● Consult doctor about prescription drug. ● Discontinue use of non-prescription drug.
● Vomiting. ● Jaundice (yellow skin or eyes).	Gallbladder or liver disorder.	● Consult doctor. ● See Acute Viral Hepatitis. ● See Gallstones.
Recent, recurrent vomiting attacks.	Several disorders.	See Recurrent Vomiting (in Symptoms section).
● Vomiting. ● Consumption of spoiled or contaminated food.	Effect of toxins in food.	● See Salmonella Infections. ● See Botulism.
● Vomiting. ● Dizziness.	Infection or disorder of inner ear.	● See Labyrinthitis. ● See Meniere's Disease.
● Vomiting. ● Excessive consumption of alcohol or rich food.	Stomach inflammation.	See Gastritis.
● Vomiting. ● Diarrhea. ● Fever.	Infection of digestive tract.	See Gastroenteritis.

*All references are to Illness section unless noted otherwise.

WEIGHT GAIN

SYMPTOMS & FACTORS	POSSIBLE PROBLEM	WHAT TO DO*
• Weight gain. • Depression.	Compensatory overeating.	See Depression.
Rapid weight gain during pregnancy	Complication of pregnancy.	See Toxemia of Pregnancy.
• Weight gain. • High blood pressure or history of heart, kidney or liver disease.	Fluid retention caused by disorder of blood vessels, heart, liver or kidney.	• See Hypertension. • See Congestive Heart Failure. • See Nephrosis. • See Cirrhosis of the Liver.
• Weight gain. • Use of prescription or non-prescription drug that causes fluid retention. such as steroids, cortisone drugs, oral contraceptives or non-steroid anti-inflammatory drugs.	Adverse reaction or side effect of drug.	Consult doctor.
• Weight gain. • Decreased tolerance for cold. • Dry skin or hair. • Fatigue. • Constipation.	Underactive thyroid gland.	See Hypothyroidism.
• Weight gain. • Change from active to sedentary lifestyle.	Calorie intake too high for current activity level.	Decrease food consumption and increase physical activity.
• Weight gain. • None of the above.	More calories consumed than burned.	See Obesity.

*All references are to Illness section unless noted otherwise.

WEIGHT GAIN, SLOW (CHILD 0 TO 5 YEARS)

SYMPTOMS & FACTORS	POSSIBLE PROBLEM	WHAT TO DO*
• Weight gain slow in young child. • Use of cortisone drugs.	Adverse reaction or side effect of drug.	Consult doctor.
• Weight gain slow in young child. • Loose, pale, bulky, bad-smelling stool.	Digestive disorder.	• See Celiac Disease. • See Lactose Intolerance.
• Weight gain slow in infant younger than 6 months. • Infant vomits after feedings.	Several disorders.	See Vomiting in Infants (in Symptoms section).
• Weight gain slow in young child. • Withdrawn personality. • Slow mental, physical and emotional development.	Effect of abuse or neglect.	• Consult doctor. • See Failure to Thrive.
• Weight gain slow in young child. • Child appears healthy and content. • Birth weight low (less than 5-1/2 pounds). OR • Parent smaller than average.	Genetic causes; no underlying disorder.	Consult doctor if worried.
• Weight gain slow in breast-fed infant younger than 1 year. • Feeding schedule rigid or allows little sucking time.	Inadequate nourishment.	• Consult doctor. • Feed on demand. • Increase sucking time.
• Weight gain slow in bottle-fed infant younger than 1 year. • Too much water added to powdered formula, or water added to ready-to-feed formula.	Inadequate nourishment.	• Prepare formula according to directions. • Do not dilute ready-to-feed formula.
• Weight gain slow in bottle-fed infant younger than 1 year. • Child empties every bottle of formula.	Inadequate nourishment.	• Tell doctor at next visit. • Increase amount offered.

*All references are to Illness section unless noted otherwise.

WEIGHT LOSS

SYMPTOMS & FACTORS	POSSIBLE PROBLEM	WHAT TO DO*
• Weight loss. • Recurrent diarrhea or constipation. • Recurrent pain in lower abdomen. • Black stool.	• Inflammation of intestine. • Tumor.	• See Crohn's Disease. • See Large-Intestine Cancer.
• Weight loss. • Recurrent pain in upper abdomen.	• Peptic-ulcer disease. • Tumor.	• See Duodenal Ulcer. • See Stomach Ulcer. • See Stomach Cancer.
• Weight loss, plus 2 or more of following: • Excessive sweating at night. • Fever. • Fatigue. • Persistent cough with blood in sputum.	Lung inflammation or infection.	• See Tuberculosis. • See Chronic Bronchitis. • See Bronchiectasis.
• Weight loss, plus 2 or more of following: • Increased hunger. • Increased thirst. • Fatigue. • Family history of diabetes. • Frequent urination. • Itching rash in genital area.	Sugar in urine.	See Diabetes Mellitus.
• Weight loss, plus 2 or more of following: • Bulging eyes. • Excessive sweating. • Fatigue. • Anxiety. • Rapid heartbeat.	Overactive thyroid gland.	See Hyperthyroidism.
• Weight loss. • Recurrent diarrhea. • Pale, bulky, bad-smelling stool that is difficult to flush.	Poor digestion.	See Malabsorption.
• Weight loss of 10 or more pounds. • Anxiety or depression.	• Effect of stress. • Psychological disorder.	• See Anxiety. • See Depression. • See Anorexia Nervosa. • See Bulimia.
• Weight loss. • Current use of prescription drug.	Adverse reaction or side effect of drug.	Consult doctor.
• Weight loss. • Increased physical activity.	Normal occurrence.	Consult doctor if weight loss continues longer than 2 weeks.

*All references are to Illness section unless noted otherwise.

WHEEZING

SYMPTOMS & FACTORS	POSSIBLE PROBLEM	WHAT TO DO*
• Wheezing. • Possible inhalation of foreign object, such as peanut.	Foreign object in larynx or bronchial tubes.	Call doctor now.
• Wheezing. • Cough with frothy pink, brownish or white sputum.	Fluid in lungs.	• Call doctor now. • See Pulmonary Edema.
• Wheezing. • Breathing difficulty.	Spasm of bronchial tubes.	• Call doctor now. • See Asthma.
• Wheezing. • Fever.	Infection of bronchial tubes.	• See Acute Bronchitis. • See Asthma. • See Bronchiolitis (young children only).
• Persistent, mild wheezing. • Cough with gray or green-yellow sputum.	Chronic infection of breathing passages.	• See Chronic Bronchitis. • See Bronchiectasis. • See Emphysema.

*All references are to Illness section unless noted otherwise.

ABRUPTIO PLACENTA

GENERAL INFORMATION

DEFINITION—Separation of the placenta from the uterus during the last third of pregnancy.

BODY PARTS INVOLVED—Uterus.

SEX OR AGE MOST AFFECTED—Females.

SIGNS & SYMPTOMS
Small separation of the placenta:
- Vaginal bleeding.
- Mild pain or discomfort.
- Fetus remains healthy.

Large separation:
- Heavy vaginal bleeding.
- Severe pain in the lower abdomen.
- Hard, tender abdomen.
- Shock (rapid heartbeat, rapid breathing and dizziness).
- Fetal distress; fetal heartbeat may be inaudible.

CAUSES—Unknown.

RISK INCREASES WITH
- Women over age 35.
- Women who have had several pregnancies.
- Women who smoke.
- A direct blow to the uterus.

HOW TO PREVENT—If pregnant, don't engage in activity more vigorous than what you were accustomed to before pregnancy.

WHAT TO EXPECT

APPROPRIATE HEALTH CARE
- Doctor's treatment.
- Hospitalization (except for mild cases).
- Surgery to deliver the fetus by cesarian section, or vaginal delivery (sometimes).

DIAGNOSTIC MEASURES
- Your own observation of symptoms.
- Medical history and physical exam by a doctor.
- Laboratory studies, such as blood counts, blood-clotting tests and ultrasound examination (see Glossary) of the uterus.

POSSIBLE COMPLICATIONS
- Shock or life-threatening bleeding in the mother.
- Fetal death.

PROBABLE OUTCOME
- With immediate medical care, the outlook for mother and fetus is excellent.
- With delay of medical care and prolonged heavy bleeding, mother and fetus may not survive.

HOW TO TREAT

NOTE—Follow your doctor's instructions. These instructions are supplemental.

GENERAL MEASURES—Abruptio placenta is an emergency, but there is usually time to obtain advice by telephone and arrange safe transportation to the hospital. Panic is not helpful.

   If the placenta separation is slight, your doctor may permit you to return home for bed rest and close observation after examination.

MEDICATION—Your doctor may prescribe:
- Oxytocin to induce labor, if immediate delivery is necessary.
- Intravenous fluids.
- Blood transfusions.

ACTIVITY—Rest in bed until bleeding and other symptoms cease, and your doctor approves a return to normal activity.

DIET—No special diet. Drink fluids only until your doctor determines that surgery is not likely. Solid food may cause risk if emergency surgery becomes necessary.

CALL YOUR DOCTOR IF

You have bleeding (anything more than slight spotting) during pregnancy. This is an emergency!

ACNE
(Acne Vulgaris)

GENERAL INFORMATION

DEFINITION—An inflammatory skin condition—common in adolescence—characterized by skin eruptions on the face, chest and back.

BODY PARTS INVOLVED—Skin.

SEX OR AGE MOST AFFECTED—Adolescents (more common in boys).

SIGNS & SYMPTOMS
- Blackheads (black spots the size of a pinhead).
- Whiteheads (white spots similar to blackheads).
- Pustules (small pus-filled lesions).
- Redness and inflammation around eruptions.

CAUSES—Oil glands in the skin become plugged for unknown reasons, but sex-hormone changes during adolescence play a role. When oil backs up, it becomes infected by bacteria normally present in glands. Contrary to myth, acne is *not* caused by dirt or masturbation. Cleanliness can lessen it, but sexual activity has no effect on it.

RISK INCREASES WITH
- Exposure to extremely hot or cold weather.
- Stress.
- Oily skin.
- Endocrine disorders.
- Use of drugs, such as cortisone, male hormones or oral contraceptives.
- Family history of acne.

HOW TO PREVENT—Cannot be prevented at present.

WHAT TO EXPECT

APPROPRIATE HEALTH CARE
- Self-care after diagnosis.
- Doctor's treatment.
- Surgery (dermabrasion) to remove unsightly scars after acne heals.

DIAGNOSTIC MEASURES
- Your own observation of symptoms.
- Medical history and physical exam by a doctor.

POSSIBLE COMPLICATIONS
- Poor self-image and psychological distress.
- Permanent facial scars.

PROBABLE OUTCOME—Most cases respond well to treatment, and the condition tends to disappear after adolescence. Despite good treatment, acne will flare up from time to time.

HOW TO TREAT

NOTE—Follow your doctor's instructions. These instructions are supplemental.

GENERAL MEASURES
- If your skin is oily, cleanse it as follows:
  Gently massage face with soap for 3 to 5 minutes. Don't massage sorest places. Cleanse skin gently—rough scrubbing spreads infection.
  Rinse soap off for 2 to 3 minutes.
  After cleansing, use an astringent, such as alcohol, to remove oil.
  Use a fresh washcloth each day. Bacteria grow in damp, wet cloths.
- Shampoo hair at least twice a week. Don't let hair hang over the face—even at night. Hair spreads oil and bacteria. Use dandruff shampoo to treat or prevent dandruff.
- After vigorous exercise, wash sweat and oil off as soon as possible.
- Don't squeeze, scratch, pick or rub the skin. Acne heals better without damage to the skin. If you *must* squeeze pimples, blackheads or whiteheads, wash your hands first. Cleanse the area with alcohol before and after squeezing.
- Don't rest your face on your hands while reading, studying or watching TV.

MEDICATION—Your doctor may prescribe:
- Antibiotics to fight infection.
- Cortisone injections into lesions.
- Skin lotions with drying agents.
- Vitamin A.
Caution: If you are pregnant, don't take oral medications for acne.

ACTIVITY—No restrictions.

DIET—Foods don't cause acne, but some foods may make it worse. Keep a record of the foods you eat. To discover any food sensitivities, eliminate all the following foods from your diet: chocolate; ice cream; nuts; peanut butter; cheese; iodized salt; seafood (especially lobster, shrimp, clams and oysters); pork and bacon; carbonated and alcoholic drinks; spicy foods; cold cuts; potato chips; popcorn; and pickles. Then reintroduce them one at a time. If acne flares up 2 or 3 days after a food is eaten, leave it out of your diet. If not, you may eat it.

Acne usually improves in the summer, so some foods that cannot be eaten in the winter may be tolerated in the summer.

CALL YOUR DOCTOR IF

- You have acne.
- New, unexplained symptoms develop. Drugs in treatment may produce side effects.

ACNE ROSACEA
("Adult Acne")

GENERAL INFORMATION

DEFINITION—Chronic inflammation of skin of the face. Severe nose involvement, mostly in men, is called rhinophyma.

BODY PARTS INVOLVED—Face, especially the nose, and surrounding areas.

SEX OR AGE MOST AFFECTED—Adults; it is more common in women, but more severe in men.

SIGNS & SYMPTOMS
- Unsightly red, thickened skin on the nose and cheeks. Small blood vessels are visible on the skin surface.
- Papules (small raised bumps) and pustules (small, white blisters with pus) on the affected skin (sometimes).

CAUSES—Unknown. The condition is worsened by stress, warm drinks, hot foods and alcohol.

RISK INCREASES WITH
- Nervousness and stress.
- Fair complexion.
- Excess alcohol consumption.

HOW TO PREVENT—No specific preventive measures.

WHAT TO EXPECT

APPROPRIATE HEALTH CARE
- Self-care after diagnosis.
- Doctor's treatment.
- Psychotherapy or counseling, if disfigurement causes distress.
- Surgery to remove excess tissue (sometimes).

DIAGNOSTIC MEASURES
- Your own observation of symptoms.
- Medical history and physical exam by a doctor.

POSSIBLE COMPLICATIONS
- Psychological distress caused by an unsightly appearance.
- Autoimmune eye disorders (rare).

PROBABLE OUTCOME—Symptoms can be controlled with treatment. Acne rosacea is a disease of remissions and frequent flare-ups.

HOW TO TREAT

NOTE—Follow your doctor's instructions. These instructions are supplemental.

GENERAL MEASURES
- Seek care early if you notice evidence of acne rosacea.
- Don't use oil-based makeup.
- See Appendix 13 for suggestions to reduce stress.

MEDICATION
- Your doctor may prescribe antibiotics such as tetracycline. These are effective for unknown reasons.
- Don't use cortisone preparations, including non-prescription preparations.

ACTIVITY—No restrictions.

DIET—No special diet. Avoid spicy foods, alcohol or anything that causes the face to flush.

CALL YOUR DOCTOR IF

You have symptoms of acne rosacea.

ADDISON'S DISEASE
(Adrenal Insufficiency)

GENERAL INFORMATION

DEFINITION—Underactive adrenal glands.

BODY PARTS INVOLVED—Adrenal glands (located over the kidneys).

SEX OR AGE MOST AFFECTED—Both sexes; all ages.

SIGNS & SYMPTOMS
- Weakness and fatigue.
- Gastrointestinal disturbances (nausea, vomiting, abdominal pain, diarrhea, and appetite and weight loss).
- Low blood pressure causing faintness and dizziness.
- Brownish skin (looks suntanned) with white patches.
- Darkening of freckles, scars and breast nipples.
- Hair loss.
- Feeling cold all the time.
- Dramatic behavior or mood changes, including aggression or depression.

CAUSES—Symptoms and signs are caused by low levels of cortisonelike hormones produced by the adrenal glands. The cause of adrenal insufficiency is usually unknown, but is sometimes a complication of:
- Tuberculosis.
- Cancer.
- Pituitary disease.
- Use of cortisone drugs for other conditions. When cortisone is withdrawn, normal adrenal function sometimes does not return.

RISK INCREASES WITH
- Stress.
- Diabetes mellitus.
- Injury to the abdomen.

HOW TO PREVENT—Don't discontinue use of cortisone drugs or change the dosage without consulting your doctor.

WHAT TO EXPECT

APPROPRIATE HEALTH CARE
- Doctor's treatment.
- Self-care after diagnosis.
- Hospitalization for an "adrenal crisis" (see Possible Complications).

DIAGNOSTIC MEASURES
- Your own observation of symptoms. "Before and after" pictures may emphasize the gradual skin change.
- Medical history and physical exam by a doctor.
- Laboratory blood counts, blood and urine measurement of adrenal hormones and a test of adrenal-gland function.

POSSIBLE COMPLICATIONS
- "Adrenal crisis" (pains, weakness, low blood pressure, high or low temperature, fainting) caused by any injury or illness.
- Misdiagnosis as a mental condition.

PROBABLE OUTCOME—Symptoms can be controlled with hormone-replacement treatment. This is fatal without treatment.

HOW TO TREAT

NOTE—Follow your doctor's instructions. These instructions are supplemental.

GENERAL MEASURES—This is a lifelong condition. Learn how to care for yourself. Strict attention to medication schedules is vital.
- Learn about adrenal crisis and its relationship to body stress (infection, surgery or injury).
- Advise any doctor and dentist who treats you that you have Addison's disease.
- Wear a Medic-Alert bracelet or pendant (see Glossary).
- Stay up-to-date on immunizations, including those for influenza and pneumonia.

MEDICATION—Your doctor may prescribe one of several types of cortisone drugs. Follow medication schedule exactly. Never change or omit medication without your doctor's advice.

ACTIVITY—No restrictions.

DIET—Eat a low-salt diet (see Appendix 9).

CALL YOUR DOCTOR IF

- You have symptoms of Addison's disease—especially an adrenal crisis. Call immediately. Adrenal crisis is an emergency!
- The following occurs after diagnosis:
  Any signs of infection, such as fever, chills muscle aches, headache and dizziness.
  Serious injury, such as bone fracture, dislocation or internal injuries.
- You are scheduled for elective surgery or require anesthesia for any reason.
- New, unexplained symptoms develop. Drugs used in treatment may produce side effects, such as:
  Protruding abdomen.
  Thin extremities.
  Puffy face and eyes.
  Acne.
  Growth of facial hair.

ILLNESSES & DISORDERS

AGRANULOCYTOSIS
(Granulocytopenia; Neutropenia)

GENERAL INFORMATION

DEFINITION—Reduction in the normal number of circulating white blood cells (granulocytes or neutrophils) in the bloodstream. These cells are the first to attack bacterial infections.

BODY PARTS INVOLVED—Blood; bone marrow.

SEX OR AGE MOST AFFECTED—Both sexes; all ages.

SIGNS & SYMPTOMS
- Fever.
- Aching.
- Sore throat.
- Ulcers (especially in the mouth and throat), which do not produce pus.
- Any sign of infection in someone who has had agranulocytosis in the past. This may signal a recurrence.

CAUSES—Increased destruction or impaired production of granulocytes (white blood cells). The most common reason for this is an adverse reaction to medications, including: anticancer drugs; anticonvulsants; antihistamines; antithyroid drugs; arsenic; chloramphenicol; dibenzapine; gold salts; indomethacin; nitrofurantoin; nitrous oxide; phenothiazines; phenylbutazone; procainamide; sulfonamides; synthetic penicillins; and thiazide diuretics.

RISK INCREASES WITH—Genetic factors. A rare form, infantile genetic agranulocytosis, is inherited.

HOW TO PREVENT—Prevent recurrences by avoiding any suspect medicine or drug that may have triggered agranulocytosis previously.

WHAT TO EXPECT

APPROPRIATE HEALTH CARE
- Doctor's treatment.
- Hospitalization for intensive treatment during the active phase, with strict reverse isolation techniques (see Glossary) and transfusions of white blood cells (sometimes).
- Self-care after diagnosis and hospitalization.

DIAGNOSTIC MEASURES
- Your own observation of symptoms.
- Medical history and physical exam by a doctor.
- Laboratory studies of blood and bone marrow, and cultures of blood, nose, throat and urine.

POSSIBLE COMPLICATIONS
- Kidney damage.
- Dangerous, sometimes fatal infections (bacterial, fungal, viral or others)—even with vigorous treatment.

PROBABLE OUTCOME—Usually curable in 6 weeks with intensive treatment.

HOW TO TREAT

NOTE—Follow your doctor's instructions. These instructions are supplemental.

GENERAL MEASURES—Hospitalization may be necessary during the acute phase. The following may be helpful after hospitalization:
- Be extra careful about personal cleanliness.
- Keep the mouth clean by rinsing frequently with warm salt water (1 teaspoon salt to 8 oz. water) or gargling with hydrogen peroxide.
- Pay particular attention to oral hygiene. Brush teeth gently with a very soft brush, avoiding irritation of the gums.
- Avoid contact with harmful materials, such as cleaning chemicals, glue, insecticide, fertilizer, paint remover and others.

MEDICATION—Your doctor may:
- Prescribe intravenous and oral antibiotics, if the white blood cell count is very low.
- Prescribe lithium to stimulate bone marrow to produce more granulocytes.
- Stop prescribing any drug that is suspected of causing agranulocytosis.

ACTIVITY—Rest in bed during the acute stage. Resume normal activities gradually after symptoms subside.

DIET—No restrictions.

CALL YOUR DOCTOR IF

- You have symptoms of agranulocytosis.
- The following occurs after treatment:
  Any sign of infection, especially fever.
  Swelling of the feet and ankles.
  Painful urination or decreased urine output in 1 day.
- New, unexplained symptoms develop.
Drugs used in treatment may produce side effects.

AIDS
(Acquired Immune Deficiency Syndrome)

 ## GENERAL INFORMATION

DEFINITION—A major failure of the body's immune system (immunodeficiency). This decreases the body's ability to fight infection and suppress multiplication of abnormal cells, such as cancer.

BODY PARTS INVOLVED—The immune system, including special blood cells (lymphocytes) and cells of the organs (bone marrow, spleen, liver and lymph glands). These cells manufacture antibodies to protect against disease and cancer.

SEX OR AGE MOST AFFECTED—Most common in men, ages 20 to 60.

SIGNS & SYMPTOMS
- Recurrent respiratory and skin infections.
- Fatigue.
- Diarrhea.
- Unexplained weight loss.
- Fever.
- Swollen lymph glands throughout the body.
- Enlarged spleen.

CAUSES—Uncertain. Evidence suggests a newly identified virus (retrovirus) invades and destroys cells of the immune system, resulting in lowered resistance to infections and some types of cancer. The virus is transmitted by:
- Homosexual activity.
- Use of contaminated needles for intravenous drug use.
- Transfusions of blood or blood products from an affected person.
- Sexual contact with an affected person. Usual non-sexual contact does not transmit the disease, so a person with AIDS is not a risk to the general population.

RISK INCREASES WITH
- Multiple homosexual sexual partners.
- Exposure of hospital workers and laboratory technicians to blood, feces and urine of AIDS patients.
- Infants born to mothers with AIDS.

HOW TO PREVENT
- Avoid sexual contact with affected persons.
- Use condoms for sexual activity with homosexual partners.
- Avoid intravenous self-administered drugs.
- If you have AIDS, don't donate blood to blood banks. You may transmit the disease to others.

OTHER—By law, AIDS must be reported to public health agencies.

 ## WHAT TO EXPECT

APPROPRIATE HEALTH CARE
- Doctor's treatment.
- Psychotherapy or counseling to cope with anxiety and depression about having the disease and the likelihood of death.
- Hospitalization. Medical schools may provide some free care if you are willing to participate in research.

DIAGNOSTIC MEASURES
- Your own observation of symptoms.
- Medical history and physical exam by a doctor.
- Laboratory blood studies of lymphocytes and blood-cell counts.

POSSIBLE COMPLICATIONS
- Serious infection in various body systems.
- Cancer.

PROBABLE OUTCOME—This condition is currently considered incurable. Complications may be fatal within 2 years. However, symptoms can be relieved or controlled.

Scientific research into causes and treatment continues, so there is hope for increasingly effective treatment and cure.

 ## HOW TO TREAT

NOTE—Follow your doctor's instructions. These instructions are supplemental.

GENERAL MEASURES
- Early diagnosis is helpful. If you are at risk, obtain a medical evaluation—even if you feel well.
- Contact social agencies in your area about AIDS support groups.

MEDICATION—Drugs are currently not effective in curing AIDS. Your doctor may prescribe antibiotics to prevent infections or control them as they develop.

ACTIVITY—No restrictions on normal activity, but refrain from sexual encounters.

DIET—No special diet.

 ## CALL YOUR DOCTOR IF

- You have symptoms of AIDS.
- Infection occurs after diagnosis.
Symptoms include: fever; cough; diarrhea; skin rash or eruption; general ill feeling.

ILLNESSES & DISORDERS

ALCOHOLISM

GENERAL INFORMATION

DEFINITION—A psychological and physiological dependence on alcohol, resulting in chronic disease and disruption of interpersonal, family and work relationships.

BODY PARTS INVOLVED—Brain; central nervous system; liver; heart.

SEX OR AGE MOST AFFECTED—Both sexes, but occurs 4 times more often in men than women. Alcoholism may develop at any age after adolescence, when drinking begins.

SIGNS & SYMPTOMS—Early stages:
- Low tolerance for anxiety.
- Need for alcohol at the beginning of the day, or at times of stress.
- Insomnia; nightmares.
- Habitual Monday-morning hangovers, and frequent absences from work.
- Preoccupation with obtaining alcohol and hiding drinking from family and friends.
- Guilt or irritability when others suggest drinking is excessive.
Late stages:
- Frequent blackouts; memory loss.
- Delirium tremens (tremors, hallucinations, confusion, sweating, rapid heartbeat). These occur most often with alcohol withdrawal.
- Liver disease (jaundice, internal bleeding, bloating).
- Neurological impairment (numbness and tingling in hands and feet, declining sexual interest and potency, confusion, coma).
- Congestive heart failure (shortness of breath, swelling of feet).

CAUSES—Not fully understood, but include:
- Personality factors, especially dependency, anger, mania, depression or introversion.
- Family influences, especially alcoholic or divorced parents.
- Social and cultural pressure to drink.
- Body-chemistry disturbances (perhaps).

RISK INCREASES WITH
- Genetic factors (perhaps). Some ethnic groups have high alcoholism rates—either for social or biological reasons.
- Use of recreational drugs.
- Crisis situations, including unemployment, frequent moves, or loss of friends or family.

HOW TO PREVENT
- Provide children with a loving, stable family environment. Use alcohol in moderation—if at all—to provide a healthy role model.
- Encourage a spouse, friend or co-worker to admit when an alcohol problem exists, and seek professional care.

OTHER—Some employers and health-insurance companies pay for treatment.

WHAT TO EXPECT

APPROPRIATE HEALTH CARE
- Self-care. The first and most difficult step of treatment is admitting the problem exists.
- Doctor's treatment.
- Psychotherapy or counseling.

DIAGNOSTIC MEASURES
- Your own observation of symptoms.
- Medical history and physical exam by a doctor.
- Laboratory studies of blood and liver function.
- EEG (see Glossary).
- Psychotherapy or counseling.

POSSIBLE COMPLICATIONS
- Chronic liver disease.
- Gastric erosion with bleeding; stomach inflammation.
- Neuritis, tremors, seizures and brain impairment.
- Inflammation of the pancreas.
- Inflammation of the heart.
- Mental and physical damage to the fetus if a woman drinks during pregnancy.

PROBABLE OUTCOME
- Without treatment:
  Progressive brain and liver disease.
  Job loss, divorce and criminal behavior.
  Painful, premature death.
- With treatment, alcoholism is often curable. Sexual function improves markedly.

HOW TO TREAT

NOTE—Follow your doctor's instructions. These instructions are supplemental.

GENERAL MEASURES
- Keep appointments with doctors and counselors.
- Join a local Alcoholics Anonymous group and attend regularly.
- Reassess your lifestyle—friends, work, family—to identify and alter factors that encourage drinking.

MEDICATION—Your doctor may prescribe disulfiram (Antabuse), which causes several extremely unpleasant physical symptoms when alcohol is consumed.

ACTIVITY—Don't drink and drive.

DIET—Normal, well-balanced diet. Vitamin supplements, such as thiamine and folic acid, are often necessary.

CALL YOUR DOCTOR IF

You or a family member have symptoms of alcoholism.

ALOPECIA AEREATA

GENERAL INFORMATION

DEFINITION—Sudden hair loss in circular patches on the scalp. Hair loss is not accompanied by other visible evidence of scalp disease. This is not contagious.

BODY PARTS INVOLVED—Hair; scalp; eyebrows; eyelashes; beard; genital area; underarm (sometimes).

SEX OR AGE MOST AFFECTED—All ages, but most likely in children (5 to 12 years).

SIGNS & SYMPTOMS
- Sudden hair loss in sharply defined circular patches. In rare cases, body hair loss may be total.
- No pain.
- No itch.

CAUSES—Unknown, but heredity and emotional factors, such as anxiety, may contribute to hair loss. The autoimmune system may also be involved.

RISK INCREASES WITH
- Stress.
- Family history of alopecia aereata.

HOW TO PREVENT—Cannot be prevented at present.

WHAT TO EXPECT

APPROPRIATE HEALTH CARE
- Self-care after diagnosis.
- Doctor's treatment.

DIAGNOSTIC MEASURES
- Your own observation of symptoms.
- Medical history and physical exam by a doctor.

POSSIBLE COMPLICATIONS
- Loss of all hair.
- Slow or incomplete regrowth.

PROBABLE OUTCOME—Usually curable, with spontaneous new growth, in 18 months. Persons with a few small patches are generally cured completely. The disorder recurs in 25% of cases.

HOW TO TREAT

NOTE—Follow your doctor's instructions. These instructions are supplemental.

GENERAL MEASURES
- Consider wearing a hairpiece or wig during the acute phase.
- Continue to bathe and shampoo as usual.
- Don't tug on normal hair close to areas of hair loss.

MEDICATION—Your doctor may prescribe topical steroids. Apply topical steroid once or twice a day unless directed otherwise. Apply immediately after bathing or shampooing for better spreading and penetration. For scalp and groin, use only low-potency steroid products without fluorine. In special cases, your doctor may inject steroids into affected areas and prescribe oral cortisone drugs for you to take on alternate days.

ACTIVITY—No restrictions.

DIET—No special diet.

CALL YOUR DOCTOR IF

- You have symptoms of alopecia aereata.
- The following occurs during treatment:
  Hair loss increases.
  Hair loss doesn't diminish in 4 weeks.
  Areas show signs of infection (redness, swelling, tenderness, warmth) after injections.

ILLNESSES & DISORDERS

ALZHEIMER'S DISEASE
(Alzheimer-type Dementia; Presenile Dementia)

 GENERAL INFORMATION

DEFINITION—A brain disorder similar to senile dementia characterized by gradual mental deterioration. A rapidly progressive form begins in adults around ages 36 to 45. A more gradual form, with slow development of symptoms, begins around ages 65 to 70.

Other disorders with similar signs and symptoms include: chronic organic brain syndrome (associated with small clots to the brain or toxic reactions to drugs); advanced syphilis; stroke; brain tumor; or hypothyroidism. These disorders may be treatable—Alzheimer's disease is not.

BODY PARTS INVOLVED—Brain.

SEX OR AGE MOST AFFECTED—Both sexes, beginning in the 40s and 50s.

SIGNS & SYMPTOMS—Early stages:
- Forgetfulness of recent events.
- Increasing difficulty performing intellectual tasks, such as accustomed work, balancing a checkbook, or maintaining a household.
- Personality changes, including poor impulse control and poor judgment.
Later stages:
- Difficulty doing simple tasks, such as choosing clothing, problem solving.
- Failure to recognize familiar persons.
- Disinterest in personal hygiene or appearance.
- Difficulty feeding self.
- Belligerence and denial that anything is wrong.
- Loss of usual sexual inhibitions.
Advanced stages:
- Complete loss of memory, speech and muscle function (including bladder and bowel control), necessitating total care and supervision.
- Extreme belligerence and hostility.

CAUSES—Irreversible damage to or loss of brain cells for unknown reasons.

RISK INCREASES WITH—Family history of Alzheimer's disease.

HOW TO PREVENT—No specific preventive measures.

 WHAT TO EXPECT

APPROPRIATE HEALTH CARE
- Doctor's treatment.
- Psychotherapy or counseling for family members.
- Nursing-home care when home care becomes impossible.

DIAGNOSTIC MEASURES
- Your own observation of symptoms.
- Medical history and physical exam by a doctor.
- X-rays of the brain, including CAT scan (see Glossary) to rule out other conditions.

POSSIBLE COMPLICATIONS
- Decreased resistance to infections, especially pneumonia and meningitis.
- Seizures.
- Coma.

PROBABLE OUTCOME—This condition is currently considered incurable and untreatable. It is usually fatal within 5 years without skillful supportive care. Scientific research into causes and treatment continues, so there is hope for eventual treatment and cure.

 HOW TO TREAT

NOTE—Follow your doctor's instructions. These instructions are supplemental.

GENERAL MEASURES
- If a family member has this disease, don't take their hostility personally.
- If you care for a family member with the disease, try to obtain help so you can get away often. Don't feel guilty about needing a respite—even if the patient resents it.
- Join or start a support group for families of Alzheimer's victims.
- Beware of persons offering treatments for large sums of money. No legitimate treatment currently exists.

MEDICATION—No medication is currently available to treat Alzheimer's disease, but many medications are being studied.

ACTIVITY—As much as possible. As the condition progresses, all activity will eventually require supervision.

DIET—Choline and lecithin supplements are under study. Feeding assistance will eventually be necessary.

 CALL YOUR DOCTOR IF

- You or some family member has symptoms of Alzheimer's disease.
- Signs of infection occur, such as fever, chills, muscle aches or headache.
- You care for someone with Alzheimer's disease, and you fear you are about to lose emotional control.

AMEBIASIS
(Amebic Dysentery; Entamebiasis)

 ## GENERAL INFORMATION

DEFINITION—Parasitic infection of the large intestine.

BODY PARTS INVOLVED—Intestinal tract, especially the colon; liver (sometimes).

SEX OR AGE MOST AFFECTED—Both sexes; all ages.

SIGNS & SYMPTOMS
- Fever.
- Intermittent diarrhea with bad-smelling stools. Diarrhea is often preceded by constipation in early stages.
- Gas and abdominal bloating.
- Abdominal cramps and tenderness.
- Mucus and blood in the stool (sometimes).
- Fatigue.
- Muscle aches.

If the liver is involved:
- Tenderness over the liver and right side of the abdomen.
- Jaundice (sometimes).

CAUSES—A microscopic parasite that is spread by flies, cockroaches and direct contact with hands or food contaminated with feces. The most common sources of infection are:
- Food handlers.
- Faulty hotel or factory plumbing.
- Raw vegetables or fruit fertilized with human feces or washed in polluted water.

RISK INCREASES WITH
- Crowded or unsanitary living conditions.
- Travel to a foreign country.
- Combination of anal-oral sex.

HOW TO PREVENT
- Wash your hands frequently—*always* before eating.
- If you are in an area where food or water may be contaminated, the following measures are necessary:
  Boil drinking water for 5 minutes.
  Don't use water for any purpose that may have raw sewage.
  Don't eat unpeeled fruit or vegetables and raw fish or shellfish.

OTHER—Many people—especially those who live in temperate climates—harbor the amoeba without symptoms. Symptoms occur when the parasite invades tissues of the colon. Symptoms may be very vague.

 ## WHAT TO EXPECT

APPROPRIATE HEALTH CARE
- Home care.
- Doctor's treatment.
- Hospitalization (severe cases only).

DIAGNOSTIC MEASURES
- Your own observation of symptoms.
- Medical history and physical exam by a doctor.
- Laboratory studies of stool and blood serum.
- Sigmoidoscopy (see Glossary).
- X-rays of lower bowel (barium enema).

POSSIBLE COMPLICATIONS
- Peritonitis.
- Hepatitis or liver abscess.
- Lung abscess.
- Infection of the pericardium.
- Brain abscess.

PROBABLE OUTCOME—In most cases without complications, amebiasis is curable in 3 weeks with treatment. In the carrier state, this disease may not cause any symptoms. In severe cases, it may cause dysentery that requires hospital treatment.

 ## HOW TO TREAT

NOTE—Follow your doctor's instructions. These instructions are supplemental.

GENERAL MEASURES—Be extra careful about personal cleanliness. Bathe frequently, and wash hands with warm water and soap after each bowel movement and before handling food.

MEDICATION—Your doctor may prescribe an antiamoeba drug such as: metronidazole; paromomycin; emetine; or diiodohydroxyquin.

ACTIVITY—Rest in bed during an acute attack. Resume normal activities when fever disappears and diarrhea improves.

DIET—Soft diet progressing to normal diet. (See Appendices 11 & 1.)

 ## CALL YOUR DOCTOR IF

- You have symptoms of amebiasis.
- The following occur during treatment:
  Abdominal cramps continue longer than 24 hours.
  Diarrhea or blood in stool increases.
  Vomiting begins.
  Pain begins over liver or jaundice occurs.
  A skin rash appears.
  Irritability or a severe headache develop.

AMENORRHEA, PRIMARY

GENERAL INFORMATION

DEFINITION—Absence of menstruation in a young woman who has passed puberty and is at least 16 years old.

BODY PARTS INVOLVED—Endocrine system; reproductive system.

SEX OR AGE MOST AFFECTED—Females over age 16.

SIGNS & SYMPTOMS—Lack of menstrual periods after puberty. Most girls begin menstruating by age 14.

CAUSES—Usually unknown. Possible causes include:
- Congenital abnormalities, such as the absence or abnormal formation of female organs (vagina, uterus, ovaries).
- Intact hymen (membrane covering the vaginal opening) that has no opening to allow passage of menstrual flow.
- Disorders (tumors, infections, or lack of maturation) of the endocrine system.
- Chromosome disorders.
- Emotional distress.
- Eating disorders, including obesity, bulimia, anorexia nervosa, excessive dieting or starvation.
- Use of certain drugs, including mind-altering drugs, sedatives and hormones.
- Participation in highly competitive, strenuous athletic activities.
- Pregnancy following intercourse prior to the first menstrual period.

RISK INCREASES WITH
- Stress.
- Use of drugs, including oral contraceptives, anticancer drugs, barbiturates, narcotics, cortisone drugs, chlordiazepoxide and reserpine.

HOW TO PREVENT
- Don't use drugs unless prescribed for you by your doctor.
- Reduce athletic activities if they are too strenuous.
- Obtain medical treatment for any underlying disorder.

WHAT TO EXPECT

APPROPRIATE HEALTH CARE
- Self-care after diagnosis.
- Doctor's treatment.
- Psychotherapy or counseling, if amenorrhea is stress-related or results from eating disorders.
- Surgery (minor) to create an opening in the hymen, if necessary.
- Surgery to correct abnormalities of the reproductive system (sometimes).

DIAGNOSTIC MEASURES
- Your own observation of symptoms.
- Medical history and physical exam by a doctor.
- Laboratory studies, such as a buccal smear (cells scraped from inside the cheek for chromosome studies) and blood tests of hormone levels.

POSSIBLE COMPLICATIONS—Psychological distress about sexual development.

PROBABLE OUTCOME—The absence of menstruation is not a health risk. It is usually curable with hormone treatment or removal of the underlying cause. Most doctors are reluctant to begin treatment before age 18 unless the cause can be identified and treated safely.

Causes which sometimes cannot be corrected include chromosome disorders and abnormalities of the reproductive system.

HOW TO TREAT

NOTE—Follow your doctor's instructions. These instructions are supplemental.

GENERAL MEASURES
- If you have emotional stress or conflicts in your life, ask family, friends or competent counselors to help you resolve them.
- Don't use mood-altering, mind-altering, stimulant or sedative drugs.

MEDICATION—Your doctor may prescribe progesterone (hormone) treatment to induce bleeding. If bleeding begins when progesterone is withdrawn, the reproductive system is functioning and the genital tract is open. This also indicates that pituitary disease is unlikely. If progesterone withdrawal does not induce bleeding, gonad stimulants such as clomiphene or gonadotrophins may be used for the same purpose.

ACTIVITY—No restrictions. Exercise regularly, but not to excess. Sleep at least 8 hours every night.

DIET
- Eat 3 well-balanced meals a day.
- Tell your doctor if you believe you are overweight. Don't try to lose weight by crash-dieting.
- Don't drink alcohol.
- Don't take vitamin and mineral supplements unless your doctor prescribes them.

CALL YOUR DOCTOR IF

- You are 16 years old and have never had a period.
- Periods don't begin in 6 months, despite treatment.

AMENORRHEA, SECONDARY

GENERAL INFORMATION

DEFINITION—Cessation of menstruation for at least 3 months in a woman who has previously menstruated.

BODY PARTS INVOLVED—Endocrine system; reproductive system.

SEX OR AGE MOST AFFECTED—Females from puberty to menopause.

SIGNS & SYMPTOMS—Absence of menstrual periods for 3 or more months in a woman who has menstruated at least once.

CAUSES
● Pregnancy (if the woman has had sexual intercourse).
● Breast-feeding an infant.
● Discontinuing use of birth-control pills.
● Menopause (if the woman is over 35 and not pregnant).
● Emotional stress or psychological disorder.
● Surgical removal of the ovaries or uterus.
● Disorder of the endocrine system, including the pituitary, hypothalamus, thyroid, parathyroid, adrenal and ovarian glands.
● Diabetes mellitus.
● Tuberculosis.
● Obesity, anorexia nervosa or bulimia.
● Strenuous program of physical exercise, such as long-distance running.

RISK INCREASES WITH
● Stress.
● Poor nutrition.
● Use of certain drugs, such as phenothiazines, reserpine or hormones.

HOW TO PREVENT—If your amenorrhea is caused by an underlying disease, such as tuberculosis, diabetes or anorexia nervosa, obtain treatment for the primary disorder.

If the cause of your amenorrhea is unknown, there are no specific preventive measures.

WHAT TO EXPECT

APPROPRIATE HEALTH CARE
● Self-care after diagnosis.
● Doctor's treatment.
● Dilatation and curettage (D & C, see Glossary).
● Psychotherapy or counseling, if amenorrhea is stress-related.

DIAGNOSTIC MEASURES
● Your own observation of symptoms.
● Medical history and physical exam by a doctor.
● Laboratory studies, such as a pregnancy test, blood studies of hormone levels and Pap smear (see Glossary).

● Surgical diagnostic procedures, such as laparoscopy or hysteroscopy (see Glossary for both).
● Therapeutic trial of progesterone. If bleeding occurs after progesterone is withdrawn, the reproduction system is functional.

POSSIBLE COMPLICATIONS—None expected if no serious underlying cause can be discovered.

PROBABLE OUTCOME—Amenorrhea is not a threat to health. Whether it can be corrected varies with the underlying cause:
● If from pregnancy or breast-feeding, menstruation will resume when these conditions cease.
● If from discontinuing use of oral contraceptives, periods should begin in 2 months to 2 years.
● If from menopause, periods will become less frequent or may never resume. Hysterectomy also ends menstruation permanently.
● If from endocrine disorders, hormone replacement usually causes periods to resume.
● If from eating disorders, successful treatment of the disorder is necessary for menstruation to resume.
● If from diabetes or tuberculosis, menstruation may never resume.
● If from strenuous exercise, periods usually resume when exercise decreases.

HOW TO TREAT

NOTE—Follow your doctor's instructions. These instructions are supplemental.

GENERAL MEASURES—See Appendix 13 for suggestions to reduce stress.

MEDICATION—Your doctor may prescribe hormone replacement therapy.

ACTIVITY—No restrictions.

DIET—No special diet.

CALL YOUR DOCTOR IF

● Your periods have ceased for 3 or more months.
● Your periods don't resume in 6 months, despite treatment.
● New, unexplained symptoms develop. Hormones used in treatment may produce side effects.

AMYOTROPHIC LATERAL SCLEROSIS
(ALS; Lou Gehrig's Disease)

 ## GENERAL INFORMATION

DEFINITION—A progressive breakdown of the cells of the spinal cord, resulting in gradual loss of muscle function. This is not contagious or cancerous.

BODY PARTS INVOLVED—Central nervous system; muscle system, especially in the hands, forearms, legs, head and neck.

SEX OR AGE MOST AFFECTED—Men over age 40.

SIGNS & SYMPTOMS—Symptoms appear in the following order:
● Muscle twitching and weakness, beginning in the hands and spreading to the arms and legs. Weakness eventually affects muscles that control breathing and swallowing.
● Stiffening and spasticity of muscle groups.

CAUSES—Unknown.

RISK INCREASES WITH—No known risk factor.

HOW TO PREVENT—Cannot be prevented at present.

 ## WHAT TO EXPECT

APPROPRIATE HEALTH CARE
● Self-care after diagnosis.
● Doctor's treatment.
● Psychotherapy or counseling to learn to cope with disability.
● Eventual hospitalization or nursing-home care.

DIAGNOSTIC MEASURES
● Your own observation of symptoms.
● Medical history and physical exam by a doctor.
● Laboratory studies, such as electromyography and muscle biopsy (see Glossary for both).

POSSIBLE COMPLICATIONS
● Pressure sores caused by immobility.
● Pneumonia caused by swallowing difficulty and choking.

PROBABLE OUTCOME—This condition is currently considered incurable. It is usually fatal within 10 years. However, pain can be relieved or controlled. Scientific research into causes and treatment continues, so there is hope for increasingly effective treatment and cure.

 ## HOW TO TREAT

NOTE—Follow your doctor's instructions. These instructions are supplemental.

GENERAL MEASURES—Obtain good nursing care to prevent pressure sores.

MEDICATION—Your doctor may prescribe antibiotics to fight infection if pneumonia develops.

ACTIVITY—Stay as active as possible. Weakness will gradually limit capability.

DIET—Soft, easy-to-swallow foods. See Appendix 11.

 ## CALL YOUR DOCTOR IF

● You have symptoms of amyotrophic lateral sclerosis.
● Coughing, choking or fever occurs after diagnosis.

ANAL FISSURE

GENERAL INFORMATION

DEFINITION—Splitting or tearing of sensitive anal tissue.

BODY PARTS INVOLVED—Anus.

SEX OR AGE MOST AFFECTED—All ages, but most common in infants, young children and adults over 60. This affects more women than men.

SIGNS & SYMPTOMS
- Sharp pain with passage of a hard or bulky stool.
- Streaks of blood on the toilet paper, underwear or diaper.
- Itching around the rectum.

CAUSES—Stretching of the anus from a large, hard stool.

RISK INCREASES WITH
- Constipation.
- Multiple pregnancies.

HOW TO PREVENT—Avoid constipation by:
- Drinking at least 8 glasses of water daily.
- Eating a diet high in fiber.
- Using stool softeners or other laxatives, if needed.

WHAT TO EXPECT

APPROPRIATE HEALTH CARE
- Home care.
- Doctor's treatment.
- Surgery to remove the fissure or to alter the muscle that contracts and prevents normal healing.

DIAGNOSTIC MEASURES
- Your own observation of symptoms.
- Medical history and physical exam by a doctor.
- Examination of the anus and rectum with an anoscope or sigmoidoscope to rule out other causes of anal or rectal bleeding.

POSSIBLE COMPLICATIONS—Permanent scarring that prevents normal bowel movements.

PROBABLE OUTCOME—Most adults recover with treatment, making surgery unnecessary. Most infants and young children recover after the stool is softened.

HOW TO TREAT

NOTE—Follow your doctor's instructions. These instructions are supplemental.

GENERAL MEASURES
- The following should be done to prevent constipation in children until the fissure heals:

  For infants: Before bedtime, fill a rubber ear syringe with plain mineral oil. Gently insert the tip and squeeze the mineral oil into the infant's rectum.

  Repeat the next morning. If no bowel movement occurs, repeat at noon. After the bowel movement, clean the anus gently with cotton and water.

  For older children: Gently squeeze 4 ounces of mineral oil into the rectum. You may use a sanitary napkin to catch oil that seeps out in the night.
- To relieve muscle spasms and pain around the anus, apply a warm towel to the area.

  Sitz baths also relieve pain. Use 8 inches of very warm water 2 or 3 times a day for 10 to 20 minutes. Be careful not to burn a young child.

MEDICATION
- For minor pain, you may use non-prescription drugs, such as acetaminophen or topical anesthetics.
- After sitz baths, apply a non-prescription ointment containing zinc oxide to help heal the fissure.
- Use mineral oil as a laxative for infants. Give the infant 1 teaspoon by mouth for each 10 pounds of body weight. Repeat each day for about 2 weeks after blood disappears from the stool.

  After giving mineral oil, wait several hours to give vitamins. Mineral oil interferes with the absorption of vitamins and other nutrients.

ACTIVITY—No restrictions. Physical activity reduces the likelihood of constipation.

DIET—Encourage a high-fiber diet and extra fluids to prevent constipation.

CALL YOUR DOCTOR IF

You or your child have symptoms of an anal fissure—especially pain—that persists despite treatment.

ILLNESSES & DISORDERS

ANAPHYLAXIS
(Allergic Shock)

 GENERAL INFORMATION

DEFINITION—A severe allergic response to medications and many other allergy-causing substances.

BODY PARTS INVOLVED—Blood vessels throughout the body; heart; lungs; skin.

SEX OR AGE MOST AFFECTED—Both sexes; all ages.

SIGNS & SYMPTOMS—Any of the following may occur within seconds or a few minutes after exposure to a substance to which you are very allergic:
- Tingling or numbness around the mouth.
- Sneezing.
- Itching all over, often accompanied by hives.
- Watery eyes.
- Tightness in the chest; difficult breathing.
- Swelling or itching in the mouth or throat.
- Pounding heart.
- Faintness.
- Loss of consciousness.

Not all symptoms occur. Seek immediate help for any.

CAUSES—Eating or receiving injections of something to which you are sensitive. The allergic response to neutralize or get rid of the material results in a life-threatening overreaction. Things which cause reactions most often include:
- Medication of all types, especially penicillin. Injections are much riskier than oral medications.
- Stings or bites from insects, such as bees, biting ants and some spiders.
- Injected chemicals used in some types of X-ray studies.
- Foods, especially eggs, beans, seafood and fruit.

RISK INCREASES WITH
- A previous mild allergic response to things listed above.
- Medical history of eczema, hayfever or asthma.

HOW TO PREVENT—If you have an allergic history:
- Tell your doctor before accepting any medication. Before you are given a shot, ask what it is.
- Keep an anaphylaxis kit, such as Ana-Kit, with you at all times. Be sure your family knows how to use the kit if you have a reaction.
- Wear a Medic-Alert (see glossary) bracelet or pendant warning that you are allergic.
- Always remain in your doctor's office 15 minutes after receiving any injection. Report any symptoms immediately.

 WHAT TO EXPECT

APPROPRIATE HEALTH CARE—Doctor's treatment.

DIAGNOSTIC MEASURES
- Your own observation of symptoms.
- Medical history and physical exam by a doctor.
- Laboratory skin tests to determine sensitivities.

POSSIBLE COMPLICATIONS—Without prompt treatment, anaphylaxis causes shock, cardiac arrest and death.

PROBABLE OUTCOME—Full recovery with prompt treatment.

 HOW TO TREAT

NOTE—Follow your doctor's instructions. These instructions are supplemental.

GENERAL MEASURES
- If you observe signs of anaphylaxis in someone and he or she stops breathing:
  Yell for help. Don't leave the victim.
  Begin mouth-to-mouth breathing immediately.
  If there is no heartbeat, give external cardiac massage.
  Have someone call 0 (operator) or 911 (emergency) for an ambulance or medical help.
  Don't stop CPR until help arrives.
- Be alert to the possibility of a reaction when taking any medicine, and be prepared to respond quickly if symptoms occur. If you have had a previous severe allergic reaction, always carry your anaphylaxis kit.

MEDICATION
- Adrenalin by injection is the only effective immediate treatment.
- Aminophylline, cortisone drugs or antihistamines, given after the adrenalin, help prevent the return of acute symptoms.

ACTIVITY—Resume your normal activities as soon as symptoms improve after an attack. Stay under someone's observation for 24 hours in case symptoms recur.

DIET—Avoid foods to which you are allergic.

 CALL YOUR DOCTOR IF

- You have symptoms of anaphylaxis. This is an emergency!
- New, unexplained symptoms develop. Drugs used in treatment may produce side effects.

ANEMIA, APLASTIC

GENERAL INFORMATION

DEFINITION—A serious disease characterized by decreased bone-marrow production of blood cells.

BODY PARTS INVOLVED—Bone marrow; lymphatic system; blood.

SEX OR AGE MOST AFFECTED—Both sexes; all ages.

SIGNS & SYMPTOMS
- Paleness.
- Weakness, tiredness, faintness and breathlessness.
- Frequent infections.
- Spontaneous bleeding from the nose, mouth, rectum, vagina, gums and other sites—including the central nervous system.
- Red dots of bleeding under the skin.
- Unexplained bruising.
- Ulcers in the mouth, throat and rectum.

CAUSES—Poor bone-marrow function. Bone marrow is often infiltrated with fat cells, which supplant areas that manufacture blood cells. Infections occur because of reduced white cells, which normally protect against infection.

Half of all cases are caused by drugs, especially immunosuppressive drugs, anticancer drugs, chloramphenicol, or chemicals such as benzene. Other cases probably result from immunodeficiency, severe illness or unidentifiable causes.

RISK INCREASES WITH
- Family history of aplastic anemia.
- Genetic factors, such as those associated with congenital hypoplastic anemia (see Glossary).
- Use of drugs listed as causes.
- Recent severe illness.

HOW TO PREVENT
- Avoid prolonged exposure to toxic compounds, such as benzene, that are used in many industrial chemicals.
- Don't use drugs that cause aplastic anemia, if substitute drugs are available.

WHAT TO EXPECT

APPROPRIATE HEALTH CARE
- Doctor's treatment.
- Surgery to transplant bone marrow.
- Hospitalization for isolation until the body can resist infection.

DIAGNOSTIC MEASURES
- Your own observation of symptoms.
- Medical history and physical exam by a doctor.
- Laboratory studies of blood and bone marrow.

POSSIBLE COMPLICATIONS—Poor response to treatment, resulting in uncontrollable infections and bleeding. Complications are fatal in 50% to 70% of those with severe aplastic anemia.

PROBABLE OUTCOME—If the cause can be identified and treated successfully, the disorder is curable. Anemia caused by immunosuppressive drugs usually improves spontaneously when drugs are withdrawn. Full recovery often requires 6 to 8 months.

HOW TO TREAT

NOTE—Follow your doctor's instructions. These instructions are supplemental.

GENERAL MEASURES
- A bone-marrow transplant requires a donor with compatible antigens. A twin, brother or sister usually makes the best donor. Donated marrow is injected gradually into the patient's veins to try to replace poorly functioning bone marrow with normal cells.

  Hair loss often accompanies treatment, and some persons wear a wig temporarily.
- Keep the mouth scrupulously clean to decrease the chance of infection. Brush often with a soft toothbrush. Rinse the mouth with a solution of equal parts hydrogen peroxide and water, or use a medicated mouthwash, if prescribed.

MEDICATION—Your doctor may prescribe:
- Immunosuppressive drugs to prevent rejection, if a bone-marrow transplant is necessary.
- Antibiotics to prevent or treat infection.
- Medicated mouthwash to suppress fungus infections.

ACTIVITY—Resume your normal activities after treatment.

DIET—No special diet. You may need iron and vitamin supplements. Ask your doctor.

CALL YOUR DOCTOR IF

- You have symptoms of aplastic anemia.
- The following occurs after a bone-marrow transplant:
  Fever.
  Any sign of infection, such as swelling anywhere in the body. Redness, tenderness or pain may not be present.
  Skin rash.
  Jaundice (yellow skin and eyes).
  Joint pain.
  Puffy feet and ankles.
  Urinary discomfort.
  Decreased urine in 1 day.

ILLNESSES & DISORDERS

ANEMIA DURING PREGNANCY

 ## GENERAL INFORMATION

DEFINITION—An inadequate level of hemoglobin during pregnancy. Hemoglobin is a protein that carries oxygen to body tissues.

BODY PARTS INVOLVED—Blood cells.

SEX OR AGE MOST AFFECTED—Pregnant females.

SIGNS & SYMPTOMS
- Breathlessness.
- Tiredness, weakness or fainting.
- Paleness.
- Palpitations or an abnormal awareness of the heartbeat.
- Inflamed, sore tongue.
- Nausea.
- Headache.
- Forgetfulness.
- Jaundice.
- Abdominal pain.

CAUSES
- Poor diet with inadequate iron.
- Folic-acid deficiency.
- Loss of blood from bleeding hemorrhoids or gastrointestinal bleeding.
- Excess cooking of food, which destroys available iron and other nutrients.
- Even if iron and folic-acid intake are sufficient, a pregnant woman may become anemic because pregnancy alters the digestive process. The fetus consumes some of the iron or folic acid normally available to the mother's body.

RISK INCREASES WITH
- Poor nutrition, especially multiple vitamin deficiencies.
- Smoking, which reduces absorption of important nutrients.
- Excess alcohol consumption, leading to poor nutrition.
- Medical history of any disorder that reduces absorption of nutrients.
- Use of anticonvulsant drugs.
- Previous use of oral contraceptives.

HOW TO PREVENT
- Eat foods rich in iron, such as liver, beef, whole-grain breads and cereals, eggs and dried fruit.
- Eat foods high in folic acid, such as wheat germ, beans, peanut butter, oatmeal, mushrooms, collards, broccoli, beef liver and asparagus.
- Eat foods high in vitamin C, such as citrus fruits and fresh, raw vegetables. Vitamin C makes iron absorption more efficient.
- Take prenatal vitamin and mineral supplements, if your doctor prescribes them.

 ## WHAT TO EXPECT

APPROPRIATE HEALTH CARE
- Self-care after diagnosis.
- Doctor's treatment.

DIAGNOSTIC MEASURES
- Your own observation of symptoms.
- Medical history and physical exam by a doctor.
- Laboratory blood studies of hemoglobin, iron, hematocrit and folic acid.

POSSIBLE COMPLICATIONS
- Premature labor.
- Dangerous anemia from normal blood loss during labor, requiring blood transfusions.
- Increased susceptibility to infection after childbirth.

PROBABLE OUTCOME—Usually curable with iron and folic-acid supplements by mouth or by injection.

 ## HOW TO TREAT

NOTE—Follow your doctor's instructions. These instructions are supplemental.

GENERAL MEASURES—If the tongue is red and sore, rinse with warm salt water 3 or 4 times a day. Use 1 teaspoon salt to 8 oz. warm water. Brush teeth with a soft toothbrush.

MEDICATION—Your doctor may prescribe iron, folic acid and other supplements. For better absorption, take iron supplements 1 hour before eating or between meals. Iron will turn bowel movements black, and often cause constipation.

ACTIVITY—No restrictions, except rest often until anemia disappears.

DIET—Eat well and take prescribed supplements. Increase fiber and fluid intake to prevent constipation. See How to Prevent for diet suggestions.

 ## CALL YOUR DOCTOR IF

- You have symptoms of anemia during pregnancy.
- The following occurs during treatment:
  Diarrhea.
  Nausea.
  Abdominal pain.
  Constipation.
  Bleeding—however slight—from any source.

ANEMIA, FOLIC-ACID DEFICIENCY
(Megaloblastic Anemia)

 GENERAL INFORMATION

DEFINITION—Anemia caused by a deficiency of folic acid. It is often accompanied by iron-deficiency anemia.

BODY PARTS INVOLVED—Blood cells, which transport oxygen to all body parts.

SEX OR AGE MOST AFFECTED—Both sexes, but most common in women over 30.

SIGNS & SYMPTOMS
- Fatigue and weakness.
- Red, sore tongue.
- Paleness.
- Shortness of breath.
- Nausea, vomiting and diarrhea.

CAUSES
- Complication of pregnancy, when the body needs 8 times more folic acid than usual.
- Inadequate intake or absorption of foods with a high folic-acid content, such as meat, poultry, fish, cheese, milk, eggs, green vegetables, yeast and mushrooms.
- Alcoholism.
- Overcooking foods, which destroys folic acid.
- Deficiency of vitamin B-12 or vitamin C.

RISK INCREASES WITH
- Adults over 60, especially those who have poor diets.
- Pregnancy.
- Illness, such as tropical sprue, psoriasis, acne rosacea, eczema or dermatitis herpetiformis.
- Fad diets or general poor nutrition, especially vitamin-C deficiency.
- Surgical removal of the stomach.
- Smoking, which decreases vitamin-C absorption. Vitamin C is necessary for folic-acid absorption.
- Use of certain drugs, such as oral contraceptives, anticonvulsants, methotrexate or triamterene.

HOW TO PREVENT
- Don't drink alcohol.
- Have regular medical checkups during pregnancy. Take prenatal vitamin supplements, if they are prescribed.
- Eat well. Include fresh vegetables, meat and other animal proteins. Avoid fad diets. Don't overcook food.
- Don't smoke. Smoking increases vitamin requirements.

 WHAT TO EXPECT

APPROPRIATE HEALTH CARE
- Self-care after diagnosis.
- Doctor's treatment.

DIAGNOSTIC MEASURES
- Your own observation of symptoms.
- Medical history and physical exam by a doctor.
- Laboratory blood studies.

POSSIBLE COMPLICATIONS
- Infertility.
- Increased susceptibility to infection.
- Congestive heart failure (severe cases only).

PROBABLE OUTCOME—Usually curable in 3 weeks with an adequate folic-acid intake.

 HOW TO TREAT

NOTE—Follow your doctor's instructions. These instructions are supplemental.

GENERAL MEASURES
- If you smoke, stop smoking.
- If you take oral contraceptives, consider using another form of contraception.

MEDICATION—Your doctor may prescribe:
- Folic-acid supplements.
- Iron supplements to take orally.

ACTIVITY—No restrictions.

DIET—No special diet. Eat foods daily that are high in folic acid. The liver can store folic acid for a limited time only.

 CALL YOUR DOCTOR IF

- You have symptoms of anemia.
- Symptoms don't improve in 2 weeks, despite treatment.
- Symptoms of infection (fever, chills and muscle aches) occur during treatment.

ILLNESSES & DISORDERS

ANEMIA, HEMOLYTIC

GENERAL INFORMATION

DEFINITION—Anemia due to the premature destruction of mature red blood cells. Bone marrow cannot produce red blood cells fast enough to compensate for those being destroyed. This is not contagious.

BODY PARTS INVOLVED—Blood; bone marrow; spleen.

SEX OR AGE MOST AFFECTED—Both sexes; all ages.

SIGNS & SYMPTOMS
- Fatigue.
- Shortness of breath.
- Irregular heartbeat.
- Jaundice (yellow skin and eyes, dark urine).
- Enlarged spleen.

CAUSES
- Inherited disorder, such as hereditary spherocytosis, G6PD deficiency, sickle-cell anemia or thalassemia.
- Antibodies produced by the body to fight infections, which for unknown reason attack red blood cells. This response is sometimes triggered by blood transfusions.
- Use of medications, including non-prescription drugs, that damage red blood cells.

RISK INCREASES WITH
- Family history of hemolytic anemia.
- Use of any medication.

HOW TO PREVENT
- Don't take any medicine that has previously triggered hemolytic anemia.
- Seek genetic counseling before having children if you have a family history of hemolytic anemia (inherited forms).

WHAT TO EXPECT

APPROPRIATE HEALTH CARE
- Doctor's treatment.
- Hospitalization for transfusions during a hemolytic crisis.
- Surgery to remove an enlarged spleen (sometimes).

DIAGNOSTIC MEASURES
- Your own observation of symptoms.
- Medical history and physical exam by a doctor.
- Laboratory blood studies, including blood count, examination of bone marrow, and measurement with radioactive chromium of red cell survival.

POSSIBLE COMPLICATIONS
- Excessive spleen enlargement, which increases destruction of red blood cells.
- Pain, shock and serious illness caused by hemolysis (red-blood-cell destruction).
- Gallstones.

PROBABLE OUTCOME
- If hemolytic anemia is acquired, it can usually be cured when the cause, such as a drug, is removed. Sometimes the spleen is removed surgically.
- If hemolytic anemia is inherited, it is currently considered incurable. However, symptoms can be relieved or controlled. Scientific research into causes and treatment continues, so there is hope for increasingly effective treatment and cure.

HOW TO TREAT

NOTE—Follow your doctor's instructions. These instructions are supplemental.

GENERAL MEASURES—If removal of the spleen is required, see Splenectomy for an explanation of surgery and postoperative care.

MEDICATION—Your doctor may prescribe:
- Immunosuppressive drugs to control the antibody response.
- Medication to reduce pain. For minor discomfort, you may use non-prescription drugs such as acetaminophen.

ACTIVITY—After treatment, resume normal activities as soon as possible.

DIET—No special diet.

CALL YOUR DOCTOR IF

- You have symptoms of hemolytic anemia.
- The following occurs during treatment:
  Fever.
  Cough.
  Sore throat.
  Swollen joints.
  Muscle aches.
  Bloody urine.
  Signs of infection in any part of the body (redness, pain, swelling, fever).
- New, unexplained symptoms develop.
Drugs used in treatment may produce side effects.

ANEMIA, IRON-DEFICIENCY

 GENERAL INFORMATION

DEFINITION—A decreased number of circulating blood cells, or insufficient hemoglobin in the cells.

Anemia is a symptom (as in fever) of other disorders. For proper treatment, the cause must be found.

BODY PARTS INVOLVED—Blood, which affects all body cells.

SEX OR AGE MOST AFFECTED—Both sexes; all ages.

SIGNS & SYMPTOMS—Signs of pronounced anemia include:
- Tiredness and weakness.
- Paleness, especially in the hands and lining of the lower eyelids.
Less common signs include:
- Tongue inflammation.
- Fainting.
- Breathlessness.
- Rapid heartbeat.
- Unusual quietness or withdrawal in a child.
- Appetite loss.
- Abdominal discomfort.
- Cravings for ice, paint or dirt.
- Susceptibility to infection.

CAUSES—Decreased absorption of iron or increased need for iron. Causes in infants and children include:
- Poor nutrition. Between 6 months and 2 years of age, children may consume large quantities of milk, to the exclusion of iron-containing foods.
- Premature birth. Premature babies often have low stores of iron at birth.
Causes in adolescents and adults:
- Rapid growth spurts.
- Heavy menstrual bleeding.
- Pregnancy.
- Malabsorption.
- Gastrointestinal disease with bleeding, including cancer.

RISK INCREASES WITH
- Poverty.
- Adults over 60.
- Recent illness, such as an ulcer, diverticulitis, colitis, hemorrhoids or gastrointestinal tumors.

HOW TO PREVENT—Maintain an adequate iron intake through a well-balanced diet or iron supplements. Provide iron-fortified formula for bottle-fed infants.

 WHAT TO EXPECT

APPROPRIATE HEALTH CARE
- Doctor's treatment.
- Self-care.

DIAGNOSTIC MEASURES
- Your own observation of symptoms.
- Medical history and physical exam by a doctor.
- Laboratory blood studies, especially of hematocrit (see Glossary), hemoglobin and red-blood-cell counts.
- X-rays of the gastrointestinal tract.

POSSIBLE COMPLICATIONS—Failure to diagnose a bleeding malignancy.

PROBABLE OUTCOME—Usually curable with iron supplements if the underlying cause can be identified and cured.

 HOW TO TREAT

NOTE—Follow your doctor's instructions. These instructions are supplemental.

GENERAL MEASURES—The most important part of treatment for iron-deficiency anemia is to correct the underlying cause. Iron deficiency can be treated well with iron supplements. Blood transfusions are sometimes prescribed, *but they should be unnecessary, except in rare instances.*

MEDICATION—Your doctor may prescribe iron supplements:
- Take iron on an empty stomach (at least 1/2 hour before meals) for best absorption. If it upsets your stomach, you may take it with a small amount of food (except milk).
- If you take other medications, wait at least 2 hours after taking iron before taking them. Antacids and tetracyclines especially interfere with iron absorption.
- Because liquid iron supplements may discolor the teeth, a child should drink any liquid iron preparation through a straw. Iron supplements may also cause black bowel movements, diarrhea or constipation.
- Continue iron supplements until 2 to 3 months after blood tests return to normal.
- Too much iron is dangerous. A bottle of iron tablets can poison a child. Keep iron supplements out of the reach of children.

ACTIVITY—No restrictions.

DIET
- Limit milk to 1 pint a day. It interferes with iron absorption.
- Eat protein- and iron-containing foods, including meat, beans and leafy green vegetables.
- Increase dietary fiber to prevent constipation.

 CALL YOUR DOCTOR IF

- You have symptoms of anemia.
- Nausea, vomiting, severe diarrhea or constipation occur during treatment.

ANEMIA, PERNICIOUS
(B-12 Deficiency Anemia)

 GENERAL INFORMATION

DEFINITION—Anemia caused by inadequate absorption of vitamin B-12.

BODY PARTS INVOLVED—Blood, which affects all body cells; stomach.

SEX OR AGE MOST AFFECTED—Adults between ages 50 and 60. This is uncommon in children.

SIGNS & SYMPTOMS
- Weakness, especially in the arms and legs.
- Sore tongue.
- Nausea, appetite loss and weight loss.
- Bleeding gums.
- Numbness and tingling in the hands and feet.
- Difficulty maintaining proper balance.
- Pale lips, tongue and gums.
- Yellow eyes and skin.
- Shortness of breath.
- Depression.
- Confusion and dementia.
- Headache.
- Poor memory.

CAUSES
- Absence of intrinsic factor, a chemical secreted by the stomach's membrane lining that makes absorption of vitamin B-12 possible. The reason for the absence of intrinsic factor is unknown, but it may be a genetic deficiency or autoimmune disorder.
- Decreased production of hydrochloric acid, especially following stomach surgery or in combination with the absence of intrinsic factor. Hydrochloric acid is also necessary for absorption of vitamin B-12.

RISK INCREASES WITH
- Improper diet, especially a vegetarian diet without supplements.
- Thyroid disease.
- Previous stomach surgery, stomach cancer or gastritis.
- Bulimia or anorexia nervosa.
- Family history of pernicious anemia.
- Genetic factors. The disorder is most common in people of Northern European ancestry. It is rare in blacks and Asians.

HOW TO PREVENT—If you have had stomach surgery or gastritis, have regular vitamin B-12 injections. See Medication.

 WHAT TO EXPECT

APPROPRIATE HEALTH CARE
- Self-care after diagnosis.
- Doctor's treatment.

DIAGNOSTIC MEASURES
- Your own observation of symptoms.
- Medical history and physical exam by a doctor.
- Laboratory blood studies.
- Radioactive studies, such as the Schilling test using radioactive vitamin B-12.

POSSIBLE COMPLICATIONS
- Congestive heart failure.
- Double vision.
- Greater susceptibility to infections.
- Impotence in males.

PROBABLE OUTCOME—This condition is currently considered incurable. However, regular vitamin B-12 injections will control symptoms indefinitely and reverse complications. Symptoms should disappear within 6 months after treatment begins.

 HOW TO TREAT

NOTE—Follow your doctor's instructions. These instructions are supplemental.

GENERAL MEASURES—Avoid very hot water and heating pads. Your nervous system may not be able to detect dangerously high temperatures.

MEDICATION—Your doctor will prescribe vitamin B-12 injections. The amount depends on the extent of your illness. The usual dosage is 1 injection a day for 7 days, then 1 injection a week for 1 month, then once a month for the rest of your life.
  Learn to give yourself vitamin B-12 injections, because oral supplements are inadequate. Lifetime treatment is essential. Even with treatment, your ability to absorb vitamin B-12 will not be normal.

ACTIVITY—No restrictions.

DIET
- No special diet. Raw meat and raw liver are no longer prescribed.
- Iron supplements may be necessary.

 CALL YOUR DOCTOR IF

- You have symptoms of pernicious anemia.
- Symptoms don't improve in 2 weeks, despite treatment.

ANEURYSM

GENERAL INFORMATION

DEFINITION—Enlargement or bulge in an artery caused by a weak artery wall.

BODY PARTS INVOLVED—Arteries. Aneurysms occur most often in the aorta (major artery in the chest and abdomen), arteries that supply the brain or legs, or arteries to the heart after a heart attack.

SEX OR AGE MOST AFFECTED—Adults of both sexes.

SIGNS & SYMPTOMS—Symptoms vary according to which artery is affected:
- Thoracic (chest) aneurysm produces pain in the chest, neck, back and abdomen. The pain may be sudden and sharp.
- Abdominal aneurysm produces back pain (sometimes severe), appetite and weight loss, and a pulsating mass in the abdomen.
- Aneurysm in a leg artery causes poor circulation in the leg, with weakness and pallor or swelling and bluish color. A pulsating mass may appear in the groin or behind the knee.
- Aneurysm in a brain artery produces headache (often throbbing), weakness, paralysis or numbness, pain behind the eye, vision change or partial blindness, and unequal pupils.
- Aneurysm in a heart muscle causes heartbeat irregularities and symptoms of congestive heart failure (see Illness section).

CAUSES
- Atherosclerosis (hardening of the arteries).
- Congenitally weak artery (especially with aneurysms in blood vessels to the brain).
- Syphilis or infection in the aorta caused by syphilis.
- Injury.

RISK INCREASES WITH
- Adults over 60.
- Previous heart attack.
- High blood pressure.
- Smoking.
- Obesity.
- Family history of atherosclerosis.

HOW TO PREVENT
- Follow prevention for atherosclerosis (in Illness section).
- Obtain early treatment for syphilis.
- Follow your treatment program to control high blood pressure.

WHAT TO EXPECT

APPROPRIATE HEALTH CARE
- Doctor's treatment.
- Hospitalization.

- Surgery to replace the diseased vessel or close off the aneurysm. An aneurysm to the brain requires emergency surgery. Surgery for other types of aneurysms may be scheduled at a convenient time.

DIAGNOSTIC MEASURES
- Your own observation of symptoms.
- Medical history and physical exam by a doctor.
- Laboratory blood studies of clotting.
- EKG (see Glossary).
- X-rays of blood vessels (angiography).
- X-rays of the head, including CAT scan or ultrasound (see Glossary for both).

POSSIBLE COMPLICATIONS
- Stroke.
- Rupture of the aneurysm. Symptoms include severe headache, severe knifelike chest, abdominal or leg pain, and loss of consciousness.

PROBABLE OUTCOME—Often curable with surgery to replace the diseased vessel with grafts (artificial vessels). Surgery on a heart aneurysm can stabilize the heartbeat and prolong life. Aneurysms sometimes recur.

HOW TO TREAT

NOTE—Follow your doctor's instructions. These instructions are supplemental.

GENERAL MEASURES—Early detection and treatment before rupture are essential. See your doctor if you have any signs of an aneurysm—especially a pulsating mass in the abdomen or leg—even if it does not cause symptoms.

MEDICATION—After surgery, your doctor may prescribe:
- Anticoagulants to prevent blood-clot formation in an aneurysm.
- Pain relievers.

ACTIVITY—Avoid heavy exertion or straining prior to surgery. After surgery, resume normal activities gradually.

DIET—Before surgery, eat a high-fiber diet so you can avoid straining during bowel movements. After surgery, no special diet is necessary.

CALL YOUR DOCTOR IF

- You have symptoms of an aneurysm, especially a pulsating mass in your abdomen or leg, or chest or abdominal pain. This is an emergency! Call for help, and rest in bed until help arrives.
- You have had a heart attack and develop heartbeat irregularity or symptoms of congestive heart failure.
- After surgery, any symptoms return.

ILLNESSES & DISORDERS

ANGINA PECTORIS

GENERAL INFORMATION

DEFINITION—Chest pain—usually under the sternum (breastbone)—brought on by exercise, emotional upset or heavy meals in a person who has a heart disorder.

BODY PARTS INVOLVED—Coronary arteries.

SEX OR AGE MOST AFFECTED—Men over age 35 and post-menopausal women.

SIGNS & SYMPTOMS—Any of the following:
- Tightness, squeezing, pressure or mild ache in the chest.
- Sudden breathing difficulty (sometimes).
- Frequent chest pain similar to indigestion.
- A choking feeling in the throat.
- Chest pain that radiates to the jaw, teeth or earlobes.
- Heaviness, numbness, tingling or ache in the arm, shoulder, elbow or hand—usually on the left side.
- Pain between the shoulder blades.

CAUSES—Insufficient blood to the heart muscle. Causes include:
- Coronary-artery disease with partial blockage or spasm of arteries that supply the heart.
- Anemia.
- Overactive thyroid gland.
- Heartbeat that is too fast.
- Heart-valve disease.

RISK INCREASES WITH
- Smoking.
- High blood pressure.
- High blood-cholesterol levels.
- Obesity.
- Excess intake of carbohydrates, fat or salt.
- Sedentary lifestyle.
- Diabetes mellitus.
- Family history of coronary-artery disease.
- Fatigue, overwork or stress.
- Exposure to cold and wind.

HOW TO PREVENT
- Obtain medical treatment for underlying causes or risks.
- Don't smoke.
- Eat a diet that is low in fat (see Appendix 8) and low in salt (see Appendix 9).
- Lose weight if you are overweight (see Appendix 10).
- Avoid activities that trigger angina attacks.
- Exercise regularly (see Appendix 20) after consulting your doctor.

WHAT TO EXPECT

APPROPRIATE HEALTH CARE
- Self-care after diagnosis.
- Doctor's treatment.
- Surgery to bypass severely blocked coronary arteries (sometimes).

DIAGNOSTIC MEASURES
- Your own observation of symptoms.
- Medical history and physical exam by a doctor.
- Laboratory studies, such as blood tests and stress tests.
- EKG (see Glossary).
- X-rays of the heart.
- Therapeutic trial of nitroglycerin. Nitroglycerin relieves symptoms of angina, but it does not affect symptoms of other disorders.

POSSIBLE COMPLICATIONS—Heart attack.

PROBABLE OUTCOME—Minor angina can be relieved with rest and use of nitroglycerin. Other treatment may be necessary to correct underlying diseases.

HOW TO TREAT

NOTE—Follow your doctor's instructions. These instructions are supplemental.

GENERAL MEASURES
- See Appendix 13 for suggestions to reduce stress and improve overall health.
- Follow suggestions under How to Prevent.

MEDICATION—Your doctor may prescribe nitroglycerin to widen arteries temporarily so more blood can reach the heart.

ACTIVITY—If angina attacks begin suddenly or increase in frequency or severity, you should rest at least 2 weeks. Rest in a chair—not in bed—except for 8 to 10 hours of sleep at night. You may read or watch TV. If you must get up, walk slowly.

After this period, resume activity slowly to a level just below that which produced pain. Gradually increase exercise time and pace. Warm up slowly before exercise.

Avoid situations that increase the heart's workload, such as anger, temperature extremes, high altitude (except in commercial airline flights), or sudden bursts of activity.

Consult your doctor about resuming sexual activity.

DIET—See diet suggestions under How to Prevent.

CALL YOUR DOCTOR IF

- You have symptoms of angina pectoris.
- The following occurs after diagnosis:
  An attack of chest pain continues longer than 10 to 15 minutes, despite rest and treatment with nitroglycerin.
  You wake from sleep with chest pain that does not go away with 1 nitroglycerin tablet. If these attacks continue, report them to your doctor—even if nitroglycerin relieves them.

ANKYLOSING SPONDYLITIS
(Marie-Strümpell Disease)

GENERAL INFORMATION

DEFINITION—Chronic, progressive disease of the joints, accompanied by inflammation and stiffening. It is characterized by a "bent forward" posture caused by stiffening of the spine and support structures.

BODY PARTS INVOLVED—Sacroiliac region; hip joints; lumbar, thoracic and cervical spines.

SEX OR AGE MOST AFFECTED—90% of all cases begin in males between ages 10 and 40.

SIGNS & SYMPTOMS—Early stages:
- Recurrent episodes of low backache. Pain can also occur along the sciatic nerve.
- Stiffness that is worse in the morning.
Later stages:
- Progressive worsening of symptoms. Pain often spreads from the low back to the middle back or higher in the neck. Joints in the arms, legs, feet and hands are sometimes affected.
- Anemia.
- Muscle stiffness.
- Fatigue.
- Weight loss.

CAUSES—Unknown, but it may be caused by genetic changes or autoimmune disorder.

RISK INCREASES WITH—Family history of ankylosing spondylitis.

HOW TO PREVENT—No specific preventive measures.

WHAT TO EXPECT

APPROPRIATE HEALTH CARE
- Self-care after diagnosis.
- Doctor's treatment.
- Surgery to replace a damaged hip or to insert bone grafts in the spine (advanced stages only).

DIAGNOSTIC MEASURES
- Your own observation of symptoms.
- Medical history and physical exam by a doctor.
- Laboratory blood studies.
- X-rays of the spine.

POSSIBLE COMPLICATIONS
- Congestive heart failure.
- Loss of vision.
- Amyloidosis.
- Heart-valve disease.
- Gastrointestinal disease.
- Lung disease.
- Permanent disability and immobilization.

PROBABLE OUTCOME—This disease is currently considered incurable. Symptoms progress unpredictably and slowly for 10 to 20 years. However, symptoms can be relieved or controlled.

Life expectancy is reduced by the likelihood of complications—not from the disease.

Medical literature cites instances of unexplained recovery. Scientific research into causes and treatment continues, so there is hope for increasingly effective treatment and cure.

HOW TO TREAT

NOTE—Follow your doctor's instructions. These instructions are supplemental.

GENERAL MEASURES
- Sleep on your back on a firm mattress. Use a small pillow or none at all.
- Take hot baths or use heat compresses before exercising or to relieve pain.
- Avoid excessive rest or exhaustion.
- Have regular massages, if possible.

MEDICATION—Your doctor may prescribe non-steroidal anti-inflammatory drugs. Don't take narcotics for pain; they are addictive.

ACTIVITY—Stay as active as your strength allows:
- Exercise to maintain good posture and retain as much upright carriage as possible. Back braces don't help.
- Swim regularly, if possible. Your buoyancy in water will allow you to move stiff, painful areas more easily.
- Avoid activity that puts stress on the back.

DIET—No special diet.

CALL YOUR DOCTOR IF

- You or your child have symptoms of ankylosing spondylitis.
- The following occurs during treatment:
Temperature of 101F (38.3C) or higher. This may indicate the recurrence of an acute phase.
Increasing pain and disability, despite measures outlined above.

ANOREXIA NERVOSA

GENERAL INFORMATION

DEFINITION—A psychological eating disorder in which a person refuses to eat adequately—in spite of hunger—and loses enough weight to become emaciated.

The illness usually begins with a normal weight-loss diet. The person eats very little, and refuses to stop dieting after a reasonable weight loss.

BODY PARTS INVOLVED—All body cells.

SEX OR AGE MOST AFFECTED—Female adolescents and young adults.

SIGNS & SYMPTOMS
- Weight loss of at least 25% of body weight without physical illness.
- High energy level despite body wasting.
- Intense fear of obesity.
- Depression.
- Appetite loss.
- Constipation.
- Cold intolerance.
- Refusal to maintain a minimum standard weight for age and height.
- Distorted body image. The person continues to feel fat—even when emaciated.
- Cessation of menstrual periods.

CAUSES—Unknown. However, all patients have family and internal conflicts, including sexual conflicts.

RISK INCREASES WITH
- Peer pressure to be thin.
- History of slight overweight.
- Perfectionistic, compulsive or overachieving personalities.
- Psychological stress.

HOW TO PREVENT—Confront personal problems realistically. Try to correct or cope with problems with the help of counselors, therapists, family and friends. See Appendix 13 for suggestions to reduce stress.

WHAT TO EXPECT

APPROPRIATE HEALTH CARE
- Doctor's treatment.
- Psychotherapy or counseling for the patient and family.
- Hospitalization during crises for intravenous or tube feeding.
- Psychiatric hospitalization for at least 2 to 3 weeks (sometimes).

DIAGNOSTIC MEASURES
- Your own observation of symptoms.
- Medical history and physical exam by a doctor.
- Laboratory blood tests for anemia and electrolyte imbalance.

POSSIBLE COMPLICATIONS
- Chronic anorexia nervosa caused by patient's resistance to treatment.
- Electrolyte disturbances or irregular heartbeat. These may be life-threatening.

PROBABLE OUTCOME—Curable if the patient recognizes the emotional disturbance, wants help and cooperates in treatment. Without treatment, this can cause permanent disability and death. Persons with anorexia nervosa have a high rate of attempted suicide due to low self-esteem.

HOW TO TREAT

NOTE—Follow your doctor's instructions. These instructions are supplemental.

GENERAL MEASURES—The goal of treatment is for the patient to establish healthy eating patterns to regain normal weight. The patient can accomplish this with behavior-modification training supervised by a qualified professional.

MEDICATION—Medicine usually is not necessary for this disorder.

ACTIVITY—No restrictions, but avoid overexertion.

DIET—No special diet. Your doctor may prescribe vitamin and mineral supplements.

CALL YOUR DOCTOR IF

- You have symptoms of anorexia nervosa or observe them in a family member.
- Life-threatening symptoms occur, including: rapid, irregular heartbeat; chest pain; or loss of consciousness. Call immediately. This is an emergency!
- Weight loss continues, despite treatment.

ANXIETY

GENERAL INFORMATION

DEFINITION—A vague, uncomfortable feeling of fear, dread or danger from an unknown source. Some persons become constantly anxious about everything.

BODY PARTS INVOLVED—Central nervous system; endocrine system.

SEX OR AGE MOST AFFECTED—Both sexes; all ages.

SIGNS & SYMPTOMS
- Feeling that something undesirable or harmful is about to happen.
- Dry mouth; swallowing difficulty or hoarseness.
- Rapid breathing and heartbeat.
- Twitching or trembling.
- Muscle tension; headaches.
- Sweating.
- Nausea; diarrhea; weight loss.
- Sleeplessness.
- Irritability.
- Fatigue.
- Nightmares.
- Memory problems.
- Sexual impotence.

CAUSES—Activation of the body's defense mechanisms for fight or flight. Excess adrenalin is discharged from the adrenal glands, and adrenalin breakdown products (catecholamines) eventually affect various parts of the body.

RISK INCREASES WITH
- Stress from any source.
- Family history of neurosis.
- Fatigue or overwork.
- Recurrence of situations that have been previously stressful or harmful.

HOW TO PREVENT—Determine what stressful or potentially harmful situation is causing the anxiety. Deal directly with it.
   Consider lifestyle changes to reduce stress. See Appendix 13.

WHAT TO EXPECT

APPROPRIATE HEALTH CARE
- Self-care.
- Doctor's treatment.
- Psychotherapy or counseling.

DIAGNOSTIC MEASURES
- Your own observation of symptoms.
- Medical history and physical exam by a doctor.
- Laboratory studies to rule out medical conditions that produce anxiety, such as hyperthyroidism.

POSSIBLE COMPLICATIONS
- Untreated anxiety may lead to neuroses, such as phobias, compulsions or hypochondriasis.
- A sudden increase in anxiety may lead to panic and violent escape behavior.

PROBABLE OUTCOME—Anxiety can be controlled with psychological therapy. Overcoming anxiety often results in a richer, more satisfying life.

HOW TO TREAT

NOTE—Follow your doctor's instructions. These instructions are supplemental.

GENERAL MEASURES
- Obtain therapy to understand the specific but unconscious threat or source of stress.
- Learn techniques, including biofeedback and relaxation therapy, to reduce muscle tension.

MEDICATION—Your doctor may prescribe tranquilizers. These are useful for a short time under the following circumstances:
- During periods of unusually intense anxiety.
- Until psychological insights prevent anxiety from developing.
- Until direct action solves the threatening problem.

ACTIVITY—Stay active. Physical exertion helps reduce anxiety.

DIET—No special diet. Avoid caffeine and other stimulants and alcohol.

CALL YOUR DOCTOR IF

- You have symptoms of anxiety and self-treatment has failed.
- You have a sudden feeling of panic.
- New, unexplained symptoms develop. Drugs used in treatment may produce side effects.

APC DISEASE
(Pharyngoconjunctival Fever)

GENERAL INFORMATION

DEFINITION—An acute, contagious viral infection that affects the eyes, throat and central nervous system. It can occur in epidemics in children.

BODY PARTS INVOLVED—Conjunctivae (whites of the eyes) and throat, including tonsils and adenoids.

SEX OR AGE MOST AFFECTED—All ages, but most common in children and adolescents from 1 to 15 years old.

SIGNS & SYMPTOMS
- Sore throat with redness and enlarged tonsils and adenoids.
- High fever—usually 102F (38.9C) to 105F (40.6C).
- Pain and redness in the whites of the eyes. The inflammation usually begins in one eye and spreads to the other.
- Runny nose.
- Cough and chest pain (rare).

CAUSES—A virus infection of the respiratory tract.
  Summer epidemics are common. They are usually associated with swimming in pools or lakes—especially in summer camps. The incubation period is 5 to 8 days.

RISK INCREASES WITH
- Crowded or unsanitary living conditions.
- Exposure to others in swimming pools and spas.

HOW TO PREVENT
- Wash hands frequently to avoid spreading the virus when touching others.
- Avoid swimming pools during epidemics.

WHAT TO EXPECT

APPROPRIATE HEALTH CARE
- Home care after diagnosis.
- Doctor's treatment.

DIAGNOSTIC MEASURES
- Your own observation of symptoms.
- Medical history and physical exam by a doctor.
- Laboratory blood counts.

POSSIBLE COMPLICATIONS—Secondary bacterial infection, especially pneumonia.

PROBABLE OUTCOME—Spontaneous recovery within 7 days. The eye inflammation may be slow to heal, lasting up to 10 days longer than other symptoms.

HOW TO TREAT

NOTE—Follow your doctor's instructions. These instructions are supplemental.

GENERAL MEASURES
- Wipe mucus away from the eyes with a cotton pad moistened with water. No other eye treatment is necessary.
- Use a cool-mist humidifier to relieve the stuffy nose.
- Don't insert cotton swabs in a child's nostrils to clear them. Instead, catch the discharge outside the nostril on a tissue.

MEDICATION
- For minor discomfort, you may use non-prescription drugs such as:
    Acetaminophen to reduce fever and aching.
    Nose drops to relieve nasal stuffiness.
    Cough medicines with decongestants.
- Your doctor may prescribe:
    Eye drops.
    Antiviral drugs.
    Antibiotics for secondary bacterial infections.

ACTIVITY
- Keep the patient isolated as long as the eyes are red. Avoiding unnecessary contact with others protects others from infection and defends the patient from further infection.
- Complete bed rest is not necessary, but extra rest is helpful. Avoid vigorous activity.

DIET—Increase fluid intake, including fruit juice, water, tea and carbonated drinks. Avoid milk, which thickens nasal secretions.

CALL YOUR DOCTOR IF

- You have symptoms of APC disease.
- The following occurs during treatment:
    Fever that lasts several days.
    Increased throat pain, or white or yellow spots on the throat.
    Cough that lasts longer than 10 days.
    Coughing episodes that last longer than non-coughing intervals, or cough that produces thick, yellow-green or gray sputum.
    Labored breathing between coughing bouts.
    Shaking chills.
    Chest pain.
    Shortness of breath.
    Earache, headache or pain in the teeth or over the sinuses.
    Skin rash.
    Extreme lethargy.
    Excessive irritability or delirium.
    Enlarged, tender neck glands.
    Bluish or gray lips, nails or skin.

APPENDICITIS

GENERAL INFORMATION

DEFINITION—Inflammation of the vermiform appendix, a small, tube that extends from the cecum, the first part of the large intestine. The appendix has no known function, but it can become diseased. Appendicitis affects 1 in 500 people each year.

BODY PARTS INVOLVED—Appendix; cecum; peritoneum (membrane covering the intestinal tract).

SEX OR AGE MOST AFFECTED—All ages, but rare in children under 2. The incidence peaks between ages 15 and 24.

SIGNS & SYMPTOMS
- Pain that begins close to the navel and migrates toward the right lower abdomen. Pain becomes persistent and well-localized. It worsens with moving, breathing deeply, coughing, sneezing, walking or being touched.
- Nausea and vomiting (sometimes).
- Constipation and inability to pass gas.
- Diarrhea (occasionally).
- Low fever, beginning after other symptoms.
- Tenderness in the right lower abdomen, usually about a third of the distance from the navel to the top of the hip bone. (This description applies only if the appendix is in its normal position. In some cases, the tip of the appendix is located elsewhere, making diagnosis difficult).
- Abdominal swelling (late stages).
- Increased white-blood-cell count.

CAUSES—Infection for unknown reason, usually with bacteria from the intestinal tract. The appendix may become obstructed from contents moving through intestinal tract, or by a constricting band of tissue. When infected, it becomes swollen, inflamed and filled with pus.

RISK INCREASES WITH—Recent illness, especially a roundworm infestation or gastrointestinal virus infection.

HOW TO PREVENT—No specific preventive measures.

WHAT TO EXPECT

APPROPRIATE HEALTH CARE
- Doctor's treatment.
- Surgery to remove the appendix. Because appendicitis can be hard to diagnose, surgery is often withheld until symptoms and signs progress enough to confirm the diagnosis.

DIAGNOSTIC MEASURES
- Your own observation of symptoms.
- Medical history and physical exam (maybe several) by a doctor.
- Laboratory blood studies. Tests usually show higher levels of white blood cells.
- Urinalysis to rule out a urinary-tract infection, which can mimic appendicitis.

POSSIBLE COMPLICATIONS
- Rupture of the appendix, abscess formation and peritonitis. This is most common in older persons.
- Misdiagnosis because of few or atypical symptoms—especially in the very young or very old.

PROBABLE OUTCOME—Usually curable with surgery. If totally untreated, a ruptured appendix is fatal.

HOW TO TREAT

NOTE—Follow your doctor's instructions. These instructions are supplemental.

GENERAL MEASURES
- While diagnosis is uncertain, take a rectal temperature every 2 hours. Keep a record for your doctor.
- For an explanation of surgery and postoperative care, see Appendectomy (in Surgery section).

MEDICATION—Don't take any laxatives, enemas or medicines for pain. Laxatives may cause rupture, and pain or fever reducers make diagnosis more difficult.

ACTIVITY—Rest in a bed or chair until surgery.

DIET—Don't eat or drink anything until appendicitis has been diagnosed. Anesthesia for surgery is much safer if the stomach is empty. If you are very thirsty, wash your mouth out with water.

CALL YOUR DOCTOR IF

- You have symptoms of appendicitis.
- The following occurs while surgery is pending:
  Fever spikes of 102F (38.9C) or over.
  Continued vomiting.
  Increased pain in the abdomen.
  Fainting.
  Blood in the stool or vomit.

ARTHRITIS, INFECTIOUS
(Septic Arthritis)

 GENERAL INFORMATION

DEFINITION—Inflammation in a joint resulting from infection.

BODY PARTS INVOLVED—Any joint, but most common in larger ones, such as the hip, or those subject to trauma, such as the knee or joints in the hands.

SEX OR AGE MOST AFFECTED—Both sexes; all ages.

SIGNS & SYMPTOMS
• Chills and fever (sometimes high).
• Redness, swelling, tenderness and pain (often throbbing) in the affected joint. Pain sometimes spreads to other joints. It worsens with movement.
• Pain in the buttocks, thighs or groin (sometimes).

CAUSES—Entry into a joint by germs, usually bacteria (streptococci, staphylococci, gonococci, hemophilus or tubercle bacillus) or fungi. Germs gain entry from:
• Infection elsewhere in the body, as with gonorrhea or tuberculosis.
• Infection next to the joint, as with skin boils, cellulitis or bone infection.
• Injury to the joint, including puncture wounds and skin abrasions.

RISK INCREASES WITH
• Adults over 60.
• Illness that has lowered resistance.
• Sexually transmitted infections.
• Diabetes mellitus.
• Rheumatoid arthritis.
• Use of immunosuppressive drugs.
• Joint surgery.
• Injections into joints.
• Excess alcohol consumption.
• Many sexual partners.
• Use of mind-altering drugs, especially those that are injected.
• Poor hygiene.

HOW TO PREVENT
• Protect exposed joints, such as the knee, during activities involving injury risks.
• Obtain prompt medical treatment for infections elsewhere in the body.

OTHER—The use of aspirin and other non-steroidal anti-inflammatory drugs for other disorders may suppress signs of joint inflammation, delaying diagnosis.

 WHAT TO EXPECT

APPROPRIATE HEALTH CARE
• Doctor's treatment.

• Hospitalization (frequently) for complete rest and intravenous antibiotics.
• Surgery to drain fluid or remove foreign material introduced by an injury.
• Physical therapy after recovery to regain full use of the joint.

DIAGNOSTIC MEASURES
• Your own observation of symptoms.
• Medical history and physical exam by a doctor.
• Laboratory studies, such as blood counts, blood culture and culture of fluid from the infected joint.
• X-rays of affected joints.

POSSIBLE COMPLICATIONS
• Misdiagnosis as gout or another non-infectious condition, delaying antibiotic treatment.
• Blood poisoning.
• Permanent joint damage.

PROBABLE OUTCOME—Usually curable with early diagnosis and treatment. Recovery takes weeks or months. Treatment delay may result in a badly damaged joint and loss of movement, requiring joint replacement.

 HOW TO TREAT

NOTE—Follow your doctor's instructions. These instructions are supplemental.

GENERAL MEASURES—No specific instructions except those listed under other headings.

MEDICATION—Your doctor may prescribe:
• Antibiotics (often intravenous). Don't discontinue antibiotics until your doctor recommends it. Infection may return after symptoms disappear.
• Codeine or narcotics for a short time to relieve pain.

ACTIVITY—Splints or casts may be necessary to rest the affected joint completely. Movement delays healing. After cure, physical therapy is often necessary to restore joint function. Resume normal activities gradually as symptoms improve.

DIET—No special diet.

 CALL YOUR DOCTOR IF

• You have symptoms of joint infection. Call immediately.
• The following occurs during the illness: Temperature spike to 103F (39.4C). Fatigue, headache, muscle aches and sweating.
• New, unexplained symptoms develop. Drugs used in treatment may produce side effects.

ARTHRITIS, JUVENILE RHEUMATOID

GENERAL INFORMATION

DEFINITION—An inflammatory disease of connective tissue—mostly joints—that affects children.

BODY PARTS INVOLVED—Joints, usually knees, elbows, ankles and neck. It may also involve adjacent muscles, cartilage and membranes lining the joints.

SEX OR AGE MOST AFFECTED—Starts at 2 to 5 years, and usually disappears by puberty. It is 4 times more frequent in girls.

SIGNS & SYMPTOMS
- Pain, swelling and stiffness in the toes, knees, ankles, elbows, shoulders or neck joints. The pain may begin suddenly or gradually, and may involve only one or many joints. The child may refuse to walk without being able to explain why.
- Daily temperature rise to about 103F (39.4C)—usually in the evening. Fever is frequently accompanied by a body rash and chills.
- Poor appetite; weight loss.
- Anemia.
- Irritability; listlessness.
- Swollen lymph glands.
- Eye pain and redness.
- Chest pain (if the disease is severe enough to affect the heart).

CAUSES—Probably caused by an autoimmune disorder, in which the body's immune system attacks its own normal tissues. The first symptoms are often associated with physical or emotional stress.

RISK INCREASES WITH—Stress.

HOW TO PREVENT—Cannot be prevented at present.

WHAT TO EXPECT

APPROPRIATE HEALTH CARE
- Home care after diagnosis.
- Doctor's treatment.
- Psychotherapy or counseling to help the family cope with the child's long-term illness. Emotional support may be the most important factor in a child's treatment.
- Surgery to correct deformed joints (sometimes).

DIAGNOSTIC MEASURES
- Your own observation of symptoms.
- Medical history and physical exam by a doctor.
- Laboratory blood studies, including autoimmune assays (ANA tests).
- X-rays of the involved joints. Changes may not appear on X-rays until the late stages.

POSSIBLE COMPLICATIONS
- Involvement of tissues other than joints, producing uveitis, an enlarged spleen, pericarditis or inflammation of the heart muscle.
- Permanent joint deformity.

PROBABLE OUTCOME—Juvenile rheumatoid arthritis is currently considered incurable. However, in 75% to 80% of cases, the disease is in complete remission by puberty.

Attacks usually last a few weeks and occur off and on throughout childhood. Symptoms can usually be controlled with treatment.

HOW TO TREAT

NOTE—Follow your doctor's instructions. These instructions are supplemental.

GENERAL MEASURES
- If the child doesn't have a firm mattress, place 3/4-inch plywood between the box springs and mattress to provide better support.
- Request eye examinations at least twice a year to detect uveitis.
- Encourage the child and family to maintain a positive outlook.

MEDICATION—Your doctor may prescribe aspirin or other non-steroidal anti-inflammatory drugs to reduce pain and inflammation.

ACTIVITY—During an attack, keep the child in bed, except to use the bathroom, until fever and other symptoms subside. Splints may be necessary to support and protect an inflamed joint.

After an attack passes, the child may gradually resume normal activities with rest periods during the day. The child should not become overtired and should sleep at least 10 to 12 hours each night.

Your doctor will probably recommend exercises when the child is well enough to do them.

DIET—No special diet.

CALL YOUR DOCTOR IF

- Your child has symptoms of juvenile rheumatoid arthritis.
- The following symptoms occur during treatment:
  Chest pain.
  Temperature of 102F (38.9C) or higher.
  Appetite loss.
- New, unexplained symptoms develop. Drugs used in treatment may produce side effects.

ARTHRITIS, RHEUMATOID

GENERAL INFORMATION

DEFINITION—An illness characterized by joint disease that involves muscles, membrane linings of the joints and cartilage.

BODY PARTS INVOLVED—Joints, including cartilage, synovial membranes, muscles and ligaments; blood vessels; eyes.

SEX OR AGE MOST AFFECTED—3 times more common in women than men. It begins between ages 20 and 60, with a peak incidence between ages 35 and 45.

SIGNS & SYMPTOMS—Slow or sudden onset of:
- Redness, pain, warmth and tenderness in any or all active joints in the hands, wrists, elbows, shoulders, feet and ankles.
- Nodules under the skin (sometimes).

CAUSES—Unknown, but probably an autoimmune disease.

RISK INCREASES WITH
- Emotional or physical stress, as from accidents, childbirth, menopause or surgery.
- Family history of rheumatoid arthritis or other autoimmune disorders.
- Genetic factors, such as autoimmune-system defects.

HOW TO PREVENT—No specific preventive measures.

WHAT TO EXPECT

APPROPRIATE HEALTH CARE
- Self-care after diagnosis.
- Doctor's treatment.
- Physical therapy.
- Time in an extended-care facility (sometimes) for physical therapy.
- Surgery (joint replacement) to correct deformities.

DIAGNOSTIC MEASURES
- Your own observation of symptoms.
- Medical history and physical exam by a doctor.
- Laboratory blood studies to detect a rheumatoid factor.
- X-rays of joints.

POSSIBLE COMPLICATIONS
- Impaired vision.
- Permanent deformity and crippling. This may develop rapidly, especially contractures (muscle shortening) or degeneration of muscles around an inflamed joint.

PROBABLE OUTCOME—The disease may be mild or severe. It is presently incurable, but pain relief, prevention of disability and an active, normal lifespan are usually possible with early diagnosis.

Conservative treatment relieves symptoms in 1 year in 75% of patients. About 5% to 10% are eventually disabled, despite treatment.

HOW TO TREAT

NOTE—Follow your doctor's instructions. These instructions are supplemental.

GENERAL MEASURES
- Splints at night may be helpful to support and protect a joint with active disease. Ask your doctor.
- Relieve pain with heat, including hot soaks (see Appendix 18), heat lamps, heating pads or whirlpool treatments.
- If you don't have a firm mattress, place 3/4-inch plywood between your bedsprings and mattress to support your back.
- Consider moving to a dry climate. Damp weather aggravates symptoms.

MEDICATION—Your doctor may prescribe: non-steroidal anti-inflammatory drugs, including aspirin and other salicylates; gold compounds; immunosuppressive drugs; penicillamine; hydrochloroquin; or cortisone.

Cortisone drugs usually relieve pain dramatically for short periods, but they are less effective for long-term use. They don't prevent progressive joint destruction, and they sometimes have hazardous side effects.

Cortisone injections into joints can temporarily relieve pain.

ACTIVITY
- Stay in bed, except to use the bathroom, until fever and other signs of an active flare-up disappear.
- Remain active, but include daily rest periods. Sleep for 10 to 12 hours each night. Don't become overtired.
- Stand, walk and sit erectly.
- When able, exercise actively to preserve strength and joint mobility. Build up slowly to the amount suggested by your doctor.
- Exercise disabled joints passively to help prevent contractures.

DIET—Eat a normal, well-balanced diet. Avoid arthritis diet fads, which are common. Lose weight if you are obese (see Appendix 10). Obesity stresses the joints.

CALL YOUR DOCTOR IF

- You have symptoms of rheumatoid arthritis.
- The following occurs during treatment: Fever rises to 101F (38.3C) or higher. Symptoms appear in previously unaffected joints.
- New, unexplained symptoms develop. Drugs in treatment may produce side effects.

ASBESTOSIS

GENERAL INFORMATION

DEFINITION—Inflammation of the lung due to breathing asbestos particles. This is not contagious. It may lead to lung cancer.

BODY PARTS INVOLVED—Lungs.

SEX OR AGE MOST AFFECTED—Men over age 40.

SIGNS & SYMPTOMS—Early symptoms:
- Shortness of breath.
- Cough that produces little or no sputum.
- General ill feeling.

Late symptoms:
- Fitful sleep.
- Appetite loss.
- Chest pain.
- Hoarseness.
- Coughing blood.
- Symptoms of congestive heart failure.
- Bluish nails.

CAUSES—Many years of exposure to small particles of asbestos at work or from a nearby asbestos plant.

RISK INCREASES WITH
- Poor nutrition.
- Smoking.
- Excess alcohol consumption.

HOW TO PREVENT
- During exposure to asbestos, wear a protective mask or external-air-supplied hood.
- Follow recommended industrial procedures to suppress asbestos dust.
- Don't smoke.
- Participate in a regular physical exercise program to maintain good cardiopulmonary fitness.

WHAT TO EXPECT

APPROPRIATE HEALTH CARE
- Self-care after diagnosis.
- Doctor's treatment.

DIAGNOSTIC MEASURES
- Your own observation of symptoms.
- Medical history and physical exam by a doctor.
- X-ray of the chest.

POSSIBLE COMPLICATIONS
- Tuberculosis (late stages of silicosis).
- Heart failure due to lung disease.
- Lung collapse.
- Pleurisy.
- Lung cancer.

PROBABLE OUTCOME—This condition is currently considered incurable. However, symptoms can be relieved or controlled. Scientific research into causes and treatment continues, so there is hope for increasingly effective treatment and cure.

HOW TO TREAT

NOTE—Follow your doctor's instructions. These instructions are supplemental.

GENERAL MEASURES—The following measures may relieve symptoms and protect against recurrent lung infections:
- Obtain medical treatment for any respiratory infection, including the common cold.
- Consider moving to a warm, dry climate if you have advanced disease.
- Practice bronchial drainage. Your physician will provide instructions.
- Use a cool-mist humidifier to loosen bronchial secretions so they can be coughed up easily.

MEDICATION
- Your doctor may prescribe:
  Antibiotics for infections.
  Bronchodilators (inhaled or oral) with inhalation therapy (supervised at first by an inhalation therapist) to open bronchial tubes to the maximum.
- For minor discomfort, you may use non-prescription drugs, such as acetaminophen or aspirin.

ACTIVITY
- Rest in bed with infections. You may read or watch TV.
- After treatment, resume normal activity as soon as symptoms improve.

DIET—No special diet.

CALL YOUR DOCTOR IF

- You have symptoms of asbestosis.
- The following occurs during treatment:
  Temperature spike of 101F (38.3C) or more.
  Increased chest pain or breathlessness.
  Blood in the sputum.
  Continuing weight loss.
- New, unexplained symptoms develop. Drugs used in treatment may produce side effects.

ILLNESSES & DISORDERS

ASTHMA

GENERAL INFORMATION

DEFINITION—A chronic disorder with recurrent attacks of wheezing and shortness of breath.

BODY PARTS INVOLVED—Lungs; bronchi; bronchioles.

SEX OR AGE MOST AFFECTED
- All ages except newborn infants.
- Affects more boys than girls in children. Affects both sexes of adults equally.

SIGNS & SYMPTOMS
- Chest tightness and shortness of breath.
- Wheezing upon breathing out.
- Coughing, especially at night, with little sputum.
- Rapid, shallow breathing that is easier with sitting up.
- Breathing difficulty—neck muscles tighten.
- Enlarged chest.
Severe late symptoms:
- Bluish skin.
- Exhaustion.
- Grunting respiration.
- Inability to speak.
- Mental changes, including restlessness or confusion.

CAUSES—Spasm of air passages (bronchi and bronchioles), followed by swelling of the passages and thickening of lung secretions (sputum). This decreases or closes off air to the lungs. These changes are caused by:
- Allergens, such as pollen, dust, animal dander, molds and some foods.
- Lung infections such as bronchitis.
- Air irritants, such as smoke and odors.
- Exercise.
- Stress.

RISK INCREASES WITH
- Other allergic conditions, such as eczema or hay fever.
- Family history of asthma or allergies.
- Exposure to air pollutants.
- Smoking.
- Use of some drugs such as aspirin.

HOW TO PREVENT
- Avoid known allergens and air pollutants.
- Take prescribed preventive medicines regularly—don't omit them when you feel well.
- See Appendix 13 for suggestions to reduce stress.

WHAT TO EXPECT

APPROPRIATE HEALTH CARE
- Self-care after diagnosis.
- Doctor's treatment.
- Emergency-room care and hospitalization for severe attacks.

- Psychotherapy or counseling, if asthma is stress-related.

DIAGNOSTIC MEASURES
- Your own observation of symptoms.
- Medical history and physical exam by a doctor.
- Laboratory blood studies and pulmonary-function test.
- Chest X-rays.

POSSIBLE COMPLICATIONS
- Respiratory failure.
- Pneumothorax.
- Lung infection.
- COPD (see Glossary) from recurrent attacks.

PROBABLE OUTCOME—Symptoms can be controlled with treatment and strict adherence to prevention measures. Children often outgrow asthma. Without treatment, severe attacks can be fatal.

HOW TO TREAT

NOTE—Follow your doctor's instructions. These instructions are supplemental.

GENERAL MEASURES
- Eliminate allergens and irritants at home and at work, if possible.
- Keep regular medications with you at all times. Ask your doctor about having emergency drugs available.
- Sit upright during attacks.
- Practice deep breathing each morning to loosen accumulated lung secretions.

MEDICATION—Your doctor may prescribe:
- Expectorants to loosen sputum.
- Bronchodilators to open air passages.
- Intravenous cortisone drugs (emergencies only) to decrease the body's allergic response.
- Cortisone drugs by nebulizer, which have fewer adverse reactions than oral forms.
- Cromolyn sodium by nebulizer. This is a preventive drug.

ACTIVITY—Stay active, but avoid sudden bursts of exercise. If an attack follows heavy exercise, sit and rest. Sip warm water.

DIET—No special diet, but avoid foods to which you are sensitive. Drink at least 3 quarts of liquid daily to keep secretions loose.

CALL YOUR DOCTOR IF

- You have symptoms of asthma.
- You have an asthma attack that doesn't respond to treatment. This is an emergency!
- New, unexplained symptoms develop. Drugs used in treatment may produce side effects.

ATELECTASIS

GENERAL INFORMATION

DEFINITION—Collapse of part or all of one lung, preventing normal oxygen absorption.

BODY PARTS INVOLVED—Lungs.

SEX OR AGE MOST AFFECTED—Both sexes; all ages.

SIGNS & SYMPTOMS
Sudden, major collapse:
- Chest pain.
- Shortness of breath; rapid breathing.
- Shock (severe weakness, paleness of skin, rapid heartbeat).
- Dizziness.
Gradual, minor collapse:
- Cough.
- Fever.
- No other symptoms.

CAUSES—Obstruction of small or large lung air passages by:
- Thick mucus plugs from infection or other disease, including cystic fibrosis.
- Tumors in the air passages.
- Tumors or blood vessels outside the air passages, causing pressure on airways.
- Inhaled objects, such as small toys or peanuts.
- Prolonged chest or abdominal surgery with general anesthetic.
- Chest injury or fractured ribs.

RISK INCREASES WITH
- Smoking.
- Illness that has lowered resistance or weakened the patient.
- Chronic obstructive lung disease, including emphysema and bronchiectasis.
- Use of drugs that depress alertness or consciousness, such as sedatives, barbiturates, tranquilizers or alcohol.

HOW TO PREVENT
- Force coughing and deep breathing every 1 to 2 hours after surgery with general anesthesia. Also change position often in bed, if possible.
- Increase fluid intake during lung illness or after surgery—by mouth or intravenously—to keep lung secretions loose.
- Keep small objects that might be inhaled away from young children (peanuts are notorious).

WHAT TO EXPECT

APPROPRIATE HEALTH CARE
- Doctor's treatment.
- Surgery to remove tumors.
- Bronchoscopy (see Glossary) to remove foreign objects or a mucus plug.

DIAGNOSTIC MEASURES
- Your own observation of symptoms.
- Medical history and physical exam by a doctor.
- Laboratory studies to measure oxygen and carbon dioxide in the blood.
- X-rays of the chest.

POSSIBLE COMPLICATIONS
- Pneumonia.
- Small lung abscess.
- Permanent lung scars and collapsed lung tissue.

PROBABLE OUTCOME—If atelectasis is caused by a mucus plug or inhaled foreign object, it is curable when the plug or object is removed. If it is caused by a tumor, the outcome depends on the nature of the tumor.

HOW TO TREAT

NOTE—Follow your doctor's instructions. These instructions are supplemental.

GENERAL MEASURES
- Cooperate with requests to turn, cough and breathe deeply after surgery. Hold a pillow tightly against surgical incisions during the coughing exercises.
- Stop smoking.
- Learn to perform postural drainage (see Glossary) after hospitalization. An inhalation therapist, nurse or doctor can demonstrate the technique.

MEDICATION
- Your doctor may prescribe:
  Antibiotics to fight infection that inevitably accompanies atelectasis.
  Pain relievers.
- Don't take sedatives. They may contribute to a recurrence.

ACTIVITY—Resume your normal activities as soon as symptoms improve.

DIET—No special diet, but drink at least 8 glasses of water or other fluid daily to thin lung secretions.

CALL YOUR DOCTOR IF

- You have symptoms of atelectasis.
- The following occurs during treatment:
  Distended abdomen.
  Sudden shortness of breath.
  Blue fingernails and lips.
  Temperature spikes to 102F (38.9C) or higher.

ILLNESSES & DISORDERS

ATHEROSCLEROSIS
(Hardening of the Arteries)

GENERAL INFORMATION

DEFINITION—A thickening of the inner lining of the arteries (blood vessels that carry oxygen and other nutrients from the heart to other body parts). Atherosclerosis may lead to kidney damage, decreased circulation to the brain and extremities, and coronary-artery disease.

BODY PARTS INVOLVED—All arterial blood vessels in the body.

SEX OR AGE MOST AFFECTED—Both sexes of adolescents and adults. Up to age 45, atherosclerosis is more common in men. After menopause, women have the same incidence.

SIGNS & SYMPTOMS—Symptoms are often absent until atherosclerosis reaches advanced stages. Symptoms depend on what part of the body has a decreased blood flow, and the extent of disease. Common symptoms include:
- Muscle cramps if atherosclerosis involves vessels in the legs.
- Angina pectoris or heart attack if it involves blood vessels to the heart.
- Stroke or transient ischemic attack if it involves vessels to the neck and brain.

CAUSES—Patches of fatty tissue that damage artery walls often collect at artery junctions. At these points, the inner lining of the artery may trap fatty substances that circulate in the blood. As fatty deposits accumulate, they reduce the blood vessel's elasticity and narrow the passageway, interfering with blood flow.

RISK INCREASES WITH
- Adults over 60.
- Stress.
- Diabetes mellitus.
- High blood pressure.
- Obesity.
- Smoking.
- Sedentary lifestyle.
- Poor nutrition, especially too much fat and cholesterol in the diet.
- Family history of atherosclerosis.

HOW TO PREVENT
- Don't smoke.
- Follow suggestions under Diet.
- Exercise regularly.
- Reduce stress to a manageable level when possible. See Appendix 13.
- If you have diabetes or high blood pressure, adhere strictly to your treatment program.

WHAT TO EXPECT

APPROPRIATE HEALTH CARE
- Self-care after diagnosis.
- Doctor's treatment.
- Psychotherapy or counseling to learn to cope with stress.

DIAGNOSTIC MEASURES
- Your own observation of symptoms.
- Medical history and physical exam by a doctor.
- Laboratory studies, including: EKG (see Glossary); exercise-tolerance test; blood studies of cholesterol and high-density lipoproteins (see Glossary); and blood-sugar tests.
- X-rays of the chest and blood vessels.

POSSIBLE COMPLICATIONS
- Heart attack.
- Stroke.
- Kidney disease.
- Loss of vision.

PROBABLE OUTCOME—This condition is currently considered incurable. However, symptoms can be controlled, and progress of the disease can be slowed with treatment. Complications are eventually fatal. Scientific research into causes and treatment continues, so there is hope for increasingly effective treatment and cure.

HOW TO TREAT

NOTE—Follow your doctor's instructions. These instructions are supplemental.

GENERAL MEASURES
- Follow instructions under How to Prevent.
- See Appendix 12 for suggestions to improve health and lengthen life.

MEDICATION—Recent studies show that lowering cholesterol levels in persons with high levels can increase life expectancy. If you have symptoms of a disorder caused by atherosclerosis—and diet and exercise fail to reduce cholesterol—your doctor may prescribe antihyperlipidemic drugs.

ACTIVITY—No restrictions.

DIET— Eat a diet that is low in fat (see Appendix 8), low in salt (see Appendix 9) and high in fiber (see Appendix 1).

CALL YOUR DOCTOR IF

You have high risk factors for athero-sclerosis and want to become involved in a prevention program.

ATHLETE'S FOOT
(Tinea Pedis; Ringworm of the Feet)

 GENERAL INFORMATION

DEFINITION—A common, contagious fungus infection of the skin on the feet.

BODY PARTS INVOLVED—Feet, especially the soles and skin between toes (usually 4th and 5th toes).

SEX OR AGE MOST AFFECTED—Both sexes and all ages, but most common in adolescents and adults.

SIGNS & SYMPTOMS
- Moist, soft, gray-white or red scales on feet, especially between toes.
- Dead skin between toes.
- Itching in inflamed areas.
- Damp, musty foot odor.
- Small blisters on the feet (sometimes).

CAUSES—Infection by a trichophyton fungus.

RISK INCREASES WITH
- Infrequent washing of the feet.
- Infrequent changes of shoes or socks.
- Use of locker rooms and public showers.
- Hot, humid weather.

HOW TO PREVENT
- Bathe feet daily. Dry thoroughly and dust with talc.
- Go barefoot when possible.
- Change shoes and socks daily.
- Wear socks made of cotton, wool or other natural, absorbent fibers. Avoid synthetics.

 WHAT TO EXPECT

APPROPRIATE HEALTH CARE
- Self-care after diagnosis.
- Doctor's treatment, if infection is severe or persistent.

DIAGNOSTIC MEASURES
- Your own observation of symptoms.
- Medical history and physical exam by a doctor.
- Laboratory culture and microscopic examination of scales.

POSSIBLE COMPLICATIONS
- Secondary bacterial infection in the affected area.
- Id reaction on hands and face (rare).

PROBABLE OUTCOME—Usually curable in 3 weeks with treatment, but recurrence is common.

 HOW TO TREAT

NOTE—Follow your doctor's instructions. These instructions are supplemental.

GENERAL MEASURES
- Remove scales and material between the toes daily.
- Keep affected areas cool and dry. Go barefoot or wear sandals during treatment.

MEDICATION
- Use non-prescription antifungal powders, creams or ointments after each bath.
- For severe cases, your doctor may prescribe an oral antifungal medication.

ACTIVITY—No restrictions.

DIET—No special diet.

 CALL YOUR DOCTOR IF

- You have severe symptoms of athlete's foot that persist, despite self-treatment.
- You develop fever or the infection seems to be spreading.

ILLNESSES & DISORDERS

ATRIAL FIBRILLATION

GENERAL INFORMATION

DEFINITION—A completely irregular heartbeat rhythm. Fibrillation means a quivering of heart-muscle fibers.

BODY PARTS INVOLVED—Heart muscles; the atrium (also called auricle), a chamber of the heart that connects to the left ventricle (main chamber); heart's electrical conduction system.

SEX OR AGE MOST AFFECTED—Adults of both sexes.

SIGNS & SYMPTOMS
- No symptoms (sometimes).
- Continuously irregular heartbeat, in which no 2 beats are of equal strength or duration.
- Weakness, dizziness or faintness (sometimes).

CAUSES
- Rheumatic heart disease caused by rheumatic fever.
- Atherosclerosis of coronary arteries, with or without a previous heart attack.
- Hyperthyroidism.
- Congestive heart failure.

RISK INCREASES WITH
- Stress.
- Heart murmur.
- Recent heart surgery.
- Electrolyte disturbances, especially low potassium.
- Pulmonary embolism.
- Excessive use of some drugs, such as thyroid hormones, caffeine or marijuana.
- Smoking.
- Excess alcohol consumption.
- Obesity.

HOW TO PREVENT—Avoid risk factors for atherosclerosis and coronary-artery disease (both in Illness section).

WHAT TO EXPECT

APPROPRIATE HEALTH CARE
- Self-care after diagnosis.
- Doctor's treatment.
- Hospitalization (sometimes).
- Electric shock (electrocardioversion), which may restore normal rhythm.

DIAGNOSTIC MEASURES
- Your own observation of symptoms.
- Medical history and physical exam by a doctor.
- EKG (see Glossary).
- Blood studies to measure levels of drugs used in treatment.

POSSIBLE COMPLICATIONS
- Acute pulmonary edema.
- Arterial thrombosis or embolus.
- Congestive heart failure.
- Other heartbeat irregularities, triggering cardiac arrest.

PROBABLE OUTCOME—A normal heartbeat rhythm can be restored with electrocardioversion in about 50% of patients. In the other 50%, some symptoms can be controlled with medication. Those whose rhythm is restored to normal have a longer life expectancy, greater strength and more energy than those who have continuing atrial fibrillation.

HOW TO TREAT

NOTE—Follow your doctor's instructions. These instructions are supplemental.

GENERAL MEASURES
- Have family members and friends learn cardiopulmonary resuscitation (CPR) in case you have cardiac arrest.
- Don't smoke, use mind-altering drugs or drink more than 1 or 2 alcoholic drinks—if any—a day.
- Learn to check your own pulse for rate (beats per minute), rhythm (regular or irregular) and strength. Call your doctor if these change.
- See Appendix 13 for suggestions to minimize stress.

MEDICATION—Your doctor may prescribe:
- Heart medications, such as digitalis, quinidine, calcium-channel blockers or beta-adrenergic blockers to regulate the heartbeat.
- Anticoagulants to prevent blood clot.

ACTIVITY—Resume your normal activities as soon as symptoms improve. Consult your doctor before resuming sexual relations.

DIET
- Lose weight if you are obese, but don't use appetite suppressants. These may worsen rhythm disturbances. A reducing diet appears in Appendix 10.
- The underlying heart condition may require a low-salt or low-fat diet (see Appendices 8 and 9) and potassium supplements.

CALL YOUR DOCTOR IF

- You have symptoms of atrial fibrillation.
- The following occurs during treatment:
  Change in heart rate, rhythm or strength.
  Chest pain, sweating and weakness.
  Shortness of breath and swollen feet and ankles.
  Pain in the calf of the leg while walking.
- New, unexplained symptoms develop. Drugs in treatment may produce side effects.

BALANITIS

GENERAL INFORMATION

DEFINITION—Inflammation of the penis of an uncircumcised male.

BODY PARTS INVOLVED—Penis and foreskin.

SEX OR AGE MOST AFFECTED—Males of all ages.

SIGNS & SYMPTOMS
- Pain, redness and swelling of the head of the penis.
- Inflammation of the foreskin.
- Chills and fever.
- Ulceration of the penis.
- Discharge from the penis.
- Burning on urination.
- Enlarged lymph glands in the groin.

CAUSES—Infection from bacteria under the foreskin of the penis that invade the head of the penis.

RISK INCREASES WITH
- Inadequate cleansing under the foreskin.
- Trauma or minor injury to the foreskin and penis, as from excessive masturbation or vigorous intercourse.

HOW TO PREVENT
- Have male infants circumcised.
- Wash daily with soap and water, especially after sexual intercourse. Cleanse under the foreskin.
- Stretch a tight foreskin with daily gentle retraction.
- Use a condom during intercourse.

WHAT TO EXPECT

APPROPRIATE HEALTH CARE
- Doctor's treatment.
- Surgery to circumcise the penis, if balanitis recurs frequently. See Circumcision (in Surgery section).

DIAGNOSTIC MEASURES
- Your own observation of symptoms.
- Medical history and physical exam by a doctor.
- Laboratory culture of the discharge from the infected area.

POSSIBLE COMPLICATIONS
- Ulceration of the penis.
- Spread of infection to deeper skin layers of the penis shaft.
- Blood poisoning.

PROBABLE OUTCOME—Usually curable in 1 to 2 weeks with medical treatment.

HOW TO TREAT

NOTE—Follow your doctor's instructions. These instructions are supplemental.

GENERAL MEASURES—Use warm-water soaks (see Appendix 18) to relieve pain.

MEDICATION—Your doctor may prescribe:
- Steroid creams to control swelling.
- Topical or oral antibiotics to fight infection.
- Aspirin or acetaminophen to relieve minor pain and fever.

ACTIVITY—Rest in bed if you have fever. You may read or watch TV. Avoid sexual intercourse during treatment. Resume your normal activities when the infection is cured.

DIET—No special diet.

CALL YOUR DOCTOR IF

- You have symptoms of balanitis.
- Symptoms don't improve in 3 days, despite treatment.
- Balanitis recurs. Consider circumcision.

ILLNESSES & DISORDERS

BALDNESS, PATTERN (MALE & FEMALE)

 GENERAL INFORMATION

DEFINITION—Gradual, painless hair loss that occurs in a distinctive pattern as a person ages. The earlier hair loss begins, the greater the eventual loss. Some persons have short periods of intense hair loss, followed by long, stable periods.

BODY PARTS INVOLVED—Hair; scalp.

SEX OR AGE MOST AFFECTED—In men, appears as early as the 20s; in women, rarely appears before the 50s.

SIGNS & SYMPTOMS
- In men, hair loss occurs on top of the head and in the temple areas of the scalp.
- In women, hair loss usually occurs only on top of the head.
- In both sexes, some diffuse loss may also occur.

CAUSES
- Genetic factors.
- Hormonal factors. Male hormones are an important factor in balding. Men castrated at a young age don't develop pattern baldness—regardless of genetic factors—unless they receive supplemental testosterone (a male hormone).
  Correspondingly, estrogen (a female hormone) may be protective in women, because hair loss rarely begins before menopause.

RISK INCREASES WITH—Family history of pattern baldness. Hair loss that occurs after illness, pregnancy or as an adverse reaction to drugs is a different form of baldness.

HOW TO PREVENT—Cannot be prevented at present.

 WHAT TO EXPECT

APPROPRIATE HEALTH CARE—Self-care.

DIAGNOSTIC MEASURES
- Your own observation of symptoms.
- Medical history and physical exam by a doctor, if diagnosis is in doubt.

POSSIBLE COMPLICATIONS—None.

PROBABLE OUTCOME—Incurable at present.

 HOW TO TREAT

NOTE—Follow your doctor's instructions. These instructions are supplemental.

GENERAL MEASURES
- Don't use medicated shampoos and ointments. They are useless.
- If you cannot accept balding as part of aging, there are 2 options:
  Consider wearing a toupeé or wig.
  Consider a hair-transplant operation. This surgery may have complications, so discuss the advantages and disadvantages with your doctor before undergoing the procedure.

MEDICATION—Medicine is not necessary for this disorder. A drug, minoxidil, has been reported to stimulate hair growth, but its safety and effectiveness are still unproven.

ACTIVITY—No restrictions.

DIET—No special diet.

 CALL YOUR DOCTOR IF

You want a medical referral for hair transplantation.

BAROTITIS MEDIA
(Barotrauma)

GENERAL INFORMATION

DEFINITION—Damage to the middle ear caused by pressure changes.

BODY PARTS INVOLVED—Middle ear; eustachian tube; nerve endings in the ear.

SEX OR AGE MOST AFFECTED—Both sexes; all ages.

SIGNS & SYMPTOMS
- Hearing loss (to varying degrees).
- A plugged feeling in the ear.
- Severe pain.
- Dizziness.
- Ringing noises in the ear.

CAUSES—Damage caused by sudden, increased pressure in the surrounding air, such as occurs in the rapid descent of an airplane or while scuba diving.

In these activities, air moves from passages in the nose into the middle ear to maintain equal pressure on both sides of the eardrum. If the tube leading from the nose to the ear (eustachian tube) doesn't function properly, pressure in the middle ear is less than outside pressure. The negative pressure in the middle ear sucks the eardrum inward. Blood and mucus may later appear in the middle ear.

This damage is more likely if you have a nose or throat infection when scuba diving or traveling by air.

RISK INCREASES WITH—Recent respiratory-tract infection.

HOW TO PREVENT
- Don't fly or scuba-dive when you have an upper-respiratory infection.
- If you must fly anyway:
  Use non-prescription decongestant tablets or sprays. Follow package instructions.
  While ascending or descending, suck on hard candy or chew gum to force frequent swallowing.
  Take a moderate-size breath, hold the nose and try to force air into the eustachian tube by gently puffing out the cheeks with the mouth closed.
  Give an infant a bottle of water or juice while ascending or descending.

WHAT TO EXPECT

APPROPRIATE HEALTH CARE
- Self-care.
- Doctor's treatment.
- Surgery to open the eardrum and release fluid trapped in the middle ear. A plastic tube may be inserted through the surgically perforated eardrum to keep it open and equalize pressure. The tube falls out spontaneously in 9 to 12 months.

DIAGNOSTIC MEASURES
- Your own observation of symptoms.
- Medical history and physical exam by a doctor.

POSSIBLE COMPLICATIONS—Without treatment, fluid may accumulate, become infected and rupture the eardrum. The rupture may affect nerve endings, causing permanent hearing loss.

PROBABLE OUTCOME—With treatment, most cases of barotitis media are reversible without permanent damage or hearing loss.

HOW TO TREAT

NOTE—Follow your doctor's instructions. These instructions are supplemental.

GENERAL MEASURES—If fluid drains from the ear, place a small piece of cotton in the outer-ear canal to absorb it.

MEDICATION
- For minor discomfort, you may use non-prescription decongestants and pain relievers, such as acetaminophen.
- Your doctor may prescribe:
  Stronger prescription decongestant nasal sprays or tablets. Use for at least 2 weeks after damage.
  Steroid nasal spray.
  Antibiotics, if infection is present.

ACTIVITY—Resume your normal activities as soon as symptoms improve.

DIET—No special diet.

CALL YOUR DOCTOR IF

- You have symptoms of barotitis media.
- The following occurs during treatment:
  Severe headache.
  Fever.
  Severe pain.
  Dizziness.
- New, unexplained symptoms develop. Drugs used in treatment may produce side effects.

ILLNESSES & DISORDERS

BED-WETTING
(Enuresis)

GENERAL INFORMATION

DEFINITION—Involuntary urination during sleep that occurs more often than once a month.

BODY PARTS INVOLVED—Urinary tract.

SEX OR AGE MOST AFFECTED—Both sexes, but more common in boys. The occurrence of bed-wetting in children is: 15% at age 5; 10% at age 6; 7% at age 8; 3% at age 12; and 1% at age 18.

SIGNS & SYMPTOMS—Bed-wetting at night. This is not significant until a child is older than 6.

CAUSES—In most cases, the cause of bed-wetting is unknown. Following are the most-common causes or popular theories:
● Underlying illness, such as diabetes or a urinary-tract infection.
● A small or weak bladder that cannot hold one night's urine production.
● Psychological problems caused by stress or separation from the mother.

RISK INCREASES WITH
● Diabetes.
● Urinary-tract infection.
● Family history of bed-wetting.

HOW TO PREVENT—Show your child love, support and understanding for this problem.

WHAT TO EXPECT

APPROPRIATE HEALTH CARE
● Self-care.
● Doctor's treatment.
● Psychotherapy or counseling.

DIAGNOSTIC MEASURES
● Your own observation of symptoms.
● Medical history and physical exam by a doctor.
● Laboratory studies of urine and blood to detect diabetes or urinary-tract infection.

POSSIBLE COMPLICATIONS—Psychological and emotional scars that may affect the child's personality for years.

PROBABLE OUTCOME—Bed-wetting may continue for several years. Your doctor will want to rule out urinary-tract infections and diabetes as causes. If these are eliminated and your child is normal in other respects, consider your child's bed-wetting a minor variation of the age at which bladder control is socially expected.

HOW TO TREAT

NOTE—Follow your doctor's instructions. These instructions are supplemental.

GENERAL MEASURES
● Prepare the bed and the child:
Protect the mattress with a heavy plastic cover.
Provide the child with extra-thick underwear and pajamas.
Discontinue diapers or plastic pants by age 4; they inhibit the child's motivation to improve.
Put an extra pair of underwear and pajama bottoms by the bed in case the child needs them during the night.
● Have the child urinate at bedtime.
● Awaken the child to urinate after he has been asleep for several hours. If the child is old enough, he may be able to set the alarm clock to awaken himself and empty his bladder during the night.
● Reward the child for staying dry. Praise him, hug him, and tell of his success to people who are important to him, such as brothers and sisters. Use gold stars or happy faces to mark dry nights on a calendar if the child likes it.
● Respond gently to accidents. Don't blame, criticize, restrict or punish the child who has wet the bed. This can cause him to give up, or lead to emotional problems.
● Follow instructions if your doctor suggests bladder-stretching or stream-interruption exercises or behavior-modification devices.

MEDICATION—Medicine usually is not necessary for this disorder, but your doctor may prescribe antidepressant drugs as a last resort.

ACTIVITY—No restrictions.

DIET—No special diet. Encourage your child to drink as much fluid as possible during the day. Decrease fluid intake during the 2 hours before bedtime.

CALL YOUR DOCTOR IF

● You are concerned about your child's bed-wetting, and your child is older than 6.
● The child dribbles urine, has a weak urinary stream, has pain when urinating or must strain to urinate.
● Medication is prescribed for the child, and new, unexplained symptoms develop. Drugs used in treatment may produce side effects.

BELL'S PALSY

GENERAL INFORMATION

DEFINITION—Paralysis on one side of the face. This is named after the physician who first described it.

BODY PARTS INVOLVED—7th cranial nerve and facial muscles supplied by that nerve.

SEX OR AGE MOST AFFECTED—All ages, but most common in adults.

SIGNS & SYMPTOMS
- Sudden paralysis on one side of the face, including muscles to the eyelid.
- Pain behind the ear on the affected side.
- Flat, expressionless features on one side of the face.
- Distorted smiles and frowns.
- Changes in taste, salivation or tear formation (sometimes).

CAUSES—Unknown. The paralysis is probably caused by swelling of the facial nerve. The swelling may be caused by a virus; an autoimmune disease; or a decrease in blood flow and pressure on the facial nerve as it passes through the temporal bone of the skull.

RISK INCREASES WITH—Unknown.

HOW TO PREVENT—Cannot be prevented at present.

WHAT TO EXPECT

APPROPRIATE HEALTH CARE
- Self-care after diagnosis.
- Doctor's treatment.
- Surgery (rare).

DIAGNOSTIC MEASURES
- Your own observation of symptoms.
- Medical history and physical exam by a doctor.
- CAT scan (see Glossary) to rule out other causes of pressure on the facial nerve.

POSSIBLE COMPLICATIONS—Eye irritation or injury because the eye does not close properly and is exposed to dust. If unprotected, the eye may develop ulcers on the cornea.

PROBABLE OUTCOME—Bell's palsy is distressing, but it is not dangerous.

The extent of nerve damage determines the extent of recovery. Improvement is gradual and recovery time varies, sometimes requiring many months.

Patients with mild facial paralysis usually recover completely within several months. Patients with severe facial paralysis recover completely in 80% to 90% of cases.

Surgery can sometimes improve facial appearance and muscle function in patients who do not recover fully.

HOW TO TREAT

NOTE—Follow your doctor's instructions. These instructions are supplemental.

GENERAL MEASURES
- If you have pain, apply heat to the painful area twice a day. Use an electric heating pad or wring out a towel soaked in hot water and apply for 15 minutes. Cover or close the eye during heat treatments.
- If you cannot wink or close your eye well, buy a pair of wrap-around, plastic bubble goggles. Wear them to protect your eye from dirt, dust and dryness. You may buy goggles from a sporting goods store or optician.
- At night, apply an eye patch to shut the lid so the eye stays moist and protected.
- As muscle strength returns, use facial massage and exercises. Massage muscles of the forehead, cheek, lips and eyes using cream or oil. Exercise the weak muscles in front of a mirror. Open and close the eye, wink, smile and bare your teeth. Perform the massage and exercise for 15 or 20 minutes several times a day.
- Brush and floss teeth more often to keep the mouth healthy.

MEDICATION—Your doctor may prescribe:
- Methylcellulose eye drops for comfort and protection of the exposed eye.
- Cortisone drugs for 2 weeks to reduce swelling and inflammation of the affected nerve.

ACTIVITY—Maintain your normal activities. Rest does not help Bell's palsy.

DIET—A soft diet (see Appendix 11) is often necessary.

CALL YOUR DOCTOR IF

- You have symptoms of Bell's palsy.
- Your eye becomes red or irritated, despite treatment.
- You cannot prevent saliva from drooling from your mouth.
- Pain worsens.
- Temperature rises to 101F (38.3C) or higher.

ILLNESSES & DISORDERS

BLADDER INFECTION
(Cystitis)

GENERAL INFORMATION

DEFINITION—Inflammation or infection of the urinary bladder.

BODY PARTS INVOLVED—Bladder; urethra.

SEX OR AGE MOST AFFECTED—All ages and both sexes, but more common in females.

SIGNS & SYMPTOMS
- Burning and stinging on urination.
- Frequent urination, especially at night, although the urine amount may be small.
- Increased urge to urinate.
- Pain in the abdomen over the bladder.
- Low back pain.
- Blood in the urine.
- Low fever.
- Bad-smelling urine.
- Painful sexual intercourse.
- Lack of urinary control (sometimes).

CAUSES
- Bacteria that reach the bladder from another part of the body through the bloodstream.
- Bacteria that enter the urinary tract from skin around the genitals and anal area.
- Injury to the urethra.
- Use of a urinary catheter to empty the bladder, such as following childbirth or surgery.

RISK INCREASES WITH
- Increased sexual activity. In women, the cause is often aggravated by bruising of the urethra during intercourse.
- Infection in other parts of the genitourinary system.
- Stress.
- Illness that has lowered resistance.
- Excess alcohol consumption.
- Obstruction of urine in the urinary tract in men—usually partial obstruction caused by an enlarged or inflamed prostate gland.

HOW TO PREVENT
- Drink a glass of water before sexual intercourse, and urinate within 15 minutes after intercourse.
- Use a water-soluble lubricant, such as K-Y Lubricating Jelly, during intercourse.
- Use female-superior or lateral positions in sexual intercourse to protect the female urethra from injury.
- Take showers instead of tub baths.
- Request frequent urinalyses to monitor signs of infection.
- Drink 8 glasses of water every day. Avoid caffeine, which irritates the bladder.
- Avoid the use of catheters, if possible.
- Obtain prompt medical treatment for urinary-tract infections.
- Women should not douche.

- Females should clean the anal area thoroughly after bowel movements. Wipe from the front to the rear—rather than rear to front—to avoid spreading fecal bacteria to the genital area.

WHAT TO EXPECT

APPROPRIATE HEALTH CARE—Doctor's treatment.

DIAGNOSTIC MEASURES
- Your own observation of symptoms.
- Medical history and physical exam by a doctor.
- Urinalysis and careful urine collection for bacterial culture.
- Cystoscopy (see Glossary).

POSSIBLE COMPLICATIONS—Inadequate treatment can cause chronic urinary-tract infections, leading to kidney failure.

PROBABLE OUTCOME—Curable in 2 weeks with prompt medical treatment. Recurrence is common.

HOW TO TREAT

NOTE—Follow your doctor's instructions. These instructions are supplemental.

GENERAL MEASURES—Apply heat to the bladder area with a heat lamp or heating pad.

MEDICATION—Your doctor may prescribe:
- Antibiotics to fight infection.
- Antispasmodics to relieve pain.

ACTIVITY—Avoid sexual intercourse until you have been free of symptoms for 2 weeks to allow inflammation to subside.

DIET
- Drink 6 to 8 glasses of water daily.
- Avoid caffeine and alcohol during treatment.
- Drink cranberry juice to acidify urine. Some drugs are more effective with acid urine.

CALL YOUR DOCTOR IF

- You have symptoms of cystitis.
- Your fever rises to 101F (38.3C) or higher during treatment.
- Blood appears in the urine.
- Discomfort and other symptoms don't improve in 1 week.
- New, unexplained symptoms develop. Drugs used in treatment may produce side effects.
- Symptoms recur after treatment.

BLADDER OR URETHRA INJURY

GENERAL INFORMATION

DEFINITION—Damage to the urinary bladder (the organ that stores urine from the kidneys) or the urethra (the tube through which urine travels from the bladder to the outside).

BODY PARTS INVOLVED—Bladder; urethra.

SEX OR AGE MOST AFFECTED—Both sexes; all ages.

SIGNS & SYMPTOMS
- Severe abdominal pain.
- Shock (sweating; faintness; nausea; panting; rapid pulse; pale, cold, moist skin).
- Painful urination or inability to urinate.
- Bloody discharge from the urethra.

CAUSES—Usually a pelvic-bone fracture that punctures the bladder or urethra.

RISK INCREASES WITH
- Excess alcohol consumption.
- Accident-proneness.
- Hazardous occupations.
- Hazardous driving conditions.
- Sexually abused children.

HOW TO PREVENT—Protect yourself from injury whenever possible. Buckle your automobile seat belt and shoulder harness to minimize internal injury in case of accident. Don't drink and drive.

WHAT TO EXPECT

APPROPRIATE HEALTH CARE
- Doctor's treatment.
- Hospitalization; emergency care.
- Surgery to repair a punctured bladder (usually). A damaged urethra may heal without surgery.

DIAGNOSTIC MEASURES
- Your own observation of symptoms.
- Medical history and physical exam by a doctor.
- Laboratory urine studies.
- X-rays of the urinary tract.

POSSIBLE COMPLICATIONS
- Internal bleeding.
- Urine leakage into the abdomen, causing abdominal inflammation or infection.
- Recurrent infections from scars in the urethra that narrow the urinary passage.

PROBABLE OUTCOME—A punctured bladder or urethra requires emergency hospital treatment. Most cases heal with bed rest, time, supportive treatment or surgery.

HOW TO TREAT

NOTE—Follow your doctor's instructions. These instructions are supplemental.

GENERAL MEASURES—No specific instructions except those under other headings.

MEDICATION—Your doctor may prescribe antibiotics to prevent infection.

ACTIVITY—Stay as active as your strength allows. Allow 1 month for recovery. Don't return to work or resume sexual relations until healing is complete.

DIET
- No special diet.
- Drink 6 to 8 glasses of fluid daily.
- Don't drink alcohol.

CALL YOUR DOCTOR IF

- You have any symptoms of bladder or urethra injury.
- During or after treatment, you develop fever of 101F (38.3C) or higher or chills.
- New, unexplained symptoms develop. Drugs used in treatment may produce side effects.

ILLNESSES & DISORDERS

BLADDER STONES
(Calculi)

 GENERAL INFORMATION

DEFINITION—Small, solid particles that form within the bladder and are too large to pass in the urine through the urethra to the outside.

BODY PARTS INVOLVED—Bladder; urethra.

SEX OR AGE MOST AFFECTED—Adults of both sexes.

SIGNS & SYMPTOMS
- Blood in the urine.
- Painful urination.
- Frequent urge to urinate, even though only small amounts of urine pass.

CAUSES
- Reduced urine volume from dehydration.
- Increased excretion by the kidney of calcium, oxalate, urate, cystine, phosphate or xanthine.
- Reduction of normal protective substances that suppress stone formation (hereditary).

RISK INCREASES WITH
- Chronic bladder infection.
- Nerve injury that impairs bladder function.
- Long-term use of urinary catheters.

HOW TO PREVENT
- Follow suggestions under Diet.
- Avoid activities that cause excessive sweating.

 WHAT TO EXPECT

APPROPRIATE HEALTH CARE
- Self-care after diagnosis.
- Doctor's treatment.
- Surgery to remove stone(s) (rare).

DIAGNOSTIC MEASURES
- Your own observation of symptoms.
- Medical history and physical exam by a doctor.
- Laboratory studies, such as: blood chemistries; urinalysis; analysis of the composition of any stone that is passed.

POSSIBLE COMPLICATIONS
- Infection.
- Urinary blockage.

PROBABLE OUTCOME—Many bladder stones pass unassisted in the urine. Those that are too large to pass must be removed surgically.

 HOW TO TREAT

NOTE—Follow your doctor's instructions. These instructions are supplemental.

GENERAL MEASURES—If you are waiting for the stone to pass, watch for it when you urinate. To trap it, urinate each time through a piece of gauze. The stone may pass without discomfort. When it passes, take it to your doctor's office for analysis.

MEDICATION—Your doctor may prescribe:
- Narcotic pain relievers during the attack.
- Antibiotics, if infection is present.
- Drugs to alkalize or acidify the urine after the attack, depending on the kind of stone.

ACTIVITY
- If you know you have bladder stones, avoid situations in which a sudden, sharp pain might cause danger, such as climbing ladders.
- During a bladder-stone episode, stay as active as your strength allows. Don't go to bed. Activity may help the stone pass more easily.

DIET
- If the stone proves to be calcium or phosphorus, avoid milk and products made with milk, chocolate or nuts.
- If the stone is a phosphate, your doctor will prescribe an acid-ash diet to keep urine slightly acid.
- If the stone is a urate or cystine stone, your doctor will prescribe an alkaline-ash diet to keep the urine slightly alkaline.
- For all types of stones, drink at least 13 glasses of fluid daily. Most of your fluid should be purified water; a small amount can be weak tea or other beverages.

 CALL YOUR DOCTOR IF

- You have symptoms of a bladder stone.
- Your temperature rises to 101F (38.3C) or higher, or you develop other symptoms of a bladder infection: stinging, burning on urination, or frequent urge to urinate.
- You develop new, unexplained symptoms during treatment. Drugs used in treatment may produce side effects.

BLADDER TUMOR

GENERAL INFORMATION

DEFINITION—Abnormal tissue growth in the bladder in which cell multiplication is uncontrolled. The tumor may be benign or malignant.

BODY PARTS INVOLVED—Urinary bladder (even malignant bladder tumors rarely spread to other body parts).

SEX OR AGE MOST AFFECTED—Adults of both sexes, but twice as common in men as women.

SIGNS & SYMPTOMS
- Blood in the urine.
- Burning on urination.
- Increased frequency of urination, but passage of only small amounts of urine.
- Pain in the pelvic area.
- Unexplained weight loss.

CAUSES—Unknown.

RISK INCREASES WITH
- Smoking.
- Family history of bladder tumors.
- Exposure to naphthylamines (dyes containing aniline) or chemicals used in the manufacture of rubber.
- Use of the drug tryptophan.

HOW TO PREVENT
- Avoid exposure to chemical or environmental hazards.
- Don't smoke.

WHAT TO EXPECT

APPROPRIATE HEALTH CARE
- Doctor's treatment.
- Surgery to remove the tumor or bladder. If the tumor is malignant, anticancer drugs may be instilled in the bladder during surgery. The operation also may include a procedure to divert the urinary stream.
- Radiation treatment.

DIAGNOSTIC MEASURES
- Your own observation of symptoms.
- Medical history and physical exam by a doctor.
- Urinalysis.
- Cystoscopy (see Glossary).
- X-rays of the bladder and urinary tract.

POSSIBLE COMPLICATIONS
- Infection in the bladder or kidneys. Symptoms include back pain, fever and vomiting.
- Urinary obstruction.

PROBABLE OUTCOME—This condition is currently considered incurable and is usually fatal within 5 years. Surgery and treatment with anticancer drugs can prolong and improve the quality of life. Pain and other symptoms can be relieved or controlled.

Medical literature cites a few instances of unexplained recovery. Scientific research into causes and treatment continues, so there is hope for increasingly effective treatment and cure.

HOW TO TREAT

NOTE—Follow your doctor's instructions. These instructions are supplemental.

GENERAL MEASURES—No specific instructions except those under other headings.

MEDICATION—Your doctor may prescribe:
- Pain relievers.
- Oral anticancer drugs.

ACTIVITY—After surgery or other treatment, resume your normal activities (including sex) as soon as possible.

DIET—No special diet.

CALL YOUR DOCTOR IF

- You have symptoms of a bladder tumor.
- New, unexplained symptoms develop. Drugs used in treatment may produce side effects.

ILLNESSES & DISORDERS

BLASTOMYCOSIS
(North American Blastomycosis; Gilchrist's Disease)

 GENERAL INFORMATION

DEFINITION—An infectious, fungus disease that starts in the lungs. Occasionally it spreads through the bloodstream to other body parts—especially the skin. Blastomycosis is not contagious from person to person.

BODY PARTS INVOLVED—Lungs; mouth; skin and tissue below the skin; prostate; epididymis.

SEX OR AGE MOST AFFECTED—Both sexes, but most common in men from ages 20 to 40.

SIGNS & SYMPTOMS—The following symptoms begin slowly:
- Cough, either dry and non-productive or with sputum.
- Chest pain.
- Chills, fever and drenching sweats.
- Shortness of breath.

CAUSES—Infection with the fungus, blastomyces dermatitidis. Skin lesions occur most commonly in gardeners or farmers, but the natural source of this fungus is unknown.

RISK INCREASES WITH
- Gardening and farming, especially in Southeastern states and the Mississippi River valley of the U.S.
- Diabetes mellitus.
- Use of immunosuppressive drugs.

HOW TO PREVENT—Cannot be prevented at present.

 WHAT TO EXPECT

APPROPRIATE HEALTH CARE
- Doctor's treatment.
- Hospitalization for intensive care, if the lung infection spreads to other body parts.
- Self-care after treatment.

DIAGNOSTIC MEASURES
- Your own observation of symptoms.
- Medical history and physical exam by a doctor.
- Laboratory cultures of pus, sputum or blood to identify the fungus.

POSSIBLE COMPLICATIONS—Spread to other body parts, with serious illness and death. If the infection spreads, the following may appear:
- Pain in long bones.
- Skin lesions that begin as small papules (small, raised bumps on the skin) or pustules (small white blisters with pus) on exposed skin surfaces. They spread slowly. When fully developed, the lesions become crusted ulcers with sloping, reddish-purple borders.
- Swelling and painful, tender nodules in the scrotum.

PROBABLE OUTCOME—This fungus can cause severe, debilitating illness that may be fatal without treatment. With intensive treatment, it is usually curable in several weeks.

 HOW TO TREAT

NOTE—Follow your doctor's instructions. These instructions are supplemental.

GENERAL MEASURES—Weigh daily and keep a weight chart. An unexplained weight loss might indicate the infection has spread.

MEDICATION—For severe cases, your doctor may prescribe potent antifungal drugs, such as ketoconazole, amphotericin B and hydroxystilbamidine isethionate.

ACTIVITY—Rest in bed during the acute stage. Resume activities gradually as your strength returns.

DIET—No special diet.

 CALL YOUR DOCTOR IF

- You have symptoms of blastomycosis.
- Any of the following occurs during treatment:
  Weight loss.
  Fever of 101F (38.3C) orally.
  Diarrhea that cannot be controlled with home remedies.
  Severe headache and stiff neck.
- New, unexplained symptoms develop. Drugs used in treatment may produce side effects.

BLEPHARITIS

GENERAL INFORMATION

DEFINITION—Inflammation of the eyelid edges.

BODY PARTS INVOLVED—Eyelids; eyelashes; meibomian glands (those which lubricate the lid); conjunctiva (white of the eye).

SEX OR AGE MOST AFFECTED—Adults of both sexes.

SIGNS & SYMPTOMS
- Redness and greasy scales on the eyelid edges.
- Eyelashes that fall out.
- Small ulcers on the eyelid. If the lid edges ulcerate, crusts will form. If crusts are removed, lids will bleed.
- Irritation of the eye if flakes from the lid fall into the eye.
- A feeling that something is in the eye. This includes itching, burning, redness, swelling of the lid, sensitivity to bright light and tearing.
- Discharge from the lids, which glues lashes together during sleep.

CAUSES
- Bacterial infection, usually staphylococcal, of the eyelash follicles and the meibomian glands.
- Allergic reaction (less serious inflammation only).
- Body lice (rare).

RISK INCREASES WITH
- Adults over 60.
- Medical history of seborrheic dermatitis of the scalp and other body parts.
- Exposure to chemical or environmental irritants.
- Crowded or unsanitary living conditions.
- Poor nutrition.

HOW TO PREVENT
- Wash hands often, and dry with clean towels.
- Avoid environments that contain dust or other irritating substances.
- Use hypoallergenic eye makeup.

WHAT TO EXPECT

APPROPRIATE HEALTH CARE
- Self-care after diagnosis.
- Doctor's treatment. If blepharitis is caused by lice, your doctor will remove them with tweezers or medication.

DIAGNOSTIC MEASURES
- Your own observation of symptoms.
- Medical history and physical exam by a doctor.
- Laboratory culture of the discharge from lids.

POSSIBLE COMPLICATIONS
- Loss of eyelashes.
- Ulceration of the cornea (covering of the eye).
- Scarred eyelids.

PROBABLE OUTCOME—Blepharitis is stubbornly resistant to treatment, but it is sometimes curable in 8 to 12 months. Recurrence is common.

HOW TO TREAT

NOTE—Follow your doctor's instructions. These instructions are supplemental.

GENERAL MEASURES
- Use warm-water soaks (see Appendix 18) to reduce inflammation and hasten healing. Apply soaks for 20 minutes, then rest at least 1 hour. Repeat as often as needed.
- Remove scales from the lids each day.
- Don't wear eye makeup until inflammation subsides.

MEDICATION—Your doctor may prescribe antibiotic ointment or eyedrops, which may contain cortisone drugs.

ACTIVITY—No restrictions.

DIET—No special diet.

CALL YOUR DOCTOR IF

- You have symptoms of blepharitis.
- You have pain in the *eye*.
- Your vision changes.
- New, unexplained symptoms develop.
Drugs used in treatment may produce side effects.

ILLNESSES & DISORDERS

BLOOD POISONING
(Septicemia)

 GENERAL INFORMATION

DEFINITION—Bacterial infection (or toxins from bacteria) in the blood.

BODY PARTS INVOLVED—Total body.

SEX OR AGE MOST AFFECTED—Both sexes; all ages.

SIGNS & SYMPTOMS
- Shaking chills.
- Rapid temperature rise.
- Rapid, pounding heartbeat.
- Warm, flushed skin.
- Confusion and other symptoms of mental impairment.
- Drop in blood pressure.
- General ill feeling.

CAUSES—Infection in some other body part, such as: appendix, tooth, sinus, pelvis, gallbladder or urinary tract. The sources may also be a burn, infected wound or open abscess.

RISK INCREASES WITH
- Adults over 60.
- Newborns and infants.
- Illness, such as diabetes, that has lowered resistance.
- Leukemia or other cancer.
- Use of immunosuppressive drugs or self-administered, intravenous drugs.

HOW TO PREVENT
- Obtain medical treatment for any infection.
- If dental procedures have produced blood poisoning in the past or you have diseased heart valves, take antibiotics before any dental treatment—including simple prophylaxis by a dentist or hygienist.

 WHAT TO EXPECT

APPROPRIATE HEALTH CARE
- Doctor's treatment.
- Hospitalization.

DIAGNOSTIC MEASURES
- Your own observation of symptoms.
- Medical history and physical exam by a doctor.
- Laboratory studies, such as: culture of the blood to identify germs responsible for the illness; urinalysis; blood count.

POSSIBLE COMPLICATIONS
- Shock, with very low blood pressure, overwhelming infection and death.
- Persistent infection of the heart valves.

PROBABLE OUTCOME—Usually curable in 1 week with intravenous antibiotics.

 HOW TO TREAT

NOTE—Follow your doctor's instructions. These instructions are supplemental.

GENERAL MEASURES—Reduce fever if it goes over 104F (40C). See Appendix 19, How to Reduce Fever. Don't reduce lower temperatures; a slight fever helps mobilize the body's defenses against infection.

MEDICATION
- Your doctor may prescribe antibiotics to fight infection.
- You may use non-prescription drugs, such as acetaminophen, to reduce fever over 104F (40C).

ACTIVITY—Resume your normal activities gradually as symptoms improve.

DIET—No special diet.

 CALL YOUR DOCTOR IF

- You have symptoms of blood poisoning.
- The following occurs during treatment: Fever higher than 103F (39.4C). Signs of infection (swelling, pain, redness) anywhere in your body.
- You plan elective surgery or a dental procedure after you have had an episode of blood poisoning.
- New, unexplained symptoms develop. Drugs used in treatment may produce side effects.

BLOOD-TRANSFUSION REACTION

GENERAL INFORMATION

DEFINITION—Symptoms triggered by a blood transfusion.

BODY PARTS INVOLVED—Blood; blood vessels; kidneys; heart; skin; central nervous system; lungs.

SEX OR AGE MOST AFFECTED—Both sexes. All ages.

SIGNS & SYMPTOMS—Less serious:
- Chills and fever.
- Backache or other aches and pains.
- Hives and itching.

More serious:
- Blood-cell destruction (hemolysis), causing shortness of breath, severe headache, chest or back pain and blood in the urine.

CAUSES—Transfusions of a different blood type than that of the patient. This may be occur from errors in matching or from the use of incompletely matched blood in an emergency.

RISK INCREASES WITH
- Blood transfusions in emergency situations, when careful typing and matching of blood must be bypassed.
- Blood transfusions from donors who carry infections.

HOW TO PREVENT
- Blood-bank and hospital personnel have safety procedures to prevent reactions except in situations that are uncontrollable (see Causes).
- Use of diphenhydramine (an antihistamine) and acetaminophen prior to transfusion may prevent minor reactions.
- If surgery is planned at least 1 month in advance, your own blood may be drawn and stored for use during surgery, if necessary. Transfusion with your own blood is least likely to produce a reaction.

WHAT TO EXPECT

APPROPRIATE HEALTH CARE
- Doctor's treatment.
- Hospitalization. Patients receiving transfusions are usually in a hospital or outpatient surgical facility, and reactions can be treated when they occur.

DIAGNOSTIC MEASURES
- Your own observation of symptoms.
- Medical history and physical exam by a doctor.
- Laboratory blood tests to recheck compatibility and detect complications.

POSSIBLE COMPLICATIONS
- Acute kidney failure.
- Anaphylaxis.
- Congestive heart failure from too rapid transfusion.
- Hypothermia from blood that is too cold.

PROBABLE OUTCOME—Most reactions clear gradually after the transfusion is halted. A few reactions are fatal.

HOW TO TREAT

NOTE—Follow your doctor's instructions. These instructions are supplemental.

GENERAL MEASURES—Stay awake and alert during a blood transfusion, if possible, so you can notify medical personnel immediately if symptoms occur.

MEDICATION—Your doctor may prescribe:
- Antihistamines to decrease hives and itching.
- Cortisone drugs to decrease the likelihood of acute kidney failure.
- Antihypertensives, if blood pressure rises too high, or hypertensives, such as ephedrine or epinephrine, if blood pressure drops too low.

ACTIVITY—Resume your normal activities as soon as symptoms improve after transfusion.

DIET—No special diet.

CALL YOUR DOCTOR IF

You have symptoms of a blood-transfusion reaction during or after a transfusion. Call immediately. This is an emergency!

ILLNESSES & DISORDERS

BOILS
(Furuncles)

 GENERAL INFORMATION

DEFINITION—A painful, deep, bacterial infection of a hair follicle. Boils are common and contagious.

BODY PARTS INVOLVED—Skin; hair follicles.

SEX OR AGE MOST AFFECTED—Both sexes; all ages.

SIGNS & SYMPTOMS
- A domed nodule that is painful, tender and red and has pus on the surface. Boils appear suddenly and ripen in 24 hours. They are usually 1-1/2cm to 3cm in diameter; some are larger.
- Fever.
- Swelling of the closest lymph glands.

CAUSES—Infection, usually from staphylococcus bacteria, that begins in the hair follicle and bores into the skin's deeper layers.

RISK INCREASES WITH
- Poor nutrition.
- Illness that has lowered resistance.
- Diabetes mellitus.
- Use of immunosuppressive drugs.

HOW TO PREVENT—Keep the skin clean.

 WHAT TO EXPECT

APPROPRIATE HEALTH CARE
- Self-care.
- Doctor's treatment, which may include incision and drainage of the boil.

DIAGNOSTIC MEASURES
- Your own observation of symptoms.
- Medical history and physical exam by a doctor.
- Laboratory culture of the pus to identify the germ.

POSSIBLE COMPLICATIONS—The infection may enter the bloodstream and spread to other body parts.

PROBABLE OUTCOME—Without treatment, a boil will heal in 10 to 20 days. With treatment, the boil should heal in less time, symptoms will be less severe, and new boils should not appear. The pus that drains when a boil opens spontaneously may contaminate nearby skin, causing new boils.

 HOW TO TREAT

NOTE—Follow your doctor's instructions. These instructions are supplemental.

GENERAL MEASURES
- Relieve pain with gentle heat from warm-water soaks (see Glossary), a heating pad, hot-water bottle or lamp close to the skin. Use 3 or 4 times daily for 20 minutes.
- Prevent the spread of boils by using clean towels only once or using paper towels and discarding them.

MEDICATION
- Your doctor may prescribe a penicillin drug, such as oxacillin, dicloxacillin or nafcillin, or erythromycin antibiotics to fight infection.
- Don't use non-prescription antibiotic creams or ointments on the boil's surface. They are ineffective.

ACTIVITY—Decrease activity until the boil heals. Avoid sweating.

DIET—No special diet.

 CALL YOUR DOCTOR IF

- You have a boil.
- The following occurs during treatment: Symptoms don't improve in 3 to 4 days, despite treatment.
  New boils appear.
  Fever rises above 100F (37.8C).
  Other family members develop boils.
- New, unexplained symptoms develop. Drugs used in treatment may produce side effects.

BONE FRACTURE

GENERAL INFORMATION

DEFINITION—Complete or incomplete break in a bone. Following are the different types of fractures:

- Complete fracture. The broken bone is completely separated.
- Incomplete (greenstick) fracture. The broken bone is not completely separated.
- Comminuted fracture. There are more than 2 bone fragments at the fracture site.
- Open fracture (compound). The fractured bone has broken the skin.
- Closed fracture (including stress fracture). The fractured bone has not broken the skin.
- Compression fracture. The break occurs from extreme pressure on the bone.
- Impacted fracture. The broken ends have been driven into each other.
- Avulsion fracture. Force has been applied to a strong tendon, causing it to pull on and break off a portion of bone.
- Pathologic fracture. A break that occurs from minor injury in bone weakened or destroyed by disease.

BODY PARTS INVOLVED—Bones.

SEX OR AGE MOST AFFECTED—Both sexes; all ages.

SIGNS & SYMPTOMS
- Pain and swelling at the fracture site.
- Tenderness close to the fracture.
- Paleness and deformity (sometimes).
- Loss of pulse below the fracture, usually in an extremity (sometimes).
- Numbness, tingling or paralysis below the fracture.
- Bleeding or bruising at the site.
- Weakness and inability to bear weight.

CAUSES—Injury.

RISK INCREASES WITH
- Osteoporosis.
- Tumors of the bone or bone marrow.
- Activities that carry the risk of injury.
- Reckless behavior that increases the chance of auto accident.

HOW TO PREVENT
- Don't drink alcohol or use mind-altering drugs and drive.
- Wear protective gear for sports.
- Use your auto seat belt or harness.
- If you have osteoporosis, adhere to your treatment program, and avoid situations in which injury is likely.

WHAT TO EXPECT

APPROPRIATE HEALTH CARE
- Doctor's treatment. Almost all fractures require immobilization with casts or splints.

- Hospitalization for anesthesia and treatment of severe fractures.
- Surgery, if the fracture must be repaired with rods, plates or screws.
- Physical therapy for rehabilitation.

DIAGNOSTIC MEASURES
- Your own observation of symptoms.
- Medical history and physical exam by a doctor.
- Laboratory studies to determine blood loss.
- X-rays of injured parts.

POSSIBLE COMPLICATIONS
- Failure to heal (non-union).
- Shock from blood loss.
- Travel of a fat embolus (clump of fat cells) from the injury site to the lungs or brain.
- Obstruction of nearby arteries.

PROBABLE OUTCOME—Usually curable with skillful first aid and aftercare. The broken bone should be manipulated, realigned and immobilized as soon as possible. Realignment is much more difficult after 6 hours.

Healing time varies. Recovery is complete when there is no bone motion at the fracture site, and X-rays show complete healing.

HOW TO TREAT

NOTE—Follow your doctor's instructions. These instructions are supplemental.

GENERAL MEASURES
- See emergency first-aid instructions on page 895.
- See Care of Casts, Appendix 17.

MEDICATION—Your doctor may prescribe:
- Pain relievers.
- Muscle relaxants.

ACTIVITY—Resume your normal activities as soon as symptoms improve.

DIET—No special diet. Take vitamin-C supplements to promote bone healing.

CALL YOUR DOCTOR IF

- You have symptoms of a bone fracture.
- The following occurs after immobilization or surgery:
  Swelling above or below the fracture site.
  Severe, persistent pain.
  Blue or gray skin below the fracture site, especially under nails.
  Numbness or loss of feeling below the fracture site.
Report any of the above signs immediately!

BOTULISM

GENERAL INFORMATION

DEFINITION—A serious, non-contagious form of food poisoning caused by eating contaminated food containing a toxin that severely affects the nervous system.

BODY PARTS INVOLVED—Central nervous system; muscular system.

SEX OR AGE MOST AFFECTED—All ages, but most common in adults.

SIGNS & SYMPTOMS—The following symptoms usually appear suddenly 18 to 36 hours after eating contaminated food:
- Blurred or double vision.
- Drooping eyelids.
- Dry mouth.
- Slurred speech.
- Swallowing difficulty.
- Vomiting and diarrhea.
- Weakness of the arms and legs, leading to paralysis.
- No fever.
- No disturbance of mental abilities.

The following symptoms appear in infants:
- Severe constipation.
- Feeble cry.
- Inability to suck.

CAUSES—Infection with bacteria, clostridium botulinum, found in contaminated or incompletely cooked, canned foods. This germ generates a powerful poison (toxin) that is absorbed from the digestive tract and spreads to the central nervous system.

Foods likely to cause botulism include home-canned vegetables and fruits and undercooked sausage, smoked meats and fish. In infants under 1 year, raw honey or other uncooked foods may cause botulism.

The bacteria also may contaminate a wound and produce the toxin.

RISK INCREASES WITH
- Infants.
- Home-canned foods. Green beans are especially susceptible to spoilage.

HOW TO PREVENT
- If a can is bulging, or the contents have a peculiar color or odor, *don't even taste the food.*
- Don't eat any foods not definitely known to be properly cooked and canned.
- Don't give infants honey in foods or cough suppressants.
- Call your local home-extension service for details about canning food and cooking it safely.

OTHER—Call your local health department if you suspect botulism. The health department can notify the news media to alert others in danger, and require retailers to remove contaminated food from store shelves.

WHAT TO EXPECT

APPROPRIATE HEALTH CARE
- Doctor's treatment.
- Hospitalization for intensive care. A respirator may be necessary.

DIAGNOSTIC MEASURES
- Your own observation of symptoms—especially if several persons eat the same food and become sick.
- Medical history and physical exam by a doctor.
- Laboratory blood tests.
- Laboratory analysis of suspected food.

POSSIBLE COMPLICATIONS
- Lung infections as a result of impaired swallowing and choking on food.
- Respiratory failure caused by weak breathing muscles.

PROBABLE OUTCOME—With prompt care, the outlook is good. The larger the toxin dose and the sooner symptoms begin, the more dangerous the condition. The overall death rate is 10% to 25%.

HOW TO TREAT

NOTE—Follow your doctor's instructions. These instructions are supplemental.

GENERAL MEASURES
- Induce vomiting, if only a few hours have passed since the poisoned food was eaten.
- If you suspect botulism, refrigerate some of the contaminated food for laboratory testing, if possible.

MEDICATION—Botulism antitoxin injections prevent the condition from worsening. The antitoxin is available through the Center for Disease Control, Atlanta, Georgia. The anti-toxin is derived from horse serum, which may be life-saving, but has serious side effects.

ACTIVITY—Bed rest is necessary during hospitalization. After treatment, resume normal activities gradually.

DIET—Intravenous fluids and foods are usually necessary during hospitalization because of swallowing difficulty. After treatment, no special diet is necessary.

CALL YOUR DOCTOR IF

- You have symptoms of botulism. Call an ambulance immediately. This is an emergency!
- Weakness, blurred vision or slurred speech occur after you return from intensive care. These may signal a need for additional treatment.

BRAIN OR EPIDURAL ABSCESS

 GENERAL INFORMATION

DEFINITION—A collection of pus caused by a bacterial infection in the brain or the outermost of 3 membranes that cover the brain and spinal cord.

BODY PARTS INVOLVED—Brain; meninges (membranes that cover the brain); skull.

SEX OR AGE MOST AFFECTED—All ages, but most common in young adults.

SIGNS AND SYMPTOMS—The following symptoms usually appear gradually over several hours. They resemble symptoms of a brain tumor or stroke:
● Pain in the back, if the infection is in the covering of the spinal cord.
● Headache.
● Nausea and vomiting.
● Weakness, numbness, or paralysis of one side of the body.
● Irregular gait.
● Convulsions.
● Fever.
● Confusion or delirium.
● Speaking difficulty.

CAUSES—The primary source of bacterial infection that causes a brain or epidural abscess often cannot be found. These 3 sources are the most common:
● An infection that spreads from an infected skull, such as in osteomyelitis, mastoiditis or sinusitis.
● An infection that is introduced by a skull injury.
● An infection that spreads through the bloodstream from other infected organs, such as the lungs, skin or heart valves.

RISK INCREASES WITH
● Head injury.
● Illness that has lowered resistance, especially diabetes mellitus.
● Recent infection, especially around the nose and face.

HOW TO PREVENT—Consult your doctor for treatment of any infection in your body—especially one around the nose or face—to prevent its spread.

 WHAT TO EXPECT

APPROPRIATE HEALTH CARE
● Doctor's treatment.
● Surgery to drain pus.
● Self-care after returning home.

DIAGNOSTIC MEASURES
● Your own observation of symptoms.
● Medical history and physical exam by a doctor.
● Laboratory studies such as blood studies, spinal-fluid studies, EEG (see Glossary), CAT scan (see Glossary).
● X-rays of the skull.

POSSIBLE COMPLICATIONS—Seizures, coma and death without treatment.

PROBABLE OUTCOME—Usually curable with antibiotic treatment and surgery to drain pus.

 HOW TO TREAT

NOTE—Follow your doctor's instructions. These instructions are supplemental.

GENERAL MEASURES—No specific instructions except those under other headings.

MEDICATION—Your doctor may prescribe:
● Antibiotics for 4 to 6 weeks to fight infection.
● Anticonvulsants to prevent seizures.

ACTIVITY—While in the hospital, you will need bed rest. After a 2- to 3-week recovery, you should be as active as your strength and feeling of well-being allow.

DIET—Eat a normal, well-balanced diet. Vitamin and mineral supplements should not be necessary unless you show evidence of deficiency or cannot eat normally.

 CALL YOUR DOCTOR IF

● You have any symptoms of a brain or epidural abscess.
● Fever rises to 101F (38.3C) or higher.
● New, unexplained symptoms develop. Drugs used in treatment may produce side effects.

ILLNESSES & DISORDERS

BRAIN TUMOR

GENERAL INFORMATION

DEFINITION—An abnormal growth in the brain that may be benign or malignant. A non-malignant brain tumor may cause as much disability as a malignant tumor unless it is treated appropriately.

BODY PARTS INVOLVED—Brain; central nervous system.

SEX OR AGE MOST AFFECTED—All ages, but most common in adults between ages 20 and 60.

SIGNS & SYMPTOMS
- Headaches that worsen when lying down.
- Vomiting with nausea, or sudden vomiting without nausea.
- Vision disturbances, including double vision.
- Weakness on one side of the body.
- Lack of balance; dizziness.
- Loss of sense of smell.
- Memory loss.
- Personality changes.
- Seizures.

CAUSES—Some tumors begin in the brain (primary tumors), but most brain tumors have spread from other cancers—especially cancer of the breast, lungs, intestines or malignant melanoma of the skin. Symptoms are caused by increasing pressure in the skull as the tumor enlarges.

RISK INCREASES WITH—The following risk factors are related to cancers in other body parts that spread to the brain:
- Poor nutrition, especially a low-fiber diet (intestinal cancer).
- Smoking (lung cancer).
- Excess alcohol consumption (liver cancer).
- Excess sun exposure (malignant melanoma).
- Previous cancer at any other body site.

HOW TO PREVENT
- Practice breast self-exam (see Appendix 14).
- Don't smoke.
- Eat a high-fiber diet (see Appendix 1).
- Protect yourself from excessive sun exposure by using sunscreens and protective clothing.

WHAT TO EXPECT

APPROPRIATE HEALTH CARE
- Self-care after diagnosis.
- Doctor's treatment.
- Surgery to remove the tumor, if possible.

DIAGNOSTIC MEASURES
- Your own observation of symptoms.
- Medical history and physical exam by a doctor.
- Laboratory studies of blood and cerebrospinal fluid.
- X-rays of the skull, bones, lungs and gastrointestinal tract.
- EEG (see Glossary).
- CAT scan (see Glossary).

POSSIBLE COMPLICATIONS—Disability and death if a tumor is inoperable because of size or location.

PROBABLE OUTCOME—Brain tumors that are not treated lead to death or permanent brain damage. Bones of the skull restrict a tumor's outward growth, so the brain is compressed as a tumor grows.

If a tumor is discovered and treated early with surgery or radiation therapy and chemotherapy, full recovery is often possible. For an explanation of this surgery, see Craniotomy (in Surgery section).

HOW TO TREAT

NOTE—Follow your doctor's instructions. These instructions are supplemental.

GENERAL MEASURES—No specific instructions except those listed under other headings.

MEDICATION—Your doctor may prescribe:
- Cortisone drugs to diminish swelling of the brain tissue.
- Anticonvulsant drugs to control seizures.
- Pain relievers.
- Anticancer drugs.

ACTIVITY—Stay as active as your strength allows. Work and exercise moderately. Rest when you tire.

DIET—Eat a normal, well-balanced diet. Vitamin and mineral supplements should not be necessary unless you cannot eat normally.

CALL YOUR DOCTOR IF

- You have symptoms of a brain tumor.
- New, unexplained symptoms develop. Drugs used in treatment may produce side effects.

BREAST ABSCESS

GENERAL INFORMATION

DEFINITION—An infected area of breast tissue that becomes filled with pus when the body fights the infection.

BODY PARTS INVOLVED—Breast tissue; nipple; milk glands; milk ducts.

SEX OR AGE MOST AFFECTED—Women between ages 20 and 40.

SIGNS & SYMPTOMS
- Breast pain, tenderness, redness or hardness.
- Fever and chills.
- A general ill feeling.
- Tender lymph glands in the underarm area.

CAUSES—Bacteria that enter the breast through the nipple—usually a cracked nipple during the early days of breast-feeding.

RISK INCREASES WITH
- Postpartum pelvic infection.
- Fatigue.

HOW TO PREVENT
- Clean the nipples and breasts thoroughly before and after nursing.
- Lubricate the nipples after nursing with lanolin or Vitamin A & D ointment.
- Avoid clothing that irritates the breasts.
- Don't allow a nursing infant to chew nipples.

WHAT TO EXPECT

APPROPRIATE HEALTH CARE
- Self-care after diagnosis.
- Doctor's treatment.
- Surgery to drain the abscess.

DIAGNOSTIC MEASURES
- Your own observation of symptoms.
- Medical history and physical exam by a doctor.
- Laboratory culture of the discharge from the abscess to identify the bacteria (usually staphylococcus).

POSSIBLE COMPLICATIONS—It may be necessary to discontinue breast-feeding if the infection is severe enough to require extensive treatment with certain antibiotics (especially tetracycline) and pain relievers.

PROBABLE OUTCOME—Usually curable in 3 to 10 days with treatment. Draining the abscess greatly hastens healing.

HOW TO TREAT

NOTE—Follow your doctor's instructions. These instructions are supplemental.

GENERAL MEASURES
- Use warm-water soaks (see Appendix 18) to relieve pain and hasten healing.
- Discontinue nursing the baby from the infected breast until it heals. Use a breast pump to express milk regularly from the infected breast until you can resume nursing on that side.

MEDICATION—Your doctor may prescribe:
- Antibiotics to fight infection.
- Pain relievers.

ACTIVITY—After treatment, resume normal activity as soon as symptoms improve.

DIET—No special diet.

CALL YOUR DOCTOR IF

- You have symptoms of a breast abscess.
- Any of the following occurs during treatment:
  Fever rises to 103F (39.4C) or higher.
  Pain becomes unbearable.
  Infection seems to be spreading, despite treatment.
  Symptoms don't improve in 72 hours.
- New, unexplained symptoms develop. Drugs used in treatment may produce side effects.

ILLNESSES & DISORDERS

BREAST CANCER

GENERAL INFORMATION

DEFINITION—A malignant growth of breast tissue.

BODY PARTS INVOLVED—Nipple or fatty tissue of the breast. Breast cancer spreads to nearby lymph glands, lungs, pleura, bone (especially the skull), pelvis and liver.

SEX OR AGE MOST AFFECTED—Women, but it may affect males in rare cases. Breast cancer is rare before age 30. The incidence increases after menopause.

SIGNS & SYMPTOMS
- Swelling or lump in the breast.
- Vague discomfort in the breast without true pain.
- Retraction of the nipple.
- Bloody discharge from the nipple (rare).
- Distorted breast contour.
- Dimpled or pitted skin in the breast.
- Enlarged nodes under the arm.

CAUSES—Unknown.

RISK INCREASES WITH
- Women over 50.
- Women who have not had children or who conceived in the late fertile years.
- Family history of breast cancer.
- Previous benign tumors of the breast (fibrocystic disease).

HOW TO PREVENT
- Examine breasts monthly for signs of cancer (see Appendix 14).
- Visit your doctor regularly for a professional examination.
- Obtain a baseline mammogram (see Glossary) between ages 35 to 40. Have mammograms every year thereafter if you have risk factors mentioned above.
- Eat a well-balanced diet that is low in fat.
- If you are pregnant, consider breast-feeding your baby. Women who have breast-fed have a lower incidence of breast cancer.

WHAT TO EXPECT

APPROPRIATE HEALTH CARE
- Self-treatment.
- Doctor's care.
- Surgery to remove the lump, or breast, lymph glands, and lymphatic channels and muscles under the breast.
- Radiation therapy.

DIAGNOSTIC MEASURES
- Your own observation of symptoms.
- Medical history and physical exam by a doctor.
- X-rays of the breast and bones.
- Laboratory blood studies of hormones.
- Biopsy (see Glossary).

POSSIBLE COMPLICATIONS
- Spread to vital organs if not treated early.
- Adverse reactions to anticancer drugs.

PROBABLE OUTCOME—Most breast cancer is curable if diagnosed and treated early. The 10-year survival rate among all women with breast cancer is less than 50%.

HOW TO TREAT

NOTE—Follow your doctor's instructions. These instructions are supplemental.

GENERAL MEASURES—For an explanation of breast-cancer surgery and postoperative care, see Mastectomy.

MEDICATION
- For minor discomfort during treatment, you may use non-prescription drugs such as acetaminophen or aspirin.
- Your doctor may prescribe:
  Pain relievers.
  Anticancer drugs, such as fluorouracil, cyclophosphamide, methotrexate, chlorambucil, vincristine, doxorubicin or melphalan.
  Hormones (male and female).
  Cortisone drugs.

ACTIVITY—After surgery, resume your normal activities gradually. Exercise for rehabilitation following surgery will depend on how much tissue has been removed and your general physical condition.

DIET—No special diet.

CALL YOUR DOCTOR IF

- You discover a lump or other change in the breast.
- The following occurs after surgery:
  Nausea or vomiting.
  Fever.
  Pain that is not controlled by medication.
  Swelling in the arm.
- New, unexplained symptoms develop. Drugs used in treatment may produce side effects.

BRONCHIECTASIS

GENERAL INFORMATION

DEFINITION—A lung disease in which the bronchial tubes become blocked and accumulate thick secretions. Frequent secondary infections occur. It is not contagious unless associated with tuberculosis.

BODY PARTS INVOLVED—Lungs; bronchial tubes.

SEX OR AGE MOST AFFECTED—All ages, but most common in adults.

SIGNS & SYMPTOMS
- Frequent coughing with bad-smelling, green or yellow sputum (sometimes flecked with blood).
- Repeated lung infections.
- Shortness of breath.
- General ill feeling.
- Frequent fatigue.
- Anemia (frequently).

CAUSES—Damage to the small bronchial tubes, which may develop over years. Common sources of damage include:
- Repeated infections.
- Chronic bronchitis.
- Allergies.
- Smoke or dust.
- Inhalation of a foreign object.
- Tuberculosis.
- Fungus infection.

RISK INCREASES WITH
- Poor nutrition.
- Repeated pneumonia.
- Family history of tuberculosis.
- Obesity.
- Smoking.
- Fatigue or overwork.
- Exposure to allergens.
- Cold, humid weather.

HOW TO PREVENT
- Obtain medical treatment for lung infections.
- Avoid as many risks as possible.

WHAT TO EXPECT

APPROPRIATE HEALTH CARE
- Self-care after diagnosis.
- Doctor's treatment.
- Surgery to remove isolated areas of damaged lung tissue.

DIAGNOSTIC MEASURES
- Your own observation of symptoms.
- Medical history and physical exam by a doctor.
- X-rays of the lung, including a bronchogram (see Glossary).

POSSIBLE COMPLICATIONS
- COPD (chronic obstructive pulmonary disease).
- Repeated pneumonia.
- Destruction of lung tissue.

PROBABLE OUTCOME—With treatment, most patients with bronchiectasis can lead nearly normal lives without major disability.

HOW TO TREAT

NOTE—Follow your doctor's instructions. These instructions are supplemental.

GENERAL MEASURES
- Don't smoke.
- Learn and practice postural drainage (see Glossary) twice a day.
- Sleep with 3- to 5-inch blocks under the foot of the bed to prevent mucus from collecting in the lower lobes of the lungs.
- If you work around heavy air pollution, do everything possible to limit your exposure—including changing jobs.
- Install air conditioning with a filter and humidity control in your home.
- Avoid sudden temperature changes.
- Avoid loud talking, loud laughing, crying, exertion or sudden temperature changes, if these trigger coughing episodes.
- Keep the teeth and mouth in excellent condition.
- If you have an allergic background, avoid allergens.

MEDICATION—Your doctor may prescribe:
- Antibiotics for 10 days every month if bacterial infections have caused bronchiectasis or triggered episodes of pneumonia or acute bronchitis.
- Bronchodilators to enlarge airways.
- Expectorants to loosen secretions.

ACTIVITY—Remain as active as possible.

DIET—Increase fluid intake. Drink a minimum of 8 glasses of fluid a day. This thins lung secretions so they can be coughed out more easily.

CALL YOUR DOCTOR IF

- You have symptoms of bronchiectasis.
- After diagnosis, you have symptoms of a respiratory infection or bronchitis.
- Temperature rises to 101F (38.3C).
- Blood appears in the sputum, sputum thickens despite treatment, or postural drainage reveals a change in color, amount or character of sputum.
- Chest pain increases.
- Shortness of breath occurs without coughing or when at rest.

BRONCHIOLITIS

GENERAL INFORMATION

DEFINITION—Inflammation of the bronchioles, the smallest branches of the respiratory tree. These carry air from the large bronchial tubes to microscopic air sacs in the lungs. The air sacs transfer oxygen to the bloodstream.

BODY PARTS INVOLVED—Bronchioles.

SEX OR AGE MOST AFFECTED—Children under age 6.

SIGNS & SYMPTOMS—Sudden breathing difficulty, usually preceded by a mild common cold and cough, and characterized by the following:
- Wheezing.
- Rapid, shallow breathing (60 to 80 times a minute).
- Retractions (see-saw movements) of the chest and abdomen.
- Fever.
- Blue skin or nails (severe cases).

CAUSES—Viral or bacterial infection, or a combination of the two. Some young children develop this disorder after every cold. Bronchiolitis is contagious and often becomes epidemic.

RISK INCREASES WITH
- Illness that has lowered resistance, especially respiratory infection.
- Family history of allergies.
- Obese infants.

HOW TO PREVENT
- Use a cool-mist humidifier in the child's room. Use it every night during and after a respiratory infection for a child who is subject to bronchiolitis.
- Observe and avoid any activities that seem to trigger attacks in the child, such as active play in cool night air.
- Decrease the child's exposure to groups of people, especially other children, to avoid colds.

WHAT TO EXPECT

APPROPRIATE HEALTH CARE
- Home care.
- Doctor's treatment.
- Hospitalization for intensive care and oxygen (severe cases).

DIAGNOSTIC MEASURES
- Your own observation of symptoms.
- Medical history and physical exam by a doctor.
- Laboratory blood studies.
- X-rays of the lungs.

POSSIBLE COMPLICATIONS—Permanent lung damage leading to chronic bronchitis, collapse of a small portion of the lung, bronchiectasis, repeated pneumonia, and rarely, chronic obstructive pulmonary disease (COPD).

PROBABLE OUTCOME—Usually curable in 7 days with treatment. Some studies indicate that infants who have 2 or more episodes of bronchiolitis before age 2 are more likely to develop allergies and asthma.

HOW TO TREAT

NOTE—Follow your doctor's instructions. These instructions are supplemental.

GENERAL MEASURES—Keep the humidity in the child's room as high as possible, preferably with a cool-mist humidifier.
  If you don't have a humidifier, run cold or hot water in the shower with windows and doors closed to produce a high-humidity room. Hold the child in this room for 20 minutes several times a day, especially at bedtime. If the child awakens at night with wheezing or shortness of breath, repeat the process.

MEDICATION—Your doctor may prescribe antibiotics to fight bacterial infections.

ACTIVITY—Have the child rest until symptoms have subsided for 48 hours. Then normal activities may be resumed gradually.

DIET—Offer the child clear fluids frequently. Give water, tea, carbonated drinks, lemonade, weak bouillon, diluted fruit juice or gelatin. Don't offer milk; it may thicken mucus secretions.

CALL YOUR DOCTOR IF

- Symptoms don't improve in 4 hours, despite treatment.
- Temperature (rectal) rises to 101F (38.3C) or higher.
- Breathing becomes more difficult.
- A cough begins that produces colored phlegm.
- The skin, lips or nails turn dark blue.
- The child becomes lethargic.

BRONCHITIS, ACUTE

GENERAL INFORMATION

DEFINITION—Inflammation of the air passages of the lungs.

BODY PARTS INVOLVED—Trachea; bronchi; bronchioles.

SEX OR AGE MOST AFFECTED—Both sexes; all ages.

SIGNS & SYMPTOMS
- Cough that produces little or no sputum.
- Low fever (usually less than 101F or 38.3C).
- Burning chest discomfort or feeling of pressure behind the breastbone.
- Wheezing or uncomfortable breathing (sometimes).

CAUSES
- Infection from one of many respiratory viruses. Most cases of acute bronchitis begin with a cold virus in the nose and throat that spreads to the airways. A secondary bacterial infection is common.
- Lung inflammation from breathing air that contains irritants, such as chemical fumes (ammonia), acid fumes, dust or smoke.

RISK INCREASES WITH
- Chronic obstructive pulmonary disease (COPD).
- Smoking.
- Cold, humid weather.
- Poor nutrition.
- Recent illness that has lowered resistance.

HOW TO PREVENT
- Avoid close contact with persons who have bronchitis.

WHAT TO EXPECT

APPROPRIATE HEALTH CARE
- Self-care, if you are in good overall health.
- Doctor's treatment, if you have chronic lung disease or complications develop.

DIAGNOSTIC MEASURES
- Your own observation of symptoms.
- Medical history and physical exam by a doctor.
- Laboratory blood counts to detect complicating infections and cultures of sputum and blood to identify the bacteria.
- X-rays of the chest (for complications only).

POSSIBLE COMPLICATIONS
- Bacterial lung infection (various kinds of pneumonia).
- Chronic bronchitis from recurrent episodes of acute bronchitis.

PROBABLE OUTCOME—Usually curable with treatment in 1 week. Cases with complications are usually curable in 2 weeks with medication.

HOW TO TREAT

NOTE—Follow your doctor's instructions. These instructions are supplemental.

GENERAL MEASURES
- If you are a smoker, don't smoke during your illness. This delays recovery and makes complications more likely.
- Increase air moisture. Take frequent hot showers. Use a cool-mist humidifier by your bed.

MEDICATION
- For minor discomfort, you may use: Acetaminophen to reduce fever. Non-prescription cough suppressants. Use only if your cough is non-productive (without sputum). It may be dangerous to stop a cough entirely—this traps excess mucus and irritants in bronchial tubes, leading to pneumonia and poor oxygen exchange in the lungs.
- Your doctor may prescribe: Antibiotics to fight bacterial infections. Expectorants to thin mucus so it can be coughed up more easily. Cough suppressants.

ACTIVITY—Rest in bed until temperature returns to normal. Then resume normal activity gradually as symptoms improve.

DIET—No special diet. Drink at least 8 to 10 glasses of fluid each day to help thin mucus secretions so they can be coughed up more easily.

CALL YOUR DOCTOR IF

- You have symptoms of bronchitis.
- The following occurs during the illness: High fever and chills.
Chest pain.
Thickened, discolored or blood-streaked sputum.
Shortness of breath, even when the body is at rest.
Vomiting.

BRONCHITIS, CHRONIC

GENERAL INFORMATION

DEFINITION—Chronic inflammation and degeneration of the bronchial tubes, with or without active infection. This is not contagious or cancerous.

BODY PARTS INVOLVED—Bronchial tubes (bronchi).

SEX OR AGE MOST AFFECTED—All ages, but most common in men.

SIGNS & SYMPTOMS
- Frequent cough or coughing spasms.
- Shortness of breath.
- Sputum that is thick and difficult to cough up. Sputum production varies according to whether infection is present.
- Barrel chest (in the late stages).

CAUSES—Repeated irritation or infection in the bronchial tubes, causing them to thicken, narrow and lose elasticity. Underlying irritants include allergens, air pollution and tobacco smoke.

RISK INCREASES WITH
- Smoking (the greatest risk factor).
- Any lung illness that has lowered resistance.
- Family history of tuberculosis or other disease of the respiratory tract.
- Exposure to air pollutants.
- Poor nutrition.
- Obesity.
- Crowded living conditions.

HOW TO PREVENT
- Don't smoke. This is the most reversible risk.
- Avoid irritating fumes in the environment.
- Obtain prompt medical treatment for respiratory infections.

WHAT TO EXPECT

APPROPRIATE HEALTH CARE
- Self-care after diagnosis.
- Doctor's treatment. Many lung and heart disorders cause symptoms identical to those of chronic bronchitis. Your doctor must exclude these possibilities to make a diagnosis.

DIAGNOSTIC MEASURES
- Your own observation of symptoms.
- Medical history and physical exam by a doctor.
- Laboratory studies of sputum and pulmonary function.
- X-rays of the chest.

POSSIBLE COMPLICATIONS
- Recurrent pneumonia.
- Chronic obstructive pulmonary disease (COPD). COPD is incurable. It is characterized by purple lips and nails and congestive heart failure.

PROBABLE OUTCOME—Chronic bronchitis is usually curable with treatment—if you are a non-smoker and don't have an underlying chronic disease, such as congestive heart failure, bronchiectasis or tuberculosis.

Chronic bronchitis usually reduces life expectancy if you smoke and don't stop, or if you have an underlying chronic disease.

HOW TO TREAT

NOTE—Follow your doctor's instructions. These instructions are supplemental.

GENERAL MEASURES
- Stop smoking.
- If you work or live in an area with heavy air pollution, do everything you can to avoid or reduce it. Consider changing jobs and installing air-conditioning with a filter and humidity control in your home.
- Avoid sudden temperature changes or exposure to cold, wet weather.
- Avoid talking loudly, laughing loudly, crying and exertion, if these trigger coughing episodes.
- Practice bronchial drainage and deep-breathing techniques. Your physician will provide instructions.
- Sleep with 5-inch blocks under the foot of your bed.

MEDICATION
- Don't take cough suppressants; they make chronic bronchitis worse.
- Your doctor may prescribe:
  Antibiotics to fight chronic or recurrent infection.
  Expectorants to loosen secretions.
  Bronchodilators to open bronchial tubes.

ACTIVITY—No restrictions. Remain as active as possible.

DIET—No special diet. Increase fluid intake to 8 to 10 glasses a day.

CALL YOUR DOCTOR IF

- You have symptoms of chronic bronchitis.
- You develop fever of 101F (38.3C).
- Blood appears in the sputum.
- Chest pain increases.
- Shortness of breath occurs even when you are resting or not coughing.
- Sputum thickens despite efforts to thin it.
- Vomiting occurs.

BRUCELLOSIS
(Undulant Fever; Bang's Disease)

 GENERAL INFORMATION

DEFINITION—A bacterial infection transmitted to humans from infected cows, pigs, sheep or goats. It is not contagious from person to person.

BODY PARTS INVOLVED—Blood-producing organs, including bone marrow, lymph glands, liver and spleen.

SEX OR AGE MOST AFFECTED—Both sexes and all ages, but most common in men between ages 20 and 60.

SIGNS & SYMPTOMS—The disease has an acute form and a chronic form. In the acute form, the following symptoms appear suddenly:
- Chills, intermittent fever, sweating.
- Marked fatigue.
- Tenderness along the spine.
- Headache.
- Enlarged lymph glands.

In the chronic form, the following symptoms appear gradually:
- Fatigue
- Muscle pain.
- Backache.
- Constipation.
- Weight loss.
- Depression.
- Sexual impotence.
- Abscesses in the ovaries, kidney and brain (rare).

CAUSES—Infection from the bacteria, brucella, which is transmitted to humans through unpasteurized milk or milk products (butter, cheese) or meat products.

RISK INCREASES WITH
- Pernicious anemia or previous stomach surgery. These conditions result in reduced stomach acid; stomach acid decreases the chance of infection.
- Persons with occupations involving animals, such as farmers, butchers, veterinarians or ranchers.

HOW TO PREVENT
- Don't drink unpasteurized milk from any source.
- Use gloves and aprons when working around animals.

 WHAT TO EXPECT

APPROPRIATE HEALTH CARE
- Doctor's treatment.
- Hospitalization.
- Self-care after treatment of the acute phase.

DIAGNOSTIC MEASURES
- Your own observation of symptoms.
- Medical history and physical exam by a doctor.
- Laboratory blood studies.

POSSIBLE COMPLICATIONS
- Heart, bone, brain or liver infection (rare).
- Chronic illness and disability from inadequate treatment and care.

PROBABLE OUTCOME—Usually curable in 3 to 4 weeks with treatment.

 HOW TO TREAT

NOTE—Follow your doctor's instructions. These instructions are supplemental.

GENERAL MEASURES
- It usually is not necessary to isolate the ill person.
- All family members who may have been exposed to the same infected milk products should have medical checkups and diagnostic tests.

MEDICATION—Your doctor may prescribe:
- Antibiotics to fight infection, such as tetracycline, for a minimum of 3 weeks.
- Cortisone drugs to reduce the inflammatory response in severe cases.
- Pain relievers for muscle pain.

ACTIVITY—Rest in bed until fever and other symptoms subside. Resume your normal activities gradually.

DIET—No special diet. Increase calories if weight loss has been significant.

 CALL YOUR DOCTOR IF

- You have symptoms of undulant fever.
- Fever or other symptoms recur after treatment.

ILLNESSES & DISORDERS

BUERGER'S DISEASE
(Thromboangiitis Obliterans)

GENERAL INFORMATION

DEFINITION—Blockage of small and medium arteries—usually in the legs and feet—from inflammation of blood vessels. This causes clot formation.

Cigarette-smoking is a very important factor in developing this disease. It is extremely rare among non-smokers.

BODY PARTS INVOLVED—Arteries (and sometimes veins) in the extremities.

SEX OR AGE MOST AFFECTED—Both sexes, but most common in cigarette-smoking men between ages 20 and 40.

SIGNS & SYMPTOMS
- Intermittent pain in the instep or the leg when exercising. The pain improves with rest.
- Pain, blueness, heat and tingling in the legs when exposed to cold.
- Painful ulcers on the toes and fingertips (sometimes).

CAUSES—Unknown, but the disease is probably triggered by nicotine. Cigarette-smoking causes blood-vessel spasms, leading to obstruction of the essential blood vessels in the extremities.

RISK INCREASES WITH
- Collagen disease or atherosclerosis.
- Stress.
- Cold weather.
- Family history of Buerger's disease.

HOW TO PREVENT
- Don't smoke.
- Avoid exposure to the cold. This also causes blood vessels to constrict and deprives extremities of a normal blood supply.

WHAT TO EXPECT

APPROPRIATE HEALTH CARE
- Self-care after diagnosis.
- Doctor's treatment.
- Surgery (sympathectomy) to cut sympathetic nerves to the area (sometimes).

DIAGNOSTIC MEASURES
- Your own observation of symptoms.
- Medical history and physical exam by a doctor.
- Laboratory studies, such as Doppler ultrasonography and arteriography (see Glossary for both).

POSSIBLE COMPLICATIONS—Gangrene in the foot or leg caused by a loss of blood supply. This may result in amputation.

PROBABLE OUTCOME—This condition is currently considered incurable. However, symptoms can be controlled for a while, but the disease causes increasing disability—especially if amputation is necessary. Life expectancy is reduced.

Scientific research into causes and treatment continues, so there is hope for increasingly effective treatment and cure.

HOW TO TREAT

NOTE—Follow your doctor's instructions. These instructions are supplemental.

GENERAL MEASURES
- Stop smoking.
- Avoid exposure to the cold. Wear warm footwear and gloves.
- Clip nails carefully to avoid injuring the skin.
- Wear well-fitting shoes and cotton or wool socks. Don't wear socks made of synthetic material.
- Insert soft padding in your shoes to protect your feet.
- Don't go barefoot outdoors.
- Consult a podiatrist or have a visiting nurse see you regularly for foot and hand care.

MEDICATION—Your doctor may prescribe vasodilator drugs, but they are usually useless if you continue smoking.

ACTIVITY—Avoid cold weather, but stay active. Begin a conditioning program to become as physically fit as possible. See Appendix 20.

DIET—No special diet.

CALL YOUR DOCTOR IF

- You have symptoms of Buerger's disease.
- Uncontrollable pain begins.
- Ulcers develop on your toes or feet.

BULIMIA
(Binge-Eating Syndrome; Binge-Purge Syndrome; Bulimarexia)

GENERAL INFORMATION

DEFINITION—A psychological eating disorder characterized by abnormal, constant craving for food and binge eating, followed by self-induced vomiting or laxative use.

BODY PARTS INVOLVED—Brain and central nervous system; kidneys; liver; endocrine system; gastrointestinal tract.

SEX OR AGE MOST AFFECTED—Adolescents or young adults, usually female.

SIGNS & SYMPTOMS—Recurrent episodes of binge eating (rapid consumption of a large amount of food in a short time, usually less than 2 hours), plus at least 3 of the following:
- Preference for high-calorie, convenience foods during a binge.
- Secretive eating during a binge. Patients are aware that the eating pattern is abnormal, and they fear being unable to stop eating.
- Termination of an eating binge with purging measures, such as laxative use or self-induced vomiting.
- Depression and guilt following an eating binge.
- Repeated attempts to lose weight with severely restrictive diets, self-induced vomiting and use of laxatives or diuretics.
- Frequent weight fluctuations greater than 10 pounds from alternately fasting and gorging.
- No underlying physical disorder.

CAUSES—Unknown. The disorder often begins during or after stringent dieting and may be caused by stress related to insufficient food intake.

RISK INCREASES WITH
- Anorexia nervosa.
- Depression.
- Stress, including lifestyle changes, such as moving or starting a new school or job.
- Neurotic preoccupation with being physically attractive.

HOW TO PREVENT—Raise children in a wholesome family environment with emphasis on caring and good communication rather than on external appearances.

WHAT TO EXPECT

APPROPRIATE HEALTH CARE
- Doctor's treatment.
- Psychotherapy or counseling that may include hypnosis or biofeedback training.
- Hospitalization (severe cases).

DIAGNOSTIC MEASURES
- Your own observation of symptoms. Many patients are secretive, and parents may be unaware of this condition.
- Medical history and physical exam by a doctor.
- Laboratory blood studies, including measurement of electrolyte levels.

POSSIBLE COMPLICATIONS—Fluid and electrolyte imbalance from vomiting.

PROBABLE OUTCOME—Most patients can control the behavior with counseling, psychotherapy, biofeedback training and individual or group psychotherapy. Without treatment, complications can be fatal.

HOW TO TREAT

NOTE—Follow your doctor's instructions. These instructions are supplemental.

GENERAL MEASURES—See Appendix 13 for suggestions to reduce stress and improve overall health.

MEDICATION—Medication is usually not necessary for this disorder. However, some doctors have successfully treated bulimia with antidepressants.

ACTIVITY—No restrictions.

DIET—If hospitalization is necessary, your doctor may prescribe intravenous fluids. During recovery, vitamin and mineral supplements will be necessary until signs of deficiency disappear and normal eating patterns are established.

CALL YOUR DOCTOR IF

- You have symptoms of bulimia or you suspect your child has bulimia.
- The following occurs during treatment:
  Rapid, irregular heartbeat or chest pain.
  Loss of consciousness.
  Cessation of menstrual periods.
  Repeated vomiting or diarrhea.
  Continued weight loss, despite treatment.

ILLNESSES & DISORDERS

BUNION
(Hallux Valgus)

GENERAL INFORMATION

DEFINITION—Inflammation, swelling and protrusion of the base of the great toe. Bunions may be congenital or hereditary.

BODY PARTS INVOLVED—Great (big) toe.

SEX OR AGE MOST AFFECTED—Female adolescents and adults.

SIGNS & SYMPTOMS
- An inward-turned great toe that may overlap the second—and sometimes the third—toe.
- Thickened skin over the bony protrusion at the base of the great toe.
- Fluid accumulation under the thickened skin (sometimes).
- Foot pain and stiffness.

CAUSES
- Arthritis.
- Narrow-toed, high-heeled shoes that compress toes together.

RISK INCREASES WITH—Family history of foot abnormalities.

HOW TO PREVENT
- Exercise daily to keep muscles of the feet and legs in good condition.
- Wear wide-toed shoes that fit well. Don't wear high heels or shoes without room for toes in their normal position.

WHAT TO EXPECT

APPROPRIATE HEALTH CARE
- Self-care in the early stages. This may prevent a bunion from worsening.
- Doctor's (orthopedist's or podiatrist's) treatment.
- Surgery to remove the overgrown tissue (bunion) and correct the position of the bones.

DIAGNOSTIC MEASURES
- Your own observation of symptoms.
- Medical history and physical exam by a doctor.
- X-rays of the foot.

POSSIBLE COMPLICATIONS
- Infection of the bunion, especially in persons with diabetes mellitus.
- Inflammation and arthritic changes in other joints caused by walking difficulty, which places abnormal stress on the foot, hip and spine.

PROBABLE OUTCOME—Usually curable with treatment and preventive measures to guard against recurrence.

HOW TO TREAT

NOTE—Follow your doctor's instructions. These instructions are supplemental.

GENERAL MEASURES
- Before bedtime, separate the great toe from the others with a foam-rubber pad.
- Wear a thick, ring-shaped adhesive pad over the bunion.
- Use arch supports to relieve pressure on the bunion. These are available in shoe-repair shops.

MEDICATION—Medicine usually is not necessary for this disorder unless infection develops.

ACTIVITY—If surgery is necessary, resume your normal activities gradually afterward. Walk on your heels until the surgical site heals. Elevate the foot of the bed to reduce swelling.

DIET—No special diet.

CALL YOUR DOCTOR IF

- You have a bunion that is interfering with normal activities.
- Signs of infection, such as fever, heat, tenderness or pain, develop after treatment or surgery.

BURNS

GENERAL INFORMATION

DEFINITION—Injury to the skin, and sometimes other organs, from contact with heat, radiation, electricity or chemicals.

BODY PARTS INVOLVED—Skin; underlying tissue and respiratory system (sometimes).

SEX OR AGE MOST AFFECTED—Both sexes; all ages. The risk of damage is greatest with infants and young children.

SIGNS & SYMPTOMS—Burns are of 3 types:
- 1st-degree burns are limited to the upper skin layer. They produce redness, tenderness, pain, swelling and slight fever.
- 2nd-degree burns affect deeper skin layers. Symptoms are more severe and include blisters.
- 3rd-degree burns involve all skin layers. Skin is white (appears cooked), and there may be no pain in the initial stages.

CAUSES
- Rise in skin temperature from heat sources, such as fire, steam or electricity.
- Tissue injury caused by chemicals or radiation, including sunlight.

RISK INCREASES WITH
- Stress, carelessness, smoking in bed or excess alcohol consumption, all of which make accidents more likely.
- Occupations involving exposure to heat or radiation, such as firefighting, police work or defense-factory work.

HOW TO PREVENT
- Wear sun-screen lotions outdoors.
- Fireproof your home. Install smoke alarms and plan emergency exits.
- Wear protective gear and observe safety precautions around heat or radiation.
- Don't touch uncovered electric wires.
- Teach children safety rules for matches, fires and electrical outlets.
- Discard extension cords with a pronged plug on one end and a bulb socket on the other. These are hazardous.
- If you have small children, put safety caps on unused outlets. Discard frayed cords.

WHAT TO EXPECT

APPROPRIATE HEALTH CARE
- Self-care for most 1st-degree burns.
- Doctor's treatment for more severe burns.
- Hospitalization for all large 3rd-degree burns and some 2nd-degree burns. Special burn centers exist for the worst cases.
- Surgery to graft skin over 3rd-degree burns.

DIAGNOSTIC MEASURES
- Your own observation of symptoms.

- Medical history and physical exam by a doctor.
- Laboratory blood and urine tests, and studies of kidney and liver function (severe burns).

POSSIBLE COMPLICATIONS
- Infection at the burn site.
- Pneumonia.
- Shock due to loss of fluids and electrolytes (severe burns).
- Permanent scars.
- Vision impairment, if eyes are injured.

PROBABLE OUTCOME—Most persons recover if the extent of burns (including 3rd-degree burns) is limited to 50% of the body surface. For less-severe burns, skin usually repairs itself in 1 to 3 weeks.

HOW TO TREAT

NOTE—Follow your doctor's instructions. These instructions are supplemental.

GENERAL MEASURES—For severe burns see instructions on page 894. For less-severe burns:
- Apply non-prescription body lotion to cool 1st-degree burns.
- Immerse small 2nd- or 3rd-degree burn areas in cold water for 10 minutes to reduce pain and swelling.
- Keep the burn area clean. Soak in a tub or use lukewarm compresses once a day. You may add 2 tablespoons of powdered detergent to the tub to help soak off crusting areas. Use plain water for compresses.
- Prop the burn area higher than the rest of the body, if possible.
- You may use dressings on the burn.

MEDICATION
- To treat minor burns, you may use non-prescription antibiotic ointments, topical anesthetics and aspirin.
- To treat severe burns, your doctor may prescribe pain relievers, antibiotics and tetanus booster shots.

ACTIVITY—Depends on location and extent of the burn. Ask your doctor.

DIET—No special diet for minor burns. More severe burns require intravenous feeding.

CALL YOUR DOCTOR IF

- You have a 2nd- or 3rd-degree burn, or a 1st-degree burn over a large area.
- An infant has a burn, even if it seems minor.
- The following occurs during treatment:
  No healing in 6 days.
  Chills and fever.
  Increased pain, redness, swelling or pus in the burn area.

BURSITIS

GENERAL INFORMATION

DEFINITION—Inflammation of a soft sac (bursa) filled with lubricating liquid that protects a joint.

BODY PARTS INVOLVED—Bursas, especially near the shoulders, elbows, knees, pelvis, hips or Achilles tendons.

SEX OR AGE MOST AFFECTED—Adults of all ages.

SIGNS & SYMPTOMS—Pain, tenderness and limited movement in the affected area.

CAUSES
- Injury to a joint.
- Acute or chronic infection.
- Arthritis.
- Gout.
- Unknown (frequently).

RISK INCREASES WITH—Unknown.

HOW TO PREVENT—Avoid injuries whenever possible. Wear seat belts in autos and protective gear for contact sports.

WHAT TO EXPECT

APPROPRIATE HEALTH CARE
- Self-care after diagnosis.
- Doctor's treatment.

DIAGNOSTIC MEASURES
- Your own observation of symptoms.
- Medical history and physical exam by a doctor.
- X-rays of the affected area.

POSSIBLE COMPLICATIONS—Frozen joint or permanent limitation of a joint's mobility.

PROBABLE OUTCOME—This is a common—but not serious—problem. Symptoms usually subside in 7 to 14 days with treatment.

HOW TO TREAT

NOTE—Follow your doctor's instructions. These instructions are supplemental.

GENERAL MEASURES
- Apply ice packs to the affected area during a flare-up or after receiving injections in the joint.
- After the acute stage, many doctors recommend continued ice treatment until inflammation subsides. Others recommend heat. If you use heat, take hot showers, use a heat lamp, apply hot compresses or a heating pad, or rub in deep-heating ointment.

MEDICATION—Your doctor may prescribe:
- Non-steroidal anti-inflammatory drugs.
- Cortisone injections into the bursa to reduce inflammation.
- Pain relievers.

ACTIVITY—Rest the inflamed area as much as possible. If you must resume normal activity immediately, wear a sling until the pain becomes more bearable. To prevent a frozen joint (especially in the shoulder), begin normal, slow joint movement as soon as possible.

DIET—No special diet.

CALL YOUR DOCTOR IF

- You have symptoms of bursitis.
- Pain increases, despite treatment.
- New, unexplained symptoms develop. Drugs used in treatment may produce side effects.

CALCIUM IMBALANCE

GENERAL INFORMATION

DEFINITION—Calcium is a component of blood that helps regulate the heartbeat, transmit nerve impulses, contract muscles and form bone and teeth. Too much *or* too little can cause serious—sometimes life-threatening—medical problems.

BODY PARTS INVOLVED—Membranes of all body cells; muscles; bones; parathyroid glands and parathyroid hormones (these regulate calcium absorption and utilization).

SEX OR AGE MOST AFFECTED—Both sexes; all ages.

SIGNS & SYMPTOMS—Too little calcium:
- Muscle spasms and twitching.
- Numbness and tingling in the arms, legs, hands and feet.
- Seizures.
- Irregular heartbeat.
- High blood pressure.

Too much calcium;
- Lethargy.
- Appetite loss.
- Vomiting and diarrhea.
- Dehydration and thirst.
- Irregular heartbeat.
- Low blood pressure.
- Seizures or coma (worst cases only).

CAUSES—Too little calcium:
- Underactive parathyroid glands from disease or damage during neck surgery.
- Inadequate dietary intake of calcium and vitamin D.
- Malabsorption from the gastrointestinal tract (usually for unknown reasons).
- Severe burns.
- Severe infections.
- Chronic pancreatitis.
- Kidney failure.
- Decreased blood levels of magnesium.

Too much calcium:
- Overactive parathyroid glands.
- Multiple fractures and prolonged bed rest.
- Multiple myeloma.
- Tumors—benign *or* malignant—that destroy bone.

RISK INCREASES WITH—Too little calcium:
- Use of certain drugs, including thiazide diuretics and calcium-channel blockers.
- Injury, cancer or surgery of the thyroid gland or parathyroid glands.
- Excess alcohol consumption leading to poor nutrition.

Too much calcium:
- Improper diet, especially overconsumption of milk products or non-prescription antacids that contain calcium.
- Repeated transfusions with citrated blood.

Either:
- Chronic kidney disease.

HOW TO PREVENT
- Eat a normal, balanced diet.
- Don't drink more than 1 or 2 alcoholic drinks—if any—a day.
- Don't use non-prescription antacids on a regular basis.

WHAT TO EXPECT

APPROPRIATE HEALTH CARE
- Doctor's treatment.
- Hospitalization.
- Self-care after hospitalization.

DIAGNOSTIC MEASURES
- Your own observation of symptoms.
- Medical history and physical exam by a doctor.
- Laboratory blood studies of calcium levels.
- EKG (see Glossary).
- X-rays of bones.

POSSIBLE COMPLICATIONS
- Cardiac arrest.
- Fractures of weak bones.

PROBABLE OUTCOME—Unless calcium imbalance is caused by cancer, most cases are curable with treatment in 1 week.

HOW TO TREAT

NOTE—Follow your doctor's instructions. These instructions are supplemental.

GENERAL MEASURES—The underlying cause must be corrected before you can follow a treatment program to prevent a recurrence.

MEDICATION—Your doctor may prescribe:
- Intravenous calcium gluconate or calcium carbonate for too little calcium.
- Intravenous saline solution and loop diuretics (furosemide and ethacrynic acid) for too much calcium.

ACTIVITY—After treatment, resume your normal activities as symptoms improve.

DIET
- For a mild, low calcium level, take calcium supplements and vitamin D. Increase your intake of protein, milk and milk products.
- For a mild, high calcium level, restrict consumption of dairy products and calcium-containing antacids.

CALL YOUR DOCTOR IF

- You have symptoms of a calcium imbalance.
- Symptoms recur after treatment.

CANDIDIASIS OF INTERTRIGINOUS SKIN
(Moniliasis)

 GENERAL INFORMATION

DEFINITION—A yeast infection in skin folds or areas of adjacent skin that come in contact with each other, such as in the groin or under the breasts. This is contagious from person to person and from place to place on the same person.

BODY PARTS INVOLVED—Skin of the scrotum, vagina and vaginal lips; underarm area; spaces between fingers and toes; inner thighs; under the breasts; and over the base of the spine (sacrum).

SEX OR AGE MOST AFFECTED—Adolescents and adults.

SIGNS & SYMPTOMS—Plaques (patches or flat areas) with the following characteristics:
- Bright red patches with poorly defined borders. They are often 6cm to 12cm in diameter or larger.
- Some plaques appear to have pus.
- Skin appears moist and crusted.
- Itching is usually severe.
- Smaller plaques sometimes surround larger plaques. Smaller plaques are less than 1mm in size. They form small pustules (small white blisters with pus inside).

CAUSES—Yeast infection of the skin caused by candida fungus (usually candida albicans).

The spore form of this organism normally grows in the intestinal tract and the vagina. Skin signs do not begin until yeast changes from its spore form to another growth phase, the mycelial phase. Damaged skin, moisture and warmth are all necessary for the infection to take over.

RISK INCREASES WITH
- Use of oral antibiotics.
- Use of steroids (oral, injectable or topical).
- Diabetes.
- Poor nutrition.
- Excessive sweating.
- Crowded or unsanitary living conditions.

HOW TO PREVENT
- If you must take antibiotics, consult your doctor about eating yogurt, buttermilk or sour cream, or taking acidophilus tablets. These help prevent yeast infections that may result as an adverse effect of the drugs.
- Keep skin cool and dry.

 WHAT TO EXPECT

APPROPRIATE HEALTH CARE
- Self-care after diagnosis.
- Doctor's treatment.

DIAGNOSTIC MEASURES
- Your own observation of symptoms.
- Medical history and physical exam by a doctor.
- Laboratory culture to identify the yeast organism.

POSSIBLE COMPLICATIONS
- Secondary bacterial infections.
- Id reactions (in Illness section).
- Blood poisoning.

PROBABLE OUTCOME—Usually curable in 2 weeks with treatment. Without treatment, healing may be slow (4 to 5 years). Recurrence is common.

 HOW TO TREAT

NOTE—Follow your doctor's instructions. These instructions are supplemental.

GENERAL MEASURES
- Keep skin cool and dry. Expose affected areas to sunlight as much as possible.
- Wear loose cotton clothing. Avoid synthetic or wool fabrics.
- Protect skin from injury.
- If you have a vaginal infection as well as infection of the surrounding skin, obtain treatment for the vaginitis (see Vaginitis, Monilial).

MEDICATION—Your doctor may prescribe antifungal topical medications such as nystatin, haloprigin, miconazole or clotrimazole. Gently massage a small amount into the affected area 3 or 4 times a day. Use only enough to cover. Larger amounts don't help.

ACTIVITY—No restrictions, except to avoid heat and sweating.

DIET—No special diet.

 CALL YOUR DOCTOR IF

- You have symptoms of candidiasis.
- The following occurs during treatment:
  Infection continues to spread, despite treatment.
  You develop signs of secondary bacterial infection (pain, tenderness, redness, warmth, oozing).
- New, unexplained symptoms develop. Drugs used in treatment may produce side effects.

CANKER SORES
(Aphthous Ulcers)

GENERAL INFORMATION

DEFINITION—Painful ulcers that occur in the lining of the mouth. Ulcers are not cancerous, but may be contagious.

BODY PARTS INVOLVED—Mouth and adjacent areas.

SEX OR AGE MOST AFFECTED—Both sexes, but more common in women.

SIGNS & SYMPTOMS—Mouth ulcers with the following characteristics:
● Ulcers are small, painful, shallow and covered by a gray membrane. Borders are surrounded by an intense red halo.
● Ulcers appear on lips, gums, inner cheeks, tongue, palate and throat. 2 or 3 ulcers usually appear during an attack, but 10 to 15 ulcers are not uncommon.
● Ulcers may be so painful during first 2 or 3 days that they interfere with eating or speaking.
● Ulcers are preceded by tingling or burning for 24 hours (sometimes).

CAUSES—Unknown, but following are the most likely causes:
● Emotional or physical stress, anxiety or premenstrual tension.
● Injury to the mouth lining caused by rough dentures, hot food, toothbrushing or dental work.
● Irritation from foods, such as chocolate, citrus, acid foods (vinegar, pickles), salted nuts or potato chips.
● Virus infection.

RISK INCREASES WITH—Recent dental treatment.

HOW TO PREVENT
● Brush teeth at least twice a day and floss regularly to keep the mouth clean and healthy.
● Avoid stress if possible. See Appendix 13.
● Observe if canker sores develop after eating specific foods. Don't eat foods that seem to trigger attacks.

WHAT TO EXPECT

APPROPRIATE HEALTH CARE
● Self-care.
● Doctor's treatment.

DIAGNOSTIC MEASURES
● Your own observation of symptoms.
● Medical history and physical exam by a doctor.
● Laboratory culture of the sores.

POSSIBLE COMPLICATIONS—Dehydration in severe cases where eating and drinking are limited.

PROBABLE OUTCOME—Most ulcers heal without scarring in 2 weeks. Recurrent attacks are common. They vary from a single lesion 2 or 3 times a year to an uninterrupted succession of multiple lesions.

HOW TO TREAT

NOTE—Follow your doctor's instructions. These instructions are supplemental.

GENERAL MEASURES
● Rinse the mouth 3 or more times a day with a salt solution (1/2 teaspoon salt to 8 oz. water).
● Clean sores frequently with 2% hydrogen peroxide on a cotton applicator.
● If a canker sore is caused by a rough tooth, braces or dentures, consult your dentist. The sore won't heal until the cause is eliminated.

MEDICATION—Your doctor may prescribe:
● Topical anesthetics to relieve pain.
● Antibiotics, such as tetracycline, to fight infection. Tetracycline is effective if the liquid form is held in the mouth for 2 to 5 minutes to coat the ulcers before swallowing. If started early, it prevents pain.
● Protective dental paste with a steroid derivative, such as Orabase with triamcinolone acetonide. If applied as soon as the ulcer begins, this prevents pain.
  Keep medicine prescribed by your doctor for the first attack. Use it immediately at the sign of a recurrent attack. The sooner treatment starts, the milder the attack.

ACTIVITY—No restrictions.

DIET—No restrictions, except to avoid foods that aggravate ulcers. Drink as many fluids and eat as well-balanced a diet as possible while healing. To minimize pain, sip liquids through straws. Foods that cause the least pain are milk, liquid gelatin, yogurt, ice cream and custard.

CALL YOUR DOCTOR IF

● Temperature rises to 102F (38.9C) or higher.
● Ulcers don't improve in 3 days, despite treatment.
● Pain is unbearable and isn't relieved by treatment.
● A child with canker sores loses weight.

ILLNESSES & DISORDERS

CARCINOID SYNDROME

GENERAL INFORMATION

DEFINITION—Malignant tumors in the wall of the intestine. Carcinoids secrete serotonin, histamine, prostaglandins and hormones—powerful chemicals which cause carcinoid symptoms.

BODY PARTS INVOLVED—Primary tumors appear in the appendix, ileum, rectum, ovaries or stomach. The malignancy may spread and cause symptoms that affect the skin, blood vessels, kidney, gastrointestinal tract and liver.

SEX OR AGE MOST AFFECTED—Adults of both sexes.

SIGNS & SYMPTOMS—Carcinoids are slow-growing, and many persons with these tumors have no symptoms. The primary tumor may cause intestinal obstruction, characterized by painful cramps in the middle of the abdomen, vomiting and abdominal swelling.

In a few cases, carcinoid cells spread to other body parts and produce secondary, hormone-producing (serotonin) tumors. Heavy exercise, alcohol consumption, or eating bananas, tomatoes, plums, avocados, pineapple or walnuts may trigger symptoms of these secondary tumors. These symptoms include:
- Flushed skin on the head and neck.
- Watery eyes.
- Diarrhea with abdominal cramps.
- Respiratory symptoms similar to asthma.
- Congestive heart failure.
- Irregular heartbeat.
- Nausea and vomiting.
- Low blood pressure.
- Unexplained weight loss.

CAUSES—Unknown.

RISK INCREASES WITH
- Adults over 60.
- Obesity.
- Smoking.
- Excess alcohol consumption.

HOW TO PREVENT—Cannot be prevented at present.

WHAT TO EXPECT

APPROPRIATE HEALTH CARE
- Self-care after diagnosis.
- Doctor's treatment.

DIAGNOSTIC MEASURES
- Your own observation of symptoms.
- Medical history and physical exam by a doctor.
- Laboratory urine studies.
- X-rays of the abdominal organs.
- Sigmoidoscopy and CAT scan of the colon (see Glossary for both).
- Biopsy (see Glossary).

POSSIBLE COMPLICATIONS—Malignancy may spread to other body parts.

PROBABLE OUTCOME—This condition is currently considered incurable. However, symptoms can be relieved or controlled, and survival is possible for 10 to 15 years.

Scientific research into causes and treatment continues, so there is hope for increasingly effective treatment and cure.

HOW TO TREAT

NOTE—Follow your doctor's instructions. These instructions are supplemental.

GENERAL MEASURES—No special instructions except those listed under other headings.

MEDICATION—For minor diarrhea, you may use non-prescription drugs, such as Pepto-Bismol.
Your doctor may prescribe:
- Anticancer drugs to kill malignant cells.
- Methyldopa to prevent formation of serotonins.
- Phenothiazines to prevent flushed skin.
- Cortisone drugs to reduce inflammation anywhere in the body.

ACTIVITY—Resume your normal activities as soon as symptoms improve, but avoid strenuous exercise.

DIET
- Include at least 2 protein servings a day.
- Take niacin and tryptophan supplements.
- Avoid foods that trigger symptoms of secondary tumors.
- Don't drink alcohol.

CALL YOUR DOCTOR IF

- You have symptoms of carcinoid syndrome.
- Symptoms become disabling, despite treatment.
- New, unexplained symptoms develop.
Drugs used in treatment may produce side effects.

CARDIAC ARREST

GENERAL INFORMATION

DEFINITION—Total loss of heart-pumping action. Delay of treatment for only 3 to 5 minutes may cause death or permanent brain damage.

BODY PARTS INVOLVED—Heart.

SEX OR AGE MOST AFFECTED—More common in men until age 45, then the incidence is equal in men and women.

SIGNS & SYMPTOMS
- Brief dizziness, followed by fainting and unconsciousness.
- No pulse.
- No breathing.
- Bluish-white skin.
- Dilated pupils.
- Seizures.
- Loss of bowel and bladder control (sometimes).
Simple fainting may resemble cardiac arrest, but pulse and breathing continue.

CAUSES
- Heartbeat irregularities.
- Heart attack (myocardial infarction, atherosclerotic heart disease).
- Lack of blood circulation and profound shock caused by a hemorrhage.
- Loss of oxygen from drowning, choking or anesthesia.
- Major changes in the blood's electrolyte composition, as with a potassium or fluid imbalance.

RISK INCREASES WITH
- Stress.
- Diabetes mellitus.
- Use of drugs, such as:
  Digitalis. Even a minor excess of this powerful drug can disturb heart rhythm.
  Diuretics. These can cause low potassium in the blood.
  Adrenalin or any drug that raises blood pressure in a heart patient, including cold capsules, decongestant tablets and nasal sprays.

HOW TO PREVENT
- Obtain immediate medical treatment for any conditions listed as Causes. Refer to appropriate chart in Illness section.
- If you have heart disease, learn all you can about *all* the drugs you take, including non-prescription drugs.

WHAT TO EXPECT

APPROPRIATE HEALTH CARE—Emergency care by others present when cardiac arrest occurs.

DIAGNOSTIC MEASURES—Your observation of symptoms. See Signs & Symptoms.

POSSIBLE COMPLICATIONS
- Death or permanent brain damage if heart action cannot be resumed in 3 to 5 minutes.
- Mistaking a faint or other causes of unconsciousness for cardiac arrest. Check for a neck pulse before starting cardiopulmonary resuscitation (CPR).

PROBABLE OUTCOME—Bystanders skilled in recognizing cardiac arrest and performing CPR can often restore heartbeat. The final outcome, however, depends on the underlying cause of the cardiac arrest. The victim must be taken to the nearest emergency facility as soon as the heartbeat is restored. Cardiac arrest may recur.

HOW TO TREAT

NOTE—Follow your doctor's instructions. These instructions are supplemental.

GENERAL MEASURES
- Learn CPR. Call your local Red Cross or hospital for information. You may save a life.
- If you have heart trouble, or are at risk, wear a Medic-Alert bracelet or pendant (see Glossary).

MEDICATION—Administer oxygen, if available, after CPR has restored a heartbeat. (Emergency oxygen may be available in welder's shops.)
   The doctor may later prescribe medications to treat the underlying cause of cardiac arrest.

ACTIVITY—After recovery, activities should be resumed gradually. Sexual relations should be resumed only after medical clearance from the doctor.

DIET—Don't give fluid or foods to anyone with signs of cardiac arrest. He or she could choke.

CALL YOUR DOCTOR IF

If the victim is unconscious and *not* breathing:
- Yell for help. Don't leave the victim.
- Begin mouth-to-mouth breathing immediately.
- If there is no heartbeat, give external cardiac massage.
- Have someone call 0 (operator) or 911 (emergency) for an ambulance or medical help.
- Don't stop CPR until help arrives.

CARDIOMYOPATHY
(Hypertrophic Cardiomyopathy; Nutritional Cardiomyopathy)

 GENERAL INFORMATION

DEFINITION—A disorder of the heart muscle usually associated with alcoholism. The heart muscle is weakened and cannot pump blood efficiently.

BODY PARTS INVOLVED—Heart muscle. Decreasing heart function eventually affects the lungs, liver and circulatory system.

SEX OR AGE MOST AFFECTED
- Both sexes, but more common in males.
- All ages, but most common in adults.

SIGNS & SYMPTOMS—If cardiomyopathy is extensive enough to cause congestive heart failure, the following symptoms may occur:
- Irregular or rapid heartbeat.
- Shortness of breath with activity.
- Swelling of the feet and ankles.
- Fatigue.
- Cough with frothy, bloody sputum.
- Appetite loss.
- Loss of sex drive.

CAUSES
- Nutritional deficiency, especially of vitamin B-4 (thiamine).
- Mineral deficiency, especially of potassium.
- Fat tissue in the heart that replaces muscle fibers.
- Amyloid deposits (see Glossary) due to other disorders.
- Tuberous sclerosis (see Glossary).
- Hemochromatosis (see Glossary).
- Severe anemia.
- Friedreich's ataxia (see Glossary).
- Stress.
- Virus infection (rare).

RISK INCREASES WITH
- Adults over 60.
- Obesity.
- Smoking.
- Alcoholism.
- Family history of cardiomyopathy.
- Use of certain drugs, such as diuretics.

HOW TO PREVENT
- Drink alcohol moderately (1 or 2 drinks a day or none at all).
- Eat a well-balanced diet.

 WHAT TO EXPECT

APPROPRIATE HEALTH CARE
- Self-care after diagnosis.
- Doctor's treatment.

DIAGNOSTIC MEASURES
- Your own observation of symptoms.
- Medical history and physical exam by a doctor.
- EKG (see Glossary).
- X-rays of the heart and lungs.

POSSIBLE COMPLICATIONS—Congestive heart failure.

PROBABLE OUTCOME
- If the underlying disorder can be corrected, cardiomyopathy may be curable.
- If the underlying cause can't be corrected, cardiomyopathy is incurable. Some patients are candidates for a heart transplant.

 HOW TO TREAT

NOTE—Follow your doctor's instructions. These instructions are supplemental.

GENERAL MEASURES—Weigh daily before breakfast and record the weight. Report any marked weight change to your doctor. This may indicate excess fluid accumulation.

MEDICATION—Your doctor may prescribe:
- Digitalis to improve heart function.
- Diuretics to decrease fluid retention.
- Vitamins or potassium supplements (if the disorder is caused by a deficiency).

ACTIVITY—After treatment:
- Resume your normal activities gradually.
- Resume sexual relations when your sense of well-being allows and symptoms are controlled.

DIET—Low-salt diet (see Appendix 9).

 CALL YOUR DOCTOR IF

- You have symptoms of cardiomyopathy or symptoms recur after treatment.
- You have chest pain.
- New, unexplained symptoms develop. Drugs used in treatment may produce side effects.

CARPAL-TUNNEL SYNDROME

 ## GENERAL INFORMATION

DEFINITION—A nerve disorder in the hand that causes pain and loss of feeling, especially in the thumb and first 3 fingers.

BODY PARTS INVOLVED—Median nerve at the wrist joint; blood vessels, nerves and tendons of the hand.

SEX OR AGE MOST AFFECTED—Both sexes, but most common in women between ages 29 and 62.

SIGNS & SYMPTOMS
- Tingling or numbness in part of the hand.
- Sharp pains that shoot from the wrist up the arm, especially at night.
- Burning sensations in the fingers.
- Thumb weakness.
- Frequent dropping of objects.
- Inability to make a fist.
- Shiny, dry skin on the hand.

CAUSES—Pressure on the median nerve caused by swollen, inflamed or scarred tissue. The sources of pressure include:
- Inflammation of the tendon sheaths, frequently from arthritis.
- Fracture of the forearm.
- Sprain or dislocation of the wrist.

RISK INCREASES WITH
- Diabetes mellitus.
- Hypothyroidism.
- Menopause.
- Raynaud's disease.
- Pregnancy.
- Work that requires strong hand or wrist action.

HOW TO PREVENT—Cannot be prevented at present.

 ## WHAT TO EXPECT

APPROPRIATE HEALTH CARE
- Self-care after diagnosis.
- Doctor's treatment.
- Surgery to free the pinched nerve.

DIAGNOSTIC MEASURES
- Your own observation of symptoms.
- Medical history and physical exam by a doctor.
- Electromyograms (see Glossary).
- X-rays of the hand and wrist.

POSSIBLE COMPLICATIONS—Permanent numbness and a weak thumb or fingers in the affected hand.

PROBABLE OUTCOME—Usually curable—sometimes spontaneously, sometimes with surgery.

 ## HOW TO TREAT

NOTE—Follow your doctor's instructions. These instructions are supplemental.

GENERAL MEASURES
- Discomfort improves by shaking hands or dangling arms. If you awaken at night with pain in your hand, hang it over the side of the bed; rub or shake it.
- Consult your doctor about wearing a splint on the affected wrist at night.

MEDICATION—Your doctor may prescribe:
- Diuretics to decrease fluid retention that causes swollen tissue.
- Anti-inflammatory drugs to reduce inflammation.
- Cortisone injections at the wrist to reduce inflammation.

ACTIVITY—Stay as active as your strength allows. If surgery has been necessary, allow 4 weeks for recovery. Exercises may be prescribed for the hand.

DIET—Eat a normal, well-balanced diet that is low in sodium (see Appendix 9).

 ## CALL YOUR DOCTOR IF

Symptoms of carpal-tunnel syndrome don't disappear in 2 weeks.

CAT-SCRATCH FEVER

GENERAL INFORMATION

DEFINITION—A mild infectious disease of unknown cause resulting from a scratch by a cat. It is not contagious from person to person. More than one family member can be infected at one time.

BODY PARTS INVOLVED—Skin; lymph glands.

SEX OR AGE MOST AFFECTED—Both sexes; all ages.

SIGNS & SYMPTOMS
- A lump, with or without pus or fluid, which starts on the scratched skin 1 to 2 weeks after the cat scratch.
- Swollen lymph glands near the affected area.
- Low fever of 99F to 101F (37.2C to 38.3C).
- Fatigue.
- Headache.

CAUSES—Infection from germ—probably viral—carried on cat's claws. The infection spreads to lymph glands near the scratch by way of lymphatic vessels.

RISK INCREASES WITH—Owning or handling cats.

HOW TO PREVENT
- Have cats declawed by the veterinarian.
- Teach children to respect animals and not provoke them.
- Don't pick up strange cats.

WHAT TO EXPECT

APPROPRIATE HEALTH CARE
- Self-care.
- Doctor's treatment.
- Surgery to drain the lymph gland, if it contains pus.

DIAGNOSTIC MEASURES
- Your own observation of symptoms.
- Medical history and physical exam by a doctor. Tell your doctor of any cat scratches in the previous 2 weeks.
- Laboratory skin test to confirm the diagnosis.

POSSIBLE COMPLICATIONS—Eye inflammation (rare).

PROBABLE OUTCOME—Spontaneous recovery within 3 weeks.

HOW TO TREAT

NOTE—Follow your doctor's instructions. These instructions are supplemental.

GENERAL MEASURES
- It is not necessary to isolate the ill person because the disease is not transmitted from person to person.
- It should not be necessary to destroy the cat. Consult your veterinarian.

MEDICATION—Your doctor may prescribe antibiotics, although their effectiveness is not proven.

ACTIVITY—Rest in bed until fever subsides and energy returns. Resume your normal activities gradually.

DIET—No special diet.

CALL YOUR DOCTOR IF

- You have symptoms of cat-scratch fever.
- A swollen lymph gland becomes painful and red. This may indicate that a doctor should open and drain the infected gland.

CATARACT

GENERAL INFORMATION

DEFINITION—A clouding of the lens of the eye. The lens is a crystal-clear, flexible structure near the front of the eyeball. It helps to keep vision in focus, and screens and refracts light rays.

The lens has no blood supply. It is nourished by the vitreous (watery substance that surrounds it). If hardening of the arteries prevents proper nourishment of the vitreous—as often occurs in aging—the lens loses its nourishment also. The lens may then become less transparent and flexible, and form cataracts.

Cataracts may form in one or both eyes. If they form in both eyes, their growth rate may be very different. Cataracts are not cancerous.

BODY PARTS INVOLVED—Lens of the eye(s).

SEX OR AGE MOST AFFECTED
- Adults over 60.
- Newborns (congenital form only).

SIGNS & SYMPTOMS
- Blurred vision that may be worse in bright light. The blurring may first become apparent to one while driving at night, when lights seem to scatter or have halos.
- Double vision (occasionally).
- Opaque, milky-white pupil (advanced stages only).

CAUSES
- Natural aging.
- Injury to the eye.
- Illnesses associated with high blood sugar, such as diabetes mellitus.
- Inflammation, such as uveitis (see Glossary).
- Drugs, especially cortisone and its derivatives.
- Exposure to X-rays, microwaves and infrared radiation.
- Hereditary causes, including the effect of German measles on the unborn child of a mother who contracts the disease early in pregnancy.
- Galactosemia (see Glossary) in an infant.

RISK INCREASES WITH
- Adults over 60.
- Exposure to any causes listed above.

HOW TO PREVENT
- Women of childbearing age should be vaccinated against German measles if they have not had the disease or been immunized.
- The use of cortisone drugs or any others that affect the eye lens should be monitored carefully by a doctor.
- Eye disorders which may cause cataract formation, such as iritis and uveitis, should receive prompt medical treatment.

WHAT TO EXPECT

APPROPRIATE HEALTH CARE
- Doctor's (ophthalmologist's) treatment.
- Surgery to remove the lens.

DIAGNOSTIC MEASURES
- Your own observation of symptoms.
- Medical history and physical exam by a doctor.

POSSIBLE COMPLICATIONS
- Loss of vision.
- Postoperative complications, including rupture of the eye, adhesions, infections and retinal detachment.

PROBABLE OUTCOME—Usually curable with surgery. Some cataracts never impair vision enough to require surgery. During the time cataracts are forming, frequent eyeglass changes may help vision.

HOW TO TREAT

NOTE—Follow your doctor's instructions. These instructions are supplemental.

GENERAL MEASURES—For a description of cataract surgery and postoperative care, see Cataract Removal (in Surgery section). Special eyeglasses or contact lenses will be needed after surgery.

MEDICATION—Medicine usually is not necessary for this disorder.

ACTIVITY—No restrictions, except don't drive at night if your vision is poor.

DIET—No special diet.

CALL YOUR DOCTOR IF

You have symptoms of cataracts.

CELIAC DISEASE
(Gluten Enteropathy; Non-Tropical Sprue)

 GENERAL INFORMATION

DEFINITION—An allergic condition in the small intestine, triggered by gluten, which prevents the intestine from absorbing nutrients. Most forms are inherited. Celiac disease is not contagious or cancerous.

BODY PARTS INVOLVED—Digestive system.

SEX OR AGE MOST AFFECTED—Usually begins during infancy or early childhood (2 weeks to 1 year). Symptoms appear when the child first begins eating food with gluten. Rarely, celiac disease may appear for the first time in adults.

SIGNS & SYMPTOMS
- Weight loss or slowed weight gain in an infant following the introduction of cereal to the diet.
- Poor appetite.
- Loose, pale, bulky, bad-smelling stools; frequent gas.
- Swollen abdomen; abdominal pain.
- General undernourished appearance.
- Mouth ulcers.
- Anemia or vitamin deficiency, with fatigue, paleness, skin rash, or bone pain.
- Mildly bowed legs in children.

CAUSES—Celiac disease is a congenital disorder caused by an intolerance for gluten, a protein present in most grains.

RISK INCREASES WITH
- Family history of celiac disease.
- Pregnancy.
- Other allergies.

HOW TO PREVENT—Cannot be prevented at present.

 WHAT TO EXPECT

APPROPRIATE HEALTH CARE
- Home care.
- Doctor's treatment.

DIAGNOSTIC MEASURES
- Your own observation of symptoms.
- Medical history and physical exam by a doctor.
- Laboratory studies of stool and blood.
- X-rays of the digestive system.

POSSIBLE COMPLICATIONS—In rare cases, gluten withdrawal does not bring immediate improvement.

PROBABLE OUTCOME—With a strict, gluten-free diet, most persons with celiac disease can expect a normal life. Improvement begins in 2 to 3 weeks.

 HOW TO TREAT

NOTE—Follow your doctor's instructions. These instructions are supplemental.

GENERAL MEASURES—No special instructions except those listed under other headings.

MEDICATION—Your doctor may prescribe:
- Iron and folic acid for anemia.
- Calcium and multiple-vitamin supplements for deficiencies.
- Oral cortisone drugs to reduce the body's inflammatory response during a severe attack.

ACTIVITY—No restrictions.

DIET—Gluten-free diet (see Appendix 5). It is difficult to exclude gluten from the diet completely, so be patient while becoming familiar with the diet.

 CALL YOUR DOCTOR IF

- You or your child have symptoms of celiac disease.
- Symptoms don't decrease within 3 weeks after beginning a gluten-free diet.
- The child fails to regain lost weight or grow and develop as expected.
- Fever develops.

CELLULITIS
(Erysipelas)

GENERAL INFORMATION

DEFINITION—A non-contagious infection of connective tissue beneath the skin.

BODY PARTS INVOLVED—Skin anywhere on the body, but most likely on the face or lower legs.

SEX OR AGE MOST AFFECTED—Both sexes; all ages.

SIGNS & SYMPTOMS
- Sudden tenderness, swelling, and redness in an area of the skin. The area of cellulitis is initially 5cm to 20cm in diameter, and grows rapidly in the first 24 hours. A thin red line often extends from the middle of the cellulitis toward the heart. Cellulitis does not develop into a boil.
- Fever, sometimes accompanied by chills and sweats.
- General ill feeling.
- Swollen lymph glands nearest the cellulitis (sometimes).

CAUSES—Infection from staphylococcus or streptococcus bacteria.

RISK INCREASES WITH
- Use of immunosuppressive or cortisone drugs.
- Chronic illness, such as diabetes mellitus, or a recent infection that has lowered resistance.
- Any injury that breaks the skin.

HOW TO PREVENT
- Avoid skin damage. Use protective clothing or gear if you participate in strenuous work or sports.
- Keep the skin clean.

WHAT TO EXPECT

APPROPRIATE HEALTH CARE
- Self-care after diagnosis.
- Doctor's treatment.

DIAGNOSTIC MEASURES
- Your own observation of symptoms.
- Medical history and physical exam by a doctor.
- Laboratory blood culture, if blood poisoning is suspected.

POSSIBLE COMPLICATIONS
- Blood poisoning, if bacteria enter the bloodstream.
- Brain infection or meningitis, if cellulitis occurs on the central part of the face.

PROBABLE OUTCOME—Usually curable in 7 to 10 days with treatment, unless the patient has a chronic disease or is receiving immunosuppressive treatment. In that case, cellulitis may lead to blood poisoning and become life-threatening.

HOW TO TREAT

NOTE—Follow your doctor's instructions. These instructions are supplemental.

GENERAL MEASURES—Use warm-water soaks (see Glossary) to hasten healing and relieve pain and inflammation.

MEDICATION—Your doctor may prescribe a penicillin drug, such as oxacillin, dicloxacillin or nafcillin, or erythromycin to fight infection. Finish the prescribed dose, even if symptoms disappear.

ACTIVITY—Rest in bed until fever disappears and other symptoms improve. Resume your normal activities as soon as symptoms improve.

DIET—No special diet. Vitamin-C supplements (250mg to 500mg daily) may hasten healing.

CALL YOUR DOCTOR IF

- You have symptoms of cellulitis, especially on the face.
- The following occurs during treatment:
  Fever of 101F (38.3C) or higher.
  Drowsiness and lethargy.
  Blister over the area of cellulitis.
  Red streaks that continue to extend, despite treatment.
- New, unexplained symptoms develop. Drugs used in treatment may produce side effects.

ILLNESSES & DISORDERS

CEREBRAL PALSY (CP)

GENERAL INFORMATION

DEFINITION—A group of muscular and nervous-system disorders that begins in infancy and causes varying degrees of disability. Cerebral palsy is not inherited.

BODY PARTS INVOLVED—Central nervous system; muscular system.

SEX OR AGE MOST AFFECTED—Usually begins in infancy and remains throughout life.

SIGNS & SYMPTOMS—Number and severity of the following symptoms vary widely among children with CP:
- Early sucking difficulty with the breast or bottle.
- Lack of normal muscle tone (early).
- Slow development (walking, talking).
- Unusual body postures.
- Stiffness and muscle spasms (later).
- Purposeless body movements.
- Poor coordination or balance.
- Crossed eyes.
- Deafness.
- Convulsions.
- Various degrees of mental retardation.

CAUSES—Defects in the brain and spinal column. The reason for these defects is often unknown. Known reasons include:
- Birth injury, including prolonged oxygen deprivation.
- Use of drugs during pregnancy that damage the fetus.
- Infections, such as German measles, in the mother during pregnancy.
- Rh incompatibility or bile blockage in the newborn.
- Meningitis or encephalitis during infancy or childhood.

RISK INCREASES WITH
- Prematurity.
- Excess alcohol consumption during pregnancy.

HOW TO PREVENT
- Before becoming pregnant, obtain immunizations against German measles, if you have never had the disease or an immunization.
- Arrange for good medical care during pregnancy, labor and delivery.
- Eat a normal, well-balanced diet during pregnancy.
- Don't drink alcohol or use any drug, including non-prescription drugs, during pregnancy without consulting your doctor.

WHAT TO EXPECT

APPROPRIATE HEALTH CARE
- Home care.
- Doctor's treatment.

- Psychotherapy or counseling to help the family accept the disease and help the child achieve maximum potential.
- Surgery to correct muscular-system deformities (sometimes).
- Time in an extended-care facility for children with severe CP (sometimes).

DIAGNOSTIC MEASURES
- Your own observation of symptoms.
- Medical history and physical exam by a doctor (sometimes a neurologist). A parent's intuition is often important. Obtain a second opinion, if necessary.
- Laboratory blood studies.
- EEG (see Glossary).
- Psychological tests.

POSSIBLE COMPLICATIONS
- Hepatitis, if the child is institutionalized.
- Pressure sores, if the child is confined to bed.

PROBABLE OUTCOME—Children vary widely in the severity of this condition. A child with CP may have high intelligence despite major muscular disability. Many children can be cared for in a loving home. Those with less-severe impairment can lead near-normal, productive lives. Children with severe impairments may require special care.

HOW TO TREAT

NOTE—Follow your doctor's instructions. These instructions are supplemental.

GENERAL MEASURES
- Because early diagnosis is important, be sure your child has regular medical checkups. Failure to diagnose CP may deny the child opportunities for special programs that maximize growth and development.
- Maintain an optimistic outlook for yourself and your child. High expectations can sometimes be met.
- Seek help and advice from other parents whose children have cerebral palsy.
- Investigate resources in your community, including educational and physical-therapy programs, to obtain treatment that maximizes your child's capabilities.

MEDICATION—Your doctor may prescribe:
- Anticonvulsants to control seizures.
- Muscle relaxants to relieve spasms.

ACTIVITY—Encourage your child to do as much as he or she can do.

DIET—No special diet.

CALL YOUR DOCTOR IF

You are concerned about your child's development or suspect CP.

CERVICAL EROSION

GENERAL INFORMATION

DEFINITION—A condition in which the lining of the uterus spreads to cover the tip of the cervix. This abnormally placed tissue is more likely to become inflamed or infected. It is not cancerous.

BODY PARTS INVOLVED—Cervix; uterus lining.

SEX OR AGE MOST AFFECTED—Adolescent and adult females.

SIGNS & SYMPTOMS
- No symptoms (usually).
- Increased mucus discharge from the vagina (sometimes).
- Unexplained vaginal bleeding (sometimes).

CAUSES—Usually unknown, but may accompany pregnancy, childbirth or the use of oral contraceptives.

RISK INCREASES WITH
- Stress.
- Repeated vaginal infections.
- Obesity.

HOW TO PREVENT—Cannot be prevented at present.

WHAT TO EXPECT

APPROPRIATE HEALTH CARE
- Doctor's treatment.
- Minor surgery to cauterize or freeze the cervix (if a Pap smear is normal). Surgery is often done without anesthesia in the doctor's office or an out-patient surgical facility.
- Conization of the cervix (see Glossary) or hysterectomy (in Surgery section), if a Pap smear is not normal.

DIAGNOSTIC MEASURES
- Medical history and physical exam—including pelvic examination—by a doctor.
- Pap smear (see Glossary)

POSSIBLE COMPLICATIONS—Occasionally precedes cancer of the cervix.

PROBABLE OUTCOME—Disorder is usually curable with treatment. Allow 3 months for the cervix to return completely to normal. Cervical erosion frequently recurs.

HOW TO TREAT

NOTE—Follow your doctor's instructions. These instructions are supplemental.

GENERAL MEASURES
- Don't douche unless instructed to by your doctor.
- Obtain medical treatment for any vaginal infection you may also have.
- Use pads instead of tampons during menstruation.

MEDICATION—Your doctor may prescribe oral antibiotics or topical antibiotics to apply to the cervix.

ACTIVITY—After treatment (except following a hysterectomy), normal activity and sexual relations may be resumed immediately.

DIET—No special diet.

CALL YOUR DOCTOR IF

- You have symptoms of cervical erosion.
- The following occurs after treatment:
  Increased discharge.
  Pain with intercourse or bleeding afterward.
  Vaginal bleeding between periods.
- New, unexplained symptoms develop.
Drugs used in treatment may produce side effects.

CERVICAL POLYPS

GENERAL INFORMATION

DEFINITION—Small, fragile, bulbous growths on stalks protruding through the cervix from the lining inside the uterus. They may be single or numerous.

BODY PARTS INVOLVED—Endometrium (thin membrane lining the uterus); cervix (lower third of the uterus).

SEX OR AGE MOST AFFECTED—Women of all ages.

SIGNS & SYMPTOMS
- Unexpected spotting of blood between menstrual periods.
- Spotting of blood after sexual intercourse or bowel movements.
- Vaginal discharge.

CAUSES—Cervical polyps are caused by cervix inflammation from infection, erosion or ulceration. They frequently accompany chronic infections in the vagina or cervix, although they are not contagious. The small growths are usually benign, but in very rare cases, they represent early cancer of the cervix.

RISK INCREASES WITH
- Diabetes mellitus.
- Recurrent vaginitis or cervicitis.

HOW TO PREVENT—To prevent vaginal or cervix infections that can precede cervical polyps:
- Wear cotton panties or pantyhose with a cotton crotch to prevent accumulation of excess heat and moisture, which can make you susceptible to vaginal and cervical infections. Don't wear panties made from non-ventilating materials.
- If you must take antibiotics for any reason, eat yogurt (with active yogurt cultures rather than pasteurized) or take acidophilus tablets (available from your pharmacy without prescription). This reduces the chance that antibiotics will irritate the cervix or vagina.
- Avoid contracting gonorrhea or other sexually transmitted diseases by having your sexual partner wear a rubber condom during intercourse.

WHAT TO EXPECT

APPROPRIATE HEALTH CARE
- Self-care after diagnosis and treatment.
- Doctor's treatment, including surgery to remove cervical polyps with a wire snare, electrocautery or liquid nitrogen. This can often be done in a simple office procedure. Your doctor may cauterize the cervix after removing the polyp to prevent regrowth of the same or another polyp.

A polyp that accompanies cervicitis (inflammation or infection of the cervix) may require more extensive surgery. See Cervicitis.

DIAGNOSTIC MEASURES
- Your own observation of symptoms.
- Medical history and physical exam by a doctor.
- Laboratory studies, such as a Pap smear (see Glossary) and examination of the vaginal discharge.

POSSIBLE COMPLICATIONS—None expected, but in very rare instances, cervical polyps may become malignant.

PROBABLE OUTCOME—Usually curable with surgery. You may feel brief, mild pain during the procedure and have mild to moderate cramps for several hours. Spotting of blood from the vagina may occur for 1 or 2 days.

HOW TO TREAT

NOTE—Follow your doctor's instructions. These instructions are supplemental.

MEDICATION—Your doctor may apply medication to the affected parts during office treatment. In addition, he or she may prescribe antibiotics by mouth or in vaginal suppositories or creams to fight infection.

GENERAL MEASURES
- Don't douche unless your doctor recommends it.
- Use small sanitary pads to protect your clothing from creams or suppositories.
- Keep creams or suppositories in the refrigerator.

ACTIVITY—No restrictions. Delay sexual relations until your doctor performs a follow-up pelvic exam and determines that healing is complete.

DIET—No special diet.

CALL YOUR DOCTOR IF

- You have symptoms of cervical polyps.
- The following occur after treatment:
  Discomfort persists longer than 1 week.
  Symptoms recur.
  Unexplained vaginal bleeding or swelling develops.
- New, unexplained symptoms develop. Drugs used in treatment may produce side effects.

CERVICAL SPONDYLOSIS
(Cervical Musculoskeletal Discomfort; Cervical Radiculopathy)

 GENERAL INFORMATION

DEFINITION—Degenerative changes of bones in the neck that place pressure on nerves and muscles to the arms, legs and bladder.

BODY PARTS INVOLVED
- 7 bones of the neck.
- Disks between the bones.
- Blood vessels to the head.
- Bladder and lower legs (advanced stages).

SEX OR AGE MOST AFFECTED—Adults of both sexes.

SIGNS & SYMPTOMS—Any of the following:
- Pain in the neck, radiating to the shoulder blades, top of the shoulders, upper arms, hands or back of the head.
- Crunching sounds with movement of the neck or shoulder muscles.
- Numbness and tingling in the arms, hands and fingers; some loss of feeling in the hands.
- Muscle weakness and deterioration; diminished reflexes.
- Neck stiffness.
- Headache.
- Dizziness.
- Double vision.
- With advanced disease, loss of bladder control and leg weakness.

CAUSES
- Arthritis (inflammation of a joint).
- Injuries such as: automobile accidents with "whiplash" injury; athletic injuries; sudden jerks on the arms; falls.
- Osteoarthritis (wear and tear on joints that accompanies aging).
- Outgrowths of bone that sometimes occur with aging.

RISK INCREASES WITH
- Adults over 60.
- Fatigue or overwork.
- Neck injury

HOW TO PREVENT
- Avoid sitting in cramped positions.
- Sleep without pillows. Use a soft fabric collar or towel to support the neck.
- Avoid injury. Wear protective headgear for contact sports. Use seat belts or harnesses in vehicles.

 WHAT TO EXPECT

APPROPRIATE HEALTH CARE
- Self-care for mild symptoms.
- Doctor's treatment for signs of nerve-root pressure (symptoms in the head, arms or bladder) or pain.

- Surgery (sometimes) to fuse neck bones, remove a damaged disk or enlarge the spinal-cord space.

DIAGNOSTIC MEASURES
- Your own observation of symptoms.
- Medical history and physical exam by a doctor.
- Nerve-conduction studies.
- X-rays of the neck.

POSSIBLE COMPLICATIONS—Reduced neck flexibility after surgery or treatment.

PROBABLE OUTCOME—Minor symptoms usually respond well to treatment and subside slowly. Severe symptoms may persist indefinitely.

 HOW TO TREAT

NOTE—Follow your doctor's instructions. These instructions are supplemental.

GENERAL MEASURES
- Wear a soft fabric collar (Thomas collar) to prevent unexpected neck-muscle strain.
- Apply moist heat. Take hot showers and let the water beat on neck and shoulders for 10 to 20 minutes twice a day. Between showers, apply hot soaks to neck. Soak towel or cloth in hot water, wring out and apply.
- Use dry heat. Sit under a heat lamp for 10 to 15 minutes several times a day.
- Improve your posture. Pull in the chin and abdomen when sitting or standing. Use a firm chair and sit with buttocks against the back.
- Sleep without a pillow. Instead, use a cervical pillow, wear a soft fabric collar, or put a small rolled towel under the neck.
- If numbness or pain affects the hands or arms, buy or rent a cervical-traction apparatus. To set it up, follow directions that accompany the apparatus.

MEDICATION
- For minor discomfort or disability, you may use aspirin or acetaminophen.
- For serious discomfort, your doctor may prescribe stronger pain medicine, muscle relaxants or tranquilizers.

ACTIVITY—No restrictions.

DIET—No special diet.

 CALL YOUR DOCTOR IF

- You have symptoms of cervical spondylosis.
- Symptoms persist or worsen despite treatment.

CERVICITIS

GENERAL INFORMATION

DEFINITION—Inflammation or infection of the cervix. There are 2 types, and either may be contagious:
- Acute cervicitis is usually a bacterial or viral infection with specific symptoms.
- Chronic cervicitis is a long-term infection that may not have symptoms.

BODY PARTS INVOLVED—Cervix and mucous membranes covering the cervix.

SEX OR AGE MOST AFFECTED—Females of all ages after adolescence.

SIGNS & SYMPTOMS—Acute cervicitis:
- Pain in the vagina.
- Thick, yellow vaginal discharge.

Chronic cervicitis:
- Slight—sometimes unnoticeable—vaginal discharge.
- Backache.
- Discomfort with urination.
- Discomfort with sexual intercourse.

Extensive chronic cervicitis:
- Profuse vaginal discharge.
- Bleeding between menstrual periods.
- Spotting or bleeding after sexual intercourse.

CAUSES
- Acute cervicitis is usually caused by infection from one of many bacteria, including the one that causes gonorrhea, or herpes virus.
- Chronic cervicitis is caused by repeated episodes of acute cervicitis, or one episode that is not treated long enough to heal completely.

RISK INCREASES WITH
- Diabetes mellitus.
- Acute or recurrent vaginitis.

HOW TO PREVENT
- Wear cotton panties or pantyhose with a cotton crotch. Avoid panties made from non-ventilating materials. Synthetic materials hold in vaginal wetness and warmth, which may trigger vaginal or cervical infections.
- If you must take antibiotics for any reason, eat yogurt (with active yogurt cultures rather than pasteurized) or take acidophilus tablets (available from your pharmacy without prescription). This reduces the chance that antibiotics will allow growth of infectious organisms in the cervix or vagina.
- Avoid contracting gonorrhea or other sexually transmitted diseases by having your sexual partner wear a rubber condom for intercourse.

OTHER—If cervicitis is caused by a sexually transmitted infection, your sexual partner also needs treatment.

WHAT TO EXPECT

APPROPRIATE HEALTH CARE
- Self-care after diagnosis.
- Doctor's treatment, including destruction of abnormal cells with silver nitrate, cryosurgery or electrocautery (see Glossary for all).
- Surgery (hysterectomy) for widespread tissue destruction (rare).

DIAGNOSTIC MEASURES
- Your own observation of symptoms.
- Medical history and pelvic exam by a doctor.
- Laboratory studies, such as a Pap smear (see Glossary) and culture of the discharge.
- Biopsy of the cervix (see Glossary).

POSSIBLE COMPLICATIONS
- Cervical polyps.
- Pelvic inflammatory disease.
- Malignant change in cervix cells (rare).

PROBABLE OUTCOME—Mild cervicitis will heal without treatment.
  Acute cervicitis caused by venereal disease is contagious through sexual intercourse and is curable with medication.
  Most other cases of cervicitis can be cured with treatment in the doctor's office. All women with cervicitis need regular checkups until the condition heals.

HOW TO TREAT

NOTE—Follow your doctor's instructions. These Instructions are supplemental.

GENERAL MEASURES
- Use sanitary pads instead of tampons during treatment.
- Don't douche unless your doctor recommends it.

MEDICATION—Your doctor may prescribe antiviral or antibiotic vaginal creams or suppositories to fight infection.

ACTIVITY—No restrictions, except to avoid sexual relations until your doctor determines that the infection has healed.

DIET—No special diet.

☎ CALL YOUR DOCTOR IF

- You have symptoms of cervicitis.
- During treatment, discomfort persists longer than 1 week or symptoms worsen.
- Unexplained vaginal bleeding or swelling develops during or after treatment.
- New, unexplained symptoms develop. Drugs used in treatment may produce side effects.

CERVIX, CANCER OF

GENERAL INFORMATION

DEFINITION—A common but preventable cancer of the female reproductive system.

BODY PARTS INVOLVED—Cervix (the lower third of the uterus, which opens into the vagina).

SEX OR AGE MOST AFFECTED—Women of all ages, but most common between ages 30 and 50.

SIGNS & SYMPTOMS
In the early, easily treatable stages:
- No symptoms.

In later stages:
- Unexplained vaginal bleeding.
- Persistent vaginal discharge.
- Pain and bleeding after intercourse.

In final stages:
- Abdominal pain.
- Leaking of feces and urine through the vagina.
- Appetite and weight loss.
- Anemia.

CAUSES—Unknown.

RISK INCREASES WITH
- Frequent sexual intercourse during the teen years.
- Multiple sex partners.
- Multiple pregnancies.
- Recurrent vaginal infections (bacterial or viral, including genital herpes and genital warts).

HOW TO PREVENT
- Avoid the risks listed above as much as possible.
- Begin medical pelvic examinations at age 18 or at the beginning of regular sexual activity.
- Obtain regular Pap smears (see Glossary). Regular pelvic examinations and the Pap smear are very effective in detecting precancerous changes or cervical cancer in its symptom-free stage.

  Consult your doctor, Planned Parenthood or the public health department about how often to be examined. Many public agencies will perform a Pap smear at little or no cost to you.

WHAT TO EXPECT

APPROPRIATE HEALTH CARE
- Doctor's treatment.
- Surgery to remove the cancerous area. During early stages, this may only involve a small area of the cervix, which preserves childbearing abilities. More advanced stages may require removal of the reproductive organs and other affected tissue (see Hysterectomy in Surgery section).
- Chemotherapy and radiation therapy (advanced cancer).

DIAGNOSTIC MEASURES
- Your own observation of symptoms, especially unexplained vaginal bleeding.
- Medical history and physical exam by a doctor.
- Laboratory studies, such as a Pap smear and biopsy (see Glossary).
- Surgical diagnostic procedures, such as conization of the cervix (see Glossary).

POSSIBLE COMPLICATIONS—If cervical cancer is not treated early, it spreads beyond the uterus to other body parts—leading to death.

PROBABLE OUTCOME—Usually curable if diagnosed before the tumor has spread.

HOW TO TREAT

NOTE—Follow your doctor's instructions. These instructions are supplemental.

GENERAL MEASURES—No specific instructions except those listed under other headings.

MEDICATION—Medicine usually is not necessary for this disorder, if it is diagnosed and treated early. If radical surgery and additional treatment are required, your doctor may prescribe:
- Anticancer drugs.
- Pain relievers.

ACTIVITY—No restrictions.

DIET—No special diet.

CALL YOUR DOCTOR IF

- You have persistent vaginal bleeding or other symptoms of cervical cancer.
- You have not had a pelvic examination or Pap smear in at least 1 year.

ILLNESSES & DISORDERS

CHALAZION

GENERAL INFORMATION

DEFINITION—A mass on the eyelid resulting from chronic inflammation of a meibomian gland (gland which lubricates the lid margins).

BODY PARTS INVOLVED—Eyelid.

SEX OR AGE MOST AFFECTED—Adults of both sexes.

SIGNS & SYMPTOMS—A painless swelling on the eyelid, which at first may resemble a sty. The eyelid may swell, and the eye may feel irritated. After a few days, these early symptoms disappear, leaving a painless, slow-growing, firm lump in the eyelid. Skin over the lump can be moved loosely.

CAUSES—Blockage of a duct leading to the surface of the eyelid from the meibomian gland. The blockage may be due to infection (usually staphylococcal) around the duct opening.

RISK INCREASES WITH
- Stress.
- Fatigue or overwork.
- Use of eye cosmetics.
- Poor nutrition.

HOW TO PREVENT
- Wash hands often, and dry with clean towels.
- Avoid environments that contain dust or other irritating substances.
- Eat a normal, well-balanced diet.

WHAT TO EXPECT

APPROPRIATE HEALTH CARE
- Self-care.
- Doctor's treatment.
- Surgical removal under local anesthesia in the doctor's office, if the chalazion does not heal spontaneously in 6 weeks.

DIAGNOSTIC MEASURES
- Your own observation of symptoms.
- Medical history and physical exam by a doctor.
- Laboratory culture of the discharge from the chalazion.

POSSIBLE COMPLICATIONS—The eyelid infection may become chronic and spread to other glands in the eye.

PROBABLE OUTCOME—A chalazion may heal spontaneously. If not, it is usually curable with surgical removal.

HOW TO TREAT

NOTE—Follow your doctor's instructions. These instructions are supplemental.

GENERAL MEASURES—Use warm-water soaks (see Appendix 18) to reduce inflammation and hasten healing. Apply soaks for 20 minutes, then rest at least 1 hour. Repeat as often as needed.

MEDICATION—Your doctor may prescribe:
- Topical antibiotic ointments or creams, such as erythromycin or bacitracin. Apply a thin layer of medication to the lid edges 3 or 4 times daily. A heavy layer wastes medicine and is no more beneficial than a thin layer.
- Antibiotic eye drops to prevent the spread of infection to other parts of the eye. Oral antibiotics or antibiotic injections usually are not needed.

ACTIVITY—No restrictions.

DIET—No special diet.

CALL YOUR DOCTOR IF

- You have symptoms of a chalazion that last longer than 2 weeks.
- You have pain in the *eye*.
- Your vision changes.
- New, unexplained symptoms develop. Drugs used in treatment may produce side effects.

CHICKENPOX
(Varicella)

GENERAL INFORMATION

DEFINITION—A very contagious, mild disease caused by the herpes zoster virus.

BODY PARTS INVOLVED—Skin and mucous membranes.

SEX OR AGE MOST AFFECTED—All ages, but most common in children.

SIGNS & SYMPTOMS—The following are usually mild in children, severe in adults:
- Fever.
- Abdominal pain or a general ill feeling that lasts 1 or 2 days.
- Skin eruptions that appear almost anywhere on the body, including the scalp, penis, and inside the mouth, nose, throat or vagina. They may be scattered over large areas, and they occur least on the arms and legs. Blisters collapse within 24 hours and form scabs. New crops of blisters erupt every 3 to 4 days.

Adults have additional symptoms that resemble influenza.

CAUSES—Infection with the herpes zoster virus. Incubation after exposure is 7 to 21 days.

A newborn is protected for several months from chickenpox if the mother had the disease prior to or during pregnancy. The immunity diminishes in 10 to 12 months.

RISK INCREASES WITH—Use of immunosuppressive drugs.

HOW TO PREVENT—Cannot be prevented at present. An experimental vaccine is available for high-risk persons, such as those who take anticancer or immunosuppressive drugs.

WHAT TO EXPECT

APPROPRIATE HEALTH CARE
- Self-care after diagnosis.
- Doctor's diagnosis and treatment, if complications arise.

DIAGNOSTIC MEASURES
- Your own observation of symptoms.
- Medical history and physical exam by a doctor.

POSSIBLE COMPLICATIONS
- Secondary bacterial infection of chickenpox blisters.
- Encephalitis (rare).
- Shingles many years later in adulthood (possibly).
- Scarring (rare). This is more common if blisters become infected.

PROBABLE OUTCOME—Spontaneous recovery. Children usually recover in 7 to 10 days. Adults take longer and are more likely to develop complications.

After recovery, a person has lifelong immunity against a recurrence of chickenpox.

After chickenpox runs its course, the virus remains dormant in the body (probably in the roots of nerves near the spinal cord). The same virus may later cause shingles.

HOW TO TREAT

NOTE—Follow your doctor's instructions. These instructions are supplemental.

GENERAL MEASURES
- Use cool-water soaks (see Appendix 18) or cool-water compresses to reduce itching.
- Keep the patient as quiet and cool as possible. Heat and sweat trigger itching.
- Keep the nails short to discourage scratching, which can lead to secondary infection.

MEDICATION
- The following non-prescription medicines may decrease itching:

Steroid lotion, ointment or cream. This reduces inflammation and relieves itching in 24 to 48 hours.

Topical anesthetics and topical antihistamines, which provide quick, short-term relief. Preparations containing lidocaine and pramoxine are least likely to cause allergic skin reactions.

Lotions that contain phenol, menthol and camphor (such as calamine lotion). These are soothing, but use with care. Large amounts may be absorbed through the skin into the bloodstream, and they can be toxic.
- If you must reduce fever, use acetaminophen instead of aspirin. Aspirin may contribute to the development of Reye's syndrome, a form of encephalitis, when given to children during a viral illness.

ACTIVITY—Bed rest is not necessary. Allow quiet activity in a cool environment. A child may play outdoors in the shade during nice weather. Keep an ill child away from others until all blisters have crusted.

DIET—No special diet.

CALL YOUR DOCTOR IF

- You or your child have symptoms of chickenpox.
- Lethargy, headache or sensitivity to bright light develop.
- Fever rises over 103F (39.4C).
- Chickenpox lesions contain pus or otherwise appear infected.

CHOLECYSTITIS OR CHOLANGITIS, ACUTE

 GENERAL INFORMATION

DEFINITION—Infection or inflammation of the gallbladder (cholecystitis) or the ducts (cholangitis) that drain bile from the gallbladder to the small intestine.

BODY PARTS INVOLVED—Gallbladder (located under the liver); bile ducts in the liver, leading to the gallbladder.

SEX OR AGE MOST AFFECTED
- Both sexes, but more common in women.
- Adults, but may rarely occur in children or adolescents.

SIGNS & SYMPTOMS
- Cramping pain in the upper right of the abdomen. Pain may also occur in the chest (imitating a heart attack), in the upper back or the right shoulder. These symptoms frequently follow a meal rich in fats.
- Tenderness in the upper abdomen.
- Nausea and vomiting.
- Belching.
- Slight fever. If high fever and chills occur, a bacterial infection is present.
- Jaundice (sometimes).
- Pale stools (sometimes).
- Skin itching (sometimes).

CAUSES—Inflammation or bacterial infection, which are usually caused by gallstone formation and blockage of bile ducts.

RISK INCREASES WITH
- Diet that is high in fat.
- Gallstones, whether or not they have caused symptoms.
- Chronic or acute pancreatitis.
- Coronary-artery disease.

HOW TO PREVENT
- Avoid any food that gives you indigestion.
- Have surgery to remove gallstones, even if they cause no symptoms.

 WHAT TO EXPECT

APPROPRIATE HEALTH CARE
- Doctor's treatment.
- Surgery to remove an infected gallbladder and gallstones. Surgery is rarely an emergency.
- Hospitalization (usually).

DIAGNOSTIC MEASURES
- Your own observation of symptoms.
- Medical history and physical exam by a doctor.
- Laboratory blood studies.
- X-rays of the gallbladder.
- Ultrasonography (see Glossary) of the gallbladder and bile ducts.
- Fiber-optic study (see Glossary) of liver and pancreas ducts.

POSSIBLE COMPLICATIONS
- Gallbladder rupture and peritonitis.
- Gallbladder abscess.
- Misdiagnosis as a heart attack.

PROBABLE OUTCOME—Symptoms of some mild attacks subside spontaneously in 1 to 4 days, if no complications develop. Most episodes require hospitalization and treatment. Recurrences are common. Attacks will cease with surgery to remove the gallbladder.

 HOW TO TREAT

NOTE—Follow your doctor's instructions. These instructions are supplemental.

GENERAL MEASURES—After an acute attack of cholecystitis, consider having elective surgery to prevent a future emergency.

MEDICATION
- Don't medicate yourself with non-prescription pain relievers during an attack. These may mask symptoms of a bacterial infection—allowing it to worsen—and delay treatment.
- Your doctor may prescribe analgesics, including narcotics, to relieve pain.

ACTIVITY—Rest in bed until symptoms disappear or recovery from surgery is complete. While in bed, move your legs often to reduce the likelihood of deep-vein blood clotting. You may read or watch TV.

DIET—Because of nausea and vomiting, intravenous fluids are usually necessary during attacks.

 CALL YOUR DOCTOR IF

- You have symptoms of cholecystitis or cholangitis. If symptoms are accompanied by shortness of breath, sweating and nausea, call immediately!
- The following occurs during an attack: Temperature over 101F (38.3C). Jaundice. Recurrent vomiting. Intolerable pain.

CIRRHOSIS OF THE LIVER

GENERAL INFORMATION

DEFINITION—Chronic scarring of the liver, leading to loss of normal liver function.

BODY PARTS INVOLVED—Liver and its major blood vessels.

SEX OR AGE MOST AFFECTED—Adults of both sexes, but twice as common in men.

SIGNS & SYMPTOMS—Early stages:
- Fatigue; weakness.
- Poor appetite; nausea; weight loss.
- Enlarged liver.
- Red palms.

Late stages:
- Jaundice (yellow skin and eyes).
- Dark yellow or brown urine.
- Spider blood vessels of the skin (fine vessels which spread out from a central point).
- Hair loss.
- Breast enlargement in men.
- Fluid accumulation in the abdomen and legs.
- Enlarged spleen.
- Diarrhea; stool may be black or bloody.
- Bleeding and bruising.
- Mental confusion; coma.

CAUSES—Inflammation of the liver, accompanied by destruction of liver cells, cell regeneration and scarring. These may be preceded by:
- Prolonged, excess alcohol consumption.
- Hepatitis.
- Exposure to toxic chemicals.

RISK INCREASES WITH
- Poor nutrition.
- Hepatitis.
- Excess alcohol consumption. Individuals vary widely in the amount and duration of alcohol consumption necessary to cause cirrhosis.
- Occupational exposure to chemicals toxic to the liver.

HOW TO PREVENT
- Obtain treatment for alcoholism.
- Obtain prompt medical treatment for hepatitis.
- Survey your work environment for possible exposure to toxic chemicals.

WHAT TO EXPECT

APPROPRIATE HEALTH CARE
- Self-care after diagnosis.
- Doctor's treatment.
- Psychotherapy or counseling (for alcoholism).
- Surgery to relieve pressure of blood in abdominal veins (rare).

DIAGNOSTIC MEASURES
- Your own observation of symptoms.
- Medical history and physical exam by a doctor.
- Laboratory studies, such as blood and urine tests of liver function.

POSSIBLE COMPLICATIONS
- Life-threatening hemorrhage, especially from the esophagus and stomach.
- Liver cancer.
- Body poisoning and coma from a buildup of ammonia and other body waste.
- Sexual impotence.

PROBABLE OUTCOME—Cirrhosis can be arrested—no matter what the cause—if the underlying cause can be removed. Liver damage is irreversible, but symptoms can be relieved or controlled. A near-normal life is possible.

If the underlying cause is not removed, liver scarring will continue, resulting in death from liver failure.

HOW TO TREAT

NOTE—Follow your doctor's instructions. These instructions are supplemental.

GENERAL MEASURES—If cirrhosis is caused by alcoholism, try to stop drinking. Ask for help from family, friends and community agencies (see Alcoholism in Illness section).

MEDICATION—Your doctor may prescribe:
- Iron supplements for anemia resulting from hemorrhage or poor nutrition.
- Diuretics to reduce fluid retention.
- Antibiotics, such as neomycin, to reduce ammonia buildup.

ACTIVITY—Resume your normal activities as soon as symptoms improve.

DIET
- In the early stages, eat a well-balanced diet that is high in carbohydrates, high in protein and low in salt (see Appendix 9). Late stages may require protein reduction.
  Vitamin and mineral supplements may be necessary.
- Don't drink alcohol.

CALL YOUR DOCTOR IF

- You have symptoms of cirrhosis.
- The following occurs during treatment:
  Vomiting blood or passing black stool.
  Mental confusion or coma.
  Fever or other signs of infection (redness, swelling, tenderness or pain).

CLUBFOOT
(Talipes)

GENERAL INFORMATION

DEFINITION—An inherited deformity of the foot or feet. The condition is not painful, but if uncorrected, it prevents normal walking.

BODY PARTS INVOLVED—Feet.

SEX OR AGE MOST AFFECTED—Occurs more often in newborn boys than girls.

SIGNS & SYMPTOMS
- Foot or feet of the newborn point down, turn inward and curl under.
- Tendon from calf to heel is short.

CAUSES—A shortened Achilles tendon and deformed bones in the foot. This is an inherited condition or is caused by the position of the fetus in the uterus.

RISK INCREASES WITH—Unknown.

HOW TO PREVENT—Cannot be prevented at present. Crippling can be prevented with early diagnosis and treatment.

WHAT TO EXPECT

APPROPRIATE HEALTH CARE
- Doctor's treatment.
- Surgery to correct the deformity (rare).
- Home care after diagnosis.

DIAGNOSTIC MEASURES
- Your own observation of symptoms.
- Medical history and physical exam by a doctor.
- X-rays of the feet.

POSSIBLE COMPLICATIONS—Permanent foot deformity and crippling without treatment.

PROBABLE OUTCOME—The foot can usually be restored to normal in young children with about 3 months of treatment. For older children, treatment may improve—but not completely correct—the disorder.

HOW TO TREAT

NOTE—Follow your doctor's instructions. These instructions are supplemental.

GENERAL MEASURES—The goal of treatment is to correct the deformity and support the correction until foot muscles are strong enough to maintain it. Your doctor may prescribe stretching exercises, massage, physical therapy, various splints for day or night, casts or surgery.

Your child will need patience and encouragement with all these methods. Your attitude and the time you spend with the child are an important part of parent-child bonding.

After surgery or casting, elevate the child's feet with pillows at nap or bedtime to reduce the risk of swelling and pain.

If your child has a cast, inspect it daily for signs of infection. These include: a wet spot; bad odor; tightness; or the foot in the cast may appear blue, pale and cold compared to the other. See Care of Casts, Appendix 17.

MEDICATION—Medicine usually is not necessary for this disorder.

ACTIVITY—No restrictions. Corrective shoes will be necessary following treatment with splints or casts.

DIET—No special diet.

CALL YOUR DOCTOR IF

- Your child has signs of a foot deformity.
- Bleeding or signs of infection occur under a cast.
- Signs of muscle pulling return after treatment.

COLD, COMMON

GENERAL INFORMATION

DEFINITION—A contagious viral infection of the upper-respiratory passages.

BODY PARTS INVOLVED—Nose; throat; sinuses; ears; eustachian tubes; trachea; larynx; bronchial tubes.

SEX OR AGE MOST AFFECTED—Both sexes; all ages.

SIGNS & SYMPTOMS
- Runny or stuffy nose. Nasal discharge is watery at first, then becomes thick and greenish yellow.
- Sore throat.
- Hoarseness.
- Cough that produces little or no sputum.
- Low fever.
- Fatigue.
- Watering eyes.
- Appetite loss.

CAUSES—Any of at least 200 viruses. Virus particles spread through the air or from person-to-person contact, especially hand-shaking.

RISK INCREASES WITH
- Stress.
- Fatigue or overwork.
- Poor nutrition.
- Smoking.
- Exposure to cold, wet weather.
- Crowded or unsanitary living conditions.

HOW TO PREVENT
- To prevent spreading a cold to others, avoid unnecessary contact during the contagious phase (first 2 to 4 days).
- Wash hands frequently, especially after blowing your nose or before handling food.
- Avoid risks listed above.

WHAT TO EXPECT

APPROPRIATE HEALTH CARE
- Self-care.
- Doctor's treatment (for complications only).

DIAGNOSTIC MEASURES
- Your own observation of symptoms.
- Medical history and physical exam by a doctor.
- Laboratory throat culture.

POSSIBLE COMPLICATIONS—Bacterial infections of the ears, throat, sinuses or lungs.

PROBABLE OUTCOME—Spontaneous recovery in 7 to 14 days.

HOW TO TREAT

GENERAL MEASURES
- To relieve nasal congestion, use salt-water drops (1 teaspoon of salt to 1 quart of water).
- Use a cool-mist humidifier to increase air moisture.
- For a baby too young to blow his nose, use an infant nasal aspirator. If mucus is thick and sticky, loosen it by putting 2 or 3 drops of salt solution (see above) into each nostril.

  Don't insert cotton swabs into a child's nostrils. Instead, catch the discharge outside the nostril on a tissue or swab, roll it around and pull the discharge out of the nose.
- For an infant or very young child, lay the child on his stomach to sleep. This improves nasal drainage and breathing.

MEDICATION—No medicine, including antibiotics, can cure the common cold. To relieve symptoms, you may use non-prescription drugs, such as acetaminophen, nose drops or sprays, cough remedies and throat lozenges.

ACTIVITY—Bed rest is not necessary, but avoid vigorous activity. Rest often.

DIET—Drink extra fluids, including water, fruit juice, tea and carbonated drinks. Avoid milk because it may thicken secretions in some persons.

CALL YOUR DOCTOR IF

The following occurs during the illness:
- Increased throat pain, or white or yellow spots on the tonsils or other parts of the throat.
- Coughing episodes that last longer than intervals between coughing; cough that produces thick, yellow-green or gray sputum; cough that lasts longer than 10 days; or difficult or labored breathing between coughing bouts.
- Fever that lasts several days or rises to 101F (38.3C).
- Shaking chills.
- Chest pain or shortness of breath.
- Earache or headache.
- Skin rash.
- Pain in the teeth or over the sinuses.
- Unusual lethargy.
- Unusual irritability.
- Delirium.
- Enlarged, tender glands in the neck.
- Dusky blue or gray lips, skin or nail beds.
- Inability to bottle-feed or breast-feed in an infant.

ILLNESSES & DISORDERS

COLD SORES
(Fever Blisters; Herpes Simplex)

 GENERAL INFORMATION

DEFINITION—A common, contagious viral infection.

BODY PARTS INVOLVED—Lip; gums and mouth area; cornea (rare); genitals (occasionally).

SEX OR AGE MOST AFFECTED—Both sexes. Most persons have their first infection before age 5.

SIGNS & SYMPTOMS
- Eruptions of very small, painful blisters —usually around the mouth, but sometimes on the genitals. The blisters are grouped together and surrounded by a red ring. They fill with fluid, then dry up and disappear.
- If the eye is infected: Eye pain and redness; feeling that something is in the eye; sensitivity to light; and tearing.

CAUSES—Infection with a herpes virus that invades the skin, often remaining for months or years before causing active inflammation. Most persons develop antibodies that control the virus unless risk factors (below) develop.

The virus is transmitted by person-to-person contact or by contact with saliva, stools, urine or discharge from an infected eye. The blisters and ulcers of herpes simplex are contagious until they heal, both in the first and in succeeding flare-ups.

RISK INCREASES WITH
- Children who have eczema.
- Physical or emotional stress.
- Illness that has lowered resistance, including a cold, minor gastrointestinal upset or fever from any cause.
- Excess sun exposure.
- Menstrual periods.
- Dental treatment that stretches the mouth.
- Use of immunosuppressive drugs.

HOW TO PREVENT
- Avoid physical contact with others who have active lesions.
- Wash your hands often during a flare-up to avoid spreading the virus.

 WHAT TO EXPECT

APPROPRIATE HEALTH CARE
- Self-care after diagnosis.
- Doctor's treatment, especially if the eye is affected.

DIAGNOSTIC MEASURES
- Your own observation of symptoms.
- Medical history and physical exam by a doctor.
- Laboratory virus cultures (rare).

POSSIBLE COMPLICATIONS
- Permanent vision impairment, if herpes eye infections are untreated.
- Severe, widespread infection in patients with eczema.
- Meningitis or encephalitis (rare).

PROBABLE OUTCOME—Spontaneous recovery in a few days to a week, occasionally longer. Recurrence is common. The virus remains in the body for life, but it is usually dormant. Research continues in developing a vaccine.

 HOW TO TREAT

NOTE—Follow your doctor's instructions. These instructions are supplemental.

GENERAL MEASURES
- Drink cool liquids or suck frozen juice bars to reduce discomfort.
- Apply an ice cube for 1 hour during the first 24 hours after a lesion appears. This may make it heal more quickly.
- Don't rub or scratch an infected eye.
- To prevent flare-ups, use zinc oxide or sun-screen preparations on your lips when you spend much time outdoors.

MEDICATION
- Use acetaminophen to relieve minor pain. Don't use aspirin, especially for children and adolescents. The use of aspirin during some viral illnesses may lead to Reye's syndrome, a form of encephalitis.
- Don't try to treat an infected eye—especially with cortisone ointments or drops—without consulting your doctor. Cortisone preparations promote growth of the herpes virus in the cornea.
- Your doctor may prescribe:
  Antiviral topical or oral medication.
  Antibiotic ointment if lesions become infected with bacteria.
  Anticancer topical medication for eye infections.

ACTIVITY—No restrictions, except to avoid close contact—especially kissing or oral sex—until lesions heal.

DIET—No special diet.

 CALL YOUR DOCTOR IF

The following occurs with a cold sore:
- Signs of secondary bacterial infection, such as fever, pus instead of clear fluid in the lesions, headache and muscle aches.
- Eruption of lesions on the genitals similar to those around the mouth.
- New, unexplained symptoms. Drugs used in treatment may produce side effects.

COLIC IN INFANTS

GENERAL INFORMATION

DEFINITION—Repeated episodes of excessive crying that cannot be explained. Crying ranges from fussiness to agonized screaming. Colic is not contagious.

BODY PARTS INVOLVED—Possibly the lower intestinal tract.

SEX OR AGE MOST AFFECTED—Both sexes, but more common in boys. Colic affects infants up to 5 months old, and is most common in a first child.

SIGNS & SYMPTOMS—Excessive crying with the following characteristics:
- Crying bouts usually occur in late afternoon or evening.
- Crying bouts usually begin at 2 to 4 weeks and last through 3 or 4 months.
- The infant's abdomen may rumble, and the child may draw up the legs as if in pain.
- No specific disease, such as an ear infection, hernia, allergy or urinary infection, can be discovered.

CAUSES—Unknown. Colic may be related to physical pain or emotional upset. Some likely possibilities include: hunger; insufficient sleep; milk that is too hot; overfeeding; food allergy; reactions to tension in the home; loneliness; or tiredness.

RISK INCREASES WITH—No known risk factor.

HOW TO PREVENT—No specific preventive measures. Remove any causes that can be identified.

WHAT TO EXPECT

APPROPRIATE HEALTH CARE
- Home care.
- Doctor's treatment.

DIAGNOSTIC MEASURES
- Your own observation of symptoms.
- Medical history and physical exam by a doctor.

POSSIBLE COMPLICATIONS—None expected.

PROBABLE OUTCOME—All babies cry, and many have fussy periods. Crying is an important activity and means of communication. Colic is a distressing, but not dangerous, condition. The symptoms can sometimes be relieved. When they can't, the colic *will* disappear after the 4th or 5th month.

HOW TO TREAT

NOTE—Follow your doctor's instructions. These instructions are supplemental.

GENERAL MEASURES
- Be patient and tolerant.
- Don't feed the baby every time he cries. Look for a reason, such as: a gas bubble; cramped position; too much heat or cold; soiled diaper; open diaper pin; or a desire to be cuddled.

  If the baby stops crying when picked up, the crying is not a result of hunger or gas. If the child continues crying, offer a feeding. If the crying stops then, it is due to hunger.

  The symptoms of overfeeding can mimic gas pains. If the baby is still screaming in agony after an hour, gently insert an infant glycerine suppository into the baby's rectum as a last resort.
- During an attack of gas, hold the baby securely, and gently massage the lower abdomen. Rocking may be soothing. Apply a good heating pad, set on "low," to the abdomen; be careful not to burn.
- Offer the baby a pacifier.
- Allow the baby to cry if you are certain everything is all right (not hungry, not soiled, no fever, no open pins) and you have done all you can.
- Ask someone to take care of the baby to relieve you as often as possible.

MEDICATION—Drugs are used only as a last resort when babies and parents are both exhausted. In that event, your doctor may prescribe antispasmodics. If so, carefully follow instructions on the label. Don't use any medicine, including non-prescription medicine, without telling your doctor.

ACTIVITY—No restrictions.

DIET
- Interrupt bottle feedings after every ounce and burp the baby. Interrupt breast feedings every 5 minutes.
- Allow at least 20 minutes to feed the baby. Don't prop the baby for feedings.
- Nipple holes should not be too large. A vigorous baby may require blind nipples in which you can make small, homemade nipple holes.

CALL YOUR DOCTOR IF

- The baby's rectal temperature rises to 101F (38.3C) or higher.
- You fear that you are about to lose emotional control.
- The baby is taking a prescription drug, and new, unexplained symptoms develop. The drug may produce side effects.

COLITIS, SPASTIC
(Spastic Colon; Mucous Colitis; Irritable Bowel Syndrome)

 GENERAL INFORMATION

DEFINITION—An irritative and inflammatory disorder of the intestine. It is not contagious, inherited or cancerous.

BODY PARTS INVOLVED—Small and large intestines.

SEX OR AGE MOST AFFECTED—Twice as likely to affect women as men.

SIGNS & SYMPTOMS—The following symptoms usually begin in early adult life. Episodes may last for days, weeks or months.
- Cramp-like pain in the middle or to one side of the lower abdomen. Pain is usually relieved with bowel movements.
- Nausea.
- Bloating and gas.
- Occasional appetite loss that may lead to weight loss.
- Diarrhea or constipation, usually alternating.
- Fatigue.
- Depression.
- Anxiety.
- Concentration difficulty.

CAUSES—Stress and emotional conflict resulting in anxiety or depression. Situations that often precede an attack include: obsessive worry about everyday problems; marital tension; fear of loss of a beloved person or object; death of a loved one.
  Symptoms may also be triggered by eating, though no specific food has been identified as responsible.

RISK INCREASES WITH
- Stress.
- Improper diet.
- Smoking.
- Excess alcohol consumption.
- Use of drugs.
- Fatigue or overwork.
- Poor physical fitness.

HOW TO PREVENT—Reduce stress or try to modify your response to it. See Appendix 13.

 WHAT TO EXPECT

APPROPRIATE HEALTH CARE
- Self-care.
- Doctor's treatment.

DIAGNOSTIC MEASURES
- Your own observation of symptoms.
- Medical history and physical exam by a doctor.
- Laboratory studies, including stool studies, to exclude other disorders such as lactose intolerance, ulcers, parasites, enzyme deficiency and ulcerative colitis.
- X-ray of the colon (barium enema).

POSSIBLE COMPLICATIONS
- Poor nutrition caused by malabsorption.
- Psychological fixation on bowel function, leading to neurosis.
- Increased risk of colon cancer.

PROBABLE OUTCOME—Curable if the underlying causes can be eliminated or modified. If not, symptoms can be controlled with treatment.

 HOW TO TREAT

NOTE—Follow your doctor's instructions. These instructions are supplemental.

GENERAL MEASURES—Medication, diet changes and adequate rest can help, but the cure is more dependant on defining, confronting and solving conflicts in day-to-day living. See Appendix 13.

MEDICATION—Medication may help, but it will not cure this disorder. Your doctor may prescribe:
- Antispasmodics to relieve severe abdominal cramps.
- Tranquilizers to reduce anxiety.

ACTIVITY—No restrictions. Good physical fitness improves bowel function.

DIET
- Increase fiber in the diet to promote good bowel function. See Appendix 1.
- Don't eat foods that aggravate symptoms.

 CALL YOUR DOCTOR IF

- Fever develops.
- Stool is black or tarry-looking.
- You begin vomiting.
- Unexplained weight loss of 5 pounds or more occurs.
- Symptoms don't improve despite treatment.

COLITIS, ULCERATIVE

GENERAL INFORMATION

DEFINITION—A serious, chronic, inflammatory disease of the colon characterized by ulceration and episodes of bloody diarrhea. The ulcerated areas are inflamed and may form abscesses in the lining of the large intestine.

BODY PARTS INVOLVED—Rectum; large bowel.

SEX OR AGE MOST AFFECTED—Most common in women between ages 15 and 40.

SIGNS & SYMPTOMS—Early symptoms include:
- Pain in the left side of the abdomen that improves after bowel movements.
- Episodes of bloody diarrhea with mucus, alternating with symptom-free intervals.

During an acute attack:
- Increased bloody diarrhea (up to 10 to 20 bowel movements a day).
- Severe cramps and pain around the rectum.
- Sweating.
- Nausea.
- Appetite and weight loss.
- Bloated abdomen.
- Fever as high as 104F (40C).

CAUSES—Unknown.

RISK INCREASES WITH
- Stress, anxiety or depression.
- Family history of ulcerative colitis.
- Excess alcohol consumption.

HOW TO PREVENT—No specific preventive measures.

WHAT TO EXPECT

APPROPRIATE HEALTH CARE
- Self-care after diagnosis.
- Doctor's treatment.
- Psychological counseling.
- Surgery to remove the diseased colon (sometimes). For an explanation of this surgery and postoperative care, see Ileostomy (in Surgery section).
- Hospitalization during worst episodes.

DIAGNOSTIC MEASURES
- Your own observation of symptoms.
- Medical history and physical exam by a doctor.
- Laboratory stool and blood studies.
- X-ray of the colon (barium enema).
- Sigmoidoscopy (see Glossary).

POSSIBLE COMPLICATIONS
- Life-threatening blood loss, ulceration through the intestinal wall or peritonitis during acute attacks.
- Malnutrition, wasting of the body or chronic disability.
- Inflammation of joints, eyes and skin.
- Colon cancer; the risk is greater in persons with ulcerative colitis.

PROBABLE OUTCOME—Often curable with counseling and medical treatment or surgery. If not curable, symptoms can be controlled with treatment.

HOW TO TREAT

NOTE—Follow your doctor's instructions. These instructions are supplemental.

GENERAL MEASURES
- To reduce cramps, apply a hot-water bottle, warm moist towels or heating pad to the abdomen.
- Try to reduce stress. See Appendix 13.

MEDICATION
- Don't use aspirin. It increases the bleeding risk.
- Your doctor may prescribe:
  Antidiarrhea medication for minimal symptoms.
  Sulfa drugs, such as sulfasalazine, for moderate symptoms.
  Cortisone drugs for severe disease.

ACTIVITY—Bed rest may be necessary during acute attacks. However, resume normal activity as soon as symptoms improve.

DIET
- Don't drink alcohol.
- During early treatment, avoid milk and milk products.

CALL YOUR DOCTOR IF

- You have symptoms of ulcerative colitis.
- Fever and chills develop.
- Frequency of bowel movements or bleeding increases.
- Abdomen becomes distended.
- Jaundice (yellow eyes and skin and dark urine) develops.
- Vomiting begins or abdominal pain increases.

CONGESTIVE HEART FAILURE

GENERAL INFORMATION

DEFINITION—A complication of many serious diseases in which the heart loses its full pumping capacity. Blood backs up into other organs, especially the lungs and liver.

BODY PARTS INVOLVED—Heart; blood vessels; lungs; liver; extremities.

SEX OR AGE MOST AFFECTED—Both sexes; all ages.

SIGNS & SYMPTOMS
- Shortness of breath, especially with exertion or when lying flat in bed.
- Fatigue, weakness or faintness.
- Cough (usually with sputum).
- Swelling of the abdomen, legs and ankles.
- Rapid or irregular heartbeat.
- Low blood pressure.
- Distended neck veins.
- Enlarged liver.

CAUSES
- High blood pressure.
- Heart-valve disease.
- Heart attack.
- Heartbeat irregularities.
- Severe lung disease such as emphysema.
- Congenital heart disease.
- Cardiomyopathy.
- Hyperthyroidism.
- Severe anemia.
- Heart tumor (rare).
- Infections complicating underlying heart disease.

RISK INCREASES WITH
- Infections with high fever.
- Smoking.
- Obesity.
- Excess alcohol consumption. Alcohol depresses heart function.
- Use of certain drugs, such as beta-adrenergic blockers or excess digitalis.
- Diet that is high in fat and salt.

HOW TO PREVENT—If you have a condition that can lead to congestive heart failure, obtain medical care and adhere to your treatment program. Follow your dietary guidelines, and don't drink alcohol or smoke.

WHAT TO EXPECT

APPROPRIATE HEALTH CARE
- Self-care after diagnosis.
- Doctor's treatment.
- Surgery on heart valves, coronary arteries or ventricular aneurysms (sometimes).
- Hospitalization (severe cases).

DIAGNOSTIC MEASURES
- Your own observation of symptoms.
- Medical history and physical exam by a doctor.
- Laboratory blood studies and urinalysis.
- EKG (see Glossary).
- Heart-catheterization studies.
- X-rays of the heart, lungs and blood vessels (angiography).
- Echocardiogram (see Glossary).

POSSIBLE COMPLICATIONS—Pulmonary edema.

PROBABLE OUTCOME—Life expectancy is reduced, but many forms are well-controlled for a while with medication and sometimes surgery. Other forms cause chronic illness. Any infection may worsen the condition.

HOW TO TREAT

NOTE—Follow your doctor's instructions. These instructions are supplemental.

GENERAL MEASURES
- Weigh daily and keep a record.
- Don't smoke.

MEDICATION—Your doctor may prescribe:
- Diuretics to decrease fluid retention and swelling.
- Digitalis to strengthen and regulate heartbeat.
- Antiarrhythmic drugs to stabilize heartbeat.
- Anticoagulants to reduce blood clotting.
- Potassium replacements, if you take diuretics or digitalis.

ACTIVITY—In early stages, bed rest with the upper body elevated is as important as medication. Avoid unnecessary exertion (such as climbing stairs) until the condition is under control. Then consult your doctor about acceptable activity.

DIET
- Achieve your ideal weight to reduce the heart's workload.
- Eat a low-salt, low-fat, high-fiber diet (see Appendices 8 and 9).
- Don't drink alcohol.

CALL YOUR DOCTOR IF

- You have symptoms of congestive heart failure.
- The following occurs during treatment: Symptoms of infection, such as fever, muscle aches, headache and dizziness. Worsening of symptoms, especially rapid or irregular heartbeat or wheezing at night. Cough with increased sputum or blood. Weight gain of 3 or 4 pounds in 1 or 2 days.
- New, unexplained symptoms develop. Drugs used in treatment may produce side effects.

CONJUNCTIVITIS
(Pink Eye)

 GENERAL INFORMATION

DEFINITION—An inflammation of the eyelid's underside and white part of the eye.

BODY PARTS INVOLVED—Eye; underside of the eyelid.

SEX OR AGE MOST AFFECTED—Both sexes; all ages.

SIGNS & SYMPTOMS—The following symptoms may affect one or both eyes:
● Clear, green or yellow discharge from the eye.
● After sleeping, crusts on lashes that cause eyelids to stick together.
● Eye pain.
● Swollen eyelids.
● Sensitivity to bright light.
● Redness and gritty feeling in the eye.
● Intense itching (allergic conjunctivitis only).

CAUSES
● Viral infection. Conjunctivitis may accompany colds or childhood diseases such as measles.
● Bacterial infection. Infants up to 3 days old can be infected with pink eye from a gonococcus bacteria present in the mother's birth canal.
● Chemical irritation or wind, dust, smoke and other types of air pollution.
● Allergies caused by cosmetics, pollen or other allergens.
● A partially closed tear duct.
● Intense light, such as from sunlamps, snow reflection or electric arcs in welding.

RISK INCREASES WITH
● Newborns of mothers who are carriers of gonorrhea.
● Crowded or unsanitary living conditions.
● Exposure to others in public places.

HOW TO PREVENT
● Wash hands frequently with soap and warm water.
● Avoid exposure to eye irritants.
● Newborns in hospital deliveries are routinely given antibiotic eye drops.

 WHAT TO EXPECT

APPROPRIATE HEALTH CARE
● Self-care after diagnosis.
● Doctor's treatment.

DIAGNOSTIC MEASURES
● Your own observation of symptoms.
● Medical history and physical exam by a doctor.
● Laboratory culture of the discharge from the eye.

POSSIBLE COMPLICATIONS—If untreated, pink eye may spread and damage the cornea permanently, impairing vision.

PROBABLE OUTCOME
● Allergic conjunctivitis can be cured if the allergen is removed. It is likely to recur.
● Other forms are curable in 1 to 2 weeks with treatment.

 HOW TO TREAT

NOTE—Follow your doctor's instructions. These instructions are supplemental.

GENERAL MEASURES
● Wash hands often with antiseptic soap, and use paper towels to dry. Don't touch eyes. Gently wipe the discharge from the eye using disposable tissues.
   Infections are frequently spread by contaminated fingers, towels, handkerchiefs or wash cloths that have touched the infected eye.
● Use warm-water soaks (see Appendix 18) to reduce discomfort.
● Don't use eye makeup.

MEDICATION—Your doctor may prescribe antibiotic eye drops, sulfa eye drops, steroid eye drops or antibiotic ointment to fight infection. Use 3 times daily.
   If the infection does not improve in 2 or 3 days, it may be caused by an insensitive bacteria, virus or allergy. At this point, an ophthalmologist may need to culture the conjunctivae or make special studies to determine the cause of the conjunctivitis.
   Most ophthalmologists believe steroid eyedrops should not be used until a diagnosis is definite. If the infection is caused by herpes simplex virus, steroids may spread it from the conjunctiva to the cornea, damaging the eye.

ACTIVITY—Resume your normal activities as soon as symptoms improve.

DIET—No special diet.

 CALL YOUR DOCTOR IF

● You have symptoms of conjunctivitis.
● The infection does not improve in 48 hours, despite treatment.
● Fever occurs.
● Pain increases.
● Vision is affected.

ILLNESSES & DISORDERS

CONSTIPATION

GENERAL INFORMATION

DEFINITION—Difficult or uncomfortable bowel movements.

BODY PARTS INVOLVED—Colon.

SEX OR AGE MOST AFFECTED—Both sexes; all ages.

SIGNS & SYMPTOMS—People vary widely in bowel activity. Any of the following may be a sign of constipation:
- Infrequent bowel movements, sometimes accompanied by abdominal swelling.
- Hard feces.
- Straining during bowel movements.
- Pain or bleeding with bowel movements.
- Sensation of continuing fullness after a bowel movement.

CAUSES
- Inadequate fluid intake.
- Insufficient fiber in the diet. Fiber adds bulk, holds water and creates easily passed, soft feces.
- Inactivity.
- Hypothyroidism.
- Hypercalcemia.
- Anal fissure.
- Depression.
- Chronic kidney failure.
- Back pain.
- Colon or rectal cancer.

RISK INCREASES WITH
- Stress.
- Illness requiring complete bed rest.
- Use of certain drugs, including: belladonna; calcium-channel blockers; beta-adrenergic blockers; atropine; or aspirin.

HOW TO PREVENT
- Eat a well-balanced, high-fiber diet.
- Exercise regularly.
- Drink at least 8 glasses of water a day.

WHAT TO EXPECT

APPROPRIATE HEALTH CARE
- Self-care.
- Doctor's treatment (occasionally).

DIAGNOSTIC MEASURES
- Your own observation of symptoms. Tell your doctor of any major change in your bowel pattern that lasts longer than 1 week. It may be a sign of cancer.
- Medical history and physical exam by a doctor.
- Laboratory tests of blood and stool to detect internal bleeding.
- Sigmoidoscopy (see Glossary).

POSSIBLE COMPLICATIONS
- Hemorrhoids.
- Laxative dependency.
- Hernia from excessive straining.
- Uterine or rectal prolapse.
- Spastic colitis.

PROBABLE OUTCOME—Usually curable with exercise, diet and adequate fluids.

HOW TO TREAT

NOTE—Follow your doctor's instructions. These instructions are supplemental.

GENERAL MEASURES
- Set aside a regular time each day for bowel movements. The best time is often within 1 hour after breakfast. Don't try to hurry. Sit at least 10 minutes, whether or not a bowel movement occurs.
- If constipation persists for 3 or 4 days, use a non-prescription, disposable enema for temporary relief. If you prefer not to use a commercial enema preparation, you may give yourself an enema as follows:
  Spread a bath mat on the bathroom floor or in the tub.
  Fill an enema bag with lukewarm water. Hang the enema bag no higher than 30 inches from the floor.
  Lie on your left side on the mat.
  Insert the nozzle gently inside the rectum. Let the water flow in slowly, a little at a time. If it hurts, stop the water flow until the pain subsides. Then start the flow again.
  Use the entire quart of water.
  Hold the fluid inside until you are uncomfortable. Then sit on the toilet for a bowel movement.

MEDICATION—For *occasional* constipation, you may use stool softeners, mild non-prescription laxatives or enemas. Don't use laxatives or enemas regularly—this can cause dependency. Avoid harsh laxatives and cathartics, such as epsom salts.

ACTIVITY—Exercise and good physical fitness helps maintain healthy bowel patterns. See Appendix 20 for exercise suggestions.

DIET—Drink at least 8 glasses of water each day. Include bulk foods, such as bran and raw fruits and vegetables, in your diet. Avoid refined cereals and breads, pastries and sugar.

CALL YOUR DOCTOR IF

- You have constipation that persists, despite self-care—especially if the constipation represents a change in your normal bowel patterns.
- Constipation is accompanied by fever and severe abdominal pain. .

CONVULSION, FEBRILE

 ## GENERAL INFORMATION

DEFINITION—A seizure triggered by fever, and characterized by altered consciousness and uncontrolled muscle spasms.

BODY PARTS INVOLVED—Central nervous system; musculo-skeletal system.

SEX OR AGE MOST AFFECTED—Infants and children (6 months to 4 years).

SIGNS & SYMPTOMS—An infection with fever usually precedes the convulsions, but sometimes convulsions may be the first sign of fever. Symptoms include:
- Unconsciousness.
- Jerking or twitching of the arms, legs or face that lasts 2 to 3 minutes.
- Loss of bladder or bowel control.
- Irritability upon regaining consciousness, followed by sleep for several hours.

CAUSES—Sudden, high fever from any cause, plus an unexplained irritability of the central nervous system in some children.

RISK INCREASES WITH—Repeated infections.

HOW TO PREVENT—When fever begins in a child who has had a febrile convulsion in the past, immediately begin measures to reduce the fever. (See General Measures.)

 ## WHAT TO EXPECT

APPROPRIATE HEALTH CARE
- Doctor's treatment for diagnosis and treatment of the underlying cause.
- Home care after the seizure has subsided and after diagnosis.

DIAGNOSTIC MEASURES
- Your own observation of symptoms.
- Medical history and physical exam by a doctor.
- Laboratory studies of blood and spinal fluid.
- EEG (see Glossary).

POSSIBLE COMPLICATIONS
- Body injury during a seizure.
- Brain injury with repeated seizures.

PROBABLE OUTCOME—Despite its frightening appearance, a convulsion caused solely by fever in a child between 6 months and 4 years of age is usually not serious.

If the first convulsion occurs with fever in a child older than 4, it is probably caused by the fever. However, other causes should be investigated.

If the first convulsion with fever occurs in a child younger than 6 months, a neurological examination and other studies may be necessary.

 ## HOW TO TREAT

NOTE—Follow your doctor's instructions. These instructions are supplemental.

GENERAL MEASURES
- During the convulsion, move potentially dangerous objects away from the child.
- Write down details of the convulsion, and report them to your doctor. Information should include the following:
  When did it begin?
  How soon did the seizure occur after the fever rose?
  Were the limb movements equal on both sides or was one side twitching more than the other?
  How long did the seizure last?
  Did the child sleep afterward? If so, how long?
  Did the seizure recur after a quiet interval?
The answers will help your doctor decide whether the seizure was a febrile convulsion or an epileptic seizure triggered by fever.
- After the convulsion, try to reduce fever. See How to Reduce Fever, Appendix 19.

MEDICATION—Your doctor may prescribe anticonvulsant drugs, such as phenobarbital, to prevent a recurrence of seizures. Some doctors recommend medication after the first convulsion; others wait to see if convulsions recur. Anticonvulsant drugs are only effective if taken daily during the susceptible years (up to age 4).

ACTIVITY—Keep the child resting quietly in bed until fever and the underlying illness are gone. Then allow activity to return gradually to normal.

DIET—After the seizure ends, encourage the child to drink extra liquids, including water, tea, cola and fruit juice.

 ## CALL YOUR DOCTOR IF

- Your child has a seizure with fever. Call your doctor *immediately*.
- An injury occurs during a seizure.
- The underlying illness does not improve in 3 days.

COR PULMONALE
(Pulmonary Hypertension)

 GENERAL INFORMATION

DEFINITION—Congestive heart failure resulting from raised blood pressure in the lungs. This is a complication of disorders that slow or block blood flow in the lungs.

BODY PARTS INVOLVED—Lungs; heart; blood vessels.

SEX OR AGE MOST AFFECTED—Both sexes and all ages, but most common in men over 40.

SIGNS & SYMPTOMS—Early stages:
- No symptoms (usually).
Later stages:
- Weakness and fatigue.
- Shortness of breath with exertion.
- Frequent fainting.
- Swelling of the ankles and feet caused by fluid retention.
- Distended neck veins.
- Bluish skin.
- Chest pain.
- Enlarged liver and swollen abdomen.

CAUSES
- Severe, chronic obstructive lung disease, such as emphysema, recurrent pneumonia, bronchiectasis, silicosis, lung cancer, tuberculosis or collagen diseases.
- Blood clots that travel to the lung from another body site—usually a deep vein in the calf of the leg—and obstruct lung blood vessels.
- Primary diseases of the heart, including rheumatic heart disease and congenital heart disease.

RISK INCREASES WITH
- Prolonged bed rest for any illness. This increases the chance of blood-clot formation.
- Smoking.

HOW TO PREVENT
- Don't smoke.
- Obtain regular medical treatment for any underlying disorder that can be corrected with surgery or medical treatment.

 WHAT TO EXPECT

APPROPRIATE HEALTH CARE
- Doctor's treatment.
- Surgery to correct problems caused by congenital or acquired disorders, such as replacing damaged heart valves (sometimes).

DIAGNOSTIC MEASURES
- Your own observation of symptoms.
- Medical history and physical exam by a doctor.
- Laboratory studies of blood and lung function.
- X-rays of the lungs.

POSSIBLE COMPLICATIONS—Irreversible congestive heart failure and death.

PROBABLE OUTCOME—This condition is currently considered incurable. Many persons live 10 or 15 years after diagnosis, but disability will slowly increase. However, symptoms can be relieved or controlled.

Scientific research into causes and treatment continues, so there is hope for increasingly effective treatment and cure.

 HOW TO TREAT

NOTE—Follow your doctor's instructions. These instructions are supplemental.

GENERAL MEASURES
- You may need oxygen. Your doctor or an oxygen therapist can arrange for the type of oxygen that allows you to be up and about.
- Weigh daily and keep a record. Any sudden increase may indicate increased fluid retention.

MEDICATION—Your doctor may prescribe:
- Diuretics to prevent fluid accumulation.
- Digitalis to strengthen the force of heart-muscle contractions.
- Antibiotics for recurrent infections.

ACTIVITY—No restrictions. Be as active as your condition allows, but don't overexert. Rest between activities.

DIET—Eat a diet that is low in salt (see Appendix 9).

 CALL YOUR DOCTOR IF

- You have symptoms of cor pulmonale.
- The following occurs during treatment:
  Temperature of 101F (38.3C) or higher.
  Weight gain of 3 to 4 pounds in 1 or 2 days.
  Increased shortness of breath.
  Increased swelling of the ankles.
  Cough with sputum that is discolored or tinged with blood.

CORN OR CALLUS

GENERAL INFORMATION

DEFINITION
- A corn is a painful thickening (bump) of the outer skin layer, usually over bony areas such as toe joints.
- A callus is a painless thickening of skin caused by repeated pressure or irritation.

BODY PARTS INVOLVED
- Corn: toe joints and skin between toes.
- Callus: any part of the body, especially hands, feet or knees, that endures repeated pressure or irritation.

SEX OR AGE MOST AFFECTED—All ages except infants.

SIGNS & SYMPTOMS
- Corn: A small, painful, raised bump on the side or over the joint of a toe. Corns are usually 3mm to 10 mm in diameter and have a hard center.
- Callus: A rough, thickened area of skin that appears after repeated pressure or irritation.

CAUSES—Corns and calluses form to protect a skin area from injury caused by repeated irritation (rubbing or squeezing). Pressure causes cells in the irritated area to grow at a faster rate, leading to overgrowth.

RISK INCREASES WITH
- Shoes that fit poorly.
- Those with occupations that involve pressure on the hands or knees, such as carpenters, writers, guitar players or tile layers.

HOW TO PREVENT
- Don't wear shoes that fit poorly.
- Avoid activities that create constant pressure on specific skin areas.
- When possible, wear protective gear, such as gloves or knee pads.

WHAT TO EXPECT

APPROPRIATE HEALTH CARE
- Self-care.
- Doctor's treatment.

DIAGNOSTIC MEASURES
- Your own observation of symptoms.
- Medical history and physical exam by a doctor of medicine or podiatrist.

POSSIBLE COMPLICATIONS—Back, hip, knee or ankle pain caused by a change in one's gait due to severe discomfort.

PROBABLE OUTCOME—Usually curable if the underlying cause can be removed. Allow 3 weeks for recovery. Recurrence is likely—even with treatment—if the cause is not removed.

HOW TO TREAT

NOTE—Follow your doctor's instructions. These instructions are supplemental.

GENERAL MEASURES
- Remove the source of pressure, if possible. Discard ill-fitting shoes.
- Use corn and callus pads to reduce pressure on irritated areas.
- Peel or rub the thickened area with a pumice stone to remove it. Don't cut it with a razor. Soak the area in warm water to soften it before peeling.
- Ask the shoe repairman to sew a metatarsal bar onto your shoe to use while a corn is healing.
- Avoid surgery. It does not remove the cause. Post-surgical scarring is painful and may complicate healing.

MEDICATION
- After peeling the upper layers of the corn once or twice a day, apply ointment. Use a non-prescription 5% or 10% salicylic ointment. Cover with adhesive tape.
- Your doctor may inject a corn or callus with cortisone medicine to suppress inflammation or pain.

ACTIVITY—Resume your normal activities as soon as symptoms improve.

DIET—No special diet.

CALL YOUR DOCTOR IF

- You have corns or calluses that persist, despite self-treatment.
- Any signs of infection, such as redness, swelling, pain, heat or tenderness, develop around a corn or callus.

ILLNESSES & DISORDERS

CORNEAL ULCER

GENERAL INFORMATION

DEFINITION—An open sore in the thin transparent layers that cover the eye.

BODY PARTS INVOLVED—Cornea (covering); conjunctiva (white of the eye); iris (colored part of the eye); and aqueous humour (fluid in the eyeball).

SEX OR AGE MOST AFFECTED—Both sexes; all ages.

SIGNS & SYMPTOMS
- Eye pain.
- Sensitivity to bright light.
- Eyelid spasm.
- Tearing.
- Blurred vision.
- Redness in the white of the eye.

CAUSES
- Injury to the cornea or the embedding in the cornea of a foreign body, such as a small piece of steel, sand or glass. A bacterial infection—usually pneumococcal, streptococcal or staphylococcal—may follow the injury.
- Complications of the virus, herpes simplex, that produces cold sores on the mouth.
- Infections of the eyelids and conjunctiva.
- Defective closure of the lid.

All the above infections are contagious from person to person or from one part of the body to another—especially finger-to-eye contact after touching cold sores on the mouth.

RISK INCREASES WITH
- Recent infection or eye injury.
- Use of contact lenses, especially extended-wear lenses.
- Smoking or other environmental eye irritants.

HOW TO PREVENT
- Wash hands frequently.
- Avoid injury. Wear safety goggles to protect eyes when exposed to flying wood shavings or splinters, or metal or stone bits.
- Don't touch your eyes if you have cold sores.

WHAT TO EXPECT

APPROPRIATE HEALTH CARE
- Self-care.
- Doctor's treatment.

DIAGNOSTIC MEASURES
- Your own observation of symptoms.
- Medical history and physical exam by a doctor (ophthalmologist).
- Laboratory studies to identify the bacterium, virus or fungus responsible for the infection and ulcer.

POSSIBLE COMPLICATIONS—Neglected corneal ulcers may penetrate the cornea, allowing infection to enter the eyeball. This can cause permanent vision loss.

PROBABLE OUTCOME—A corneal ulcer is a serious eye problem. It is usually curable in 2 to 3 weeks if treated by an ophthalmologist.

If scars from previous corneal ulcers impair vision significantly, a corneal transplant (grafting a new cornea onto the eye) may make vision nearly normal.

HOW TO TREAT

NOTE—Follow your doctor's instructions. These instructions are supplemental.

GENERAL MEASURES—Apply cool-water compresses to the eye as often as they feel good.

MEDICATION
- Your doctor may prescribe antibiotic eye drops, ointments or oral antibiotics for bacterial infections. Your doctor will administer medication for viral and fungus infections.
- For minor pain, you may use non-prescription drugs such as acetaminophen.

ACTIVITY—After treatment, resume normal activity as soon as possible.

DIET—No special diet.

CALL YOUR DOCTOR IF

- You have symptoms of a corneal ulcer.
- The following occurs during treatment:
  Fever over 101F (38.3C).
  Pain that is not relieved by acetaminophen.
  Changed vision.
- New, unexplained symptoms develop. Drugs used in treatment may produce side effects.

CORONARY-ARTERY DISEASE
(Coronary Atherosclerosis; Ischemic Heart Disease; Coronary Heart Disease)

 GENERAL INFORMATION

DEFINITION—Hardening and narrowing of the coronary arteries, which provide the blood supply to the heart. There are two main coronary arteries. When they become narrowed, they can no longer provide adequate oxygen for heart cells.

BODY PARTS INVOLVED—Blood vessels to the heart.

SEX OR AGE MOST AFFECTED—Adults of both sexes over age 40. Coronary-artery disease is uncommon in women before menopause.

SIGNS & SYMPTOMS—Early stages:
- No symptoms (often).
Later stages:
- Angina pectoris.
- Heart attack.

CAUSES—Often unknown, except for association with risks listed below.
   In addition to narrowing due to hardening of the arteries, blood clots frequently form and block arteries.

RISK INCREASES WITH
- Stress.
- Poor nutrition, especially too much fat in the diet.
- Obesity.
- History of diabetes, high blood pressure or atherosclerosis.
- Previous heart attack or stroke.
- Smoking.
- Fatigue or overwork.

HOW TO PREVENT
- Don't smoke.
- Eat a low-fat, low-salt, high-fiber diet.
- Exercise regularly.
- Reduce stress to a manageable level when possible (see Appendix 13).
- If you have diabetes or hypertension, adhere strictly to the treatment schedule, including diet restrictions.

 WHAT TO EXPECT

APPROPRIATE HEALTH CARE
- Self-care after diagnosis to make necessary lifestyle changes.
- Doctor's treatment.
- Surgery to bypass coronary arteries (severe cases) or balloon angioplasty (see Glossary). Although these procedures may decrease or eliminate symptoms for a while, they do not control the underlying disease. See Coronary-Artery Bypass Graft (in Surgery section).

DIAGNOSTIC MEASURES
- Your own observation of symptoms.
- Medical history and physical exam by a doctor.
- Laboratory studies such as: EKG (see Glossary); exercise-tolerance test; blood studies to measure total fat, cholesterol and lipoproteins.
- X-rays of the chest.

POSSIBLE COMPLICATIONS—Life-threatening heart attack causing myocardial infarction (death of heart-muscle cells from inadequate blood supply).

PROBABLE OUTCOME—This condition is currently considered incurable. However, symptoms can usually be relieved or controlled. Treatment can prolong life and improve its quality.
   Scientific research into causes and treatment continues, so there is hope for increasingly effective treatment and cure.

 HOW TO TREAT

NOTE—Follow your doctor's instructions. These instructions are supplemental.

GENERAL MEASURES—Try to reduce as many risk factors as possible. Consider lifestyle changes (see Appendix 12).

MEDICATION—Your doctor may prescribe:
- Nitroglycerin, anticoagulants or beta-adrenergic blockers for angina pectoris and blood-vessel spasms.
- Vasodilator drugs to increase the blood supply to the heart muscle.

ACTIVITY—Engage in a program of moderate, daily physical exercise—especially exercise that is fun. See Appendix 20.

DIET
- Low-fat diet (see Appendix 8).
- Low-salt diet (see Appendix 9).

 CALL YOUR DOCTOR IF

- You develop deep chest discomfort (aching or pressure) with radiation to the jaw, left arm or back. Call immediately. This may be an emergency!
- You sweat and feel short of breath.
- You have high risk factors and wish to become involved in a program of prevention.
- After exertion, you develop chest, neck or jaw pain that goes away with rest.

CROHN'S DISEASE
(Regional Ileitis; Granulomatous Ileitis or Ileocolitis; Regional Enteritis)

 GENERAL INFORMATION

DEFINITION—An inflammatory disease of the ileum, the lower part of the small intestine.

BODY PARTS INVOLVED—Ileum, colon and other parts of the gastrointestinal tract; regional lymph nodes; the mesentery (outside covering of the intestines).

SEX OR AGE MOST AFFECTED—Adults between ages 20 and 40.

SIGNS & SYMPTOMS
- Cramping abdominal pain—especially after eating. The pain is sometimes in the right lower abdomen, mimicking appendicitis.
- Nausea and diarrhea.
- General ill feeling.
- Fever.
- Appetite and weight loss.
- Abdominal tenderness.
- Abdominal mass that can be felt.
- Bloody stools (sometimes).

CAUSES—Unknown.

RISK INCREASES WITH
- Medical history of food allergies.
- Family history of Crohn's disease.

HOW TO PREVENT—Cannot be prevented at present.

 WHAT TO EXPECT

APPROPRIATE HEALTH CARE
- Self-care after diagnosis.
- Doctor's treatment.
- Surgery (see Ileostomy) to resect the inflamed area (sometimes)—although non-surgical treatment is preferred.

DIAGNOSTIC MEASURES
- Your own observation of symptoms.
- Medical history and physical exam by a doctor.
- Laboratory blood studies.
- Surgical diagnostic procedures, such as sigmoidoscopy or colonoscopy (see Glossary for both).
- X-rays of the colon and small intestine.

POSSIBLE COMPLICATIONS
- Intestinal obstruction.
- Bleeding and anemia.
- Fistula between the bowel and bladder.
- Perirectal abscess.
- Perforation of the inflamed bowel.
- Increased susceptibility to cancer of the ileum.
- Vitamin-B-12 deficiency.

PROBABLE OUTCOME—Attacks begin in patients in their early 20s and may continue for years. Intervals between attacks vary from every few months to every few years. Occasionally, symptoms appear only once or twice, and the disease disappears.

If you and your doctor decide that your condition requires surgery, it can dramatically improve your condition and delay progress of the disease for many years.

 HOW TO TREAT

NOTE—Follow your doctor's instructions. These instructions are supplemental.

GENERAL MEASURES
- Use heat to relieve pain. Apply a heating pad or warm compresses to the abdomen. If abdominal cramps are continuous or severe, notify your doctor.
- Check your stool daily for signs of bleeding. Take any suspicious specimens to your doctor's office for analysis.

MEDICATION—Your doctor may prescribe:
- Pain relievers.
- Antidiarrhea medication.
- Vitamin supplements.
- Anti-inflammatory drugs, including cortisone.
- Antibiotics to fight infections.

ACTIVITY
- During acute attacks, rest in bed or a chair. Get up only to go to the bathroom, to bathe or to eat.
- During periods between attacks, rest often during the day and sleep up to 10 hours a night.

DIET
- Eat a low-residue, high-protein, high-carbohydrate diet that is high in vitamins and minerals. Meats, potatoes and their substitutes are the mainstays of the diet.
- Don't drink alcohol. It irritates the gastrointestinal tract.
- If you have possible food allergies, omit milk, wheat, eggs, nuts and other suspected foods. Omit each one—especially milk—for a short period, then try it again in a few weeks.

 CALL YOUR DOCTOR IF

- You have symptoms of Crohn's disease.
- You have black, tarry stools or blood in the stool.
- Your abdomen swells.
- Your temperature rises to 101F (38.3C) or higher.

CROUP
(Laryngo-Tracheo-Bronchitis)

 GENERAL INFORMATION

DEFINITION—Infection, inflammation and swelling of the larynx (vocal cords) and surrounding tissue. This causes labored breathing and a characteristic "barking" noise with each inhalation or cough.

BODY PARTS INVOLVED—Larynx; throat; bronchial tubes; trachea (windpipe).

SEX OR AGE MOST AFFECTED—Children under age 6.

SIGNS & SYMPTOMS
- Hoarseness.
- Barking cough and difficult breathing, especially at night.
- Chest or throat discomfort or pain.

CAUSES—Contagious viral or bacterial infection.

RISK INCREASES WITH—Allergies.

HOW TO PREVENT
- To prevent recurrent attacks, run the humidifier at the child's bedside for several nights after the first attack.
- If croup is a recurring problem in your family, consider adding a humidifier to your home's heating and air-conditioning system.

 WHAT TO EXPECT

APPROPRIATE HEALTH CARE
- Home care after diagnosis.
- Doctor's treatment.
- Emergency-room care, if the windpipe is blocked.

DIAGNOSTIC MEASURES
- Your own observation of symptoms.
- Medical history and physical exam by a doctor.
- X-rays of the chest.

POSSIBLE COMPLICATIONS—Airway obstruction and death (rare).

PROBABLE OUTCOME—Croup can be frightening, because attacks usually happen at night and the child has trouble breathing. In most cases, croup is not serious, and symptoms can be relieved. If attacks happen during the day and are accompanied by fever, the illness is more serious.

 HOW TO TREAT

NOTE—Follow your doctor's instructions. These instructions are supplemental.

GENERAL MEASURES—Home care for a mild croup attack:

- Stay calm. Anxiety increases the child's breathing difficulty.
- Take the child into the bathroom and close the door.
- Turn on the hot water full force in the sink and shower to saturate the air with moisture. Open the windows to let in cold air.
- Allow 10 minutes for the steam and cold air to relieve symptoms. If severe symptoms don't improve in 10 minutes, take the child to the nearest emergency room.
- Stay in the steamed bathroom until you are ready to leave. Don't be afraid to take the child out in the cold night air—it may lessen breathing difficulty.
- If breathing improves in 10 minutes, take the child with you while you call the doctor or wait for a return call. While waiting, use a cool-mist humidifier in the room.
- Keep the child comfortable in a semiseated position. Use TV, radio or a story to distract the child so he can relax.
- If breathing worsens again, return to the steam-filled bathroom.
- Run the humidifier by the child's bed for several nights after an attack—even if the child appears well. Simple croup often recurs.

MEDICATION—If croup is caused by a bacterial infection, your doctor may prescribe antibiotics. However, most cases are viral, so antibiotics are ineffective.

ACTIVITY—Decrease the child's activity and encourage rest as long as croup attacks are occurring. Don't allow the child to play outside in cool night air—this may trigger attacks (although cool air can help relieve symptoms *during* an attack).

DIET—Croup usually depresses appetite. Offer frequent small amounts of fluid, such as water, ginger ale, tea, juice or cola—not milk. Coughing may cause vomiting, so don't give the child solids during an attack.

 CALL YOUR DOCTOR IF

- Your child is having trouble breathing and cannot swallow saliva or water. This is an emergency! Call your doctor and ask him or her to meet you at the nearest emergency room.
- Breathing rate increases to 80 breaths a minute.
- Breathing is labored and retraction (the drawing in of neck and chest with each inhalation) is pronounced.
- Nails or lips become dark or blue.
- Mild croup symptoms don't improve with 30 to 60 minutes of cool-mist treatment.

ILLNESSES & DISORDERS

CRYPTOCOCCOSIS
(Torulosis)

GENERAL INFORMATION

DEFINITION—A fungal disease that usually begins in the lung and may spread to other body parts. It is much more serious when there are underlying illnesses or risk factors.

BODY PARTS INVOLVED—Lung; central nervous system; kidney; bone; skin.

SEX OR AGE MOST AFFECTED—Most common in men between ages 40 and 60.

SIGNS & SYMPTOMS
- Severe headache.
- Stiff neck.
- Fever.
- Blurred vision.
- Protein in the urine.
- Mental disturbances, such as confusion, depression, agitation or inappropriate speech or dress.
- Cough.

CAUSES—Infection from the fungus, cryptococcus neoformans (also called filobasidiella neoformans). The fungus is acquired by breathing air that contains spores of this organism, which comes from soil.

The serious, progressive, systemic form of this fungus disease is most apt to occur in persons who are seriously ill with other diseases or who are receiving immunosuppressive treatment.

RISK INCREASES WITH
- Geographic location. The disease is most common in the southeastern U.S.
- Use of cortisone, immunosuppressive or antimetabolite drugs.
- Illness that has lowered resistance—especially Hodgkin's disease—or others, including: uremia; diabetes; chronic lung disease; tuberculosis; leukemia; or severe burns.

HOW TO PREVENT—Obtain medical treatment for any of the serious illnesses listed as risks.

WHAT TO EXPECT

APPROPRIATE HEALTH CARE
- Doctor's treatment.
- Hospitalization for intensive care in severe cases.
- Self-care after diagnosis and hospitalization.

DIAGNOSTIC MEASURES
- Your own observation of symptoms.
- Medical history and physical exam by a doctor.
- Laboratory studies of cerebrospinal fluid, blood and urine.
- X-rays of the chest and bones.

POSSIBLE COMPLICATIONS—This fungus can cause severe, debilitating illness. In rare cases, the fungi spread from the lungs throughout the body, causing skin ulcers and bone and kidney infections.

PROBABLE OUTCOME—Usually curable if the infection remains confined to the lung, or if treatment with potent antifungal medicines is successful against complications.

HOW TO TREAT

NOTE—Follow your doctor's instructions. These instructions are supplemental.

GENERAL MEASURES
- It is usually not necessary to isolate ill persons.
- Weigh daily and keep a weight chart. An unexplained weight loss might indicate that infection has spread.

MEDICATION—If the disease remains confined to the lungs, no medication may be needed.

If complications arise, your doctor may prescribe potent antifungal drugs. These are effective for skin, bone or kidney involvement, and life-saving for cryptococcal meningitis. Treatment with these drugs requires hospitalization.

ACTIVITY—If you have a mild form of the disease that does not require strong antifungal medication, rest in bed until the cough and fever disappear.

DIET—No special diet.

CALL YOUR DOCTOR IF

- You have symptoms of cryptococcosis, especially a severe headache or stiff neck.
- The following occurs during treatment:
  Weight loss.
  Fever of 101F (38.3C) orally.
  Diarrhea that cannot be controlled.
  Severe headache and stiff neck.
- New, unexplained symptoms develop. Drugs used in treatment may produce side effects.

CUSHING'S SYNDROME

GENERAL INFORMATION

DEFINITION—An endocrine disorder caused by excess adrenal hormones.

BODY PARTS INVOLVED—Adrenal gland (located over the kidney); pituitary gland (at the base of the brain).

SEX OR AGE MOST AFFECTED
- All ages, but most common in adults.
- Both sexes, but more common in women.

SIGNS & SYMPTOMS
- Round face and puffy eyes.
- Ruddy red complexion.
- Growth of facial hair in women.
- Fat accumulation over the upper back and trunk, accompanied by red "stretch marks."
- High blood pressure.
- Mental and emotional changes, including psychosis.
- Menstrual changes, including cessation of, increased or irregular periods.
- Enlarged clitoris.
- Diabetes mellitus.
- Peptic ulcers.
- Osteoporosis.
- Low resistance to infection.

CAUSES—Symptoms and signs result from overproduction of the cortisonelike hormone produced by the adrenal glands. The overproduction may result from:
- A tumor in the adrenal glands.
- A pituitary tumor, causing production of excessive ACTH (adreno-cortico-tropic-hormone), which the pituitary gland produces to stimulate adrenal glands to secrete hormones.
- Prolonged use of cortisone drugs.

RISK INCREASES WITH—Prolonged use of ACTH for treatment of pituitary cancer.

HOW TO PREVENT—If use of ACTH or cortisone is necessary for other disorders, such as asthma, arthritis, kidney disease or Addison's disease, take the lowest dose possible for the shortest time. Consult your doctor.

WHAT TO EXPECT

APPROPRIATE HEALTH CARE
- Doctor's treatment, including consultation with an endocrinologist.
- Surgery (sometimes) to remove ACTH-producing tumors from the pituitary or to remove adrenal-gland tumors.
- Hospitalization for high voltage radiation treatment of the pituitary gland (sometimes).

DIAGNOSTIC MEASURES
- Your own observation of symptoms. Pictures taken before symptoms begin are helpful in noting changes in appearance.
- Medical history and physical exam by a doctor.
- Laboratory blood and urine studies of white-blood-cell counts, pituitary and adrenal-gland function and hormone levels.
- X-rays of the pituitary and adrenal glands.

POSSIBLE COMPLICATIONS
- Bone fractures due to osteoporosis.
- Pituitary tumor, if adrenal glands are removed (rare).

PROBABLE OUTCOME
- If caused by an adrenal-gland tumor, the disorder is curable with removal of the tumor or glands. Lifelong, carefully monitored drug therapy is essential if the glands are removed.
- If caused by a pituitary tumor, the disorder is curable with removal of the tumor, but tumors may recur.
- If caused by prolonged use of cortisone drugs or ACTH, the condition may improve if these are withdrawn *gradually under medical supervision.*

HOW TO TREAT

NOTE—Follow your doctor's instructions. These instructions are supplemental.

GENERAL MEASURES
- Learn all you can about this condition and its treatment. You must often monitor your own reactions to medications. Discontinuing drugs suddenly is dangerous.
- Wear a Medic-Alert bracelet or pendant (see Glossary).
- Protect yourself from fractures. Accidentproof your home. Wear seat belts in autos. Don't take risks.

MEDICATION—Your doctor may prescribe:
- Drugs, such as aminoglutethimide or mitotane, to suppress adrenal-gland function.
- Cortisone drugs, if adrenal glands must be removed surgically.
- Drugs to replace pituitary hormones (sometimes).
- Antihypertensive drugs to lower blood pressure.
- Calcium supplements to treat osteoporosis.

ACTIVITY—No restrictions. Energy will increase once treatment begins.

DIET—A low-salt diet (see Appendix 9) is sometimes necessary. Consult your doctor.

CALL YOUR DOCTOR IF

- You have symptoms of Cushing's syndrome.
- You have signs of infection, such as fever, chills, muscle aches, headache and dizziness.

CYSTIC FIBROSIS (CF)

GENERAL INFORMATION

DEFINITION—An inherited disease in which mucus-producing glands throughout the body—especially in the pancreas and lung—fail to produce normal enzymes and mucus.

BODY PARTS INVOLVED—Pancreas; lungs; sweat glands of the skin; gastrointestinal tract.

SEX OR AGE MOST AFFECTED—Children of both sexes.

SIGNS & SYMPTOMS—Newborn period:
• Thick, sticky stools (meconium), which may cause intestinal obstruction.
Later:
• Poor weight gain despite good appetite.
• Bad-smelling, large, fatty stools.
• Chronic cough.
• Frequent, severe respiratory infections with sticky, hard-to-cough-up sputum.
• Salty sweat.
• Enlarged liver and spleen.

CAUSES—Genetic factors. Many people carry the genes for cystic fibrosis, and 1 in 2000 newborns is born with it. The genes cause abnormal mucus in the respiratory and gastrointestinal tracts and sweat glands. This causes lung obstruction and infection, poor digestion and poor food absorption.

RISK INCREASES WITH—Family history of cystic fibrosis. If both parents come from families with cystic fibrosis, the chances are 1 in 4 that each child will have the disease.

HOW TO PREVENT—If you have a family history of cystic fibrosis, seek genetic counseling before starting a family.

WHAT TO EXPECT

APPROPRIATE HEALTH CARE
• Home care after diagnosis.
• Doctor's treatment.
• Psychotherapy or counseling to help parents and children adjust.
• Surgery to relieve intestinal obstruction (sometimes).
• Hospitalization to control serious infections, which occur frequently.

DIAGNOSTIC MEASURES
• Your own observation of symptoms. Sometimes a parent notes a salty taste when kissing a child.
• Medical history and physical exam by a doctor.
• Laboratory studies to analyze sweat, stools and digestive juices.

POSSIBLE COMPLICATIONS
• Pneumonia.
• Chronic bronchitis.
• Bronchiectasis.
• Fluid and electrolyte imbalance—especially in hot weather.
• Malnutrition.
• Nasal polyps.
• Rectal prolapse.

PROBABLE OUTCOME—This condition is currently considered incurable and is often fatal in childhood. Careful long-term care by parents and professionals can help children lead reasonably comfortable lives. Children with milder forms may live to adulthood, especially if the disorder is detected early.

HOW TO TREAT

NOTE—Follow your doctor's instructions. These instructions are supplemental.

GENERAL MEASURES
• Learn as much as possible about this condition. Diet, medication and early recognition of infection are very important.
• You will need to perform daily postural drainage to drain mucus from the lungs, and chest pounding to shake loose sticky mucus plugs. Ask your doctor for instructions.
• Use a cool-mist humidifier in your child's room whenever he or she has respiratory symptoms. Moisture helps thin mucus so it can be coughed up more easily.
• Keep your child's immunizations, including pneumonia and influenza vaccines, up to date. An immunization schedule appears in Appendix 16.
• Join a support group for parents of children with cystic fibrosis.
• Encourage your child to lead as normal and active a life as possible.

MEDICATION—Your doctor may prescribe:
• Digestive enzymes.
• Antibiotics when lung infections occur.
• Enzymes by nebulizer to help loosen lung secretions.

ACTIVITY—As much as the condition permits.

DIET—Your child should eat a low-fat diet with adequate protein. Consult a dietitian for specific instructions. Vitamin and mineral supplements may be necessary. Encourage intake of liquids, which helps thin mucus.

CALL YOUR DOCTOR IF

• You suspect your child has cystic fibrosis.
• After diagnosis, your child develops fever, a worsening cough and muscle aches.

DECOMPRESSION SICKNESS
(Caisson Disease; "The Bends")

 GENERAL INFORMATION

DEFINITION—A painful, sometimes life-threatening condition of blood gases that is caused by a sudden drop in environmental pressure.

BODY PARTS INVOLVED—Blood in all body parts.

SEX OR AGE MOST AFFECTED—Both sexes; all ages.

SIGNS & SYMPTOMS—The following may occur immediately or up to 24 hours after the pressure change:
- Mild to severe joint pain, especially in the shoulders, elbows, hips and knees.
- Chest pain; shortness of breath; "chokes" (see Glossary); coughing; a burning sensation behind the breastbone.
- Weakness; loss of normal sensation; paralysis; loss of consciousness; and coma (rare).
- Inability to speak; blindness; and deafness.
- Abdominal pain.
- Difficult urination.

CAUSES—Formation of nitrogen bubbles in the blood. Nitrogen is a normal blood component. If the pressure around the body drops rapidly—as in surfacing too quickly while scuba diving, or climbing too rapidly in a non-pressurized aircraft—the nitrogen collects in bubbles in the blood vessels, blocking them and depriving the body of essential blood nutrients.

RISK INCREASES WITH
- Commercial diving or recreational scuba diving. Repeated dives in one day increase the risk.
- Some kinds of high-performance aircraft.
- Working in compression chambers.

HOW TO PREVENT
- Obtain professional instruction before scuba diving.
- Don't dive if you are not in good general health. You are at risk if you are obese or have a medical history of:
    Lung conditions, such as asthma.
    Spontaneous pneumothorax.
    Heart disease.
    Chronic sinusitis.
    Emotional instability.
    Alcoholism.
- Allow for a slow, gradual change to normal air pressure in situations listed above. (The U.S. Navy has tested and established guidelines.)
- Avoid air travel for 24 hours after diving.

 WHAT TO EXPECT

APPROPRIATE HEALTH CARE
- Doctor's treatment.
- Hospitalization in a decompression chamber to force nitrogen bubbles to dissolve into the blood.

DIAGNOSTIC MEASURES
- Your own observation of symptoms.
- Medical history and physical exam by a doctor.

POSSIBLE COMPLICATIONS
- Permanent brain damage.
- Permanent bone destruction caused by inadequate nourishment from the blood.

PROBABLE OUTCOME—Complete recovery with treatment.

 HOW TO TREAT

NOTE—Follow your doctor's instructions. These instructions are supplemental.

GENERAL MEASURES—Self-care is impossible for this condition. If you observe someone with symptoms of decompression sickness, obtain emergency medical care immediately.

MEDICATION—Medicine usually is not necessary for this disorder. Don't take pain relievers. These may further decrease normal breathing efficiency.

ACTIVITY—Resume your normal activities as soon as symptoms improve after treatment.

DIET—No special diet.

 CALL YOUR DOCTOR IF

You develop any symptoms of decompression sickness within 24 hours after scuba diving or rapid ascent without pressurization.

ILLNESSES & DISORDERS

DEHYDRATION

GENERAL INFORMATION

DEFINITION—Loss of water and essential body salts.

BODY PARTS INVOLVED—Blood; gastrointestinal tract; kidneys.

SEX OR AGE MOST AFFECTED—Both sexes; all ages. Dehydration is most dangerous in newborns, infants and persons over 60.

SIGNS & SYMPTOMS
- Dry mouth.
- Decreased or absent urination.
- Sunken eyes.
- Wrinkled skin.
- Confusion; coma.
- Low blood pressure.

CAUSES
- Persistent vomiting or diarrhea from any cause.
- Heavy sweating.
- Use of drugs that deplete fluids and electrolytes, such as diuretics ("water pills").
- Overexposure to sun or heat.

RISK INCREASES WITH
- Newborns and infants.
- Adults over 60.
- Recent illness with high fever.
- Diabetes mellitus.
- Chronic kidney disease.

HOW TO PREVENT
- Obtain medical treatment for underlying causes of dehydration.
- If you are vomiting or have diarrhea, take small amounts of liquid with non-prescription electrolyte supplements—or drinks such as Gatorade—every 30 to 60 minutes.
- If you use diuretics, weigh daily. Report to your doctor a weight loss of more than 3 pounds in 1 day or 5 pounds in 1 week.

WHAT TO EXPECT

APPROPRIATE HEALTH CARE
- Self-care.
- Doctor's treatment.
- Hospitalization for intravenous fluids (severe or prolonged illness only).

DIAGNOSTIC MEASURES
- Your own observation of symptoms.
- Medical history and physical exam by a doctor.
- Laboratory blood studies, including blood counts and electrolyte measurement (see Glossary).

POSSIBLE COMPLICATIONS—Blood-pressure drop, shock and death from prolonged, severe dehydration.

PROBABLE OUTCOME—Curable with control of the underlying cause and replacement of necessary fluids.

HOW TO TREAT

NOTE—Follow your doctor's instructions. These instructions are supplemental.

GENERAL MEASURES
- Weigh daily on an accurate home scale and record the weight so you can be aware of fluid loss.
- If you have vomiting or diarrhea, keep a record of the number of episodes so you can estimate your fluid loss.
- For minor dehydration, take frequent small amounts of clear liquids. Large amounts may trigger vomiting.

MEDICATION—Your doctor may prescribe intravenous fluids to replace lost water.

ACTIVITY—Rest in bed until you recover. You may read or watch TV.

DIET—Depends on the underlying disorder. Salty foods decrease the effect of dehydration.

CALL YOUR DOCTOR IF

You have symptoms of dehydration.

DEMENTIA
(Chronic Brain Syndrome)

 GENERAL INFORMATION

DEFINITION—Mental impairment caused by a variety of diseases that produce permanent brain deterioration.

BODY PARTS INVOLVED—Brain.

SEX OR AGE MOST AFFECTED—Adults over 60.

SIGNS & SYMPTOMS
- Forgetfulness, especially of recent events.
- Unpredictable, sometimes violent, behavior.
- Confusion.
- Loss of interest in normal activities.
- Disorientation, especially at night.
- Poor personal hygiene and appearance.
- Depression.
- Poor judgment.

CAUSES—Degeneration and loss of the gray matter from the brain. The causes include:
- Alzheimer's disease.
- Inadequate blood supply to the brain due to blood clots, hypertension or hardening of the arteries.
- Alcoholism.
- Syphilis or other chronic infection.
- Chronic poisoning from industrial chemicals.
- Inherited condition, such as Huntington's chorea.
- Brain injury from any cause.
- Some endocrine conditions, such as diabetes or hypothyroidism.
- Brain tumor.

RISK INCREASES WITH
- Chemical or environmental exposure to heavy metals.
- Adults over 60.
- Excess alcohol consumption.
- Use of cocaine, LSD or mescaline, or glue-sniffing.
- Family history of Alzheimer's disease.

HOW TO PREVENT
- Obtain early medical treatment for underlying causes, such as syphilis, hypertension, alcoholism, diabetes and hypothyroidism.
- Protect yourself from head injury. Wear shoulder harnesses and seat belts in vehicles. Wear protective head gear for riding bicycles, motorcycles and participating in contact sports. Don't drink or use mind-altering drugs and drive.
- Survey your workplace for chemical hazards and protect yourself from exposure.
- To prevent atherosclerosis, don't smoke, eat a diet low in fat (see Appendix 8), exercise regularly (see Appendix 20) and reduce stress whenever possible.

 WHAT TO EXPECT

APPROPRIATE HEALTH CARE
- Doctor's treatment. A neurological examination will detect curable conditions.
- Nursing-home care, if the disorder is too advanced for home care.
- Psychotherapy or counseling for family members.

DIAGNOSTIC MEASURES
- Your own observation of symptoms.
- Medical history and physical exam by a doctor.
- Laboratory blood studies.
- EEG (see Glossary).
- X-rays of the head.

POSSIBLE COMPLICATIONS
- Infections, falls and injuries, and poor nutrition. These occur because the ill person cannot care for himself or herself.
- Misdiagnosis. Many curable conditions have symptoms that mimic dementia.

PROBABLE OUTCOME—This condition is currently considered incurable. Medicine may prevent the condition from worsening, but it cannot restore lost brain function.

 HOW TO TREAT

NOTE—Follow your doctor's instructions. These instructions are supplemental.

GENERAL MEASURES—Family members can help:
- Notice early behavior changes and seek prompt medical care.
- Provide simple reminders, such as a clock, daily calendar or name tag.
- Encourage social activities and contacts.
- Treat the person with respect and kindness.
- Provide a protected, non-judgmental environment when the patient cannot provide self-care. When home care is no longer possible, find a good extended-care facility.
- Visit the patient often—even if he or she doesn't seem to recognize you.

MEDICATION—Your doctor may prescribe medication appropriate to treat the underlying condition.

ACTIVITY—Encourage as much activity as possible.

DIET—Provide a well-balanced diet.

 CALL YOUR DOCTOR IF

You observe symptoms of dementia in a family member.

DENTURE PROBLEMS

 ## GENERAL INFORMATION

DEFINITION—Dentures are false teeth—either full or partial. In some cases, they may cause pain or another disorder. However, problems usually don't arise if dentures fit well, look natural, feel good and are cared for properly.

BODY PARTS INVOLVED—Gums; temporal-mandibular joints.

SEX OR AGE MOST AFFECTED—Adults over 50.

SIGNS & SYMPTOMS
- Pain with dentures in place.
- Inflamed or dark red gums that bleed easily.
- Possible hard pads at pressure points (dental granulomas).

CAUSES
- Pressure on mouth tissues from dentures.
- Jawbone deterioration.

RISK INCREASES WITH
- Adults over 60.
- Poor nutrition.

HOW TO PREVENT—Consult your dentist regularly for checkups.

 ## WHAT TO EXPECT

APPROPRIATE HEALTH CARE
- Self-care.
- Dentist's treatment.

DIAGNOSTIC MEASURES
- Your own observation of symptoms.
- Medical history and physical exam by a dentist.

POSSIBLE COMPLICATIONS
- Susceptibility to fungus infection (thrush), especially with the use of antibiotics.
- Protruding jaw and sunken cheeks after many years of wearing dentures.
- Trapped food particles in partial dentures.

PROBABLE OUTCOME—Artificial teeth are not as efficient as natural teeth, and an adjustment period is necessary. Most people adapt well to dentures, but some persons never adjust to them completely. Problems can usually be treated.

 ## HOW TO TREAT

NOTE—Follow your dentist's instructions. These instructions are supplemental.

GENERAL MEASURES
- Practice speaking aloud to gain muscle control and tone so your speech is normal. Speak slowly at first until you feel at ease.
- Remove dentures at night to rest your gums. Store dentures in a glass of water mixed with denture cleanser so they will not dry out and warp.
- Clean and massage your gums regularly with a finger, cloth or brush.
- Clean dentures daily. Use a stiff brush and regular toothpaste to clean your dentures as you would natural teeth. Tartar accumulates on dentures as on natural teeth.
- Clean dentures over a basin of water to cushion a fall if you should drop them.
- If stubborn stains appear, place the dentures in a glass of water mixed with 1 teaspoon of chlorine bleach. (Don't use bleach if your dentures contain metal. The chemical may damage the metal.)
- If you have a partial denture, clean your natural teeth and gums thoroughly, especially around the base of the teeth.

MEDICATION—Your doctor may prescribe antifungal medicine if you develop thrush.

ACTIVITY—No restrictions.

DIET—No special diet if dentures fit properly.

 ## CALL YOUR DENTIST IF

- Your dentures won't stay in place when you smile, laugh or talk.
- Sore spots develop on your gums. These are common and can be treated easily and quickly by your dentist.
- White spots develop in your mouth which become irritated when you try to brush them away.
- Your dentures break. Save all the pieces for your dentist. Your dentist can usually repair dentures quickly. Don't try to repair them yourself.

DEPRESSION

 GENERAL INFORMATION

DEFINITION—A feeling of continuing sadness, despondency or hopelessness.

BODY PARTS INVOLVED—Central nervous system.

SEX OR AGE MOST AFFECTED—Both sexes; all ages.

SIGNS & SYMPTOMS
- Loss of interest in life; boredom.
- Listlessness and fatigue.
- Insomnia or excessive sleeping.
- Social isolation.
- Appetite loss or overeating.
- Loss of sex drive.
- Constipation.
- Concentration difficulty.
- Unexplained crying bouts.
- Intense guilt feelings over minor or imaginary misdeeds.
- Difficulty making decisions.
- Irritability.
- Various pains, such as headache or chest pain, without evidence of disease.

CAUSES
- Failure in occupation, marriage or other interpersonal relationships.
- Death of a loved one.
- Loss of something important (job, home, investments).
- Job change or move to a new area.
- Surgery, such as mastectomy for cancer.
- Major illness or disability.
- Passing from one life stage to another, such as menopause or retirement.
- Use of some drugs, such as reserpine, beta-adrenergic blockers or benzodiazepines.
- Withdrawal from mood-altering drugs, such as narcotics, amphetamines or caffeine.
- Some diseases, including diabetes mellitus, cancer of the pancreas and hormonal abnormalities.

RISK INCREASES WITH
- Unexpressed anger or other emotion.
- Compulsive, rigid, perfectionist or highly dependent personalities.
- Family history of depression.
- Alcoholism.

HOW TO PREVENT
- Maintain good communication with family and close friends.
- Raise children with love and reasonable expectations in school and home.

 WHAT TO EXPECT

APPROPRIATE HEALTH CARE
- Self-care for mild depression.
- Doctor's treatment.
- Psychotherapy or counseling.
- Hospitalization for severe depression.

DIAGNOSTIC MEASURES
- Your own observation of symptoms.
- Medical history and physical exam by a doctor (sometimes a psychiatrist).
- Psychological testing.

POSSIBLE COMPLICATIONS
- Suicide. Warning signs include:
  Withdrawal from family and friends.
  Neglect of personal appearance.
  Mention of wanting "to end it all" or being "a burden to others."
  Evidence of a suicide plan, such as buying or cleaning a gun.
  Sudden cheerfulness after prolonged despondency.
- Hallucinations or psychotic behavior.
- Manic behavior, characterized by inappropriate overactivity and comic or irresponsible behavior.

PROBABLE OUTCOME—Spontaneous recovery in many cases, but professional help can shorten the duration and help you learn to cope in the future. Recurrence is common. The recovery rate is high, despite one's pessimism while depressed.

 HOW TO TREAT

NOTE—Follow your doctor's instructions. These instructions are supplemental.

GENERAL MEASURES
- Seek support groups. Contact social agencies or churches for help.
- Call your local suicide-prevention hot line if you feel suicidal.

MEDICATION—Your doctor may prescribe:
- Antidepressant drugs (often tricyclics) to accompany therapy.
- Lithium for alternating mania and depression.

ACTIVITY—No restrictions. Maintain daily activities and interests—even if you don't feel like it. Attend social functions, concerts, athletic events, plays and movies. Keep in touch with friends and loved ones.
  Engage in regular, strenuous exercise. This helps relieve depression.

DIET—Eat a normal, well-balanced diet—even if you have no appetite. Vitamin and mineral supplements may be necessary.

 CALL YOUR DOCTOR IF

- You have symptoms of depression.
- You feel suicidal or hopeless.

DERMATITIS, ATOPIC

 GENERAL INFORMATION

DEFINITION—A chronic inflammatory disease of the skin that is often associated with other allergic disorders that affect the respiratory system, such as asthma or hay fever.

BODY PARTS INVOLVED—Skin.

SEX OR AGE MOST AFFECTED—Adolescents and adults. For children, see Eczema (in Illness section).

SIGNS & SYMPTOMS
- Itching rash in areas where heat and moisture are retained, such as skin creases of elbows, knees, neck, face, hands, feet, groin, genitals and around the anus.
- Dry, thickened skin in affected areas.
- Uncontrolled scratching (frequently unconscious).
- Chronic fatigue from loss of sleep due to severe itching.

CAUSES—Unknown, but probably inherited and probably related to immune-system deficiency.

RISK INCREASES WITH
- Hay fever or asthma.
- Food allergy.
- Family history of atopic dermatitis or other allergic disorders.
- Stress. The rash and itching increase during stressful periods.
- Use of immunosuppressive drugs.

HOW TO PREVENT—Cannot be prevented at present.

 WHAT TO EXPECT

APPROPRIATE HEALTH CARE
- Self-care after diagnosis.
- Doctor's treatment.

DIAGNOSTIC MEASURES—Laboratory blood studies and patch tests to identify allergies.

POSSIBLE COMPLICATIONS
- Secondary bacterial infection in the affected area.
- Increased susceptibility to adverse drug reactions.
- Decreased resistance to fungal and viral infections.
- Permanent scarring from scratching.

PROBABLE OUTCOME—Unpredictable. Flare-ups and remissions may occur throughout life.

 HOW TO TREAT

NOTE—Follow your doctor's instructions. These instructions are supplemental.

GENERAL MEASURES
- Use cool-water soaks (see Appendix 18) for crusting, oozing lesions. These decrease itching and remove crusts.
- Bathe in cool water with cleansing agents other than soap.
- Wear loose-fitting, cotton clothing—avoid wool and synthetics.
- Don't allow yourself to be vaccinated against smallpox. It can cause a life-threatening reaction.
- Reduce stress in your life, if possible. See Appendix 13 for suggestions.

MEDICATION
- To relieve minor itching, use non-prescription topical steroids or coal-tar preparations.
- For severe itching, your doctor may prescribe:
  More potent topical steroids.
  Oral cortisone drugs (rarely, and for short periods only).
  Antihistamines or mild tranquilizers.
  Lubricating ointments for the hands.
  Antibiotics (sometimes) to fight secondary infections.

ACTIVITY—No restrictions except to keep cool. Avoid prolonged exposure to heat.

DIET—An allergy diet (see Appendix 6) may be necessary, if food allergy is suspected.

 CALL YOUR DOCTOR IF

- You have symptoms of atopic dermatitis.
- You develop fever or uncontrolled itching during a flare-up.

DERMATITIS, CONTACT
(Housewives' Eczema)

 ### GENERAL INFORMATION

DEFINITION—Skin inflammation caused by contact with an irritating substance. Contact dermatitis is not contagious.

BODY PARTS INVOLVED—Skin, especially of the hands, feet and groin.

SEX OR AGE MOST AFFECTED—All ages, but most common in women.

SIGNS & SYMPTOMS
- Itching (sometimes).
- Slight redness.
- Cracks and fissures in the skin.
- Bright red, weeping areas (severe cases).

CAUSES—Contact with irritants, such as acids or solvents. (Hot water and detergent are the most common irritants.) The irritant removes the fatty layer of skin. This causes dehydration and shrinking of surface cells.

RISK INCREASES WITH
- Constant exposure to hot water, detergents, or any irritant that changes the moisture content of skin.
- Burns from hot water or sunburn.

HOW TO PREVENT
- Avoid contact with any irritant which has caused dermatitis in the past.
- Protect skin from sunburn and other burns.

 ### WHAT TO EXPECT

APPROPRIATE HEALTH CARE
- Self-care.
- Doctor's treatment.

DIAGNOSTIC MEASURES
- Your own observation of symptoms.
- Medical history and physical exam by a doctor.

POSSIBLE COMPLICATIONS—Pain and disfigurement of hands from constant lesions.

PROBABLE OUTCOME—Symptoms can be controlled with treatment and avoidance of the irritant. Recurrence is common, so treatment may be necessary for years.

 ### HOW TO TREAT

NOTE—Follow your doctor's instructions. These instructions are supplemental.

GENERAL MEASURES
- Avoid the chemical or material causing the skin eruption.
- Use bath oil instead of soap for bathing.
- Pat skin dry rather than rubbing it.
- Reduce water temperature to lukewarm for bathing or other uses.
- Use only cream, lotion or ointment prescribed for the condition. Other commercial products may aggravate the condition. Apply ointment or cream to hands 6 or 7 times a day. For other body parts, lubricate twice a day, especially after bathing.
- Minimize the use of solvents, and wear heavy-duty vinyl gloves to prevent contact with irritating substances such as: water; soap; detergent; metal scouring pads; scouring powder; paint; paint thinner; turpentine; and polish for cars, floors, shoes, furniture or metal.
- Dry the insides of gloves after use. Discard gloves if they develop a hole.
- Wear gloves when you peel or squeeze lemons, oranges, grapefruit, tomatoes or potatoes.
- Wear leather or heavy-duty fabric gloves for housework or gardening.
- Use a dishwashing machine to wash dishes or ask someone else to do it.
- Remove rings before doing housework or washing hands.

MEDICATION—Your doctor may prescribe topical creams, ointments or lotions. These may include steroid preparations to reduce inflammation or lubricants to preserve moisture.

ACTIVITY—Resume your normal activities gradually as irritation subsides.

DIET—No special diet.

 ### CALL YOUR DOCTOR IF

- You develop fever.
- Signs of infection (swelling, tenderness, redness, warmth) develop at the site of irritation.
- Treatment does not relieve symptoms in 1 week.

ILLNESSES & DISORDERS

DERMATITIS HERPETIFORMIS

 ## GENERAL INFORMATION

DEFINITION—A chronic skin inflammation characterized by clusters of small itching blisters. The disorder is hereditary, but not contagious or cancerous.

BODY PARTS INVOLVED—Skin of the elbows, knees, shoulders, arms, legs, and over the bottom of the spine (sacrum).

SEX OR AGE MOST AFFECTED—Adolescents and adults.

SIGNS & SYMPTOMS—Lesions with the following characteristics:
● Lesions are small clusters of 5 to 20 blisters. Blisters usually measure 2mm to 6mm in diameter.
● Clusters appear on both sides of the body in the same places.
● Lesions itch, but they are not usually painful if there are no complications.

CAUSES—Unknown, but may be a disorder of the autoimmune system.

RISK INCREASES WITH—Exposure to heat and humidity.

HOW TO PREVENT—Cannot be prevented at present. To prevent a recurrence of symptoms, continue to take medication as directed and prevent injury to normal skin.

 ## WHAT TO EXPECT

APPROPRIATE HEALTH CARE
● Self-care after diagnosis.
● Doctor's treatment.

DIAGNOSTIC MEASURES
● Your own observation of symptoms.
● Medical history and physical exam by a doctor.
● Biopsy (see Glossary).

POSSIBLE COMPLICATIONS—People with dermatitis herpetiformis also may have disease of the small bowel (without symptoms), which pathologically resembles that of patients who are intolerant to gluten. The only way to diagnose this is with biopsy.

PROBABLE OUTCOME—This is a chronic disease. Treatment can control symptoms—including itching—but it will not cure the disease.

 ## HOW TO TREAT

NOTE—Follow your doctor's instructions. These instructions are supplemental.

GENERAL MEASURES—Soak in cool water or use cool-water compresses to reduce itching.

MEDICATION
● For itching, you may use non-prescription drugs such as:
   Low-dose steroid lotion, ointment and cream. These reduce inflammation and itching in 24 to 48 hours.
   Topical anesthetics and topical antihistamines. These provide quick, short-term relief. Many cause skin sensitivity, but lidocaine and pramoxine usually do not.
   Lotions containing phenol, menthol and camphor (such as calamine lotion). These are soothing, but use with care. Large amounts may be absorbed through the skin into the bloodstream; they can be toxic.
● To control blistering, your doctor may prescribe two oral medications, sulfapyridine or dapsone. If either one is needed, it will be required indefinitely.

ACTIVITY—No restrictions, except avoid overheating and moisture.

DIET—Restricting gluten in your diet will reduce the amount of medicine you will need. For a gluten-free diet, see Appendix 5.

 ## CALL YOUR DOCTOR IF

● You have symptoms of dermatitis herpetiformis.
● New, unexplained symptoms develop. Drugs used in treatment may produce side effects.

DERMATITIS, SEBORRHEIC

GENERAL INFORMATION

DEFINITION—A skin condition characterized by greasy cr dry, white scales. Dandruff and cradle cap are both forms of seborrheic dermatitis. This is not contagious.

BODY PARTS INVOLVED—Skin of the scalp, eyebrows, forehead, face, folds around the nose, behind ears, external ear canal or skin of the trunk, especially over the breastbone (sternum) or in skin folds.

SEX OR AGE MOST AFFECTED—Both sexes; all ages.

SIGNS & SYMPTOMS—Flaking, white scales over reddish patches on the skin. Scales anchor to hair shafts. They may itch, but they are usually painless unless complicated by infection.

CAUSES—Unknown.

RISK INCREASES WITH
- Stress.
- Hot, humid weather or cold, dry weather.
- Infrequent shampoos.
- Oily skin.
- Other skin disorders, such as acne rosacea, acne or psoriasis.
- Obesity.
- Parkinson's disease.
- Use of drying lotions that contain alcohol.

HOW TO PREVENT—Cannot be prevented. To minimize severity or frequency of flare-ups:
- Shampoo frequently.
- Dry skin folds thoroughly after bathing.
- Wear loose, ventilating clothing.

WHAT TO EXPECT

APPROPRIATE HEALTH CARE
- Self-care after diagnosis.
- Doctor's treatment.

DIAGNOSTIC MEASURES
- Your own observation of symptoms.
- Medical history and physical exam by a doctor.

POSSIBLE COMPLICATIONS
- Embarrassment and social discomfort.
- Secondary bacterial infection in affected areas.

PROBABLE OUTCOME—This is a chronic condition, but it is often characterized by long periods of inactivity. During active phases, symptoms can be controlled with treatment.

HOW TO TREAT

NOTE—Follow your doctor's instructions. These instructions are supplemental.

GENERAL MEASURES—Shampoo vigorously and as often as once a day. The shampoo you use is not as important as the way you scrub your scalp. Loosen scales with your fingernails while shampooing, and scrub at least 5 minutes.

MEDICATION
- For minor dandruff, you may use non-prescription dandruff shampoos and lubricating skin lotion.
- For severe problems, your doctor may prescribe:
  Shampoos that contain coal tar or scalp creams that contain cortisone. To apply medication to the scalp, part the hair a few strands at a time, and rub the ointment or lotion vigorously into the scalp.
  Topical steroids for other affected parts.

ACTIVITY—No restrictions. Outdoor activities in summer may help.

DIET—No special diet. Avoid foods that seem to worsen your condition.

CALL YOUR DOCTOR IF

- You have symptoms of seborrheic dermatitis that don't respond to self-care.
- Patches of seborrheic dermatitis ooze, form crusts or drain pus.

ILLNESSES & DISORDERS

DIABETES INSIPIDUS

 GENERAL INFORMATION

DEFINITION—Temporary disorder of the hormone system, centered in the pituitary gland.

BODY PARTS INVOLVED—Pituitary gland; endocrine system.

SEX OR AGE MOST AFFECTED—Both sexes; all ages.

SIGNS & SYMPTOMS
- Excessive thirst that is difficult to satisfy.
- Passage of large amounts (up to 15 quarts a day) of diluted, colorless urine.
- Dry hands.
- Constipation.

CAUSES—Deficiency of an antidiuretic (ADH) hormone normally secreted by the pituitary gland. The deficiency may result from the following:
- Head injury, with damage to the pituitary gland.
- Tumor of the pituitary gland.
- Other brain tumor that applies pressure to the pituitary gland.
- Infection in the brain, such as encephalitis or meningitis.
- Bleeding inside the skull.
- Aneurysm.
- Kidney disease.

RISK INCREASES WITH
- Preceding illness or injury in the brain.
- Atherosclerosis (hardening of the arteries).
- Family history of diabetes insipidus.

HOW TO PREVENT—No specific preventive measures.

 WHAT TO EXPECT

APPROPRIATE HEALTH CARE
- Doctor's treatment.
- Surgery if a tumor or aneurysm is present.

DIAGNOSTIC MEASURES
- Your own observation of symptoms.
- Medical history and physical exam by a doctor.
- Laboratory studies, such as water-deprivation tests to determine levels of ADH.

POSSIBLE COMPLICATIONS—Electrolyte imbalance, especially increased sodium or potassium deficiency. Either of these can cause heartbeat irregularity, fatigue and congestive heart failure.

PROBABLE OUTCOME
- If the disorder is caused by a tumor or aneurysm, it can be cured by surgery.
- If the disorder is caused by a head injury, spontaneous recovery is likely within a year.
- If the disorder is caused by a preceding brain infection, symptoms may persist indefinitely.

 HOW TO TREAT

NOTE—Follow your doctor's instructions. These instructions are supplemental.

GENERAL MEASURES—If brain surgery is necessary, see Craniotomy (in Surgery section) for an explanation of surgery and postoperative care.

MEDICATION—Your doctor may prescribe synthetic ADH in nose drops, powder or injection form.

ACTIVITY—No restrictions.

DIET—No special diet. Drink as much water as you feel you need.

 CALL YOUR DOCTOR IF

- You have symptoms of diabetes insipidus.
- Symptoms don't improve, despite treatment.
- New, unexplained symptoms develop. Drugs used in treatment may produce side effects.

DIABETES MELLITUS, INSULIN-DEPENDENT

GENERAL INFORMATION

DEFINITION—A chronic disease of metabolism characterized by the body's inability to produce enough insulin to process carbohydrates, fat and protein efficiently. Treatment requires injections of insulin. Insulin-dependent diabetes is often called *ketosis-prone diabetes* if it begins in adulthood and *juvenile diabetes* if it begins in childhood.

BODY PARTS INVOLVED
● Islet cells of the pancreas that produce insulin.
● All body cells that need insulin to convert food into chemicals the body can use.

SEX OR AGE MOST AFFECTED—Usually begins before age 30, but may begin at any age.

SIGNS & SYMPTOMS
● Fatigue.
● Excess thirst.
● Increased appetite *and* weight loss.
● Frequent urination.
● Itching around the genitals.
● Increased susceptibility to infections, especially urinary-tract infections and yeast infections of the skin, mouth or vagina.
● Deterioration of vision (advanced stages).

CAUSES
● Too little insulin produced by the islet cells of the pancreas for unknown reasons.
● Interference with insulin use in the body cells for unknown reasons.
● Virus infection of the pancreas.

RISK INCREASES WITH
● Family history of diabetes mellitus. It often skips one generation.
● Pregnancy.

HOW TO PREVENT—Cannot be prevented.

WHAT TO EXPECT

APPROPRIATE HEALTH CARE
● Self-care after diagnosis.
● Doctor's treatment.
● Hospitalization for severe complications.
● Surgery for treatment of some complications, such as failing eyesight, gangrene or coronary-artery disease.

DIAGNOSTIC MEASURES
● Your own observation of symptoms.
● Medical history and physical exam by a doctor.
● Laboratory urine and blood studies to measure glucose, cholesterol and insulin.

POSSIBLE COMPLICATIONS
● Cardiovascular disease, especially stroke, atherosclerosis, and coronary-artery disease.
● Kidney failure.
● Blindness.
● Peripheral vascular disease, with gangrene in legs and feet and sexual impotence in men.
● Life-threatening hypoglycemia (low blood sugar) if too much insulin is used.
● Life-threatening ketoacidosis (very high blood sugar) with breakdown of body cells.

PROBABLE OUTCOME—This disease is presently considered incurable, but symptoms and progress of the disease can be controlled with rigid adherence to a treatment program. Life expectancy is somewhat reduced, but many persons with diabetes have a nearly normal life span.

HOW TO TREAT

NOTE—Follow your doctor's instructions. These instructions are supplemental.

GENERAL MEASURES
● Learn all you can about controlling diabetes and recognizing signs and symptoms of ketoacidosis or hypoglycemia.
● Keep a vial of glucagon available at all times to use if hypoglycemia occurs.
● Learn to give yourself insulin injections. They will be necessary every day for life.
● Wear a Medic-Alert bracelet or pendant (see Glossary).
● Seek medical treatment for any infection.

MEDICATION—Your doctor will prescribe insulin by injection. The dosage must be individualized and occasionally adjusted.

ACTIVITY—No restrictions. Regular daily exercise is an important part of controlling diabetes. Consult your doctor.

DIET—A special diet will be prescribed by your doctor.

CALL YOUR DOCTOR IF

● You have symptoms of diabetes mellitus.
● The following occurs during treatment:
  Inability to think clearly; weakness; sweating; paleness; rapid heartbeat; seizures; or coma (may indicate hypoglycemia).
  Orange odor on the breath; changes in breathing pattern; or stupor (may indicate ketoacidosis).
  Several days of illness or weakness.
  Numbness, tingling or pain in the feet or hands.
  Chest pain.

DIABETES MELLITUS, NON-INSULIN-DEPENDENT

GENERAL INFORMATION

DEFINITION — A disease of metabolism characterized by the body's inability to produce enough insulin to process carbohydrates, fat and protein efficiently. Non-insulin-dependent diabetes mellitus is most prevalent among obese adults. It is often called *maturity-onset diabetes.*

BODY PARTS INVOLVED
- Islet cells of the pancreas that produce insulin.
- All body cells that need insulin to convert food into chemicals the body can use.

SEX OR AGE MOST AFFECTED — Both sexes of adults.

SIGNS & SYMPTOMS
- Overweight.
- Fatigue.
- Excess thirst.
- Increased appetite.
- Frequent urination.
- Decreased resistance to infection, especially urinary-tract infections and yeast infections of the skin, mouth or vagina.

CAUSES
- Insufficient insulin produced by the pancreas to sustain normal function of body cells.
- Interference with insulin utilization in body cells for unknown reasons.

RISK INCREASES WITH
- Obesity in adults.
- Stress.
- Pregnancy.
- Use of certain drugs, including oral contraceptives, thiazide diuretics, cortisone or phenytoin.
- Family history of diabetes mellitus.

HOW TO PREVENT — Control your weight to avoid becoming obese.

WHAT TO EXPECT

APPROPRIATE HEALTH CARE
- Self-care after diagnosis.
- Doctor's treatment.
- Surgery for treatment of some complications, such as gangrene or heart disease.

DIAGNOSTIC MEASURES
- Your own observation of symptoms.
- Medical history and exam by a doctor.
- Laboratory urine and blood studies to measure glucose, cholesterol and insulin levels.

POSSIBLE COMPLICATIONS
- Cardiovascular disease, especially atherosclerosis, stroke and coronary-artery disease.
- Vision impairment.
- Peripheral vascular disease, with gangrene in legs and feet and sexual impotence in men (sometimes).
- Hypoglycemia, if oral hypoglycemic medication is used (rare).

PROBABLE OUTCOME — This form of diabetes can often be controlled with weight loss. Good control decreases the chance of complications. In some cases, it progresses to insulin-dependent diabetes, a more serious form.

HOW TO TREAT

NOTE — Follow your doctor's instructions. These instructions are supplemental.

GENERAL MEASURES
- Learn to test your urine for glucose (sugar).
- Learn all you can about controlling diabetes and recognizing signs and symptoms of complications.
- Wear a Medic-Alert pendant or bracelet (see Glossary).
- Lose weight to a normal level.
- Obtain prompt medical treatment for any infection or injury.

MEDICATION — Your doctor may prescribe oral medicines to reduce blood sugar (hypoglycemics). These are not always necessary. They can often be discontinued when body weight becomes normal.

ACTIVITY — No restrictions. Regular daily exercise is an important part of controlling diabetes. Consult your doctor.

DIET — A special diet will be necessary to: reduce weight; limit refined carbohydrates; balance unrefined carbohydrates, protein and fat; and increase plant fiber. Your doctor will provide instructions.

CALL YOUR DOCTOR IF

- You have symptoms of diabetes mellitus.
- The following occurs during treatment:
  Inability to think clearly; weakness; sweating; paleness; rapid heartbeat; seizures; coma (may indicate hypoglycemia).
  Numbness, tingling or pain in the feet or hands.
  Infection that does not improve in 3 days.
  Chest pain.
  Worsening of original symptoms, despite adherence to treatment.

DIAPER RASH

GENERAL INFORMATION

DEFINITION—A form of contact dermatitis that causes skin irritation in the diaper area of infants.

BODY PARTS INVOLVED—Skin around the genitals, rectum and abdomen in the area covered by diapers.

SEX OR AGE MOST AFFECTED—Infants and young children who wear diapers.

SIGNS & SYMPTOMS
- Moist, painful, red, spotty and itchy (sometimes) skin in the diaper area. The skin may be cracked and fissured.
- In male infants, a red, raw and occasionally bloody area may appear around the meatus (the opening at the tip of the penis).
- In female infants, a thin adhesive membrane may form between the vaginal lips.

CAUSES
- Excessive ammonia on the wet diaper and skin caused by bacterial action. (Urine does not naturally contain ammonia).
- Monilia fungus infection—the same fungus that causes thrush.
- Allergy to soap, detergent, fabric softener, lotion, powder or other chemicals.

RISK INCREASES WITH
- Infrequent diaper changes.
- Improper laundering of diapers.
- Family history of skin allergies.
- Hot, humid weather.

HOW TO PREVENT
- Change diapers frequently.
- Don't use waterproof diapers at night.
- Keep diapers clean. After washing, rinse them twice to remove detergents and other chemicals.

WHAT TO EXPECT

APPROPRIATE HEALTH CARE
- Self-care after diagnosis.
- Doctor's treatment, if home treatment fails to cure the rash.

DIAGNOSTIC MEASURES
- Your own observation of symptoms.
- Medical history and physical exam by a doctor.
- Urinalysis to rule out urinary-tract infection, which may complicate healing.

POSSIBLE COMPLICATIONS—Secondary bacterial infection in the rash area.

PROBABLE OUTCOME—Usually curable with treatment. Recurrence is common.

HOW TO TREAT

NOTE—Follow your doctor's instructions. These instructions are supplemental.

GENERAL MEASURES
- Expose the buttocks to air as much as possible.
- Don't use waterproof pants during treatment—either in the day or at night. They keep skin wet and subject to rash or infection.
- Change diapers frequently—even at night if the rash is extensive.
- Don't use soap or boric acid to wash the rash area. Cleanse with cotton dipped in mineral oil.
- Discontinue using baby lotion, powder, ointment or baby oil (except zinc oxide) unless prescribed by your doctor.
- Apply small amounts of non-prescription zinc-oxide ointment to the rash at the earliest sign of diaper rash, and 2 or 3 times a day thereafter.
- Add 1 cup of vinegar to the washing machine when it is half-full of rinse water. This neutralizes detergent residue. If you use a diaper service, add 1 oz. of vinegar to 1 gallon of water, rinse laundered diapers and dry before using.

MEDICATION—Your doctor may prescribe medicated anti-inflammatory ointments or creams, such as hydrocortisone, nystatin or myconazole, to apply to the skin.

ACTIVITY—No restrictions.

DIET—No special diet.

CALL YOUR DOCTOR IF

- Home treatment doesn't cure the rash in 1 week.
- The following occurs during treatment:
  Fever.
  Pustules in the rash area.
  Male infant has a weak urinary stream.
  Female infant develops adhesions of the vaginal lips.
- New, unexplained symptoms develop. Medicine used in treatment may produce side effects.

ILLNESSES & DISORDERS

DIARRHEA, ACUTE

 GENERAL INFORMATION

DEFINITION—The passage of many loose, watery or unformed bowel movements. This is a symptom, not a disease.

BODY PARTS INVOLVED—Colon; small intestine.

SEX OR AGE MOST AFFECTED—Both sexes; all ages.

SIGNS & SYMPTOMS
- Cramping abdominal pain.
- Loose, watery or unformed bowel movements.
- Lack of bowel control (sometimes).
- Fever (sometimes).

CAUSES
- Emotional upsets.
- Food poisoning.
- Infections (viral, parasitic or bacterial).
- Regional enteritis.
- Malabsorption syndromes.
- Disease or tumor of the pancreas (malignant or benign).
- Diverticulitis.
- Foods, such as prunes or beans.
- Excess alcohol consumption.
- Use of drugs, such as laxatives, antacids, antibiotics, quinine or anticancer drugs.
- Food allergy.
- Radiation treatments for cancer.

RISK INCREASES WITH
- Stress.
- Recent illness.
- Excess alcohol consumption.
- Crowded or unsanitary living conditions.

HOW TO PREVENT—If diarrhea is recurrent and a cause can be identified, treatment or avoidance of the cause should prevent recurrence.

OTHER—Everyone is likely to have bouts of diarrhea occasionally from insignificant causes which disappear and leave no lasting effects. Most cases of acute diarrhea last a short time and a search for the cause may not be necessary.

 WHAT TO EXPECT

APPROPRIATE HEALTH CARE
- Self-care.
- Doctor's treatment (if symptoms persist longer than 2 to 3 days).

DIAGNOSTIC MEASURES
- Your own observation of symptoms.
- Medical history and physical exam by a doctor.
- Laboratory stool studies (for prolonged diarrhea).

POSSIBLE COMPLICATIONS—Dehydration if diarrhea is prolonged, especially in infants.

PROBABLE OUTCOME—Spontaneous recovery in 24 to 48 hours.

 HOW TO TREAT

NOTE—Follow your doctor's instructions. These instructions are supplemental.

GENERAL MEASURES—If cramps are present, place hot compresses, a hot-water bottle or an electric heating pad on the abdomen.

MEDICATION—For minor discomfort, you may use non-prescription drugs such as Pepto-Bismol or Kaopectate.

ACTIVITY—Decrease activity until diarrhea stops.

DIET—If diarrhea is accompanied by nausea, suck ice chips only.

If you are not nauseated, drink small amounts of clear liquid, such as herbal tea, ginger ale, broth or gelatin until diarrhea stops.

After symptoms disappear, eat soft foods, such as cooked cereal, rice, eggs, custard, baked potato and yogurt for 1 or 2 days.

Resume a normal diet 2 or 3 days after the diarrhea stops. Avoid fruit, alcohol and highly seasoned foods for several more days.

 CALL YOUR DOCTOR IF

- Diarrhea lasts more than 48 hours.
- Mucus, blood or worms appear in the stool.
- Fever rises to 101F (38.3C) or higher.
- Severe pain develops in the abdomen or rectum.
- Dehydration develops. Signs include: dry mouth; wrinkled skin; excess thirst; little or no urination.

DIARRHEA, CHRONIC, NON-SPECIFIC OF CHILDHOOD

 ## GENERAL INFORMATION

DEFINITION—Chronic diarrhea (more than 5 watery or loose stools a day) in a healthy child.

BODY PARTS INVOLVED—Colon.

SEX OR AGE MOST AFFECTED—Young children (1-1/2 to 3-1/2 years).

SIGNS & SYMPTOMS
● Frequent, loose stools that often contain undigested vegetable fibers or mucus and occur primarily during the morning.
● Occasional irritation of the anal area caused by frequency of bowel movements.

CAUSES—Unknown.

RISK INCREASES WITH—Family history of intestinal problems.

HOW TO PREVENT—Cannot be prevented at present.

 ## WHAT TO EXPECT

APPROPRIATE HEALTH CARE
● Doctor's treatment.
● Home care after diagnosis.

DIAGNOSTIC MEASURES
● Your own observation of symptoms.
● Medical history and physical exam by a doctor.
● Laboratory stool studies.

POSSIBLE COMPLICATIONS—Possible psychological fixation on bowel function because of excessive parental attention to bowel habits.

PROBABLE OUTCOME—Despite the chronic diarrhea, affected children develop normally and show no signs of malnutrition. The frequent stools have no special significance. Bowel movements eventually become normal, but it may take 2 to 3 years.

 ## HOW TO TREAT

NOTE—Follow your doctor's instructions. These instructions are supplemental.

GENERAL MEASURES—Don't blame or criticize your child for this problem. Don't expect toilet training to be successful as soon as with other children. Treat your child as normal and try to ignore the problem. Avoid tension. If the child becomes anxious about diarrhea, the problem may become worse or psychological problems may arise.

MEDICATION—Medicine usually is not necessary for this disorder. Don't give your child any non-prescription antidiarrheal drugs. Side effects may be harmful.

ACTIVITY—No restrictions. Insist on full normal activity for your child's age group.

DIET
● No special diet, but vitamin and mineral supplements may be helpful.
● The child should drink at least 6 to 8 glasses of fluid each day to replace fluid lost in stools.

 ## CALL YOUR DOCTOR IF

● Your child has chronic diarrhea or stools with mucus that haven't been diagnosed.
● There is blood in the stool.
● Your child's rectal temperature is 102F (38.9C) or higher.
● Your child becomes listless, refuses to eat, or cries loudly and persistently, even when picked up.
● Your child's growth and development are not normal.

ILLNESSES & DISORDERS

DIC
(Disseminated Intravascular Coagulation; Defibrinogenation Syndrome; Coagulopathy)

 GENERAL INFORMATION

DEFINITION—A serious disruption of blood-clotting mechanisms, resulting in hemorrhaging or internal bleeding. This disorder is a complication of an underlying disorder.

BODY PARTS INVOLVED—Blood vessels and blood in all parts of the body.

SEX OR AGE MOST AFFECTED—Both sexes; all ages.

SIGNS & SYMPTOMS
- Bleeding and hemorrhage from any or several body parts. Bleeding may be heavy. Common signs of bleeding include:
  Bloody vomit or red or black stools.
  Vaginal bleeding.
  Red or cloudy urine.
  Unexplained bruising.
- Severe abdominal or back pain caused by bleeding into body organs.
- Convulsions (rare).
- Coma (rare).

CAUSES—Depletion of blood-clotting components, causing widespread bleeding. This condition can be the result of:
- Pregnancy abnormalities, such as placenta previa, abruptio placenta or toxemia.
- Widespread or major infection.
- Widespread cancer.
- Some kinds of surgery.
- Widespread tissue destruction, as with extensive burns.
- Poisonous snakebite.
- Transfusion of mismatched blood.

RISK INCREASES WITH
- Poor nutrition.
- Illness that has lowered resistance.

HOW TO PREVENT—Obtain prompt medical treatment for the underlying causes.

 WHAT TO EXPECT

APPROPRIATE HEALTH CARE
- Doctor's treatment.
- Hospitalization.
- Surgery to correct the underlying disorder (sometimes).
- Self-care after treatment.

DIAGNOSTIC MEASURES
- Your own observation of symptoms.
- Medical history and physical exam by a doctor.
- Laboratory blood tests, especially of the blood-clotting mechanism.

POSSIBLE COMPLICATIONS
- Kidney failure.
- Brain damage, with seizures or coma.
- Shock.
- Death.

PROBABLE OUTCOME—Depends on the severity. If the underlying cause of DIC is treated promptly, full recovery is likely.

 HOW TO TREAT

NOTE—Follow your doctor's instructions. These instructions are supplemental.

GENERAL MEASURES
- Patients with this condition are often desperately ill and require intensive hospital care. Family members can help by maintaining a positive, hopeful attitude.
- During recovery, don't scrub or take scabs off sores. This may trigger new bleeding.

MEDICATION—Your doctor may prescribe:
- Blood transfusions or blood-component infusions.
- Heparin (an anticoagulant administered by injection).

ACTIVITY—Rest in bed until your doctor approves a return to normal activity. You may read or watch TV.

DIET—No special diet.

 CALL YOUR DOCTOR IF

- You have symptoms of DIC.
- Any bleeding recurs or the abdomen swells rapidly during treatment.

DIPHTHERIA

GENERAL INFORMATION

DEFINITION—A highly contagious throat infection.

BODY PARTS INVOLVED—Throat; skin; heart; central nervous system.

SEX OR AGE MOST AFFECTED—Older children (5 years and up), adolescents and adults.

SIGNS & SYMPTOMS—Early stages:
- Sore throat.
- Low fever.
- Swollen neck glands.
Late stages:
- Airway obstruction and breathing difficulty.
- Shock (low blood pressure; rapid heartbeat; paleness; cold skin; sweating; anxious appearance).

CAUSES—A bacterial germ, corynebacterium diphtheriae, infects the throat and sometimes the skin. The incubation period is 5 to 9 days following exposure. The germ produces poisons that spread to the heart, central nervous system and other organs.

RISK INCREASES WITH
- Adults over 60.
- Poor nutrition.
- Outbreak in the community.
- Crowded or unsanitary living conditions.
- Lack of up-to-date immunizations.

HOW TO PREVENT
- Immunization with diphtheria vaccine. See Appendix 16 for an immunization schedule.
- Improved nutrition and standard of living.

OTHER—Notify the local health department of any case of diphtheria. Anyone having contact with the patient must be examined and treated.

WHAT TO EXPECT

APPROPRIATE HEALTH CARE
- Doctor's treatment. This is a medical emergency.
- Hospitalization.

DIAGNOSTIC MEASURES
- Your own observation of symptoms.
- Medical history and physical exam by a doctor.
- Laboratory studies, such as throat culture and blood counts.

POSSIBLE COMPLICATIONS
- Heart inflammation and heart failure.
- Suffocation.
- Nerve inflammation.
- Misdiagnosis as a less-serious infection, resulting in dangerous delay of treatment.

PROBABLE OUTCOME—Usually curable in 1 week, followed by slow recovery for several weeks. A delay in treatment may result in death or long-term heart disease.

HOW TO TREAT

NOTE—Follow your doctor's instructions. These instructions are supplemental.

GENERAL MEASURES
- Quarantine the patient until fully recovered. Protect susceptible individuals (the non-immunized, very young or elderly) from exposure.
- Dispose of all secretions (nose and mouth) and excretions (urine and feces) in an acceptable manner. Call the local health department for instructions.

MEDICATION—Your doctor may prescribe:
- Diphtheria antitoxin to neutralize the diphtheria toxin.
- Antibiotics to fight remaining diphtheria germs.

ACTIVITY—Prolonged bed rest (2 to 3 months or until fully recovered), especially if the heart is involved. The patient may watch TV or read.

DIET—No special diet, except to eat heartily.

CALL YOUR DOCTOR IF

- You have symptoms of diphtheria or observe them in someone else.
- Anyone in your family is exposed to diphtheria.
- Your immunizations are not current.
- The following occurs during treatment: Temperature spikes to 102F (38.9C). Increasing breathing difficulty. Increasing shortness of breath. Confusion.

DISK, RUPTURED
(Herniated Disk; Slipped Disk)

 GENERAL INFORMATION

DEFINITION—Sudden or gradual break in the supportive ligaments surrounding a spinal disk (cushions separating bony spinal vertebrae).

BODY PARTS INVOLVED—Disks of the neck or lower spine (most common sites).

SEX OR AGE MOST AFFECTED—Adults of both sexes.

SIGNS & SYMPTOMS—Lower back:
• Severe pain in the low back or back of one leg, buttock or foot (sciatica). Pain usually affects one side and worsens with movement, coughing, sneezing, lifting or straining.
• Weakness, numbness or muscular wasting of the affected leg.
Neck:
• Pain in the neck, shoulder or down one arm. Pain worsens with movement.
• Weakness, numbness or muscular wasting of the affected arm.

CAUSES—Weakening and rupture of the disk material, creating pressure on nearby spinal nerves. Rupture of the disk is caused by sudden injury or chronic stress, such as from constant lifting or obesity.

RISK INCREASES WITH
• Heavy lifting.
• Poor physical condition.

HOW TO PREVENT
• Practice proper posture when lifting.
• Exercise regularly to maintain good muscle tone.

 WHAT TO EXPECT

APPROPRIATE HEALTH CARE
• Self-care after diagnosis.
• Doctor's treatment.
• Traction at home or in the hospital (sometimes).
• Surgery to relieve nerve pressure if bed rest does not relieve symptoms.
• Injection of chymopapain enzymes into the disk (sometimes).
• Rehabilitation to strengthen muscles.
• Psychotherapy or counseling to learn coping methods for enduring pain and frustration.

DIAGNOSTIC MEASURES
• Your own observation of symptoms.
• Medical history and physical exam by a doctor.
• X-rays of the neck or lower spine, including myelogram (see Glossary).
• CAT scan (see Glossary).

POSSIBLE COMPLICATIONS
• Loss of bladder and bowel function.
• Paralysis.
• Muscle wasting and weakness.

PROBABLE OUTCOME—Spontaneous recovery in many cases. At least 2 weeks in bed should be tried before considering other therapy, unless complications occur. When necessary, a ruptured disk is curable with surgery.

 HOW TO TREAT

NOTE—Follow your doctor's instructions. These instructions are supplemental.

GENERAL MEASURES
• Apply ice packs to the painful area during the first 72 hours and occasionally thereafter, if they provide relief. Alternately, try to relieve pain with a heat lamp, hot showers or baths, compresses or a heating pad.
• See Appendix 15 for suggestions for back care.

MEDICATION
• For minor discomfort, you may use non-prescription drugs such as aspirin.
• Your doctor may prescribe:
  Pain relievers.
  Muscle relaxants, such as diazepam or methocarbamol.
  Non-steroidal anti-inflammatory drugs to reduce inflammation around the rupture.
  Laxatives or stool softeners to prevent constipation.

ACTIVITY—Rest in bed at least 2 weeks during the acute phase. You may read or watch TV. Resume your normal activities, including sexual relations, when symptoms improve.

DIET—No special diet. Increase consumption of dietary fiber and drink at least 8 glasses of fluid a day to prevent constipation or fecal impaction.

 CALL YOUR DOCTOR IF

• You have symptoms of a ruptured disk.
• The following occurs during treatment:
  Increased pain or weakness in the extremities.
  Loss of bladder or bowel control.
• New, unexplained symptoms develop.
Drugs used in treatment may produce side effects.

DISLOCATION OR SUBLUXATION

GENERAL INFORMATION

DEFINITION—Dislocation is injury to a joint so that adjoining bones no longer touch each other.

Subluxation is a minor dislocation. Joint surfaces still touch, but not in normal relation to each other.

BODY PARTS INVOLVED—Bones in joints, especially the jaw, shoulder, knee and spine. Some infants are born with a hip dislocation.

SEX OR AGE MOST AFFECTED—Both sexes; all ages.

SIGNS & SYMPTOMS
- Sudden joint pain, swelling or deformity after an injury.
- Limited or absent movement around a joint.

CAUSES
- Injury that stretches or tears ligaments that surround a joint and hold the bones together.
- Shallow or abnormally formed joint surfaces (congenital).
- Rheumatoid arthritis or other diseases of ligaments and tissue around a joint.

RISK INCREASES WITH
- Rheumatoid arthritis.
- Family history of congenital hip dislocation.
- Repeated injury to a joint.

HOW TO PREVENT—If you are involved in heavy work or strenuous sports, learn to protect the involved joints. Use protective devices, such as wrapped elastic bandages, tape wraps, knee or shoulder pads, and special support stockings.

WHAT TO EXPECT

APPROPRIATE HEALTH CARE
- Self-care after diagnosis.
- Doctor's treatment. This may include manipulating the joint to reposition the bones.
- Surgery to restore the joint to its normal position (sometimes). Recurring dislocation may require surgical reconstruction or replacement of the joint.

DIAGNOSTIC MEASURES
- Your own observation of symptoms.
- Medical history and physical exam by a doctor. (Infants should be examined for congenital hip dislocation at birth and at "well-baby" checkups.)
- X-rays of the joint and adjacent bones.

POSSIBLE COMPLICATIONS—Damage to nearby nerves or major blood vessels, causing numbness, coldness and paleness.

PROBABLE OUTCOME—Usually curable with prompt treatment. After the dislocation has been corrected, the joint may require immobilization with a cast or sling for 2 to 8 weeks.

HOW TO TREAT

NOTE—Follow your doctor's instructions. These instructions are supplemental.

GENERAL MEASURES—Immediately after injury:
- Apply ice packs to the involved joint to prevent swelling.
- Use a splint or sling to prevent movement while transporting the injured person to the doctor.
- If your doctor puts a cast on the joint, see Appendix 17 (Care of Casts).

MEDICATION—Your doctor may prescribe:
- General anesthesia or muscle relaxants to make joint manipulation possible.
- Acetaminophen or aspirin to relieve moderate pain.
- Narcotic pain relievers for severe pain.

ACTIVITY—Resume your normal activities gradually after treatment.

DIET—Drink only water before manipulation or surgery to correct the dislocation. Solid food makes general anesthesia more hazardous.

CALL YOUR DOCTOR IF

- You have difficulty moving a joint after injury.
- Any extremity becomes numb, pale or cold after injury. This is an emergency!
- Dislocations occur repeatedly that you can "pop" back into normal position.

ILLNESSES & DISORDERS

DIVERTICULAR DISEASE
(Diverticulosis; Diverticulitis)

 GENERAL INFORMATION

DEFINITION—Diverticulosis is the presence of small, saclike swellings (diverticulae) in the wall of the colon. Diverticulae may be present without any symptoms. Diverticulitis is the inflammation of diverticulae. It is not contagious or cancerous.

BODY PARTS INVOLVED—Left side of the large intestine.

SEX OR AGE MOST AFFECTED—Adults. Diverticulae are present in 30% to 40% of persons over age 50. They increase with each decade of life.

SIGNS & SYMPTOMS—Diverticulosis symptoms:
- Mild cramping or tenderness in the left side of the abdomen that is relieved by passing gas or moving bowels.
- Occasional bright red blood in the stool. Non-infected diverticulae sometimes bleed.
- Constipation (sometimes).
- No symptoms (usually).
Diverticulitis symptoms:
- Intermittent cramping, abdominal pain that becomes constant. Pain may be disabling from the onset, or may not become disabling for several days.
- Fever.
- Nausea.
- Tenderness over the affected area of the colon.

CAUSES—Unknown, but the tendency is inherited.
Recent evidence suggests that the highly refined, low-residue diet common in the U.S. and other developed countries may contribute to the formation of diverticulae. Pressure builds up inside the sigmoid colon as a result of spasm due to lack of dietary bulk. The inner lining eventually pushes through to form the small pouches.

RISK INCREASES WITH
- Improper diet that lacks fiber.
- Family history of diverticulosis.
- Coronary-artery disease or gallbladder disease.
- Obesity.

HOW TO PREVENT—Cannot be prevented at present, but risk can be reduced by:
- Eating a diet high in fiber throughout life.
- Maintaining good cardiovascular fitness. This disease may be related to blood-vessel disorders.

 WHAT TO EXPECT

APPROPRIATE HEALTH CARE
- Self-care after diagnosis.
- Doctor's treatment.
- Hospitalization (complications only).
- Surgery to remove part of the colon if diverticulae become infected or bleed significantly.

DIAGNOSTIC MEASURES
- Your own observation of symptoms.
- Medical history and physical exam by a doctor.
- X-rays of the lower intestinal tract (barium enema).
- Sigmoidoscopy (see Glossary).

POSSIBLE COMPLICATIONS—If diverticulae become infected, they may bleed profusely or perforate (erode through the intestinal wall) and cause peritonitis. Both are medical and surgical emergencies.

PROBABLE OUTCOME—Diverticulosis is dangerous only if the diverticulae become infected or bleed. Diverticulitis is curable with surgery.

 HOW TO TREAT

NOTE—Follow your doctor's instructions. These instructions are supplemental.

GENERAL MEASURES
- Try to have a bowel movement at about the same time each day. Allow at least 10 minutes, and don't strain.
- Check your stool daily for bleeding. If the stool is black, remove it from the toilet and take it to your doctor's office for analysis.
- To relieve mild pain and spasms, apply a heating pad to the abdomen.

MEDICATION—Your doctor may prescribe:
- Antibiotics, if the diverticulae are infected.
- Bulk-producing laxatives, if you are unable to eat a high-fiber diet. Don't take laxatives unless prescribed.

ACTIVITY—If you have fever or severe pain, stay in bed. Resume normal activity as soon as symptoms improve.

DIET—Eat a well-balanced diet that is high in fiber, low in salt and low in fat (see Appendices 1, 8 and 9).

 CALL YOUR DOCTOR IF

- Temperature rises to 101F (38.3C).
- Severe pain continues despite treatment.
- Blood appears in the stool.
- Vomiting or abdominal swelling occurs.

DOWN'S SYNDROME
(Mongolism; Trisomy 21)

 GENERAL INFORMATION

DEFINITION—Retardation and abnormalities in many organs caused by a major chromosome abnormality that is inherited.

BODY PARTS INVOLVED—Central nervous system; heart; skeletal system.

SEX OR AGE MOST AFFECTED—Newborns.

SIGNS & SYMPTOMS—Shortly after birth:
- Lack of normal muscle tone. The child seems "floppy."
- Head and face abnormalities, including: a small or odd-shaped skull; slanting, almond-shaped eyes; small mouth and protruding tongue.
- Broad hands with large, unusual palm creases. The little finger curves inward (sometimes).
- Heart murmur.
Later:
- Retarded growth and development. The child never reaches full stature.
- Mental retardation. The IQ is usually between 30 and 50.

CAUSES—An extra chromosome in the fertilized egg creates abnormalities as the fetus develops. In 1/3 of cases, the extra chromosome comes from the father.

RISK INCREASES WITH
- Pregnancy in females under age 16 or over 35.
- Family history of Down's syndrome.
- Mother's exposure to drugs, radiation, chemicals or infections before pregnancy.

HOW TO PREVENT
- If you are pregnant and over age 35, or you or your partner have a family history of Down's syndrome, request amniocentesis (see Glossary). This can detect whether the fetus has Down's syndrome.
- If you or your partner have a family history of Down's syndrome, obtain genetic counseling before starting a family.

 WHAT TO EXPECT

APPROPRIATE HEALTH CARE
- Doctor's treatment.
- Psychotherapy or counseling for the parents. Many parents blame themselves and need help to cope with unnecessary, harmful guilt.
- Surgery to correct congenital heart or intestinal disorders.
- Nursing-home or group-home care, if home care is not feasible.

DIAGNOSTIC MEASURES
- Parent's observation of symptoms.
- Medical history and physical exam by a doctor.
- Laboratory studies of chromosomes.

POSSIBLE COMPLICATIONS
- Increased susceptibility to leukemia.
- Increased susceptibility to infections.
- Congestive heart failure caused by congenital heart abnormalities.

PROBABLE OUTCOME—Special education and training allow many children with Down's syndrome to lead happy, loving and useful lives. Life expectancy is reduced—few persons with Down's syndrome reach age 40.

 HOW TO TREAT

NOTE—Follow your doctor's instructions. These instructions are supplemental.

GENERAL MEASURES—Learn all you can about programs and resources in your community to help children with Down's syndrome.

MEDICATION—Your doctor may prescribe antibiotics for frequent, complicating infections. There is no medication to cure Down's syndrome.

ACTIVITY—Encourage the child to be as active as possible in a protected environment.

DIET—No special diet. Extra patience may be necessary in feeding an infant with Down's syndrome. Some have difficulty sucking or are not eager to eat.

 CALL YOUR DOCTOR IF

- Your infant seems "floppy" or does not seem to be developing normally.
- A child with Down's syndrome develops signs of infection (fever, warmth or pain).

ILLNESSES & DISORDERS

DROWNING, NEAR-

GENERAL INFORMATION

DEFINITION—The immediate aftereffects of prolonged submersion under water.

BODY PARTS INVOLVED—Lungs; blood; heart.

SEX OR AGE MOST AFFECTED—Both sexes; all ages.

SIGNS & SYMPTOMS
- Confusion or unconsciousness.
- Little or no breathing or heartbeat.
- Bluish-white paleness.

CAUSES—Submersion under water results in either:
- Spasm of the larynx (the tube from the throat to the lungs). After rescue, this spasm prevents oxygen from reaching the lungs.
- Water in the lungs, causing life-threatening changes in the circulating blood.

RISK INCREASES WITH
- Excess alcohol consumption.
- Accidents—especially head injury—while swimming.
- Suicidal persons.

HOW TO PREVENT
- Learn cardiopulmonary resuscitation (CPR).
- Encourage all family members—including infants—to learn to swim.
- Install a fence around your home swimming pool.
- Never swim alone.
- Don't drink alcohol and swim.

WHAT TO EXPECT

APPROPRIATE HEALTH CARE
- Immediate cardiopulmonary resuscitation (CPR).
- Hospitalization for observation for delayed, serious reactions.

DIAGNOSTIC MEASURES
- Your own observation of symptoms.
- Medical history and physical exam by a doctor.
- Laboratory blood tests.

POSSIBLE COMPLICATIONS
- Pulmonary edema (body fluid in the lungs).
- Permanent brain damage.
- Heart irregularities, including cardiac arrest and death.
- Lung infection.

PROBABLE OUTCOME—Depends on the length of time under water. With early rescue and treatment, full recovery is possible. Special body mechanisms may permit full recovery from near-drowning in icy water.

HOW TO TREAT

NOTE—Follow your doctor's instructions. These instructions are supplemental.

GENERAL MEASURES
- If the victim is unconscious and *not* breathing, yell for help. Don't leave the victim.
- Begin mouth-to-mouth breathing immediately.
- If there is no heartbeat, give external cardiac massage.
- Have someone call 0 (operator) or 911 (emergency) for an ambulance or medical help.
- Don't stop CPR until help arrives.
- The near-drowning victim should be taken to the nearest hospital for intensive care—even if the victim has regained consciousness. Complications or death may occur 24 to 48 hours after the accident due to heart-rhythm disturbances.
- Remain with a recovering patient to provide support and reassurance. Near-drowning is a traumatic experience.

MEDICATION—The doctor may prescribe:
- Oxygen.
- Cortisone drugs to prevent or treat lung inflammation.
- Antibiotics to prevent lung infection.
- Bronchodilators to enable oxygen to enter the lungs.

ACTIVITY—Complete bed rest until activity is permitted by the doctor.

DIET—Intravenous nutrients, if the victim is unconscious upon hospitalization. After recovery, no special diet is necessary.

CALL YOUR DOCTOR IF

- Someone appears to have drowned. Call for emergency help immediately! See General Measures for additional emergency information.
- Signs of infection (fever, cough, muscle aches and fatigue) appear after apparent recovery.

DRUG ABUSE & ADDICTION

 GENERAL INFORMATION

DEFINITION—A psychological or physiological need for chemical substances that produce temporary, pleasant mood changes.

BODY PARTS INVOLVED—Central nervous system; liver; kidneys; blood.

SEX OR AGE MOST AFFECTED—All ages, except early childhood.

SIGNS & SYMPTOMS—Depends on the substance of abuse. Most produce:
- A temporary, pleasant mood.
- Relief from anxiety.
- False feelings of self-confidence.
- Increased sensitivity to sights and sounds (including hallucinations).
- Altered activity levels—either stupor and sleeplike states *or* frenzies.
- Unpleasant or painful symptoms when the abused substance is withdrawn.

CAUSES—Substances of abuse may produce addiction (a physiological need) or dependence (a psychological need). The most common substances of abuse include:
- Nicotine.
- Alcohol.
- Marijuana.
- Amphetamines.
- Barbiturates.
- Cocaine.
- Opiates, including codeine, heroin, methadone, morphine and opium.
- Psychedelic drugs, including PCP ("angel dust"), mescaline and LSD.
- Volatile substances, such as glue, solvents and paints.

RISK INCREASES WITH
- Illness that requires prescription pain relievers or tranquilizers.
- Family history of drug abuse.
- Genetic factors (possibly). Some persons may be more susceptible to addiction.
- Excess alcohol consumption.
- Fatigue or overwork.
- Poverty.
- Psychological problems, including depression, dependency or poor self-esteem.

HOW TO PREVENT
- Don't socialize with persons who use and abuse drugs.
- Seek counseling for mental-health problems, such as depression or chronic anxiety, before they lead to drug problems.
- Develop wholesome interests and leisure activities.
- After surgery, illness or injury, discontinue the use of prescription pain relievers and tranquilizers as soon as possible. Don't use more than you need.

 WHAT TO EXPECT

APPROPRIATE HEALTH CARE
- Doctor's treatment.
- Psychotherapy or counseling.
- Hospitalization for drug-withdrawal symptoms.

DIAGNOSTIC MEASURES
- Your own observation of symptoms.
- Medical history and physical exam by a doctor.
- Laboratory blood tests.

POSSIBLE COMPLICATIONS
- Sexually transmitted diseases, which are more likely among addicts.
- Severe infections, such as endocarditis, hepatitis or blood poisoning, from intravenous injections with non-sterile needles.
- Malnutrition.
- Accidental injury to oneself or others while in a drug-induced state.
- Loss of job or family.
- Irreversible damage to body organs.
- Death caused by overdose.

PROBABLE OUTCOME—Curable with strong motivation, good medical care and support from family and friends.

 HOW TO TREAT

NOTE—Follow your doctor's instructions. These instructions are supplemental.

GENERAL MEASURES
- Admit you have a problem.
- Seek professional help.
- Be open and honest with your family and good friends, and ask their help.
- Avoid friends who tempt you to resume your habit.
- Join self-help groups.

MEDICATION—Your doctor may prescribe:
- Disulfiram (Antabuse) for alcoholism. This drug produces severe illness when alcohol is consumed.
- Methadone for narcotic abuse. This drug is a less-potent narcotic used to decrease the severity of physical withdrawal symptoms.

ACTIVITY—No restrictions.

DIET—Eat a normal, well-balanced diet that is high in protein. Vitamin supplements may be necessary if you suffer from malnutrition.

 CALL YOUR DOCTOR IF

- You abuse or are addicted to drugs and want help.
- New, unexplained symptoms develop. Drugs in treatment may produce side effects.

DRUG HYPERSENSITIVITY

 ## GENERAL INFORMATION

DEFINITION—A variety of allergic responses caused by medication.

BODY PARTS INVOLVED—Skin; blood vessels; lungs.

SEX OR AGE MOST AFFECTED—Both sexes; all ages.

SIGNS & SYMPTOMS
- Rash, itching or hives.
- Flushed skin.
- Anxiety.
- Serum sickness (fever, rash, joint pain and nerve damage).
- Anaphylaxis (wheezing and breathing difficulty). For signs and symptoms, see Anaphylaxis (in Illness section).
- Various blood disorders, such as hemolytic anemia.
- Peripheral neuropathy (nerve damage).
- Vasculitis (blood vessel inflammation).

The following reactions to medications are usually *not* the result of allergy:
   - Vomiting or diarrhea.
   - Fever.
   - Photosensitivity (a skin reaction to sunlight).

CAUSES—Medications are "foreign" materials. When injected—or less often, when taken orally—the body develops antibodies to the medication. Subsequent exposure to the medication causes an allergic reaction in the body.

RISK INCREASES WITH
- Use of the following drugs:
   Penicillin and cephalosporin antibiotics.
   Sulfa drugs.
   Animal serums.
   Vaccines.
   Local anesthetics.
   Allergy extracts.
   Iodine-containing compounds, such as those used in some X-rays.
- Injected medications, especially in high doses.
- Medical history of other allergies, such as hay fever, asthma or eczema.
- Current infectious illness (probably because infection increases immune-system functions).

HOW TO PREVENT
- Tell your doctor about any drug reactions you have had.
- Learn the name of any medication you are given. If it causes a reaction, you must avoid it in the future.
- Don't take medication—including non-prescription drugs—for minor illness, if possible.

 ## WHAT TO EXPECT

APPROPRIATE HEALTH CARE
- Self-care.
- Doctor's treatment.

DIAGNOSTIC MEASURES
- Your own observation of symptoms.
- Medical history and physical exam by a doctor.

POSSIBLE COMPLICATIONS
- Death from severe anaphylaxis reactions.
- Disability for many months from serum sickness.

PROBABLE OUTCOME—Most reactions disappear once the medication is permanently discontinued.

 ## HOW TO TREAT

NOTE—Follow your doctor's instructions. These instructions are supplemental.

GENERAL MEASURES
- See page 893 for treatment of anaphylaxis.
- Wear a Medic-Alert pendant or bracelet (see Glossary) if you have drug hypersensitivity.
- Keep an anaphylaxis kit at home for emergency use if anyone in the family has had a severe drug reaction. Ask your doctor how to obtain one.

MEDICATION—Your doctor may prescribe:
- Cortisone drugs to decrease the inflammatory reaction.
- Antihistamines to decrease the body's allergic response.

ACTIVITY—Resume your normal activities as soon as symptoms improve.

DIET—No special diet.

 ## CALL YOUR DOCTOR IF

You have symptoms of drug hypersensitivity or observe them in someone else.

DUMPING SYNDROME

GENERAL INFORMATION

DEFINITION—A group of symptoms that are a complication of surgical removal of all or part of the stomach. Most patients experience the problem to a minor degree for 1 to 6 months after surgery. It becomes a serious problem in 1% or 2% of patients.

The symptoms are of 2 types—early dumping syndrome and late dumping syndrome. Symptoms of the first begin a few minutes to 45 minutes after every meal. Symptoms of the second begin 2 to 3 hours after eating. Most persons experience late dumping syndrome—one person does not have both forms.

BODY PARTS INVOLVED—Gastrointestinal system; cardiovascular system.

SEX OR AGE MOST AFFECTED—Both sexes of adults following surgery on the stomach.

SIGNS & SYMPTOMS—Early dumping syndrome:
- Weakness and fainting.
- Sweating.
- Irregular or rapid heartbeat.
- Decreased blood pressure.
- Flushing of skin.
- Dizziness.
- Shortness of breath.
- Vomiting.
- Explosive diarrhea and abdominal cramps.
Late dumping syndrome:
- Sweating, anxiety and tremors.
- Exhaustion and faintness.
- Decreased blood pressure.
- Headache.

CAUSES
- Early dumping syndrome: Rapid entry of food and fluids directly into the small intestine, producing decreased blood pressure and increased blood flow to the intestines.
- Late dumping syndrome: Low blood sugar caused by excess insulin produced in response to sudden dumping of food and fluids into the intestine.

RISK INCREASES WITH—The larger the amount of stomach removed, the more severe the dumping syndrome.

HOW TO PREVENT—Some degree cannot be prevented, but recurrence and severity can be minimized with dietary changes (see Diet).

WHAT TO EXPECT

APPROPRIATE HEALTH CARE
- Self-care after diagnosis.
- Doctor's treatment.

DIAGNOSTIC MEASURES
- Your own observation of symptoms.
- Medical history and physical exam by a doctor.
- Laboratory studies of blood sugar levels.

POSSIBLE COMPLICATIONS
- Malnutrition and weight loss.
- Anxiety.

PROBABLE OUTCOME—Spontaneous recovery for most patients. Early dumping syndrome usually lasts 3 to 4 months. Late dumping syndrome usually lasts 1 year, but it may persist for many years.

HOW TO TREAT

NOTE—Follow your doctor's instructions. These instructions are supplemental.

GENERAL MEASURES
Early syndrome: Lie down for 45 minutes until symptoms pass.
Late syndrome: Eat small amounts of sugar candy or drink sweetened orange juice.

MEDICATION—Your doctor may prescribe:
- Anticholinergics to block the dumping-syndrome reflex.
- Pectin to reduce the severity of diarrhea.
- Vitamin and mineral supplements to compensate for poor absorption.

ACTIVITY
- Between symptoms: no restrictions.
- With symptoms: rest until they pass.

DIET
- Early dumping syndrome: Diet control is the most important treatment. Eat a diet low in sugar and other simple carbohydrates. Increase fat and protein consumption. Eat 6 small, evenly spaced meals a day. Take meals dry—without water or beverages—and drink fluids only between meals.
- Late dumping syndrome: Avoid refined sugar.

CALL YOUR DOCTOR IF

- You have symptoms of dumping syndrome not relieved by measures outlined above.
- You vomit blood, have black, tarry stools or other signs of gastrointestinal bleeding.
- New, unexplained symptoms develop. Drugs used in treatment may produce side effects.

DYSENTERY, BACILLARY
(Shigellosis)

GENERAL INFORMATION

DEFINITION—A bacterial infection of the surface layers of the intestinal tract. This is contagious with close personal contact and occurs in epidemics. It has a 1- to 3-day incubation period.

BODY PARTS INVOLVED—Lower small intestine (ileum); large intestine (colon).

SEX OR AGE MOST AFFECTED—Both sexes; all ages.

SIGNS & SYMPTOMS
- Abdominal cramps.
- Fever.
- Diarrhea (up to 20 or 30 watery bowel movements in 1 day).
- Blood, mucus or pus in the stool.
- Nausea or vomiting.
- Muscle aches or pain.
- White-blood-cell count lower than normal at the onset (sometimes).

CAUSES—Bacteria called shigella bacillus, a germ that invades the lining of the colon. It spreads from person to person, usually from contaminated hands to mouth.

RISK INCREASES WITH
- Travel to foreign countries.
- Crowded or unsanitary living conditions.

HOW TO PREVENT
- Wash hands after bowel movements and before handling food.
- Isolate anyone with symptoms of bacillary dysentery.
- Immerse soiled clothes and bedclothes in covered buckets of soap and water until they can be boiled.

WHAT TO EXPECT

APPROPRIATE HEALTH CARE
- Home care.
- Doctor's treatment.
- Hospitalization of persons (especially small children with dehydration) who are severely ill. Hospital care will include isolation and intravenous fluid supplements.

DIAGNOSTIC MEASURES
- Your own observation of symptoms.
- Medical history and physical exam by a doctor.
- Laboratory stool culture.

POSSIBLE COMPLICATIONS
- Dangerous dehydration, especially in children.

- In rare cases, the bacteria may enter the bloodstream from the digestive tract and infect other body organs, such as kidneys, gallbladder, liver or heart and joints. This may cause shock and death.

PROBABLE OUTCOME—Usually curable in 7 days with treatment. Most shigella infections are mild and don't require drastic treatment. However, in a severe attack, excessive dehydration can be fatal (especially in infants and young children) if treatment is unsuccessful.

HOW TO TREAT

NOTE—Follow your doctor's instructions. These instructions are supplemental.

GENERAL MEASURES
- Isolate the patient from others.
- Use a heating pad or hot-water bottle on the abdomen to relieve pain.

MEDICATION
- Your doctor may prescribe antibiotics, such as ampicillin or trimethoprim with sulfamethoxazole.
- Don't use paregoric preparations or other antidiarrhea drugs unless your doctor prescribes them. These may prolong the illness. If used, discontinue them as soon as possible.

ACTIVITY—Bed rest is necessary, except for trips to the bathroom, until fever, diarrhea and other symptoms have been gone for at least 3 days. The legs should be exercised regularly in bed.

DIET—Liquid or soft diet until diarrhea stops, then return to normal diet. For infants and children, see diet instructions in Gastroenteritis in Infants & Children (in Illness section).

CALL YOUR DOCTOR IF

- You or your child have symptoms of bacillary dysentery.
- The following occurs during treatment:
  Fever of 102F (38.9C) or more.
  Sore throat, headache or earache.
  Shortness of breath or severe cough.
  Traces of blood in the sputum.
  Severe abdominal pain or abdominal swelling.
  Rectal bleeding.
  Pain in the calf or leg.
  Swollen joints.
  Signs of dehydration (lethargy, sunken eyes, rapid weight loss or dry skin) appear.

DYSHIDROSIS

GENERAL INFORMATION

DEFINITION—A skin condition, characterized by small blisters on the hands or feet—apparently related to stress.

BODY PARTS INVOLVED—Tips and sides of the fingers, toes, palms and soles.

SEX OR AGE MOST AFFECTED—Both sexes and all ages, but most common in men between ages 20 and 50.

SIGNS & SYMPTOMS—Small blisters with the following characteristics:
- Blisters are very small (1mm or less in diameter). They appear on the tips and sides of fingers, toes, palms and soles.
- Blisters are opaque and deep-seated; they are either flush with the skin or slightly elevated. They don't break easily. Eventually, small blisters come together and form large blisters.
- Blisters may itch, cause pain or produce no symptoms. They worsen after contact with soap, water or irritating substances.

CAUSES—Unknown, but they are probably related to periods of anxiety, stress and frustration in ambitious people who internalize their emotions. Persons with dyshidrosis have difficulty relaxing—even during non-stressful periods.

This problem is not caused by sweat retention, as was once believed.

RISK INCREASES WITH
- Stress and internalized frustration or irritation.
- Obsessive-compulsive personalities.

HOW TO PREVENT—Follow instructions under General Measures. These are helpful in preventing recurrences, as well as in treating active episodes.

WHAT TO EXPECT

APPROPRIATE HEALTH CARE
- Self-care after diagnosis.
- Doctor's treatment.
- Psychotherapy or counseling to learn to cope with stress more effectively.

DIAGNOSTIC MEASURES
- Your own observation of symptoms.
- Medical history and physical exam by a doctor.

POSSIBLE COMPLICATIONS—Secondary bacterial infection (sometimes).

PROBABLE OUTCOME—Symptoms can be controlled with treatment, but recurrence is common. Persons with mild problems have occasional attacks, and the skin returns to normal between episodes. Persons with severe problems have more severe symptoms—sometimes with persistent peeling and fissuring of the involved skin.

HOW TO TREAT

NOTE—Follow your doctor's instructions. These instructions are supplemental.

GENERAL MEASURES—Keep heat and moisture away from the affected areas whenever possible:
- Wear cotton socks and leather-soled shoes. Don't wear tennis shoes or other footwear made of man-made materials.
- Remove shoes and socks frequently to allow sweat to evaporate.
- Wear heavy-duty vinyl gloves to prevent contact with irritating substances, such as: water; soap; detergent; metal scrubbing pads; scouring powder; and other chemicals.
- Dry insides of gloves after use. Discard gloves if they develop a hole.
- Wear gloves when you peel or squeeze acid fruits and vegetables.
- Wear leather or heavy-duty fabric gloves for housework or gardening.
- Use a dishwashing machine to wash dishes if possible. If not, ask someone else to wash them.
- Avoid contact with irritating chemicals, such as: paint; paint thinner; and polish for cars, floors, shoes, furniture and metal.
- Remove rings before doing housework or washing hands.
- Use lukewarm water and very little mild soap to shower or bathe.

MEDICATION—You may use non-prescription topical steroid preparations to reduce inflammation and decrease itching. Apply once or twice a day after bathing, unless directed otherwise. If these are not effective, your doctor may prescribe stronger steroid preparations.

ACTIVITY—No restrictions.

DIET—No special diet.

CALL YOUR DOCTOR IF

- You have symptoms of dyshidrosis.
- Signs of infection (swelling, redness, tenderness or warmth) appear around blisters.
- Symptoms don't improve after 1 week, despite treatment.
- Improvement begins, and then symptoms recur.

DYSMENORRHEA
(Menstrual Cramps)

 GENERAL INFORMATION

DEFINITION—Severe, painful cramps during menstruation. Primary dysmenorrhea means pain has recurred regularly since periods began. Secondary dysmenorrhea means pain began years after periods started. Women with dysmenorrhea are generally fertile —cramps indicate that ovulation occurred 12 to 14 days earlier. Dysmenorrhea usually is less severe after a woman has a baby.

BODY PARTS INVOLVED—Female reproductive system, especially the uterus.

SEX OR AGE MOST AFFECTED—Women of childbearing age.

SIGNS & SYMPTOMS
- Cramping and sometimes sharp pains in the lower abdomen, lower back and thighs.
- Nausea and vomiting (sometimes).
- Diarrhea (occasionally).
- Sweating.
- Lack of energy.
Severity of symptoms varies greatly from woman to woman, and from one time to the next in the same woman.

CAUSES
- Strong or prolonged contractions of the muscular wall of the uterus. These may be caused by concentration of prostaglandins (hormones manufactured by the body). Research shows that women with dysmenorrhea produce and excrete more prostaglandins than those who don't have as much discomfort.
- Dilation of the cervix to allow passage of blood clots from the uterus to the vagina.
- Organic causes include:
  Pelvic infections.
  Endometriosis, especially if dysmenorrhea begins after age 20.
  Benign tumors of the uterus.
  Poor posture.
  An underdeveloped uterus.

RISK INCREASES WITH
- Use of caffeine.
- Stress. The degree of dysmenorrhea may vary according to general health or mental state. While emotional or psychological factors don't *cause* the pain, they can worsen pain or cause some women to be less responsive to treatment.

HOW TO PREVENT—Take female hormones that prevent ovulation, such as oral contraceptives.

 WHAT TO EXPECT

APPROPRIATE HEALTH CARE
- Self-care after diagnosis.
- Doctor's treatment.
- Psychotherapy or counseling, if dysmenorrhea is stress-related.

DIAGNOSTIC MEASURES
- Your own observation of symptoms.
- Medical history and physical exam, including a pelvic examination, by a doctor.

POSSIBLE COMPLICATIONS—Severe pain that regularly interferes with normal activity.

PROBABLE OUTCOME—Symptoms can be controlled with treatment.

 HOW TO TREAT

GENERAL MEASURES
- Heat helps relieve pain. Use a heating pad or hot-water bottle on the abdomen or back, or take hot baths. Sit in a tub of hot water for 10 to 15 minutes as often as necessary.
- See Appendix 13 for suggestions to reduce stress.

MEDICATION
- For minor discomfort, you may use non-prescription drugs such as acetaminophen.
- Your doctor may prescribe:
  Antiprostaglandins, including non-steroidal, anti-inflammatory drugs.
  Oral contraceptives, which prohibit ovulation.

ACTIVITY—No restrictions. When resting in bed, elevate your feet or bend your knees and lie on your side.

DIET—No special diet. Your doctor may prescribe vitamin-B supplements. These help relieve symptoms in some persons.

 CALL YOUR DOCTOR IF

- You have symptoms of dysmenorrhea you cannot control by yourself.
- Your bleeding becomes excessive (you saturate a pad or tampon more frequently than once each hour).
- You develop signs of infection, such as fever, a general ill feeling, headache, dizziness or muscle aches.
- New, unexplained symptoms develop. Drugs used in treatment may produce side effects.

DYSPAREUNIA

GENERAL INFORMATION

DEFINITION—Difficult or painful sexual intercourse for a female.

BODY PARTS INVOLVED—Vaginal muscles; hymen (sometimes); uterus (sometimes); brain.

SEX OR AGE MOST AFFECTED—Sexually active females of all ages.

SIGNS & SYMPTOMS—Pain in the genital area during sexual activity, including foreplay, intercourse or attempted intercourse. Pain may be mild or severe, and it may vary with different intercourse positions.

CAUSES—Physical causes include:
- Infection of the genitals, including herpes and others involving the vagina, cervix, Fallopian tubes or ovaries.
- Pressure against the vaginal wall caused by scarring from operations or radiation treatment.
- A tight episiotomy scar from vaginal repair after childbirth.
- A fibroid or other uterine tumor.
- Endometriosis.
- A hymen that is torn or thicker than normal.
- A bruised opening to the urethra.
- Inadequate vaginal or condom lubrication.
- Allergic reactions to diaphragms, condoms or contraceptive foams and jellies.
- Dryness and thinness of the vaginal wall after menopause.
- Pelvic inflammatory disease.

Psychological and emotional causes include:
- Fear of pregnancy.
- Fear of injury to the unborn child during pregnancy.
- Lack of sexual arousal and vaginal lubrication caused by inadequate or insufficient sexual foreplay, aversion to a sexual partner, fatigue or anxiety.
- Lack of sexual experience or information.
- Past sexual injury or psychological trauma.
- Temporary lack of desire for a particular sexual partner.

RISK INCREASES WITH
- Stress.
- Recent illness.
- Fatigue or overwork.

HOW TO PREVENT
- Obtain prompt medical treatment if you have symptoms of infection of the reproductive organs.
- Discontinue use of contraceptive foams or jellies that produce allergic reactions.
- Obtain professional counseling to resolve feelings about past sexual trauma.

- Discuss the lack of sexual arousal with your partner, including ways to improve foreplay. Enlist your partner's support and patience to overcome the problem. Use a lubricant, if necessary.

WHAT TO EXPECT

APPROPRIATE HEALTH CARE
- Doctor's treatment.
- Psychotherapy or counseling (sometimes), if the cause is psychological.

DIAGNOSTIC MEASURES
- Your own observation of symptoms.
- Medical history and physical exam by a doctor.
- Laboratory studies, such as a Pap smear (see Glossary) and culture of any vaginal discharge.

POSSIBLE COMPLICATIONS—Damage to personal relationships, permanent inability to enjoy sexual experiences and loss of self-esteem.

PROBABLE OUTCOME—Depends on the cause. Medical disorders are usually curable with treatment. Psychological problems can often be cured with therapy, and interpersonal problems can improve with communication and patience.

HOW TO TREAT

NOTE—Follow your doctor's instructions. These instructions are supplemental.

GENERAL MEASURES
- Sitz baths frequently relieve tenderness. Sit in a tub of hot water for 10 to 15 minutes. Repeat baths as often as 3 or 4 times a day.
- Use a non-prescription lubricant, such as baby oil or K-Y Lubricating Jelly, during sexual intercourse.
- Your doctor may provide instructions for exercises or techniques to dilate the vagina.
- Try different positions for sexual intercourse to discover new ones that might reduce penile penetration and be pain-free.

MEDICATION—Your doctor may prescribe antibiotic, antiviral, or antifungal medications for underlying infection.

ACTIVITY—No restrictions. Resume sexual relations as soon as possible.

DIET—No special diet.

CALL YOUR DOCTOR IF

- You have symptoms of dyspareunia.
- Pain worsens, despite treatment.
- Symptoms don't disappear after 3 months of treatment.

EAR INFECTION, MIDDLE-
(Otitis Media)

 GENERAL INFORMATION

DEFINITION—Infection in the middle ear. This is not contagious from person to person, but the preceding respiratory infection causing it may be infectious.

BODY PARTS INVOLVED—Middle-ear space where nerves and small bones connect to the eardrum on one side and the eustachian tube on the other side.

SEX OR AGE MOST AFFECTED—All ages, but most common in infants and children.

SIGNS & SYMPTOMS
- Irritability.
- Earache.
- Feeling of fullness in the ear.
- Hearing loss.
- Fever.
- Discharge or leakage from the ear.
- Diarrhea (sometimes).
- Pulling at the ear (small children).

CAUSES
- Bacterial or viral infections which spread to the middle ear by way of the eustachian tube. These are usually upper-respiratory virus infections in the nose or throat.
- Sinus and eustachian-tube blockage caused by nasal allergies or enlarged adenoids.
- A ruptured eardrum.

RISK INCREASES WITH
- Recent illness, such as a respiratory infection, that has lowered resistance.
- Crowded or unsanitary living conditions.
- Genetic factors. Some American Indians—especially the Navajo—seem more susceptible.
- High altitude.
- Cold climate.

HOW TO PREVENT
- If your child has an ear infection followed by a hearing loss or enlarged adenoids, ask your doctor about using a steroid nasal spray, preventive antibiotics or decongestants during future respiratory infections. This may prevent fluid accumulation.
- Bottle-feed infants in a sitting position—never lying down.

 WHAT TO EXPECT

APPROPRIATE HEALTH CARE
- Doctor's treatment.
- Home care after diagnosis.
- Surgery to insert plastic tubes through the eardrum to drain pus or fluid from the middle ear (rare).

DIAGNOSTIC MEASURES
- Your own observation of symptoms.
- Medical history and physical exam by a doctor.

POSSIBLE COMPLICATIONS
- Eardrum rupture.
- Hearing impairment—usually temporary, but sometimes permanent—leading to delay of normal language development in children.
- Enlarged adenoids in children from repeated middle-ear infections, causing chronic middle-ear infections.
- Mastoiditis.
- Meningitis.

PROBABLE OUTCOME—Usually curable with treatment.

 HOW TO TREAT

NOTE—Follow your doctor's instructions. These instructions are supplemental.

GENERAL MEASURES—Apply heat to the area around the ears to relieve pain.

MEDICATION
- Use ear drops to relieve pain. You may use non-prescription drops or those prescribed for a previous infection. They will not cure the infection.
- Use non-prescription nasal sprays or drops to help open the eustachian tube and relieve pressure in the middle ear.
- Use non-prescription drugs, such as acetaminophen, to reduce pain and fever.
- Your doctor may prescribe antibiotics if the infection appears to be bacterial rather than viral. Finish the medication. The infection may remain active for several days after symptoms disappear.

ACTIVITY—Rest in bed or reduce activity until fever and pain subside.

DIET—No special diet.

 CALL YOUR DOCTOR IF

- You or your child have symptoms of a middle-ear infection.
- The following occurs during treatment:
  Fever above 102F (38.9C), despite treatment.
  Severe headache.
  Earache that persists longer than 2 days, despite treatment.
  Swelling around the ear.
  Convulsions.
  Twitching of the face muscles.
  Dizziness.

EAR INFECTION, OUTER-
(Otitis Externa; Swimmer's Ear)

 GENERAL INFORMATION

DEFINITION—Inflammation or infection of the ear canal that extends from the eardrum to the outside.

BODY PARTS INVOLVED—Skin of the ear canal.

SEX OR AGE MOST AFFECTED—Both sexes; all ages.

SIGNS & SYMPTOMS
- Ear pain that worsens when the earlobe is pulled.
- Slight fever (sometimes).
- Discharge of pus from the ear.
- Temporary loss of hearing on the affected side.

CAUSES—Bacterial or fungal infection of the delicate skin lining of the ear canal. Infection may develop because of:
- Swimming in dirty, polluted water.
- Excessive swimming in chlorinated pools. Chlorinated water dries out the ear canal, allowing bacteria or fungi to enter the skin.
- Excess moisture from any cause.
- Irritation from: swabs; metal objects, such as bobby pins; or ear plugs, especially if they are left in a long time.
- Inadequate production of protective ear wax (cerumen).

RISK INCREASES WITH
- Previous ear infections.
- Skin allergies.
- Diabetes mellitus or other disorders that predispose to infection.

HOW TO PREVENT
- Don't clean your ears with any object or chemical.
- Don't use ear plugs, alcohol in the ears, lamb's wool or anything else to keep ears dry. These are not only useless—they may be harmful.

 WHAT TO EXPECT

APPROPRIATE HEALTH CARE
- Self-care after diagnosis.
- Doctor's treatment. Severe cases may require treatment by an ear, nose and throat specialist.

DIAGNOSTIC MEASURES
- Your own observation of symptoms.
- Medical history and physical exam by a doctor.

POSSIBLE COMPLICATIONS
- Severe pain.
- Chronic inflammation that is difficult to cure.
- A boil in the ear canal.
- Cellulitis (deep-tissue infection).

PROBABLE OUTCOME—Usually curable with treatment in 7 to 10 days.

 HOW TO TREAT

NOTE—Follow your doctor's instructions. These instructions are supplemental.

MEDICATION
- You may use non-prescription drugs, such as acetaminophen or aspirin, for minor pain.
- Your doctor may prescribe:
  Ear drops that contain antibiotics and cortisone drugs to control inflammation and fight infection.
  Oral antibiotics for severe infection.
  Codeine or narcotics for a short time to relieve severe pain.

GENERAL MEASURES
- Your doctor will probably cleanse the ear canal and insert a cotton wick. The wick allows medication to reach all infected parts.
  Moisten the wick with medication every hour for the first 24 hours. Continue to use drops according to your doctor's instructions after the wick is removed.
  Clean the tip of the dropper with alcohol after each use. Don't let other persons use the medicine.
- After you have had otitis externa, keep the prescription ear drops on hand. If the ear canals get wet for any reason, such as swimming or shampooing, put drops in both ears at bedtime.

ACTIVITY—Resume your normal activities as soon as symptoms improve. Avoid getting water in the ears for 3 weeks after all symptoms disappear. Any moisture—even from showering or washing hair—can trigger a recurrence.

DIET—No special diet.

 CALL YOUR DOCTOR IF

- You have symptoms of otitis externa.
- The following occurs during treatment:
  Pain persists, despite treatment.
  You feel your ears need cleaning.
  Remember that a small amount of ear wax helps protect against infection.

EARDRUM, RUPTURED
(Tympanic-Membrane Perforation)

 GENERAL INFORMATION

DEFINITION—A perforation of the thin membrane (tympanic membrane) that separates the inner ear from the outer ear.

BODY PARTS INVOLVED—Eardrum (tympanic membrane); middle ear.

SEX OR AGE MOST AFFECTED—Both sexes; all ages.

SIGNS & SYMPTOMS
- Sudden pain in the ear.
- Partial hearing loss.
- Bleeding or discharge from the ear. The discharge may resemble pus within 24 to 48 hours after rupture.
- Ringing in the ear.
- Dizziness.

CAUSES
- Perforation of the eardrum when a sharp object is inserted in the ear, such as: a cotton swab to clean the ear or relieve an itch; an unseen twig on a tree; hot slag from an industrial site.
- Sudden inward pressure in the ear, such as with: a slap; a swimming or diving accident; a nearby explosion.
- Sudden outward pressure or suction, such as with a kiss over the ear.
- Severe middle-ear infection.

RISK INCREASES WITH
- Recent middle-ear infection.
- Head injury.

HOW TO PREVENT
- Don't put any object into the ear canal.
- Avoid injuries that may cause a rupture (see Causes).
- Obtain prompt medical treatment for middle-ear infections.

 WHAT TO EXPECT

APPROPRIATE HEALTH CARE
- Self-care.
- Doctor's treatment.
- Microsurgery to repair the perforation (rare).

DIAGNOSTIC MEASURES
- Your own observation of symptoms.
- Medical history and physical exam by a doctor. When the eardrum ruptures, contents of the middle ear (primarily bones) can be seen with a special instrument called an otoscope. A healthy eardrum is almost transparent.

POSSIBLE COMPLICATIONS
- Ear infection, with fever, vomiting and diarrhea.
- Significant blood loss (rare).
- Meningitis.
- Mastoiditis (see Glossary).
- Permanent hearing loss (rare).

PROBABLE OUTCOME—If the ruptured eardrum does not become infected, it will usually repair itself in 2 months. If it becomes infected, the infection is curable with treatment, and hearing is usually not affected permanently.

 HOW TO TREAT

NOTE—Follow your doctor's instructions. These instructions are supplemental.

GENERAL MEASURES
- Don't blow your nose, if possible. If you must, blow gently.
- Keep the ear canal dry. Don't swim, take showers or get caught in the rain. Insert a wisp of cotton in the ear canal to keep moisture out of it when bathing.

MEDICATION—Your doctor may prescribe:
- Antibiotics to prevent or treat infections.
- Sedatives or tranquilizers to reduce apprehension.
- Pain relievers. For minor pain, you may use non-prescription drugs such as acetaminophen.

ACTIVITY—Resume your normal activities as soon as symptoms improve.

DIET—No special diet.

 CALL YOUR DOCTOR IF

- You have symptoms of a ruptured eardrum, especially a puslike discharge.
- The following occurs during treatment:
  Fever.
  Pain that persists, despite treatment.
  Dizziness that continues longer than 12 to 24 hours.
- New, unexplained symptoms develop. Drugs used in treatment may produce side effects.

EARWAX BLOCKAGE
(Cerumen Impaction)

 GENERAL INFORMATION

DEFINITION—Overproduction of earwax, causing blockage of the external ear canal. Wax is produced by the ear to protect the canal leading from the eardrum to the outside.

BODY PARTS INVOLVED—External ear canal on one or both sides.

SEX OR AGE MOST AFFECTED—Both sexes; all ages.

SIGNS & SYMPTOMS
- Decreased hearing.
- Ear pain.
- Plugged feeling in the ear.
- Ringing in the ear.

CAUSES—Overproduction of wax by glands in the external-ear canal.

RISK INCREASES WITH
- Exposure to dust or debris.
- Family history of overproduction of earwax.

HOW TO PREVENT—Avoid areas where the air is dusty or filled with debris. This stimulates overproduction of earwax.

 WHAT TO EXPECT

APPROPRIATE HEALTH CARE
- Self-care. Sometimes wax can be removed easily at home with ear drops and irrigation of the ear canal.
- Doctor's treatment if the wax is difficult to remove.

DIAGNOSTIC MEASURES
- Your own observation of symptoms.
- Medical history and physical exam by a doctor.

POSSIBLE COMPLICATIONS
- Ear infection.
- Eardrum damage.

PROBABLE OUTCOME—Earwax can be removed, but stubborn cases require patience.

 HOW TO TREAT

NOTE—Follow your doctor's instructions. These instructions are supplemental.

GENERAL MEASURES—To remove earwax at home:
- Buy non-prescription wax-softening ear drops.
- Lie down with the affected ear toward the ceiling.
- Pull the top of the ear gently up and back toward the back of the head.
- Instill the ear drops; use the amount given in the package directions.
- Leave the drops in the ear for 20 minutes. Continue to lie down, if possible. Plug the ear with cotton.
- Sit up, leaning a little toward the affected side.
- Use a soft rubber bulb syringe to irrigate the ear canal gently with plain warm water or equal parts warm water and hydrogen peroxide.
- Repeat irrigations until the ear feels clear. If the ear doesn't clear, consult your doctor.
- Don't try to remove wax with a stick or cotton swab. You may damage the eardrum or cause infection in the ear canal.

MEDICATION
- For minor pain, you may use non-prescription drugs such as acetaminophen.
- After treatment, your doctor may prescribe wax-softening ear drops to use when needed.

ACTIVITY—No restrictions.

DIET—No special diet.

 CALL YOUR DOCTOR IF

- You have symptoms of an earwax blockage that does not clear, despite treatment described above.
- A child younger than 4 has an earwax blockage.
- Fever and ear pain accompany an earwax blockage. Do *not* irrigate the ear in this case.

ILLNESSES & DISORDERS

ECTOPIC PREGNANCY

GENERAL INFORMATION

DEFINITION—A pregnancy that develops outside the uterus. The most common site is in one of the narrow tubes that connect each ovary to the uterus (Fallopian tube). Other sites include the ovary or outside the reproductive organs in the abdominal cavity.

BODY PARTS INVOLVED—Female reproductive system; abdominal cavity.

SEX OR AGE MOST AFFECTED—Females of childbearing age.

SIGNS & SYMPTOMS—Early stages:
- Missed menstrual period or a heavy, painful period.
- Unexplained vaginal spotting or bleeding.
- Lower abdominal pain and cramps.
- Pain in the shoulder.
Late stages:
- Sudden, sharp, severe abdominal pain caused by rupture of the Fallopian tube.
- Dizziness, fainting and shock (paleness, rapid heartbeat, drop in blood pressure and cold sweats). These may precede or accompany pain (sometimes).

CAUSES—An egg from the ovary is fertilized and becomes implanted outside the uterus—usually in the Fallopian tube. As the fertilized egg enlarges, the Fallopian tube stretches and ruptures, causing life-threatening internal bleeding.

RISK INCREASES WITH
- Use of an intrauterine device (IUD) for contraception.
- Previous pelvic infections.
- Adhesions (bands of scar tissue) from previous abdominal surgery.

HOW TO PREVENT
- Use a contraceptive method other than IUD.
- Obtain prompt treatment for any pelvic infection.

WHAT TO EXPECT

APPROPRIATE HEALTH CARE
- Doctor's treatment.
- Surgery (exploratory laparotomy) to remove the growing fertilized ovum and control internal bleeding.

DIAGNOSTIC MEASURES
- Your own observation of symptoms.
- Medical history and physical exam by a doctor.
- Laboratory studies, such as a pregnancy test and blood count.
- Surgical diagnostic procedures, such as laparoscopy and culdocentesis (see Glossary for both).

- Ultrasound to outline the fetus (see Glossary).

POSSIBLE COMPLICATIONS—Shock and death from internal bleeding.

PROBABLE OUTCOME—An ectopic pregnancy cannot progress to full term or produce a viable fetus. Rupture of an ectopic pregnancy is an emergency requiring immediate hospitalization and surgery. Full recovery is likely with early diagnosis and surgery. Subsequent pregnancies are usually normal.

HOW TO TREAT

NOTE—Follow your doctor's postoperative instructions. These instructions are supplemental.

GENERAL MEASURES—After surgery:
- You may wash normally over the stitches in your incision.
- Use heat to relieve pain. Apply a heating pad or hot-water bottle to the abdomen or back.
  Hot baths also relieve discomfort and relax muscles. Sit in a tub of hot water (106F to 110F or 41.1C to 43.3C) for 10 to 15 minutes. Repeat as often as needed.

MEDICATION—Medicine usually is not necessary for this disorder.

ACTIVITY—Resume your normal activities, including sexual relations, as soon as possible. Frequent, satisfying sexual activity helps you feel closer to your mate and promotes healing.
  Attempt sexual intercourse soon, but provide adequate lubrication. Spend extra time touching, conversing intimately and caressing. During early encounters, the woman must decide how much penile penetration and vigorous thrusting is comfortable. At first, it may be best if the man only inserts his penis partially into the vagina.

DIET—No special diet.

CALL YOUR DOCTOR IF

- You have symptoms of ectopic pregnancy, especially a rupture. Call immediately. This is an emergency!
- The following occurs after surgery:
  Excessive vaginal bleeding (soaking a pad or tampon every hour).
  Signs of infection, such as fever, chills, headache, dizziness or muscle aches.
  Increased urinary frequency that lasts longer than 1 month. This may be a sign of bladder irritation or infection resulting from surgery.

ECTROPION

GENERAL INFORMATION

DEFINITION—A disorder of the lower eyelid in which it weakens and turns outward (inside out).

BODY PARTS INVOLVED—Eyelid (one or both).

SEX OR AGE MOST AFFECTED—Adults over 40.

SIGNS & SYMPTOMS
● Turning out of the lower eyelid, causing an unattractive facial appearance.
● Inflammation (pain, redness and swelling) in the affected eyelid.
● Inadequate eye lubrication, caused when lubricating tears run down the cheek instead of into the eye.

CAUSES
● Weakening of the muscles and tissues that normally support the lid against the eye.
● Paralysis of the nerve that supplies the eyelid muscles.

RISK INCREASES WITH—Adults over 60.

HOW TO PREVENT—Cannot be prevented at present.

WHAT TO EXPECT

APPROPRIATE HEALTH CARE
● Doctor's treatment.
● Minor surgery to restore normal tension to the eyelid.

DIAGNOSTIC MEASURES
● Your own observation of symptoms.
● Medical history and physical exam by a doctor.

POSSIBLE COMPLICATIONS—Cornea damage caused by dryness.

PROBABLE OUTCOME—Usually curable with surgery.

HOW TO TREAT

NOTE—Follow your doctor's instructions. These instructions are supplemental.

GENERAL MEASURES
● Apply warm compresses to the eyelids several times a day to relieve inflammation and discomfort. To prepare compresses:
    Pour warm water in a clean bowl.
    Soak a clean cloth in the water. Wring it out almost dry.
    Apply the warm, moist cloth to the closed eye for 10 to 15 minutes.
    Remoisten the cloth frequently.
● Wear protective glasses or goggles if you are exposed to wind or pollutants.

MEDICATION—Your doctor may prescribe:
● Artificial tears until surgery can be performed.
● Antibiotics if infection is present.

ACTIVITY—No restrictions.

DIET—No special diet.

CALL YOUR DOCTOR IF

● You have symptoms of ectropion.
● The following occurs after surgery:
    Eye pain, redness and photosensitivity.
    Your vision changes in any way.

ILLNESSES & DISORDERS

ECZEMA
(Atopic Dermatitis; Infantile Eczema; Neurodermatitis)

 GENERAL INFORMATION

DEFINITION—A chronic allergic skin disorder of childhood.

BODY PARTS INVOLVED—Skin, especially of the scalp, face, back of the neck or skin creases of elbows and knees.

SEX OR AGE MOST AFFECTED—May begin between 1 month and 1 year. It usually subsides somewhat by age 3, but it may flare again at ages 10 to 12 and last through puberty.

SIGNS & SYMPTOMS—Skin affected by eczema has the following characteristics:
- Itching (sometimes severe).
- Small blisters with oozing.
- Thickening and scaling from chronic inflammation.

CAUSES—An allergic reaction to a wide variety of things, including:
- Foods, such as eggs, wheat, milk or seafood.
- Wool clothing.
- Skin lotions and ointments.

RISK INCREASES WITH
- Stress.
- Medical history of other allergic conditions, such as hay fever, asthma or sensitivity to certain drugs.
- Clothing made of synthetic fabric, which traps perspiration.
- Weather extremes, including humidity, severe cold and severe heat (especially with increased sweating).

HOW TO PREVENT—No specific preventive measures.

 WHAT TO EXPECT

APPROPRIATE HEALTH CARE
- Home care.
- Doctor's treatment.
- Hospitalization (rare).

DIAGNOSTIC MEASURES
- Your own observation of symptoms.
- Medical history and physical exam by a doctor.
- Laboratory studies, such as blood and skin tests to identify allergies.

POSSIBLE COMPLICATIONS
- Bacterial infections caused by injury to the skin.
- Life-threatening infection from a smallpox vaccination.
- Cataracts (for unknown reason).

PROBABLE OUTCOME—Variable. Some children outgrow eczema. Others are resistant to treatment, and eczema may persist through puberty. However, symptoms can usually be controlled with treatment.

Skin irritation from any other cause can trigger a flare-up or aggravate existing eczema.

 HOW TO TREAT

NOTE—Follow your doctor's instructions. These instructions are supplemental.

GENERAL MEASURES
- Provide loose, cotton clothing to help absorb perspiration.
- Minimize stress in the child's life whenever possible.
- Don't allow the child to have a smallpox vaccination or to be exposed to someone who has recently had one.
- Keep the child's fingernails short and put soft gloves on at night to minimize scratching. Scratching worsens eczema.
- Bathe the child less frequently to avoid excessive skin dryness. Soap and water may trigger flare-ups. When bathing, use special non-fat soaps and tepid water. Use *no* soap on inflamed areas.
- Lubricate the skin after bathing.
- Protect the child from extreme temperature changes.
- Avoid anything that has previously worsened the condition.

MEDICATION—Your doctor may prescribe:
- Ointments containing coal tar or cortisone drugs to decrease inflammation. These may help more if used at night under occlusive plastic wrap. Ask your doctor.
- Antihistamines to decrease itching.
- Antibiotics for complicating infections, if they occur.
- Sedatives or tranquilizers to calm the child.

ACTIVITY—No restrictions.

DIET—No special diet. Eliminate any foods known to cause flare-ups of eczema.

 CALL YOUR DOCTOR IF

- Your child has symptoms of eczema.
- New, unexplained symptoms develop.
Drugs used in treatment may produce side effects. Excessive use of cortisone drugs is dangerous, and antihistamines frequently cause drowsiness.

ELECTRIC SHOCK

GENERAL INFORMATION

DEFINITION—Injury caused by electricity passing through the body.

BODY PARTS INVOLVED—Total body.

SEX OR AGE MOST AFFECTED—Both sexes; all ages.

SIGNS & SYMPTOMS—Depends on where the current enters the body and the kind of electrical current. Following are the most common:
- Burns at areas of contact. The burns are often deep.
- Heart damage, including cardiac arrest.
- Severe muscle spasms that may cause fractures.
- Breathing paralysis.

CAUSES—Contact with electricity from downed power lines, exposed appliance wires, faulty electrical equipment, lightning strikes or other electrical sources.

RISK INCREASES WITH
- Standing on wet ground or under a tree during an electrical storm.
- Mishandling of electrical equipment.
- Occupations that involve electrical machinery or lines.

HOW TO PREVENT
- Inspect your house, especially the kitchen, bathroom and workshop, for hazards.
- Don't use hair dryers or radios in the bathroom where they can fall into a tub or sink.
- Use safety plugs in empty electrical outlets to prevent children from inserting metal objects.
- Don't try to repair electrical equipment unless you know how.
- Wear protective gloves and clothing for work that involves exposure to electricity.
- Replace worn cords or wiring at home or work.
- Go indoors during electrical storms.

WHAT TO EXPECT

APPROPRIATE HEALTH CARE
- Self-care after diagnosis (minor burns only).
- Emergency cardiopulmonary resuscitation (CPR) at the time of injury, if the victim is unconscious and not breathing. See General Measures.
- Doctor's treatment.
- Hospitalization.

DIAGNOSTIC MEASURES—Diagnosis is usually obvious from the circumstances.

POSSIBLE COMPLICATIONS
- Pneumonia.
- Permanent brain damage.
- Severe burns of the skin and underlying muscle.
- Death from heart damage.

PROBABLE OUTCOME—Depends on the extent of injury. Full recovery is likely if major brain or heart damage does not occur.

HOW TO TREAT

NOTE—Follow your doctor's instructions. These instructions are supplemental.

GENERAL MEASURES
- If the victim is touching live electrical wires, shut off the power or remove the wires with a non-metal object before giving aid. Don't electrocute yourself trying to help someone else.
- If the victim is unconscious and not breathing:
  Yell for help. Don't leave the victim.
  Begin mouth-to-mouth breathing immediately.
  If there is no heartbeat, give external cardiac massage.
  Have someone call O (operator) or 911 (emergency) for an ambulance or medical help.
  Don't stop cardiopulmonary resuscitation (CPR) until help arrives.

MEDICATION—Medicine usually is not necessary for electric shock.

ACTIVITY—No restrictions, if the shock is mild. If the shock is severe, the victim may resume activities gradually as injuries heal.

DIET—No special diet following electric shock.

CALL YOUR DOCTOR IF

- You or someone around you receives an electric shock severe enough to cause injury.
- The following occurs during convalescence:
  Irregular heartbeat.
  Fever.
  Cough with sputum.

EMPHYSEMA

GENERAL INFORMATION

DEFINITION—A chronic lung condition in which air sacs in the lungs become overstretched, destroying the elasticity of fibers that open and close the air sacs during breathing.

BODY PARTS INVOLVED—Alveoli (microscopic-sized air sacs in the lungs).

SEX OR AGE MOST AFFECTED—Usually begins between ages 55 and 75.

SIGNS & SYMPTOMS
- No symptoms in the early stages (often).
- Shortness of breath that increases in severity over several years.
- Wheezing and coughing that produces scant sputum.
- Occasional recurrent infections of the lungs or bronchial tubes.

CAUSES
- Many years of cigarette smoking.
- Air pollution.
- Inflammation of the air sacs in the lungs.
- Inherited trypsin deficiency.

RISK INCREASES WITH
- Occupations that require exceptional forced breathing, such as glass blowing or playing a wind musical instrument.
- Repeated lung infections that decrease lung-tissue function.
- Allergies or a family history of allergies.

HOW TO PREVENT
- Don't smoke.
- Avoid places with polluted air.
- Exercise moderately in fresh clean air.
- Prevent flu and pneumonia with immunizations.
- Avoid persons with respiratory infections.
- Obtain antibiotic treatment for lung infections.

WHAT TO EXPECT

APPROPRIATE HEALTH CARE
- Self-care after diagnosis.
- Doctor's treatment.
- Hospitalization for complications.

DIAGNOSTIC MEASURES
- Your own observation of symptoms.
- Medical history and physical exam by a doctor.
- Laboratory studies, such as blood tests and spirometry (see Glossary).

POSSIBLE COMPLICATIONS
- Susceptibility to lung infections.
- Chronic obstructive pulmonary disease (COPD).
- Respiratory failure.
- Congestive heart failure.

PROBABLE OUTCOME—Incurable, but symptoms can be controlled to retard progress and severity of the disease. Although emphysema reduces life expectancy, many persons live many years with it. Without treatment, complications can be fatal.

HOW TO TREAT

NOTE—Follow your doctor's instructions. These instructions are supplemental.

GENERAL MEASURES
- Don't smoke.
- Avoid breathing irritating substances.
- If you work in an area with severe air pollution, do all you can to decrease your exposure. Change jobs, if necessary.
- Install air conditioning with a filter and humidity control in your home.
- Treat any accompanying allergies to minimize aggravation of emphysema.
- Avoid sudden temperature or humidity changes, loud talking, laughing, crying or exertion, if these trigger coughing episodes.
- Floss and brush your teeth regularly to reduce the chance of oral infection.
- Elevate the foot of your bed with 4- or 5-inch blocks. This helps prevent mucus from accumulating in the lower parts of the lungs.
- Learn and practice breathing exercises. Ask your doctor for instructions.

MEDICATION
- Your doctor may prescribe:
  Antibiotics to fight or prevent secondary infections.
  Bronchodilators to relax spasms of the bronchial tubes.
- Arrange for immunizations against influenza and pneumonia.

ACTIVITY—Activity will be limited, but stay as active as your strength allows.

DIET—Unless you have congestive heart failure, drink at least 8 glasses of fluid a day. This thins lung secretions so they can be coughed up more easily.

CALL YOUR DOCTOR IF

- You have symptoms of emphysema.
- The following occurs after diagnosis:
  Temperature over 101F (38.3C).
  Blood in the sputum.
  Increased shortness of breath, or shortness of breath without coughing or when at rest.
  Chest pain.
  Sputum that increases, thickens or changes color, despite treatment.

EMPYEMA

GENERAL INFORMATION

DEFINITION—An accumulation of pus between layers of infected pleura (thin membranes that cover the lung).

BODY PARTS INVOLVED—Lung; pleura.

SEX OR AGE MOST AFFECTED—Both sexes; all ages.

SIGNS & SYMPTOMS
- Chest pain. Pain varies from vague discomfort to stabbing pain. It is often worse with coughing or breathing. Pain may extend to the lower chest wall or abdomen.
- Rapid, shallow breathing.
- Chills.
- Fever.
- Extreme fatigue.
- Bad breath.
- Weight loss.

CAUSES—A complication of:
- Lung or chest infections, such as pneumonia or tuberculosis.
- Collapsed lung or chest injury.
- Malignancy in other parts of the body.
- Collagen vascular disease, such as systemic lupus erythematosus.
- Infection in another part of the body that has spread to the chest.
- Congestive heart failure.
- Kidney disorders.
- Liver disorders.

RISK INCREASES WITH
- Poor nutrition.
- Recent illness (see Causes).
- Smoking.
- Fatigue or overwork.
- Wet, cold climates.
- Crowded or unsanitary living conditions.

HOW TO PREVENT—Obtain medical treatment for any serious disorder or infection that may cause empyema.

WHAT TO EXPECT

APPROPRIATE HEALTH CARE
- Self-care after diagnosis.
- Doctor's treatment.
- Hospitalization.

DIAGNOSTIC MEASURES
- Your own observation of symptoms.
- Medical history and physical exam by a doctor.
- Laboratory culture of pus from the empyema cavity.
- X-ray of the chest.

POSSIBLE COMPLICATIONS
- Meningitis.
- Pericarditis.
- Endocarditis.
- Brain abscess.

PROBABLE OUTCOME—Successful treatment depends on discovery and treatment of the underlying disorder. Draining the pus from the infected space hastens healing. High doses of antibiotics are needed, and hospitalization is usually required.

HOW TO TREAT

NOTE—Follow your doctor's instructions. These instructions are supplemental.

GENERAL MEASURES
- To reduce chest pain, wrap the entire chest *loosely* with 2 or 3 non-adhesive, 6-inch elastic bandages.
- Use a cool-mist humidifier to loosen bronchial secretions so they may be coughed up more easily.
- Practice these breathing exercises: Purse your lips and breathe forcefully against resistance (as if blowing out a candle) 10 times. Repeat every hour. Take 10 deep breaths every hour.
- Don't smoke.

MEDICATION
- Your doctor may prescribe antibiotics to fight infection. The type of antibiotic will depend on the type of germ responsible and sensitivity studies (see Glossary).
- For minor pain, you may use non-prescription drugs such as acetaminophen.

ACTIVITY—Reduce activity until the pain and fever are gone. Gradually return to normal activity. Allow 2 months for recovery.

DIET—No special diet. Take vitamin supplements. Increase fluid intake.

CALL YOUR DOCTOR IF

- You have symptoms of empyema.
- The following occurs during treatment:
  Fever rises rapidly over 101F (38.3C).
  Pain increases.
  Breathlessness worsens.
  Cough becomes dry and non-productive.
  Fingernails or toenails turn blue or dark.
  Blood appears in the sputum.

ILLNESSES & DISORDERS

ENCEPHALITIS, VIRAL OR ASEPTIC
(Acute Viral Encephalitis; Aseptic Encephalitis)

GENERAL INFORMATION

DEFINITION—An acute inflammation in the brain caused by a contagious viral infection.

BODY PARTS INVOLVED—Brain; sometimes meninges (membranes that cover the brain).

SEX OR AGE MOST AFFECTED—Both sexes; all ages.

SIGNS & SYMPTOMS—Mild cases:
- No symptoms (sometimes).
- Fever.
- General ill feeling.

Severe cases:
- Vomiting.
- Headache.
- Stiff neck.
- Pupils of different size.
- Unconsciousness.
- Personality changes.
- Seizures.
- Occasional weakness or paralysis of an arm or leg.
- Double vision.
- Speech impairment.
- Hearing loss.
- Drowsiness that progresses to coma.

CAUSES
- Viruses that cause other illnesses, including: polio; herpes; measles; mumps; chickenpox; infectious mononucleosis; infectious hepatitis; German measles; smallpox; coxsackie virus; echovirus diseases; and Eastern & Western equine virus.
- Viruses carried by mosquitoes or other insects.
- Lead poisoning.
- Vaccine reactions.
- Leukemia.

RISK INCREASES WITH
- Newborns and infants.
- Adults over 60.
- Illness that has lowered resistance.
- Crowded or unsanitary living conditions.

HOW TO PREVENT
- Avoid contact with anyone who has encephalitis.
- Consult your doctor for treatment of any infection in your body—especially those mentioned as causes—to attempt to prevent the spread of infection.

WHAT TO EXPECT

APPROPRIATE HEALTH CARE
- Doctor's treatment.
- Hospitalization (worst cases only).
- Self-care after diagnosis or hospitalization.

DIAGNOSTIC MEASURES
- Your own observation of symptoms.
- Medical history and physical exam by a doctor.
- Laboratory studies of blood and cerebrospinal fluid.

POSSIBLE COMPLICATIONS—A very small percentage of patients suffer permanent brain damage that impairs mental or muscle functions.

PROBABLE OUTCOME—Mild viral encephalitis is common and may go unnoticed. Severe cases usually require hospitalization.

Complications and fatalities from encephalitis are most common in infants and the elderly. People in other age groups usually recover completely. Unless the attack is severe, you can expect full recovery within 2 to 3 weeks.

HOW TO TREAT

NOTE—Follow your doctor's instructions. These instructions are supplemental.

GENERAL MEASURES—No specific instructions except those listed under other headings.

MEDICATION—Antibiotics are not helpful with viral diseases such as this. Your doctor may prescribe:
- Antiviral drugs, such as amantadine.
- Cortisone drugs to suppress inflammation (rare).

ACTIVITY—You will need bed rest in a darkened room. After a 2- to 3-week recovery, you should be as active as your strength and feeling of well-being allow.

DIET—No special diet.

CALL YOUR DOCTOR IF

- You have any symptoms of encephalitis.
- Temperature rises to 101F (38.3C) or higher.
- New, unexplained symptoms develop. Drugs used in treatment may produce side effects.

ENCOPRESIS

GENERAL INFORMATION

DEFINITION—Lack of bowel control in a child who has previously been toilet-trained and does not have diarrhea or constipation. A child cannot be expected to have complete bowel control until at least 2-1/2 years of age.

BODY PARTS INVOLVED—Bowels.

SEX OR AGE MOST AFFECTED—Both sexes of children over age 2-1/2.

SIGNS & SYMPTOMS—Bowel movements in underwear.

CAUSES
● Physical or emotional crisis in the child's life, such as birth of a sibling or recent illness with diarrhea.
● Resistance to using the toilet because of too much pressure to do so.
● If the problem is long-term, the original cause may be forgotten, and the behavior may persist as a habit.

RISK INCREASES WITH
● Stress.
● Recent illness that brought the child increased attention.

HOW TO PREVENT
● Don't lavish attention on a child for being ill.
● Avoid undue emphasis on toilet-training. Approach it calmly with realistic expectations. Don't shame or blame the child for accidents.
● Be sensitive to stressful situations your child faces. Talk together about the child's feelings.

WHAT TO EXPECT

APPROPRIATE HEALTH CARE
● Home care.
● Doctor's treatment, if home care fails.
● Psychotherapy or counseling (sometimes).

DIAGNOSTIC MEASURES
● Your own observation of symptoms.
● Medical history and physical exam by a doctor, if necessary.

POSSIBLE COMPLICATIONS—None expected. The symptoms frequently trigger more emotional difficulties than the initial cause.

PROBABLE OUTCOME—Usually curable, unless there is a serious underlying physical problem.

HOW TO TREAT

NOTE—Follow your doctor's instructions. These instructions are supplemental.

GENERAL MEASURES
● Let your child decide when it is time to go to the bathroom. Don't remind him or make him sit on the toilet against his will. This fosters a negative attitude.
● Praise your child for having bowel movements in the toilet—he deserves positive reinforcement for success. Other family members may also praise the child.
● Provide a prearranged reward if the child stays clean all day. The favorite reward of many children is 30 minutes of free time with either parent, doing whatever the child chooses. Incentives build motivation to succeed.
● Respond gently to accidents. When the child is soiled, he should clean himself and change into clean underwear. For younger children (under age 5), the parent will probably have to do this.
● Don't blame, criticize, restrict or punish the child for accidents. This may cause him to give up, as well as lead to secondary emotional problems.
● Don't allow siblings or others to tease the child.
● Never put the child back in diapers.
● Ask for the school's cooperation. The child needs quick access to the bathroom at school, especially if he is shy or new at school. Remind him that there should be nothing embarrassing about leaving the classroom to go to the bathroom.

MEDICATION—Don't use:
● Laxatives and stool softeners. These will probably cause diarrhea in addition to the original problem.
● Enemas and suppositories. These may make the child resistant and uncooperative.

ACTIVITY—No restrictions.

DIET—No special diet.

CALL YOUR DOCTOR IF

Your child has encopresis, and it persists longer than 2 months, despite your efforts.

ILLNESSES & DISORDERS

ENDOCARDITIS
(Bacterial Endocarditis; Infective Endocarditis)

 GENERAL INFORMATION

DEFINITION—A non-contagious infection of the valves or lining of the heart.

BODY PARTS INVOLVED—Heart muscle; heart valves; endocardium (lining of the heart chambers and valves).

SEX OR AGE MOST AFFECTED—Both sexes; all ages.

SIGNS & SYMPTOMS—Early symptoms:
- Fatigue and weakness.
- Intermittent fever, chills and excessive sweating, especially at night.
- Weight loss.
- Vague aches and pains.
- Heart murmur.
Late symptoms:
- Severe chills and high fever.
- Shortness of breath on exertion.
- Swelling of the feet, legs and abdomen.
- Rapid or irregular heartbeat.

CAUSES—Bacteria or fungi that enter the blood and infect the valves and heart lining of persons with damaged hearts (see risks below). Bacteria or fungi further damage the heart valves, muscles and linings.

RISK INCREASES WITH—Risk of heart-valve damage increases with:
- Rheumatic fever.
- Congenital heart disease.
Risk of endocarditis following heart-valve damage increases with:
- Pregnancy.
- Injections of contaminated materials into the bloodstream, such as with self-administered intravenous drugs.
- Excess alcohol consumption.
- Use of immunosuppressive drugs.
- Artificial heart valves.

HOW TO PREVENT—If you have heart-valve damage or a heart murmur:
- Request antibiotics prior to medical procedures that may introduce bacteria into the blood. These include dental work, childbirth and surgery of the urinary or gastrointestinal tract.
- Don't drink more than l or 2—if any—alcoholic drinks in 1 day.
- Consult your doctor before becoming pregnant.
- Don't use mind-altering drugs.

 WHAT TO EXPECT

APPROPRIATE HEALTH CARE
- Doctor's treatment.
- Hospitalization.
- Self-care after the acute illness.

DIAGNOSTIC MEASURES
- Medical history and physical exam by a doctor.
- Your own observation of symptoms.
- Laboratory blood counts and blood cultures.
- EKG (see Glossary).
- X-rays of the heart and lungs, including echocardiogram (see Glossary).

POSSIBLE COMPLICATIONS
- Blood clots that may travel to the brain, kidneys or abdominal organs, causing infections, abscesses or stroke.
- Heart-rhythm disturbances (atrial fibrillation is most common).

PROBABLE OUTCOME—Usually curable with early diagnosis and treatment. If treatment is delayed, heart function deteriorates, resulting in congestive heart failure and death.

 HOW TO TREAT

NOTE—Follow your doctor's instructions. These instructions are supplemental.

GENERAL MEASURES
- If you have damaged heart valves, tell any doctor or dentist who treats you.
- Once you have had endocarditis, stay under a doctor's care to prevent a relapse.

MEDICATION—Your doctor may prescribe antibiotics for many weeks to fight infection. Antibiotic treatment is often intravenous.

ACTIVITY—Rest in bed until you are fully recovered. While in bed, flex your legs often to prevent clots from forming in deep veins.

Resume your normal activities, including sexual relations, when strength allows.

DIET—No special diet, unless you have an underlying heart disorder. In that case, follow a low-salt diet (see Appendix 9).

 CALL YOUR DOCTOR IF

- You have symptoms of endocarditis.
- The following occurs during or after treatment:
  Weight gain without diet changes.
  Blood in the urine.
  Chest pain.
  Sudden weakness or numbness in muscles of the face, trunk or limbs.

ENDOMETRIAL HYPERPLASIA
(Adenomatous Hyperplasia of the Uterus)

 GENERAL INFORMATION

DEFINITION—An overgrowth of tissue in the endometrium (inner lining of the uterus). This is not cancerous.

BODY PARTS INVOLVED—Endometrium.

SEX OR AGE MOST AFFECTED—Women over age 35.

SIGNS & SYMPTOMS
- Bleeding between normal menstrual periods.
- Heavy menstrual flow (saturating a tampon or pad once every hour).
- Bleeding after menopause.

CAUSES—Excessive estrogen, a female hormone. This is caused internally or from the use of hormone-containing medications. Endometrial hyperplasia rarely occurs in women who have a normal menstrual cycle.

RISK INCREASES WITH—Use of oral contraceptives or estrogen replacement therapy after menopause.

HOW TO PREVENT—No specific preventive measures.

 WHAT TO EXPECT

APPROPRIATE HEALTH CARE
- Doctor's treatment.
- D & C (dilatation and curettage, see Glossary) to obtain tissue for microscopic examination to rule out malignancy.
- Hysterectomy (surgery to remove the uterus) sometimes.

DIAGNOSTIC MEASURES
- Your own observation of symptoms.
- Medical history and physical exam by a doctor.
- Laboratory tests, such as blood tests of hormone levels and Pap smear (see Glossary).

POSSIBLE COMPLICATIONS
- Perforation of the uterus and peritonitis as a complication of surgery (rare).
- Excessive, uncontrollable bleeding.

PROBABLE OUTCOME—Often curable with D & C or hysterectomy. If a woman chooses not to have surgery, hormone therapy usually controls symptoms.

 HOW TO TREAT

NOTE—Follow your doctor's instructions. These instructions are supplemental.

GENERAL MEASURES
- Try to reduce psychological stress that can complicate your illness and delay your recovery. If you can't resolve the stress, ask for help from family, friends or competent counselors.
- Use heat to relieve pain. Place a heating pad or hot-water bottle on your abdomen or back.
- Take frequent hot baths to relax muscles and relieve discomfort. Sit in a tub of hot water for 10 to 15 minutes.
- Don't douche unless your doctor recommends it.
- For an explanation of surgery and postoperative care, see Hysterectomy.

MEDICATION—If the D & C does not relieve symptoms and you don't want a hysterectomy, your doctor will probably prescribe progesterone, a female hormone.

ACTIVITY—No restrictions unless you have surgery. Then resume your activities gradually.
  Ask your doctor about resuming sexual relations following surgery or D & C. Don't hesitate to discuss this—it is an important part of your life.

DIET—No special diet.

 CALL YOUR DOCTOR IF

- You have symptoms of endometrial hyperplasia.
- The following symptoms occur during hormone treatment or after surgery or D & C:
  Excessive bleeding (saturating more than 1 pad or tampon every hour).
  Signs of infection, such as fever, general ill feeling, headache, dizziness or muscle aches.
- New, unexplained symptoms develop. Hormones used in treatment may produce side effects.

ENDOMETRIOSIS

GENERAL INFORMATION

DEFINITION—A disorder in which tissue resembling the inner lining of the uterus (endometrium) appears at unusual locations in the lower abdomen. This tissue may be found: on the ovary surfaces; behind the uterus, low in the pelvic cavity; on the intestinal wall; and rarely, at other sites far away.

BODY PARTS INVOLVED—Uterus; ovaries; Fallopian tubes; outer layer of the intestines.

SEX OR AGE MOST AFFECTED—Females between puberty and menopause, but most common between ages 20 and 30.

SIGNS & SYMPTOMS—The following symptoms may begin abruptly or develop over many years:
- Increased pelvic pain during menstrual periods, especially the last days.
- Pain with sexual intercourse.
- Blood in the urine.
- Back pain.
- Pain with intestinal contractions.
- Blood in the stool (sometimes).

CAUSES—Unknown, but the following theory is most accepted among doctors:

Normally during ovulation, the uterus lining thickens to prepare for implantation of a fertilized egg. If this does not occur, the lining tissue peels away from the uterus and is expelled in the menstrual flow.

In some cases, this material builds up and passes backward out of the Fallopian tubes into the pelvic cavity. Here it floats freely and attaches itself to other tissues.

The transplanted tissue reacts each month as if it were still in the uterus, thickening and peeling away. New bits of peeled-off tissue create new implants. The growing endometrial tissue between pelvic organs may cause them to adhere together, producing pain and other symptoms.

RISK INCREASES WITH—Adult women who don't become pregnant.

HOW TO PREVENT—Have children while you are young. Pregnancy permanently cures some people with endometriosis.

WHAT TO EXPECT

APPROPRIATE HEALTH CARE
- Self-care after diagnosis.
- Doctor's treatment. Diagnosing the disorder may be difficult, requiring repeated examinations or surgical diagnostic procedures.

- Surgery to remove implants, or a hysterectomy to remove the uterus, Fallopian tubes and ovaries in women who don't want to become pregnant.

DIAGNOSTIC MEASURES
- Your own observation of symptoms.
- Medical history and physical exam by a doctor.
- Laboratory blood studies.
- Surgical diagnostic procedures, such as laparoscopy (see Glossary).
- X-rays of the lower intestines (barium enema).

POSSIBLE COMPLICATIONS
- Sterility from tissue implants that constrict the Fallopian tubes.
- Disabling, but never life-threatening, pain.

PROBABLE OUTCOME—Without treatment, endometriosis becomes increasingly severe. It subsides after menopause when estrogen production decreases.

Symptoms can be relieved with medication, and it is usually curable with surgery.

HOW TO TREAT

NOTE—Follow your doctor's instructions. These instructions are supplemental.

GENERAL MEASURES
- If you want children, consider pregnancy as soon as possible. Pregnancy often cures the disorder. Delaying pregnancy may cause infertility.
- Use sanitary napkins instead of tampons. Tampons may make backward menstrual flow more likely.
- Use heat to relieve pain. Place a heating pad or hot-water bottle on your abdomen or back, or take hot baths to relax muscles and relieve discomfort.

MEDICATION
- You may use non-prescription drugs, such as acetaminophen, to relieve minor pain.
- Your doctor may prescribe:
  Pain relievers.
  Hormones, including oral contraceptives.

ACTIVITY—No restrictions.

DIET—No special diet.

CALL YOUR DOCTOR IF

- You have symptoms of endometriosis.
- The following occurs during treatment:
  Intolerable pain.
  Unusual or excessive vaginal bleeding.
- New, unexplained symptoms develop. Drugs used in treatment may produce side effects.
- Symptoms recur after treatment.

ENTROPION

GENERAL INFORMATION

DEFINITION—A disorder of the eyelid (usually the lower) in which it curls inward toward the eye.

BODY PARTS INVOLVED—Eyelid.

SEX OR AGE MOST AFFECTED—Adults over 40.

SIGNS & SYMPTOMS—Inflammation of the eye (swelling, redness, pain and excessive tears) caused when the inward-turning eyelid and lashes rub against the cornea.

CAUSES—Several different factors may cause entropion:
- Relaxation of the eyelid's supporting tissue, coupled with the inward pull of the eyelid muscles.
- Chronic eye inflammation (including allergy), creating scar tissue in the eyelid.

RISK INCREASES WITH—Aging.

HOW TO PREVENT—Obtain prompt medical attention for any eye infection.

WHAT TO EXPECT

APPROPRIATE HEALTH CARE
- Self-care after diagnosis.
- Doctor's treatment. Your doctor may attach a small strip of adhesive tape to the lower lid as a temporary measure before surgery.
- Minor surgery (usually) to correct the condition.

DIAGNOSTIC MEASURES
- Your own observation of symptoms.
- Medical history and physical exam by a doctor.

POSSIBLE COMPLICATIONS—Ulceration of the cornea from eyelash and eyelid irritation.

PROBABLE OUTCOME—Usually curable with surgery.

HOW TO TREAT

NOTE—Follow your doctor's instructions. These instructions are supplemental.

GENERAL MEASURES
- Apply warm compresses to the eyelids several times a day to relieve inflammation and discomfort. To prepare compresses:
  Pour warm water in a clean bowl.
  Soak a clean cloth in the water. Wring it out almost dry.
  Apply the warm, moist cloth to the closed eye for 10 to 15 minutes.
  Remoisten the cloth frequently.
- Wear protective glasses or goggles if you are exposed to wind or pollutants.

MEDICATION—Your doctor may prescribe:
- Artificial tears until surgery can be performed.
- Antibiotics if infection is present.

ACTIVITY—No restrictions.

DIET—No special diet.

CALL YOUR DOCTOR IF

- You have symptoms of entropion.
- The following occurs after surgery:
  Eye pain, redness and photosensitivity.
  Your vision changes in any way.

ILLNESSES & DISORDERS

EPIDIDYMITIS

 GENERAL INFORMATION

DEFINITION—An inflammation and infection of the epididymis, an oblong structure attached to the upper part of each testis.

BODY PARTS INVOLVED—Epididymis.

SEX OR AGE MOST AFFECTED—Males between puberty and old age.

SIGNS & SYMPTOMS
- Enlarged, hardened testicle.
- Fever.
- Tender scrotal contents.
- Tenderness of the second testicle (sometimes).
- Acute urethritis (often).

CAUSES—Usually a complication of a bacterial infection elsewhere in the body, such as: gonococcal infection of the urethra; prostate infection; or bladder or kidney infection.
Epididymitis may also complicate an infection of the scrotum or be caused by scrotal injury.

RISK INCREASES WITH—Recent illness, especially acute or chronic prostatitis, urethritis, or urinary-tract infection.

HOW TO PREVENT
- Use rubber condoms during intercourse to protect from venereal disease. Don't engage in sexual activity with persons who have venereal disease.
- Avoid urethral catheters if possible.

 WHAT TO EXPECT

APPROPRIATE HEALTH CARE
- Self-care after diagnosis.
- Doctor's treatment.

DIAGNOSTIC MEASURES
- Your own observation of symptoms.
- Medical history and physical exam by a doctor.
- Laboratory studies, such as urinalysis and culture of prostate secretions, to identify the germ responsible.

POSSIBLE COMPLICATIONS
- Constipation (sometimes) because bowel movements aggravate pain.
- Sterility or narrowing and blockage of the urethra if the epididymitis involves both testicles. This requires surgery.

PROBABLE OUTCOME—Usually curable with treatment.

 HOW TO TREAT

NOTE—Follow your doctor's instructions. These instructions are supplemental.

GENERAL MEASURES
- Support the weight of the scrotum and tender testicles. Roll a soft bath towel and place it between the legs under the inflamed area.
- Apply either an ice bag or warm compresses, electric heating pad or hot water bottle to the inflamed parts. Use whichever relieves pain best.
- Wear an athletic supporter or two pairs of athletic briefs when you resume normal activity.

MEDICATION—Your doctor may prescribe:
- Antibiotics to fight infection.
- Pain relievers.
- Stool softeners.
- Hormones to decrease sexual tension, if necessary.

ACTIVITY—Rest in bed until fever, pain and swelling improve. Don't engage in sexual intercourse. If sexual desire and erections become a problem, consult your doctor for medication. Wait at least 1 month after *all* symptoms disappear before resuming sexual relations.

DIET
- Don't drink alcohol, tea, coffee or carbonated beverages. These irritate the urinary system.
- Eat natural laxative foods, such as prunes, fresh fruit, whole-grain cereals and nuts, to prevent constipation.

 CALL YOUR DOCTOR IF

- You have symptoms of epididymitis.
- Pain is not relieved by measures outlined above.
- Your temperature reaches 103F (39.4C).
- You become constipated.
- Symptoms don't improve within 4 days after treatment begins.

EPIGLOTTITIS, ACUTE

GENERAL INFORMATION

DEFINITION—A sudden, life-threatening childhood infection of the epiglottis (a small flap of tissue in the back of the throat that guards the airway entrance to the lung). Epiglottitis is contagious.

BODY PARTS INVOLVED—Epiglottis and surrounding tissue.

SEX OR AGE MOST AFFECTED—Children (2 to 12 years).

SIGNS & SYMPTOMS—Sudden onset of the following:
- Sore throat.
- Fever.
- Hoarseness.
- Drooling caused by difficulty swallowing saliva.
- Increasing breathing difficulty.
- Noisy, high-pitched, squeaky inhalations.
- Purple skin and nails.
- Odd head posture. The child tilts the neck back and leans forward with the tongue stuck out and the nostrils flared, trying to inhale more air.

CAUSES—Infection of the epiglottis by a bacteria (usually hemophilus influenza, pneumococcus or streptococcus). The swollen epiglottis blocks the trachea (the main lung airway).

RISK INCREASES WITH
- Illness that has lowered resistance.
- Crowded or unsanitary living conditions.

HOW TO PREVENT—If your child has had epiglottitis previously, treat all respiratory infections early and with medical supervision.

WHAT TO EXPECT

APPROPRIATE HEALTH CARE
- Doctor's treatment.
- Hospitalization for oxygen and other intensive care.
- Surgery to make an opening in the windpipe (trachea) or to place a tube in the trachea to permit breathing. Usually the tube is withdrawn or the opening is closed in 4 to 7 days.

DIAGNOSTIC MEASURES
- Your own observation of symptoms.
- Medical history and physical exam by a doctor.
- Laboratory studies, such as blood counts and a throat culture.
- X-rays of the throat to determine the amount of airway obstruction.

POSSIBLE COMPLICATIONS—Without treatment, complete airway obstruction and death within hours.

PROBABLE OUTCOME—Full recovery with prompt diagnosis and treatment.

HOW TO TREAT

NOTE—Follow your doctor's instructions. These instructions are supplemental.

GENERAL MEASURES
- Have the child sit up rather than lie down.
- Keep the child calm and still until reaching the hospital. Panic increases breathing difficulty.
- After hospitalization, use a cool-mist humidifier at night in the child's room for 2 to 3 weeks.

MEDICATION—Your doctor may prescribe antibiotics to control infection. Continue for a minimum of 10 days.

ACTIVITY—Bed rest is necessary until all symptoms disappear. Activities may then be resumed gradually.

DIET—Fluids only (usually intravenous) until the child can swallow. After hospitalization, encourage extra fluids and provide a normal diet.

CALL YOUR DOCTOR IF

- Your child has symptoms of epiglottitis, especially signs of breathing difficulty. This is an emergency!
- Your child has had epiglottitis in the past, and symptoms of respiratory infection appear.

ILLNESSES & DISORDERS

EPILEPSY

 GENERAL INFORMATION

DEFINITION—A disorder of brain function characterized by sudden seizures, brief attacks of inappropriate behavior, change in one's state of consciousness or bizarre movements. Seizures—also called fits or convulsions—are a symptom, not a disease. Epilepsy is not contagious.

BODY PARTS INVOLVED—Brain.

SEX OR AGE MOST AFFECTED—Both sexes; all ages. Seizures usually begin between ages 2 and 14.

SIGNS & SYMPTOMS—There are several forms of epilepsy (listed below), each with its own characteristics:
- Petit mal epilepsy, which mostly affects children. The person stops activity and stares blankly around for a minute or so—unaware of what is happening.
- Grand mal epilepsy, which affects all ages. The person loses consciousness, stiffens, then twitches and jerks uncontrollably. He or she may lose bladder control. The seizure lasts several minutes, and is often followed by deep sleep or mental confusion. Prior to the seizure, the person may have warning signals: a tense feeling; visual disturbances; smelling a bad odor; or hearing strange noises.
- Focal epilepsy, in which a small part of the body begins twitching uncontrollably. The twitching spreads until it may involve the whole body. The person does not lose consciousness.
- Temporal-lobe epilepsy, in which the person suddenly behaves out of character or inappropriately, such as: becoming suddenly violent or angry; laughing for no reason; or making agitated or bizarre body movements, including odd chewing movements.

CAUSES—More than 50 brain disorders, but the organic cause can be determined in only 25% of cases. Common causes include:
- Brain damage at birth.
- Drug or alcohol abuse.
- Severe head injury.
- Brain infection.
- Brain tumor or an expanding lesion that compresses the brain (occasionally).

RISK INCREASES WITH
- Family history of seizure disorders.
- Excess alcohol consumption.
- Use of mind-altering drugs.
- Exposure to toxic fumes.
- Low blood sugar.

HOW TO PREVENT—No specific preventive measures.

 WHAT TO EXPECT

APPROPRIATE HEALTH CARE
- Self-care after diagnosis.
- Doctor's treatment.
- Surgery to remove any tumor, scar, or abscess, if one is causing epilepsy.
- Psychotherapy or counseling to learn to understand and live with the disorder.

DIAGNOSTIC MEASURES
- Your own observation of symptoms.
- Medical history and physical exam by a doctor.
- Laboratory blood studies.
- EEG (see Glossary).
- X-rays of the head.
- CAT scan (see Glossary).

POSSIBLE COMPLICATIONS—Continuing seizures (despite treatment), and mental deterioration (rare).

PROBABLE OUTCOME—Epilepsy is incurable, except in relatively rare cases where epilepsy is caused by treatable brain damage, tumors or infection. However, anticonvulsant drugs can prevent most seizures and allow a near-normal life.

 HOW TO TREAT

NOTE—Follow your doctor's instructions. These instructions are supplemental.

GENERAL MEASURES
- Request and carry a Medic-Alert bracelet or pendant that shows you have epilepsy in case you have a seizure.
- Avoid any circumstance that has triggered a seizure previously.

MEDICATION—Your doctor will prescribe anticonvulsant drugs. Your response to treatment will be monitored. Medication changes or adjustments are often necessary.

Learn as much as you can about your medication. The drugs used cause significant side effects, in addition to suppressing seizures.

ACTIVITY—No restrictions. Most states allow persons with epilepsy to drive a vehicle after being seizure-free for 1 year.

DIET—No special diet. Don't drink alcohol. It may decrease the effectiveness of your medication and provoke seizures.

 CALL YOUR DOCTOR IF

- You or your child have a seizure.
- New, unexplained symptoms develop during treatment for epilepsy. Drugs used in treatment may produce side effects.

ERYTHEMA NODOSUM

GENERAL INFORMATION

DEFINITION—An inflammatory disease of the skin and tissue under the skin, characterized primarily by painful red nodules on the legs. It is not contagious.

BODY PARTS INVOLVED—Skin of the legs, especially areas over the large bone in the lower leg. The disease occasionally involves the arms or other areas.

SEX OR AGE MOST AFFECTED—Both sexes and all ages, but more likely in females (ages 12 to 40).

SIGNS & SYMPTOMS—Nodules with the following characteristics:
- Nodules are red, painful or tender, and warm.
- Nodules are large (4cm to 10cm). Usually no more than 6 nodules appear at one time.
- Nodules usually occur on the front of the lower legs. They appear on one side and then the other.
- Nodules usually appear suddenly. They are often accompanied by fever and swollen, red, tender ankles and knees.
- Nodules change color from pink to red to blue to brown over 7 to 10 days.

CAUSES—Sometimes unknown. Known causes include:
- Use of drugs, such as birth-control pills (especially those high in estrogen), sulfonamides, iodides and bromides.
- Preceding infection, including: streptococcus (most common), coccidioidomycosis, histoplasmosis, sarcoidosis, blastomycosis, tuberculosis and yersinia infections (see Glossary).
- Autoimmune disease.
- Chronic bowel inflammation.
- Dysproteinemia (see Glossary).
- Consumption of foods with food dyes or preservatives.

RISK INCREASES WITH—Pregnancy.

HOW TO PREVENT—Remove or treat the cause, if it can be identified.

WHAT TO EXPECT

APPROPRIATE HEALTH CARE
- Doctor's treatment.
- Self-care after diagnosis.

DIAGNOSTIC MEASURES
- Medical history and physical exam by a doctor.
- Laboratory studies, such as antistreptococcal titre (see Glossary).
- X-rays of the chest to detect sarcoidosis or tuberculosis.

POSSIBLE COMPLICATIONS—Rarely, erythema nodosum can indicate a hidden malignancy in the gastrointestinal tract, liver or lung.

PROBABLE OUTCOME—Individual nodules diminish in size and tenderness and heal in 10 to 20 days. However, others may begin. The disease may last several months. Once it disappears, erythema nodosum probably will not return. Treatment hastens recovery.

HOW TO TREAT

NOTE—Follow your doctor's instructions. These instructions are supplemental.

GENERAL MEASURES
- Elevate the legs whenever possible.
- Use elastic wrap or support stockings.
- Use wrapped or immersion soaks (see Appendix 18) to hasten healing and relieve discomfort. Warm-water soaks are usually more soothing for pain or inflammation. Cool-water soaks feel better for itching.

MEDICATION
- For minor discomfort, you may use non-prescription drugs such as acetaminophen.
- Your doctor may prescribe a non-steroidal anti-inflammatory drug or cortisone drugs to reduce inflammation.

ACTIVITY—Rest in bed as much as possible with the legs elevated. Overexertion will cause lesions to recur. When symptoms subside, resume normal activity slowly. Allow 3 weeks for recovery.

DIET—No special diet.

CALL YOUR DOCTOR IF

- You have symptoms of erythema nodosum.
- The following occurs during treatment: Symptoms don't improve after 3 days of treatment.
  Temperature rises to 101F (38.3C).
- Any new symptoms arise which you think may be due to the disorder or the medications prescribed.

ESOPHAGEAL STRICTURE OR CORROSIVE ESOPHAGITIS

 GENERAL INFORMATION

DEFINITION
- Esophageal stricture is narrowing of the esophagus (the tube connecting the mouth to the stomach) caused by inflammation. The narrowing interferes with swallowing.
- Corrosive esophagitis is narrowing of the esophagus caused by chemical damage.

BODY PARTS INVOLVED—Esophagus.

SEX OR AGE MOST AFFECTED—Both sexes; all ages.

SIGNS & SYMPTOMS
- Sudden or gradual decrease in the ability to swallow. Gradual swallowing difficulty affects solid foods first, then liquids.
- Pain in the mouth and chest after eating.
- Increased salivation.
- Rapid breathing.
- Vomiting, sometimes with mucus or blood. Cancer of the esophagus often causes similar symptoms.

CAUSES—Scarring of the esophagus following inflammation or damage caused by:
- Chronic heartburn or hiatal hernia.
- Prolonged use of feeding tubes.
- Accidental swallowing of lye or other corrosive chemicals by a child.
- Deliberate swallowing of lye or other corrosive chemicals by a suicidal person.

RISK INCREASES WITH—Careless storage of corrosive chemicals, such as lye, kerosene, harsh detergent or bleach.

HOW TO PREVENT
- Store all chemicals out of the reach of young children.
- Avoid prolonged use of feeding tubes.

 WHAT TO EXPECT

APPROPRIATE HEALTH CARE
- Doctor's treatment.
- Hospitalization for supportive care and intravenous nutrition.
- Surgery to remove stricture if other measures fail.
- Psychotherapy or counseling for suicidal persons.

DIAGNOSTIC MEASURES
- Your own observation of symptoms.
- Medical history and physical exam by a doctor.
- Surgical diagnostic procedures such as endoscopy (see Glossary).
- X-rays of the esophagus (barium swallow).

POSSIBLE COMPLICATIONS
- Malnutrition from inability to eat normally.
- Perforation of the damaged esophagus. This may be life-threatening.

PROBABLE OUTCOME—Usually curable with treatment. Normal swallowing can be maintained with regular treatment to stretch the stricture.

 HOW TO TREAT

NOTE—Follow your doctor's instructions. These instructions are supplemental.

GENERAL MEASURES—The stricture must be stretched regularly (about once a month) with large, heavy dilators. Your doctor will provide specific instructions. The stricture will eventually return if regular treatments are not continued.

MEDICATION—Your doctor may prescribe:
- Cortisone drugs to reduce inflammation and diminish the possibility of scarring.
- Antibiotics to prevent infection.

ACTIVITY—Resume normal activities gradually.

DIET
- Eat a soft or liquid diet (see Appendix 11) after treatment until normal swallowing is possible. Avoid spicy foods that irritate the esophagus.
- Don't drink alcohol.

 CALL YOUR DOCTOR IF

- You have symptoms of esophageal stricture or corrosive esophagitis.
- The following occurs during treatment:
  Chest pain.
  Fever.
  Inability to speak.
  Feeling of air bubbles under the skin of the chest.

ESOPHAGUS CANCER

GENERAL INFORMATION

DEFINITION—A new growth of tissue in the esophagus (tube connecting the mouth to the stomach) in which cells multiply in an uncontrolled fashion.

BODY PARTS INVOLVED—Cancer that begins in the esophagus (primary) usually occurs in the lower third of the esophagus where it passes through the chest.

SEX OR AGE MOST AFFECTED
- Adults (age 50 and over).
- Both sexes, but more likely in men.

SIGNS & SYMPTOMS
- Swallowing difficulty or pain.
- Rapid weight loss.
- Regurgitation of bloody mucus.

CAUSES—Unknown. Most esophagus cancers are primary (begin there), but some spread from other body parts. It is not inherited.

RISK INCREASES WITH
- Smoking.
- Excess alcohol consumption.
- Previous head and neck tumors.
- Celiac disease.

HOW TO PREVENT
- Don't smoke.
- Don't drink more than 1 or 2 alcoholic drinks—if any—a day.
- Obtain medical treatment for any gastrointestinal disorder that lasts longer than 5 days.

WHAT TO EXPECT

APPROPRIATE HEALTH CARE
- Doctor's treatment.
- Surgery to remove cancer.
- Radiation treatment (sometimes).

DIAGNOSTIC MEASURES
- Your own observation of symptoms.
- Medical history and physical exam by a doctor.
- Biopsy (see Glossary) of tumor.
- X-ray of the upper-intestinal tract.

POSSIBLE COMPLICATIONS—If treatment doesn't begin immediately, esophagus cancer spreads rapidly to the lungs and liver.

PROBABLE OUTCOME—This condition is currently considered incurable. Early diagnosis and aggressive treatment offer the only chance of survival. In any case, symptoms can be relieved or controlled.

Medical literature cites a few instances of unexplained recovery. Scientific research into causes and treatment continues, so there is hope for increasingly effective treatment and cure.

HOW TO TREAT

NOTE—Follow your doctor's instructions. These instructions are supplemental.

GENERAL MEASURES—No specific treatment except that listed under other headings.

MEDICATION—Your doctor may prescribe:
- Medicine to relieve pain.
- Tranquilizers to reduce anxiety.
- Anticancer drugs (sometimes).

ACTIVITY—Remain as active as possible.

DIET—Your doctor may prescribe a special diet, depending on the treatment chosen.

CALL YOUR DOCTOR IF

- You have symptoms of cancer of the esophagus.
- Pain becomes intolerable despite treatment.
- New, unexplained symptoms develop. Drugs used in treatment may produce side effects.

EXOPHTHALMOS
(Proptosis)

 GENERAL INFORMATION

DEFINITION—A protrusion or bulging of one or both eyes.

BODY PARTS INVOLVED—Eyes.

SEX OR AGE MOST AFFECTED—Both sexes; all ages.

SIGNS & SYMPTOMS
- Bulging eyes, which creates a staring or frightened look.
- Double vision.
- Pain (sometimes).
- Infrequent blinking (sometimes).

CAUSES—Swelling of tissue behind the eye. Swelling may be caused by:
- Overactive thyroid gland (most common cause).
- Infection or tumor in the supportive tissues behind the eye.
- Aneurysm, blood clot or hemorrhage in the veins or arteries behind the eye.
- Injury to the eye or face.
- Congenital deformity of the head.

RISK INCREASES WITH—Unknown.

HOW TO PREVENT—Obtain prompt medical treatment for the underlying disorder.

 WHAT TO EXPECT

APPROPRIATE HEALTH CARE
- Doctor's treatment.
- Surgery to:
  Remove a tumor, blood clot or aneurysm.
  Return the eyes to their normal position, if necessary, after the underlying cause is corrected.
  Correct congenital abnormalities.

DIAGNOSTIC MEASURES
- Your own observation of symptoms.
- Biopsy (see Glossary) of tissue behind the eyes.
- X-rays of the head.
- CAT scan (see Glossary).

POSSIBLE COMPLICATIONS—Injury to the eye and impaired vision.

PROBABLE OUTCOME—Spontaneous recovery in most cases after the underlying cause is treated. If not, surgery can often correct any remaining protrusion.

 HOW TO TREAT

NOTE—Follow your doctor's instructions. These instructions are supplemental.

GENERAL MEASURES
- If the disorder is caused by injury, see a doctor immediately.
- If your vision is affected, don't drive or engage in dangerous activity.
- If eyelids don't blink properly, wear goggles to protect them from wind or dust.

MEDICATION
- If the lids don't blink properly, you should use non-prescription, lubricating eye drops.
- Your doctor may prescribe drugs to treat the underlying cause, such as:
  Antithyroid drugs for hyperthyroidism.
  Antibiotics to fight infection.
  Cortisone drugs to reduce inflammation.

ACTIVITY—No restrictions.

DIET—No special diet.

 CALL YOUR DOCTOR IF

- You have symptoms of exophthalmos.
- Symptoms don't improve within 5 days after treatment begins.
- New, unexplained symptoms develop. Drugs used in treatment may produce side effects.

EXTRADURAL HEMORRHAGE
(Epidural Hemorrhage)

 GENERAL INFORMATION

DEFINITION—Bleeding between the skull and the outermost of 3 membranes that cover the brain (meninges).

BODY PARTS INVOLVED—Skull; meninges; brain.

SEX OR AGE MOST AFFECTED—Both sexes; all ages.

SIGNS & SYMPTOMS—These symptoms develop within 24 to 96 hours after a head injury:
- Headache that steadily worsens.
- Drowsiness or unconsciousness.
- Nausea or vomiting.
- Inability to move arms and legs.
- Change in the size of eye pupils.

CAUSES—Head injury.

RISK INCREASES WITH
- Use of anticoagulant drugs.
- Bleeding disorders, such as hemophilia, ITT or aplastic anemia.
- Injuries. These occur more often after excess alcohol consumption or use of mind-altering drugs.

HOW TO PREVENT—Avoid head injury in the following ways:
- Use seat belts in cars.
- Wear protective head gear during contact sports, or while riding a bicycle or motorcycle.
- Don't drink alcohol or use mind-altering drugs and drive.

 WHAT TO EXPECT

APPROPRIATE HEALTH CARE
- Doctor's treatment. Extradural hemorrhage is an emergency that requires rapid treatment to prevent permanent brain damage or death.
- Surgery to stop bleeding and remove blood clots.
- Home-care after surgery.

DIAGNOSTIC MEASURES
- Your own observation of symptoms.
- Medical history and physical exam by a doctor.
- Laboratory studies of blood and cerebrospinal fluid.
- Hospital diagnostic tests, such as X-rays of the head, arteriography, radioscopic scan and CAT scan (see Glossary for all).

POSSIBLE COMPLICATIONS—Fatal compression of the brain if bleeding lasts longer than 24 hours.

PROBABLE OUTCOME—Quick diagnosis and prompt surgery usually bring complete recovery.

 HOW TO TREAT

NOTE—Follow your doctor's instructions. These instructions are supplemental.

GENERAL MEASURES—No specific instructions except those under other headings.

MEDICATION—Your doctor may prescribe cortisone drugs to reduce swelling inside the skull.

ACTIVITY—Stay as active as your strength allows. Work and exercise moderately. Rest when you tire. If speech or muscle control has been damaged, you may need physical therapy or speech therapy.

DIET—Eat a normal, well-balanced diet. Vitamin and mineral supplements should not be necessary unless you cannot eat normally.

 CALL YOUR DOCTOR IF

- You have had a head injury—even if it seems minor—and you develop any symptoms of extradural hemorrhage.
- The following occurs during treatment:
  Temperature rises to 101F (38.3C) or higher.
  Surgical wound becomes red, swollen or tender.
  Headache worsens.

ILLNESSES & DISORDERS

EYE CONTUSION OR LACERATION

GENERAL INFORMATION

DEFINITION—Eye injury, including blunt injury (contusion) or cut (laceration).

BODY PARTS INVOLVED—Eyeball; eyelid; bones around the eyeball (eye socket); muscles attached to the eyeball.

SEX OR AGE MOST AFFECTED—Both sexes; all ages.

SIGNS & SYMPTOMS
- Swelling, redness, tenderness, pain, bleeding or bruising ("black eye") in or around the eye.
- Change in ability to see clearly.

CAUSES—A blunt or sharp blow or cut to the eye or surrounding structures.

RISK INCREASES WITH
- Eye injuries often occur in fights. Fights are more likely with alcohol consumption or in hostile environments that foster aggression.
- Occupations that expose the eye to injury, such as athletics, bartending (opening champagne bottles), carpentry or steel-construction work.

HOW TO PREVENT—Wear protective eye coverings, if possible, for any exposure to eye injury.

WHAT TO EXPECT

APPROPRIATE HEALTH CARE
- Doctor's treatment, which may include suturing a laceration.
- Self-care after treatment.

DIAGNOSTIC MEASURES
- Your own observation of symptoms.
- Medical history and physical exam by a doctor.
- X-rays of bone surrounding the eye.

POSSIBLE COMPLICATIONS
- Permanent vision loss.
- Infection.

PROBABLE OUTCOME—Usually curable with treatment to prevent infection and suture of lacerations in and around the eye. Sutures are usually removed in about 7 days. Allow 2 weeks for complete healing.

HOW TO TREAT

NOTE—Follow your doctor's instructions. These instructions are supplemental.

GENERAL MEASURES
- Protect eyes from bright light or sunlight by wearing dark glasses temporarily.
- Use ice packs or warm moist compresses to relieve discomfort. Prepare a compress by folding a clean cloth in several layers. Dip in warm water, wring out slightly, and apply to the eye. Dip the compress often to keep it moist. Apply the compress for an hour, rest an hour and repeat.
- Sleep with the head elevated with 2 pillows until symptoms subside.

MEDICATION—Your doctor may prescribe:
- Antibiotic eye drops or ointments to prevent infection.
- Pain relievers.
- Eye drops to dilate the eye pupil and rest the eye muscles (sometimes).

ACTIVITY—Resume normal activities gradually after treatment.

DIET—No special diet.

CALL YOUR DOCTOR IF

- You have a cut or other eye injury.
- The following occurs after eye injury:
  Fever.
  Severe eye pain that persists, despite treatment.
  Vision changes.

EYE, FOREIGN BODY IN

 ## GENERAL INFORMATION

DEFINITION—Embedding of a small speck of metal, wood, stone, sand, paint or other foreign material in the eye.

BODY PARTS INVOLVED—Eye, usually the conjunctiva (outer eye covering).

SEX OR AGE MOST AFFECTED—Both sexes; all ages.

SIGNS & SYMPTOMS
- Severe pain, irritation and redness in the eye.
- Foreign body visible with the naked eye (usually). Sometimes the foreign body is very small, trapped under the eyelid and invisible except with medical examination.

CAUSES—Accident.

RISK INCREASES WITH
- Windy weather.
- Occupations or activity, such as carpentry, in which fine particles of wood or other materials fly loose in the air.

HOW TO PREVENT—Wear protective eye coverings if your occupation or hobby involves the risk of eye injury.

 ## WHAT TO EXPECT

APPROPRIATE HEALTH CARE
- Doctor's treatment.
- Emergency-room care (sometimes).
- Self-care after removal of the particle.

DIAGNOSTIC MEASURES
- Your own observation of symptoms.
- Medical history and physical exam by a doctor. This may include staining the eye with a harmless substance (flourescein) to outline the object and examine the eye through a magnifying lens.

POSSIBLE COMPLICATIONS
- Infection, especially if the foreign body is not removed completely.
- Severe, permanent vision damage caused by penetration of deeper eye layers.

PROBABLE OUTCOME—Most objects can be removed simply under local anesthesia in a doctor's office or emergency room.

 ## HOW TO TREAT

NOTE—Follow your doctor's instructions. These instructions are supplemental.

GENERAL MEASURES
- Ask someone else to drive you to the doctor's office. Don't try to drive yourself.
- Don't rub the eye.
- Keep the eye closed, if possible, until you are examined.
- Wear an eye patch to keep the eye closed, or dark glasses, for 24 hours after removal to protect your eye from bright light.
- Use moist compresses to relieve discomfort after removal. Prepare by folding a clean cloth in several layers. Dip in warm water, wring out slightly and apply to the eye. Dip the compress often to keep it moist. Apply the compress for 1 hour, rest 1 hour and repeat.

MEDICATION—Your doctor may prescribe:
- Antibiotic eye drops or ointment to prevent infection.
- Pain relievers.
- Local anesthetic eye drops.

ACTIVITY—Resume your normal activities gradually after removal of the foreign body and the patch, if one is applied.

DIET—No special diet.

 ## CALL YOUR DOCTOR IF

- You have a foreign body in the eye.
- The following occurs after removal:
  Pain increases or does not disappear in 2 days.
  You develop a fever.
  Your vision changes.

ILLNESSES & DISORDERS

EYE TUMOR

 GENERAL INFORMATION

DEFINITION—A growth in the eye in which cell multiplication is uncontrolled and progressive. Eye tumors are of 3 types: retinoblastoma, malignant melanoma or secondary tumors that have spread from other parts of the body.

BODY PARTS INVOLVED—Usually one eye. Retinoblastoma invades both eyes in 25% of cases.

SEX OR AGE MOST AFFECTED
- Melanoma: Adults over 60.
- Retinoblastoma: Young children between ages 1 and 5.
- Secondary tumors: All ages.

SIGNS & SYMPTOMS—The following are characteristic of all 3 types:
- Possibly no signs in the early stages.
- Gradual loss of vision.
- Bulging eyes (sometimes).
Retinoblastoma may have the following additional signs:
- Crossed eyes.
- A tumor that is visible through the pupil.

CAUSES
- Melanoma and secondary tumors: Unknown.
- Retinoblastoma: Inherited tendency.

RISK INCREASES WITH—Family history of retinoblastoma. The genetic trait is dominant, but it does not affect all children.

HOW TO PREVENT—Cannot be prevented at present. If the family has a history of retinoblastoma, obtain genetic counseling before having children.

 WHAT TO EXPECT

APPROPRIATE HEALTH CARE—One of the following:
- Surgery to remove the tumor.
- Radiation therapy.
- Cryotherapy (see Glossary).
- Treatment with laser beams.

DIAGNOSTIC MEASURES
- Your own observation of symptoms.
- Medical history and physical exam by a doctor.
- Echography (see Glossary).
- Fluorescein dye tests (see Glossary) to outline blood vessels in the eye.
- X-rays of the skull.

POSSIBLE COMPLICATIONS
- Spread to other parts of the body.
- Partial or complete loss of vision.

PROBABLE OUTCOME—Some eye tumors are curable in 6 months with medical treatment.
　　Other eye tumors are considered incurable. A fatal spread to other body parts usually occurs rapidly. However, medical literature cites a few instances of unexplained recovery. Scientific research into causes and treatment continues, so there is hope for increasingly effective treatment and cure.

 HOW TO TREAT

NOTE—Follow your doctor's instructions. These instructions are supplemental.

GENERAL MEASURES—The surgeon will provide instructions for postoperative care.

MEDICATION—Your doctor may prescribe:
- Pain relievers.
- Anticancer drugs.

ACTIVITY—After treatment, resume your normal activities as soon as possible.

DIET—No special diet.

 CALL YOUR DOCTOR IF

- You have symptoms of an eye tumor.
- Pain becomes intolerable during treatment.
- New, unexplained symptoms develop that may indicate the malignancy has spread to other body parts.

FACIAL BONES, FRACTURE OF

GENERAL INFORMATION

DEFINITION—Broken bones in the face.

BODY PARTS INVOLVED—Facial nerves, blood vessels, skin and bones. Facial bones include those of the upper jaw (maxilla), lower jaw (mandible), cheek (zygoma), around the eyes (orbital) and nose (see Nose Fracture in Illness section).

SEX OR AGE MOST AFFECTED—Both sexes; all ages.

SIGNS & SYMPTOMS—The following apply to the site of injury:
- Swelling.
- Tenderness, crepitation (a crackly feeling upon touching) or pain.
- Redness that becomes multicolored soon after injury.
- Loss of sensation in the lips and nose from nerve damage.
- Double or blurred vision.

CAUSES—Injury, especially from auto or bicycle accidents, sports injuries and fist fights.

RISK INCREASES WITH
- Excess alcohol consumption.
- Hostile, aggressive personalities.
- Participation in contact sports.

HOW TO PREVENT—Avoid injury whenever possible. Wear protective headgear for contact sports or when riding motorcycles or bicycles. Use auto seat belts. Don't drink or use mind-altering drugs and drive.

WHAT TO EXPECT

APPROPRIATE HEALTH CARE
- Doctor's treatment. A plastic surgeon, oral surgeon, opthalmologist, or ear, nose and throat specialist may be consulted.
- Surgery to realign fractured bones and reconstruct normal facial contours.

DIAGNOSTIC MEASURES
- Your own observation of symptoms.
- Medical history and physical exam by a doctor.
- Laboratory blood studies to measure blood loss.
- X-rays of the skull and facial bones.

POSSIBLE COMPLICATIONS
- Infection in the injured area.
- Permanent disfigurement.

PROBABLE OUTCOME—Surgery usually produces good cosmetic results and a return to normal function. It should be done as soon as possible after injury.

Teeth that have been knocked out can sometimes be replanted. A broken jaw is corrected by securing the teeth with wire or plastic splints so the jaw heals in its proper position. Speech will be changed while the wires are in place, but it should return to normal when they are removed. Normal vision should return if the eye is not injured.

Allow about 6 weeks for recovery.

HOW TO TREAT

NOTE—Follow your doctor's instructions. These instructions are supplemental.

GENERAL MEASURES
- Don't exercise to the point that you must pant for breath because breathing may be difficult for a while.
- Protect the face from pressure. Sleep on your back.
- Don't blow your nose hard or use makeup until healing is complete.
- If your jaws are wired, learn how to release them quickly in case of emergency, such as severe coughing or vomiting.

MEDICATION—Your doctor may prescribe:
- Pain relievers.
- Antibiotics to fight infection, if necessary.

ACTIVITY—Rest quietly for about 2 days, then resume your normal activities as strength returns.

DIET—Eat a high-protein, liquid diet (see Appendix 7) for several days. If your jaw is wired, the liquid diet will be necessary for up to 8 weeks. Add soft solid foods when able. Take vitamin and mineral supplements to hasten healing.

CALL YOUR DOCTOR IF

- You have a facial-bone fracture.
- The following occurs during treatment:
  Fever.
  Impaired vision.
  Severe headache.
  Loss of sensation in face.
  Intolerable pain.
  Illness of any kind during healing.
  Loosening of wires or splints.
- New, unexplained symptoms develop. Drugs used in treatment may produce side effects.

FAILURE TO THRIVE

GENERAL INFORMATION

DEFINITION—Failure of infants, children, and adolescents to grow and develop normally. This is different from morasmus, in which infants in emotionally deprived environments become listless, weaken and sometimes die.

BODY PARTS INVOLVED—All.

SEX OR AGE MOST AFFECTED—Young children (1 to 5 years).

SIGNS & SYMPTOMS
- Persistent vomiting in an infant between 0 and 6 months.
- Height, weight and head circumference do not progress normally, as measured on doctors' growth charts.
- Physical skills are slow to develop. Such skills include:
  Turning over in bed.
  Sitting.
  Standing and walking.
- Mental and social skills are delayed. These skills include:
  Talking.
  Social interaction.
  Self-feeding.
  Toilet training.
Normal growth and development vary widely. The *rate of change*—as measured at regular medical checkups—is more significant.

CAUSES
- Parental inexperience.
- A negative emotional environment (neglect, abuse or rejection).
- Malnutrition.
- Chronic disease, such as kidney failure or chronic infection.
- Genetic disorders, such as Down's Syndrome or cystic fibrosis.
- Endocrine diseases, including disorders of the thyroid, pituitary, adrenal, pancreas and sexual glands.

RISK INCREASES WITH
- Poverty.
- Parents who were raised in a negative emotional environment or are poorly educated.
- Crowded or unsanitary living conditions.

HOW TO PREVENT
- Arrange for parenting classes if you are an expectant mother or father.
- Take your child regularly to the doctor for "well-baby" checkups.

WHAT TO EXPECT

APPROPRIATE HEALTH CARE
- Doctor's treatment.
- Psychotherapy or counseling, if parents have emotional problems that prevent a healthy relationship with the child.
- Hospitalization (short-term), if complicated diagnostic procedures are necessary or food intake must be verified.

DIAGNOSTIC MEASURES
- Your own observation of symptoms.
- Medical history and physical exam by a doctor.
- Psychological tests, such as the Denver Developmental test, which measures growth and development.
- Laboratory blood tests, including hormone studies.
- X-rays of the hands, which provide a good measure of body growth.

POSSIBLE COMPLICATIONS—Permanent mental, emotional or physical disability.

PROBABLE OUTCOME
- If failure to thrive is caused by parental inexperience or psychological problems, recovery is possible with education and counseling for the parents.
- If failure to thrive is caused by an underlying physical illness or disorder, including malnutrition, recovery depends on whether the condition can be corrected.

HOW TO TREAT

NOTE—Follow your doctor's instructions. These instructions are supplemental.

GENERAL MEASURES
- Read books and pamphlets on child-rearing or attend parenting classes.
- Ask a visiting nurse to visit your home for guidance.
- Provide as much love and support as possible for your child. Examine your feelings and behavior toward your child. If you don't think they are what they should be, arrange for psychological counseling.

MEDICATION—If an underlying disorder is causing failure to thrive, your doctor may prescribe medication to treat the condition.

ACTIVITY—No restrictions.

DIET
- Provide your child with an adequate, well-balanced diet. See Appendix 1.
- If malnutrition is causing failure to thrive, your doctor may prescribe a special diet.

CALL YOUR DOCTOR IF

You are concerned that your child is not developing properly. Trust your instincts—obtain a second doctor's opinion, if necessary.

FAINTING
(Syncope)

GENERAL INFORMATION

DEFINITION—Sudden, temporary loss of consciousness.

BODY PARTS INVOLVED—Circulatory system (heart and blood vessels); brain.

SEX OR AGE MOST AFFECTED—Both sexes; all ages.

SIGNS & SYMPTOMS
- Sudden lightheadedness.
- Blurred vision (sometimes).
- Nausea (sometimes).
- General weakness, then falling.
- Paleness and sweating.
- Rapid heartbeat and rapid breathing. If heartbeat or breathing is not present, this may be cardiac arrest rather than fainting.

CAUSES—A sudden decrease in blood pressure, which temporarily deprives the brain of blood. The drop in blood pressure may result from:
- Heartbeat abnormalities—too fast, too slow or irregular.
- Prolonged straining, such as from severe coughing or attempted bowel movements when constipated.
- Sudden emotional stress.
- Heart diseases that limit the amount of blood the heart pumps.
- Getting out of bed or a chair suddenly (orthostatic hypotension).
- Epilepsy.
- Low blood sugar.
- Heart attack (rare).
- Anemia (rare).

RISK INCREASES WITH
- Stress.
- Heart disease.
- Use of certain drugs, such as heart medications that slow the heartbeat. These include digitalis, beta-adrenergic blockers and other antihypertensive drugs.
- Hot, humid weather.

HOW TO PREVENT
- Avoid sudden changes in physical activity.
- If fainting episodes are caused by medication, consult your doctor about changing drugs.

WHAT TO EXPECT

APPROPRIATE HEALTH CARE
- Care from bystanders.
- Self-care after regaining consciousness.
- Doctor's treatment, if fainting is caused by other conditions (see Causes).

DIAGNOSTIC MEASURES
- Observation of symptoms by those nearby.
- Medical history and physical exam by a doctor.

POSSIBLE COMPLICATIONS
- Injury while fainting.
- Mistaking cardiac arrest for fainting.

PROBABLE OUTCOME—Simple fainting disappears in 1 or 2 minutes.

HOW TO TREAT

NOTE—Follow your doctor's instructions. These instructions are supplemental.

GENERAL MEASURES
- If someone faints, check for breathing and a neck pulse. If neither is present:
  Dial 0 (operator) or 911 (emergency) for an ambulance or medical help. Then give first aid immediately.
  Begin cardiac massage and mouth-to-mouth breathing (CPR). Don't stop until help arrives.
- If someone faints, is breathing and has a pulse, leave the person on the ground and elevate both legs. This helps return blood to the heart.
- If you feel faint, sit down immediately and bend over, or lie down.
- If you are subject to frequent fainting spells, avoid activities in which fainting may endanger your life, such as climbing to high places, driving vehicles or operating dangerous machinery.

MEDICATION—Medication usually is not necessary for fainting. Medication may be necessary for underlying disorders.

ACTIVITY—Resume your normal activities as soon as you regain consciousness.

DIET—No special diet unless fainting episodes are caused by low blood sugar. If so, eat 5 or 6 small meals a day. The meals should be high in protein, high in complex carbohydrates and low in simple carbohydrates (sugar).

CALL YOUR DOCTOR IF

- An unconscious person has no pulse and is not breathing. Give CPR first.
- Someone faints and does not regain consciousness in 2 minutes.
- Fainting is a symptom of another condition (see Causes).

FARMER'S LUNG

GENERAL INFORMATION

DEFINITION—Inflammation of the lung due to inhalation of fungus germs from moldy hay or grain. This is an allergic response and is not contagious or cancerous.

BODY PARTS INVOLVED—Lungs.

SEX OR AGE MOST AFFECTED—Male adults.

SIGNS & SYMPTOMS—In persons sensitive to the fungus, the following appear 4 to 8 hours after exposure to hay. They usually diminish in a few hours, but may last up to 2 weeks:
- Breathlessness (sometimes with wheezing).
- Dry cough.
- Chest pain.
- Chills and fever.
- Headache.
- Abnormal chest X-ray.
- Decreased breathing ability (shown with respiratory-function tests).

The following occur with repeated episodes over many years. All these are similar to emphysema and chronic obstructive pulmonary disease (COPD) from any cause:
- Increasing shortness of breath with wheezing on exertion.
- Cough with sputum.
- Fatigue.
- Weight loss.

CAUSES—Allergy to the fungus in moldy hay called micropolyspora faeni or thermoactinomyces vulgaris. The time it takes to develop the allergy varies from person to person.

RISK INCREASES WITH
- Family history of allergy.
- Smoking.

HOW TO PREVENT
- Avoid exposure to the fungus. If you cannot avoid exposure, wear masks or hoods during exposure.
- Don't smoke.
- Treat hay in silos with chemicals that prevent growth of fungus spores.

WHAT TO EXPECT

APPROPRIATE HEALTH CARE
- Self-care after diagnosis.
- Doctor's treatment.

DIAGNOSTIC MEASURES
- Your own observation of symptoms.
- Medical history and physical exam by a doctor.
- Laboratory studies of lung function.
- X-ray of the chest.

POSSIBLE COMPLICATIONS—Continued exposure can lead to chronic obstructive pulmonary disease (COPD) or respiratory failure.

PROBABLE OUTCOME—Usually curable—even in late stages of the disease—if exposure can be avoided.

HOW TO TREAT

NOTE—Follow your doctor's instructions. These instructions are supplemental.

GENERAL MEASURES
- Avoid exposure to moldy hay.
- Obtain medical treatment for any respiratory infection, including the common cold.

MEDICATION
- For minor discomfort, you may use non-prescription drugs such as:
  Cough preparations to loosen secretions.
  Acetaminophen for pain.
- For serious symptoms, your doctor may prescribe:
  Cortisone drugs to suppress the inflammatory response.
  Antibiotics to fight any secondary infections.

ACTIVITY—Resume your normal activities as soon as symptoms improve.

DIET—No special diet.

CALL YOUR DOCTOR IF

- You have symptoms of farmer's lung.
- The following occurs during or after treatment:
  Temperature spikes to over 101F (38.3C).
  Chest pain increases.
  Breathlessness worsens.
  Blood appears in sputum.
  You have an unexplained weight loss.
- New, unexplained symptoms develop. Drugs used in treatment may produce side effects.

FECAL IMPACTION

GENERAL INFORMATION

DEFINITION—A severe form of constipation in which a large mass of feces cannot be passed. Fecal impaction is not a serious condition, but it complicates other illnesses.

BODY PARTS INVOLVED—Lower colon; rectum.

SEX OR AGE MOST AFFECTED—Both sexes; all ages.

SIGNS & SYMPTOMS
- Absence of normal bowel movements.
- Thin, watery discharge from the rectum.
- Sense of fullness in the rectum, but inability to pass stool.
- Lack of urinary control.
- A firm mass in the lower left abdomen (sometimes).
- Pain or cramps (sometimes). Impaction often develops slowly without discomfort.
- Low fever (sometimes).

CAUSES
- Rectal disorders that make normal bowel movements uncomfortable, such as painful hemorrhoids or anal fissure.
- Rectal or colon tumors.
- Barium that is swallowed for X-rays of the intestinal tract.
- Loss of nerve supply to the colon or rectum, as with a spinal-cord injury.
- Insufficient fiber and liquid in the diet.

RISK INCREASES WITH
- Bed rest for any condition, such as a recent heart attack, surgery or fracture.
- Back disorders with nerve pressure.
- Decreased fluid and fiber intake.
- Use of some drugs, such as narcotic pain killers, antiparkinsonism drugs, atropine, phenothiazines or tricyclic antidepressants.

HOW TO PREVENT
- If confined to bed, drink extra fluids and increase consumption of dietary fiber.
- If simple constipation develops, use a mild laxative, such as milk of magnesia, a stool softener or an enema.

WHAT TO EXPECT

APPROPRIATE HEALTH CARE
- Self-care.
- Doctor's treatment to remove feces manually or by enema.

DIAGNOSTIC MEASURES
- Your own observation of symptoms.
- Medical history and physical exam, including a rectal exam, by a doctor.

POSSIBLE COMPLICATIONS
- Persons who have had a previous heart attack may suffer fatal rupture of the heart muscle while straining to pass a fecal impaction.
- Rectal prolapse (protrusion outside the body).
- Aggravation of hemorrhoids.

PROBABLE OUTCOME—Usually curable with treatment, but recurrence is common unless the underlying cause is removed.

HOW TO TREAT

NOTE—Follow your doctor's instructions. These instructions are supplemental.

GENERAL MEASURES
- If your doctor prescribes it, use an oil-retention enema before and after manual removal of the impaction. Follow instructions on the package.
- See Constipation (in Illness section) for suggestions to improve bowel habits.

MEDICATION—After removal of the impaction, your doctor may prescribe laxatives or stool softeners.

ACTIVITY—No restrictions. Be as active as possible. Good physical fitness improves bowel function.

DIET
- Eat a normal, well-balanced diet high in fiber (see Appendix 1).
- Drink at least 8 glasses of fluid each day.

CALL YOUR DOCTOR IF

- You have symptoms of a fecal impaction.
- Your normal bowel pattern changes.
- You cannot pass feces while under treatment for other conditions.

ILLNESSES & DISORDERS

FERTILITY PROBLEMS IN MEN

GENERAL INFORMATION

DEFINITION—The inability to impregnate a female after 1 year of sexual activity without contraception. Infertility occurs in 10% of all couples.

BODY PARTS INVOLVED—Genitals; endocrine system; brain.

SEX OR AGE MOST AFFECTED—Males after puberty.

SIGNS & SYMPTOMS—Inability to impregnate a fertile woman.

CAUSES—Infertility in men is caused by an absence of sperm, defective sperm or not enough sperm in each ejaculation. Reasons for this include:
- Anatomical abnormalities of the penis or testicles, including undescended testicles.
- Excessive alcohol intake.
- Urinary-tract infection.
- Hormone disturbance.
- Mumps.
- Use of some drugs, such as antihypertensives, cytotoxic drugs, male hormones and MAO inhibitors.
- Sexually transmitted disease, especially syphilis and non-specific urethritis that causes scarring.
- Injury to the genitals.
- Varicose veins in the testicles.
- Psychological reasons, such as fear of infertility.
- Overheating of the testicles caused by vigorous, repetitive exercise or underwear that is too tight and holds the testicles too close to the body.

RISK INCREASES WITH
- Diabetes mellitus.
- Poor nutrition.
- Family history of Klinefelter's syndrome (see Glossary).

HOW TO PREVENT—No specific preventive measures.

WHAT TO EXPECT

APPROPRIATE HEALTH CARE
- Self-care after diagnosis.
- Doctor's treatment.
- Psychotherapy or counseling for marital problems or alcoholism.
- Surgery to correct anatomical abnormalities of the reproductive system.

DIAGNOSTIC MEASURES
- Your own observation of symptoms.
- Medical history and physical exam by a doctor.
- Laboratory studies, such as blood studies of hormones and semen analysis.
- Surgical diagnostic procedures such as testicular biopsy (see Glossary).

POSSIBLE COMPLICATIONS—Psychological distress caused by feelings of guilt, inadequacy and loss of self-esteem.

PROBABLE OUTCOME—Many fertility problems are minor and reversible. Approach treatment with optimism.

HOW TO TREAT

NOTE—Follow your doctor's instructions. These instructions are supplemental.

GENERAL MEASURES—Heat may decrease sperm production in the testicles. To prevent this:
- Don't wear tight underwear or athletic supporters that hold the testicles too close to the body.
- Don't take hot baths.
- Avoid long bicycle rides.
- Have sexual intercourse during the time your partner is ovulating. Don't ejaculate for 3 days prior.

MEDICATION—Your doctor may prescribe the following to stimulate sperm production and activity:
- Vitamin supplements (B & E).
- Human chorionic gonadotrophins, a hormone replacement.

ACTIVITY—Work and exercise moderately. Overexercising can be a factor in infertility. Rest when you tire.

DIET—Eat a normal, well-balanced diet (see Appendix 1).

CALL YOUR DOCTOR IF

- You have symptoms of infertility and want help.
- Conception doesn't occur within 6 months, despite recommendations and treatment.
- New, unexplained symptoms develop. Drugs used in treatment may produce side effects.

FERTILITY PROBLEMS IN WOMEN

GENERAL INFORMATION

DEFINITION—The inability to become pregnant after 1 year of sexual activity without contraception. Infertility occurs in 10% of all couples.

BODY PARTS INVOLVED—Genitals; endocrine system; brain.

SEX OR AGE MOST AFFECTED—Females between puberty and menopause.

SIGNS & SYMPTOMS—Inability to conceive.

CAUSES
- Minor anatomic abnormalities of the reproductive system.
- Emotional stress.
- Repeated weight-gain/weight-loss cycles.
- Hormone dysfunction, especially thyroid disorders.
- Vaginitis.
- Disorders of the cervix, such as infection, laceration from previous childbirth or narrowing of the cervical opening for any reason.
- Amenorrhea (lack of menstrual periods) caused by strenuous exercise programs or nutritional disorders (bulimia or anorexia nervosa).
- Chemical changes in the cervical mucus.
- Ovarian cysts.
- Endometriosis.
- Tumors.
- The use of some medications, including oral contraceptives. Many women cannot conceive for many months after discontinuing use.
- Disorders probably *not* related to infertility include: a tilted uterus; small fibroid tumors of the uterus; or inability to achieve sexual orgasm.

RISK INCREASES WITH
- Stress.
- Marital discord and infrequent sexual intercourse.

HOW TO PREVENT
- Obtain treatment for any treatable disorder that causes infertility.
- Avoid preventable causes of infertility, especially poor nutrition.

WHAT TO EXPECT

APPROPRIATE HEALTH CARE
- Self-care after diagnosis.
- Doctor's treatment.
- Psychotherapy or counseling, if marital problems exist.
- Surgery to correct anatomical abnormalities of the reproductive system.

DIAGNOSTIC MEASURES
- Your own observation of symptoms.
- Medical history and physical exam by a doctor.
- Laboratory studies, such as: blood studies; Rubin's insufflation tests (see Glossary); culdoscopy (see Glossary); and studies of mucus of the cervix.
- Surgical diagnostic procedures, such as laparoscopy or hystoscopy (see Glossary).

POSSIBLE COMPLICATIONS—Psychological distress, including feelings of guilt, inadequacy and loss of self-esteem.

PROBABLE OUTCOME—Many fertility problems are minor and reversible. Approach treatment with optimism.

HOW TO TREAT

NOTE—Follow your doctor's instructions. These instructions are supplemental.

GENERAL MEASURES
- Keep a basal body-temperature chart to become familiar with your ovulation pattern. Ask your doctor for instructions.
- Have intercourse during ovulation, which can be determined from the chart.
- Don't use a lubricant (except saliva) during sexual relations. Lubricants may interfere with sperm mobility.
- Your partner should withdraw his penis quickly from your vagina after ejaculation. If left in, it reduces the number of sperm that can swim toward the egg.
- After your partner's ejaculation, place pillows under your buttocks to provide an easier downhill swim for the sperm.
- Avoid physical exhaustion prior to intercourse.
- Maintain a positive attitude. Worry and tension contribute to infertility.

MEDICATION—Your doctor may prescribe:
- Hormones for a hormone imbalance.
- Clomiphene, a gonad stimulant.

ACTIVITY—Work and exercise moderately. Overexercising contributes to infertility.

DIET—Eat a normal, well-balanced diet. If you are overweight, try to achieve your ideal weight. See Appendix 10 for a reducing diet.

CALL YOUR DOCTOR IF

- You have symptoms of infertility and want help.
- Conception doesn't occur within 6 months, despite recommendations and treatment.
- New, unexplained symptoms develop. Hormones used in treatment may produce side effects.

FEVER OF UNDETERMINED ORIGIN (FUO)

GENERAL INFORMATION

DEFINITION—Prolonged (2 to 3 weeks) temperature above normal for which no cause is evident.

BODY PARTS INVOLVED—Any body organs or system may be the source of a fever-producing condition.

SEX OR AGE MOST AFFECTED—Both sexes; all ages.

SIGNS & SYMPTOMS—Fever (measured rectally) for at least 2 weeks. Fever may be intermittent.

CAUSES—In infants and children:
- Infections.
- Collagen or autoimmune diseases.
- Tumors and cancer, especially leukemia.

In adults:
- Infections.
- Collagen or autoimmune diseases.
- Tumors and cancer, especially kidney cancer and leukemia.
- Self-induced in some psychologically unstable persons.

RISK INCREASES WITH
- Poor nutrition.
- Illness that has lowered resistance.
- Chemical or environmental exposure to polluted water or air.
- Travel in areas with unsanitary conditions.
- Exposure to others with contagious diseases.

HOW TO PREVENT—No specific preventive measures.

WHAT TO EXPECT

APPROPRIATE HEALTH CARE
- Self-care after diagnosis.
- Doctor's treatment.

DIAGNOSTIC MEASURES
- Your own observation of symptoms.
- Medical history and physical exam by a doctor. Because fever may be the first evidence of a serious condition in an early stage, your doctor may recommend thorough diagnostic testing.
- Laboratory studies, such as blood studies and a urine culture (see Glossary).
- X-rays of the chest.

POSSIBLE COMPLICATIONS—Depends on the underlying condition causing fever.

PROBABLE OUTCOME—Spontaneous recovery in about 10% of cases. In other cases, the outcome depends on successful detection and treatment of the underlying disorder.

HOW TO TREAT

NOTE—Follow your doctor's instructions. These instructions are supplemental.

GENERAL MEASURES—Until the fever's cause has been diagnosed, keep a daily temperature chart.

MEDICATION—For minor discomfort, you may use non-prescription drugs such as acetaminophen. Until the underlying cause is determined, your doctor may withhold prescription drugs to avoid masking symptoms of the underlying disorder. Occasionally, in critically ill patients awaiting results of laboratory studies, the doctor may recommend a therapeutic trial of antibiotics or other drugs.

ACTIVITY—Bed rest may be advisable.

DIET—No special diet.

CALL YOUR DOCTOR IF

- You have unexplained fever that lasts longer than 24 hours.
- New symptoms develop. They may provide a clue about the underlying cause of the fever.

FIBROCYSTIC BREAST DISEASE
(Chronic Cystic Mastitis; Breast Lumps)

GENERAL INFORMATION

DEFINITION—A disorder of the female breast characterized by non-malignant lumps.

BODY PARTS INVOLVED—Breasts.

SEX OR AGE MOST AFFECTED—Females from puberty to old age. This affects about 20% of premenopausal women. It usually disappears after menopause unless estrogen-replacement therapy is used.

SIGNS & SYMPTOMS—Lumps in the breasts with the following characteristics:
- Lumps are usually on both sides. Solitary lumps may occur, but multiple lumps are common.
- Lumps offer resistance when pressed with fingertips; they may be tender.
- Lumps may be accompanied by generalized breast pain, especially before menstrual periods.
- Lumps often enlarge before menstrual periods and shrink afterward.
- Lumps come in different sizes. When the lumps are relatively large and near the surface, they can be moved freely within the breast.
- Lumps deep within the breast may be indistinguishable from breast cancer.

CAUSES—Unknown, but probably related to estrogen and other hormones produced by the ovaries. This is not inherited.

RISK INCREASES WITH—Preliminary studies indicate that drinking coffee and smoking cigarettes are associated with a higher incidence and greater extent of fibrocystic breast disease.

HOW TO PREVENT—Until research is conclusive, avoid smoking and drinking coffee.

WHAT TO EXPECT

APPROPRIATE HEALTH CARE
- Self-care to check breasts for lumps and to check for changes in lumps after diagnosis.
- Doctor's supervision.

DIAGNOSTIC MEASURES
- Your own observation of symptoms.
- Medical history and physical exam by a doctor.
- Mammogram (see Glossary).
- Surgical diagnostic procedures such as biopsy or cyst aspiration (see Glossary).

POSSIBLE COMPLICATIONS—Misdiagnosis. Some lumps appear benign, but are cancerous. Diagnostic studies, including biopsy, are often necessary to rule out malignancy.

PROBABLE OUTCOME—Women with fibrocystic breast disease continue to have breast lumps that appear and dissolve; some remain permanently. The disorder is presently incurable, but it does not jeopardize health.

Some cysts can be aspirated in a doctor's office, causing the lump to disappear. If the lump does not disappear completely after aspiration, it may be cancerous and should be diagnosed by biopsy and microscopic analysis.

HOW TO TREAT

NOTE—Follow your doctor's instructions. These instructions are supplemental.

GENERAL MEASURES
- Examine your breasts carefully each month just prior to or at the onset of menstruation (see Appendix 14). Report any changes in lumps that have been diagnosed previously.
- Visit your doctor at least every 6 months for a breast exam or other studies.

MEDICATION—To decrease the size of lumps or inhibit the formation of new lumps, your doctor may prescribe:
- Vitamin E.
- Female hormones.

ACTIVITY—No restrictions.

DIET—No special diet, but avoid caffeine.

CALL YOUR DOCTOR IF

- You have undiagnosed lumps in the breast.
- You detect a change in a lump, or new lumps appear.
- You have not had a breast exam in 2 years.
- New, unexplained symptoms develop. Hormones used in treatment may produce side effects.

FIBROID TUMORS OF THE UTERUS
(Myomas; Leiomyomas)

 ## GENERAL INFORMATION

DEFINITION—An abnormal growth of cells in the muscular wall of the uterus (myometrium). The term "fibroids" is misleading. The tumor cells are not fibrous; they are composed of abnormal muscle cells. Uterine fibroids are almost always benign (not cancerous).

BODY PARTS INVOLVED—Uterus; cervix (sometimes).

SEX OR AGE MOST AFFECTED—Fibroids affect 18% to 24% of all women over 35. They don't develop after menopause.

SIGNS & SYMPTOMS
- No symptoms (often).
- More frequent menstruation.
- Increased menstrual flow and discomfort.
- Bleeding between periods.
- Painful sexual intercourse or bleeding after intercourse.
- Anemia (weakness, fatigue and paleness).
- Feelings of pressure on the urinary bladder or rectum.
- Increased vaginal discharge.

CAUSES—Unknown; however, fibroids may be hereditary. Some studies indicate that:
- Women with fibroids may have higher levels of the human growth hormone.
- Birth-control pills, especially those with large amounts of estrogen, may stimulate the growth of fibroid tumors.

RISK INCREASES WITH
- Use of oral contraceptives.
- Genetic factors. Fibroid tumors are 3 to 5 times more common in black women than Caucasian women.

HOW TO PREVENT—Cannot be prevented at present, but avoiding the use of oral contraceptives decreases the risk of developing fibroids.

 ## WHAT TO EXPECT

APPROPRIATE HEALTH CARE
- Self-care after diagnosis.
- Doctor's treatment.
- Hospitalization, if surgery is necessary. Fibroids are generally removed surgically if they cause excessive bleeding, become malignant, or produce symptoms that interfere with conception or pregnancy.

DIAGNOSTIC MEASURES
- Your own observation of symptoms.
- Medical history and physical exam by a doctor.
- Laboratory studies, such as sonography, laparoscopy or hystosalpingogram (see Glossary for all).

POSSIBLE COMPLICATIONS—Malignant change in the fibroid tumor (occurs in less than 0.5%). This rare complication is usually signaled by very rapid growth.

PROBABLE OUTCOME—If surgery is not necessary prior to menopause, these tumors usually decrease in size without treatment after menopause.

Fibroids can often be removed surgically without removing the entire uterus. The ability to conceive continues as long as the uterus remains.

 ## HOW TO TREAT

NOTE—Follow your doctor's instructions. These instructions are supplemental.

GENERAL MEASURES
- If your doctor recommends surgery, ask for a full explanation and discussion before making a decision.
- Record dates of bleeding and number of pads used each day.

MEDICATION
- If you have a small fibroid, don't take contraceptive pills with a high estrogen content. Estrogen may cause fibroids to enlarge. Consider other forms of contraception, such as a diaphragm, cervical cap, IUD, condom, or contraceptive foam, sponge or jelly.
- Your doctor may prescribe iron supplements if you are anemic from excessive blood loss.

ACTIVITY—No restrictions.

DIET—No special diet.

 ## CALL YOUR DOCTOR IF

- You have symptoms of a fibroid tumor.
- A fibroid tumor has been diagnosed, and symptoms become more severe.
- You saturate a pad or tampon more often than once an hour.

FIBROSITIS
(Fibromyositis)

GENERAL INFORMATION

DEFINITION—Inflammation of muscles, muscle sheaths and connective-tissue layers of tendons, muscles, bones and joints.

BODY PARTS INVOLVED—Muscular areas of the low back, neck, shoulder, chest, arms, hips and thighs.

SEX OR AGE MOST AFFECTED—Adults (usually begins between ages 30 and 60).

SIGNS & SYMPTOMS
- Stiffness and weakness.
- Sudden, painful muscle spasms ("charley horse") that worsen with activity.
- Nodules or localized areas that are tender to the touch (trigger points).
- Fatigue.
- Difficulty remaining asleep.

CAUSES—Unknown.

RISK INCREASES WITH
- Stress.
- Muscle injury.
- Exposure to dampness or cold.
- Medical history of disorders that produce joint inflammation, such as rheumatoid arthritis or polyarteritis.
- Viral infections.
- Poor nutrition.
- Fatigue or overwork.

HOW TO PREVENT—Avoid risk factors when possible.

WHAT TO EXPECT

APPROPRIATE HEALTH CARE
- Self-care after diagnosis.
- Doctor's treatment.

DIAGNOSTIC MEASURES
- Your own observation of symptoms.
- Medical history and physical exam by a doctor.
- Laboratory blood studies to measure inflammation and tests to rule out rheumatoid arthritis or polymyalgia.

POSSIBLE COMPLICATIONS—Muscle atrophy.

PROBABLE OUTCOME—Spontaneous recovery in some persons. Other persons may have flare-ups and remissions indefinitely. The disease is uncomfortable, but not life-threatening. Symptoms can be controlled with treatment.

HOW TO TREAT

NOTE—Follow your doctor's instructions. These instructions are supplemental.

GENERAL MEASURES
- Heat relieves pain. Take hot showers, and let the water beat on painful areas. Use heat lamps, electric heating pads, whirlpool or plain tub baths in hot water and hot compresses.
- Have someone gently massage painful areas.

MEDICATION
- For minor discomfort, you may use non-prescription drugs such as aspirin, acetaminophen or ibuprofen.
- Your doctor may prescribe:
  Cortisone injections into "trigger points."
  Non-steroidal anti-inflammatory drugs.

ACTIVITY—Stay as active as possible, even when you are in pain.

DIET—No special diet.

CALL YOUR DOCTOR IF

- You have symptoms of fibrositis that last more than 2 or 3 days.
- New, unexplained symptoms develop. Drugs used in treatment may produce side effects.

FLUID & ELECTROLYTE DISORDERS
(Fluid & Electrolyte Imbalance)

 GENERAL INFORMATION

DEFINITION—An imbalance in the mixture of water and salts (electrolytes) needed for normal body function. Necessary salts contain sodium, potassium, calcium, bicarbonate and phosphate.

BODY PARTS INVOLVED—Total body. All body parts—even hard bone—are bathed in a precise blend of water and natural salts.

SEX OR AGE MOST AFFECTED—Both sexes; all ages.

SIGNS & SYMPTOMS—Depends on whether water or salts are out of proportion. The following may indicate either:
- Dry mouth.
- Wrinkled skin.
- Increased, decreased or absent urination.
- Fatigue.
- Puffy legs, hands, face or abdomen.
- Lung congestion.
- Weakness and confusion.
- Heartbeat irregularities.

CAUSES—Fluid and salts may be *lost* by:
- Vomiting.
- Diarrhea.
- Heavy perspiration.
- Some medications, such as diuretics.
- Nasogastric tubes during hospitalization.

Fluid and salts may *accumulate* from:
- Congestive heart failure.
- Excess intravenous fluids.
- Acute or chronic kidney failure.
- Diabetes insipidus.
- Adrenal disease.
- Chronic lung disease.
- Use of cortisone drugs, female hormones or sodium bicarbonate.

RISK INCREASES WITH
- Fever.
- Kidney disease.
- Diabetes mellitus.
- Heart disease.
- Anorexia nervosa or bulimia.
- Alcoholism.
- Use of diuretics.
- Infants, young children and persons over 60. These people lose fluid very quickly when sick.

HOW TO PREVENT
- For vomiting or diarrhea, take small amounts of clear liquids every 30 minutes.
- During serious illness, keep a fluid-balance record (see General Measures).

 WHAT TO EXPECT

APPROPRIATE HEALTH CARE
- Doctor's treatment.
- Self-care after diagnosis of a minor imbalance.
- Hospitalization for intravenous fluids and treatment of a serious imbalance, including the underlying cause.

DIAGNOSTIC MEASURES
- Your own observation of symptoms.
- Medical history and physical exam by a doctor.
- Laboratory studies of urine, stool, blood and electrolytes—especially sodium, chloride and potassium.
- Radioactive studies of total body water.

POSSIBLE COMPLICATIONS
- Heartbeat irregularities.
- Cardiac arrest and death.

PROBABLE OUTCOME—Usually curable in 24 to 48 hours with early treatment, depending on the underlying cause.

 HOW TO TREAT

NOTE—Follow your doctor's instructions. These instructions are supplemental.

GENERAL MEASURES
- Keep a fluid-balance record during serious illnesses at home. Record liquids taken in each day; use a measuring cup to estimate. Measure and record how much urine is passed each day. Ask your doctor if he wants a specimen for testing.
- Weigh yourself daily on an accurate home scale. Any sudden weight increase or decrease may indicate fluid changes.

MEDICATION
- For fluid loss, your doctor may prescribe: Salt-containing drinks to make at home. Intravenous fluids during hospitalization.
- For fluid accumulation and sodium overload, your doctor may prescribe diuretics and potassium supplements.

ACTIVITY—Rest in bed until your strength returns.

DIET—For a serious fluid imbalance, your doctor may withhold solid food until the fluid imbalance returns to normal.

 CALL YOUR DOCTOR IF

- You have symptoms of a fluid and electrolyte imbalance.
- Your weight increases or decreases 4 or more pounds in 1 day.

FOLLICULITIS, BACTERIAL

GENERAL INFORMATION

DEFINITION—A superficial or deep bacterial irritation and infection of hair follicles of the skin. This is contagious.

BODY PARTS INVOLVED—Skin anywhere on the body, but usually the exposed areas of arms, legs and beard area of the face.

SEX OR AGE MOST AFFECTED—Both sexes; all ages.

SIGNS & SYMPTOMS—Pustules (small white blisters with pus inside) with the following characteristics:
- Pustules are yellow-white and surrounded by narrow red rings.
- Pustules are 1mm to 2mm in size; there may be few or many.
- Pustules discharge a blood-stained pus made from dead cells.
- Some pustules are pierced by hair; others may be adjacent to hair follicles.

CAUSES
- Infection of the hair follicles with staphylococcus bacteria, usually after minor skin injury. Infection spreads to other parts of the body by fingernails, frequently from staphylococcus in the nose.
- Infection with pseudomonas bacteria following the use of contaminated hot tubs or spas. This is rare but increasing.

RISK INCREASES WITH
- Recent illness such as a nose infection.
- Diabetes.
- Eczema or dermatitis.
- Crowded or unsanitary living conditions.

HOW TO PREVENT
- Keep skin clean.
- Avoid hot, humid environments, which foster bacterial growth.

WHAT TO EXPECT

APPROPRIATE HEALTH CARE
- Self-care after diagnosis.
- Doctor's treatment.

DIAGNOSTIC MEASURES
- Your own observation of symptoms.
- Medical history and physical exam by a doctor.
- Laboratory culture of the discharge from the pustule.

POSSIBLE COMPLICATIONS—The infection may enter the bloodstream and spread to other body parts.

PROBABLE OUTCOME—Without treatment, an individual pustule heals in 7 days—but as some heal, new ones appear. Without treatment, boils or deep skin infections may develop. Treatment will shorten the course of the infection. Healing should be complete in 2 weeks. Recurrence is common.

HOW TO TREAT

NOTE—Follow your doctor's instructions. These instructions are supplemental.

GENERAL MEASURES
- Don't scratch pustules. The germs that cause them can be transferred from under the fingernails to other parts of the body.
- Use warm-water soaks (see Appendix 18) to relieve itching and hasten healing.

MEDICATION
- If there are only a few pustules, you may use non-prescription antibiotics, such as bacitracin, mycitracin or neomycin. Apply and gently massage a small amount into the affected areas 3 or 4 times a day. Use only the small amount needed to cover—larger quantities don't help.
- If there are many pustules, your doctor may prescribe injections or oral antibiotics, such as erythromycin or dicloxacillin, to fight infection.

ACTIVITY—Resume your normal activities as soon as symptoms improve.

DIET—No special diet.

CALL YOUR DOCTOR IF

- The pustules spread, despite treatment.
- Your temperature rises to 101F (38.3C).
- Your ankles swell.
- You develop a boil or signs of spreading infection.
- Symptoms of bacterial folliculitis recur after treatment.

ILLNESSES & DISORDERS

FOLLICULITIS, FUNGAL

GENERAL INFORMATION

DEFINITION—A superficial or deep fungal irritation and infection of hair follicles of the skin. It is contagious.

BODY PARTS INVOLVED—Skin on hands, arms, legs, face and scalp.

SEX OR AGE MOST AFFECTED—Both sexes; all ages.

SIGNS & SYMPTOMS—Plaques (patches or flat areas) with clearly defined borders and pustules (small, white blisters with pus inside) on top. Pustules are 1mm to 2mm in diameter and frequently appear in clusters.

CAUSES—A fungus infection that causes a small abscess next to the hair follicle.

RISK INCREASES WITH
- Illness that has lowered resistance.
- Diabetes.
- Eczema or dermatitis.
- Exposure to heat and high humidity.

HOW TO PREVENT
- Protect skin as much as possible from minor injury.
- Avoid hot, humid environments.

WHAT TO EXPECT

APPROPRIATE HEALTH CARE
- Self-care after diagnosis.
- Doctor's treatment.

DIAGNOSTIC MEASURES
- Your own observation of symptoms.
- Medical history and physical exam by a doctor.
- Laboratory culture of the pustule.

POSSIBLE COMPLICATIONS—Bacterial folliculitis and fungal folliculitis are difficult to differentiate. Fungal folliculitis may be misdiagnosed and treated with steroid creams, which aggravate the disorder.

PROBABLE OUTCOME—Usually curable in 6 weeks with treatment.

HOW TO TREAT

NOTE—Follow your doctor's instructions. These instructions are supplemental.

GENERAL MEASURES
- Avoid injury to the skin.
- Women should use depilatory creams instead of razors.
- Men should not shave during treatment until lesions on the face heal.

MEDICATION—Your doctor may prescribe griseofulvin (an oral antifungal medication) and topical antifungal agents. Follow directions on the label.

These medications may cause side effects or adverse reactions. Side effects usually disappear when your body adjusts to the drug or the drug is discontinued.

Don't use any medicine, including non-prescription medicine, without telling your doctor.

ACTIVITY—No restrictions.

DIET—No special diet.

CALL YOUR DOCTOR IF

- You have symptoms of fungal folliculitis.
- The following occurs during treatment:
  Signs of spreading infection (redness, swelling, warmth, pain).
  Fever over 101F (38.3C).
- New, unexplained symptoms develop. Drugs used in treatment may produce side effects.

FROSTBITE

 GENERAL INFORMATION

DEFINITION—Temporary or permanent tissue damage from exposure to subfreezing temperature.

BODY PARTS INVOLVED—Arms and legs (especially fingers and toes); face (especially nose and ears).

SEX OR AGE MOST AFFECTED—Both sexes; all ages.

SIGNS & SYMPTOMS—During exposure:
- Gradual numbness, hardness and paleness in the affected area.
Upon rewarming:
- Pain and tingling or burning (sometimes severe) in the affected area, with color change from white to red, then purple.
- Blisters (severe cases).
- Shivering.
- Slurred speech.
- Memory loss.

CAUSES—Formation of ice crystals in skin and blood vessels, leading to tissue injury or tissue death, depending on temperature and length of exposure.

RISK INCREASES WITH
- Diabetes mellitus.
- Blood-vessel disease such as Raynaud's phenomena.
- Peripheral neuropathy.
- Smoking.
- Excess alcohol consumption.
- Windy weather, which increases the chill factor.

HOW TO PREVENT
- Anticipate sudden temperature changes and carry a jacket, gloves, socks, hat and scarf.
- Don't drink or smoke prior to anticipated exposure.

 WHAT TO EXPECT

APPROPRIATE HEALTH CARE
- Self-care until medical help is available.
- Doctor's treatment.
- Hospitalization (sometimes).
- Surgery to remove permanently damaged (gangrenous) tissue (sometimes).

DIAGNOSTIC MEASURES
- Your own observation of symptoms.
- Medical history and physical exam by a doctor.
- X-rays of damaged areas.

POSSIBLE COMPLICATIONS
- Amputation of dead or infected tissue, especially fingers, toes, nose or ears, following severe exposure.
- Cardiac arrest, if frostbite is accompanied by total body hypothermia.

PROBABLE OUTCOME—For mild cases, full recovery is possible with treatment. Severe cases usually require amputation of the affected part.

 HOW TO TREAT

NOTE—Follow your doctor's instructions. These instructions are supplemental.

GENERAL MEASURES—The following instructions apply to emergency care until medical care is available:
- Upon reaching shelter, remove clothing from the frostbitten parts.
- *Never* massage damaged tissue.
- Immerse the affected parts in warm water (about 100F or 37.8C). Use a thermometer, if available. Higher temperatures may cause further injury.
- Drink warm fluids with a high sugar content, if available.
- Don't smoke.
- After rewarming, cover the affected areas with soft cloth bandages.
- Don't use affected limbs until you have medical attention. If feet are involved, don't walk.

MEDICATION
- Your doctor may prescribe:
  Analgesics, including narcotics, to relieve severe pain. Don't use strong pain killers longer than 4 to 7 days.
  Antibiotics to fight infection.
- You may use non-prescription drugs, such as acetaminophen, for minor pain.

ACTIVITY—Resume normal activities after treatment.

DIET—No special diet.

 CALL YOUR DOCTOR IF

- You have symptoms of frostbite or observe them in someone else.
- The following occurs during treatment:
  Increased pain, swelling, redness or drainage at the site of injury.
  Fever, muscle aches, dizziness or a general ill feeling.
- New, unexplained symptoms develop. Drugs used in treatment may produce side effects.

ILLNESSES & DISORDERS

GALLSTONES
(Cholelithiasis)

 GENERAL INFORMATION

DEFINITION—Stones in the gallbladder (the organ under the liver that stores bile). Most gallstones are composed primarily of cholesterol. They are not cancerous.

BODY PARTS INVOLVED—Gallbladder; bile ducts.

SEX OR AGE MOST AFFECTED—Adolescents and adults of both sexes, but more common in women. 10% of the U.S. population—and 20% of those over 40—have gallstones.

SIGNS & SYMPTOMS
● Colicky pain in the upper right abdomen or between the shoulder blades.
● Nausea and vomiting.
● Bloating or belching.
● Intolerance for fatty foods (indigestion, bloating and belching).
● Jaundice.
● No symptoms in about 40% of cases.

CAUSES—Unknown, but following are the most common theories:
● Failure of the gallbladder to empty competently.
● Alterations in bile mucus.
● Increased bilirubin (see Glossary) concentration in bile.
● Infection in the tubes that carry bile out of the liver.

RISK INCREASES WITH
● Recent illness, such as coronary-artery disease, cirrhosis of the liver or disorder of the small intestine.
● Family history of gallstones.
● Genetic factors. Some ethnic groups are more susceptible. About 70% of American Indians have gallstones.
● Obesity.
● Excess alcohol consumption.

HOW TO PREVENT—No specific preventive measures, except a low-fat diet (see Appendix 8).

 WHAT TO EXPECT

APPROPRIATE HEALTH CARE
● Self-care.
● Doctor's treatment.
● Surgery to remove the gallbladder and stones in the bile ducts.

DIAGNOSTIC MEASURES
● Your own observation of symptoms.
● Medical history and physical exam by a doctor.
● Laboratory studies, such as: blood count; blood chemistry; CAT scan (see Glossary); and ultrasound (see Glossary).
● X-rays of the gallbladder.

POSSIBLE COMPLICATIONS—Infection or rupture of the gallbladder.

PROBABLE OUTCOME—Many persons with gallstones have no symptoms. For those who do, the disorder is curable with surgery.

 HOW TO TREAT

NOTE—Follow your doctor's instructions. These instructions are supplemental.

GENERAL MEASURES—If you know you have gallstones and experience pain in the upper right abdomen, apply heat to the area. If pain worsens or continues more than 3 hours, call your doctor.

MEDICATION
● For minor discomfort, you may use non-prescription drugs such as acetaminophen.
● Your doctor may prescribe oral medication to try to dissolve stones. This treatment is still experimental.

ACTIVITY—No restrictions, except to rest during attacks of gallbladder colic.

DIET
● During an attack, sip water occasionally, but don't eat.
● At other times, eat a low-fat diet (see Appendix 8).

 CALL YOUR DOCTOR IF

● You have symptoms of gallstones.
● Your temperature rises to 101F (38.3C) or higher.

GANGRENE

 GENERAL INFORMATION

DEFINITION—Dead tissue. Gangrene develops when a wound becomes infected or tissue is destroyed by an accident.

BODY PARTS INVOLVED—Any body part, but the most common sites are toes, feet, legs, fingers, hands and arms. The most dangerous sites are abdominal organs.

SEX OR AGE MOST AFFECTED—Both sexes; all ages.

SIGNS & SYMPTOMS
- Black skin with dead underlying muscle and bone.
- Crepitation of the skin. This feels like pressing on air bubbles under the skin.
- Swelling.
- Pain.
- Bad-smelling discharge from ulcers in dead tissues.
- Moderate fever up to 101F (38.3C).

CAUSES—Gangrene occurs when blood flow to a body part is blocked or severely reduced. The following may interrupt blood flow and cause gangrene:
- Infection with clostridia perfringens germs.
- Tissue injury caused by accidents, surgery or deep puncture wounds.
- Crushing injury that cuts off blood supply.
- Blood clot in an artery.
- Hardening of the arteries.
- Prolonged frostbite.

RISK INCREASES WITH
- Diabetes mellitus.
- Smoking, which impairs blood circulation.
- Excess alcohol consumption, which interferes with blood-vessel function.

HOW TO PREVENT
- If you have diabetes, adhere closely to your treatment program to control diabetes. Examine your feet often for signs of unhealthy tissue. Keep your nails trimmed. Wear comfortable, well-fitting shoes.
- If you have hardening of the arteries, see Atherosclerosis (in Illness section) for preventive measures.
- Consult your doctor for signs of infection (warmth, swelling, redness, pain or tenderness) in a skin injury.

 WHAT TO EXPECT

APPROPRIATE HEALTH CARE
- Doctor's treatment.
- Self-care during convalescence.
- Time in a decompression chamber to halt the progress of gangrene.
- Surgery to remove dead tissue, sometimes by amputation.
- Physical therapy, if amputation is necessary.

DIAGNOSTIC MEASURES
- Your own observation of symptoms.
- Medical history and physical exam by a doctor.
- Laboratory blood cultures from the gangrene site.
- X-rays of any suspicious area to detect gas in tissues.

POSSIBLE COMPLICATIONS
- Blood poisoning.
- Shock.
- DIC (disseminated intravascular coagulation), a blood-clotting disorder.
- Limb amputation to prevent death.

PROBABLE OUTCOME—Usually curable in the early stages with antibiotic treatment and surgery to remove dead tissue. Without treatment, gangrene is fatal.

 HOW TO TREAT

NOTE—Follow your doctor's instructions. These instructions are supplemental.

GENERAL MEASURES—After surgery or intensive hospital care:
- Don't smoke!
- Wear sterile gloves to change dressings.
- Place any material that touches ulcerated areas in double plastic bags and burn it.
- Have whirlpool treatments and massages to increase circulation.

MEDICATION—Your doctor may prescribe:
- Antibiotics—usually intravenously in the early stages—to fight infection.
- Pain relievers.
- Anticoagulants to prevent blood clotting.

ACTIVITY—Rest in bed until gangrene stops progressing and healing begins. Then resume activity gradually. Move legs frequently while in bed to prevent blood clots in deep veins. You may read or watch TV.

DIET
- Eat a high-protein, high-calorie diet while your body is repairing damaged tissue.
- Take vitamin and mineral supplements, including zinc. Take 220mg of zinc orally twice a day.
- Drink adequate fluids (6 to 8 glasses daily).

 CALL YOUR DOCTOR IF

- You have symptoms of gangrene.
- You have persistent pain, despite medication and treatment.
- During convalescence, your temperature rises to 102F (38.9C) or higher.

GASTRIC EROSION

GENERAL INFORMATION

DEFINITION—A slight ulceration of the stomach lining. This is not contagious or cancerous.

BODY PARTS INVOLVED—Stomach.

SEX OR AGE MOST AFFECTED—All ages, but most common in men.

SIGNS & SYMPTOMS
- Vomiting blood. Blood may be bright red or resemble black coffee grounds.
- Blood in stool. Blood will appear black or "tarry."

CAUSES—Probably caused by drugs that irritate the stomach lining. Most likely drugs are: alcohol; caffeine; tobacco; aspirin; non-steroidal anti-inflammatory drugs used to treat arthritis and gout; and cortisone drugs used to treat asthma, Addison's disease or other conditions.

RISK INCREASES WITH
- Stress.
- Use of *any* oral medication.

HOW TO PREVENT
- Don't take medicines without enteric (protective) coatings.
- Don't drink alcohol if you have had gastric erosion. It may trigger bleeding.

WHAT TO EXPECT

APPROPRIATE HEALTH CARE
- Self-care after diagnosis.
- Doctor's treatment.

DIAGNOSTIC MEASURES
- Your own observation of symptoms.
- Medical history and physical exam by a doctor.
- Laboratory studies of stool and blood tests for anemia.
- X-rays of the upper digestive tract.

POSSIBLE COMPLICATIONS—Bleeding is an uncommon but dangerous complication, especially in the elderly. Another major complication is perforation, in which the erosion penetrates the stomach wall. Surgery is necessary to correct either complication. It involves little risk except for those over 70 years of age.

PROBABLE OUTCOME—Curable in 2 weeks with treatment if the cause is eliminated. Recurrence is common.

HOW TO TREAT

NOTE—Follow your doctor's instructions. These instructions are supplemental.

GENERAL MEASURES
- Check your stool every day for signs of bleeding. If the stool is black, remove a stool portion from the toilet bowl and take it to your doctor's office for examination.
- Avoid stressful situations (see Appendix 12).
- Don't smoke or drink alcoholic beverages.

MEDICATION
- Your doctor may prescribe H-2 blockers to reduce production of stomach acid.
- For minor pain, you may use non-prescription antacids.

ACTIVITY—Resume normal activities as soon as symptoms improve.

DIET—Avoid hot and spicy foods. Eat small frequent meals for 2 weeks. Don't drink alcohol.

CALL YOUR DOCTOR IF

- You have signs of bleeding described in Signs & Symptoms.
- You develop diarrhea. This may represent an adverse reaction to drugs used in treatment. The prescription may need adjustment.
- You have severe pain that is not relieved by treatment.
- You are unusually weak, pale or lightheaded.
- Symptoms of gastric erosion recur after treatment.

GASTRITIS

GENERAL INFORMATION

DEFINITION—Irritation, inflammation or infection of the stomach lining.

BODY PARTS INVOLVED—Stomach.

SEX OR AGE MOST AFFECTED—Both sexes; all ages.

SIGNS & SYMPTOMS
- Mild nausea and diarrhea.
- Vomiting (occasionally).
- Abdominal pain and cramps.
- Appetite loss.
- Fever.
- Weakness.
- Swollen abdomen.
- Sharp, dull or annoying pain in the chest.
- Acid taste in the mouth.
- Belching or gas.

CAUSES
- Excess stomach acid caused by heavy drinking, smoking or overeating (especially foods you don't digest easily).
- Food allergy.
- Virus infection. This form may be contagious.
- Adverse reaction to alcohol, caffeine or drugs.
- Unknown (sometimes).

RISK INCREASES WITH
- Stress.
- Improper diet.
- Illness that has lowered resistance.
- Smoking.
- Use of drugs, such as aspirin, non-steroidal anti-inflammatories, cortisone, caffeine, and many more.
- Excess alcohol consumption.
- Fatigue or overwork.

HOW TO PREVENT
- Eat and drink moderately.
- Avoid foods you find hard to digest.
- Don't smoke.
- Discuss with your doctor all medicines you take. Avoid medicines that irritate your stomach, if possible.

WHAT TO EXPECT

APPROPRIATE HEALTH CARE
- Self-care.
- Doctor's treatment.

DIAGNOSTIC MEASURES
- Your own observation of symptoms.
- Medical history and physical exam by a doctor.
- Laboratory studies to measure stomach acid.

POSSIBLE COMPLICATIONS—Bleeding is an uncommon but dangerous complication, especially in the elderly. Another major complication is ulceration or perforation, in which stomach acid erodes into or through the stomach wall. Surgery is necessary to correct either complication. Gastritis involves little risk except for those over 70 years of age.

PROBABLE OUTCOME—Usually curable in 1 week if the cause is eliminated.

HOW TO TREAT

NOTE—Follow your doctor's instructions. These instructions are supplemental.

GENERAL MEASURES—Consider lifestyle changes (see Appendix 12).

MEDICATION
- For minor discomfort, you may use non-prescription antacids.
- Your doctor may prescribe additional medication, depending on the cause of your gastritis.

ACTIVITY—Resume normal activities as soon as symptoms improve.

DIET—Don't eat solid food on the first day of the attack. Drink liquids frequently, preferably milk or water. Resume a normal diet slowly, but avoid hot and spicy foods until symptoms disappear. For a well-balanced diet, see Appendix 1.

CALL YOUR DOCTOR IF

- You vomit blood.
- Bowel movements become black or tarry.
- Pain becomes severe.
- Signs of dehydration, such as a dry mouth, wrinkled skin, excess thirst or decreased urination, develop.

ILLNESSES & DISORDERS

GASTROENTERITIS

GENERAL INFORMATION

DEFINITION—Irritation and infection of the digestive tract.

BODY PARTS INVOLVED—Stomach; small intestine; colon.

SEX OR AGE MOST AFFECTED—All ages, but most severe in young children (1 to 5 years) and adults over 60.

SIGNS & SYMPTOMS
- Nausea that sometimes causes vomiting.
- Diarrhea that ranges from 2 or 3 loose stools to many watery stools.
- Abdominal cramps, pain or tenderness.
- Appetite loss.
- Fever.
- Weakness.

CAUSES
- Food poisoning.
- Food allergy.
- Emotional upset.
- Infection (viral, bacterial or parasitic).
- Excess alcohol consumption.
- Use of harsh laxatives.
- Use of drugs that affect the brain's vomiting center.
- Change in bacteria that normally live in the intestinal tract.

RISK INCREASES WITH
- Adults over 60.
- Newborns and infants.
- Improper diet.
- Excess alcohol consumption.
- Use of drugs, such as aspirin, non-steroidal anti-inflammatories, antibiotics, laxatives, cortisone or caffeine.
- Travel to foreign countries.

HOW TO PREVENT
- Wash hands frequently if you or someone around you has gastroenteritis.
- Avoid as many causes and risks mentioned above as possible.

WHAT TO EXPECT

APPROPRIATE HEALTH CARE
- Self-care.
- Doctor's treatment.
- Hospitalization, if dehydration is severe.

DIAGNOSTIC MEASURES
- Your own observation of symptoms.
- Medical history and physical exam by a doctor.
- Laboratory studies, such as blood counts and stool studies.

POSSIBLE COMPLICATIONS
- Serious dehydration that requires intravenous fluids.
- Serious illness that may be overlooked because symptoms of gastroenteritis mimic other disorders.

PROBABLE OUTCOME—Vomiting and diarrhea usually disappear in 2 to 5 days, but adults may feel weak, fatigued and depressed for about 1 week.

HOW TO TREAT

NOTE—Follow your doctor's instructions. These instructions are supplemental.

GENERAL MEASURES—It is not necessary to isolate persons with gastroenteritis.

MEDICATION—Medicine is usually not necessary. If gastroenteritis is severe or prolonged, your doctor may prescribe antinausea and antidiarrhea medication.

ACTIVITY—Rest in bed until nausea, vomiting, diarrhea and fever are gone.

DIET
- Suck ice chips only until vomiting stops.
- After diarrhea and vomiting stop, drink small amounts of clear liquids, such as tea, "flat" ginger ale or lemon-lime soda, broth and gelatin.
- If you tolerate liquids for 12 hours, eat small amounts of soft foods, such as cooked cereal, rice, eggs, custard, baked potato and yogurt.
- If you tolerate soft food for 2 or 3 days, gradually return to a normal diet. Avoid alcohol, spicy food (pizza, spaghetti, onions), gravy, raw vegetables, raw fruit, salad dressing, cream soup, coffee and milk for several more days.

CALL YOUR DOCTOR IF

- Symptoms of gastroenteritis persist longer than 2 days.
- The following occurs during treatment:
  Mucus or blood in the stool.
  Fever of 101F (38.3C) or higher.
  Abdominal swelling.
  Severe pain in the abdomen or rectum, especially pain that begins in the center and moves to the lower right side.
- Vomiting and diarrhea recur after treatment.
- Signs of dehydration, such as a dry mouth, wrinkled skin, excess thirst or decreased urination, develop.

GASTROENTERITIS IN INFANTS & CHILDREN

GENERAL INFORMATION

DEFINITION—Irritation or infection of the digestive tract.

BODY PARTS INVOLVED—Stomach; small intestine; large intestine.

SEX OR AGE MOST AFFECTED—Newborns, infants and children (0 to 5 years).

SIGNS & SYMPTOMS
- Vomiting.
- Diarrhea.
- Irritability.
- Poor appetite.
- Fever.

CAUSES
- Virus.
- Bacterial infection.
- Intestinal parasites.

RISK INCREASES WITH
- Poor or improper diet.
- Illness that has lowered resistance.
- Crowded or unsanitary living conditions.

HOW TO PREVENT—Wash hands often with warm water and soap, especially before eating or handling the child, to avoid passing germs from hand to mouth.

WHAT TO EXPECT

APPROPRIATE HEALTH CARE
- Home care.
- Doctor's treatment.
- Hospitalization if dehydration is severe and intravenous fluid is needed.

DIAGNOSTIC MEASURES
- Your own observation of symptoms.
- Medical history and physical exam by a doctor.
- Laboratory stool and blood studies.

POSSIBLE COMPLICATIONS—Possible dehydration with 10 or more liquid bowel movements in 1 day. Signs of dehydration include: lethargy; sunken eyes; dry mouth; sunken fontanels (soft spots on baby's head); wrinkled skin; little or no urination.

PROBABLE OUTCOME—Condition should improve in 48 hours if the bowel is allowed to rest. If diarrhea or vomiting is so severe that the child cannot retain fluids, serious dehydration can occur.

HOW TO TREAT

NOTE—Follow your doctor's instructions. These instructions are supplemental.

GENERAL MEASURES
- Check the child's rectal temperature once or twice a day. Don't check more often to avoid stimulating diarrhea.
- Observe the child for signs of dehydration.
- Wash hands after handling the child or before preparing food.

MEDICATION—Don't use *any* non-prescription, antidiarrhea drugs without consulting your doctor. They can harm the child.

ACTIVITY—Reduce the child's activity until illness improves. The child may resume normal activity 24 hours after vomiting stops.

DIET—Fluids are necessary, but the bowel needs rest.
- For a bottle-fed infant, prepare a mixture of 16 oz. (1 pint) water, 1/4 teaspoon salt and 1 tablespoon sugar.
- For a breast-fed infant, consult your doctor for diet instructions.
- For an older child, offer the following clear liquids: apple, grape or cranberry juice; sweetened herbal tea; "flat" cola or lemon-lime soda; gelatin and gelatin water; bouillon.

  For an infant under 1 year, give 1/2 oz. of fluid every 20 minutes. For a child over 1 year, give 1 oz. every 30 minutes. Don't exceed these amounts during the first day or two, even if the child is not satisfied. Offer only as much as you intend the child to have. Don't supplement clear fluids with milk or solid food.

  When the child has been free of diarrhea for 1 day, offer one of the following low-residue foods: applesauce; banana; bread; cooked carrots; cooked cherries; eggs; ground meat; melon; noodles; cooked peaches; cooked pears; cooked peas; potatoes; rice; sugar cookies.

  If diarrhea doesn't recur within 2 hours after the solid feeding, continue feeding the child from the preceding list for 24 hours. Gradually work back to a normal diet.

CALL YOUR DOCTOR IF

- The child's rectal temperature rises to 103F (39.4C) or higher.
- The child shows signs of dehydration listed under Possible Complications.
- The child doesn't improve in 48 hours despite treatment.
- An infant under 2 months old has symptoms of gastroenteritis.

GIARDIASIS

GENERAL INFORMATION

DEFINITION—Bowel inflammation caused by a parasite found in contaminated water.

BODY PARTS INVOLVED—Gastrointestinal tract, especially the small bowel.

SEX OR AGE MOST AFFECTED—All ages, but most common in children.

SIGNS & SYMPTOMS
- Sudden diarrhea and abdominal cramping. Some persons have only mild diarrhea and indigestion.
- Loose, bulky, bad-smelling stools.
- Slight fever.

CAUSES—Infestation by a microscopic parasite, giardia lamblia. Giardia parasites enter the body through food or water, and multiply in the small intestine. Local inflammation, causing diarrhea and other symptoms, occurs in 1 to 3 weeks.

RISK INCREASES WITH
- Crowded or unsanitary living conditions, especially a substandard water supply and poor sanitation system.
- Drinking stream water while camping.
- Previous stomach surgery. Stomach acid normally provides some protection against this infection.
- Oral-anal sexual practices.

HOW TO PREVENT
- Boil water that is not known to be safe or treat it with commercial chemical purifiers.
- Avoid uncooked foods that may have been rinsed in contaminated water.
- Wash hands often, especially before meals, to avoid catching infection from other persons.

WHAT TO EXPECT

APPROPRIATE HEALTH CARE—Doctor's treatment.

DIAGNOSTIC MEASURES
- Your own observation of symptoms.
- Medical history and physical exam by a doctor. Tell your doctor if you have been traveling or camping in the previous month.
- Laboratory stool studies to detect parasites.

POSSIBLE COMPLICATIONS
- Chronic bowel inflammation.
- Malabsorption and weight loss.
- Dehydration.

PROBABLE OUTCOME—Spontaneous recovery in about 1 month for most persons. Medication hastens recovery.

HOW TO TREAT

NOTE—Follow your doctor's instructions. These instructions are supplemental.

GENERAL MEASURES
- Prevention is the best treatment. Be cautious when away from normal water supplies.
- Practice careful personal hygiene if you have diarrhea or are around those who do.

MEDICATION
- Don't use non-prescription drugs for gastrointestinal problems. These can mask symptoms.
- Your doctor may prescribe an antiparasite drug, metronidazole, which is very effective. Alcohol interacts with metronidazole to cause abdominal cramps and nausea, so don't drink alcohol during treatment.

ACTIVITY—No restrictions.

DIET—Maintain an adequate fluid intake (at least 8 glasses of water or liquid a day).

CALL YOUR DOCTOR IF

- You have symptoms of giardiasis.
- New, unexplained symptoms develop. Drugs used in treatment may produce side effects.

GILBERT'S SYNDROME
(Hyperbilirubinemia)

 GENERAL INFORMATION

DEFINITION—Increased blood levels of bilirubin (a yellow chemical byproduct of red-blood-cell breakdown).

BODY PARTS INVOLVED—Blood.

SEX OR AGE MOST AFFECTED—Both sexes and all ages, but most common in men between ages 20 and 45.

SIGNS & SYMPTOMS
- Slight jaundice (yellow skin and eyes).
- No other symptoms (usually).

CAUSES—The liver is inefficient in changing bilirubin to bile, leaving above-normal levels of bilirubin in the blood. This causes jaundice. Any liver abnormality associated with this disorder is minor.

RISK INCREASES WITH
- Stress.
- Poor nutrition, especially fasting.
- Genetic factors. This disorder is probably inherited.

HOW TO PREVENT—No specific preventive measures.

 WHAT TO EXPECT

APPROPRIATE HEALTH CARE—Doctor's diagnosis.

DIAGNOSTIC MEASURES
- Your own observation of symptoms (sometimes). The minor jaundice may be unnoticeable.
- Medical history and physical exam by a doctor.
- Laboratory blood studies of bilirubin and liver function.

POSSIBLE COMPLICATIONS—Misdiagnosis of a serious liver disease as Gilbert's syndrome.

PROBABLE OUTCOME—The condition is harmless.

 HOW TO TREAT

NOTE—Follow your doctor's instructions. These instructions are supplemental.

GENERAL MEASURES—If you or others notice a yellowing of your eyes or skin—it may seem like a good suntan—see your doctor for a diagnosis. Some more serious conditions also begin with mild jaundice.

MEDICATION—Medicine is not necessary for this disorder.

ACTIVITY—No restrictions.

DIET—No special diet.

 CALL YOUR DOCTOR IF

You or anyone else thinks your skin looks a bit yellow.

GINGIVITIS

 GENERAL INFORMATION

DEFINITION—Inflammation or infection of the gums.

BODY PARTS INVOLVED—Gum tissue around teeth.

SEX OR AGE MOST AFFECTED—All ages, but most common in adults.

SIGNS & SYMPTOMS
- Gums that are swollen, red and soft around the teeth.
- Gums that bleed easily.
- Bad breath.
- Fever (sometimes).
- No pain.

CAUSES
- Poor nutrition, especially vitamin deficiencies that cause diseases such as scurvy or pellagra.
- Plaque (food particles, germs and mucus at the base of the teeth).
- Blood disorders, including leukemia.
- Adverse reactions to drugs, such as anticonvulsants (primarily phenytoin and barbiturates).
- Exposure to lead and bismuth.

RISK INCREASES WITH
- Diabetes.
- Poor nutrition, especially vitamin deficiency.
- Infections.
- Pregnancy.

HOW TO PREVENT
- Practice good oral hygiene, (see General Measures) to prevent plaque formation.
- Have regular dental checkups twice a year.
- Eat a well-balanced diet. Take vitamin supplements if you cannot eat well-balanced meals.

 WHAT TO EXPECT

APPROPRIATE HEALTH CARE
- Self-care after diagnosis.
- Doctor's or dentist's treatment.
- Surgery to remove infected gum tissue, if other treatment fails.

DIAGNOSTIC MEASURES
- Your own observation of symptoms.
- Medical history and physical exam by a doctor or dentist.
- Laboratory culture of the plaque to identify the bacteria responsible for the infection.

POSSIBLE COMPLICATIONS—Extensive involvement may require painful, prolonged gum surgery.

PROBABLE OUTCOME—Usually curable in 2 weeks with treatment.

 HOW TO TREAT

NOTE—Follow your doctor's or dentist's instructions. These instructions are supplemental.

GENERAL MEASURES
- Brush your teeth properly. Scrub clear, sticky plaque off the teeth daily with a soft tooth brush. Place the brush at the gum line and gently rotate it, pointing bristles toward the gum. Brush one section of teeth at a time. A soft brush is less likely to damage teeth and gums than a hard brush.
- Floss your teeth at least once a day. Use waxed or unwaxed dental floss. Wind most of it around the middle finger of each hand. Use index fingers as guides to force the floss between the teeth gently. Gently clean adjacent tooth surfaces with a back-and-forth, sawing motion at the gum line. Floss between all lower teeth. Loosen floss and place it on the tops of the thumbs. Floss between all upper teeth, using the thumbs as guides.
- Use a fluoride toothpaste.
- Make regular appointments with your dentist for cleaning and treatment of cavities.

MEDICATION—Your doctor or dentist may prescribe:
- Antibiotics to fight infection.
- Fluoride mouthwash.
- Vitamins, if you have a deficiency.

ACTIVITY—No restrictions.

DIET—No special diet. Avoid candy, sweet drinks or sweet snacks. Sugar stimulates the production of acid, which attacks normal teeth. The best desserts are fruit and cheese, rather than ice cream or other high-sugar desserts.

 CALL YOUR DOCTOR OR DENTIST IF

- You have symptoms of gingivitis.
- The following occurs during treatment:
  Bleeding increases.
  Pain becomes intolerable.
  Temperature rises to 101F (38.3C) or higher.
  Neck or face becomes swollen.
  Swallowing becomes difficult.
- New, unexplained symptoms develop. Drugs used in treatment may produce side effects.

GLAUCOMA, ACUTE
(Angle-Closure Glaucoma)

 GENERAL INFORMATION

DEFINITION—A condition of the eye in which the fluid that normally drains into and out of the eye is suddenly obstructed. The obstruction causes severe pain and loss of vision.

BODY PARTS INVOLVED—Eye.

SEX OR AGE MOST AFFECTED—Adults of both sexes.

SIGNS & SYMPTOMS
- Severe, throbbing eye pain and headache.
- Redness in the eye.
- Blurred vision or halos around lights.
- Vomiting and weakness.
- Tender, firm eyeball.
- Dilated, fixed pupil.
- Swollen upper eyelid.

CAUSES—Unknown.

RISK INCREASES WITH
- Adults over 60.
- Family history of glaucoma or farsightedness.
- Emotional upsets.
- Smoking.

HOW TO PREVENT—Consult your doctor regularly for checkups to detect glaucoma before symptoms begin. If you are over 40, have pressure inside the eye checked at least once a year. The test is simple and painless.

 WHAT TO EXPECT

APPROPRIATE HEALTH CARE
- Doctor's treatment.
- Hospitalization during the attack until pressure in the eye decreases.
- Surgery (iridectomy with laser beam) to prevent further attacks—if other treatment is unsuccessful.

DIAGNOSTIC MEASURES
- Your own observation of symptoms.
- Medical history and physical exam by a doctor.
- Laboratory studies such as tonometry (measurement of pressure within the eyeball).

POSSIBLE COMPLICATIONS—Total blindness in the affected eye, if treatment is delayed or unsuccessful.

PROBABLE OUTCOME—Symptoms can be controlled if treatment begins quickly.

 HOW TO TREAT

NOTE—Follow your doctor's instructions. These instructions are supplemental after hospitalization—or if hospitalization is not required.

GENERAL MEASURES
- Avoid emotional upset, which raises pressure in the eye.
- Don't smoke. Tobacco constricts blood vessels, reducing the blood supply to the eye.

MEDICATION—Your doctor may prescribe:
- Eye drops to lower pressure inside the eye. Follow the instructions and schedule carefully, even if symptoms subside or the eye drops are occasionally uncomfortable.
- Diuretics to decrease fluid pressure in the eye.
- Pain relievers.

ACTIVITY—After treatment, resume your normal activities gradually—but avoid fatigue. Resume sexual relations when eye pressure is under control.

DIET—Low-salt diet (see Appendix 9).

 CALL YOUR DOCTOR IF

- You have symptoms of acute glaucoma. This is an emergency!
- New, unexplained symptoms develop. Drugs used in treatment may produce side effects.

ILLNESSES & DISORDERS

GLAUCOMA, CHRONIC
(Open-Angle Glaucoma)

 GENERAL INFORMATION

DEFINITION—A condition of the eye in which the fluid that normally drains into and out of the eye is gradually obstructed. This causes loss of vision. Chronic glaucoma—unlike acute glaucoma—usually causes no pain.

BODY PARTS INVOLVED—Eye.

SEX OR AGE MOST AFFECTED—Adults over 30.

SIGNS & SYMPTOMS
Early stages:
- Loss of peripheral vision in small areas.
- Blurred vision on one side toward the nose.
Later stages:
- Larger areas of vision loss, usually in both eyes.
Late stages:
- Hard eyeball.
- Halos around lights.
- Blind spots.
- Poor night vision.

CAUSES—Symptoms are caused by pressure in the eyeball that damages fibers in the optic nerve.

Glaucoma is probably hereditary, but it may be suspected in any person who requires frequent lens changes, has mild headaches or vague visual disturbances, sees halos around electric lights, or whose vision does not adapt well from light to dark.

RISK INCREASES WITH
- Adults over 60.
- Family history of acute or chronic glaucoma.
- Emotional stress.
- Smoking.
- Fatigue or overwork.

HOW TO PREVENT
- Make sure that tension in the eyeball is measured with every eye examination (at least once a year after age 40).
- Tell your doctor of any changes in your ability to see.

 WHAT TO EXPECT

APPROPRIATE HEALTH CARE
- Self-care after diagnosis.
- Doctor's treatment.
- Surgery (if other treatment is unsuccessful or unfeasible).

DIAGNOSTIC MEASURES
- Your own observation of symptoms.
- Medical history and physical exam by a doctor.
- Laboratory studies such as tonometry (measurement of pressure within the eyeball).

POSSIBLE COMPLICATIONS—Loss of vision before other symptoms begin.

PROBABLE OUTCOME—Symptoms can usually be controlled with treatment. Glaucoma treatment is lifelong. Vision is usually not impaired permanently, if glaucoma is treated.

 HOW TO TREAT

NOTE—Follow your doctor's instructions. These instructions are supplemental.

GENERAL MEASURES
- Avoid emotional upheavals and fatigue, which increase pressure in the eye.
- Don't smoke. Tobacco constricts blood vessels, restricting the blood supply to the eye.

MEDICATION—Your doctor may prescribe:
- Eye drops to lower pressure inside the eye. Follow the instructions and schedule carefully, even if symptoms subside or eye drops are occasionally uncomfortable. Use drops 4 to 5 times daily.
- Diuretics to reduce excess fluid.

ACTIVITY—Resume your normal activities gradually.

DIET—Low-salt diet (see Appendix 9).

 CALL YOUR DOCTOR IF

- You have symptoms of chronic glaucoma.
- Medicine in the eye becomes intolerable.
- Any sign of eye infection, such as fever, develops.
- Pain begins in the eye.
- Redness occurs in the eye.
- Vision changes suddenly.

GLOMERULONEPHRITIS
(Post-infectious, Acute or Chronic Glomerulonephritis)

 GENERAL INFORMATION

DEFINITION—Inflammation of the glomeruli (small, round filters in the kidney). Damaged glomeruli cannot effectively filter waste products from the bloodstream.

BODY PARTS INVOLVED—Kidneys.

SEX OR AGE MOST AFFECTED—All ages, but most common in children (1 to 11 years).

SIGNS & SYMPTOMS—Mild glomerulonephritis produces no symptoms. Diagnosis is possible only with urine studies. Severe glomerulonephritis produces the following:
- Smoky or slightly red urine.
- General ill feeling.
- Drowsiness.
- Nausea or vomiting.
- Headaches.
- Fever (sometimes).
- Appetite loss.
- Decreased urination.
- Fluid accumulation in the body, especially puffy eyes and ankles.
- Shortness of breath.
- High blood pressure.
- Protein in the urine.
- Disturbed vision.

CAUSES
- Classic acute glomerulonephritis follows a streptococcal infection. The most common infection sites are the throat and skin. Kidney symptoms usually begin 2 or 3 weeks after the strep infection.
- Chronic glomerulonephritis is rare and may have different causes than acute glomerulonephritis.

RISK INCREASES WITH—Exposure to people in public places where strep infections can be transmitted.

HOW TO PREVENT
- Avoid exposure to people with strep infection.
- Consult your doctor for antibiotic treatment of any infection that may be strep.

 WHAT TO EXPECT

APPROPRIATE HEALTH CARE
- Self-care after diagnosis.
- Doctor's treatment.
- Hospitalization (severe cases).

DIAGNOSTIC MEASURES
- Your own observation of symptoms.
- Medical history and physical exam by a doctor.
- Laboratory studies, such as: blood counts; repeated urinalyses to determine the presence of protein or other abnormal elements; and streptococcal antibody titer (a sophisticated blood study).
- Kidney-function tests.

POSSIBLE COMPLICATIONS—Kidney failure, which may require dialysis or other dramatic treatment.

PROBABLE OUTCOME—Symptoms subside in 2 weeks to several months. 90% of children recover without complications. Adults recover also—but more slowly.

 HOW TO TREAT

NOTE—Follow your doctor's instructions. These instructions are supplemental.

GENERAL MEASURES
- Record temperature 3 times a day.
- Collect and record the amount of urine passed in each 24-hour period. Some of this collection will be analyzed in the doctor's office.

MEDICATION—Your doctor may prescribe:
- Cortisone or cytotoxic drugs, if the illness is severe.
- Diuretics to increase urination.
- Antihypertensives, if high blood pressure accompanies the illness.
- Iron and vitamin supplements, if anemia develops.

ACTIVITY—Stay in bed, except to go to the bathroom, until all signs of illness have passed. This may be several weeks or months. Bed rest ensures an adequate blood flow to the kidney; blood flow is best when lying down. You may read or watch TV.
  Resume normal activities after recovery. Your doctor will determine when all signs and symptoms have disappeared.

DIET—As long as your kidneys function properly, you may eat a normal, well-balanced diet. Greatly decrease the sodium in your diet.

 CALL YOUR DOCTOR IF

- You have symptoms of glomerulonephritis.
- The following occur during treatment:
  Severe headache or convulsion.
  Failure to pass at least 22 ounces of urine in a 24-hour period.
  Fever.
  Skin rash.
  Increased fluid retention.
  Increased nausea, vomiting or diarrhea.

ILLNESSES & DISORDERS

GONORRHEA

GENERAL INFORMATION

DEFINITION—An infectious disease of the reproductive organs that is sexually transmitted (venereal disease).

BODY PARTS INVOLVED
- Males—urethra.
- Females—urethra; reproductive system.
- Both sexes—rectum; throat; joints; eyes (sometimes).

SEX OR AGE MOST AFFECTED—Both
sexes and all ages—even young children—of persons who have sexual contact with infected persons. The peak incidence is between ages 20 and 30.

SIGNS & SYMPTOMS
- Burning urination.
- Thick green-yellow discharge from the penis or vagina.
- Little or no fever.
- Pain or tenderness with sexual intercourse (sometimes).
- Rectal discomfort and discharge (sometimes).
- Mild sore throat (sometimes).

Females often have few or no symptoms. Males usually have more pronounced symptoms.

CAUSES—Infection from gonococcus bacteria that grow well on delicate, moist tissue. The bacteria is usually transmitted sexually, but some cases are of unknown origin. Sexual activity involving the rectum or mouth may transmit infection to those areas if either partner is infected.

RISK INCREASES WITH
- Many sexual partners, whether heterosexual or homosexual.
- Prostitution.
- Child sexual abuse.

HOW TO PREVENT
- Avoid sexual partners whose health practices and status are uncertain.
- Use a rubber condom during sexual intercourse.
- Women: Never use someone else's douche equipment.

OTHER—This condition must be reported to the local health department to prevent its spread. It sometimes occurs simultaneously with syphilis. Your cooperation is important, and your confidentiality will be maintained.

WHAT TO EXPECT

APPROPRIATE HEALTH CARE
- Doctor's treatment.
- Hospitalization for complications.

DIAGNOSTIC MEASURES
- Your own observation of symptoms.
- Medical history and physical exam by a doctor.
- Blood studies.
- Laboratory culture and microscopic analysis of the discharge from the reproductive organs, rectum or throat.

POSSIBLE COMPLICATIONS
- Gonococcal eye infection. This may cause blindness in children.
- Blood poisoning (gonococcal septicemia).
- Infectious arthritis.
- Pelvic inflammatory disease.
- Epididymitis.
- Endocarditis.
- Sexual impotence in men, if untreated (sometimes).

PROBABLE OUTCOME—Usually curable in 1 to 2 weeks with treatment.

HOW TO TREAT

NOTE—Follow your doctor's instructions. These instructions are supplemental.

GENERAL MEASURES
- Use separate linens and disposable eating utensils during treatment.
- Wash hands frequently—especially after urination and bowel movements.
- Don't touch eyes with hands.
- Inform all sexual contacts so they can seek treatment.

MEDICATION
- Your doctor will prescribe antibiotics to fight the infection.
- You may take non-prescription drugs, such as acetaminophen or aspirin, to reduce discomfort—but not in place of antibiotics. Home remedies or folk-medicine treatments are ineffective.

ACTIVITY—No restrictions, except don't resume sexual activity until a follow-up culture shows the infection is cured.

DIET—No special diet. Reduce consumption of caffeine and alcohol during treatment. These irritate the urethra.

CALL YOUR DOCTOR IF

- You have symptoms of gonorrhea.
- You develop chills, fever, abdominal pain, swelling of the testicles, genital sores or joint pain—either before or during treatment.
- New, unexplained symptoms develop. Drugs used in treatment may produce side effects.

GOUT

GENERAL INFORMATION

DEFINITION—Recurrent attacks of joint inflammation caused by deposits of uric-acid crystals in the joints.

BODY PARTS INVOLVED—Joints, especially the base of the big toe. Gout may also involve the elbow, knee, hand, foot, ankle, arm or shoulder.

SEX OR AGE MOST AFFECTED—Adults of both sexes, but 20 times more frequent in men than women.

SIGNS & SYMPTOMS
- Severe pain in the inflamed joint, usually at the base of the big toe.
- Involved joints are red, hot, swollen, and very tender. Skin over the joint is red and shiny.
- Fever (sometimes).

CAUSES
- Genetic transmission.
- A high level of uric acid in the blood due to increased production of uric acid or decreased elimination of uric acid by the kidneys.
- Use of diuretic drugs (water pills) such as furosemide and hydroclorothiazide.
- Use of some antibiotics.
- Some blood diseases, such as polycythemia and leukemia.

RISK INCREASES WITH
- Men over 60.
- Family history of gout.
- Use of drugs, such as diuretics or antibiotics.

HOW TO PREVENT—Cannot be prevented at present. Recurrent attacks can usually be prevented with medication.

OTHER—Excess consumption of rich food and alcohol does not cause gout, as was once believed, but it may trigger attacks.

WHAT TO EXPECT

APPROPRIATE HEALTH CARE
- Self-care after diagnosis.
- Doctor's treatment.
- Nursing-home care (only with crippling complications).

DIAGNOSTIC MEASURES
- Laboratory studies to determine blood levels of uric acid.
- Therapeutic trial with antigout medications.

POSSIBLE COMPLICATIONS—If untreated, may cause:
- Crippled, deformed joints.
- Kidney stones.
- Inflammation of bones, ligaments and tendons.

PROBABLE OUTCOME—The first attack may last a few days, but recurrent attacks are common without treatment to reduce the uric-acid level in the blood. Symptoms can be eliminated with treatment.

HOW TO TREAT

NOTE—Follow your doctor's instructions. These instructions are supplemental.

GENERAL MEASURES
- Use warm or cold compresses on painful joints.
- Keep the weight of bedclothes off any painful joint by making a frame that raises sheets off the feet.

MEDICATION—Your doctor may prescribe:
- Pain relievers.
- Non-steroidal anti-inflammatory drugs to control inflammation in painful joints.
- Lifelong medication, such as allopurinol to decrease uric-acid production or probenecid to increase the kidneys' excretion of uric acid.
These medications have significant side effects and adverse reactions. Obtain as much information as possible regarding their use.

ACTIVITY—Acute attacks will end sooner with complete rest.

DIET
- Don't eat liver, sweetbreads, kidney or sardines.
- Drink 8 to 10 glasses of water daily.
- Don't drink alcoholic beverages.

CALL YOUR DOCTOR IF

- You have symptoms of gout.
- The following occurs during treatment:
  Fever of 101F (38.3C) or higher.
  Skin rash, sore throat, red tongue or bleeding gums.
  Marked swelling of feet or abrupt weight increase.
  Diarrhea or vomiting.
- Symptoms are not relieved in 3 days despite treatment.
- New, unexplained symptoms develop that may indicate an adverse reaction of the drug or interactions between drugs.

ILLNESSES & DISORDERS

GRANULOMA ANNULARE

 GENERAL INFORMATION

DEFINITION—A chronic skin disorder characterized by lesions that appear in the shape of a ring. This is not malignant or contagious.

BODY PARTS INVOLVED—Skin on the bottoms of feet and backs of fingers, hands, arms, elbows, legs and knees.

SEX OR AGE MOST AFFECTED—All ages, but most common in children (4 to 12 years).

SIGNS & SYMPTOMS—Papules (small, raised bumps on the skin) with the following characteristics:
- Papules have a domed or slightly flat shape, 3mm to 6mm in diameter.
- Papules are non-scaling.
- Papules are pink or violet. Those on the lower extremities are darker than ones on other parts of the body.
- Papules don't itch or hurt.
- Multiple papules cluster in a ring. Ring diameters range from 1cm to 10cm. Papules around the ring border are close, but don't grow completely together. This gives the border a beaded appearance. The ring's center is often darker than the edge. Ringed lesions change in size and shape over a period of several weeks to 6 months.

CAUSES—Unknown.

RISK INCREASES WITH—Injury to the skin, including sunburn.

HOW TO PREVENT—Avoid injury to the skin. Protect skin from sunburn with sunscreen or clothing.

 WHAT TO EXPECT

APPROPRIATE HEALTH CARE
- Self-care after diagnosis.
- Doctor's treatment, which may include injections of steroid medications into lesions.

DIAGNOSTIC MEASURES
- Your own observation of symptoms.
- Medical history and physical exam by a doctor.
- Biopsy (see Glossary) to confirm diagnosis.

POSSIBLE COMPLICATIONS
- Papules and nodules occasionally ulcerate.
- Body temperature may rise if a large part of the body is covered with plastic dressing (see How to Treat). If fever occurs, stop treatment.

PROBABLE OUTCOME—Spontaneous recovery within 2 years, but therapy hastens recovery.

 HOW TO TREAT

NOTE—Follow your doctor's instructions. These instructions are supplemental.

GENERAL MEASURES—Protect involved areas from injury.

MEDICATION—Your doctor may prescribe topical steroids with occlusion to hasten healing. To use steroids:
- Gently rub a small amount of the steroid drug into the affected area.
- Reapply a small amount.
- Cover the affected area with clear kitchen plastic wrap. If skin becomes dry and itchy, provide additional moisture by covering the affected area with a damp, clean cloth before applying plastic. You may also soak the affected area briefly in water after applying medicine.
- Ask your doctor how often to change the plastic dressing.
- Reapply medicine every time you change the plastic dressing.

ACTIVITY—No restrictions.

DIET—No special diet.

 CALL YOUR DOCTOR IF

- You have symptoms of granuloma annulare.
- Lesions ulcerate.
- New lesions occur during treatment.
- Signs of infection, such as redness, swelling, pain or tenderness, develop around the lesions.
- You become sensitive to the occlusive plastic dressing.
- New, unexplained symptoms develop. Steroid drugs used in treatment may produce side effects.

GRANULOMA, PYOGENIC

 GENERAL INFORMATION

DEFINITION—Skin lesions composed of small blood vessels. These are not contagious or cancerous.

BODY PARTS INVOLVED—Skin anywhere on the body, but most commonly on the face and shoulder.

SEX OR AGE MOST AFFECTED
- Children of both sexes (ages 5 to 15).
- Pregnant women.

SIGNS & SYMPTOMS—Papules (small, raised bumps on the skin) with the following characteristics:
- Papules appear first as pinhead-sized, but grow rapidly within weeks to full size (2mm to 20mm).
- Papules bleed easily when injured.
- Papules don't hurt or itch.

CAUSES—Unknown. Pyogenic refers to an infectious process, but these lesions are misnamed. Because they frequently appear in late childhood or pregnancy, hormonal changes may be a factor in their development.

RISK INCREASES WITH—Pregnancy.

HOW TO PREVENT—Cannot be prevented at present.

OTHER—Because pyogenic granuloma resembles melanoma (skin cancer), medical diagnosis is important.

 WHAT TO EXPECT

APPROPRIATE HEALTH CARE
- Doctor's treatment.
- Surgery or cryotherapy (see Glossary) to remove papule.
- Self-care after surgery.

DIAGNOSTIC MEASURES
- Your own observation of symptoms.
- Medical history and physical exam by a doctor.
- Biopsy (see Glossary).

PROBABLE OUTCOME—Spontaneous recovery, usually within 2 to 6 months. Recurrence is common.

POSSIBLE COMPLICATIONS—None expected.

 HOW TO TREAT

NOTE—Follow your doctor's instructions. These instructions are supplemental.

GENERAL MEASURES—After surgery:
- Apply rubbing alcohol to the scab twice a day.
- Apply an adhesive bandage to the scab during the day. Leave it uncovered at night.
- Wash the wound as usual. Dry gently and completely after bathing or swimming.

MEDICATION
- For minor pain, you may use non-prescription drugs, such as acetaminophen or aspirin.
- If the scab cracks or oozes, apply a non-prescription antibiotic ointment several times a day.

ACTIVITY—No restrictions.

DIET—No special diet.

 CALL YOUR DOCTOR IF

- You have symptoms of pyogenic granuloma.
- The wound bleeds after surgery, and bleeding cannot be stopped by applying pressure for 10 minutes.
- The wound shows signs of infection, such as redness, swelling, pain or increased tenderness.

ILLNESSES & DISORDERS

GUILLAIN-BARRÉ SYNDROME
(Infectious Polyneuritis; Acute Idiopathic Polyneuritis)

 GENERAL INFORMATION

DEFINITION—An inflammatory condition of nerves and muscles that causes rapid weakness and loss of sensation.

BODY PARTS INVOLVED—Central nervous system; muscles.

SEX OR AGE MOST AFFECTED—All ages, but most common between 30 and 50.

SIGNS & SYMPTOMS—Early stages:
- Muscle weakness in hands and feet, arms and legs, abdomen and chest. The weakness spreads within 72 hours; it may create life-threatening breathing difficulty.
- Shock (weakness; faintness; cold hands and feet; rapid heartbeat; sweating).
Later stages:
- Complete paralysis (sometimes) for weeks or months.

CAUSES—Unknown, but may be an autoimmune disorder. It sometimes follows an immunization or minor surgery.

RISK INCREASES WITH
- Recent surgery.
- Recent immunization.
- Recent illness, such as a minor respiratory infection, gastroenteritis, Hodgkin's disease or lupus erythematosus.

HOW TO PREVENT—Cannot be prevented at present.

 WHAT TO EXPECT

APPROPRIATE HEALTH CARE
- Doctor's treatment.
- Hospitalization.

DIAGNOSTIC MEASURES
- Your own observation of symptoms.
- Medical history and physical exam by a doctor.
- Laboratory study of spinal fluid.

POSSIBLE COMPLICATIONS
- Paralysis of eyelid muscles, resulting in eye damage.
- Thrombophlebitis.
- Pneumonia.
- Respiratory failure.
- Pressure sores, if the person is immobilized.
- Constipation or fecal impaction.

PROBABLE OUTCOME—Complete recovery without residual effects in most cases. Some persons recover in 15 to 20 days, others require a year or more. Many mechanical devices can aid mobility until the person recovers.

 HOW TO TREAT

NOTE—Follow your doctor's instructions. These instructions are supplemental.

GENERAL MEASURES
- Remain mentally and socially active during recovery.
- Encourage coughing to rid lungs of mucus.

MEDICATION—Your doctor may prescribe:
- Laxatives to prevent constipation.
- Cortisone drugs, although they are not always effective.

ACTIVITY—Remain as active as muscle strength permits. Have a family member or visiting nurse passively move and stretch muscles.

DIET—No special diet. Drink at least 8 glasses of fluid a day to prevent constipation.

 CALL YOUR DOCTOR IF

- You have symptoms of Guillain-Barré syndrome.
- The following occurs during treatment:
  Fever.
  Breathing difficulty.
  Sores on the skin.
  Vision changes.
  Swollen or tender calves.
  Constipation.
- New, unexplained symptoms develop. Drugs used in treatment may produce side effects.

HAND, FOOT & MOUTH DISEASE

 GENERAL INFORMATION

DEFINITION—Virus infection that begins in the throat.

BODY PARTS INVOLVED—Throat; tonsils; skin; gastrointestinal tract; central nervous system.

SEX OR AGE MOST AFFECTED—Infants and young children (2 weeks to 3 years).

SIGNS & SYMPTOMS
- Sudden fever.
- Sore throat with blisters and ulcers in the mouth and throat lining.
- Headache.
- Rash with blisters on the hands, feet and groin.
- Appetite loss.
- Abdominal pain (sometimes).

CAUSES—Infection from the coxsackievirus A-16, which is transmitted from person to person.

RISK INCREASES WITH—Summer and fall seasons.

HOW TO PREVENT—Prevent exposure of infants and young children to anyone with a respiratory illness.

 WHAT TO EXPECT

APPROPRIATE HEALTH CARE
- Home care.
- Doctor's treatment.

DIAGNOSTIC MEASURES
- Your own observation of symptoms.
- Medical history and physical exam by a doctor.

POSSIBLE COMPLICATIONS
- Convulsions with high fever (sometimes, especially in infants).
- Permanent brain damage caused by spread of infection to the central nervous system.

PROBABLE OUTCOME—Spontaneous recovery in 4 to 5 days.

 HOW TO TREAT

NOTE—Follow your doctor's instructions. These instructions are supplemental.

GENERAL MEASURES
- Dip a cotton applicator in 2% hydrogen peroxide, and apply to the blisters in the mouth.
- Rinse the mouth with salt water (1/2 teaspoon salt to 1 cup water) after eating, if the child is old enough to rinse without swallowing.
- Boil eating utensils and other items that touch the mouth or saliva—or use disposable utensils—to avoid transmitting the disease.
- Boil bottle nipples separately for 20 minutes before sterilizing formula in the bottles.

MEDICATION—To reduce high fever, you may use non-prescription drugs such as acetaminophen. Antibiotics are not effective against this disease.

ACTIVITY—Keep the child in bed until fever and other symptoms disappear. Normal activities may be resumed gradually.

DIET—Encourage the child to increase fluid intake, including milk, liquid gelatin, ice cream, custard or drinks made with syrup of wild cherry (available from your druggist). If drinking is painful, older children may use a straw.

 CALL YOUR DOCTOR IF

- Your child has symptoms of hand, foot and mouth disease.
- The following occurs during treatment:
  Fever of 101F (38.3C) or higher.
  Skin lesions.
  Significant weight loss (10% of body weight).
  Signs of dehydration (wrinkled skin, weight loss, irritability, lethargy and dry-looking tongue).
  Pain in the neck or extremities.
  Convulsion.
  Decreased urination or dark urine.

ILLNESSES & DISORDERS

HAY FEVER
(Allergic Rhinitis)

GENERAL INFORMATION

DEFINITION—An allergic response to airborne allergens that affects the eyes and upper respiratory tract.

BODY PARTS INVOLVED—Nose; eyes; sinuses; throat; mouth; lungs.

SEX OR AGE MOST AFFECTED—Both sexes; all ages.

SIGNS & SYMPTOMS
- Itching, watery eyes.
- Frequent sneezing; stuffy nose with a clear discharge.
- Itching in the roof of the mouth.
- Wheezing (sometimes).

CAUSES—An allergic sensitivity to airborne allergens such as:
- Pollen from weeds, flowers, grasses and trees.
- Mold.
- Dust.
- Mites.
- Tobacco smoke and other air pollutants.

RISK INCREASES WITH
- Medical history of allergic reactions, such as eczema or asthma.
- Smoking.
- Spring and autumn. Most plants produce pollen during these seasons.

HOW TO PREVENT
- Change furnace or air-conditioner filters often.
- Wear a filter face mask during exposure to allergens.
- Install an air-purification unit in your home's heating and air-conditioning system.

WHAT TO EXPECT

APPROPRIATE HEALTH CARE
- Self-care.
- Doctor's treatment.

DIAGNOSTIC MEASURES
- Your own observation of symptoms.
- Medical history and physical exam by a doctor.
- Laboratory tests such as a blood count and allergy skin tests (see Glossary).

POSSIBLE COMPLICATIONS
- Sleeping difficulty and chronic fatigue.
- Sinus infection.

PROBABLE OUTCOME—Symptoms can be controlled with treatment.

HOW TO TREAT

NOTE—Follow your doctor's instructions. These instructions are supplemental.

GENERAL MEASURES—Eliminate as many allergens in your environment as possible. Prepare your bedroom as follows:
- Empty the room of furniture, rugs or carpet, and drapes or curtains.
- Clean the walls, woodwork and floors with a damp mop. Wax the floor.
- Take the mattress and box springs outside and vacuum or clean them.
- Cover the box springs, mattress and pillows with plastic covers.
- Use only rugs that can be washed once a week.
- Use bedclothes that can be washed often, such as cotton sheets, washable mattress pads and synthetic fiber blankets. Don't use chenille bedspreads, quilts or comforters.
- Use wood or plastic chairs. Don't used stuffed chairs.
- Use plastic curtains, if possible. Dust them daily.
- Use a vacuum cleaner, damp rags, and a damp or oiled mop to clean the bedroom thoroughly once a week.
- Keep windows and doors closed as much as possible.
- Don't handle objects that are very dusty, such as books or stored clothing.
- Don't keep stuffed animals or toys in the house.
- Remove *all pets* (except fish) from the house.

MEDICATION—To reduce the body's allergic response, your doctor may prescribe:
- Antihistamines; decongestants; cortisone eye drops or nasal spray; cortisone tablets (severe cases only); or cromolyn nasal spray. These medications relieve symptoms, but they don't cure hay fever.
- Desensitization injections for known allergens.

ACTIVITY—No restrictions.

DIET—Avoid foods that cause allergic reactions.

CALL YOUR DOCTOR IF

- You have severe symptoms of hay fever that are interfering with your normal activities.
- Signs of infection, such as fever, headache, muscle aches, or thick, discolored nasal discharge, appear. A sinus infection may be complicating the allergy.
- New, unexplained symptoms develop. Drugs in treatment may produce side effects.

HEAD INJURY

GENERAL INFORMATION

DEFINITION—Injury to the head, with or without unconsciousness or other visible signs.

BODY PARTS INVOLVED—Head.

SEX OR AGE MOST AFFECTED—Both sexes; all ages.

SIGNS & SYMPTOMS—Depends on the extent of injury. The presence or absence of swelling at the injury site is not related to the seriousness of injury. Signs and symptoms include any or all of the following:
- Drowsiness or confusion.
- Vomiting and nausea.
- Blurred vision.
- Pupils of different size.
- Loss of consciousness—either temporarily or for long periods.
- Amnesia or memory lapses.
- Irritability.
- Headache.
- Bleeding of the scalp, if the skin is broken.

CAUSES—Injury. The worst injuries usually result from motor-vehicle accidents.

RISK INCREASES WITH
- Excess alcohol consumption.
- Contact sports, especially football or boxing.
- Seizure disorders.

HOW TO PREVENT
- Don't drink or use mind-altering drugs and drive.
- Wear protective headgear for contact sports and cycling.
- Use your auto seat belt or shoulder harness. Place young children in safety car seats.

WHAT TO EXPECT

APPROPRIATE HEALTH CARE
- Home care.
- Doctor's treatment.
- Hospitalization for observation, if signs and symptoms are severe.

DIAGNOSTIC MEASURES
- Your own observation of symptoms.
- Medical history and physical exam by a doctor.
- Laboratory studies of blood and cerebrospinal fluid.
- X-rays of the skull and neck.
- CAT scan (see Glossary) of the head.

POSSIBLE COMPLICATIONS
- Bleeding under the skull (subdural hemorrhage and hematoma).
- Bleeding into the brain.

PROBABLE OUTCOME—Usually curable with early recognition of danger signs and medical treatment. Complications can be life-threatening or cause permanent disability.

HOW TO TREAT

NOTE—Follow your doctor's instructions. These instructions are supplemental.

GENERAL MEASURES—The extent of injury can be determined only with careful examination and observation. After a doctor's examination, the injured person may be sent home—but a responsible person must stay with the person and watch for serious symptoms. The first 24 hours after injury are critical, although serious aftereffects can appear later.

If you are watching the patient, awaken him or her every hour for 24 hours. Report to the doctor immediately if you can't awaken or arouse the person. Report also any of the following:
Vomiting.
Inability to move arms and legs equally well on both sides.
Temperature above 100F (37.8C).
Stiff neck.
Pupils of unequal size or shape.
Convulsions.
Noticeable restlessness.
Severe headache that persists longer than 4 hours after injury.
Confusion.

MEDICATION—Don't give *any* medicine—including non-prescription acetaminophen or aspirin—until the diagnosis is certain.

ACTIVITY—The patient should rest in bed until the doctor determines the danger is over. Normal activity may then be resumed as symptoms improve.

DIET—Full liquid diet (see Appendix 7) until the danger passes.

CALL YOUR DOCTOR IF

You have symptoms of a head injury or observe them in someone else.

ILLNESSES & DISORDERS

HEADACHE, MIGRAINE

GENERAL INFORMATION

DEFINITION—An intense, incapacitating headache, accompanied by other symptoms, that occurs repeatedly in some persons.

BODY PARTS INVOLVED—Blood vessels leading to the scalp and brain.

SEX OR AGE MOST AFFECTED
- Both sexes, but more common in females.
- Adolescents and adults.

SIGNS & SYMPTOMS—The nature of attacks varies between persons and from time to time in the same person. Symptoms of a classic migraine attack appear in the following sequence:
- Inability to see clearly, followed by seeing bright spots and zig-zag patterns. Visual disturbances may last several minutes or several hours, but they disappear once the headache begins.
- Dull, boring pain in the temple that spreads to the entire side of the head. Pain becomes intense and throbbing.
- Nausea and vomiting.

In other types of migraine attack, the above symptoms (vision disturbances, headache or vomiting) may be absent, or other symptoms may be present. Some persons become pale, with bloodshot eyes and a runny nose or eyes.

CAUSES—Constriction, then dilation and inflammation of blood vessels that go to the scalp and brain. Vision disturbances occur when blood vessels narrow. Headache begins when they widen again. Attacks may be triggered by:
- Tension. Emotional problems are probably the most common reason for migraine attacks, but headaches don't necessarily coincide with emotional upset. They often occur on weekends when stress is decreased.
- Menstruation.
- Use of oral contraceptives.
- Fatigue.
- Consumption of alcohol or certain foods.

RISK INCREASES WITH
- Stress.
- Family history of migraines.
- Smoking.
- Excess alcohol consumption.
- Use of many prescription and non-prescription drugs.

HOW TO PREVENT
- See Appendix 13 for suggestions to reduce stress.
- 1 aspirin a day may prevent migraine attacks in adults.
- Use of the drug propranolol prevents attacks in some persons.

WHAT TO EXPECT

APPROPRIATE HEALTH CARE
- Self-care after diagnosis.
- Doctor's treatment.

DIAGNOSTIC MEASURES
- Your own observation of symptoms.
- Medical history and physical exam by a doctor.
- Laboratory blood studies.
- CAT scan (see Glossary) of the head.

POSSIBLE COMPLICATIONS—None expected.

PROBABLE OUTCOME—Symptoms can be controlled with treatment.

HOW TO TREAT

NOTE—Follow your doctor's instructions. These instructions are supplemental.

GENERAL MEASURES—At the first sign of a migraine attack:
- Apply a cold cloth or ice pack to your head, or splash your face with cold water.
- Take pain relievers, such as aspirin or acetaminophen.
- Lie down in a quiet, dark room for several hours. Relax if possible. Listen to music, sleep or meditate.
- Don't read.

MEDICATION—Your doctor may prescribe:
- Antihistamines to expand blood vessels.
- Antiemetics to decrease nausea and vomiting.
- Vasoconstrictors to narrow blood vessels.
- Pain relievers.
- Beta-adrenergic blockers to prevent attacks, if headaches are so frequent or severe that you can't function normally. This medication may have undesirable side effects and it does not help everyone.

ACTIVITY—Rest during attacks. Between attacks, exercise to achieve maximum fitness.

DIET—Because some attacks are caused by foods, such as cheese or chocolate, keep a record of what you ate before each attack. Avoid foods that seem to trigger migraine attacks. Otherwise, no special diet is necessary.

CALL YOUR DOCTOR IF

- You have a migraine attack that persists longer than 24 hours, despite treatment.
- Frequent migraine attacks interfere with normal life.

HEADACHE, TENSION OR VASCULAR

 ## GENERAL INFORMATION

DEFINITION—Simple tension or vascular headaches are of 3 types:
- Pain from muscle strain in the scalp, neck and face.
- Pain from constricted blood vessels in the head that cause pressure on blood-vessel walls.
- Pain from dilated blood vessels in the brain.

BODY PARTS INVOLVED—Sensory nerves in the skin, scalp, blood vessels and muscles of the head.

SEX OR AGE MOST AFFECTED—Both sexes; all ages.

SIGNS & SYMPTOMS—Any of the following:
- Moderate pain in the front or back of the head, accompanied by tight muscles in the neck or scalp.
- Constant pain over the temples, accompanied by the feeling that a vise is over the back of the head.
- Throbbing pain all over the head.

CAUSES
- Tension, producing strain on muscles of the neck, scalp, face and jaw.
- Sleep disturbances.
- Excessive eating or drinking.
- Physically exhausting work.
- Anxiety or depression.
- Eye strain, including sun glare.
- Use of drugs or alcohol.
- Low blood sugar.
- Hormone changes during the menstrual cycle.
- Allergic reactions.

RISK INCREASES WITH
- Stress, either mental or physical.
- Environments that are noisy, stuffy, hot, poorly lit, or have irritating odors.
- Exposure to or consumption of nitrites, sulfites, monosodium glutamate or other food additives.

HOW TO PREVENT
- Get enough sleep—an average of 8 hours for men and 7 hours for women.
- Don't skip meals, especially breakfast.
- Don't overeat.
- Exercise regularly (see Appendix 20) to reduce tension and improve circulation.
- Drink alcohol moderately—no more than 1 or 2 drinks a day, if at all.
- Don't smoke cigarettes, and avoid smoky environments.
- Don't use mood-altering, mind-altering, stimulant or sedative drugs.
- Avoid foods that contain nitrites or other additives to which you are sensitive.

 ## WHAT TO EXPECT

APPROPRIATE HEALTH CARE
- Self-care.
- Doctor's treatment, if headache persists or worsens despite self-care.
- Biofeedback training or counseling for chronic headaches caused by stress.

DIAGNOSTIC MEASURES
- Your own observation of symptoms.
- Medical history and physical exam by a doctor.
- Laboratory studies, such as a CAT scan (see Glossary) for unrelenting pain.

POSSIBLE COMPLICATIONS—None expected for a simple headache.

PROBABLE OUTCOME—Most tension or vascular headaches can be relieved with simple treatment (see How to Treat).

 ## HOW TO TREAT

NOTE—Follow your doctor's instructions. These instructions are supplemental.

GENERAL MEASURES—If possible, stop what you are doing and try to relax:
- Massage shoulders, neck, jaw and scalp.
- Take a hot bath.
- Lie down. Place a warm or cold cloth, whichever feels better, over the aching area.

MEDICATION—You may take acetaminophen or aspirin to relieve pain.

ACTIVITY—Rest in a quiet room.

DIET
- Most persons feel better if they don't eat, unless the headache is from low blood sugar.
- Don't drink alcohol.

 ## CALL YOUR DOCTOR IF

You have a headache and any of the following:
- Fever of 101F (38.3C) or higher.
- Recent head injury.
- Drowsiness.
- Nausea and vomiting.
- Pain in one eye.
- Blurred vision.
- High blood pressure.
- Pain and tenderness around the eyes and cheekbones that worsens when you lean forward.
- Vision disturbances and vomiting prior to the headache.
- Persistent headache pain for longer than 24 hours without other symptoms.
- You suspect a prescription or non-prescription drug caused the headache.

ILLNESSES & DISORDERS

HEARING IMPAIRMENT OR LOSS

 ## GENERAL INFORMATION

DEFINITION—Decreased ability or complete inability to hear. Classifications include:
- Conductive loss, in which middle-ear bones degenerate and don't transmit sound waves. See Otosclerosis in Illness section.
- Sensorineural loss, in which the 8th cranial nerve (the acoustic nerve) is damaged—often for unknown reasons.
- Mixed loss, involving both conductive and sensorineural disabilities.

BODY PARTS INVOLVED—Middle-ear bones that conduct sound; branches of the 8th cranial nerve that transmit sound to the brain.

SEX OR AGE MOST AFFECTED—Both sexes; all ages.

SIGNS & SYMPTOMS—In an infant:
- Lack of response to environmental sounds—especially startling sounds.
In older persons:
- Difficulty in discriminating (listening selectively) to environmental sounds.
- Ringing in the ears.

CAUSES
- Congenital, transmitted as a dominant or recessive genetic trait.
- Chronic middle-ear infections or spread of infection to the inner ear.
- Blood-vessel disorders, including hypertension.
- Head injury.
- Brain tumor.
- Blood clot that travels to the acoustic nerve.
- Multiple sclerosis.
- Syphilis.
- Blood-coagulation disorders.
- Prolonged exposure to sound levels of 85 decibels or above.
- Aging. Most persons over 65 have some hearing loss of high-pitched tones.

RISK INCREASES WITH
- Family history of congenital or acquired deafness.
- Use of drugs, such as streptomycin, tobramycin, quinine, furosemide, ethacrynic acid or heavy doses of aspirin.
- Persons with occupations or hobbies involving high noise levels, such as rock musicians or jackhammer operators.

HOW TO PREVENT
- Avoid prolonged use or overdosage of drugs that cause hearing loss.
- Obtain medical treatment for underlying disorders that cause hearing loss.
- Avoid prolonged exposure to loud noise. If exposure is unavoidable, protect your ears with ear plugs.

 ## WHAT TO EXPECT

APPROPRIATE HEALTH CARE
- Doctor's treatment.
- Surgery for conductive-type deafness (sometimes).
- Speech therapy and rehabilitation, if necessary.

DIAGNOSTIC MEASURES
- Your own observation of symptoms.
- Medical history and physical exam by a doctor.
- Laboratory studies, such as blood studies, audiogram, Weber test, Rinne test (see Glossary for all).

POSSIBLE COMPLICATIONS
- Permanent deafness.
- Delayed language development in a child.

PROBABLE OUTCOME—Some conductive hearing loss is curable with surgery. Hearing loss caused by prolonged exposure to loud noise sometimes disappears when the noise is eliminated. Other types of hearing loss are usually permanent.

 ## HOW TO TREAT

NOTE—Follow your doctor's instructions. These instructions are supplemental.

GENERAL MEASURES
- Contact local rehabilitation facilities to learn sign-language and lip-reading skills.
- Learn to use and wear a hearing aid, if one is prescribed.
- Consult your phone company about special audio equipment for your phone.
- Resist the temptation to withdraw socially because of your hearing difficulty. Isolation will increase your communication problems and frustration, and make adjustment more difficult.

MEDICATION—Medicine usually is not necessary for this disorder.

ACTIVITY—No restrictions.

DIET—No special diet.

 ## CALL YOUR DOCTOR IF

- Your child shows signs of hearing impairment.
- You suspect you have a hearing loss, especially if you must ask others often to repeat themselves or family members frequently ask you if your hearing is all right.

HEART ATTACK
(Myocardial Infarction)

 GENERAL INFORMATION

DEFINITION—Death of heart-muscle cells from reduced or obstructed blood flow through the coronary arteries.

BODY PARTS INVOLVED—Coronary arteries; heart muscle; platelets and clotting factors circulating in the blood.

SEX OR AGE MOST AFFECTED—Adults over 40. This is more common in men, but the incidence is rising for women.

SIGNS & SYMPTOMS
- Chest pain or "heavy, squeezing or crushing" feeling in the chest.
- Sweating.
- Pain that radiates from the chest to the jaw, neck, left arm, the area between the shoulder blades or upper abdomen (sometimes).
- Feeling of impending doom.
- Shortness of breath.
- Nausea and vomiting.

CAUSES—Partial or complete blockage of coronary arteries. Symptoms are often triggered by an emotional crisis, a heavy meal or heavy exercise.

RISK INCREASES WITH
- Smoking.
- High blood-cholesterol levels.
- High blood pressure.
- Diet that is high in fat, sugar and salt.
- Obesity.
- Stress.
- Diabetes mellitus.
- Family history of coronary-artery disease.
- Sedentary lifestyle.
- Fatigue or overwork.
- Exercise in heat or cold and wind.

HOW TO PREVENT—Follow suggestions for prevention of Atherosclerosis (in Illness section).

 WHAT TO EXPECT

APPROPRIATE HEALTH CARE
- Hospitalization.
- Surgery (pacemaker insertion, balloon angioplasty or coronary-artery bypass graft. See Surgery section).

DIAGNOSTIC MEASURES
- Your own observation of symptoms.
- Medical history and physical exam by a doctor.
- Laboratory blood studies.
- EKG (see Glossary).
- Radioactive technetium 99 scan (see Glossary).

POSSIBLE COMPLICATIONS
- Irregular heart rhythms.
- Shock.
- Congestive heart failure.
- Pericarditis.
- Pleural effusion (see Glossary).
- Deep-vein thrombosis.
- Pulmonary embolism.
- Rupture of the heart septum or wall.
- Ventricular aneurysm (see Glossary).

PROBABLE OUTCOME—With immediate emergency care and hospitalization in a coronary-care unit, most persons recover from a first heart attack. Treatment delay is often fatal. Survivors should allow 6 to 8 weeks for recovery.

 HOW TO TREAT

NOTE—Follow your doctor's instructions. These instructions are supplemental.

GENERAL MEASURES—If a heart-attack victim is unconscious and *not* breathing:
- Yell for help. Don't leave the victim.
- Begin mouth-to-mouth breathing immediately.
- If there is no heartbeat, give external cardiac massage.
- Have someone call O (operator) or 911 (emergency) for help.
- Don't stop CPR until help arrives.

MEDICATION—Your doctor may prescribe:
- Pain relievers.
- Antiarrhythmic and antianginal drugs, such as beta-adrenergic blockers or calcium-channel blockers, to stabilize an irregular heartbeat.
- Anticoagulants to prevent blood clots.
- Nitroglycerin to widen arteries and increase blood supply to the heart.
- Digitalis to strengthen heart-muscle contractions and stabilize the heartbeat.

ACTIVITY—Resume your normal activities gradually during recovery. Consult your doctor before resuming sexual relations.

DIET—Eat a low-fat, low-salt, high-fiber diet (see Appendices 8 and 9).

 CALL YOUR DOCTOR IF

- You have symptoms of a heart attack. This is a life-threatening emergency!
- The following occurs during recovery:
  Chest pain that is not relieved by prescribed medication.
  Shortness of breath or cough while at rest.
  Nausea, vomiting or diarrhea.
  Fever over 100F (37.8C).
  Bleeding from the gums or other sites.

HEART BLOCK
(Atrioventricular Block)

GENERAL INFORMATION

DEFINITION—A chronic disruption (either mild or major) in transmission of electrical signals between the heart's upper and lower chambers. Contractions of the atria (upper heart chambers) lose synchronization with those of the ventricles (lower heart chambers). The heartbeat is no longer regulated normally to quicken under exertion or stress and slow down at other times.

BODY PARTS INVOLVED—Heart's electrical-transmission system that coordinates contractions of heart-muscle cells. The heart's natural pacemaker initiates the electrical system.

SEX OR AGE MOST AFFECTED—All ages, but most common in men over 40 and women after menopause.

SIGNS & SYMPTOMS
- No symptoms (sometimes) for less-severe forms.
- Slow, irregular heartbeat.
- Sudden loss of consciousness.
- Convulsions (sometimes).

CAUSES
- Coronary-artery disease, a sign of atherosclerosis (hardening of the arteries).
- Congenital heart abnormalities.
- Excessive digitalis dosage.

RISK INCREASES WITH
- Adults over 60.
- Stress.
- Improper diet that is high in fat and salt.
- Obesity.
- Smoking.
- Diabetes mellitus.
- Heart disease, including atherosclerosis, congestive heart failure or heart-valve disease.
- High blood pressure.
- Previous electrolyte imbalance.
- Use of some drugs, such as digitalis, quinidine or beta-adrenergic blockers.
- Sick-sinus syndrome (see Glossary).

HOW TO PREVENT
- Obtain medical treatment for any underlying disease.
- Don't smoke.
- Exercise regularly (see Appendix 20).
- Eat a diet that is low in fat (see Appendix 8) and low in salt (see Appendix 9).

WHAT TO EXPECT

APPROPRIATE HEALTH CARE
- Self-care after diagnosis.
- Doctor's treatment.

- Surgery to implant an artificial pacemaker (sometimes).

DIAGNOSTIC MEASURES
- Your own observation of symptoms.
- Medical history and physical exam by a doctor.
- EKG (see Glossary).
- Holter monitor, a 12- or 24-hour continuous EKG monitor (see Glossary).

POSSIBLE COMPLICATIONS—Uncontrolled rapid, irregular heartbeat and cardiac arrest.

PROBABLE OUTCOME—Symptoms can be controlled with surgery to implant a pacemaker.

HOW TO TREAT

NOTE—Follow your doctor's instructions. These instructions are supplemental.

GENERAL MEASURES
- Wear a Medic-Alert bracelet or pendant (see Glossary) in case you suddenly lose consciousness.
- Don't smoke.

MEDICATION—There are no medications that cure heart block, but there are some that make it worse. Don't take medications to relieve allergy or nasal congestion, including antihistamines, or any stimulant, including caffeine, cocaine or marijuana.

ACTIVITY—Don't think of yourself as an invalid. Unless your doctor advises against it, mild exercise is helpful and not to be feared. Begin a regular exercise program—walking is ideal—and increase the amount daily.

DIET
- Lose weight if you are overweight. A reducing diet appears in Appendix 10. Don't use amphetamines or other appetite suppressants to curb your appetite.
- Avoid excessive use of alcoholic beverages. Alcohol depresses the heartbeat.
- Avoid caffeine in all forms. It is in coffee, tea, cocoa, cola drinks and chocolate.

CALL YOUR DOCTOR IF

- You have symptoms of heart block, especially an episode with loss of consciousness.
- After diagnosis, stress increases in your life.

HEART-RHYTHM IRREGULARITY
(Arrhythmia)

 GENERAL INFORMATION

DEFINITION—Occasional or constant abnormalities in the rhythm of the heartbeat.

BODY PARTS INVOLVED—Heart; nerves that transmit impulses to coordinate heart-muscle contractions.

SEX OR AGE MOST AFFECTED—All ages, but most likely over age 65.

SIGNS & SYMPTOMS
- Awareness of one's own heartbeat, including whether it skips, is always fast, slow, irregular, or suddenly changes rhythm.
- Shortness of breath.
- Sudden faintness or weakness.
- No symptoms (frequently).

CAUSES
- Heart diseases, such as: rheumatic fever; congenital heart disease; cardiomyopathy; previous heart attack; or heart-muscle inflammation.
- Endocrine disorders, especially thyroid and adrenal-gland diseases.
- Fluid and electrolyte imbalance, especially too little or too much potassium.
- Side effects of certain drugs, especially digitalis, beta-adrenergic blockers, stimulants and diuretics.
- Overdose of certain drugs, including antidepressants, marijuana and cocaine.
- Postoperative effects following chest or heart surgery.

RISK INCREASES WITH
- Stress.
- Chronic kidney disease.
- Hypertension.
- Use of certain drugs, such as caffeine, alcohol, amphetamines, and many non-prescription cough and cold remedies.
- Smoking.
- Fatigue or overwork.

HOW TO PREVENT—If you have any disorders listed as causes or risks, follow your treatment program carefully to control the disease. If medication is part of your treatment, consult your doctor about having blood levels monitored and electrolytes measured periodically.

 WHAT TO EXPECT

APPROPRIATE HEALTH CARE
- Doctor's treatment.
- Psychotherapy or counseling, if stress is a major factor.
- DC cardioversion (see Glossary) in a hospital or outpatient surgical facility.

- Surgery to correct some heart problems (coronary-artery bypass, damaged valve replacement or insertion of a pacemaker).

DIAGNOSTIC MEASURES
- Your own observation of symptoms.
- Medical history and physical exam by a doctor (sometimes a cardiologist).
- Laboratory blood studies.
- EKG and 24-hour Holter monitor (see Glossary for both).
- X-rays of the heart, including echocardiogram (see Glossary).

POSSIBLE COMPLICATIONS
- Fainting.
- Congestive heart failure.
- Death from prolonged (more than 3 to 6 minutes) cardiac arrest.

PROBABLE OUTCOME—Most rhythm disturbances can be controlled with treatment.

 HOW TO TREAT

NOTE—Follow your doctor's instructions. These instructions are supplemental.

GENERAL MEASURES
- Consider lifestyle changes. See Appendix 13.
- Wear a Medic-Alert bracelet or pendant (see Glossary) showing the name of your condition.
- A few arrhythmias are fatal unless cardiopulmonary resuscitation (CPR) is performed immediately. Take a course to learn CPR, especially if someone in your home or neighborhood has heart disease.

MEDICATION—Your doctor may prescribe antiarrhythmic medications. You may need to try several to find the most effective one.

ACTIVITY—Resume most normal activities as soon as symptoms improve. Consult your doctor about exercise.

DIET
- Some heart medicines require extra potassium, found mostly in citrus fruits, bananas, dried apricots or peaches, raisins, lentils and whole-grain cereals. Ask your doctor if you need to eat more of these.
- Don't drink caffeine-containing beverages, such as coffee, tea, cola or chocolate.

 CALL YOUR DOCTOR IF

- You have symptoms of heart-rhythm irregularity.
- New, unexplained symptoms develop. Drugs used in treatment may produce side effects.

HEART-VALVE DISEASE
(Valvular Heart Disease)

 GENERAL INFORMATION

DEFINITION—A complication of diseases that distort or destroy valves of the heart.

BODY PARTS INVOLVED—Heart valves (aortic, mitral, tricuspid and pulmonic valves).

SEX OR AGE MOST AFFECTED—Both sexes; all ages.

SIGNS & SYMPTOMS
- No symptoms (sometimes).
- Fatigue and weakness.
- Dizziness or fainting.
- Chest pain.
- Shortness of breath.
- Lung congestion.
- Heart-rhythm irregularities.
- Heart murmurs (abnormal heart sounds heard by the doctor through a stethoscope).
- Abnormal blood pressure (high or low).

CAUSES—The heart has 4 valves. The mitral and tricuspid valves (main heart valves) control blood flow into the ventricles. The aortic and pulmonic valves control blood flow out of the heart. Heart-valve disease can be either narrowed valves (stenosis), which obstructs blood flow, or widened or scarred valves, which allow blood to leak backward into the heart (insufficiency). The disorder may be inherited or caused by any of the following:
- Rheumatic fever.
- Atherosclerosis.
- High blood pressure.
- Congenital heart defects.
- Endocarditis.
- Syphilis (rare).

RISK INCREASES WITH
- Persons over 60.
- Family history of heart-valve disease.
- Pregnancy.
- Fatigue or overwork.

HOW TO PREVENT
- Obtain medical treatment for diseases that cause heart-valve damage, such as high blood pressure, endocarditis and syphilis.
- Take antibiotics for streptococcal infections to prevent rheumatic fever.
- If you have a family history of congenital heart disease, obtain genetic counseling before starting a family.

 WHAT TO EXPECT

APPROPRIATE HEALTH CARE
- Self-care after diagnosis.
- Doctor's treatment.
- Hospitalization.
- Surgery to replace or open defective valves (sometimes).

DIAGNOSTIC MEASURES
- Your own observation of symptoms.
- Medical history and physical exam by a doctor.
- Laboratory blood tests.
- EKG (see Glossary).
- Heart catheterization (see Glossary).
- X-rays of the heart, lungs and blood flow (angiography).

POSSIBLE COMPLICATIONS
- Infection of the valves.
- Congestive heart failure.

PROBABLE OUTCOME—Depends on the underlying condition. Many complications of valvular disease can be controlled with medication or cured with surgery.

 HOW TO TREAT

NOTE—Follow your doctor's instructions. These instructions are supplemental.

GENERAL MEASURES—Tell any doctor, dentist or anesthesiologist who treats you that you have heart-valve disease. Remind those involved, even if you think they know the details of your medical history.

MEDICATION—Your doctor may prescribe:
- Antibiotics to treat or prevent bacterial infection of abnormal heart valves.
- Antiarrhythmic drugs to stabilize heartbeat irregularities.
- Digitalis medication to strengthen or regulate the heartbeat.

ACTIVITY—As much as can be tolerated. No restrictions are necessary with some forms of heart-valve disease.

DIET—Eat a low-fat, low-salt diet (see Appendices 8 and 9).

 CALL YOUR DOCTOR IF

- You have symptoms of heart-valve disease.
- During treatment, you develop signs of infection, such as fever, chills, muscle aches, headache, fatigue and a general ill feeling.

HEARTBEAT, RAPID
(Tachycardia; Paroxysmal Tachycardia)

 GENERAL INFORMATION

DEFINITION—Heartbeat that is much more rapid than usual and is not caused by overexertion. Normal heartbeat ranges are 70 to 90 beats per minute in adults and 80 to 110 beats per minute in children. Tachycardia ranges from 150 to 300 beats per minute. A person with no heart disease may exercise and raise the heartbeat to 160 or more. This is normal and is not a medical problem.

BODY PARTS INVOLVED—Heart muscle; electrical system of the heart.

SEX OR AGE MOST AFFECTED—Both sexes; all ages.

SIGNS & SYMPTOMS
- Heart pounding or palpitations. The pulse at the wrist or neck will be 100 to 180 beats per minute, which is much faster than normal.
- Faintness or a feeling of impending death.
- Increased urination.
- Chest pain.
- Involuntary cough.
- Breathlessness.

CAUSES—Unknown. This usually occurs in young persons with no evidence of disease, but it may also occur in older patients who have coronary-artery disease.

RISK INCREASES WITH
- Heart disease.
- Stress.
- Smoking.
- Use of some drugs, such as caffeine, ephedrine or other sympathomimetic drugs.
- Fatigue or overwork.

HOW TO PREVENT
- Don't smoke.
- Reduce stress, if possible. See Appendix 13.

 WHAT TO EXPECT

APPROPRIATE HEALTH CARE
- Doctor's treatment.
- Self-care after diagnosis.
- Hospitalization if the attack persists, despite treatment.
- DC electrocardioversion, a controlled electric shock (rarely necessary).

DIAGNOSTIC MEASURES
- Your own observation of symptoms.
- Medical history and physical exam by a doctor.
- EKG (see Glossary).

POSSIBLE COMPLICATIONS—Uninterrupted tachycardia can lead to life-threatening congestive heart failure, heart attack or cardiac arrest.

PROBABLE OUTCOME—Rapid heartbeat can usually be controlled with treatment.

 HOW TO TREAT

NOTE—Follow your doctor's instructions. These instructions are supplemental.

GENERAL MEASURES—The following sometimes reduce heartbeat:
- Hold your breath briefly.
- Pinch the skin on your arm enough to cause pain.
- Bathe your face in cold water, submerge your head briefly in a sink of cool water or take a cool shower and let the water beat on your head.
- Hold your nostrils closed and blow gently through the nose, making the eardrums pop.
- Massage the carotid area in the neck, *if you have been taught to do this safely.* Ask your doctor for instructions.

MEDICATION—For repeated attacks, your doctor may prescribe medication to control heart rhythm. These include: digitalis; quinidine; calcium-channel blockers; procainamide; and beta-adrenergic blockers.

ACTIVITY—Lie down during an attack until your heartbeat returns to normal, then resume your activities. Between attacks, exercise regularly (see Appendix 20) with your doctor's approval. Physical fitness helps prevent tachycardia.

DIET—No special diet.

 CALL YOUR DOCTOR IF

- You have an episode of rapid, irregular heartbeat that does not end in 4 or 5 minutes.
- You develop shortness of breath.
- You have chest pain.

ILLNESSES & DISORDERS

HEADBURN

GENERAL INFORMATION

DEFINITION—Discomfort in the upper digestive tract. Heartburn is a symptom—not a disease—and has nothing to do with the heart.

BODY PARTS INVOLVED—Stomach; lower esophagus.

SEX OR AGE MOST AFFECTED—All ages, but most common in adults over 60.

SIGNS & SYMPTOMS—The following signs are worse at night:
- Belching or slight regurgitation of stomach contents into the mouth, producing an acid taste.
- Heavy, uncomfortable sensation in the chest.
- Swallowing difficulty.
- Mild abdominal pain.
- Vomiting (rarely).

CAUSES
- Hiatal hernia (part of stomach protrudes into the chest).
- Ulcers of the esophagus.
- Irritation of the lower esophagus caused by stomach acid spilling into the esophagus.

RISK INCREASES WITH
- Stress.
- Improper diet.
- Obesity.
- Smoking.
- Excess alcohol consumption.
- Use of drugs, such as aspirin, arthritis medicine or cortisone.

HOW TO PREVENT—No specific preventive measures. Consider lifestyle changes (see Appendix 12).

WHAT TO EXPECT

APPROPRIATE HEALTH CARE
- Self-care.
- Doctor's treatment.
- Hospitalization for special studies or surgery (rarely).

DIAGNOSTIC MEASURES
- Your own observation of symptoms.
- Medical history and physical exam by a doctor.
- Laboratory studies, such as blood studies, EKG (see Glossary) to exclude chance of heart disease; esophagoscopy (see Glossary).
- X-rays of the upper digestive tract.

POSSIBLE COMPLICATIONS
- Misdiagnosis of a heart attack that produces symptoms similar to heartburn.
- If heartburn is caused by a large hiatal hernia, surgery may be necessary to repair the hernia.
- If heartburn is caused by ulcers in the esophagus, surgery may be necessary to remove scar tissue. Scar tissue forms with repeated ulceration and healing and may interfere with swallowing.

PROBABLE OUTCOME—Symptoms can be controlled with treatment, but recurrence is common.

HOW TO TREAT

NOTE—Follow your doctor's instructions. These instructions are supplemental.

GENERAL MEASURES
- Elevate the head of the bed 4 to 6 inches with blocks.
- Don't smoke.
- Lose weight if you are overweight.
- Don't bend over, lie down or exercise immediately after eating.
- Don't wear tight pantyhose, girdles, belts or pants.

MEDICATION—For minor discomfort, you may use non-prescription liquid antacids. These preparations coat the inside of the esophagus and neutralize stomach acid. Follow instructions on the bottle. The usual dose is 1 tablespoon taken 1 hour after meals and at bedtime.

ACTIVITY—Resume normal activities as soon as symptoms subside.

DIET—Avoid foods and beverages that stimulate heavy stomach-acid secretion, such as spicy dishes, coffee, acid fruit juice or alcohol. Avoid chocolate, and reduce your consumption of fatty foods.

CALL YOUR DOCTOR IF

- Swallowing becomes more difficult.
- You regurgitate blood when you have heartburn.
- Heartburn continues despite self-care.
- The following symptoms accompany heartburn:
  Shortness of breath.
  Sweating.
  Pain in the jaw, neck and arm.
  Nausea.

HEARTBURN DURING PREGNANCY

GENERAL INFORMATION

DEFINITION—Burning pain in the chest and upper abdomen during pregnancy.

BODY PARTS INVOLVED—Stomach; esophagus.

SEX OR AGE MOST AFFECTED—Occurs in at least half of all pregnant women.

SIGNS & SYMPTOMS
- Burning pain in the center of the chest and upper abdomen, frequently accompanied by an unpleasant taste in the mouth.
- Belching.

CAUSES—Heartburn is not associated with a heart disorder. It is caused by a backflow of acid from the stomach into the esophagus. The muscles that close off the upper stomach become lax, allowing stomach juices to enter the esophagus and irritate its lining. During late pregnancy, the enlarged womb presses on the stomach and causes this.

RISK INCREASES WITH
- Overeating or eating before lying down.
- Smoking.
- Excess alcohol consumption.

HOW TO PREVENT—Avoid risk factors listed above.

WHAT TO EXPECT

APPROPRIATE HEALTH CARE
- Doctor's diagnosis.
- Self-care after diagnosis.

DIAGNOSTIC MEASURES
- Your own observation of symptoms.
- Medical history and physical exam by a doctor.

POSSIBLE COMPLICATIONS—Inflammation and ulcer in the lower esophagus (rare).

PROBABLE OUTCOME—This is an uncomfortable—but harmless—condition. It disappears after the baby is born unless its cause is not related to pregnancy.

HOW TO TREAT

NOTE—Follow your doctor's instructions. These instructions are supplemental.

GENERAL MEASURES
- Avoid stooping, especially after eating.
- Don't wear tight girdles or belts.
- Place books or blocks under the head of your bed to raise it about 4 inches.
- Don't smoke.

MEDICATION—Medicine usually is not necessary for this disorder. Avoid *all* medicines while pregnant, if possible. If your doctor prescribes one, question him or her. Be sure the benefit outweighs the risk. As long as you can live with the symptoms, endure the discomfort without drugs or medicines.

ACTIVITY—Stay active. Avoid abdominal exercises that require bending.

DIET
- Eat small, frequent meals.
- Don't eat before bedtime.
- Avoid highly seasoned food.
- Don't drink alcohol.
- Avoid very hot or very cold beverages.

CALL YOUR DOCTOR IF

- You have symptoms of heartburn during pregnancy. This should be diagnosed.
- The following occurs after diagnosis:
  Simple measures don't bring relief.
  You begin vomiting late in pregnancy.
  You vomit material that has blood in it or looks life coffee grounds.
  You have black or tarry stools.

HEATSTROKE OR HEAT EXHAUSTION
(Sunstroke or Heat Prostration)

 GENERAL INFORMATION

DEFINITION—Illness caused by prolonged exposure to hot temperatures.

BODY PARTS INVOLVED—Total body.

SEX OR AGE MOST AFFECTED—All ages, but most common in the elderly.

SIGNS & SYMPTOMS—Heatstroke:
- Sudden dizziness, weakness, faintness and headache.
- Skin that is hot and dry.
- No sweating.
- High body temperature—frequently 102F (38.9C) or higher.
- Rapid heartbeat.
- Muscle cramps.

Heat exhaustion:
- Skin that is cool and moist.
- Pale or gray skin color.
- Slow pulse.
- Confusion.
- Muscle cramps.
- Low or normal body temperature.
- Dark yellow or orange urine.

CAUSES—Heatstroke:
Failure of the body's heat-regulating mechanisms, leading to a heat buildup in the body. The failure may be a result of:
- General effects of aging.
- Alcoholism.
- Chronic illness.
- Diabetes.
- Blood-vessel disease.

Heat exhaustion:
- Loss of body fluids from sweating and failure to drink enough replacement fluid.

RISK INCREASES WITH
- Adults over 60.
- Sweating and inadequate fluid intake.
- Recent illness involving fluid loss from vomiting or diarrhea.
- Hot, humid weather.
- Working in a hot environment.

HOW TO PREVENT
- Wear light, loose-fitting clothing in hot weather.
- Drink extra water if you sweat heavily. Be guided by your urine output. If the output decreases, increase your water intake.
- If you become overheated, improve your ventilation. Open a window or use a fan or air conditioner. This promotes sweat evaporation, which cools the skin.

 WHAT TO EXPECT

APPROPRIATE HEALTH CARE
- Self-care after diagnosis (mild cases).
- Doctor's treatment.
- Hospitalization to lower body temperature and provide intravenous replacement fluids.

DIAGNOSTIC MEASURES
- Your own observation of symptoms.
- Medical history and physical exam by a doctor.
- Laboratory studies of blood and urine to measure electrolyte levels.

POSSIBLE COMPLICATIONS
- Shock.
- Brain damage caused by prolonged, high body temperature (106F or 41.1C).

PROBABLE OUTCOME—Prompt treatment usually brings full recovery in 1 to 2 days.

 HOW TO TREAT

NOTE—Follow your doctor's instructions. These instructions are supplemental.

GENERAL MEASURES
- If someone with symptoms is very hot and *not sweating:*
  Cool the person rapidly. Use a cold-water bath or wrap in wet sheets.
  Arrange for transportation to the nearest hospital. This is an emergency!
- If someone is faint *but sweating:*
  Give the person liquids (water, soft drinks or fruit juice). Don't give salt pills.
  Arrange for transportation to the hospital, except in mild cases. Call your doctor for advice.

MEDICATION—Medicine usually is not necessary for this disorder.

ACTIVITY—Activity may be resumed as soon as symptoms improve.

DIET—No special diet.

 CALL YOUR DOCTOR IF

You have symptoms of heatstroke or heat exhaustion, or observe them in someone else. Call immediately! These conditions may be serious or fatal.

HEEL SPUR
(Calcaneal Spur)

 GENERAL INFORMATION

DEFINITION—A hard, bony growth in the tissue of the heel that causes pain and difficulty walking.

BODY PARTS INVOLVED—Heel, including the calcaneus (the major bone in the heel).

SEX OR AGE MOST AFFECTED—Adults (20 to 60 years).

SIGNS & SYMPTOMS—Pain and tenderness in the sole of the foot, under the heel bone.

CAUSES—Stress or injury to the heel tissues, which causes inflammation and calcification of ligaments in the foot.

RISK INCREASES WITH
- Running or jogging. The condition is less likely with vigorous walking.
- Prolonged standing.

HOW TO PREVENT
- Avoid activities that put constant strain on the foot.
- Wear a shoe with a rubber or felt heel cushion.

 WHAT TO EXPECT

APPROPRIATE HEALTH CARE
- Self-care after diagnosis.
- Doctor's treatment.
- Surgery to remove the spur (rare).

DIAGNOSTIC MEASURES
- Your own observation of symptoms.
- Medical history and physical exam by a doctor.
- X-rays of the heel.

POSSIBLE COMPLICATIONS—Lower-back or knee disorders caused by constant limping.

PROBABLE OUTCOME—Usually curable with conservative treatment (see How to Treat). If not, heel spurs are curable with surgery.

 HOW TO TREAT

NOTE—Follow your doctor's instructions. These instructions are supplemental.

GENERAL MEASURES—Place a doughnut-shaped rubber or felt insert in the shoe to relieve pressure on the heel.

MEDICATION
- To relieve minor pain, you may use non-prescription drugs, such as acetaminophen or aspirin.
- Your doctor may inject steroids into the inflamed area to reduce inflammation.

ACTIVITY—Stay off your feet as much as possible, especially at the beginning of treatment.

DIET—No special diet, unless you are overweight. If so, lose weight to reduce stress on the foot. A reducing diet appears in Appendix 1.

 CALL YOUR DOCTOR IF

- You have symptoms of a heel spur.
- Pain or disability persists, despite treatment.

ILLNESSES & DISORDERS

HEMIPLEGIA

GENERAL INFORMATION

DEFINITION—Partial or complete paralysis of one side of the body.

BODY PARTS INVOLVED—Brain.

SEX OR AGE MOST AFFECTED—Both sexes; all ages.

SIGNS & SYMPTOMS—Because of the anatomy of the brain and spinal cord, injury to one side of the brain affects the opposite side of the body. The following signs and symptoms vary greatly between individuals:
- Weakness or paralysis of the arm and leg on the affected side.
- Difficulty speaking, understanding or recognizing words.
- Altered or lost sensation on the affected side.
- Difficulty with self-feeding.
- Urinary incontinence.
- Blurred, double or decreased vision.

CAUSES—Brain injury in an area that controls one side of the body. Injury may result from:
- Stroke (the most common). Stroke may be caused by bleeding in the brain, or a blood clot or other obstruction of a blood vessel to the brain.
- Brain tumor.
- Head injury.
- Multiple sclerosis.

RISK INCREASES WITH
- Hypertension.
- Diabetes.

HOW TO PREVENT
- Obtain medical treatment to control hypertension or diabetes.
- Protect yourself from head injury:
  Use seat belts in cars.
  Wear protective headgear during contact sports, or while riding a bicycle or motorcycle.
  Don't drink alcohol or use mind-altering drugs and drive.

WHAT TO EXPECT

APPROPRIATE HEALTH CARE
- Doctor's treatment.
- Hospitalization.
- Psychotherapy or counseling for depression, and to learn to cope with disability.
- Physical therapy.
- Long-term nursing-home care (sometimes).

DIAGNOSTIC MEASURES
- Your own observation of symptoms.
- Medical history and physical exam by a doctor.
- Laboratory studies of blood, urine and cerebrospinal fluid.
- EKG (see Glossary).
- X-rays of the brain and neck.

POSSIBLE COMPLICATIONS
- Pressure sores.
- Shortening of the muscles (contractures).
- Slow deterioration of the musculo-skeletal system.

PROBABLE OUTCOME—Depends on the extent of injury. Brain tissue does not repair itself, but other parts of the brain can take over lost functions.

HOW TO TREAT

NOTE—Follow your doctor's instructions. These instructions are supplemental.

GENERAL MEASURES
- Ask family and friends for support, and obtain professional help in readjusting your life.
- Sleep on an egg-crate foam mattress or a waterbed to prevent pressure sores.

MEDICATION—No medication can repair damaged brain tissue, but your doctor may prescribe:
- Medications to control hypertension, diabetes or other underlying disorders.
- Anticoagulants to prevent blood-clot formation, if a stroke resulting from a clot caused the paralysis.

ACTIVITY—Resume your normal activities gradually. With rehabilitation, many lost functions can be compensated for or restored.
   Use passive exercise for paralyzed or partially paralyzed muscles to prevent contractures.

DIET—No special diet for hemiplegia, but diabetes or hypertension may require special diets. Consult your doctor.

CALL YOUR DOCTOR IF

- You have symptoms of hemiplegia.
- The following occurs during treatment:
  Signs of infection, such as fever, muscle aches, chills and headache.
  Difficulty in emptying the bladder.
- New, unexplained symptoms develop. Drugs used in treatment may produce side effects.

HEMOPHILIA

 GENERAL INFORMATION

DEFINITION—An inherited deficiency of a blood-clotting factor that results in dangerous bleeding.

BODY PARTS INVOLVED—All body parts.

SEX OR AGE MOST AFFECTED—Affects 1 in 10,000 males, and appears early in childhood.

SIGNS & SYMPTOMS
- Painful, swollen joints or swelling in the leg or arm (especially the knee or elbow) when bleeding occurs.
- Frequent bruises.
- Excessive bleeding from minor cuts.
- Spontaneous nosebleeds.
- Blood in the urine.

CAUSES—The deficiency of a coagulation factor passed by a female carrier to male children in an X-linked recessive gene.

RISK INCREASES WITH—No known risk factor.

HOW TO PREVENT—Cannot be prevented at present. If your family has a history of hemophilia, obtain genetic counseling before having children.

 WHAT TO EXPECT

APPROPRIATE HEALTH CARE
- Doctor's treatment. Doctor should be a qualified hematologist (blood specialist).
- Hospitalization or care in an outpatient facility for transfusions of plasma and various blood factors.
- Self-care.

DIAGNOSTIC MEASURES
- Your own observation of symptoms.
- Medical history and physical exam by a doctor.
- Laboratory blood studies.

POSSIBLE COMPLICATIONS
- Dangerous bleeding episodes requiring emergency treatment.
- Permanent joint disability caused by persistent bleeding.
- Hepatitis or AIDS from blood transfusions.

PROBABLE OUTCOME—This condition is currently considered incurable, but not fatal. If bleeding can be controlled, patients can expect a nearly normal life span.

Scientific research into causes and treatment continues, so there is hope for increasingly effective treatment and cure.

 HOW TO TREAT

NOTE—Follow your doctor's instructions. These instructions are supplemental.

GENERAL MEASURES
- For bleeding at any accessible site, apply direct pressure by hand or elastic bandage or apply ice and elevate the limb. Call your doctor immediately.
- In case of emergency, wear a bracelet or pendant that identifies you as a person who has hemophilia.

MEDICATION
- Your doctor may prescribe:
  Medication to reduce joint pain.
  Transfusions of plasma or clotting factors.
- Don't take aspirin. It may increase bleeding.

ACTIVITY—Avoid activities that can cause injury, such as contact sports. Swim, bicycle or walk instead. Otherwise, no restrictions.

DIET—No special diet.

 CALL YOUR DOCTOR IF

- You have symptoms of hemophilia.
- The following occurs after diagnosis:
  Injury with swelling. This may indicate bleeding under the skin.
  Bleeding that isn't quickly controlled.
  Tender, painful, swollen joint.

ILLNESSES & DISORDERS

HEMORRHOIDS
(Piles)

 GENERAL INFORMATION

DEFINITION—Dilated (varicose) veins of the rectum or anus.

BODY PARTS INVOLVED—Veins under the rectal or anal membrane.

SEX OR AGE MOST AFFECTED—Adults of both sexes.

SIGNS & SYMPTOMS
- Rectal bleeding. Bright-red blood may appear as streaks on toilet paper adhering to fecal residue, or it may be a slow trickle for a short while following bowel movements.
- Pain, itching or mucus discharge after bowel movements.
- A lump that can be felt in the anus.
- A sensation that the rectum has not emptied completely after a bowel movement (large hemorrhoids only).

CAUSES
- Repeated pressure in the anal or rectal veins—usually caused by straining during bowel movements.
- Abdominal or rectal tumors—benign or malignant.

RISK INCREASES WITH
- Diet that lacks fiber; constipation.
- Obesity.
- Pregnancy.

HOW TO PREVENT
- Don't try to hurry bowel movements.
- Lose weight if you are overweight.

OTHER—Straining during bowel movements increases pain.

 WHAT TO EXPECT

APPROPRIATE HEALTH CARE
- Self-care.
- Doctor's treatment.
- Surgery to remove hemorrhoids (sometimes).

DIAGNOSTIC MEASURES
- Your own observation of symptoms.
- Medical history and physical exam by a doctor.
- Anoscopy (see Glossary) or sigmoidoscopy (see Glossary).
- X-rays of the lower intestinal tract.

POSSIBLE COMPLICATIONS
- Iron-deficiency anemia if blood loss is significant.
- Severe pain caused by a blood clot in a hemorrhoid.
- Infection or ulceration of a hemorrhoid.

 HOW TO TREAT

NOTE—Follow your doctor's instructions. These instructions are supplemental.

GENERAL MEASURES
- Clean the anal area gently with soft, moist paper after each bowel movement.
- To relieve pain, sit in 8 to 10 inches of hot water for 10 to 20 minutes several times a day.
- To reduce pain and swelling of a blood clot or protruding hemorrhoid, stay in bed for 1 day and apply ice packs to the anal area.

MEDICATION
- For minor pain, you may use non-prescription drugs that contain zinc oxide or low-strength steroids.
- Your doctor may prescribe a stool softener or bulk laxative.

ACTIVITY—No restrictions. Bowel function improves with good physical conditioning.

DIET—To prevent constipation, eat a well-balanced diet that contains many high-fiber foods such as fresh fruit, vegetables and whole-grain cereals. See Appendix 1.

 CALL YOUR DOCTOR IF

- A hard lump develops where a hemorrhoid has been.
- Hemorrhoids cause severe pain that isn't relieved by treatment above.
- Rectal bleeding is excessive (more than a trace or streak on toilet paper or stool).

HEPATITIS, ACUTE VIRAL

 GENERAL INFORMATION

DEFINITION—Inflammation of the liver caused by a virus.

BODY PARTS INVOLVED—Liver.

SEX OR AGE MOST AFFECTED—Both sexes; all ages.

SIGNS & SYMPTOMS—Early stages:
- Flulike symptoms, such as fever, fatigue, nausea, vomiting, diarrhea and loss of appetite.
Several days later:
- Jaundice (yellow eyes and skin) caused by a buildup of bile in the blood.
- Dark urine from bile spilling over into the urine.
- Light, "clay-colored" or whitish stools.

CAUSES—Any of 3 different but related viruses that may infect the liver:
- Type A: Usually enters the body through water or food, especially raw shellfish, that has been contaminated by sewage.
- Type B: Usually enters the body through blood transfusions contaminated with the virus or from injections with non-sterile needles or syringes.
- Type Non-A, Non-B: Usually enters the body by contaminated blood transfusions.

RISK INCREASES WITH
- Travel to areas with poor sanitation.
- Oral-anal sexual practices.
- Use of intravenous, mind-altering drugs.
- Alcoholism.
- Blood transfusions.
- Hospital workers.
- Kidney-dialysis treatment.
- Poor nutrition.
- Illness that has lowered resistance.

HOW TO PREVENT
- Avoid risks listed above.
- If you are exposed to someone with hepatitis, consult your doctor about receiving gamma-globulin injections to prevent or decrease the risk of hepatitis.
- If you are in a high-risk group, such as hospital workers or male homosexuals, consult your doctor about having a vaccine for Type-B hepatitis. Vaccines are not available for other forms.

 WHAT TO EXPECT

APPROPRIATE HEALTH CARE
- Self-care after diagnosis (mild cases).
- Doctor's treatment.
- Hospitalization (severe cases).

DIAGNOSTIC MEASURES
- Your own observation of symptoms.
- Medical history and physical exam by a doctor.
- Laboratory blood tests to identify infection (Type A and Type B) and study liver function.
- Urinalysis.

POSSIBLE COMPLICATIONS—Liver failure in severe cases.

PROBABLE OUTCOME—Jaundice and other symptoms peak and then gradually disappear over 3 to 16 weeks. Most people in good general health recover fully in 1 to 4 months. A small percentage (1% to 2%) may proceed to chronic hepatitis. Recovery from viral hepatitis usually provides permanent immunity against it.

 HOW TO TREAT

NOTE—Follow your doctor's instructions. These instructions are supplemental.

GENERAL MEASURES
- Most persons with hepatitis can be cared for at home without undue risk. Strict isolation is not necessary, but the ill person should have separate eating and drinking utensils, or use disposable ones.
- If you have hepatitis or are caring for someone with it, wash your hands carefully and often, especially after bowel movements.

MEDICATION—Your doctor may prescribe cortisone drugs for severe cases to reduce liver inflammation.

ACTIVITY—Bed rest is necessary until jaundice disappears and appetite returns. People differ widely in the rate at which they can return to normal activity.

DIET—Despite poor appetite, small well-balanced meals help promote recovery. At least 8 glasses of water are necessary each day. *Don't drink alcohol.*

 CALL YOUR DOCTOR IF

- You have symptoms of hepatitis, or have been exposed to someone who has it.
- The following occurs during treatment:
  Increasing loss of appetite.
  Excessive drowsiness or mental confusion.
  Vomiting, diarrhea or abdominal pain.
  Deepening jaundice.
  Skin rash or itching.

HEPATITIS IN CHILDREN

 GENERAL INFORMATION

DEFINITION—Inflammation of the liver. Hepatitis has several forms. The most common are infectious hepatitis (hepatitis A) and serum hepatitis (hepatitis B). All forms are contagious.

BODY PARTS INVOLVED—Liver.

SEX OR AGE MOST AFFECTED—Infants and young children (2 weeks to 5 years).

SIGNS & SYMPTOMS—Symptoms vary greatly between children. Early symptoms are non-specific and include:
- Fever.
- Headache.
- Muscle aches.
- Loss of appetite.
- General ill feeling.

Later symptoms include:
- Nausea; vomiting.
- Abdominal pain.
- Foul breath; bitter taste.
- Jaundice (yellow whites of eyes and skin; dark urine).
- Swollen, tender liver (sometimes).

CAUSES—Viruses cause several types:
- Hepatitis A is spread by person-to-person contact. Eating or drinking contaminated food or water, including shellfish from polluted waters, also spreads infectious hepatitis.
- Hepatitis B is spread primarily by inoculation of serum or blood from an individual with the virus. It can occur with blood transfusions or with the use of contaminated syringes or improperly sterilized instruments or needles.
   Blood-sucking insects are also suspected as sources of hepatitis B.
- Other forms of hepatitis are spread by any of the above methods.

RISK INCREASES WITH
- Crowded or unsanitary living conditions.
- Exposure to others in public places.

HOW TO PREVENT
- Don't eat shellfish from areas with poor sanitation systems.
- Isolate a child with hepatitis.
- When caring for a child with hepatitis, wash your hands often. Use care in disposing of bowel movements.
- If you have intimate contact with a child with hepatitis, consult your doctor about immunization with gamma globulin (GG) or other immuno-globulins. GG can suppress—but not prevent—infectious hepatitis after exposure.
- If you are traveling where infectious hepatitis is endemic (constantly present), consult your doctor or health department about a vaccine or GG injection.

 WHAT TO EXPECT

APPROPRIATE HEALTH CARE
- Doctor's treatment.
- Home care after diagnosis.
- Hospitalization (severe cases only).

DIAGNOSTIC MEASURES
- Your own observation of symptoms.
- Medical history and physical exam by a doctor.
- Laboratory studies of blood, stool and liver function.

POSSIBLE COMPLICATIONS—Liver failure (very rare).

PROBABLE OUTCOME—This is a common infection that is usually mild in children. It is usually curable in 2 to 3 weeks. Wait 2 more weeks before sending the child to school or other public places.

 HOW TO TREAT

NOTE—Follow your doctor's instructions. These instructions are supplemental.

GENERAL MEASURES
- Use disposable eating utensils.
- Have the child wash hands with warm water and soap after every bowel movement.
- Keep the child isolated from others at least 1 week. The child should sleep alone.

MEDICATION—Medicine usually is not necessary for this disorder.

ACTIVITY—Keep the child in bed, except to use the bathroom, until fever is gone and jaundice improves. With improvement, the child may sit in a chair, read or watch TV.

DIET—No restrictions. Encourage the child to eat as much as he or she wants of whatever is appetizing. Hard candy may taste good and be nourishing to the liver.

 CALL YOUR DOCTOR IF

- Your child has symptoms of hepatitis.
- The following occurs during treatment:
   Excessive drowsiness or confusion.
   Vomiting, diarrhea or abdominal pain.
   Skin rash or itching.
   Increased jaundice.
   Increased appetite loss.

HEPATOMA
(Malignant Liver Tumor; Hepatocellular Carcinoma)

 GENERAL INFORMATION

DEFINITION—A malignant tumor that begins in the liver (primary), as opposed to liver cancer that has spread from another site.

BODY PARTS INVOLVED—Liver.

SEX OR AGE MOST AFFECTED—Adults of both sexes, but more common in men.

SIGNS & SYMPTOMS
- Hard mass in the right upper abdomen.
- Unexplained weight loss and appetite loss.
- Jaundice (yellow skin and eyes).
- Abdominal discomfort that resembles a pulled muscle.
- Low blood sugar (weakness, sweating, hunger, tremor and headache).
- Fever.
- Fluid in the abdomen.
- Enlarged spleen.
- Bleeding tendency in the gastrointestinal tract and other sites.

CAUSES
- Pre-existing cirrhosis of the liver. 50% of persons with hepatoma have cirrhosis.
- Possible slow virus.

RISK INCREASES WITH
- Medical history of hepatitis.
- Alcoholism.
- Geographic locations. This is especially common in South Africa and Southeast Asia.

HOW TO PREVENT
- Don't drink more than 1 or 2 alcoholic drinks—if any—a day.
- Immunization against hepatitis B may be helpful.

 WHAT TO EXPECT

APPROPRIATE HEALTH CARE
- Doctor's treatment.
- Surgery to remove the tumor, if possible. Only 25% can be removed successfully. Liver transplants have been successful in a few patients.
- Psychotherapy or counseling to help in coping with incurable illness.

DIAGNOSTIC MEASURES
- Your own observation of symptoms.
- Medical history and physical exam by a doctor.
- Laboratory blood studies of liver function and hepatitis B antigen.
- CAT scan (see Glossary) of the liver.
- X-rays of the abdomen, including angiography (see Glossary) of liver blood vessels.

POSSIBLE COMPLICATIONS
- Liver failure.
- Spread to other organs, especially the lungs, adrenal glands and bones.

PROBABLE OUTCOME—This condition is currently considered incurable. Only 15% to 20% of patients survive 5 years following surgery. However, symptoms can be relieved or controlled, and medical literature cites a few instances of unexplained recovery.

Scientific research into causes and treatment continues, so there is hope for increasingly effective treatment and cure.

 HOW TO TREAT

NOTE—Follow your doctor's instructions. These instructions are supplemental.

GENERAL MEASURES—No specific instructions except those listed under other headings.

MEDICATION
- For minor discomfort, you may use non-prescription drugs such as acetaminophen. Your doctor may prescribe pain relievers, if necessary.
- Anticancer drugs have produced disappointing results so far.

ACTIVITY—Stay as active as your strength allows.

DIET—No special diet. Don't drink alcohol.

 CALL YOUR DOCTOR IF

- You have symptoms of hepatoma.
- You develop signs of bleeding, especially from the gastrointestinal tract. Signs include bloody vomit or vomit that contains black material resembling coffee grounds, blood in the stool or black, tarry stools.

ILLNESSES & DISORDERS

HERNIA

GENERAL INFORMATION

DEFINITION—Protrusion of an internal organ through a weakness or abnormal opening in the muscle around it. The most-common types include: inguinal hernia; incisional hernia; femoral hernia; umbilical hernia; and hiatus hernia (this has a separate chart in Illness section).

BODY PARTS INVOLVED
● Umbilical: muscles around the navel.
● Inguinal or femoral: connective tissue in the groin.
● Incisional: muscles at the site of previous surgery.

SEX OR AGE MOST AFFECTED—Both sexes; all ages.

SIGNS & SYMPTOMS
● A lump that usually returns to its normal position with gentle pressure or by lying down.
● Mild discomfort or pain at the site of the lump (sometimes).
● Scrotal swelling, with or without pain.
● Vomiting in young infants.

CAUSES—Weakness in connective tissue or a muscle wall. This may be present at birth or acquired later in life. Incisional hernias result from previous surgery.

RISK INCREASES WITH
● Premature infants.
● Adults over 60.
● Obesity.
● Pregnancy.
● Straining.

HOW TO PREVENT—A weak area may not herniate until it ruptures with heavy lifting or straining.
　If you must lift something, lift properly. Bend your knees, lift the object and rise using your leg muscles. Keep the object close to your body. Don't lift by bending from the waist and lifting using your back muscles.
　If constipation is a problem, see Constipation (in Illness section) for treatment.

WHAT TO EXPECT

APPROPRIATE HEALTH CARE
● Doctor's treatment.
● Surgery to repair the opening caused by weakened muscle or connective tissue.

DIAGNOSTIC MEASURES
● Your own observation of symptoms.
● Medical history and physical exam by a doctor.
● Laboratory blood studies.
● X-rays of the abdomen.

POSSIBLE COMPLICATIONS—If the hernia becomes strangulated (loses its blood supply), the protruding part may cause intestinal obstruction with fever, severe pain and shock.

PROBABLE OUTCOME—Umbilical hernias usually heal spontaneously by age 4 and rarely require surgery. Other hernias are usually curable with surgery.

HOW TO TREAT

NOTE—Follow your doctor's instructions. These instructions are supplemental.

GENERAL MEASURES
● For an explanation of surgery and postoperative care, see Hernia (in Surgery section).
● Whenever you lie down prior to surgery, push your hernia gently into place if it protrudes visibly.
● Don't wear a hernia truss. It injures or weakens tissues, making surgery difficult or impossible.

MEDICATION—For minor discomfort, you may use non-prescription drugs such as acetaminophen.

ACTIVITY—Avoid heavy lifting—either before or after surgery.

DIET—No special diet.

CALL YOUR DOCTOR IF

You have symptoms of a hernia. If you have fever or severe pain, call immediately!

HERPANGINA

 GENERAL INFORMATION

DEFINITION—A viral inflammation of the mouth and throat.

BODY PARTS INVOLVED—Soft palate (back of the mouth and tonsil area).

SEX OR AGE MOST AFFECTED—Young children (1 to 10 years).

SIGNS & SYMPTOMS
- Fever.
- Sudden sore throat, with redness, inflammation and painful swallowing.
- General ill feeling.
- Vomiting and abdominal pain (sometimes).
- Tiny blisters (vesicles) in the affected areas. The blisters become small ulcers.

CAUSES—Infection from a virus (coxsackievirus) that is spread from person to person.

RISK INCREASES WITH—Summer and early fall seasons.

HOW TO PREVENT—Cannot be prevented at present, but wash hands carefully to prevent its spread.

 WHAT TO EXPECT

APPROPRIATE HEALTH CARE
- Home care.
- Doctor's treatment.

DIAGNOSTIC MEASURES
- Your own observation of symptoms.
- Medical history and physical exam by a doctor.

POSSIBLE COMPLICATIONS—Febrile convulsions.

PROBABLE OUTCOME—Spontaneous recovery in a few days to a week.

 HOW TO TREAT

NOTE—Follow your doctor's instructions. These instructions are supplemental.

GENERAL MEASURES—Try to reduce fever if it rises above 105F (40.6C) rectally. See How to Reduce Fever, Appendix 19.

MEDICATION—Medicine usually is not necessary for this disorder. You may use non-prescription drugs, such as acetaminophen, to relieve pain and fever.

ACTIVITY—Bed rest is necessary until the fever and sore throat disappear.

DIET—No special diet. Encourage extra fluids, such as water, fruit ices, ice chips or cool-gelatin solutions. Avoid acid fruit juices, which irritate inflamed tissues.

 CALL YOUR DOCTOR IF

Your child has symptoms of herpangina.

ILLNESSES & DISORDERS

HERPES, GENITAL

GENERAL INFORMATION

DEFINITION—A virus infection of the genitals transmitted by sexual relations (intercourse or oral sex). Genital herpes may increase the risk of cervical cancer.

BODY PARTS INVOLVED—Penis; vagina; cervix; thighs; buttocks (sometimes).

SEX OR AGE MOST AFFECTED—Both sexes and all ages of sexually active persons.

SIGNS & SYMPTOMS
- Painful blisters, preceded by itching and irritation, on the vaginal lips or penis. In women, the blisters may extend into the vagina to the cervix and urethra. After a few days, the blisters rupture and leave painful, shallow ulcers which last 1 to 3 weeks.
- Difficult, painful urination.
- Enlarged lymph glands.
- Fever and a general ill feeling.

CAUSES—Herpes Type 2 virus (HSV-2). (Herpes Type 1 virus causes common cold sores, which appear around the mouth.) Genital herpes is transmitted by a sexual partner who has active herpes lesions. Lesions may be on the genitals, hands, lips or mouth (including Type 1 virus). The virus lies dormant inside infected cells until conditions for multiplication are right; then the infected cells grow.

RISK INCREASES WITH
- Serious illness that has lowered resistance.
- Use of immunosuppressive or anticancer drugs.
- Stress (increases susceptibility to a primary infection or a recurrence). Stress may lead to diminished efficiency of the immune responses that usually suppress growth of the virus.

HOW TO PREVENT
- Avoid sexual intercourse if either partner has blisters or sores.
- Use a rubber condom during intercourse if either sex partner has inactive genital herpes.
- Avoid oral sex with a partner who has cold sores on the mouth.
- If you are pregnant, tell your doctor if you have had herpes or any genital lesions in the past. Precautions should be taken to prevent infection of the baby.

WHAT TO EXPECT

APPROPRIATE HEALTH CARE
- Self-care after diagnosis.
- Doctor's treatment.

DIAGNOSTIC MEASURES
- Your own observation of symptoms.
- Medical history and physical exam by a doctor.

POSSIBLE COMPLICATIONS
- Generalized disease and death in persons who must take anticancer drugs or immunosuppressive drugs.
- Transmittal of life-threatening systemic herpes to a newborn infant from an infected mother.
- Secondary bacterial infection.

PROBABLE OUTCOME—Genital herpes is currently considered incurable, but symptoms can be relieved with treatment.

During symptom-free periods, the virus returns to its dormant state. Symptoms recur when the virus is reactivated. Recurrent symptoms are not new infections.

The discomfort varies from person to person and from time to time in the same person. The first herpes infection is much more uncomfortable than following ones.

HOW TO TREAT

NOTE—Follow your doctor's instructions. These instructions are supplemental.

GENERAL MEASURES
- Women should wear cotton panties or pantyhose with a cotton crotch—not panties made from non-ventilating materials.
- Women should not douche unless told to by a doctor.
- To reduce pain during urination, women may urinate in a bath or shower, or urinate through a tubular device, such as a toilet-paper roll or plastic cup with the end cut out.

MEDICATION—Your doctor may prescribe an antiviral drug, such as acyclovir, in oral or topical form. This new drug reduces the intensity and duration of the first attack. It does not prevent recurrent attacks.

ACTIVITY
- Reduce normal activities until fever diminishes and you feel well.
- Don't resume sexual relations until at least 1 month after full recovery.

DIET—No special diet.

CALL YOUR DOCTOR IF

- You have symptoms of genital herpes.
- Symptoms don't improve in 1 week, despite treatment.
- Symptoms worsen, despite treatment.
- Unusual vaginal bleeding or swelling occurs.
- Fever returns during treatment or you become generally ill.
- Symptoms of herpes recur after treatment.

HERPETIC WHITLOW

GENERAL INFORMATION

DEFINITION—An inflammation of skin folds around the fingernails caused by a contagious herpes virus.

BODY PARTS INVOLVED—Fingernail or toenail bed.

SEX OR AGE MOST AFFECTED—All ages, but most common in adults.

SIGNS & SYMPTOMS
- Sudden pain around the nail.
- Redness, swelling and warmth around the nail.
- Swelling of the lymph glands nearby, such as in the elbow or armpit.
- Groupings of tiny blisters that are barely visible around the nail.

CAUSES—Herpes virus hominus, Type 1 or Type 2. Herpetic whitlow is often transmitted to the fingers from cold sores (herpes simplex) on the mouth.

RISK INCREASES WITH
- Occupational exposure to constant wetness, such as with dishwashers or maintenance personnel.
- Occupational exposure to herpes infection, such as with nurses, dentists or dental assistants who provide mouth care.

HOW TO PREVENT
- Avoid exposure to people who have active herpes infections.
- Keep hands warm and dry.

WHAT TO EXPECT

APPROPRIATE HEALTH CARE
- Self-care after diagnosis.
- Doctor's treatment.

DIAGNOSTIC MEASURES
- Your own observation of symptoms.
- Medical history and physical exam by a doctor.
- Laboratory culture of discharge from the infected area.

POSSIBLE COMPLICATIONS—Spread of herpes infection to other body parts, such as the lips or genitals.

PROBABLE OUTCOME—The first episode is usually curable in 2 months with treatment. However, recurrent attacks are common.

HOW TO TREAT

NOTE—Follow your doctor's instructions. These instructions are supplemental.

GENERAL MEASURES
- Protect your hands to prevent further injury or spread of the infection to others. Wear heavy-duty vinyl gloves to avoid contact with irritating substances, such as water, soap, detergent, metal scrubbing pads, scouring pads, scouring powder and other chemicals.
- Don't touch other persons until inflammation clears.

MEDICATION—Your doctor may prescribe:
- Topical steroid preparations to reduce inflammation. They include creams, ointments and lotions. Apply the topical steroid only once or twice a day unless directed otherwise. Apply immediately after bathing for better spreading and penetration.
- Oral antiviral medications. These are still experimental, but they may prove safe and effective.

ACTIVITY—No restrictions.

DIET—No special diet.

CALL YOUR DOCTOR IF

- You have symptoms of herpetic whitlow.
- Temperature rises over 101F (38.3C).
- Symptoms don't improve in 3 days, despite treatment.
- Herpes lesions appear elsewhere on the body.

ILLNESSES & DISORDERS

HIATAL HERNIA

GENERAL INFORMATION

DEFINITION—An abnormal weakness or opening in the diaphragm, the big, thin muscle that separates the chest cavity from the abdominal cavity.

BODY PARTS INVOLVED—Esophagus; stomach; diaphragm.

SEX OR AGE MOST AFFECTED—All ages, but most common in adults over 50.

SIGNS & SYMPTOMS—The following symptoms usually develop within 1 hour or more after eating:
- "Heartburn" (a burning sensation in the area of the heart and behind the breastbone).
- Belching.
- Swallowing difficulty (rare).

CAUSES
- Congenital weakness in the muscular ring of the diaphragm through which the esophagus passes and empties into the stomach.
- Abdominal injury, causing tremendous pressure that tears a hole in some part of the diaphragm.

Either of the above can allow gastric (stomach) acid to flow backward from the stomach into the esophagus, irritating the esophagus. The hernia weakens the sphincter that controls the opening between the two—the stomach may even protrude into the lower chest. Lying flat or abdominal pressure (like straining) may push the stomach upward.

RISK INCREASES WITH
- Chronic constipation and straining during bowel movements.
- Obesity.
- Pregnancy.
- Constant straining or lifting with tightening of the abdominal muscles.
- Smoking.

HOW TO PREVENT—No specific preventive measures.

WHAT TO EXPECT

APPROPRIATE HEALTH CARE
- Self-care after diagnosis.
- Doctor's treatment.
- Surgery to close the weakness in the diaphragm and keep the stomach in its natural place (rare).

DIAGNOSTIC MEASURES
- Your own observation of symptoms.
- Medical history and physical exam by a doctor.
- X-rays of the esophagus and stomach.

- Gastroscopy with a flexible gastroscope (see Glossary) to view the esophagus and stomach.

POSSIBLE COMPLICATIONS
- Bleeding from the esophagus. This can be excessive, leading to shock.
- Misdiagnosis as a heart attack.

PROBABLE OUTCOME—Symptoms can usually be controlled with the suggestions listed under How to Treat. If symptoms cannot be controlled and it appears that irritation of the esophagus is causing scarring and ulceration, the condition can be corrected with surgery.

HOW TO TREAT

NOTE—Follow your doctor's instructions. These instructions are supplemental.

GENERAL MEASURES
- Raise the head of your bed 4 to 6 inches. This allows gravity to keep stomach acid away from the hernia.
- Avoid large meals. Eat 4 or 5 small meals a day instead. Don't eat anything for at least 2 hours before bedtime.
- Lose weight, if you are overweight. A reducing diet appears in Appendix 10.
- Don't smoke.
- Don't wear tight pantyhose, girdles, belts or pants.
- Don't strain during bowel movements, urination or lifting.

MEDICATION—Your doctor may prescribe:
- Antacids. These are most effective for some persons when they take them 1 hour before meals and at bedtime. Others find them more helpful 1 to 2 hours after meals and at bedtime. Try both ways to find the best schedule for you.
- Stool softeners.

ACTIVITY—No restrictions.

DIET—Avoid alcoholic beverages, caffeine-containing beverages (coffee, tea, cocoa, cola drinks) and any other food, juice or spice that aggravates symptoms. Eat slowly.

CALL YOUR DOCTOR IF

- You have symptoms of a hiatal hernia, especially the sensation that food stops beneath the breastbone. Call immediately if pain is accompanied by shortness of breath, sweating or nausea.
- You vomit blood or have recurrent vomiting.
- Temperature rises over 100F (37.8C).
- Symptoms don't improve with treatment in 1 month.

HICCUP
(Hiccough; Singultus)

 GENERAL INFORMATION

DEFINITION—Repeated, involuntary spasmodic contractions of the diaphragm. Hiccups are a symptom—not a disease.

BODY PARTS INVOLVED
- Diaphragm (big muscle which separates the chest from the abdomen).
- Phrenic nerve (nerve that connects the diaphragm to the brain).

SEX OR AGE MOST AFFECTED—Both
sexes, but more common in men.

SIGNS & SYMPTOMS—A sharp, quick
sound produced from the mouth by a spasm of the diaphragm. The spasm closes muscles in the back of the throat during inhalation.

CAUSES—Irritation of nerves from the brain that control breathing muscles, especially the diaphragm. The cause of short hiccup episodes is usually unknown. Prolonged or recurrent hiccup episodes may be caused by:
- Swallowing hot or irritating substances.
- Diseases of the pleura (thin membrane layers that cover the lung).
- Pneumonia.
- Uremia.
- Alcoholism.
- Use of certain prescription or non-prescription drugs.
- Disorders of the stomach, esophagus, bowel or pancreas.
- Pregnancy.
- Bladder irritation.
- Hepatitis.
- Spread of cancer from another part of the body to the liver or part of the pleura.
- Recent surgery, especially abdominal surgery.
- Emotional causes.

RISK INCREASES WITH
- Illness that has diminished health.
- Recent abdominal surgery.
- Use of drugs, especially those that irritate the stomach.

HOW TO PREVENT—Cannot be prevented at present.

 WHAT TO EXPECT

APPROPRIATE HEALTH CARE
- Self-care.
- Doctor's treatment (prolonged hiccups).
- Surgery to cut phrenic nerve (severe, prolonged cases only).

DIAGNOSTIC MEASURES
- Your own observation of symptoms.
- Medical history and physical exam by a doctor.

POSSIBLE COMPLICATIONS—None unless hiccups are prolonged, which may indicate serious disease.

PROBABLE OUTCOME—Short hiccup episodes usually don't indicate disease. They will subside with the treatment discussed below. Continued hiccups can be debilitating and require medical attention to determine the cause.

 HOW TO TREAT

NOTE—Follow your doctor's instructions. These instructions are supplemental.

GENERAL MEASURES—These instructions are for short hiccup episodes. Prolonged hiccups require medical care.
- Hold your breath and count to 10.
- Breathe into a paper bag, and rebreathe air in the bag. Don't use a plastic bag because it may cling to nostrils.
- Insert your thumb between your teeth and upper lip; press the upper lip with your index finger just below the right nostril.
- Drink a glass of water rapidly.
- Swallow dry bread or crushed ice.
- Pull gently on the tongue.
- Close eyelids and apply gentle pressure to the eyeballs.
- Swallow a teaspoon of dry sugar.

MEDICATION—For prolonged or recurrent hiccups, your doctor may prescribe a mild tranquilizer or sedative.

ACTIVITY—No restrictions.

DIET—No special diet.

 CALL YOUR DOCTOR IF

- Hiccups persist longer than 8 hours.
- You suspect a prescription drug may be causing hiccups.

HIDRADENITIS SUPPURATIVA

GENERAL INFORMATION

DEFINITION—A skin disorder characterized by nodules in the armpit.

BODY PARTS INVOLVED—Armpits. It appears rarely on buttocks, groin or under breasts.

SEX OR AGE MOST AFFECTED—Both sexes, but more common in females (13 to 16 years).

SIGNS & SYMPTOMS—Nodules with the following characteristics:
- Nodules are firm, tender and domed.
- Nodules are 1cm to 3cm in diameter.
- Larger nodules soften in the center and become painful. When pressed, they feel like an overfilled inner tube.
- Nodules open and drain pus spontaneously.
- Individual nodules (with or without drainage) heal slowly over 10 to 30 days.
- Nodules leave scars.
- Severity of the disorder varies from a few lesions per year to a constant succession of lesions that form as old ones heal. Lesions frequently recur at the same site.

CAUSES—Hormonal influences that activate the apocrine glands under the arms. Secretions in these glands enlarge the gland. The outlets become blocked, probably by heat, sweat or incomplete gland development. The secretions that are dammed in the glands force sweat and bacteria into surrounding tissue, which becomes infected.

RISK INCREASES WITH
- Obesity.
- Exposure to environmental heat and moisture.
- Genetic factors. This disorder is most common in black females.

HOW TO PREVENT—No specific preventive measures.

WHAT TO EXPECT

APPROPRIATE HEALTH CARE
- Self-care after diagnosis.
- Doctor's treatment.
- Surgery to open and drain abscesses or to remove involved skin (desperate cases only).

DIAGNOSTIC MEASURES
- Your own observation of symptoms.
- Medical history and physical exam by a doctor.
- Laboratory culture of the discharge from the draining abscess.

POSSIBLE COMPLICATIONS—Scarring.

PROBABLE OUTCOME—This disorder may last many years—from puberty through the following 10 to 20 years. Symptoms can be controlled with treatment.

HOW TO TREAT

NOTE—Follow your doctor's instructions. These instructions are supplemental.

GENERAL MEASURES
- Don't use commercial underarm deodorants.
- Minimize heat and sweating.
- Avoid constrictive clothing.
- Lose weight, if your overweight.
- Use soaks (see Appendix 18) to relieve itching and hasten healing. Warm-water soaks are usually more soothing for pain or inflammation. Cool-water soaks feel better for itching.

MEDICATION—Your doctor may:
- Inject cortisone drugs directly into the lesions.
- Prescribe antibiotics to fight infection.
- Prescribe hormones to help subdue inflammation.
- Provide instructions for acceptable deodorant protection.
- Prescribe pain medication. For minor discomfort, you may use non-prescription drugs such as acetaminophen.

ACTIVITY—Restrict your activity in hot weather, and avoid hot jobs if possible. Swimming is excellent, especially swimming in the ocean.

DIET—No special diet unless you need to lose weight. See Appendix 10 for a reducing diet.

CALL YOUR DOCTOR IF

- You have symptoms of hidradenitis suppurativa.
- Lesions don't improve after 5 days of treatment.
- Your temperature rises to 101F (38.3C).
- Lesions appear that become soft and seem to have pus, but don't drain spontaneously.
- New, unexplained symptoms develop. Drugs used in treatment may produce side effects.

HIP DISLOCATION, CONGENITAL

GENERAL INFORMATION

DEFINITION—A disorder in which the head of the thigh bone doesn't fit properly into, or is outside of, the hip socket.

BODY PARTS INVOLVED—One or both hip joints.

SEX OR AGE MOST AFFECTED—About 1 of every 60 newborns has a possible hip dislocation. About 85% are girls.

SIGNS & SYMPTOMS—The earliest symptom may be a clicking sound in a newborn when the legs are pulled apart. However, this symptom is not always present.

After the newborn period, partial dislocation may become full dislocation. Then the thigh bone (femur) rides up behind or to the side of its hip socket. The limb will appear shorter than its mate. Skin folds of the buttocks will not be symmetrical; the side with the dislocated hip will have more creases than the other.

When the child is old enough to walk, he or she may limp or favor one side.

CAUSES—Unknown. Congenital hip dislocations seem more common after breech deliveries than following head-first or Cesarean deliveries. Theories about the reasons include: hormonal changes in the mother during pregnancy; abnormal fetal position in the uterus; or birth injury.

RISK INCREASES WITH—Unknown.

HOW TO PREVENT—Cannot be prevented at present.

WHAT TO EXPECT

APPROPRIATE HEALTH CARE
- Home care after diagnosis.
- Doctor's treatment.
- Surgery (sometimes).

DIAGNOSTIC MEASURES
- Your own observation of symptoms.
- Medical history and physical exam by a doctor.
- X-rays of the hip.

POSSIBLE COMPLICATIONS—Late detection and treatment can lead to permanent crippling.

PROBABLE OUTCOME—If congenital hip dislocation is detected early, it can often be cured. Surgery is used only when conservative treatment fails or the disorder has not been discovered until late in childhood.

HOW TO TREAT

NOTE—Follow your doctor's instructions. These instructions are supplemental.

GENERAL MEASURES
- To correct the dislocation, the head of the thigh bone must be returned to its socket in the pelvic bone and held firmly in place.

For mild forms, use triple diapers to immobilize the child and arrange for frequent medical exams.

For more severe forms, splints, casts or traction are used to immobilize the ball and socket until it heals. Plaster casts may be necessary for several months. They must be replaced every 1-1/2 to 2 months. See Care of Casts, Appendix 17.
- While an infant or young child is immobilized, he or she will require more physical care than normal. Soiled diapers, especially, should not be left on the child for any length of time.
- During the first few days that the child is in a cast, splints, or traction, stay as close by as possible to give reassurance and love.
- Remove braces or splints for bathing, but replace them immediately afterward.
- Turn the child in bed at least every 2 hours during the day and every 4 hours at night.

MEDICATION—Medicine usually is not necessary for this disorder.

ACTIVITY
- If traction is required, the child must stay in bed until the dislocation is corrected. The child may read or watch TV.
- If a cast or splints are used and the child's condition allows it, put the child on the floor for short play periods—either alone or with other children. Car rides are acceptable.

DIET—No special diet.

CALL YOUR DOCTOR IF

- Your child has signs of a congenital hip dislocation.
- The following occurs during treatment:
  Rectal temperature rises to 101F (38.3C) or higher, which may indicate infection of the skin or urinary tract.
  The cast, bar or other immobilization device does not seem to hold the hip in position.
  A dent appears in the cast, which might cause a pressure sore.
  The child shows signs of severe pain.
  Color or mobility of the child's legs and feet change.
  The child loses appetite.

ILLNESSES & DISORDERS

HIP FRACTURE

GENERAL INFORMATION

DEFINITION—A complete or partial break in the femur, the major bone in the hip joint.

BODY PARTS INVOLVED—Femur, including muscles and tendons that attach the head of the femur to the acetabulum (hip socket in the bony pelvis).

SEX OR AGE MOST AFFECTED
- Breaks from common injuries affect both sexes and all ages.
- Spontaneous breaks or breaks from minor injuries affect mostly adults over 60.

SIGNS & SYMPTOMS
- Intolerable pain when trying to walk.
- Swelling, tenderness and bruising in the hip area.
- Deformed hip appearance.

CAUSES—Injury.

RISK INCREASES WITH
- Activities that increase the risk of injury.
- Osteoporosis, especially post-menopausal osteoporosis.
- Bone cancer.
- Osteogenesis imperfecta (see Glossary).
- Calcium imbalance.
- Poor nutrition, especially insufficient calcium and protein.

HOW TO PREVENT
- Ensure an adequate calcium intake (1000mg to 1500mg a day) with milk and milk products or calcium supplements.
- Protect yourself against falls, especially in the home.
- Women should consult a doctor about taking estrogen after menopause begins.

WHAT TO EXPECT

APPROPRIATE HEALTH CARE
- Doctor's treatment.
- Surgery to reattach broken fragments, usually by nailing them together.
- Physical therapy and rehabilitation.

DIAGNOSTIC MEASURES
- Your own observation of symptoms.
- Medical history and physical exam by a doctor.
- X-rays of the hip.

POSSIBLE COMPLICATIONS
- Surgical-wound infection.
- Nerve and blood-vessel damage at the fracture site.
- Accompanying dislocation.
- Inadequate blood supply to the injured area, causing tissue death of the bone.
- Poor healing (non-union) of the fracture.

PROBABLE OUTCOME—Usually curable with surgery and rehabilitation.

HOW TO TREAT

NOTE—Follow your doctor's instructions. These instructions are supplemental.

GENERAL MEASURES—Self-care is not appropriate—surgery is the only treatment. The surgeon reattaches fractured bone parts, and secures them with surgical steel pins. Unlike most fractures, hip fractures usually don't require casts.

After surgery, bathe and shower as usual. You may wash the incision gently with mild unscented soap. Wound dressings are optional.

Heat relieves incision pain. Use an electric heating pad, a heat lamp or a towel wrung out in warm water.

MEDICATION—Your doctor may prescribe:
- Pain relievers.
- Antibiotics to fight infection, if necessary.
- Stool softeners to prevent constipation.

ACTIVITY—After awakening from anesthesia, move the unaffected leg often to decrease the possibility of deep-vein blood clots. Most surgeons urge patients to get up and move about as soon as possible. Resume your normal activities gradually as healing progresses.

DIET—Clear liquids for the 1st day after surgery, then no special diet. Ask your doctor if you should take calcium supplements.

CALL YOUR DOCTOR IF

- You have symptoms of a hip fracture. Call immediately if you have numbness or loss of feeling below the fracture site. This is an emergency!
- The following occurs after surgery: Swelling above or below the fracture site. Chills, fever, muscle aches or headache. Increased pain, swelling, redness or discharge at the surgical site. Constipation.

HISTOPLASMOSIS

GENERAL INFORMATION

DEFINITION—A fungus infection confined mostly to people who live in eastern and midwestern parts of the U.S.

BODY PARTS INVOLVED—Lungs; central nervous system; gastrointestinal system.

SEX OR AGE MOST AFFECTED—Both sexes; all ages.

SIGNS & SYMPTOMS
- Cough and other symptoms similar to a cold.
- Loss of appetite, diarrhea and weight loss.
- Fever.
- Headache.
- Irritability.
- Paleness.
- Abdominal swelling.
- Breathing difficulty (rare).

CAUSES—Infection by the fungus, histoplasma capsulatum. People become infected by breathing dust that contains fungus spores. The fungus is found in soil contaminated by feces of birds and bats that carry the fungus. Contaminated soil is most often in pigeon lofts, barns, chicken houses, damp areas under bridges, along streams and in caves.

RISK INCREASES WITH
- Recent severe illness, especially uremia, diabetes mellitus, chronic lung disease, cancer or severe burns.
- Geographic location. The disease occurs most often in the western Appalachian slopes and the Mississippi, Missouri and Ohio River valleys.
- Use of immunosuppressive, anticancer or cortisone drugs.

HOW TO PREVENT—Avoid areas where the soil is likely to be infected with histoplasma spores.

WHAT TO EXPECT

APPROPRIATE HEALTH CARE
- Self-care after diagnosis.
- Doctor's treatment.
- Hospitalization for complications.

DIAGNOSTIC MEASURES
- Your own observation of symptoms.
- Medical history and physical exam by a doctor.
- Laboratory studies, such as a sputum culture, blood studies and skin tests.

POSSIBLE COMPLICATIONS—Spread of infection to the heart, spleen, adrenal glands and meninges (membranes that cover the brain). This is rare, but it can be fatal.

PROBABLE OUTCOME—Usually curable—even with complications—with intensive care and 10 to 12 weeks of treatment with antifungal drugs. Most people only feel tired or "bad" for several weeks.

HOW TO TREAT

NOTE—Follow your doctor's instructions. These instructions are supplemental.

GENERAL MEASURES
- Isolation is not necessary. The disease is not transmitted from person to person.
- Use a cool-mist humidifier with pure water and no medicine in it to increase air moisture. This helps thin lung secretions so they can be coughed up more easily.
- Don't smoke.
- Use a heating pad on the chest to relieve pain.
- Weigh daily and keep a record.

MEDICATION
- Your doctor may prescribe antifungal drugs that must be given intravenously in a hospital.
- Don't suppress the cough with cough medicine if it produces sputum. It is ridding the lungs of mucus. If the cough is painful and non-productive, consult your doctor about a prescription cough suppressant.
- You may use non-prescription drugs, such as acetaminophen or aspirin, to relieve pain.

ACTIVITY—Stay in bed until fever, pain and shortness of breath disappear for at least 48 hours. Then resume your normal activities gradually. Many people are fatigued and weak after recovery. Don't expect too much too soon.

DIET—No special diet.

CALL YOUR DOCTOR IF

- You have symptoms of histoplasmosis.
- The following occurs during treatment:
  Weight loss continues.
  Fever rises to 101F (38.3C) orally.
  Diarrhea is uncontrollable.
  Severe headache and stiff neck begin.

HIVES
(Urticaria; Giant Urticaria; Angioneurotic Edema)

 GENERAL INFORMATION

DEFINITION—An allergic disorder characterized by skin changes with raised areas, redness and itching.

BODY PARTS INVOLVED—Skin anywhere, including the scalp, lips, palms and soles.

SEX OR AGE MOST AFFECTED—Both sexes; all ages.

SIGNS & SYMPTOMS—Itchy skin papules (small, raised bumps) with the following characteristics:
● They swell and produce pink or red lesions called wheals. Wheals have clearly defined edges and flat tops. They measure 1cm to 5cm in diameter.
● Wheals join together quickly and form large, flat plaques (larger areas of raised, skin-colored lesions).
● Wheals and plaques change shape, resolve and reappear in minutes or hours. This rapid change is unique to hives.

CAUSES—Release of histamines, sometimes for unknown reason. Following are the most common causes:
● Medications. Nearly every drug causes hives in some persons.
● Insect bites.
● Viral infections.
● Autoimmune disease.
● Dysproteinemias.
● Exposure to cold, heat, water or sunlight.
● Cancer, especially leukemia.
● Exposure to animals, especially cats.
● Eating eggs, fruits, nuts and shellfish. Other foods sometimes cause hives in infants, but not in adults.
● Food dyes and preservatives (possibly).

RISK INCREASES WITH
● Stress.
● Other allergies or a family history of allergies.

HOW TO PREVENT—If you have had hives and identified the cause, avoid the source.

 WHAT TO EXPECT

APPROPRIATE HEALTH CARE
● Self-care after diagnosis.
● Doctor's treatment.
● Emergency-room care for life-threatening reactions.

DIAGNOSTIC MEASURES
● Your own observation of symptoms.
● Medical history and physical exam by a doctor.
● Allergy skin tests and desensitization injections.

POSSIBLE COMPLICATIONS
● Swelling of the larynx and inability to breathe.
● Hives may be the first sign of life-threatening anaphylaxis. If so, it will be followed by itching, runny nose, wheezing, paleness, cold sweats and low blood pressure. Without prompt treatment, coma and cardiac arrest can occur.

PROBABLE OUTCOME—Unpredictable, depending on the cause. If a medication or acute viral infection is responsible, hives usually disappear within hours or days. Some cases become chronic and last for months or years. Most eventually go into spontaneous remission—even if the cause is not identified.

 HOW TO TREAT

NOTE—Follow your doctor's instructions. These instructions are supplemental.

GENERAL MEASURES
● Don't take drugs (including aspirin, laxatives, sedatives, vitamins, antacids, pain killers or cough syrups) not prescribed for you.
● Don't wear tight underwear or foundation garments. Any skin irritation may trigger new outbreaks.
● Don't take hot baths or showers.
● Apply cold-water compresses or soaks (see Appendix 18) to relieve itching.

MEDICATION—Your doctor may prescribe:
● Antihistamines, ephedrine, terbutaline or cortisone drugs to relieve itching and rash.
● Sedatives or tranquilizers for anxiety.
● Epinephrine by injection for severe symptoms.

ACTIVITY—Decrease activities until several days after hives disappear. Avoid getting hot, sweaty or excited.

DIET
● If foods are suspected as a cause, keep a food diary to help identify the offending food.
● Avoid alcohol and coffee or other caffeine-containing beverages. These may trigger outbreaks.

 CALL YOUR DOCTOR IF

● The following occurs during an episode of hives:
  Swollen lips.
  Shortness of breath or wheezing.
  A tight or constricted feeling in the throat. This is an emergency!
● New, unexplained symptoms develop. Drugs used in treatment may produce side effects.

HODGKIN'S DISEASE

GENERAL INFORMATION

DEFINITION—Malignant tumor of the lymph glands. This is less common than lymphoma (non-Hodgkin's disease).

BODY PARTS INVOLVED
- Lymphocytes (white blood cells).
- Lymph glands (glands which check infection and produce immune substances).
- Spleen (a large lymph gland).

SEX OR AGE MOST AFFECTED—All ages, but most common in men between ages 20 and 40, and over age 60. Hodgkin's disease is rare in children under 10.

SIGNS & SYMPTOMS
- Itching all over the body.
- Swollen, non-tender, rubbery, distinct lymph glands anywhere in the body—but most commonly in the armpit or groin.
- Intermittent fever.
- Pain in the diseased area after drinking alcohol.
- Weight loss.
- Jaundice (yellow skin and eyes).
- General ill feeling.
- Anemia.
- Bleeding from the gastrointestinal tract.

CAUSES—Unknown, but research suggests a virus infection may be a factor.

RISK INCREASES WITH—No known risk factor.

HOW TO PREVENT—No specific preventive measures.

WHAT TO EXPECT

APPROPRIATE HEALTH CARE
- Doctor's treatment.
- Hospitalization for short periods of treatment.
- Surgery to discover the extent of disease.
- Radiation therapy.

DIAGNOSTIC MEASURES
- Your own observation of symptoms.
- Medical history and physical exam by a doctor.
- Laboratory studies of blood and bone marrow.
- Lymphangiogram (see Glossary).
- Biopsy (see Glossary) of lymph node.
- X-rays of various body parts that may be involved.

POSSIBLE COMPLICATIONS—Spread of malignancy to other parts of the body.

PROBABLE OUTCOME—Usually curable with radiation therapy and anticancer drugs. With treatment, the 10-year survival rate is about 80%. The potential for cure varies according to the cell type discovered from biopsy of the lymph node.

HOW TO TREAT

NOTE—Follow your doctor's instructions. These instructions are supplemental.

GENERAL MEASURES—Try to remain optimistic about your treatment and chances for cure. A good mental attitude is a powerful ally.

MEDICATION—Your doctor may prescribe anticancer drugs. Medication may cause side effects or adverse reactions in some people. New symptoms may be caused by the medicine, original disorder or a new illness. Side effects caused by medicine usually disappear when the body adjusts to the drug or when the drug is discontinued.

ACTIVITY—Remain as active as your strength allows.

DIET—No special diet.

CALL YOUR DOCTOR IF

- You have symptoms of Hodgkin's disease.
- The following occurs during treatment:
  Fever.
  Signs of infection (redness, swelling, pain or tenderness) anywhere in the body.
  Swelling of the feet and ankles.
  Discomfort when urinating or decreased urination in 1 day.
- You think your medicine is causing symptoms.

HYPERALDOSTERONISM

GENERAL INFORMATION

DEFINITION—An endocrine disease caused by overproduction of aldosterone, a hormone manufactured by the adrenal gland. Excess aldosterone causes the kidneys to absorb too much sodium and water, and eliminate too much potassium.

BODY PARTS INVOLVED—Adrenal glands, which are attached at the upper part of the kidneys; kidneys; fluids and electrolytes in the bloodstream and body cells.

SEX OR AGE MOST AFFECTED
- Both sexes, but more common in females.
- All ages, but most common in adults between ages 30 and 50.

SIGNS & SYMPTOMS
- Fatigue and weakness.
- Temporary paralysis (sometimes).
- Tingling sensations in the arms, legs, hands and feet.
- Urinary frequency, especially at night.
- Thirst.
- Severe muscle spasms.
- Vision disturbances.

The following are apparent with diagnostic tests:
- Low blood levels of potassium.
- High blood levels of sodium.
- High blood pressure.

CAUSES—Increased adrenal secretion of aldosterone. This is caused by:
- A tumor of the adrenal gland.
- High blood pressure or kidney disease, causing increased production in the kidneys of a hormone (renin) that controls aldosterone levels.

RISK INCREASES WITH
- Diet that contains large amounts of licorice.
- Kidney disease.
- Congestive heart failure.
- Cirrhosis of the liver.
- Use of oral contraceptives.
- Use of diuretic drugs that cause potassium loss.
- Pregnancy.

HOW TO PREVENT—If you have kidney disease or high blood pressure, remain under a doctor's care, and adhere strictly to your treatment program—even if you have no symptoms.

WHAT TO EXPECT

APPROPRIATE HEALTH CARE
- Self-care after diagnosis.
- Doctor's treatment.
- Hospitalization.
- Surgery to examine the adrenal glands and remove any tumors.

DIAGNOSTIC MEASURES
- Your own observation of symptoms.
- Medical history and physical exam by a doctor.
- Laboratory blood studies of electrolyte levels.
- EKG (see Glossary).
- Surgical diagnostic procedures such as laparoscopy (see Glossary).
- X-rays of the kidneys.
- CAT scan (see Glossary) of the kidneys.

POSSIBLE COMPLICATIONS
- Congestive heart failure.
- Atherosclerosis.
- Kidney failure.

PROBABLE OUTCOME—If the disorder is caused by an adrenal tumor, it is usually curable with surgery. If it is caused by kidney disease or high blood pressure, medical treatment for these disorders will control symptoms of hyperaldosteronism.

HOW TO TREAT

NOTE—Follow your doctor's instructions. These instructions are supplemental.

GENERAL MEASURES
- Weigh daily and keep a record. Report a gain of 3 or more pounds in a 24-hour period.
- Wear a Medic-Alert bracelet or pendant (see Glossary).

MEDICATION—Your doctor may prescribe:
- Cortisone drugs to replace adrenal hormones, if the adrenal gland is removed. This is essential for life. Don't discontinue or change your dose without consulting your doctor.
- Spironolactone to decrease the aldosterone effect, if surgery is not performed. This drug may cause breast enlargement and sexual impotence in men.

ACTIVITY—No restrictions, if surgery is not necessary. If it is, resume your normal activities gradually.

DIET—Eat a diet that is low in sodium (see Appendix 9) and high in potassium. Foods rich in potassium include dried apricots and peaches, raisins, citrus fruits, lentils and whole-grain cereals. Don't eat licorice.

CALL YOUR DOCTOR IF

- You have symptoms of hyperaldosteronism.
- New, unexplained symptoms develop. Drugs used in treatment may produce side effects.

HYPEREMESIS GRAVIDARUM

GENERAL INFORMATION

DEFINITION—Severe nausea and vomiting in a pregnant woman, causing dehydration and drastic changes in body chemistry. This is different and much more serious than morning sickness during pregnancy.

BODY PARTS INVOLVED—Gastrointestinal tract; vomiting center in the brain.

SEX OR AGE MOST AFFECTED—Pregnant females.

SIGNS & SYMPTOMS
- Severe nausea.
- Vomiting, first of mucus, then of bile and finally of blood.
- Dehydration.
- Failure to gain weight, or weight loss to less than prepregnancy weight.
- Pale, waxy, dry and sometimes yellow skin.
- Rapid heartbeat.
- Headache, confusion or lethargy.

CAUSES—Unknown. The most common theories include:
- Multiple pregnancy (more than one fetus), producing high levels of a hormone, human chorionic gonadotrophin.
- Inflammation of the pancreas.
- Bile-duct disease.
- Psychological factors, such as depression or a poor response to stress.

RISK INCREASES WITH
- Poor nutrition, especially deficiency of vitamin B-6.
- Use of any drug that may interfere with normal pregnancy.

HOW TO PREVENT
- Don't use any drugs, including non-prescription drugs or alcohol, during pregnancy without consulting your doctor.
- Maintain an adequate diet during all stages of pregnancy (see Appendix 3).

WHAT TO EXPECT

APPROPRIATE HEALTH CARE
- Self-care after diagnosis.
- Doctor's treatment.
- Hospitalization to replace fluid and electrolytes intravenously, if needed.

DIAGNOSTIC MEASURES
- Your own observation of symptoms.
- Medical history and physical exam by a doctor.
- Laboratory studies of blood and urine to measure electrolytes and detect anemia.

POSSIBLE COMPLICATIONS
- Severe dehydration.
- Liver disease.
- Coma.
- Miscarriage or damage to the fetus.
- Death of the mother.

PROBABLE OUTCOME—Usually curable with treatment.

HOW TO TREAT

NOTE—Follow your doctor's instructions. These instructions are supplemental.

GENERAL MEASURES—Reduce stress whenever possible. See Appendix 13.

MEDICATION
- Your doctor may prescribe:
  Intravenous fluid and electrolyte replacement if your condition is serious.
  Therapeutic trial of vitamin B-6.
- If other drugs are prescribed for you, carefully follow instructions on the label.
- Don't use *any* medicine, including non-prescription medicine to prevent vomiting, without telling your doctor.

ACTIVITY—Stay as active as your strength allows. Work and exercise moderately. Rest often.

DIET—If the condition has not reached the point to warrant hospitalization for intravenous fluids, follow these instructions:
- If you feel nauseated in the morning, eat dry toast or saltine crackers before you get out of bed.
- Eat small, frequent meals.
- Don't eat fried foods; they increase nausea.
- Sit upright for 45 minutes after eating.
- Obtain additional dietary instructions from your doctor or nutritionist.
If intravenous fluids are necessary, you will probably progress from them to a clear liquid diet, full liquid diet and then regular diet with small, frequent meals.

CALL YOUR DOCTOR IF

- You have symptoms of hyperemesis gravidarum.
- Nausea, vomiting or weight loss increase, despite treatment.

ILLNESSES & DISORDERS

HYPERHIDROSIS

GENERAL INFORMATION

DEFINITION—Excessive sweating. Sweating is a normal body function that helps maintain even body temperature. Excess sweat serves no purpose and often creates social embarrassment because of odor or stained clothes. In extreme cases, excess sweat can ruin clothes and shoes.

BODY PARTS INVOLVED—Skin, especially of the underarms, palms and soles.

SEX OR AGE MOST AFFECTED—Both sexes and all ages, except young children.

SIGNS & SYMPTOMS
- Heavy perspiration from underarm area, soles and palms—and to a lesser degree, from other body parts.
- Unpleasant odor, which is caused by bacteria in sweat.

CAUSES
- Stress or chronic anxiety.
- Fever and infection.
- Malignancy, such as lymphoma.
- Hyperthyroidism.
- Heart attack.
- Menopause.
- Some drugs and medicines, such as narcotics.
- Withdrawal from addicting drugs.
- Unknown in some cases.

RISK INCREASES WITH
- Stress.
- Strenuous activity.
- Hot weather.

HOW TO PREVENT—Resolve tension-causing conditions. See Appendix 13.

WHAT TO EXPECT

APPROPRIATE HEALTH CARE
- Self-care.
- Doctor's treatment for underlying conditions, or if self-care is unsuccessful.
- Psychotherapy or counseling, if stress is a major factor.
- Surgery to remove sweat glands or sever nerves to major sweat areas (rare).

DIAGNOSTIC MEASURES
- Your own observation of symptoms.
- Medical history and physical exam by a doctor.

POSSIBLE COMPLICATIONS
- Psychological distress caused by social embarrassment.
- Rashes from deodorants or antiperspirants.
- Dehydration if water intake is insufficient to replace water lost in sweat.

PROBABLE OUTCOME—Symptoms can be controlled with treatment.

HOW TO TREAT

NOTE—Follow your doctor's instructions. These instructions are supplemental.

GENERAL MEASURES
- Bathe frequently.
- Change clothes frequently.
- Wear loose-fitting clothes of natural fibers, such as cotton.
- Use underarm sweat shields.
- Use antiperspirants and deodorants.
- Use drying powders.
- Wear cotton socks.
- Wear leather shoes or sandals. Don't use man-made materials.

MEDICATION—Your doctor may prescribe:
- Tranquilizers or anticholinergics to reduce activity of the central nervous system. Don't use these if you have glaucoma or prostate disease.
- Special solutions to reduce sweating, such as topical applications of aluminum chloride.

ACTIVITY—No restrictions.

DIET—No special diet. Drink at least 8 glasses of water a day—more in hot weather.

CALL YOUR DOCTOR IF

Excessive sweating is causing you problems at work or in social situations.

HYPERLIPIDEMIA, TYPES I, II, III, IV, V
(Hyperlipoproteinemia)

 GENERAL INFORMATION

DEFINITION—Above-normal levels of fat in the blood.

BODY PARTS INVOLVED—Blood and arteries.

SEX OR AGE MOST AFFECTED—All ages, but most common in adults. Different types appear at different ages.

SIGNS & SYMPTOMS
- Yellowish nodules of fat in the skin beneath eyes, elbows and knees, and in tendons.
- Enlarged spleen and liver (some types).
- Whitish ring around the eye pupil (some types).

CAUSES—The blood contains a variety of fats (lipids) joined to blood proteins, forming lipoproteins. These include cholesterol, triglycerides and high-density lipoproteins (HDL). They provide energy and are "building blocks" for some tissues and hormones. In excess, they filter out and are deposited in blood vessels, tendons and other tissues, where they cause symptoms and disease.

RISK INCREASES WITH
- Improper diet that is high in fat and cholesterol.
- Family history of hyperlipidemia.
- Use of oral contraceptives or estrogen.
- Diabetes mellitus.
- Hypothyroidism.
- Nephrosis.
- Alcoholism.

HOW TO PREVENT
- Eat a diet that is low in fat. See Appendix 8.
- If you have diabetes, adhere closely to your treatment program.

 WHAT TO EXPECT

APPROPRIATE HEALTH CARE
- Self-care after diagnosis.
- Doctor's treatment.
- Surgery to remove fat deposits in the skin and tendons.

DIAGNOSTIC MEASURES
- Medical history and physical exam by a doctor.
- Laboratory blood studies to measure blood lipids.

POSSIBLE COMPLICATIONS
- Heart attack.
- Stroke.
- Acute pancreatitis.

PROBABLE OUTCOME—Usually curable with lifelong dietary control and medication.

 HOW TO TREAT

NOTE—Follow your doctor's instructions. These instructions are supplemental.

GENERAL MEASURES—See Appendix 13 for suggestions to reduce stress and improve health. Stress increases the risk of heart disease, a major complication of hyperlipidemia.

MEDICATION
- Your doctor may prescribe:
  Medications to control blood lipids, such as niacin, clofibrate or cholestyramine.
  Medications to treat underlying diseases, such as diabetes or thyroid conditions.
- Don't take oral contraceptives. Use other forms of birth control.

ACTIVITY—No restrictions unless tendons are weakened by fat deposits.

DIET
- Eat a diet that is low in fat. See Appendix 8.
- Lose weight if you are overweight. See Appendix 10 for a reducing diet.
- Don't drink alcohol.

 CALL YOUR DOCTOR IF

- You have symptoms or a family history of hyperlipidemia.
- New, unexplained symptoms develop. Drugs used in treatment may produce side effects.

HYPERNEPHROMA
(Kidney Tumor)

 GENERAL INFORMATION

DEFINITION—A form of kidney cancer with uncontrolled growth of malignant cells in the kidney.

BODY PARTS INVOLVED—Kidney.

SEX OR AGE MOST AFFECTED—Men over age 40.

SIGNS & SYMPTOMS
- Firm mass in an enlarged abdomen.
- Appetite and weight loss.
- Persistent low-grade fever.
- Vomiting.
- Mild abdominal pain.
- Red or smoky urine caused by bleeding from the tumor.

If the tumor grows large enough to cause kidney failure, symptoms include:
- Increasing fatigue and weakness.
- Headache
- Bad breath.
- Nausea, vomiting or diarrhea.
- Shortness of breath.
- Chest pain.
- Itching skin.

CAUSES—Unknown.

RISK INCREASES WITH—Multiple congenital abnormalities.

HOW TO PREVENT—Cannot be prevented at present. If you are a woman of childbearing age with a family history of kidney tumors, seek genetic counseling before becoming pregnant.

 WHAT TO EXPECT

APPROPRIATE HEALTH CARE
- Doctor's treatment.
- Radiation therapy.
- Surgery to remove the tumor.
- Self-care after surgery.

DIAGNOSTIC MEASURES
- Your own observation of symptoms.
- Medical history and physical exam by a doctor.
- Laboratory blood and urine studies of kidney function and to detect blood in the urine.
- X-rays of the kidneys and urinary tract.
- Surgical diagnostic procedures, such as a needle biopsy (see Glossary) of the kidney.

POSSIBLE COMPLICATIONS
- Spread to other organs, especially the liver, lungs, brain and bones, before discovery of the primary tumor.
- Softening of the bones (osteoporosis or osteomalacia).
- Increased susceptibility to urinary-tract infections.

PROBABLE OUTCOME—Usually curable with surgery, if the tumor is detected before it spreads to other body parts.

 HOW TO TREAT

NOTE—Follow your doctor's instructions. These instructions are supplemental.

GENERAL MEASURES—If kidney tumors run in your family, consult your doctor for tests. Even if you feel well and don't have the disease, get regular checkups.

MEDICATION
- Your doctor may prescribe anticancer drugs.
- Most medicines are excreted by the kidney. If chronic kidney failure develops and you take any medications, consult your doctor. Dosages may need adjustment.

ACTIVITY—Take short, frequent rests during the day. Otherwise, stay as active as your strength allows.

DIET
- Eat a low-protein diet. Because of dietary restrictions, multiple-vitamin and mineral supplements may be necessary.
- Increase fluid intake to several pints a day.

 CALL YOUR DOCTOR IF

- You have symptoms of hypernephroma.
- The following occurs during treatment: Fever rises to 101F (38.3C) or higher. Urination decreases.
- New, unexplained symptoms develop. Anticancer drugs used in treatment may produce side effects.
- Symptoms recur after treatment.

HYPERPARATHYROIDISM

GENERAL INFORMATION

DEFINITION—Excess parathyroid hormone circulating in the blood. The excess amounts increase blood levels of calcium (hypercalcemia) and decrease blood levels of phosphorous (hypophosphatemia).

BODY PARTS INVOLVED—Parathyroid glands in the neck; teeth; blood, which affects all body tissues—especially the heart, blood vessels, bones, kidneys, gastrointestinal tract, central nervous system and skin.

SEX OR AGE MOST AFFECTED—Both sexes and all ages, but most common in women between ages 30 and 50.

SIGNS & SYMPTOMS
- Severe flank pain caused by kidney stones.
- Chronic low-back pain caused by bone softening.
- Easy bone fractures caused by decreased calcium in the bones.
- Upper abdominal pain caused by a peptic ulcer or pancreatitis.
- Depression.

CAUSES—Benign tumors of the parathyroid glands, which are located next to the thyroid gland in the neck.

RISK INCREASES WITH
- Recent illness, especially endocrine disorders.
- Medical history of rickets or vitamin-D deficiency.
- Kidney failure.
- Use of laxatives.
- Use of digitalis.

HOW TO PREVENT—No specific preventive measures.

WHAT TO EXPECT

APPROPRIATE HEALTH CARE
- Doctor's treatment.
- Surgery to remove parathyroid tumors, if they are present.
- Self-care after treatment or surgery.

DIAGNOSTIC MEASURES
- Your own observation of symptoms.
- Medical history and physical exam by a doctor.
- Laboratory studies of blood and urine.
- X-rays of bones.

POSSIBLE COMPLICATIONS
- Cataracts.
- Kidney damage.
- Psychosis.
- Hypoparathyroidism caused by removal of too much parathyroid tissue during surgery.
- Hypothyroidism if the thyroid gland is injured inadvertently during surgery on the parathyroid glands.

PROBABLE OUTCOME—Curable with surgery.

HOW TO TREAT

NOTE—Follow your doctor's instructions. These instructions are supplemental.

GENERAL MEASURES—To prevent fractures:
- Use a walker or cane until blood studies return to normal. This may take up to 6 months.
- Install safety rails near the tub, shower and toilet.
- Tape rugs down around the edges.
- Keep the house—especially stairs—brightly lit to avoid stumbling.

MEDICATION
- Your doctor may prescribe: Diuretics to force sodium and calcium excretion. Vitamin D.
- *Don't take* antacids that contain calcium.

ACTIVITY—No restrictions.

DIET
- Limit calcium-containing foods, such as milk and cheese.
- Avoid highly seasoned or spicy foods, especially if you have an ulcer.

CALL YOUR DOCTOR IF

- You have symptoms of hyperparathyroidism.
- The following occurs during treatment: Muscle cramps, numbness or weakness. Breathing difficulty. Persistent heartburn or pain in the upper abdomen. Drastic mood or behavior changes.

HYPERTENSION
(High Blood Pressure)

 GENERAL INFORMATION

DEFINITION—An increase in the force against arteries (blood vessels) as blood circulates through them. Hypertension is sometimes called "the silent killer" because it often has no symptoms in the early stages.

BODY PARTS INVOLVED—Heart; blood vessels; kidneys and eyes (advanced stages).

SEX OR AGE MOST AFFECTED—All ages, but most common in adults.

SIGNS & SYMPTOMS—Usually no symptoms unless disease is severe. Following are symptoms of a hypertensive crisis:
- Headache.
- Drowsiness.
- Confusion.
- Numbness and tingling in the hands and feet.
- Coughing blood.
- Severe shortness of breath.

CAUSES—Usually unknown. A small number of cases result from:
- Chronic kidney disease.
- Severe narrowing of the aorta (major artery of the heart).
- Tumors of the adrenal gland.
- Hardening of the arteries.

RISK INCREASES WITH
- Adults over 60.
- Obesity.
- Smoking.
- Stress.
- Diet that is high in salt or saturated fat.
- Sedentary lifestyle.
- Genetic factors. Hypertension is most common among blacks.
- Family history of hypertension, stroke, heart attack or kidney failure.
- Use of contraceptive pills.

HOW TO PREVENT—Essential hypertension (from unknown causes) cannot be prevented at present. If you have a family history of hypertension, obtain frequent blood-pressure checks. If hypertension is detected early, treatment that includes diet, exercise, stress management and medication can usually prevent complications.

 WHAT TO EXPECT

APPROPRIATE HEALTH CARE
- Self-care after diagnosis.
- Doctor's treatment.

DIAGNOSTIC MEASURES
- Your own observation of symptoms.
- Medical history and physical exam by a doctor.
- Laboratory studies such as blood studies of kidney function, urinalysis and EKG (see Glossary).
- X-rays of the chest and kidneys.

POSSIBLE COMPLICATIONS
- Stroke.
- Heart attack.
- Congestive heart failure and pulmonary edema.
- Kidney failure.
- Blindness caused by ruptured blood vessels.

PROBABLE OUTCOME
- With treatment, complications are preventable (except for possible side effects of drugs). Life expectancy is normal.
- Without treatment, life expectancy is reduced because of the likelihood of heart attack or stroke.

 HOW TO TREAT

NOTE—Follow your doctor's instructions. These instructions are supplemental.

GENERAL MEASURES
- Consider lifestyle changes to reduce stress. See Appendix 13.
- Learn to take your own blood pressure. Your doctor or nurse can teach you.

MEDICATION
- Many antihypertensive medications can reduce blood pressure. Your doctor will prescribe the type appropriate for you. Don't stop taking them without consulting your doctor.
- Don't take non-prescription cold and sinus remedies. These contain chemicals, such as ephedrine and pseudoephedrine, that raise blood pressure.

ACTIVITY—Exercise at least 3 times a week. This helps reduce stress and maintain normal body weight; it may lower blood pressure. See Appendix 20.

DIET
- Low-salt diet (see Appendix 9).
- Reducing diet if overweight (see Appendix 10).

 CALL YOUR DOCTOR IF

- You have symptoms of a hypertensive crisis.
- Chest pain occurs.

HYPERTHYROIDISM

GENERAL INFORMATION

DEFINITION—Overactivity of the thyroid, an endocrine gland that regulates all body functions.

BODY PARTS INVOLVED—Thyroid gland and most other body organs, especially the endocrine system, which includes the pituitary gland, parathyroid glands, pancreas, adrenal glands, and ovaries or testicles.

SEX OR AGE MOST AFFECTED—Adults between ages 20 and 50, mostly women.

SIGNS & SYMPTOMS
- Hyperactivity.
- Feeling warm or hot all the time.
- Tremors.
- Sweating.
- Itching skin.
- Pounding, rapid, irregular heartbeat.
- Weight loss, despite overeating. Older persons may gain weight.
- Marked anxiety and restlessness.
- Sleeplessness.
- Fatigue and weakness.
- Protruding eyes (exophthalmos) and double vision (sometimes).
- Diarrhea (sometimes).
- Hair loss (sometimes).
- Goiter (sometimes).

CAUSES
- Thyroid nodules or tumors.
- Pituitary disorders.
- Ovarian disorders.

RISK INCREASES WITH
- Family history of hyperthyroidism.
- Stress.

HOW TO PREVENT—No specific preventive measures.

WHAT TO EXPECT

APPROPRIATE HEALTH CARE
- Self-care after diagnosis.
- Doctor's treatment.
- Surgery to remove part of the thyroid, if medication does not control the disorder.

DIAGNOSTIC MEASURES
- Your own observation of symptoms.
- Medical history and physical exam by a doctor.
- Laboratory blood studies.
- EKG (see Glossary).
- Radioactive studies such as I131 uptake (see Glossary).

POSSIBLE COMPLICATIONS
- Congestive heart failure.
- "Thyroid storm"—a sudden worsening of all symptoms. This is a life-threatening emergency.
- Misdiagnosis as a psychiatric anxiety reaction.

PROBABLE OUTCOME—Usually curable with medication or surgery. Allow 6 months of treatment for the condition to stabilize.

HOW TO TREAT

NOTE—Follow your doctor's instructions. These instructions are supplemental.

GENERAL MEASURES—Since this condition develops gradually, symptoms may be difficult to recognize. If family and friends mention changes in your behavior or appearance, consult your doctor.

MEDICATION—Your doctor may prescribe:
- Antithyroid drugs to depress thyroid activity.
- Beta-adrenergic blockers to decrease a rapid heartbeat.
- Radioactive iodine, which selectively destroys thyroid cells.

ACTIVITY—Rest in bed as much as possible until the disorder is cured.

DIET—Eat a diet high in protein to replace tissue lost from thyroid overactivity.

CALL YOUR DOCTOR IF

- You have symptoms of hyperthyroidism.
- Symptoms worsen suddenly, especially after surgery.
- New, unexplained symptoms develop. Drugs used in treatment may produce side effects.

ILLNESSES & DISORDERS

HYPERVENTILATION SYNDROME
(Panic Attack)

 GENERAL INFORMATION

DEFINITION—Breathing so fast that carbon-dioxide levels in the blood are decreased, temporarily upsetting normal blood chemistry.

BODY PARTS INVOLVED—Central nervous system; lungs; skin; hands; feet.

SEX OR AGE MOST AFFECTED—All ages, but most common in young adults.

SIGNS & SYMPTOMS
- Rapid breathing.
- Numbness and tingling around the mouth, hands and feet.
- Weakness or faintness.
- Muscle spasm or contractions in the hands and feet.
- Fainting (occasionally).

CAUSES—A change in the normal ratio of acid to other elements in the blood caused by breathing out too much carbon dioxide.

Hyperventilation can accompany fever, disease of the heart and lungs, or severe injury.

If disease or injury is not present, hyperventilation is caused by anxiety.

RISK INCREASES WITH
- Stress.
- Feelings of guilt.
- Fatigue or overwork.
- Illness, such as those listed above.
- Smoking.
- Excess alcohol consumption.

HOW TO PREVENT
- Avoid anxiety-producing situations.
- See Appendix 13 for suggestions to reduce stress.

 WHAT TO EXPECT

APPROPRIATE HEALTH CARE
- Self-care.
- Doctor's treatment, if the cause is organic or symptoms are prolonged.
- Psychotherapy or counseling, if hyperventilation occurs often and is caused by anxiety.

DIAGNOSTIC MEASURES
- Your own observation of symptoms.
- Medical history and physical exam by a doctor.

POSSIBLE COMPLICATIONS
- Seizures.
- Fainting.

PROBABLE OUTCOME—Symptoms can be controlled with the instructions below.

If hyperventilation is caused by a disease, it will stop when the disease is cured.

Recurrent attacks caused by anxiety should stop if underlying stress can be eliminated.

 HOW TO TREAT

GENERAL MEASURES—During an attack, the following instructions will increase carbon dioxide in the blood and relieve symptoms:
- Cover your mouth and nose completely with a paper bag.
- Breathe slowly into the bag and rebreathe the air. The air in the bag contains additional carbon dioxide.
- Breathe slowly in and out of the bag at least 10 times.
- Put the bag aside and breathe normally a few minutes.
- Repeat the process until the symptoms diminish or disappear.
- If symptoms return, repeat the process as often as needed.

MEDICATION—Medicine usually is not necessary for this disorder.

ACTIVITY—After treatment, resume normal activity as soon as possible.

DIET—No special diet.

 CALL YOUR DOCTOR IF

- You have symptoms of hyperventilation that don't diminish with self-treatment.
- The following occurs during an attack:
  Fainting.
  Seizure.
  Sudden fever.

HYPOCHONDRIASIS

 GENERAL INFORMATION

DEFINITION—A person's conviction that he or she has a serious or fatal disease, despite evidence to the contrary from medical examinations and tests.

BODY PARTS INVOLVED—Brain.

SEX OR AGE MOST AFFECTED—Both sexes; all ages.

SIGNS & SYMPTOMS—Anxiety and persistent reports of symptoms involving any body part. Concern about heart disease or cancer is common. Symptoms may change, but the person's belief that a serious condition exists does not. Frequently reported symptoms include insomnia, sexual dysfunction and gastrointestinal discomfort, such as bloating, belching and cramps.

CAUSES
● Overly protective parents in childhood.
● Lack of social outlets and contacts.
● Guilt feelings and an imagined need for punishment.
● Extreme need for attention.

RISK INCREASES WITH
● Stress.
● Major life changes, such as a divorce, job change, marriage, move, loss of a valued person or object, menopause or retirement.
● Depression.
● Psychosis.

HOW TO PREVENT—In childhood, don't reward illness by giving a child special privileges and undue attention for being sick. Provide adequate love and support during healthy periods.

 WHAT TO EXPECT

APPROPRIATE HEALTH CARE
● Doctor's treatment.
● Psychotherapy or counseling. This offers the best hope for cure. However, few persons with hypochondriasis accept the conclusion that their health problem is psychological.

DIAGNOSTIC MEASURES
● Your own observation of symptoms.
● Medical history and physical exam by a doctor. After a thorough medical evaluation, repeat testing should be avoided.

POSSIBLE COMPLICATIONS
● Wasting money on unnecessary—and sometimes dangerous—medical care.
● Insisting on unnecessary surgical procedures or medications.
● Failure of a doctor to take symptoms of real disease seriously when they do develop.

PROBABLE OUTCOME—Generally resistant to treatment. Most patients maintain a lifelong belief that they have a serious disease, and they change doctors frequently.

 HOW TO TREAT

NOTE—Follow your doctor's instructions. These instructions are supplemental.

GENERAL MEASURES—Persons with hypochondriasis are often difficult to live with because of their constant worry and demands for attention. Realize that the person really suffers, and try to be supportive. Reward positive behavior that is not related to physical complaints. Don't encourage the "sick role."

MEDICATION—Medicine usually is not necessary for this disorder. Your doctor may prescribe mild tranquilizers for a short time while therapy is being arranged.

ACTIVITY—No restrictions.

DIET—No special diet.

 CALL YOUR DOCTOR IF

● You have symptoms of hypochondriasis and want professional help to overcome the problem.
● New, unexplained symptoms develop. Tranquilizers used in treatment may produce side effects or dependence.

ILLNESSES & DISORDERS

HYPOGLYCEMIA, FUNCTIONAL

 GENERAL INFORMATION

DEFINITION—Low blood sugar caused by abnormal function—not disease—of the pancreas.

BODY PARTS INVOLVED—Pancreas; this eventually involves all body cells.

SEX OR AGE MOST AFFECTED—Both sexes; all ages.

SIGNS & SYMPTOMS—The following vary greatly among people in frequency and severity:
- Weakness or faintness.
- Sweating.
- Excessive hunger.
- Nervousness and trembling hands.
- Heartbeat irregularities.
- Headache.
- Confusion.
- Personality changes.
- Loss of consciousness.
- Seizures (sometimes).

CAUSES—Functional hypoglycemia probably results when the pancreas produces too much insulin in response to sugars and other carbohydrates, heavy exercise, pregnancy or unknown causes.

The following drugs decrease blood-sugar levels in some persons: tobacco; caffeine; alcohol; aspirin; sulfonurea medications; phenformin; haloperidol; propoxyphene; chlorpromazine.

Some doctors believe functional hypoglycemia may be the first indication that diabetes mellitus is developing.

RISK INCREASES WITH
- Stress.
- Improper diet.
- Smoking.
- Use of drugs, such as those listed above.
- Fatigue or overwork.

HOW TO PREVENT
- Follow instructions under Diet. Don't skip meals.
- Avoid stress.
- Don't smoke.
- Don't drink alcohol.

 WHAT TO EXPECT

APPROPRIATE HEALTH CARE
- Self-care after diagnosis.
- Doctor's treatment.
- Psychotherapy or counseling to learn to cope with stress.

DIAGNOSTIC MEASURES
- Your own observation of symptoms.
- Medical history and physical exam by a doctor.
- Laboratory studies, such as blood-sugar and glucose-tolerance tests.

POSSIBLE COMPLICATIONS—Repeated attacks can cause personality changes.

PROBABLE OUTCOME—Symptoms can be controlled with treatment.

 HOW TO TREAT

NOTE—Follow your doctor's instructions. These instructions are supplemental.

GENERAL MEASURES—Consider lifestyle changes. See Appendix 13.

MEDICATION—Medicine usually is not necessary for this disorder.

ACTIVITY—No restrictions.

DIET—Eat 5 or 6 small meals a day that are low in simple carbohydrates, moderate in fats and high in protein. Between-meals snacks should include protein, such as chicken, eggs, cheese or skim milk, rather than carbohydrates. Avoid highly concentrated sweets, such as candy.

 CALL YOUR DOCTOR IF

You have symptoms of functional hypoglycemia.

HYPOGLYCEMIA OF DIABETES

 ## GENERAL INFORMATION

DEFINITION—Low blood sugar in a patient taking medication, such as insulin or oral antidiabetic drugs, for diabetes.

BODY PARTS INVOLVED—Brain; this quickly involves all body cells.

SEX OR AGE MOST AFFECTED—Both sexes; all ages.

SIGNS & SYMPTOMS—Mild hypoglycemic reaction:
- Excessive hunger.
- Weakness.
- Nervousness.
- Emotional instability.
- Difficulty concentrating.
- Sweating.
- Headache.

Moderate hypoglycemic reaction:
- Increased weakness.
- Excessive sweating.
- Cold, clammy skin.
- Numbness around the mouth or fingers.
- Pounding heartbeat.
- Memory loss.
- Double vision.
- Staring expression.
- Difficulty walking.
- Unawareness of surroundings.

Severe hypoglycemic reaction:
- Muscle twitching.
- Unconsciousness.
- Convulsions.
- Lack of urinary control.

CAUSES—Too much insulin or oral antidiabetic drug or not enough food for the condition your body is in. Factors which affect this include:
- More exercise than usual.
- Irregular meals, skipped meals or partial meals.
- Loose bowel movements, diarrhea or vomiting of the last meal.
- Infection.
- Anger or excitement.

RISK INCREASES WITH
- Stress.
- Illness with fever.
- Smoking. Smoking decreases blood sugar.
- Use of other drugs which may also reduce blood sugar, such as diuretics, caffeine or alcohol.
- Liver or pancreas disorder.

HOW TO PREVENT
- Follow diabetic diet, exercise and medication instructions carefully.
- Keep hard candy available for early symptoms.
- Request glucagon and an injection kit from your doctor.

 ## WHAT TO EXPECT

APPROPRIATE HEALTH CARE
- Self-care.
- Doctor's treatment.

DIAGNOSTIC MEASURES
- Your own observation of symptoms.
- Medical history and physical exam by a doctor.
- Laboratory studies of blood sugar.

POSSIBLE COMPLICATIONS—Repeated attacks can cause permanent brain damage.

PROBABLE OUTCOME—Disorder is curable in 10 to 15 minutes if glucose can be given orally or by injection.

 ## HOW TO TREAT

NOTE—Follow your doctor's instructions. These instructions are supplemental.

GENERAL MEASURES
- Wear a Medic-Alert bracelet or pendant (see Glossary).
- For a mild hypoglycemic reaction: Drink 1/2 cup of orange juice or a non-dietetic soft drink, or eat 1/2 candy bar, 6 or 7 hard candies, or 2 teaspoons of honey, syrup or sugar. Repeat, if necessary, in 10 to 15 minutes.
- For a moderate hypoglycemic reaction: Eat or drink something sugary as above, but follow it with a carbohydrate that is absorbed more slowly, such as a banana, apple, cereal, bread or crackers.
- For a severe hypoglycemic reaction: If the person is unconscious, inject glucagon (1/2 to 1cc) deeply into a muscle and at right angles to the big muscle in the arm or leg.
  After the person regains consciousness, give sweet foods as above.
  Prop the person in a sitting position as soon as possible. Call the doctor.

MEDICATION—Always carry hard candy. Your doctor may prescribe glucagon to have available for emergencies.

ACTIVITY—After treatment, resume normal activity as soon as possible.

DIET—Ask your doctor if the basic diet plan needs changing.

 ## CALL YOUR DOCTOR IF

- You have diabetes, take medication and have symptoms of hypoglycemia—especially severe symptoms.
- Symptoms don't disappear with treatment above.
- Hypoglycemic reactions occur frequently.

HYPOPARATHYROIDISM

GENERAL INFORMATION

DEFINITION—Decreased production of hormones by the parathyroid glands, causing a low level of calcium in the blood.

BODY PARTS INVOLVED—Parathyroid glands in the neck; teeth; blood, which affects all body tissues, especially the heart, blood vessels, bones, kidneys, gastrointestinal tract, central nervous system and skin.

SEX OR AGE MOST AFFECTED—Both sexes; all ages.

SIGNS & SYMPTOMS—Acute phase:
- Tingling fingertips.
- Muscle tension and spasms in the hands and feet.
- Spasms of the larynx and throat muscles, causing breathing difficulty.
- Scaling skin.
- Splitting nails.
Chronic phase:
- Poor tooth development.
- Seizures.
- Mental retardation in children.
- Psychosis in adults.

CAUSES
- Complication of surgery on the parathyroid glands, the thyroid glands or other neck tissues.
- Genetic autoimmune disorder (possibly).
- Radiation of the thyroid gland.
- Hemochromatosis (see Glossary).
- Tuberculosis.
- Neck injury.

RISK INCREASES WITH
- Recent infection of any kind.
- Pregnancy.
- Use of diuretic drugs.

HOW TO PREVENT—No specific preventive measures.

WHAT TO EXPECT

APPROPRIATE HEALTH CARE
- Doctor's treatment during the acute stage.
- Self-care after diagnosis during the chronic stage.
- Hospitalization for severe muscle spasms.

DIAGNOSTIC MEASURES
- Your own observation of symptoms.
- Medical history and physical exam by a doctor.
- Laboratory blood and urine studies.
- EKG (see Glossary).
- X-rays of bones to detect increased bone density.

POSSIBLE COMPLICATIONS
- Cataracts.
- Brain damage.
- Heartbeat abnormalities and congestive heart failure.

PROBABLE OUTCOME—This condition is currently considered incurable. It requires lifelong replacement therapy to control symptoms. Without treatment, it is fatal.

Scientific research into causes and treatment continues, so there is hope for increasingly effective treatment and cure.

HOW TO TREAT

NOTE—Follow your doctor's instructions. These instructions are supplemental.

GENERAL MEASURES
- If muscle cramps start, place a paper bag over your mouth. Blow into it and rebreathe your breath. This will raise carbon-dioxide levels in the blood and decrease muscle spasms.
- Apply lubricating creams or ointments to dry, scaling skin.
- Keep nails trimmed to prevent splitting.

MEDICATION—Your doctor may prescribe:
- Vitamin-D and calcium supplements in high doses.
- Intravenous calcium supplements during hospitalization for severe muscle spasms.
- Sedatives and anticonvulsants for frequent muscle spasms.

ACTIVITY—No restrictions.

DIET—High calcium, low-phosphorous diet. Your doctor or dietitian will provide specific instructions.

CALL YOUR DOCTOR IF

- You have unexplained muscle spasms of the hands, feet or throat, or numbness or tingling in the hands or feet.
- Muscle spasms don't decrease in 1 week, despite treatment.

HYPOTHERMIA

 ## GENERAL INFORMATION

DEFINITION—Dangerous cooling of the body from exposure to cold air or water.

BODY PARTS INVOLVED—All major organ systems, including decreased blood flow through the kidneys and brain.

SEX OR AGE MOST AFFECTED—All ages, but most common in adults over 60.

SIGNS & SYMPTOMS—Early symptoms:
- Poor muscle coordination.
- Mental confusion and amnesia.
- Shivering and low body temperature (95F to 98F or 35C to 36.7C) rectally.
- Slow pulse.
Late symptoms:
- Rigid muscles.
- Temperature drop to 77F to 84F (25C to 28.9C).
- Purple fingers, toes and nail beds.
- Loss of consciousness.

CAUSES—Prolonged exposure to cold temperatures, especially outdoors with a high wind-chill factor.

RISK INCREASES WITH
- Adults over 60.
- Thin or wet clothing.
- Slender body size. Slender persons lose heat more rapidly than obese persons.
- Smoking, which decreases circulation to extremities.
- Excess alcohol consumption.
- Mental impairment.

HOW TO PREVENT
- Obtain warm housing and adequate clothing before winter.
- In cold weather, wear windproof clothing in many layers, including a scarf, hat and mittens.
- Don't leave your home during a severe winter storm.
- Don't skate or fish on ice unless you have determined the ice is safe.
- Persons who are unable to care for themselves fully, such as the elderly, mentally impaired or alcoholic, should be visited or supervised during cold weather.

 ## WHAT TO EXPECT

APPROPRIATE HEALTH CARE
- Doctor's treatment.
- Hospitalization. Arrange transportation to the nearest emergency center immediately.

DIAGNOSTIC MEASURES
- Your own observation of symptoms.
- Medical history and physical exam by a doctor.
- Laboratory studies, such as kidney-function studies.

POSSIBLE COMPLICATIONS
- Shock.
- Pneumonia.
- Death.

PROBABLE OUTCOME—Sometimes fatal, depending on the length and amount of temperature loss. Chances of survival are excellent if the patient is conscious on arrival at the emergency center.

 ## HOW TO TREAT

NOTE—Follow your doctor's instructions. These instructions are supplemental.

GENERAL MEASURES—The following may be helpful while waiting for emergency help:
- Place the person in bed and cover with a blanket or electric blanket at normal body temperature.
- A warm (not hot) bath may be helpful—but call the nearest emergency center for advice.
- If the person is outdoors, cover with blankets or shield from the wind.

MEDICATION—The doctor may prescribe medicine to support blood pressure if the person's condition is critical.

ACTIVITY—After treatment, normal activity should be resumed gradually.

DIET—Don't give alcohol to a person with hypothermia. It is of no help and may be harmful.

 ## CALL YOUR DOCTOR IF

You observe symptoms of hypothermia in someone.

HYPOTHYROIDISM

GENERAL INFORMATION

DEFINITION—Underactive thyroid gland.

BODY PARTS INVOLVED—Thyroid gland (located in the neck below the Adam's apple); endocrine system.

SEX OR AGE MOST AFFECTED—Both sexes of adults, but more common in women.

SIGNS & SYMPTOMS—It is unlikely one person will have all the following symptoms, but most will have several:
- Decreased tolerance for cold.
- Decreased sweating.
- Decreased appetite.
- Constipation.
- Chest pain.
- Coarse or slow-growing hair.
- Slow, rapid or irregular heartbeat.
- Weight gain or extreme thinness.
- Placidity or nervousness.
- Sleepiness or insomnia.
- Mental impairment, including depression, psychosis or poor memory.
- Fluid retention, especially around the eyes.
- Dull facial expression and droopy eyelids.
- Coarse skin.
- Decreased tolerance for medication.
- Decreased sex drive and infertility.
- Menstrual disorders.
- Anemia.
- Numbness and tingling of the hands and feet.
- Deepened or hoarse voice.

CAUSES—Sometimes unknown. Following are the most common causes:
- Autoimmune disease, in which the body's immune system functions abnormally and attacks the thyroid gland.
- Radioactive iodine treatment.
- Surgery for hyperthyroidism.
- Iodine deficiency in the diet.
- Decreased activity of the pituitary gland, which secretes a thyroid-stimulating hormone.
- Use of drugs, such as lithium, that may depress thyroid function.

RISK INCREASES WITH
- Adults over 60.
- Obesity.
- Surgery for hyperthyroidism.
- X-ray treatments.

HOW TO PREVENT
- Use iodized salt.
- Take replacement thyroid for life after thyroid surgery or destruction of the thyroid gland by radiation treatment.

WHAT TO EXPECT

APPROPRIATE HEALTH CARE
- Self-care after diagnosis.
- Doctor's treatment.

DIAGNOSTIC MEASURES
- Your own observation of symptoms.
- Medical history and physical exam by a doctor.
- Laboratory blood studies of thyroid hormones. Lab studies can confirm the diagnosis of hypothyroidism, but they cannot indicate how much replacement therapy is needed.

POSSIBLE COMPLICATIONS—None expected.

PROBABLE OUTCOME—Usually curable with careful thyroid-replacement therapy. The goal of treatment is to provide the body with enough thyroid substance for efficient body function. Medical evaluation may be necessary for several months to establish the correct dose of thyroid replacement.

HOW TO TREAT

NOTE—Follow your doctor's instructions. These instructions are supplemental.

GENERAL MEASURES—No special instructions except those listed under other headings.

MEDICATION—Your doctor will prescribe thyroid-replacement hormones.

ACTIVITY—No restrictions.

DIET—No special diet.

CALL YOUR DOCTOR IF

- You have symptoms of hypothyroidism.
- Symptoms don't improve within 3 weeks after treatment begins.
- New, unexplained symptoms develop. Drugs used in treatment may produce side effects.

ID REACTION
(Autoeczematization; Autosensitization)

 GENERAL INFORMATION

DEFINITION—An allergic response to a skin disorder of the feet, groin or other area, producing an itching rash somewhere else in the body.

BODY PARTS INVOLVED
- Parts with the original disorder: groin, ears, hands, feet.
- Parts with the allergic response: hands, feet, arms, legs or trunk.

SEX OR AGE MOST AFFECTED—Both sexes; all ages.

SIGNS & SYMPTOMS
- Itching (often severe).
- Vesicles (fluid-filled, small blisters) of varying size on the skin.

CAUSES—Unknown. An id reaction may be a disorder of the body's immunological response to the original ailment. They occur most often with some forms of dermatitis, outer-ear infections and eczema of the hand or foot.

RISK INCREASES WITH
- Recent skin rash anywhere.
- Stress.
- Medical history of allergies.

HOW TO PREVENT—Treat all skin disorders thoroughly until they disappear.

 WHAT TO EXPECT

APPROPRIATE HEALTH CARE
- Doctor's treatment.
- Self-care after diagnosis.

DIAGNOSTIC MEASURES
- Your own observation of symptoms.
- Medical history and physical exam by a doctor.
- Laboratory culture of the original skin disorder.

POSSIBLE COMPLICATIONS—Adverse reaction to medication used in treatment.

PROBABLE OUTCOME—Usually curable in 2 weeks. Recurrence is rapid if treatment is discontinued before the id reaction and original disorder are completely gone.

 HOW TO TREAT

NOTE—Follow your doctor's instructions. These instructions are supplemental.

GENERAL MEASURES
- Treat the original skin disorder until it heals completely to prevent a recurrence of the id reaction. For instructions, consult your doctor or refer to the disorder in this book.
- Minimize stress, if possible. (See Appendix 13.)

MEDICATION—Your doctor may prescribe topical or oral cortisone drugs. Oral steroids quickly control the id reaction, but slow healing of the underlying disorder.

ACTIVITY—No restrictions.

DIET—No special diet.

 CALL YOUR DOCTOR IF

- You have symptoms of an id reaction.
- The following occurs during treatment: Fever higher than 101F (38.3C). Heat, redness, pain or tenderness in any of the lesions. This indicates infection.
- New, unexplained symptoms develop. Drugs used in treatment may produce side effects.

ILLNESSES & DISORDERS

IDIOPATHIC HYPERTROPHIC SUBAORTIC STENOSIS (IHSS)

 GENERAL INFORMATION

DEFINITION—A chronic heart condition that produces an enlarged heart muscle, restricting the amount of blood the heart pumps.

BODY PARTS INVOLVED—Heart.

SEX OR AGE MOST AFFECTED—Both sexes; all ages.

SIGNS & SYMPTOMS
- Chest pain (angina pectoris).
- Heart-rhythm irregularity.
- Fainting.
- Shortness of breath.
- Swollen feet and ankles.
- Distended neck veins.
- Enlarged and tender liver (under the rib cage).
- Heart murmur (see Glossary).

CAUSES—Thickening of the left chamber (ventricle) of the heart for unknown reason. This obstructs the flow of blood, and the heart may be unable to pump enough blood during exertion. In some cases, this condition is inherited as a dominant genetic trait.

RISK INCREASES WITH—Family history of IHSS.

HOW TO PREVENT—If you have a family history of IHSS, obtain genetic counseling before starting a family.

 WHAT TO EXPECT

APPROPRIATE HEALTH CARE
- Doctor's treatment, including consultation with a cardiologist.
- Surgery to reduce the obstruction, if medication does not control the problem.
- DC electrocardioversion (electric shock to the heart) for treatment of life-threatening heartbeat irregularities.

DIAGNOSTIC MEASURES
- Your own observation of symptoms.
- Medical history and physical exam by a doctor.
- Laboratory studies, such as cardiac catheterization to measure blood flow through heart chambers.
- X-rays of the heart.
- EKG and echocardiogram (see Glossary for both) of the heart.

POSSIBLE COMPLICATIONS—Fatal heartbeat irregularity.

PROBABLE OUTCOME—Usually curable with medication or surgery.

 HOW TO TREAT

NOTE—Follow your doctor's instructions. These instructions are supplemental.

GENERAL MEASURES
- Stay under close medical supervision.
- Wear a Medic-Alert bracelet or pendant (see Glossary).
- Family members, close friends and business acquaintances should learn cardiopulmonary resuscitation (CPR), in case cardiac arrest occurs.

MEDICATION—Your doctor may prescribe:
- Beta-adrenergic blockers or calcium-channel blockers to prevent heartbeat irregularities.
- Don't use nitroglycerin for angina pain. It dilates arteries, which may be harmful.
- If digitalis is prescribed for you, discuss the risks with your doctor. It may trigger heartbeat irregularities.

ACTIVITY—Your doctor should guide you about how much physical activity is ideal. Your ability to increase activity is dependent on your response to therapy. Don't regard yourself as an invalid.

DIET—A low-salt diet (see Appendix 9) may be necessary, if you have fluid accumulation (a possible sign of congestive heart failure).

 CALL YOUR DOCTOR IF

- You have symptoms of IHSS, or symptoms worsen during treatment.
- New, unexplained symptoms develop. Drugs used in treatment may produce side effects.

IMMUNODEFICIENCY DISEASE

GENERAL INFORMATION

DEFINITION—Defects in the body's immune system. A healthy immune system protects the body against germs (bacteria, viruses and fungi), cancer (partial protection) and any foreign material that enters the body. When the system fails, the body becomes susceptible to infection and cancer.

BODY PARTS INVOLVED—Immune system (blood, bone marrow, lymph tissue, liver, spleen and thymus gland).

SEX OR AGE MOST AFFECTED—Both sexes; all ages.

SIGNS & SYMPTOMS—Recurrent, severe infections and illnesses. The most common include:
- Ear or respiratory infections, such as otitis media and pneumonia.
- Yeast infections, especially candidiasis.
- Cancer, especially leukemia and lymphoma.
- Bleeding disorders.
- Eczema.
- Meningitis or encephalitis.

CAUSES
- Birth defects that involve an incomplete or absent immune system.
- Surgical removal of the spleen before age 2.
- Use of immunosuppressive drugs.
- Radiation treatment.
- Some cancers, such as Hodgkin's disease.
- Hypogammaglobulinemia (see Glossary).
- Viral infections, such as AIDS (acquired immunodeficiency syndrome).

RISK INCREASES WITH
- Poor nutrition.
- Male homosexual activity, blood transfusions or intravenous drug use (AIDS only).
- Family history of immunodeficiency disease.

HOW TO PREVENT—If you have a family history of immunodeficiency disease, seek genetic counseling before starting a family.

WHAT TO EXPECT

APPROPRIATE HEALTH CARE
- Doctor's treatment.
- Surgery to transplant bone marrow or the thymus gland (occasionally).
- Hospitalization for treatment of serious infection.

DIAGNOSTIC MEASURES
- Your own observation of symptoms, especially repeated infections in children.
- Medical history and physical exam by a doctor.
- Laboratory blood studies of antibodies, microscopic examination of blood and tissue cells and skin tests.
- Chest X-rays of the thymus gland.
- Radioactive studies of immune function.

POSSIBLE COMPLICATIONS
- Uncontrolled bacterial, viral or fungal infections that don't respond to treatment.
- Cancer.
- Infectious arthritis.

PROBABLE OUTCOME—Severe forms of immunodeficiency are usually fatal. Minor forms can be treated successfully.

HOW TO TREAT

NOTE—Follow your doctor's instructions. These instructions are supplemental.

GENERAL MEASURES
- Avoid exposure to persons with contagious illnesses.
- Don't take *any* type of vaccine without medical advice.
- Don't take cortisone or immunosuppressive drugs prescribed for you without getting a second medical opinion.

MEDICATION—Your doctor may prescribe:
- Antibiotics to fight infections.
- Injections of antibodies.
- Transfusions of blood components.
- Injections of gamma globulin (sometimes).

ACTIVITY—Bed rest is usually necessary during acute illnesses. Otherwise, there are no restrictions on activity.

DIET—No special diet.

CALL YOUR DOCTOR IF

- You have symptoms of immunodeficiency disease.
- After diagnosis, you have signs of infection, such as: chills; fever; muscle aches; headache; dizziness; and cough with thick, discolored or blood-streaked sputum.

ILLNESSES & DISORDERS

IMPETIGO
(Pyoderma)

 GENERAL INFORMATION

DEFINITION—A contagious, common bacterial skin infection that affects the superficial layers of the skin.

BODY PARTS INVOLVED—Skin of the face, arms and legs.

SEX OR AGE MOST AFFECTED—All ages, but most common in infants and children.

SIGNS & SYMPTOMS
- A red rash with many small blisters. Some blisters contain pus, and yellow crusts form when they break. The blisters don't hurt, but they may itch.
- Slight fever (sometimes).

CAUSES—Staphylococci or streptococci bacteria growing in the upper skin layers.

RISK INCREASES WITH
- Fair complexion.
- Skin that is sensitive to sun and irritants, such as soap and makeup.
- Poor nutrition.
- Illness that has lowered resistance.
- Warm, moist weather.
- Crowded or unsanitary living conditions.
- Poor hygiene.

HOW TO PREVENT
- Bathe daily with soap and water.
- Keep fingernails short. Don't scratch impetigo blisters.
- If there is an outbreak in the family, urge all members to use antibacterial soap.
- Use separate towels for each family member, or substitute paper towels temporarily.

 WHAT TO EXPECT

APPROPRIATE HEALTH CARE
- Home care after diagnosis.
- Doctor's treatment.

DIAGNOSTIC MEASURES
- Your own observation of symptoms.
- Medical history and physical exam by a doctor.
- Laboratory skin culture to identify the germ causing the infection.

POSSIBLE COMPLICATIONS
- Penetration of the infection to deeper skin layers (ecthyma or cellulitis). This may cause scarring. Treatment is the same as for impetigo.
- Acute glomerulonephritis.

PROBABLE OUTCOME—Curable in 10 days with treatment.

 HOW TO TREAT

NOTE—Follow your doctor's instructions. These instructions are supplemental.

GENERAL MEASURES
- Follow the suggestions listed under How to Prevent.
- Scrub lesions with gauze and antiseptic soap. Break any pustules. Remove all crusts, and expose and cleanse all lesions. If crusts are difficult to remove, soak them in warm soapy water and scrub gently.
- Cover impetigo sores with gauze and tape to keep hands away from them.
- Treat new lesions the same way, even if you are not sure they are impetigo.
- Separate and boil bed linen, if possible, and towels, clothes and other items that have touched sores.
- Men should shave around sores on the face, not over them. Use an aerosol shaving cream and change razor blades each day. Don't use a shaving brush—it may harbor germs.

MEDICATION—Your doctor may prescribe:
- Oral antibiotics, such as dicloxacillin or erythromycin. To avoid complications, take antibiotics for 10 days even if symptoms disappear.
- Antibiotic ointments for very small areas of infection. Rub antibiotic ointment into the lesions for 60 seconds at least 4 times a day. If your doctor has not prescribed an ointment, you may use a non-prescription ointment containing neomycin and bacitracin.

ACTIVITY—No restrictions.

DIET—No special diet.

 CALL YOUR DOCTOR IF

- You or your child have symptoms of impetigo.
- Fever of 101F (38.3C) or higher orally develops.
- The sores continue to spread or don't begin to heal in 3 days, despite treatment.

IMPOTENCE, MALE SEXUAL
(Erectile Dysfunction)

 GENERAL INFORMATION

DEFINITION—Inability to have or maintain an erection of the penis necessary for satisfactory sexual intercourse.

BODY PARTS INVOLVED—Male reproductive system; central nervous system.

SEX OR AGE MOST AFFECTED—Male adolescents and adults, but most common in men over 45.

SIGNS & SYMPTOMS—Absent penile erections, or erections that are too weak, brief or painful for sexual intercourse.

CAUSES—About 80% of cases have psychological causes. These include:
- Guilt feelings.
- A poor relationship with the sexual partner.
- Psychological disorders, including depression, anxiety and psychosis.
- Lack of sexual information, including an understanding of the emotional aspects of sexuality and information about female anatomy and physiology.

Physiological causes include:
- Temporary fatigue.
- Diabetes mellitus.
- Atherosclerosis (hardening of the arteries).
- Use of some antihypertensive medications.
- Disorders of the central nervous system, such as spinal-cord injury, multiple sclerosis, stroke or syphilis.
- Endocrine disorders that involve the pituitary, thyroid, adrenal or sexual glands.
- Alcoholism.
- Drug abuse, especially of marijuana, cocaine, narcotics, tranquilizers, sedatives, hypnotics and hallucinogenics.

RISK INCREASES WITH
- Stress.
- Recent illness that has lowered strength.
- Recent major surgery, especially cardiovascular or prostate surgery.
- Excess alcohol consumption.
- Use of drugs—including necessary prescription drugs and illicit drugs.

HOW TO PREVENT
- Maintain good communication with your partner. Don't be hesitant about discussing the problem, exploring your needs and asking for help. Your partner's understanding is critical to solving the problem.
- Don't drink more than 1 or 2 alcoholic drinks—if any—a day. Don't use other drugs that can be abused.
- If you have diabetes, adhere closely to your treatment program.

 WHAT TO EXPECT

APPROPRIATE HEALTH CARE
- Self-care after diagnosis.
- Doctor's treatment.
- Psychotherapy or counseling from a qualified, professional sex therapist.
- Surgery to implant an inflatable or non-inflatable penile prosthesis (sometimes).

DIAGNOSTIC MEASURES
- Your own observation of symptoms.
- Medical history and physical exam by a doctor.
- Laboratory blood studies of hormone levels.

POSSIBLE COMPLICATIONS
- Depression and loss of self-esteem.
- Marital problems or breakdown of close personal relationships.

PROBABLE OUTCOME—Spontaneous recovery or recovery after brief counseling in many cases with psychological origins.

For other cases with physical origins, treatment and improvement in the underlying disorder may improve sexual performance.

 HOW TO TREAT

NOTE—Follow your doctor's instructions. These instructions are supplemental.

GENERAL MEASURES—See Appendix 13 for suggestions to reduce stress and improve overall health.

MEDICATION
- Medication is not helpful for impotence caused by psychological factors. Be wary of persons who offer cures with shots or pills.
- Medication may be prescribed to treat the underlying medical condition.
- If you suspect that a medication is causing impotence, consult your doctor about changing your prescription or dosage.

ACTIVITY—No restrictions. Resume sexual relations when potency returns or surgery heals.

DIET—Eat a well-balanced diet, and take vitamin and mineral supplements.

 CALL YOUR DOCTOR IF

You have symptoms of impotence, especially if you take medications or have disorders listed as causes.

INCONTINENCE, STRESS

GENERAL INFORMATION

DEFINITION—An involuntary loss of urine in women that accompanies any action that suddenly increases pressure in the abdomen.

BODY PARTS INVOLVED—Urinary bladder; urethra.

SEX OR AGE MOST AFFECTED—Females of all ages, but most common in older women.

SIGNS & SYMPTOMS—Unintentional loss of urine with lifting, sneezing, singing, coughing, laughing, crying or straining to have a bowel movement.

CAUSES—Shortening of the urethra and loss of the normal muscular support for the bladder and floor of the pelvis. These changes occur during pregnancy and after childbirth, particularly repeated childbirth. They may also occur as a natural consequence of aging.

RISK INCREASES WITH
- Repeated childbirth.
- Adults over 60.
- Obesity.
- Chronic lung disease with a cough.

HOW TO PREVENT
- Eat a normal, well-balanced diet and exercise regularly to build and maintain muscle strength.
- Learn and practice Kegel exercises (see General Measures) after childbirth, before symptoms of stress incontinence begin.

WHAT TO EXPECT

APPROPRIATE HEALTH CARE
- Self-care.
- Doctor's treatment.
- Surgery to tighten relaxed or damaged muscles that support the bladder.

DIAGNOSTIC MEASURES
- Your own observation of symptoms.
- Medical history and physical exam by a doctor.
- Urinalysis to determine if a urinary-tract infection is causing the symptoms.

POSSIBLE COMPLICATIONS
- Complete loss of urinary control. This requires surgery (see Anterior and Posterior Repair).
- Urinary-tract infections.

PROBABLE OUTCOME—If the stress incontinence is not severe enough to require surgery, exercise can improve the muscle function. If it is severe, it can be cured with surgery.

HOW TO TREAT

NOTE—Follow your doctor's instructions. These instructions are supplemental.

GENERAL MEASURES—Learn to recognize, control and develop the muscles of the pelvic floor. These are the ones you use to interrupt urination in mid-stream. The following exercises (Kegel exercises) strengthen these muscles so you can control or relax them completely:
- To identify which muscles are involved, alternately start and stop urinating when using the toilet.
- Practice tightening and releasing these muscles while sitting, standing, walking, driving, watching TV or listening to music.
- Tighten the muscles a small amount at a time, "like an elevator going up to the 10th floor." Then release very slowly, "one floor at a time."
- Tighten the muscles from front to back, including the anus, as in the previous exercise.
- Practice exercises every morning, afternoon and evening. Start with 5 times each, and gradually work up to 20 or 30 each time.

MEDICATION—Medicine usually is not necessary for this disorder, but your doctor may prescribe:
- Antibiotics if you have a complicating urinary-tract infection.
- A pessary (support device) made of rubber or other material to fit inside the vagina to support the uterus and lower muscular layer of the bladder.

ACTIVITY—No restrictions.

DIET—Lose weight if you are obese. A reducing diet appears in Appendix 1.

CALL YOUR DOCTOR IF

- You have symptoms of stress incontinence.
- Any sign of infection develops, such as fever, pain on urination, frequent urination or a general ill feeling.
- Symptoms don't improve after 3 months of Kegel exercises, or symptoms become intolerable and you wish to consider surgery.

INDIGESTION
(Dyspepsia)

GENERAL INFORMATION

DEFINITION—Vague chest or abdominal discomfort—with no apparent organic cause—that occurs during or soon after eating or drinking.

BODY PARTS INVOLVED—Stomach; esophagus; small intestine.

SEX OR AGE MOST AFFECTED—Both sexes; all ages.

SIGNS & SYMPTOMS
- Mild nausea.
- Heartburn.
- Upper abdominal pain.
- Gas or belching.
- Bloated or full feeling.
- Acid taste.

CAUSES—Symptoms seem related to eating, drinking, or swallowing air while talking or chewing gum. They occur most often with: emotional upset while eating; excessive smoking; constipation; eating improperly cooked food; eating food with a high fat content; poor digestion of gas-forming foods such as beans, cucumbers, cabbage, turnips and onions; food allergy; or overindulgence in alcohol.

RISK INCREASES WITH
- Stress.
- Smoking.
- Excess alcohol consumption.
- Use of drugs that may irritate the stomach.
- Fatigue or overwork.

HOW TO PREVENT
- Avoid foods you don't digest well.
- Don't smoke.
- Relax after meals.
- Avoid emotional situations during meals.
- Don't eat fast.

OTHER—Persistent symptoms can indicate disease in the digestive tract or other body parts. Occasionally, symptoms occur in patients with no apparent disease. This indicates an abnormal function in a normal part of the body.

WHAT TO EXPECT

APPROPRIATE HEALTH CARE
- Self-care.
- Doctor's care (severe, recurrent indigestion only).

DIAGNOSTIC MEASURES
- Your own observation of symptoms.
- Medical history and physical exam by a doctor.

- X-rays of the upper digestive tract.
- Gastroscopy (see Glossary).

POSSIBLE COMPLICATIONS—Indigestion may mimic signs of a heart attack or serious disease of the esophagus or stomach, causing the serious disorder to be ignored.

PROBABLE OUTCOME—Symptoms can be controlled with treatment, but recurrence is likely.

HOW TO TREAT

NOTE—Follow your doctor's instructions. These instructions are supplemental.

GENERAL MEASURES—Treatment and prevention are similar:
- Allow time for leisurely meals. Chew food carefully and thoroughly. Avoid conflicts during meals.
- Don't smoke immediately before a meal.
- Avoid excitement or exercise immediately after a meal.
- Avoid situations than make you swallow air, such as chewing gum.
- Observe episodes of indigestion for changes in symptoms. If character, timing, frequency or severity changes, a more serious disorder may be responsible. These include heartburn from irritation of the lower esophagus, gallbladder disease, ulcers or stomach cancer.

MEDICATION
- For minor discomfort, you may use non-prescription antacids.
- For serious discomfort, your doctor may prescribe H-2 blockers, antispasmodics or tranquilizers to relieve tension.

ACTIVITY—No restrictions.

DIET—No special diet. Avoid foods—especially those listed under causes—if they cause discomfort.

CALL YOUR DOCTOR IF

- The pattern of indigestion symptoms changes markedly.
- You develop the following:
  Vomiting, weight loss or appetite loss.
  Black, tarry stool or vomiting of blood.
  Fever.
  Severe pain in the upper right abdomen.
  Discomfort that continues unrelated to meals, eating or chewing gum.
- Indigestion is accompanied by:
  Shortness of breath.
  Sweating.
  Pain radiating to the jaw, neck or arm.

INFLUENZA
(Flu; Grippe)

 GENERAL INFORMATION

DEFINITION — A common, contagious respiratory infection caused by a virus. Incubation after exposure is 24 to 48 hours.

BODY PARTS INVOLVED — Upper- respiratory system.

SEX OR AGE MOST AFFECTED — Both sexes; all ages except infants.

SIGNS & SYMPTOMS
- Chills and moderate to high fever.
- Muscle aches, including backache.
- Cough, usually with little or no sputum.
- Sore throat.
- Hoarseness.
- Runny nose.
- Headache.
- Fatigue.

CAUSES — Infection by viruses of the myxovirus class. The viruses spread by personal contact.

RISK INCREASES WITH
- Stress.
- Fatigue or overwork.
- Poor nutrition.
- Recent illness that has lowered resistance.
- Chronic illness, especially chronic lung disease.

HOW TO PREVENT
- Avoid risks listed above.
- Have a yearly influenza vaccine injection if you are over age 65 or have chronic heart or lung disease. A vaccine only protects against a few — not all — types of flu.
- Avoid unnecessary contact with persons who have upper-respiratory infections during the flu season (winter).

 WHAT TO EXPECT

APPROPRIATE HEALTH CARE
- Self-care after diagnosis.
- Doctor's treatment.

DIAGNOSTIC MEASURES
- Your own observation of symptoms.
- Medical history and physical exam by a doctor.
- Laboratory studies, such as blood tests and sputum culture (only for complications).
- X-rays of the chest.

POSSIBLE COMPLICATIONS — Bacterial infections, including middle-ear infection, bronchitis or pneumonia. These can be especially dangerous for chronically ill persons or those over age 65.

PROBABLE OUTCOME — Spontaneous recovery in 7 to 14 days if no complications occur. If complications arise, treatment with antibiotics is usually necessary, and recovery may take 3 to 6 weeks.

 HOW TO TREAT

NOTE — Follow your doctor's instructions. These instructions are supplemental.

GENERAL MEASURES
- To relieve nasal congestion, use salt-water drops (1 teaspoon of salt to 1 quart of water).
- To relieve a sore throat, gargle often with warm or cold, double-strength tea.
- Use a cool-mist humidifier to increase air moisture. This thins lung secretions so they can be coughed up more easily. Don't put medicine in the humidifier; it does not help.
- To avoid spreading germs to others, wash your hands frequently — especially after blowing your nose or before handling food.

MEDICATION
- For minor discomfort, you may use non-prescription drugs, such as acetaminophen, cough syrups, nasal sprays or decongestants.
- Don't give aspirin to a person younger than 19. Some research shows a link between the use of aspirin in children during a virus illness and the development of Reye's syndrome (a type of encephalitis).
- Your doctor may prescribe an antiviral drug, amantadine, for seriously ill persons or for those at greatest risk from complications.

ACTIVITY — Rest is the best medicine. If you are in good general health, rest helps your body fight the virus.

DIET — No special diet. If you have a high fever, drink extra fluids — at least 8 glasses of water a day. Extra fluids, including fruit juice, tea and carbonated drinks, also help thin lung secretions. Avoid milk because it thickens secretions in some persons.

 CALL YOUR DOCTOR IF

- You have symptoms of influenza.
- The following occurs during treatment:
  Increased fever or cough.
  Blood in the sputum.
  Earache.
  Shortness of breath or chest pain.
  Thick discharge from the nose, sinuses or ears.
  Sinus pain.
  Neck pain or stiffness.
- New, unexplained symptoms develop. Drugs in treatment may produce side effects.

INSECT BITES & STINGS

 GENERAL INFORMATION

DEFINITION—Skin eruptions and other symptoms caused by insect bites or stings. The victim often doesn't remember being bitten or stung.

BODY PARTS INVOLVED
- Skin on any part of the body.
- Lymph glands in the neck, armpit, groin or elbow.

SEX OR AGE MOST AFFECTED—Both sexes; all ages.

SIGNS & SYMPTOMS—Red lumps in the skin. The lumps usually appear within minutes after the bite or sting, but some don't appear for 6 to 12 hours. Skin reactions fall into 2 categories:
- A toxic reaction with pain, such as from bee stings.
- A toxic reaction with itching due to the body's release of histamine at the bite site, such as from mosquitoes.

CAUSES—Bites or stings from mosquitoes, fleas, chiggers, bedbugs, ants, spiders, bees and other insects.

RISK INCREASES WITH
- Areas with heavy insect infestations.
- Warm weather in spring and summer.

HOW TO PREVENT
- After identifying the cause, remove it if possible. Treat animals for fleas and exterminate the house or kennel.
- If you cannot avoid exposure, apply insect repellents with diethyltoluamide (DEET).
- Recent evidence indicates that vitamins in the B-vitamin group may be a deterrent to insect bites.

 WHAT TO EXPECT

APPROPRIATE HEALTH CARE
- Self-care.
- Doctor's treatment (sometimes).

DIAGNOSTIC MEASURES
- Your own observation of symptoms.
- Medical history and physical exam by a doctor.

POSSIBLE COMPLICATIONS
- Secondary bacterial infection at the site of the bite. This may cause swollen lymph glands in the neck, armpit, groin or elbow.
- Anaphylaxis (for hypersensitive persons). See Anaphylaxis (in Illness section).

PROBABLE OUTCOME—Most troublesome symptoms disappear in 2 to 3 days, but scratching may prolong symptoms for several weeks. Treatment helps, but it doesn't cure quickly.

 HOW TO TREAT

NOTE—Follow your doctor's instructions. These instructions are supplemental.

GENERAL MEASURES
- Use immersion or wrapped soaks (see Appendix 18) to relieve itching and hasten healing. Warm-water soaks are usually more soothing for pain or inflammation. Cool-water soaks feel better for itching.
- If you have had anaphylaxis (severe allergic reaction) following an insect bite, ask your doctor for an anaphylaxis kit to treat it in the future.

MEDICATION
- For minor discomfort, you may use: Non-prescription oral antihistamines to decrease itching. Non-prescription topical steroid preparations to reduce inflammation and decrease itching. Use according to label directions. For face and groin, use only low-potency steroid products without fluorine.
- For serious symptoms, your doctor may: Prescribe stronger topical steroids or oral steroids if the reaction is severe. Inject epinephrine or cortisone to prevent or diminish anaphylaxis symptoms.

ACTIVITY—No restrictions.

DIET—No special diet.

 CALL YOUR DOCTOR IF

- You have symptoms of anaphylaxis. This is an emergency!
- Self-care does not relieve symptoms, or symptoms don't improve after 2 to 3 days of medical treatment.
- A bitten area becomes red, swollen, warm and tender, indicating infection.
- Temperature rises to 101F (38.3C).

ILLNESSES & DISORDERS

INSOMNIA

GENERAL INFORMATION

DEFINITION—Sleep disturbance—difficulty either falling asleep or remaining asleep.

BODY PARTS INVOLVED—All body cells, especially the central nervous system.

SEX OR AGE MOST AFFECTED—Both sexes; all ages.

SIGNS & SYMPTOMS
- Restlessness when trying to fall asleep.
- Brief sleep followed by wakefulness.
- Normal sleep until very early in the morning (3 a.m. or 4 a.m.), then wakefulness (often with frightening thoughts).
- Periods of sleeplessness, alternating with periods of excessive sleep or sleepiness at inconvenient times.

CAUSES
- Depression. This is usually characterized by early-morning wakefulness.
- Overactivity of the thyroid gland.
- Anxiety caused by stress.
- Sexual problems, such as impotence or lack of a sex partner.
- Noisy environment (including a snoring partner).
- Allergies and early-morning wheezing.
- Heart or lung conditions that cause shortness of breath when lying down.
- Painful disorders, such a fibromyositis or arthritis.
- Urinary or gastrointestinal problems that require urination or bowel movements during the night.
- Consumption of stimulants, such as coffee, tea or cola drinks.
- Use of some medications, including dextroamphetamines or cortisone drugs.
- Erratic work hours.
- New environment or location.
- Jet lag after travel.
- Lack of physical exercise.
- Alcoholism.
- Drug abuse, including overuse of sleep-inducing drugs.
- Withdrawal from addictive substances.

RISK INCREASES WITH
- Stress.
- Obesity.
- Smoking.

HOW TO PREVENT—Establish a lifestyle that fosters healthy sleep patterns (see General Measures).

WHAT TO EXPECT

APPROPRIATE HEALTH CARE
- Self-care after diagnosis.
- Doctor's treatment.
- Psychotherapy or counseling, if the cause is psychological.

DIAGNOSTIC MEASURES
- Your own observation of symptoms.
- Medical history and physical exam by a doctor.
- Laboratory thyroid studies.
- EEG (see Glossary).
- Tests in a sleep-study laboratory.

POSSIBLE COMPLICATIONS
- Impaired relationships.
- Poor work performance.
- Lower resistance to disease.
- Injury from falling asleep around machinery or while driving.

PROBABLE OUTCOME—Most persons can establish good sleep patterns if the underlying cause of insomnia is treated or eliminated.

HOW TO TREAT

NOTE—Follow your doctor's instructions. These instructions are supplemental.

GENERAL MEASURES
- Seek ways to minimize stress. See Appendix 13.
- Obtain medical treatment for any underlying medical disorder.
- Don't use stimulants for several hours before bedtime.
- Relax in a warm bath before bedtime.

MEDICATION—Your doctor may prescribe sleep-inducing drugs for a short time if:
- Temporary insomnia is interfering with your daily activities.
- You have a medical disorder that regularly disturbs sleep.
- You need to establish regular sleep patterns.

Long-term use of sleep inducers may be counter-productive or addictive. Don't use sleeping pills given to you by friends, and don't take non-prescription sleeping pills.

ACTIVITY
- Exercise regularly (see Appendix 20) to create healthy fatigue.
- Have sexual relations before going to sleep.

DIET—No special diet, but don't eat within 3 hours of bedtime if indigestion has previously disturbed your sleep. Drinking a glass of warm milk before bedtime helps some people.

CALL YOUR DOCTOR IF

- You have insomnia.
- New, unexplained symptoms develop. Drugs used in treatment may produce side effects.

INTESTINAL OBSTRUCTION

GENERAL INFORMATION

DEFINITION—Partial or complete blockage of the intestines.

BODY PARTS INVOLVED—Small and large bowel.

SEX OR AGE MOST AFFECTED—Both sexes; all ages.

SIGNS & SYMPTOMS
- Abdominal pain and cramps.
- Nausea and vomiting. In the advanced stage, vomit resembles feces.
- Weakness, dizziness or fainting.
- Little or no urine, due to fluid loss.
- Audible noises from the abdomen in early stages. Later, *no* sounds are audible.
- Abdominal bloating, swelling and gas.
- Fever (sometimes).
- Diarrhea (partial obstruction only).
- Rectal bleeding (sometimes).

CAUSES
- Adhesions (constricting bands of fibrous tissue that result from previous surgery).
- Intestinal hernias.
- Intestinal inflammation or tumors—either benign or cancerous.
- Tumors in adjacent organs that cause pressure on the intestines.
- Foreign objects inside the intestines (swallowed objects or parasites such as worms).
- Twisted bowel (volvulus, see Glossary).
- Severe constipation (fecal impaction).

RISK INCREASES WITH—Previous abdominal surgery.

HOW TO PREVENT
- Eat a diet high in fiber and drink at least 6 to 8 glasses of liquid a day to avoid constipation or fecal impaction.
- Obtain prompt medical treatment for repair of hernias.
- See your doctor if your bowel habits change significantly for longer than 7 days. This may be an early symptom of bowel cancer.

WHAT TO EXPECT

APPROPRIATE HEALTH CARE
- Doctor's treatment.
- Surgery to remove the obstruction (usually).
- Hospitalization for diagnosis and replacement of lost fluids prior to surgery.

DIAGNOSTIC MEASURES
- Your own observation of symptoms.
- Medical history and physical exam by a doctor.
- Laboratory blood studies to measure fluids and electrolytes and to detect bleeding or infection.
- X-rays of the intestinal tract and abdomen (upper and lower GI series).

POSSIBLE COMPLICATIONS
- Dehydration and shock.
- Bowel gangrene.
- Peritonitis.

PROBABLE OUTCOME—Surgery can usually correct the obstruction, but it may not correct the underlying cause, such as cancer. Without treatment, complications can be fatal.

HOW TO TREAT

NOTE—Follow your doctor's instructions. These instructions are supplemental.

GENERAL MEASURES—Intestinal obstruction usually develops rapidly into an emergency. Home remedies are of no value, and some—such as enemas or laxatives—may be harmful.

MEDICATION—Medication is not helpful for intestinal obstruction. However, your doctor may prescribe medication appropriate for the underlying disorder.

ACTIVITY—Rest in bed until the obstruction is corrected. If surgery is necessary, resume normal activities gradually.

DIET—Don't eat anything until the obstruction is corrected. You will probably receive intravenous nourishment until then.

CALL YOUR DOCTOR IF

- Your bowel habits change.
- You have early symptoms of intestinal obstruction.

INTUSSUSCEPTION

GENERAL INFORMATION

DEFINITION—An intestinal obstruction in which the bowel telescopes (folds back on itself).

BODY PARTS INVOLVED—Intestine, usually the large intestine.

SEX OR AGE MOST AFFECTED—All ages, but most common in infants and children between 2 months and 6 years. It is more common in boys.

SIGNS & SYMPTOMS—Early stages:
- Cramping abdominal pain. Infants cry out, bring the legs up to the abdomen, and become pale and sweaty during an attack.
- Vomiting.
Later stages:
- Rectal bleeding. This may be dark red material that resembles jelly.
- Swollen abdomen.
- Mass in the abdomen that can be felt.

CAUSES—Unknown factors cause a loop of bowel to turn in on itself. This blocks the bowel's blood supply, causing gangrene and peritonitis. The disorder may be caused by a virus infection, but that is unproven.

RISK INCREASES WITH
- Family history of intussusception.
- The seasons (for unknown reasons). It is most common in late spring, early summer and midwinter.

HOW TO PREVENT—No specific preventive measures.

WHAT TO EXPECT

APPROPRIATE HEALTH CARE
- Doctor's treatment.
- Surgery to remove the strangulated bowel and rejoin healthy sections.
- Hospitalization until the obstruction is corrected.
- Home care during convalescence.

DIAGNOSTIC MEASURES
- Your own observation of symptoms.
- Medical history and physical exam by a doctor.
- Laboratory blood tests.
- X-rays of the abdomen and intestinal tract (barium enema, see Glossary). The radiologist may manipulate the barium and clear the obstruction.

POSSIBLE COMPLICATIONS
- Dehydration and shock.
- Intestinal perforation and peritonitis.
- Gangrene.

PROBABLE OUTCOME—Spontaneous recovery in 24 hours (sometimes). If not, this is curable with early diagnosis and surgery or barium treatment. Without treatment, complications are life-threatening. The disorder sometimes recurs.

HOW TO TREAT

NOTE—Follow your doctor's instructions. These instructions are supplemental.

GENERAL MEASURES—Observe your child carefully if symptoms develop. Prevent complications by seeking medical treatment during early stages.

MEDICATION—Medicine usually is not necessary for this disorder unless infection develops. Then your doctor may prescribe antibiotics.
  Don't use home remedies or non-prescription drugs, such as laxatives, for this condition. They may be dangerous.

ACTIVITY—The child should rest in bed until the obstruction is cleared. Activities may then be resumed gradually.

DIET—Don't feed a child with signs of intestinal obstruction. Intravenous fluids are necessary until the obstruction is removed. No special diet is required then.

CALL YOUR DOCTOR IF

Your child has signs or symptoms of intestinal obstruction. This condition changes quickly from a curable one to a life-threatening one.

IRITIS

GENERAL INFORMATION

DEFINITION—Inflammation of the tissues that support the iris (the ring of colored tissue around the pupil of the eye).

BODY PARTS INVOLVED—Eye.

SEX OR AGE MOST AFFECTED—Adults between ages 20 and 60.

SIGNS & SYMPTOMS—Acute iritis of sudden onset:
- Severe eye pain.
- Photophobia (sensitivity to light).
- Eye redness.
- Smaller pupil in the affected eye (sometimes).
- Tears.
- Blurred vision.

Iritis of gradual onset:
- Eye pain.
- Photophobia.
- Floating spots in the field of vision.
- Blurred vision.

CAUSES
- Infection that spreads to the eye from other body parts. Common causes include:
  - Toxoplasmosis.
  - Tuberculosis.
  - Histoplasmosis.
  - Syphilis.
  - Sarcoidosis.
  - Viruses.
- Injury to the eye.
- Autoimmune reaction (possibly).
- Unknown in many cases.

RISK INCREASES WITH
- Rheumatoid arthritis.
- Ulcerative colitis.

HOW TO PREVENT—Cannot be prevented at present.

WHAT TO EXPECT

APPROPRIATE HEALTH CARE
- Self-care after diagnosis.
- Doctor's treatment.

DIAGNOSTIC MEASURES
- Your own observation of symptoms.
- Medical history and physical exam by a doctor (ophthalmologist).

POSSIBLE COMPLICATIONS
- Glaucoma.
- Cataracts.
- Permanent, partial vision loss.

PROBABLE OUTCOME—Vision can usually be preserved with prompt treatment.

HOW TO TREAT

NOTE—Follow your doctor's instructions. These instructions are supplemental.

GENERAL MEASURES—Wear dark glasses—even indoors—until treatment is complete.

MEDICATION—Your doctor may prescribe:
- Eye drops (mydriatics) that dilate the pupil and prevent scarring. You may need to use eye drops for a long time. Ask your doctor how to instill them in the eye correctly.
- Oral cortisone drugs or cortisone eye drops to reduce inflammation. Discuss the side effects of cortisone drugs with your doctor.

ACTIVITY—Rest in bed until symptoms subside. Allow 1 to 2 weeks.

DIET—No special diet.

CALL YOUR DOCTOR IF

- You have symptoms of iritis—either sudden or gradual. Call immediately.
- Your vision changes in any way.
- New, unexplained symptoms develop. Drugs used in treatment may produce side effects.

JAW DISLOCATION
(Temporo-Mandibular Joint Dislocation)

GENERAL INFORMATION

DEFINITION—Temporo-mandibular joints connect the lower jaw (mandible) with the skull. They are just forward of the ears.

With dislocation, one cannot close the mouth because the head of the mandible (the condyle) slides backward into a depression in the skull.

BODY PARTS INVOLVED—Jaw.

SEX OR AGE MOST AFFECTED—Both sexes; all ages.

SIGNS & SYMPTOMS
- Inability to close the mouth.
- Pain and swelling in the jaw.
- Bleeding under the skin of the jaw.
- Obvious asymmetry of the face.
- Numbness of the chin and lower lip (sometimes).

CAUSES
- Injury inflicted in a fight, auto accident or contact sports.
- Some persons dislocate mandibles with little provocation, as with yawning, yelling, biting large pieces of food, or opening the mouth very wide for any reason.

RISK INCREASES WITH—Injuries are most often associated with:
- Accident-proneness.
- Excess alcohol consumption or use of mind-altering drugs.
- Non-use of seat belts.

HOW TO PREVENT
- Avoid opening your mouth widely, if possible, when you yawn, bite large pieces of food, yell or scream during excitement, call out loudly, or sing.
- Use seat belts and shoulder harnesses in vehicles. Don't drink alcohol or use mind-altering drugs and drive.

WHAT TO EXPECT

APPROPRIATE HEALTH CARE
- Doctor's or dentist's treatment. Muscles tighten and pain increases within 15 to 30 minutes after dislocation, so a dislocated jaw should be treated quickly.
- Self-care after diagnosis and treatment.

DIAGNOSTIC MEASURES
- Your own observation of symptoms.
- Medical history and physical exam by a doctor.
- X-rays of the jaw.

POSSIBLE COMPLICATIONS—Obstruction of the airway and inhalation of mucus and blood into the lungs, leading to pneumonia. This occurs most often with dislocation and fracture.

PROBABLE OUTCOME—Usually curable with treatment.

HOW TO TREAT

NOTE—Follow your doctor's or dentist's instructions. These instructions are supplemental.

GENERAL MEASURES
- Make sure an injured person with a fractured or dislocated jaw has no breathing obstruction. If there is an obstruction, seek emergency help immediately.
- If your jaw is injured, don't panic. Stay calm. Go to the nearest dental office or emergency facility for help.
- Don't try to talk with a dislocated jaw—write messages instead. Don't try to push or force your mouth closed. Your mouth cannot close normally until the dislocation is corrected.

MEDICATION—Your doctor may prescribe:
- Pain relievers.
- Muscle relaxants.

ACTIVITY—Rest in bed with the head turned to one side. You may read or watch TV. Resume your normal activities in 2 to 3 days. Allow 6 weeks for muscles and tendons attached to the joint to heal.

DIET—A liquid diet (see Appendix 7) may be necessary for up to 4 weeks. Start with clear liquids, then graduate to a full liquid diet, including blenderized foods, milk shakes and juices. Don't chew solid foods without your doctor's or dentist's permission.

CALL YOUR DOCTOR OR DENTIST IF

- You have symptoms of a dislocated jaw.
- Pain is intolerable.

KERATITIS

GENERAL INFORMATION

DEFINITION—Inflammation of the cornea (the clear central portion of the eye that covers the pupil).

BODY PARTS INVOLVED—Eye.

SEX OR AGE MOST AFFECTED—Both sexes; all ages.

SIGNS & SYMPTOMS
- Eye pain.
- Photophobia (sensitivity to light).
- Tears.

CAUSES
- Bacterial, viral or fungal infections. The most common is herpes simplex virus, Type I.
- Drying of the eye caused by an eyelid disorder or insufficient tear formation.
- Foreign object in the eye.
- Intense light, such as from welding arcs or the reflection of intense sunlight from snow or water. (Symptoms may not appear for 24 hours after exposure.)
- Vitamin-A deficiency.
- Allergy or sensitivity to eye cosmetics, air pollution, airborne particles (pollen, dust, mold or yeasts) and other allergens.

RISK INCREASES WITH
- Poor nutrition, especially insufficient vitamin A.
- Illness that has lowered resistance.
- Crowded or unsanitary living conditions.
- Viral infections elsewhere in the body, especially cold sores or genital herpes.

HOW TO PREVENT
- Wear protective glasses, if your work involves eye hazards.
- Eat a well-balanced diet that contains sufficient vitamin A or take multiple-vitamin supplements containing vitamin A.

WHAT TO EXPECT

APPROPRIATE HEALTH CARE
- Doctor's (ophthalmologist's) treatment.
- Surgery to replace the cornea (severe cases only).

DIAGNOSTIC MEASURES
- Your own observation of symptoms.
- Medical history and physical exam by a doctor.
- Laboratory culture of the discharge from the eye.

POSSIBLE COMPLICATIONS
- Glaucoma.
- Ulceration of the cornea.
- Permanent scarring in the eye.
- Vision loss.

PROBABLE OUTCOME—Depends on the cause. With early treatment, most types of keratitis are curable.

HOW TO TREAT

NOTE—Follow your doctor's instructions. These instructions are supplemental.

GENERAL MEASURES—A temporary eye patch is often necessary. It may limit your ability to take care of yourself.

MEDICATION
- Your doctor may prescribe:
  Antibiotic or antiviral eye drops and ointments.
  Artificial tears.
- Don't treat any eye inflammation without consulting your doctor. *Don't use non-prescription eye drops containing topical corticosteroids.* These may worsen the condition or cause eyeball perforation.

ACTIVITY—Eye patching will restrict activity. Resume your normal activities gradually.

DIET—No special diet.

CALL YOUR DOCTOR IF

- You have symptoms of keratitis.
- Your vision diminishes in any way.

KERATOSES, SEBORRHEIC

GENERAL INFORMATION

DEFINITION—A non-contagious, inflammatory, scaling disease of the skin.

BODY PARTS INVOLVED—Chest; back; face; arms.

SEX OR AGE MOST AFFECTED—Adults of both sexes. By age 60, almost everyone has a few seborrheic keratoses.

SIGNS & SYMPTOMS—Papules (small, raised bumps) with the following characteristics:
- Papules are flat-topped with well-defined borders.
- Young papules are relatively flat and light brown. More-advanced papules are dark brown or black.
- Papules are wider than tall, and they appear "stuck on."
- Papules measure 5mm to 20mm in diameter. They are distributed on the chest, back, face and arms.
- Papules don't itch or hurt.
- There may be only 1 or 2 papules, or there may be up to 100.

CAUSES—Unknown.

RISK INCREASES WITH
- Aging.
- Family history of the disorder.
- Excessive sun exposure or other skin injury.

HOW TO PREVENT—No specific preventive measures.

WHAT TO EXPECT

APPROPRIATE HEALTH CARE
- Self-care.
- Doctor's diagnosis to rule out skin cancer.
- Removal of lesions if they are unsightly, are irritated by clothing or interfere with grooming. Removal methods include cryosurgery, chemocautery, light electrosurgery or shave biopsy (see Glossary for all).

DIAGNOSTIC MEASURES
- Your own observation of symptoms.
- Medical history and physical exam by a doctor.
- Biopsy (see Glossary).

POSSIBLE COMPLICATIONS—Seborrheic keratoses on the eyelid borders may require special treatment.

PROBABLE OUTCOME—The number of lesions increases with time. Each lesion is permanent unless removed. Seborrheic keratoses are harmless and require no treatment, but most people want them removed.

HOW TO TREAT

GENERAL MEASURES—After removal, a blister (sometimes with blood) will develop at the treatment site. The top of the blister will come off spontaneously in about 2 weeks. You should have little or no scarring. Wash and use make-up or cosmetics as usual. If clothing irritates the blister, cover it with a small adhesive bandage.

MEDICATION—Medicine usually is not necessary for this disorder.

ACTIVITY—No restrictions.

DIET—No special diet.

CALL YOUR DOCTOR IF

- You have symptoms of seborrheic keratoses.
- You want unsightly seborrheic keratoses removed.
- Treated areas become infected, as evidenced by pain, tenderness, redness, swelling or heat.

KERATOSIS, ACTINIC

GENERAL INFORMATION

DEFINITION—A small area of sun-damaged skin that is precancerous.

BODY PARTS INVOLVED—Skin of exposed areas, especially the scalp, face, ears, lips, arms and hands.

SEX OR AGE MOST AFFECTED—Adults.

SIGNS & SYMPTOMS—Brownish or reddish scaly patches on exposed areas of skin. The patches are painless.

CAUSES—Prolonged exposure to the sun's radiation.

RISK INCREASES WITH
- Outdoor occupations such as farming.
- Outdoor sports.
- Light complexion.

HOW TO PREVENT—Protect yourself against direct sun exposure. When outdoors, wear a hat and protective clothing. Use sunscreen lotions and creams.

WHAT TO EXPECT

APPROPRIATE HEALTH CARE
- Self-care after diagnosis.
- Doctor's treatment.

DIAGNOSTIC MEASURES
- Your own observation of symptoms.
- Medical history and physical exam by a doctor.

POSSIBLE COMPLICATIONS
- Skin damage.
- Skin cancer (including malignant melanoma, basal-cell carcinoma and squamous-cell carcinoma).

PROBABLE OUTCOME—An individual keratosis will disappear with treatment, but new lesions are likely to recur. If neglected, actinic keratosis can lead to skin cancer.

HOW TO TREAT

NOTE—Follow your doctor's instructions. These instructions are supplemental.

GENERAL MEASURES
After diagnosis:
- Minimize direct sun exposure.
- See your doctor for checkups every 6 months to ensure early detection and treatment of skin cancers.

MEDICATION—Your doctor may use:
- Liquid nitrogen to freeze the affected tissue.
- Applications of 5-fluorocil to the affected area. This causes uncomfortable inflammation, but it is very effective.
- Vitamin A, which is still experimental.

ACTIVITY—No restrictions.

DIET—No special diet.

CALL YOUR DOCTOR IF

You have signs of actinic keratosis. Even though this causes no symptoms, it is precancerous.

ILLNESSES & DISORDERS

KERATOSIS PILARIS

 GENERAL INFORMATION

DEFINITION—A common skin disorder in which the openings of the hair follicles become filled with hard plugs. These are not contagious.

BODY PARTS INVOLVED—Skin on the backs of upper arms, fronts of thighs or buttocks.

SEX OR AGE MOST AFFECTED—Children and young adults.

SIGNS & SYMPTOMS—Papules (small, raised bumps) with the following characteristics:
- Papules are small, firm and white, with a dry "sandpaper" feeling.
- Papules are clustered. Each one is about 1mm in size.
- Papules are at the openings of hair follicles. They can be scooped out with the fingernails.
- When scooped out, a papule usually contains a coiled hair inside of white, semisolid material.
- Papules don't itch or hurt.

CAUSES—Unknown, but it may be hereditary. These commonly occur in association with allergic dermatitis and several types of ichthyosis, both of which have strong hereditary links.
Lesions similar—possibly identical—to those of keratosis pilaris appear in persons with vitamin-A deficiency.

RISK INCREASES WITH
- History of skin allergies.
- Family history of keratosis pilaris.
- Poor nutrition, especially vitamin-A deficiency.

HOW TO PREVENT—Cannot be prevented at present.

 WHAT TO EXPECT

APPROPRIATE HEALTH CARE.
- Self-care.
- Doctor's diagnosis.

DIAGNOSTIC MEASURES
- Your own observation of symptoms.
- Medical history and physical exam by a doctor.
- Biopsy (see Glossary).

POSSIBLE COMPLICATIONS—Secondary infection of papules.

PROBABLE OUTCOME—Keratosis pilaris is a chronic, harmless skin problem with no permanent cure. Individual papules may come and go over a matter of weeks. All gradually disappear by age 30.

 HOW TO TREAT

NOTE—Follow your doctor's instructions. These instructions are supplemental.

GENERAL MEASURES
- Take long soaking tub baths.
- Use mild, unscented soap.
- Scrub gently with a stiff brush to remove the plugs in the follicles temporarily.
- Apply lubricating ointments or creams to the affected areas 6 or 7 times a day. The most useful time is immediately after bathing when lubrication helps the skin retain moisture.

MEDICATION—Medicine usually is not necessary for this disorder.

ACTIVITY—No restrictions.

DIET—No special diet.

 CALL YOUR DOCTOR IF

Signs of infection develop around the keratoses pilaris. Signs include pain or tenderness, redness, swelling and fever of 101F (38.3C) or higher.

KIDNEY CANCER

GENERAL INFORMATION

DEFINITION—Uncontrolled growth of malignant cells in the kidney. The cancer may begin in the kidney (primary) or spread to the kidney from other sites.

BODY PARTS INVOLVED—One or both kidneys.

SEX OR AGE MOST AFFECTED—Both sexes of adults over 40, but twice as common in men as women.

SIGNS & SYMPTOMS
- Blood in the urine.
- Pain in the flank (lower back on either side of the spine).
- Unexplained fever, usually low.
- Swelling or mass in the abdomen.
- Hypertension (sometimes).

CAUSES—Unknown.

RISK INCREASES WITH—Adults over 60.

HOW TO PREVENT—Cannot be prevented at present. Seek early medical care if you have urinary symptoms, pain or unexplained fever.

WHAT TO EXPECT

APPROPRIATE HEALTH CARE
- Doctor's treatment.
- Surgery to remove the affected kidney.
- Postoperative radiation treatment, if cancer has spread. Otherwise, radiation is usually not helpful.
- Self-care after surgery.

DIAGNOSTIC MEASURES
- Your own observation of symptoms.
- Medical history and physical exam by a doctor.
- Laboratory studies of blood and urine to measure kidney function.
- X-rays of the kidneys, associated blood vessels and surrounding tissue.
- CAT scan of the abdomen.

POSSIBLE COMPLICATIONS—Spread of cancer (metastasis) to nearby tissues or through the bloodstream to the lungs, bone, liver or lymph glands.

PROBABLE OUTCOME—Depends on how early kidney cancer is discovered. The 5-year survival rate is 50% to 60% if the cancer is diagnosed and treated before it spreads from the kidney. Survival for 5 years is unlikely if the cancer is discovered after it spreads. However, medical literature cites instances of unexplained recovery.

HOW TO TREAT

NOTE—Follow your doctor's instructions. These instructions are supplemental.

GENERAL MEASURES—For an explanation of surgery and postoperative care, see Nephrectomy (in Surgery section).

MEDICATION
- Chemotherapy is currently not effective against kidney cancer.
- Your doctor may prescribe pain relievers.

ACTIVITY—No restrictions.

DIET—No special diet.

CALL YOUR DOCTOR IF

You have symptoms of kidney cancer.

KIDNEY FAILURE, ACUTE

 GENERAL INFORMATION

DEFINITION—Sudden failure of the kidneys to function. This usually has a short, relatively severe course, but it is curable.

BODY PARTS INVOLVED—Kidneys.

SEX OR AGE MOST AFFECTED—Both sexes; all ages.

SIGNS & SYMPTOMS—Early stages:
- Little or no urine output.
Later stages:
- Nausea, vomiting, diarrhea and appetite loss.
- Mental changes, including irritability, drowsiness, stupor or coma.
- Convulsions.
- Severe itching.
- High or low blood pressure.
- Unexplained bruising, bleeding spots under the skin or spontaneous bleeding. The symptoms of the underlying cause (see below) will also be present.

CAUSES—Conditions in the kidney, or in other areas of the body, that cause the kidneys to stop functioning. This leads to a buildup of waste products in the blood and tissues. Underlying conditions include:
- Shock with very low blood pressure.
- Blood poisoning (septicemia).
- Congestive heart failure.
- Fluid and electrolyte imbalance.
- Blood-transfusion reaction.
- Severe accident with extensive muscle injury.
- Acute glomerulonephritis.
- Multiple myeloma.
- Obstruction of blood vessels that supply the kidney.
- Kidney stones that obstruct both ureters or the urethra.
- Prostate enlargement.
- Use of certain medications, including anticancer drugs, kanamycin, amphotericin B, anticonvulsants or excessive vitamin D.
- Overdose of many poisons or drugs, especially mind-altering drugs.

RISK INCREASES WITH
- Persons with one kidney.
- Recent surgery.
- Accidents with severe injuries.
- Medical history of conditions affecting the kidney, such as diabetes or gout.

HOW TO PREVENT—No specific preventive measures. Avoid causes and risk factors when possible.

 WHAT TO EXPECT

APPROPRIATE HEALTH CARE
- Doctor's treatment.
- Surgery, if the cause can be corrected by surgery.
- Hospitalization for fluid and electrolyte therapy and kidney dialysis (sometimes).

DIAGNOSTIC MEASURES
- Your own observation of symptoms.
- Medical history and physical exam by a doctor.
- Laboratory blood counts, and blood and urine tests that measure kidney function and fluid and electrolyte balance.
- EKG (see Glossary).
- Needle biopsy (see Glossary) of kidneys.
- X-rays of the abdomen, kidneys, ureters and bladder to detect kidney stones.

POSSIBLE COMPLICATIONS
- Congestive heart failure.
- Increased risk of infections.
- Chronic kidney failure.

PROBABLE OUTCOME—If the underlying condition can be controlled and the kidney failure can be treated promptly, complete recovery is likely. If not, the disorder can lead to chronic kidney failure or death.

 HOW TO TREAT

NOTE—Follow your doctor's instructions. These instructions are supplemental.

GENERAL MEASURES—No specific instructions except those listed under other headings.

MEDICATION—Your doctor may prescribe:
- Medications appropriate to control the underlying condition.
- Antibiotics if infection develops.

ACTIVITY—Rest in bed until the condition is cured. Then resume your normal activities as soon as symptoms improve.

DIET—Food and water intake is rigorously controlled to prevent fluid and electrolyte imbalance, and to minimize buildup of body wastes.

 CALL YOUR DOCTOR IF

- You have symptoms of kidney failure.
- The following occurs during treatment:
  Chills, fever, headache or muscle aches.
  Shortness or breath.
  Unexpected bleeding from any body opening.

KIDNEY FAILURE, CHRONIC
(Uremia)

GENERAL INFORMATION

DEFINITION—Inability of the kidneys to eliminate the body's nitrogen waste products. Uremia usually develops gradually.

BODY PARTS INVOLVED—Kidneys, which eventually affect all body systems.

SEX OR AGE MOST AFFECTED—Both sexes; all ages.

SIGNS & SYMPTOMS—None or few symptoms until 60% to 75% of kidney filtration fails. Then, 1 or more of the following:
- Listlessness, mental confusion and drowsiness.
- High blood pressure.
- Shortness of breath.
- Bad breath.
- Inflamed, bleeding gums and mouth ulcers.
- Abdominal pain.
- Itching skin.
- Numbness, tingling and burning in the legs and feet.
- Muscle cramps.
- Decreased sex drive.
- Cessation of menstruation.
- Anemia, with paleness and fatigue.
- Unusual bleeding.
- Muscle and bone pain. Bones break easily.

CAUSES
- Collagen diseases, such as systemic lupus erythematosus.
- Chronic glomerulonephritis.
- Chronic urinary-tract infections.
- Congenital kidney abnormalities, such as polycystic kidney disease.
- Kidney damage due to diabetes mellitus.
- Urinary-tract obstruction.
- Overdose of many drugs and chemicals, especially phenacetin or streptomycin.
- Blood-vessel diseases, such as hardening of the arteries in or leading to the kidney.

RISK INCREASES WITH—Use of mind-altering drugs.

HOW TO PREVENT—Obtain medical treatment for underlying diseases that lead to uremia *before* uremia results.

WHAT TO EXPECT

APPROPRIATE HEALTH CARE
- Doctor's treatment.
- Kidney transplant, if possible.
- Kidney dialysis (see Glossary), if available.
- Hospitalization for complications and care in final stages.

DIAGNOSTIC MEASURES
- Laboratory blood and urine studies of kidney function.
- X-rays of kidneys.
- Kidney biopsy (see Glossary).

POSSIBLE COMPLICATIONS
- Pericarditis.
- Myocarditis.
- Pneumonia.
- Pancreatitis.
- Hormone deficiencies.
- Fluid and electrolyte imbalance.
- Gastrointestinal ulcers.

PROBABLE OUTCOME—Kidney transplants can sometimes cure younger patients. Otherwise, kidney failure is a condition that worsens gradually and causes death. Kidney dialysis treatment can improve and prolong life for several years.

HOW TO TREAT

NOTE—Follow your doctor's instructions. These instructions are supplemental.

GENERAL MEASURES
- To decrease itching, add 1 cup of oatmeal to your daily bath.
- Brush your teeth and use mouthwash often to minimize gum and mouth problems.
- Weigh daily and keep a record.
- Measure the fluids you drink and the urine you pass each day. Keep a record, and take it with you to doctor visits.

  You should pass about 2500cc or more of urine a day. If you pass less, decrease fluid intake so intake does not exceed output by more than 800cc a day. For example, if you pass 2000cc in 24 hours, don't drink more than 2800cc in the next 24 hours.

MEDICATION—Your doctor may prescribe:
- Diuretics to reduce fluid accumulation.
- Iron and folic-acid supplements for anemia.
- Stool softeners to prevent constipation.
- Digitalis for congestive heart failure.

ACTIVITY—You must reduce activity. Don't become overheated or fatigued. Sleep more at night, and take rests during the day. If you are confined to bed, flex your legs often to reduce the chance of blood clots in leg veins.

DIET—Eat a low-salt, low-potassium, low-protein diet with added fiber. Eat frequent small, high-calorie meals.

CALL YOUR DOCTOR IF

- You have symptoms of uremia.
- The following occurs during treatment:
  Fever.
  Vomiting or diarrhea.
  Urine output of less than 2000cc.
  Severe headache.
  Convulsion.

ILLNESSES & DISORDERS

KIDNEY INFECTION, ACUTE
(Acute Pyelonephritis)

 GENERAL INFORMATION

DEFINITION—A non-contagious bacterial infection of the kidneys.

BODY PARTS INVOLVED—Kidneys; urinary tract.

SEX OR AGE MOST AFFECTED—Both sexes, but more common in females of all ages.

SIGNS & SYMPTOMS—Sudden onset of:
- Fever and shaking chills.
- Burning, frequent urination.
- Cloudy urine or blood in the urine.
- Aching (sometimes severe) in one or both sides of the lower back.
- Abdominal pain.
- Marked fatigue.

Note: Young children and the elderly may not have typical symptoms or signs.

CAUSES—Bacteria (most commonly escherichia coli) invade one or both kidneys. The infection may begin in the bladder. The most common sources of bacterial infection are:
- Vigorous sexual activity in women, which allows bacteria to enter the urethra and bladder.
- Infections elsewhere in the body that travel to the kidneys through the bloodstream or lymph glands.
- Blockage or abnormality of the urinary system, caused by stones, obstructions, bladder dysfunction from nerve diseases, tumors or congenital abnormalities.
- Catheters, tubes or surgical procedures used for other medical conditions.

RISK INCREASES WITH
- Diabetes mellitus.
- Chronic urinary-bladder infection or tumor.
- Paralysis from spinal-cord injury or tumor.
- Pregnancy.

HOW TO PREVENT—No specific preventive measures for males. For females:
- After bowel movements, always wipe from the vaginal area toward the rectum.
- Avoid prolonged moistness around the urethra, such as that caused by nylon underpants or wet swim suits.
- Avoid sexual positions that irritate or hurt the urethra or bladder.
- Urinate within 15 minutes after sexual intercourse.

OTHER—Acute kidney infections in males of any age may indicate a serious underlying disease, such as a tumor, obstruction or prostate disorder. Consult your doctor even if symptoms disappear spontaneously.

 WHAT TO EXPECT

APPROPRIATE HEALTH CARE
- Self-care after diagnosis.
- Doctor's treatment.

DIAGNOSTIC MEASURES
- Your own observation of symptoms.
- Medical history and physical exam by a doctor.
- Urinalysis and urine culture (see Glossary).

POSSIBLE COMPLICATIONS
- Chronic kidney infection.
- Hypertension.

PROBABLE OUTCOME—Usually curable in 10 to 14 days with treatment. Make a return doctor visit to assure complete cure.

 HOW TO TREAT

NOTE—Follow your doctor's instructions. These instructions are supplemental.

GENERAL MEASURES—To collect urine for urinalysis or culture:
- Females: Clean the vaginal area with warm, soapy water; sponge dry. Spread the vaginal lips with one hand and urinate briefly into the toilet bowl. Then urinate into the container.
- Males: Pull back the foreskin of the penis if you are not circumcised. Clean the end of the penis with soapy water. Urinate briefly into the toilet bowl, then into the special container.

MEDICATION—Your doctor may prescribe:
- Oral antibiotics. Take all the antibiotics prescribed, even if symptoms disappear.
- Antibiotics (intravenous or by injection), if oral antibiotics don't cure the infection.
- Urinary analgesics to relieve pain.

ACTIVITY—Rest in bed until high fever and discomfort subside. Don't resume sexual relations until you finish the antibiotic treatment.

DIET—No special diet. Drink at least 2 quarts of liquid daily; include cranberry juice to acidify the urine.

 CALL YOUR DOCTOR IF

- You have symptoms of a kidney infection.
- The following occurs during treatment: Symptoms and fever persist after 48 hours of antibiotic treatment. Occasionally a different antibiotic is needed. Symptoms return (especially if accompanied by fever) after antibiotic treatment.
- New, unexplained symptoms develop. Drugs in treatment may produce side effects.

KIDNEY INFECTION, CHRONIC
(Chronic Pyelonephritis)

 GENERAL INFORMATION

DEFINITION—Infection of the kidneys that develops slowly and lasts for months or years. It leads to scarring and eventual loss of kidney function.

BODY PARTS INVOLVED—Kidneys.

SEX OR AGE MOST AFFECTED—Adults of both sexes, but more common in women.

SIGNS & SYMPTOMS—Usually no signs or symptoms, unlike acute kidney infection. The following occur if chronic kidney failure develops:
- Anemia.
- Weakness.
- Loss of appetite.
- Hypertension.
- Pain in one or both sides of the lower back.
- Protein and blood in the urine.

CAUSES—Frequent, acute bacterial kidney infections.

RISK INCREASES WITH
- History of diabetes mellitus.
- Urinary obstruction, such as stones or tumors.
- Long-term use of catheters.

HOW TO PREVENT
- Obtain prompt medical treatment for acute kidney infections, including 2 or more weeks of antibiotic treatment. Don't discontinue prescribed medication even if symptoms disappear after a few days of treatment.
- Obtain treatment for any abnormality of the urinary tract that causes infection.

 WHAT TO EXPECT

APPROPRIATE HEALTH CARE
- Self-care after diagnosis.
- Doctor's treatment.
- Surgery to relieve obstruction in the urinary tract, if one exists.

DIAGNOSTIC MEASURES
- Medical history and physical exam by a doctor.
- Laboratory blood studies of kidney function, urinalysis and urine culture (see Glossary).
- X-rays of kidneys.

POSSIBLE COMPLICATIONS
- Kidney-caused hypertension.
- Chronic kidney failure.

PROBABLE OUTCOME—Symptoms can be controlled with treatment. If only one kidney is chronically infected and antibiotic treatment is unsuccessful, surgical removal of the affected kidney may prevent complications.
   If chronic kidney failure develops in both kidneys, a kidney transplant or kidney dialysis (see Glossary) can be life-saving.

 HOW TO TREAT

NOTE—Follow your doctor's instructions. These instructions are supplemental.

GENERAL MEASURES—Follow your treatment plan carefully. This may not be easy for an illness that causes few symptoms in the early stages.

MEDICATION—Your doctor may prescribe:
- Antibiotics for months or years.
- Drugs to keep the urine slightly acid.

ACTIVITY—No restrictions.

DIET—No special diet. Drink 2 quarts of liquid daily; include cranberry juice to acidify the urine.

 CALL YOUR DOCTOR IF

- You have symptoms of chronic kidney failure.
- You have symptoms of an acute kidney infection, such as: urgent, frequent or burning urination; fever and chills; fatigue; cloudy urine.

ILLNESSES & DISORDERS

KIDNEY OR URETER INJURY

GENERAL INFORMATION

DEFINITION—Bruising or tearing of the kidney or ureter. Kidneys filter waste material from the bloodstream and produce urine. Ureters are the tubes that carry urine from the kidneys to the bladder.

BODY PARTS INVOLVED—Kidney; ureter.

SEX OR AGE MOST AFFECTED—Both sexes; all ages.

SIGNS & SYMPTOMS
- Pain or tenderness in the back, just below the ribs on the injured side.
- Fever less than 101F (38.3C).
- Blood in the urine.
If you have severe pain with large amounts of blood in your urine, one or both kidneys may be seriously injured.

CAUSES—A blow or penetrating wound to the side of the body under the ribs.

RISK INCREASES WITH
- Excess alcohol consumption.
- Accident-proneness.
- Hazardous occupations.
- Hazardous driving conditions.

HOW TO PREVENT—Protect yourself from injury whenever possible. Buckle your automobile seat belt and shoulder harness to minimize internal injury in case of accident. Don't drink and drive.

WHAT TO EXPECT

APPROPRIATE HEALTH CARE
- Doctor's treatment.
- Hospitalization for shock or internal bleeding.
- Surgery to repair the ureter or remove the kidney, if other treatment fails.

DIAGNOSTIC MEASURES
- Your own observation of symptoms.
- Medical history and physical exam by a doctor.
- Laboratory urine studies.
- X-rays of the urinary tract.

POSSIBLE COMPLICATIONS
- Internal bleeding.
- Shock (sweating; faintness; nausea; panting; rapid pulse; pale, cold, moist skin).
- Urine leakage into the abdomen, causing abdominal inflammation or infection.
- Scarring and narrowing of the injured ureter.

PROBABLE OUTCOME—Usually curable with time, bed rest and surgery or protection against infection. The surgery to remove an injured kidney (if it does not heal with other measures) is not complicated. After recovery, you can lead a normal life with one kidney.

HOW TO TREAT

NOTE—Follow your doctor's instructions. These instructions are supplemental.

GENERAL MEASURES—No special instructions except those listed under other headings.

MEDICATION—Your doctor may prescribe:
- Pain relievers.
- Antibiotics to treat or protect against infection.

ACTIVITY—You will need bed rest for 1 to 2 weeks after the injury. After recovery, resume normal activities gradually.

DIET
- No special diet.
- Drink 6 to 8 glasses of fluid daily.
- Don't drink alcohol.

CALL YOUR DOCTOR IF

- You have any symptoms of kidney or ureter injury.
- Symptoms recur after treatment, especially blood in the urine.
- New, unexplained symptoms develop. Drugs used in treatment may produce side effects.

KIDNEY, POLYCYSTIC

GENERAL INFORMATION

DEFINITION—An inherited kidney disorder in which cysts develop in the kidneys. The cysts enlarge the kidney and reduce its function. This is not cancerous.

Most cases show no symptoms until adulthood. Then symptoms progress slowly for up to 20 years.

BODY PARTS INVOLVED—Kidneys.

SEX OR AGE MOST AFFECTED—Both sexes; all ages.

SIGNS & SYMPTOMS—Early stages:
● Blood in the urine that may be visible only by microscopic examination.
● Repeated kidney infections.
● A mass in the abdomen.
● No symptoms (frequently) until the cysts replace so much normal kidney structure that kidney failure occurs.
Symptoms of kidney failure are:
● Pain in the lower back.
● Frequent urination.
● Increasing fatigue and weakness.
● Headache.
● Bad breath.
● Hypertension.
● Nausea, vomiting or diarrhea.
● Fluid retention, especially swelling around the ankles or eyes.
● Shortness of breath.
● Chest pain.
● Itching skin.
● Cessation of menstruation in women of childbearing age.

CAUSES—This disease is inherited; the cause is unknown.

RISK INCREASES WITH—Family history of polycystic disease.

HOW TO PREVENT—Cannot be prevented at present. If polycystic kidney disease runs in your family, consult your doctor for tests to discover if you have kidney cysts. Even if you feel well and don't have the disease, get regular checkups. If you have a family history of polycystic kidney, seek genetic counseling before starting a family.

WHAT TO EXPECT

APPROPRIATE HEALTH CARE
● Self-care after diagnosis.
● Doctor's treatment.
● Surgery to perform a kidney transplant (rare).
● Hospitalization for dialysis (rare).

DIAGNOSTIC MEASURES
● Your own observation of symptoms.

● Medical history and physical exam by a doctor.
● X-rays and ultrasonography of kidneys and other parts of the urinary tract.

POSSIBLE COMPLICATIONS
● Urinary-tract infections.
● Chronic kidney failure.

PROBABLE OUTCOME—Polycystic kidney disease is currently considered incurable, but persons with it have a normal life expectancy. Your doctor may slow the progressive kidney damage by treating complications as they arise.

Scientific research into causes and treatment continues. This offers hope for increasingly effective treatment and eventual cure.

HOW TO TREAT

NOTE—Follow your doctor's instructions. These instructions are supplemental.

GENERAL MEASURES—There is no specific treatment for polycystic kidney disease. The treatment described below applies primarily to patients with polycystic disease who have chronic kidney failure.

MEDICATION—Without complications, medicine usually is not necessary for this disorder.

If necessary, your doctor may prescribe antibiotics for infection or antihypertensives to control high blood pressure.

Most drugs are excreted by the kidney. If you have chronic kidney failure and take prescription drugs, the dose may need adjustment because of this disorder.

ACTIVITY—Take short, frequent rest periods during the day. Otherwise, stay as active as your strength allows.

DIET
● Eat a low-salt, low-protein diet (see Appendix 9).
● Drink at least 8 glasses of fluid every day.
● Iron and multiple-vitamin supplements may be necessary to ensure good nutrition because of the dietary restrictions. Your doctor may also prescribe calcium and vitamin-D supplements to prevent softening of the bones (osteoporosis).

CALL YOUR DOCTOR IF

● You have symptoms of polycystic kidney.
● You have symptoms of kidney failure.
● You have fever or other signs of infection.
● Urination decreases.

KIDNEY STONES
(Renal Calculi; Urinary Calculi; Urinary Stones)

 GENERAL INFORMATION

DEFINITION—Small, solid particles that form in one or both kidneys and sometimes travel into the ureter. Stones vary from the size of a grain of sand to a golf ball, and there may be one or several.

BODY PARTS INVOLVED—Kidneys; ureters; bladder; urethra.

SEX OR AGE MOST AFFECTED—Both sexes, but most likely in men. Kidney stones affect adults over age 30.

SIGNS & SYMPTOMS
- Episodes of severe, colicky (intermittent) pain every few minutes. The pain usually appears first in the back, just below the ribs. Over several hours or days, the pain follows the stone's course through the ureter toward the groin. Pain stops when the stone passes.
- Frequent nausea.
- Traces of blood in the urine.

CAUSES
- Excess calcium in the urine caused by: Disturbance in the parathyroid gland, which upsets calcium metabolism. Excess calcium or vitamin-D intake.
- Gout (uric-acid stones).
- Blockage of urine from any cause.

RISK INCREASES WITH
- Decreased urine volume caused by dehydration or hot, dry weather.
- Improper diet (too much calcium).
- Family history of kidney stones.
- Excess alcohol consumption.
- Bed confinement for any reason.

HOW TO PREVENT
- Drink 3 quarts of fluid, mostly purified water, every day.
- Avoid milk and milk products if you have had a calcium or phosphorus kidney stone.
- Avoid excessive sweating.

 WHAT TO EXPECT

APPROPRIATE HEALTH CARE
- Self-care after diagnosis.
- Doctor's treatment.
- Surgery or ultrasound treatment to remove stones, if they don't pass spontaneously.

DIAGNOSTIC MEASURES
- Your own observation of symptoms.
- Medical history and physical exam by a doctor.
- Urinalysis and blood studies for calcium and phosphorus.

POSSIBLE COMPLICATIONS
- Urinary-tract infection.
- Damage to the kidney, necessitating surgical removal.

PROBABLE OUTCOME—Large stones usually remain in the kidney without symptoms, although they damage the kidney. Small stones pass easily into the ureter through the urine. Stones that are big enough to pass—but not small enough to pass with ease—cause excruciating pain. These usually pass in a few days. If the stone stops and blocks urine, it must be removed to prevent further kidney damage.

 HOW TO TREAT

NOTE—Follow your doctor's instructions. These instructions are supplemental.

GENERAL MEASURES—Strain all urine through gauze to detect passage of the stone. Take it to the doctor for composition analysis.

MEDICATION—Your doctor may prescribe:
- Pain relievers.
- Antispasmodics to relax the ureter muscles and help the stone pass.

ACTIVITY
- If you know you have kidney stones, avoid situations in which a sudden pain might cause danger, such as climbing ladders or working on roofs or girders.
- During a kidney-stone episode, stay as active as possible. Don't go to bed. Activity may help the stone pass.

DIET
- If the stone proves to be calcium or phosphorus, avoid products made with milk, chocolate and nuts.
- If the stone is a phosphate, your doctor will prescribe an acid-ash diet to keep the urine slightly acid.
- If the stone is a urate or cystine stone, your doctor will prescribe an alkaline-ash diet to keep the urine slightly alkaline.
- For all types of stones, drink at least 13 glasses of fluid daily. Most of the fluid should be purified water.

 CALL YOUR DOCTOR IF

- You have symptoms of a kidney stone.
- Your temperature rises to 101F (38.3C).
- You develop symptoms of a kidney infection: stinging, burning on urination or a frequent urge to urinate.
- New, unexplained symptoms develop. Drugs used in treatment may produce side effects.

LABYRINTHITIS

GENERAL INFORMATION

DEFINITION—Inflammation of the semicircular canals in the inner ear.

BODY PARTS INVOLVED—Semicircular canals of the inner ear. The fluid-filled canals help maintain balance.

SEX OR AGE MOST AFFECTED—Adults.

SIGNS & SYMPTOMS
- Extreme dizziness—especially with head movement—that begins gradually and peaks in 48 hours.
- Involuntary eye movement.
- Nausea and vomiting.
- Loss of balance, especially falling toward the affected side.
- Temporary hearing loss.

CAUSES
- Virus infection (usually) in the inner ear.
- Bacterial infection in the inner ear.
- Spread of a chronic middle-ear infection.
- Ingestion of toxic drugs.
- Allergy.
- Cholesteatoma (an accumulation of debris covered by skin in the outer-ear canal).

RISK INCREASES WITH
- Stress.
- Recent viral illness, especially respiratory infection.
- Family history of allergies.
- Smoking.
- Excess alcohol consumption.
- Use of some prescription or non-prescription drugs, especially aspirin.
- Fatigue or overwork.

HOW TO PREVENT
- Obtain prompt medical treatment for ear infections.
- Don't take medication that has produced dizziness without consulting your doctor.

WHAT TO EXPECT

APPROPRIATE HEALTH CARE
- Self-care after diagnosis.
- Doctor's treatment.
- Surgery to remove cholesteatoma, if necessary.

DIAGNOSTIC MEASURES
- Your own observation of symptoms.
- Medical history and physical exam by a doctor.
- Laboratory culture of any discharge that leaks from the infected ear.
- Audiometry (see Glossary).

POSSIBLE COMPLICATIONS—Permanent hearing loss on the affected side (rare).

PROBABLE OUTCOME—Recovery—either spontaneous or with treatment—in 1 to 6 weeks.

HOW TO TREAT

NOTE—Follow your doctor's instructions. These instructions are supplemental.

GENERAL MEASURES—No specific instructions except those listed under other headings.

MEDICATION—Your doctor may prescribe:
- Antinausea medications.
- Tranquilizers to reduce dizziness.
- Diuretics to decrease fluid accumulation in the inner ear.
- Antibiotics to fight bacterial infection.

ACTIVITY—Keep the head as still as possible. Rest in bed until dizziness subsides. Then resume your normal activities gradually. Avoid hazardous activities, such as driving, climbing or working around dangerous machinery, until 1 week after symptoms disappear.

DIET—No special diet, but decrease salt and fluid intake.

CALL YOUR DOCTOR IF

- You have symptoms of labyrinthitis.
- The following occurs during treatment:
  Decreased hearing in either ear.
  Persistent vomiting.
  Convulsions.
  Fainting.
  Fever of 101F (38.3C) or higher.
- New, unexplained symptoms develop. Drugs used in treatment may produce side effects.

LACTOSE INTOLERANCE
(Milk Intolerance; Lactase Deficiency)

 GENERAL INFORMATION

DEFINITION—Difficulty digesting cow's milk. Lactose intolerance occurs—with varying severity—in 75% of the black population, 90% of Orientals or American Indians, and less than 20% of Caucasians of northwest European origin. It is not contagious or cancerous.

BODY PARTS INVOLVED—Digestive system.

SEX OR AGE MOST AFFECTED—Both sexes; all ages.

SIGNS & SYMPTOMS—In children:
● Foamy diarrhea with diaper rash.
● Vomiting.
● Slow weight gain, growth and development.
In adults:
● Rumbling abdominal sounds, abdominal cramps and diarrhea.
● Gas and bloating.
● Nausea.

CAUSES—Deficiency or absence of the enzyme lactase. Lactase is necessary to digest all milk except mother's milk. Without it, sugars in milk absorb fluid and cause diarrhea. Although some infants are born with the disorder, lactose intolerance usually develops in adulthood.
　　Temporary lactose intolerance can occur in an infant after a severe bout of gastroenteritis that damages the intestinal lining.

RISK INCREASES WITH—Family history of enzyme-lactase deficiency.

HOW TO PREVENT—Cannot be prevented at present. If you are pregnant and there is a history of lactose intolerance in your family, consider breast-feeding your baby. If not, you may need an alternate non-milk formula.

 WHAT TO EXPECT

APPROPRIATE HEALTH CARE
● Self-care after diagnosis.
● Doctor's treatment.

DIAGNOSTIC MEASURES
● Your own observation of symptoms.
● Medical history and physical exam by a doctor.
● Laboratory studies, such as a stool exam and lactose-tolerance test.
● X-rays of the lower intestinal tract.
● Therapeutic trial with a milk-free diet.

POSSIBLE COMPLICATIONS—Infants with inherited deficiency will not thrive without treatment.

PROBABLE OUTCOME—This condition is currently considered incurable. However, symptoms can be relieved or controlled with a diet free of milk and milk products. Symptoms worsen at times for unexplained reasons.

 HOW TO TREAT

NOTE—Follow your doctor's instructions. These instructions are supplemental.

GENERAL MEASURES—No special instructions except those listed under other headings.

MEDICATION—Your doctor may prescribe a supplement to neutralize lactose in milk.

ACTIVITY—No restrictions.

DIET—If the condition is present at birth, your doctor will probably prescribe an infant formula that contains little or no lactose, such as a soybean-based formula.
　　If the lactose intolerance is temporary and caused by gastroenteritis, the substitute formula should be necessary for a short time only. Cow's milk can be introduced again later.
　　Older persons with lactose intolerance should avoid milk and milk products, such as cheese and ice cream.

 CALL YOUR DOCTOR IF

● You or your child have symptoms of lactose intolerance.
● Temperature rises to 101F (38.3C) or higher.
● Your infant fails to gain weight.
● Your infant refuses food or formula.
● Vomiting or diarrhea reappears in a child who has previously had a temporary intolerance to milk or milk products.
● A milk-free diet doesn't relieve symptoms.

LARGE-INTESTINE CANCER
(Colon Cancer; Colorectal Cancer)

 GENERAL INFORMATION

DEFINITION—Uncontrolled growth of malignant cells in the rectum or colon (large intestine).

BODY PARTS INVOLVED—Large intestine, including the cecum, ascending colon, transverse colon, descending colon and sigmoid colon; rectum (50% of all colorectal cancers occur here).

SEX OR AGE MOST AFFECTED—Adults over 40.

SIGNS & SYMPTOMS
- No symptoms in the early stages (frequently).
- Bloody or black, tarry stools.
- Cramping abdominal pain.
- Feeling of fullness.
- Change in bowel habits, such as diarrhea, constipation or small stools.
- Unexplained weight loss.
- Pain in the rectum.
- Anemia.
- Loss of bowel control (sometimes).

CAUSES—Unknown.

RISK INCREASES WITH
- Adults over 60.
- Ulcerative colitis and some other chronic disorders of the gastrointestinal tract.
- Improper diet that is low in fiber and high in fat.
- Previous rectal polyps.
- Family history of rectal polyps or colorectal cancer.

HOW TO PREVENT
- Eat a diet that is high in fiber and low in fat.
- After age 50, have annual physical examinations and request rectal and colon exams, and tests for blood in the stool.
- If you have any of the risk factors listed above, buy from your pharmacy a detection kit for blood in the stool. Check for bleeding every 2 months.

 WHAT TO EXPECT

APPROPRIATE HEALTH CARE
- Doctor's treatment.
- Surgery to remove the tumor. It is sometimes necessary to divert the bowel through a surgical opening in the abdomen (colostomy).
- Radiation treatment before and after surgery.

DIAGNOSTIC MEASURES
- Your own observation of symptoms.
- Medical history and physical exam by a doctor.
- Laboratory blood studies.
- Sigmoidoscopy; colonoscopy (see Glossary for both).
- X-rays of the colon (barium enema) and kidney (intravenous pyelogram).

POSSIBLE COMPLICATIONS—Spread to other body parts and death.

PROBABLE OUTCOME—Curable in 80% to 90% of cases with early surgery to remove the tumor. This is a high rate of cure compared to other types of cancer.

 HOW TO TREAT

NOTE—Follow your doctor's instructions. These instructions are supplemental.

GENERAL MEASURES—If you have a colostomy, you will require special instructions for care of the opening. Consult your doctor. For an explanation of surgery and postoperative care, see Colostomy.

MEDICATION—Your doctor may prescribe:
- Pain relievers.
- Medicine to regulate bowel movements.
- Anticancer drugs, although they are usually not very effective.

ACTIVITY
- Avoid sports or activities that might injure the stoma (surgical bowel opening).
- Resume your normal activities, including sexual relations, as soon as possible after surgery. A colostomy should not prevent intercourse.

DIET—Eat a low-fat, high-fiber diet (see Appendices 1 and 8).

 CALL YOUR DOCTOR IF

- You have symptoms of cancer of the large intestine, especially rectal bleeding or a significant change in bowel habits that lasts longer than 7 days.
- You develop anemia (fatigue, paleness and rapid heartbeat).

ILLNESSES & DISORDERS

LARGE-INTESTINE POLYP

GENERAL INFORMATION

DEFINITION—A benign growth shaped like a grape on a stalk or lying flat against the inner lining of the large intestine. Polyps occur singly or in groups. They are more common than malignant tumors.

BODY PARTS INVOLVED—Large intestine, most often in the rectum and sigmoid colon.

SEX OR AGE MOST AFFECTED—Adults of both sexes.

SIGNS & SYMPTOMS
- No symptoms (usually).
- Rectal bleeding (sometimes).
- Mucus discharge from the rectum (sometimes).

CAUSES—Unknown.

RISK INCREASES WITH—Family history of intestinal polyps.

HOW TO PREVENT—If you have had polyps in the past, you should have regular sigmoidoscopic (see Glossary) examinations—at least once a year or more, depending on your doctor's recommendation.

WHAT TO EXPECT

APPROPRIATE HEALTH CARE
- Doctor's treatment.
- Surgery to remove polyps.
- Self-care after surgery.

DIAGNOSTIC MEASURES
- Your own observation of symptoms.
- Medical history and physical exam by a doctor.
- Laboratory studies of blood and stool.
- Sigmoidoscopy; colonoscopy (see Glossary).

POSSIBLE COMPLICATIONS—Malignant change in about 1% of polyps.

PROBABLE OUTCOME—Usually curable with surgery, although polyps may recur.

HOW TO TREAT

NOTE—Follow your doctor's instructions. These instructions are supplemental.

GENERAL MEASURES—Surgery to remove a polyp is usually done with insertion of a proctoscope or sigmoidoscope in the anus. Polyps are snipped off or destroyed by electric cauterization. If a pathologist's report indicates the polyp is malignant, total excision of the polyp and surrounding tissue is necessary.

For multiple polyps, a portion of the colon may be removed through an abdominal incision (laparotomy).

MEDICATION—Medicine usually is not necessary for this disorder.

ACTIVITY—No restrictions.

DIET—Eat a diet that is high in fiber (see Appendix 1) and low in fat (see Appendix 8) to reduce the risk of malignant change.

CALL YOUR DOCTOR IF

- You have bleeding or mucus discharge from the rectum.
- Other members of your family have polyps or colorectal cancer. You should have periodic examinations.
- The following occurs after surgery:
  Increased rectal bleeding.
  Fever, chills or aches. This may indicate an infection at the surgical site.

LARVA MIGRANS, CUTANEOUS
(Creeping Eruptions)

 GENERAL INFORMATION

DEFINITION—Skin infestation of hookworm or roundworm larvae. These parasites usually infect dogs and cats.

BODY PARTS INVOLVED—Skin areas that come in contact with the ground, usually feet, legs or buttocks.

SEX OR AGE MOST AFFECTED—Both sexes; all ages.

SIGNS & SYMPTOMS—Skin rash or small blister, progressing to thin, raised lines on the skin leading from the parasite's entry point. The random lines create tunnel-like lesions that lengthen up to 1cm a day. Most persons have several tracks simultaneously, each of different length and pattern.

CAUSES—Infestation by larvae of hookworms and roundworms found in the intestinal tracts of dogs and cats.

RISK INCREASES WITH
● Play in warm, moist sand in which cats or dogs have defecated.
● Work that requires crawling in confined spaces and contact with infected soil, as when plumbers work under houses.

HOW TO PREVENT
● Handle cat litter carefully. Avoid touching soil.
● Don't work or play in soil used by cats and dogs for elimination.
● Have pets treated for worms.

 WHAT TO EXPECT

APPROPRIATE HEALTH CARE
● Home care after diagnosis.
● Doctor's treatment.

DIAGNOSTIC MEASURES
● Your own observation of symptoms.
● Medical history and physical exam by a doctor.

POSSIBLE COMPLICATIONS—Secondary bacterial infection of affected skin.

PROBABLE OUTCOME—Usually curable in 1 to 2 weeks with treatment.

 HOW TO TREAT

NOTE—Follow your doctor's instructions. These instructions are supplemental.

GENERAL MEASURES—No specific instructions except those listed under other headings.

MEDICATION—Your doctor may prescribe:
● Topical thiabendazole for local application in a 2% solution with dimethyl sulfoxide (DMSO). Follow instructions carefully. Apply it to the end of the track (farthest from the point of entry).
● Oral thiabendazole for serious infestations by many larvae. This form causes adverse reactions and side effects.

ACTIVITY—No restrictions.

DIET—No special diet.

 CALL YOUR DOCTOR IF

● You have symptoms of larva migrans.
● Skin lesions develop pus, indicating secondary infection.
● You take oral thiabendazole, and new, unexplained symptoms develop.

LARYNGITIS

GENERAL INFORMATION

DEFINITION—A minor inflammation of the larynx (voice box) and surrounding tissues, causing temporary hoarseness.

BODY PARTS INVOLVED—Larynx (voice box); the upper part of the neck, behind the Adam's apple.

SEX OR AGE MOST AFFECTED—Both sexes; all ages.

SIGNS & SYMPTOMS
- Hoarseness or loss of voice.
- Sore throat; tickling in the back of the throat.
- Sensation of a lump in the throat.
- Slight fever (sometimes).
- Swallowing difficulty.

CAUSES—Inflammation of the vocal cords and surrounding area caused by:
- Viruses.
- Bacteria.
- Allergies.
- Excessive use of the voice.
- Electrolyte-balance disturbances, especially low potassium, that cause muscle weakness.
- Tumors (rare).

RISK INCREASES WITH
- Exposure to irritants distributed by air-conditioning systems, such as mold, pollen and pollutants.
- Extremely cold weather.
- Smoking.
- Excess alcohol consumption.
- Recent respiratory illness, such as bronchitis or pneumonia.

HOW TO PREVENT
- Avoid yelling or straining your voice.
- Treat respiratory infections carefully.

WHAT TO EXPECT

APPROPRIATE HEALTH CARE
- Self-care after diagnosis.
- Doctor's treatment.

DIAGNOSTIC MEASURES
- Your own observation of symptoms.
- Medical history and physical exam by a doctor. Treatment by an ear, nose and throat specialist might be helpful for persistent cases.

POSSIBLE COMPLICATIONS—Total breathing obstruction, if laryngitis is part of a serious infection of the respiratory system, such as epiglottitis.

PROBABLE OUTCOME—Spontaneous recovery for viral laryngitis in 10 to 14 days. Bacterial infections are usually curable in 7 to 10 days with antibiotic treatment.

HOW TO TREAT

NOTE—Follow your doctor's instructions. These instructions are supplemental.

GENERAL MEASURES
- Don't use your voice—whisper or write notes. For most cases, resting the voice for a few days is all that is needed.
- Use a cool-mist humidifier to increase air moisture and ease the constricted feeling in the throat. Hot, steamy showers also help.

MEDICATION—For minor discomfort, you may use non-prescription drugs, such as acetaminophen, aspirin or cough syrup.

ACTIVITY—Rest more frequently.

DIET—No special diet.

CALL YOUR DOCTOR IF

- You have hoarseness or other symptoms of laryngitis that last longer than 2 weeks. This may be an early sign of cancer.
- You feel very ill, have a high fever or breathing difficulty. If these symptoms develop in a child, call your doctor immediately.

LARYNX CANCER
(Laryngeal Cancer)

 GENERAL INFORMATION

DEFINITION—Uncontrolled growth of malignant cells in the vocal cords and surrounding tissues.

BODY PARTS INVOLVED—Larynx (back of the throat and "voice box").

SEX OR AGE MOST AFFECTED—Both sexes of adults over age 40, but more common in men.

SIGNS & SYMPTOMS
- Hoarseness that does not disappear after resting the voice.
- "Lump-in-the-throat" feeling.
- Painful or difficult swallowing.
- Hard, swollen lymph glands in the neck.

CAUSES—Smoking. Other causes are unknown.

RISK INCREASES WITH
- Heavy smoking.
- Excess alcohol consumption.
- Vocal-cord polyps.
- Chronic vocal-cord inflammation from any cause.

HOW TO PREVENT
- Stop smoking.
- Don't drink more than 1 or 2 alcoholic drinks—if any—a day.
- Don't abuse your voice.

 WHAT TO EXPECT

APPROPRIATE HEALTH CARE
- Doctor's treatment (ear, nose and throat specialist).
- Hospitalization for radiation treatment.
- Surgery to remove cancer and involved tissue (sometimes).
- Speech therapy to learn to speak without vocal cords, if surgery is necessary.

DIAGNOSTIC MEASURES
- Your own observation of symptoms. Be alert to hoarseness which persists beyond 2 weeks.
- Medical history and physical exam by a doctor.
- Biopsy (see Glossary) of the vocal cords or other affected tissue.

POSSIBLE COMPLICATIONS—Life-threatening spread to other body parts.

PROBABLE OUTCOME—Often curable with early diagnosis and treatment. In the late stages, this condition is currently considered incurable. However, symptoms can be relieved or controlled.

Scientific research into causes and treatment continues, so there is hope for increasingly effective treatment and cure.

 HOW TO TREAT

NOTE—Follow your doctor's instructions. These instructions are supplemental.

GENERAL MEASURES
- Early diagnosis and treatment—as with other cancers—are the best hope for complete cure.
- If your vocal cords are removed, join a support group for persons like you who have faced the same situation. This helps minimize stress and adjustment.

MEDICATION—Medicine usually is not necessary for this disorder. Anticancer drugs are not often prescribed; radiation therapy is used instead.

ACTIVITY—Resume your normal activities gradually after treatment or surgery.

DIET—No special diet, unless surgery is performed. In that case, a liquid diet (see Appendix 7) is necessary until the affected area heals.

 CALL YOUR DOCTOR IF

You have symptoms of larynx cancer.

LEGG-PERTHES DISEASE
(Slipped Femoral Epiphysis; Coxa Plana)

 GENERAL INFORMATION

DEFINITION—Gradual weakening of the upper end of the thigh bone where it meets the pelvis.

BODY PARTS INVOLVED—Either leg at the hip joint (occasionally both).

SEX OR AGE MOST AFFECTED—Older children (5 to 11 years) of both sexes, but more common in boys.

SIGNS & SYMPTOMS
- Pain and stiffness in the hip and thigh.
- Pain in the leg—often the *knee*—even though the disorder is in the hip.
- Limping.

CAUSES—Unknown. Injury is usually not a factor.

RISK INCREASES WITH
- Family history of hip disorders.
- Use of cortisone drugs for other disorders.
- Overweight.
- Periods of rapid growth.

HOW TO PREVENT—Help an overweight youngster lose weight. A reducing diet appears in Appendix 10.

 WHAT TO EXPECT

APPROPRIATE HEALTH CARE
- Doctor's treatment, including consultation with an orthopedist.
- Surgery to reinforce the bone's attachment to the joint and prevent further deformity (sometimes).
- Hospitalization (sometimes) for traction (a steady pull on the leg).
- Home care after diagnosis or hospitalization.

DIAGNOSTIC MEASURES
- Your own observation of symptoms, especially a limp or knee pain in your child.
- Medical history and physical exam by a doctor.
- X-ray of the hip.

POSSIBLE COMPLICATIONS
- Bone infection.
- Permanent damage to the thigh bone and hip joint.

PROBABLE OUTCOME—Often curable in 3 to 4 years with early treatment. Delayed treatment may cause permanent bone injury and require surgery to replace the hip.

 HOW TO TREAT

NOTE—Follow your doctor's instructions. These instructions are supplemental.

GENERAL MEASURES
- Youngsters often have difficulty accepting the need for bed rest, casts, braces or other treatment. Enlist the help of your doctor, a counselor, school nurse, or other significant persons, if necessary, to discuss the situation with your child.
- Help your child find activities and interests that don't involve athletics.
- Use heat to relieve pain. Warm compresses, heating pads, whirlpool baths, heat lamps, diathermy and ultrasound are effective.

MEDICATION—For minor discomfort, you may use non-prescription drugs, such as aspirin, acetaminophen or ibuprofen.

ACTIVITY—Bed rest may be necessary for 6 months to 1 year until the condition improves, or until after surgery. When the bones can bear weight, crutches, braces or casts are usually necessary. After that, activities may be resumed gradually. See Appendix 17, Care of Casts.

DIET—No special diet, unless the child is overweight. See Appendix 10.

 CALL YOUR DOCTOR IF

- Your child has hip pain, knee pain, stiffness or a limp.
- The following occurs during treatment:
  Symptoms don't improve in 4 weeks, despite treatment.
  Pain increases.
  Temperature rises to 101F (38.3C).

LEGIONNAIRE'S DISEASE
(Legionella Pneumophilia Bronchopneumonia)

 GENERAL INFORMATION

DEFINITION—A form of lung infection (bronchopneumonia) named after an epidemic that affected 182 people attending an American Legion Convention in 1976.

BODY PARTS INVOLVED—Bronchial tubes; lungs.

SEX OR AGE MOST AFFECTED—Both sexes, but more common in men over age 40.

SIGNS & SYMPTOMS
- General ill feeling.
- Headache.
- Chills and fever up to 105F (40.6C).
- Muscle aches.
- Cough without sputum that progresses to one with gray or blood-streaked sputum.
- Nausea and vomiting.
- Disorientation.

CAUSES—Infection from bacteria (legionella pneumophilia) that is not contagious between persons. The germ is transmitted through the air, and the incubation period after exposure is 2 to 10 days.

In the 1976 epidemic, the germ was transmitted through the cooling and evaporating elements of a large, central air-conditioning system. The bacteria are also found in excavation sites and newly plowed soil.

RISK INCREASES WITH
- Chronic, debilitating illness including diabetes mellitus, chronic kidney failure or emphysema.
- Smoking. This increases the risk 3 to 4 times.
- Excess alcohol consumption.
- Use of immunosuppressive drugs, including cortisone and anticancer drugs.

HOW TO PREVENT
- Have cooling and heating systems cleaned and inspected regularly. Change filters often.
- Don't smoke.
- Don't drink more than 1 or 2 alcoholic drinks—if any—a day.

 WHAT TO EXPECT

APPROPRIATE HEALTH CARE
- Doctor's treatment.
- Hospitalization for intensive care and oxygen (severe cases).
- Self-care for mild cases or during convalescence after hospitalization.

DIAGNOSTIC MEASURES
- Your own observation of symptoms.
- Medical history and physical exam by a doctor.
- Laboratory blood studies and culture of sputum.

POSSIBLE COMPLICATIONS
- Shock or delirium.
- Congestive heart failure.
- Kidney failure.
- Heart-rhythm disturbances.

PROBABLE OUTCOME—Usually curable with prompt diagnosis and treatment. If untreated, 15% of cases are fatal.

 HOW TO TREAT

NOTE—Follow your doctor's instructions. These instructions are supplemental.

GENERAL MEASURES—The following apply to mild cases or to care after hospitalization:
- Use a cool-mist humidifier to increase air moisture and thin lung secretions so they can be coughed up more easily.
- Use a heating pad on the chest to relieve chest pain.
- Practice deep-breathing exercises as often as your strength allows.
- Avoid loud talking, laughing or singing. They may trigger excessive coughing.
- Keep warm. If you become chilled, the germ can become more virulent.

MEDICATION
- Your doctor may prescribe antibiotics, such as erythromycin or a combination of rifampin and tetracycline.
- If the cough is painful and doesn't produce sputum, you may use non-prescription medicine to suppress it. If the cough produces sputum, don't suppress it.
- You may take aspirin or acetaminophen to reduce fever.

ACTIVITY—Rest in bed until completely well. You may read or watch TV. Allow 2 to 4 weeks for recovery.

DIET—No special diet.

 CALL YOUR DOCTOR IF

- You have symptoms of Legionnaire's disease.
- The following occurs during or after treatment:
    Temperature spike to 102F (38.9C).
    Severe chest pain, despite treatment.
    Increased shortness of breath.
    Dark or bluish nails, lips or skin.
    Blood in the sputum.
- New, unexplained symptoms develop. Drugs in treatment may produce side effects.

LEUKEMIA, ACUTE

GENERAL INFORMATION

DEFINITION—A malignant overgrowth of white blood cells in bone marrow or tissues that are part of the lymphatic system (lymph glands, spleen, liver). These excess cells accumulate and spill into the bloodstream, eventually involving other tissues.

Common forms of leukemia include: acute lymphocytic leukemia (especially prevalent in children), acute myelogenous leukemia and acute monocytic leukemia. Acute leukemia is the most common form of cancer in children.

BODY PARTS INVOLVED—Bone marrow and lymph tissue in early stages. The disease eventually affects all body tissues.

SEX OR AGE MOST AFFECTED
● Both sexes, but more common in males.
● All ages. Acute lymphocytic leukemia has a peak incidence between ages 2 and 5.

SIGNS & SYMPTOMS
● Low fever.
● Tiredness.
● Anemia.
● Increasing paleness.
● General ill feeling.
● Easy bruising and spontaneous bleeding (nosebleeds, bleeding from the gums or prolonged menstruation).
● Enlarged spleen and abdominal pain.
● Susceptibility to infection, especially pneumonia.
● Mouth infections with ulcers and sores.
● Headache and lethargy, if meninges (brain membranes) are affected.

CAUSES—Unknown, but there are many suspected predisposing factors—especially viruses and radiation.

RISK INCREASES WITH
● Family history of leukemia.
● Excess exposure to X-rays.
● Congenital disorders, especially Down's syndrome.
● Identical twins.
● Exposure to benzenes, which are used in many industrial chemicals.
● Use of cytotoxic drugs.

HOW TO PREVENT—Cannot be prevented. If you have a family history of leukemia, seek genetic counseling before starting a family.

WHAT TO EXPECT

APPROPRIATE HEALTH CARE
● Doctor's treatment.
● Home care after diagnosis and treatment and during remission.
● Hospitalization for treatment in the initial stage or for relapse.

DIAGNOSTIC MEASURES
● Your own observation of symptoms.
● Medical history and physical exam by a doctor.
● Laboratory studies of blood, bone marrow and cerebrospinal fluid.

POSSIBLE COMPLICATIONS
● Hemorrhage.
● Death from destruction of the body's defenses against infection.

PROBABLE OUTCOME—Treatment brings remission in 90% of patients and cure in 50% for some forms of leukemia—especially in children. Other forms are eventually fatal.

HOW TO TREAT

NOTE—Follow your doctor's instructions. These instructions are supplemental.

GENERAL MEASURES
● Avoid ill persons and crowds to prevent dangerous exposure to infection.
● Rinse the mouth often with a warm salt-water solution to decrease mouth ulcers. Use 1 tablespoon salt in 8 oz. water.
● Use a soft toothbrush to prevent gum abrasion.

MEDICATION—Your doctor may prescribe:
● Anticancer drugs.
● Cortisone drugs.
● Pain relievers.
● Antibiotics to fight infection.
● Uricosuric drugs to increase excretion of uric acid that may accumulate as a side effect of anticancer drugs.

ACTIVITY—No restrictions during remissions. Bed rest is usually necessary during active phases.

DIET—Drink extra fluids. Adults should drink 8 to 10 glasses of fluid daily, and children should drink 4 to 6 glasses of fluid. During chemotherapy, eat and drink high-calorie foods and beverages, such as milkshakes or eggnog.

CALL YOUR DOCTOR IF

● You or your child have symptoms of leukemia.
● The following occurs during active stages *or* remissions:
Fever, chills, cough or sore throat.
Abnormal bleeding. Apply pressure and ice while awaiting your doctor's return call.
Constipation.

LEUKEMIA, CHRONIC LYMPHOCYTIC

GENERAL INFORMATION

DEFINITION—A very slow-growing cancer of the blood-forming organs of older persons. About 1/3 of leukemia victims have this form. It is often discovered in a routine blood test for unrelated purposes.

BODY PARTS INVOLVED—Blood-forming organs: bone marrow; lymph glands; liver; spleen.

SEX OR AGE MOST AFFECTED—Both sexes, but more common in men over 50.

SIGNS & SYMPTOMS—In early stages, the following appear gradually:
- Fatigue and general weakness.
- Mild to moderate anemia.
- Firm, enlarged lymph nodes.
- Unexplained weight loss.
- Enlarged liver and spleen.
- Susceptibility to infection.
- Skin nodules (sometimes).
In late stages:
- Inability to resist bacterial, viral or fungal infections.
- Incapacitating weakness.

CAUSES—Unknown. Unlike some forms of leukemia, excess exposure to radiation does *not* seem to be a factor in chronic lymphocytic leukemia.

RISK INCREASES WITH
- Adults over 60.
- Family history of chromosome or immunological defects. (This is a suspected—but unproven—risk factor).

HOW TO PREVENT—No specific preventive measures.

WHAT TO EXPECT

APPROPRIATE HEALTH CARE
- Self-care after diagnosis.
- Doctor's treatment.
- Hospitalization for anticancer drugs and radiation treatment.
- Psychotherapy or counseling for the patient and family.

DIAGNOSTIC MEASURES
- Your own observation of symptoms.
- Medical history and physical exam by a doctor.
- Laboratory studies of blood and bone marrow.

POSSIBLE COMPLICATIONS
- Bleeding.
- Severe anemia.
- Infections.
- Gout.

PROBABLE OUTCOME—This condition is currently considered incurable. However, symptoms can be relieved or controlled. Many patients live for years with few or no symptoms, and medical literature cites a few instances of unexplained recovery.

Scientific research into causes and treatment continues, so there is hope for increasingly effective treatment and cure.

HOW TO TREAT

NOTE—Follow your doctor's instructions. These instructions are supplemental.

GENERAL MEASURES—Be extra careful about avoiding illness:
- Wash hands frequently.
- Don't become chilled.
- Avoid contact with all obviously ill people, especially children with infections.
- Avoid crowds during cold and flu seasons.

MEDICATION—Many persons with this disorder require little treatment. Treatment plans are highly individualized.
- Your doctor may prescribe:
  Anticancer medications, including cortisone drugs.
  Antigout drugs.
- *Don't take aspirin* or any product containing aspirin. Aspirin increases the likelihood of bleeding.

ACTIVITY—No restrictions.

DIET—No special diet. Eat as heartily as possible.

CALL YOUR DOCTOR IF

- You have symptoms of chronic lymphocytic leukemia.
- The following occurs after diagnosis and treatment:
  Recurrence or worsening of symptoms.
  Signs of infection, such as fever and chills.
  Black, tarry stools, bleeding gums or nosebleed.

LEUKOPLAKIA

 GENERAL INFORMATION

DEFINITION—A thickened area in the delicate lining of the mouth or tongue. This is not contagious, but it may be premalignant.

BODY PARTS INVOLVED—Inside of cheek; floor of mouth; tongue; palate; roof of mouth.

SEX OR AGE MOST AFFECTED—All ages, but most common in adults over 60.

SIGNS & SYMPTOMS
- Sensitivity to hot and spicy food.
- A small white patch in the mouth. The patch feels firm, rough and stiff.
- No symptoms in the early stages.

CAUSES
- Deficiency of vitamins A or B.
- Deficiency of male or female hormones.
- Syphilis.
- Chronic irritation in the mouth. The irritation may be from jagged teeth, ill-fitting dentures, hot or spicy food, excess alcohol consumption or nicotine.

RISK INCREASES WITH
- Use of tobacco products, including cigarettes, chewing tobacco, snuff, pipe or cigars.
- Dentures.

HOW TO PREVENT
- Don't smoke or use tobacco products.
- Inspect the mouth regularly if you wear dentures or smoke.
- Decrease consumption of hot or highly seasoned foods if suspicious lesions develop.

 WHAT TO EXPECT

APPROPRIATE HEALTH CARE
- Doctor's treatment.
- Surgery to remove the lesions.

DIAGNOSTIC MEASURES
- Your own observation of symptoms.
- Medical history and physical exam by a doctor or dentist.
- Biopsy (see Glossary).

POSSIBLE COMPLICATIONS—The lesion may become cancerous if untreated.

PROBABLE OUTCOME—Usually curable with surgery and removal of the source of irritation, such as tobacco.

 HOW TO TREAT

NOTE—Follow your doctor's instructions. These instructions are supplemental.

GENERAL MEASURES—Following surgery or biopsy:
- If bleeding occurs, press cotton gauze gently for 5 minutes against the operation site.
- 24 hours after the operation, rinse the mouth with a warm salt-water solution. Use 1/2 teaspoon salt in 8 oz. warm water. Repeat every 1 or 2 hours.
- Brush and floss teeth often and use antiseptic mouthwash during the healing process. A clean mouth heals faster.
- Return to the doctor or dentist for removal of sutures 5 to 7 days after the operation. By then, the laboratory report may be complete.

MEDICATION—For minor pain, you may use non-prescription drugs such as acetaminophen.

ACTIVITY—No restrictions.

DIET—Liquid or soft diet for 24 hours; then no special diet.

 CALL YOUR DOCTOR OR DENTIST IF

- You have symptoms of leukoplakia.
- The following occurs after surgery: Bleeding after 12 hours or more. Severe pain.

LICE
(Pediculosis; Head Lice; Body Lice; "Crabs")

 GENERAL INFORMATION

DEFINITION—Skin inflammation caused by tiny parasites (lice) which live on the body or in clothing.

BODY PARTS INVOLVED—Hairy areas anywhere, especially the scalp, eyebrows or genital area; skin, especially areas in which clothing is in close contact with skin, such as the shoulders, waist, genital area or buttocks.

SEX OR AGE MOST AFFECTED—Both sexes; all ages.

SIGNS & SYMPTOMS
- Itching and scratching, sometimes intense and usually in hair-covered areas.
- Eggs ("nits") on hair shafts.
- Scalp inflammation and matted hair.
- Enlarged lymph glands at the back of the scalp or in the groin (sometimes).
- Red bite marks and hives.

CAUSES—Tiny (3mm to 4mm) parasites that bite through skin to obtain nourishment (blood). The bites cause itching and inflammation. Some lice live on skin, although they are difficult to see. Others live in clothing near skin. Eggs (nits) adhere to hairs.

RISK INCREASES WITH
- Crowded or unsanitary living conditions.
- Family history of lice.
- Sexual intercourse with an infected person.

HOW TO PREVENT
- Bathe and shampoo often.
- Avoid wearing the same clothing more than a day or two.
- Change bed linens often.
- Don't share combs, brushes or hats with others.

 WHAT TO EXPECT

APPROPRIATE HEALTH CARE
- Self-care after diagnosis.
- Doctor's treatment.

DIAGNOSTIC MEASURES
- Your own observation of symptoms. You may see nits (like tiny footballs) on the side of hairs.
- Medical history and physical exam by a doctor.

POSSIBLE COMPLICATIONS—Infection at the site of deep scratching may cause diseases such as typhus (rare).

PROBABLE OUTCOME—Usually curable with medicated creams, lotions and shampoos. Allow 5 days after treatment for symptoms to disappear. Lice often recur.

 HOW TO TREAT

NOTE—Follow your doctor's instructions. These instructions are supplemental.

GENERAL MEASURES—The following measures apply to all members of the household, and to any sexual partners of household members:
- Use medicated shampoo, cream or lotion prescribed by your doctor.
- Machine-wash *all* clothing and linen in hot water. Dry in the dryer's hot-air cycle. Iron the clothing and linen, if possible. Washing removes the lice, and ironing destroys nits.
- If you don't have a washing machine, iron the clothes and linen, or seal for 10 days in a plastic bag to kill lice and nits.
- Dry-clean non-washable items or seal in a plastic bag for 10 days.
- Boil articles such as combs, curlers, hairbrushes and barrettes.
- Hair does not have to be shaved.

MEDICATION—Your doctor may prescribe anti-lice (pediculocide) cream, lotion or shampoo. Apply creams or lotions to infected body parts according to instructions. To use the shampoo:
- Wet the hair. Apply 1 tablespoon of shampoo. Lather for 4 minutes, working the lather well into the scalp.
- If shampoo gets in eyes, wash out immediately with water.
- Rinse hair thoroughly and towel dry. Don't use this towel again without laundering.
- Comb the hair with a fine comb dipped in hot vinegar to remove the lice. The comb must run through the hair repeatedly from the scalp outward until the hair is completely free of nits.
- A single application of shampoo is effective in more than 90% of cases. Don't use more frequently than recommended, because the shampoo may cause skin irritation or be absorbed into the body.
- If the lice infect eyelashes, they must be removed carefully by your doctor. The prescribed medications should *not* go into the eye or on the eyelashes. You may apply petroleum jelly to the eyelashes for 7 or 8 days after removal.

ACTIVITY—No restrictions.

DIET—No special diet.

 CALL YOUR DOCTOR IF

You, your sexual partner, or anyone in your household have symptoms of lice—or symptoms recur after treatment.

ILLNESSES & DISORDERS

LICHEN PLANUS

GENERAL INFORMATION

DEFINITION—A chronic skin eruption that is not cancerous or contagious.

BODY PARTS INVOLVED
- Skin of the legs, trunk, arms, wrists, scalp or penis.
- Lining of the mouth or vagina.
- Toenails and fingernails (around or partially under the nailbed).

SEX OR AGE MOST AFFECTED—All ages, but most common in adults over 40.

SIGNS & SYMPTOMS
- Small, slightly raised bumps that itch. The bumps are purplish with a whitish surface.
- An irregular whitish line inside the mouth or vagina.
- Sudden hair loss in patches on the head.

CAUSES—Unknown, but may be caused by a virus. In a few cases, lichen planus may be an adverse reaction to certain drugs.

RISK INCREASES WITH
- Stress.
- Fatigue or overwork.

HOW TO PREVENT—Cannot be prevented at present.

WHAT TO EXPECT

APPROPRIATE HEALTH CARE
- Self-care after diagnosis.
- Doctor's treatment.

DIAGNOSTIC MEASURES
- Your own observation of symptoms.
- Medical history and physical exam by a doctor.
- Biopsy of questionable papules (raised bumps).

POSSIBLE COMPLICATIONS—None expected.

PROBABLE OUTCOME—Symptoms can be controlled with treatment, but the disorder lasts months or years. Be patient and persist with your treatment, even if results are disappointing or slow.

HOW TO TREAT

NOTE—Follow your doctor's instructions. These instructions are supplemental.

GENERAL MEASURES—Use cool-water soaks (see Appendix 18) to relieve itching.

MEDICATION—Your doctor may prescribe:
- Antihistamines for their sedative effect to control itching.
- Cortisone creams or ointments to reduce inflammation and decrease itching. Use only once or twice a day unless directed otherwise. Apply immediately after bathing for better spreading and penetration. For the face and groin, use only low-potency steroid products without fluorine.
- Cortisone tablets for severe cases.

ACTIVITY—No restrictions.

DIET—No special diet.

CALL YOUR DOCTOR IF

- You have symptoms of lichen planus.
- New, unexplained symptoms develop. Drugs used in treatment may produce side effects.

LIPOMAS

GENERAL INFORMATION

DEFINITION—Benign tumors of fat cells.

BODY PARTS INVOLVED—Trunk; neck; back; upper thighs; arms.

SEX OR AGE MOST AFFECTED—Both sexes of persons from puberty to old age.

SIGNS & SYMPTOMS—Nodules under the skin with the following characteristics:
- Nodules are dome-shaped and about 2cm to 10cm in diameter. Some grow larger.
- Nodules feel "doughy."
- Only one—or many—lipomas may occur at one time.

CAUSES—Unknown, but the tendency is probably inherited. Minor injury may trigger growth.

RISK INCREASES WITH—Family history of lipomas.

HOW TO PREVENT—Cannot be prevented at present. If you are obese, you can reduce the size of lipomas by losing weight.

WHAT TO EXPECT

APPROPRIATE HEALTH CARE
- Doctor's treatment.
- Surgery to remove the lipoma (sometimes).

DIAGNOSTIC MEASURES
- Your own observation of symptoms.
- Medical history and physical exam by a doctor.

POSSIBLE COMPLICATIONS—Large lipomas may interfere with muscle function.

PROBABLE OUTCOME—These tumors are benign and require no treatment, but they may be removed if they are unsightly or interfere with muscle function. Surgical removal is usually done in a doctor's office.

HOW TO TREAT

NOTE—Follow your doctor's instructions. These instructions are supplemental.

GENERAL MEASURES—After surgical removal:
- Apply rubbing alcohol to the scab twice a day.
- Apply an adhesive bandage to the scab during the day. Leave it uncovered at night.
- Wash the wound as usual. Dry gently and completely after bathing or swimming.
- If the scab cracks or oozes, apply non-prescription antibiotic ointment several times a day.
- Return to your doctor for removal of sutures in 5 to 10 days.

MEDICATION—Medication usually is not necessary for this disorder.

ACTIVITY—After surgical removal, resume your normal activities gradually. Allow 1 month for complete healing.

DIET—No special diet.

CALL YOUR DOCTOR IF

The following occurs after surgery:
- Fever.
- Bleeding which does not respond to moderate pressure.
- Signs of infection (warmth, swelling or redness) at the surgical site.

ILLNESSES & DISORDERS

LIVER CANCER

GENERAL INFORMATION

DEFINITION—Uncontrolled growth of malignant cells in the liver. Liver cancer may be primary—resulting from abnormal liver or bile-duct cells—or it may result from spread of cancer from another site. The most common sources are cancers of the rectum, colon, lung, breast, pancreas, esophagus or skin (malignant melanoma).

BODY PARTS INVOLVED—Liver; bile ducts.

SEX OR AGE MOST AFFECTED—All ages, but most common in men over 60.

SIGNS & SYMPTOMS
- Loss of appetite and weight loss.
- Tender mass in the right upper abdomen.
- Pain in the upper abdomen.
- Low fever, usually less than 101F (38.3C).
- Yellow eyes and skin (sometimes).
- Swollen abdomen from fluid retention (sometimes).

CAUSES—Unknown.

RISK INCREASES WITH
- Cirrhosis of the liver.
- Excess alcohol consumption.
- Previous hepatitis B infection.

HOW TO PREVENT—No specific preventive measures.

WHAT TO EXPECT

APPROPRIATE HEALTH CARE
- Self-care after diagnosis.
- Doctor's treatment.
- Surgery to confirm the diagnosis.
- Radiation therapy.
- Liver transplant. These are available at a few medical centers in the U.S.

DIAGNOSTIC MEASURES
- Your own observation of symptoms.
- Medical history and physical exam by a doctor.
- Laboratory blood studies.
- CAT scan.
- X-rays of the chest.

POSSIBLE COMPLICATIONS
- Sodium retention, leading to life-threatening fluid accumulation in the abdomen and lower body parts.
- Kidney failure.
- Death from loss of liver function.

PROBABLE OUTCOME—This condition is currently considered incurable and fatal within a short time. However, pain can be controlled. Treatment is usually attempted, although it is not likely to be successful.

Scientific research into causes and treatment continues, so there is hope for increasingly effective treatment and cure.

HOW TO TREAT

NOTE—Follow your doctor's instructions. These instructions are supplemental.

GENERAL MEASURES—See Liver Transplant (in Surgery section) for information about the procedure.

MEDICATION—Your doctor may prescribe:
- Anticancer drugs.
- Pain relievers.

ACTIVITY—No restrictions. Stay as active as your strength allows.

DIET—Low-salt diet (see Appendix 9).

CALL YOUR DOCTOR IF

- You have symptoms of liver cancer, especially unexplained weight loss, low fever or a mass in the abdomen.
- You develop a swollen abdomen during treatment.
- New, unexplained symptoms develop. Drugs used in treatment may produce side effects.

LUNG ABSCESS

GENERAL INFORMATION

DEFINITION—An infected area of lung tissue, surrounded by lung inflammation. The infected lung tissue dies and is replaced with pus. The infection is not contagious from person to person.

BODY PARTS INVOLVED—Lung.

SEX OR AGE MOST AFFECTED—Both sexes; all ages.

SIGNS & SYMPTOMS
- Cough with sputum. The sputum is puslike, often blood-streaked and sometimes smells bad.
- Bad breath.
- Sweating.
- Fever to 101F (38.3C) or higher.
- Chills.
- Weight loss.
- Chest pain (sometimes).

CAUSES—Usually a complication of pneumonia. A lung abscess sometimes occurs when an unconscious or sedated person inhales infected material from the upper-breathing passages. The patient may be unconscious from a head injury, an anesthetic (including dental anesthesia), intoxicated from alcohol or heavily sedated. Lung abscesses are generally caused by virulent bacteria, such as klebsiella, pseudomona, staphylococcus or beta-hemolytic streptococcus.

RISK INCREASES WITH
- Recent illness, especially pneumonia that has been slow to heal.
- Alcoholism.
- Recent general anesthesia or injury causing unconsciousness.

HOW TO PREVENT
- Obtain prompt medical treatment for respiratory infections, especially pneumonia.
- Keep the teeth and mouth in good condition to prevent oral infections that could result In a lung abscess.

WHAT TO EXPECT

APPROPRIATE HEALTH CARE
- Doctor's treatment.
- Surgery (sometimes) to aspirate pus from the abscess or to remove the abscess and part of the lung, if the abscess does not heal.
- Self-care during convalescence.

DIAGNOSTIC MEASURES
- Your own observation of symptoms.
- Medical history and physical exam by a doctor.

- Laboratory blood tests and a culture of pus from the abscess to determine what antibiotic to use.
- X-rays of the lung.

POSSIBLE COMPLICATIONS
- Chronic abscess, leading to weight loss, anemia, bronchiectasis or chronic lung disease, if the abscess does not respond well to antibiotic treatment.
- Rupture of the abscess, causing empyema or massive bleeding in the lung.
- Spread of infection to other body parts, especially the brain.

PROBABLE OUTCOME—Usually curable with prolonged antibiotic treatment (up to 6 months).

HOW TO TREAT

NOTE—Follow your doctor's instructions. These instructions are supplemental.

GENERAL MEASURES
- Don't smoke.
- Practice deep-breathing exercises as often as possible.
- Learn postural drainage to help rid the lung of bronchial secretions. Lie on the bed on your stomach with your head and chest hanging over the edge. Force yourself to cough. Continue until you cannot raise any more sputum. Practice this twice a day for 5 to 10 minutes.

MEDICATION—Your doctor may prescribe antibiotics for prolonged periods to fight infection and prevent a recurrence.

ACTIVITY—No restrictions.

DIET—No special diet. Increase your fluid intake to a minimum of 1 glass of fluid at least 8 times a day. By drinking extra liquids, the body is forced to eliminate part of the fluid through the lungs. This makes thick lung secretions thinner, so they can be coughed up more easily.

CALL YOUR DOCTOR IF

- You have symptoms of a lung abscess.
- The following occurs during treatment: Fever rises to 101F (38.3C) or higher. Sputum thickens, despite treatment. Postural drainage reveals a change in color, amount or consistency of the sputum.
- Symptoms of a lung infection recur after treatment, especially a sputum-producing cough, fever or general ill feeling.

ILLNESSES & DISORDERS

LUNG CANCER
(Bronchogenic Carcinoma)

 GENERAL INFORMATION

DEFINITION—Malignant tissue growth in the lung.

BODY PARTS INVOLVED—Bronchial tubes and lungs. Cancer spreads to the larynx, liver, brain, bones and kidneys.

SEX OR AGE MOST AFFECTED—Adults of both sexes between ages 40 and 70, but more common in men.

SIGNS & SYMPTOMS
- Intense, persistent cough.
- Sputum that may contain blood.
- Wheezing.
- Chest pain.
- Fatigue and weakness.
- Weight loss.

CAUSES
- Cigarette smoking.
- Air pollution.
- Unknown (some forms).
- Spread of cancer from somewhere else in the body.

RISK INCREASES WITH
- Adults over 60.
- Smoking. A smoker is 22 times more likely to develop lung cancer than a non-smoker.
- Environmental exposure to asbestos, uranium ore, nickel, chromates, bischloromethyl ether or air pollution.

HOW TO PREVENT
- Avoid pollutants. Wear a protective mask if you work with pollutants.
- Don't smoke. Because tumors don't develop for a long time, smokers can quit at any time and greatly reduce the risk of developing lung cancer.
- Visit your doctor for regular health checkups that include a chest X-ray.

OTHER
Lung cancer causes more deaths than any other form of cancer. Its incidence is increasing. It is related almost exclusively to cigarette smoking.

 WHAT TO EXPECT

APPROPRIATE HEALTH CARE
- Doctor's care.
- Surgery for diagnosis (bronchoscopy), biopsy (see Glossary) or removal of cancerous lung tissue.
- About 2 weeks in an extended-care facility for physical therapy to regain lost lung function after surgery.
- Radiation treatment (sometimes).

DIAGNOSTIC MEASURES
- Your own observation of symptoms.
- Medical history and physical exam by a doctor.
- Laboratory studies of cells in sputum and pleural fluid.
- X-rays of lungs.

POSSIBLE COMPLICATIONS
- Destructive spread to other body parts, including the brain.
- Lung collapse.
- Fluid on the lung.
- Club-shaped fingers.

PROBABLE OUTCOME—Without surgery, this condition is currently considered incurable. Only 25% of tumors can be removed surgically. However, symptoms can be relieved or controlled. The survival rate after 5 years is less than 10%.

 HOW TO TREAT

NOTE—Follow your doctor's instructions. These instructions are supplemental.

GENERAL MEASURES—For an explanation of lung-cancer surgery and post-operative care, see Lung Resection.

MEDICATION
- For minor pain, you may use non-prescription drugs such as acetaminophen or aspirin.
- Your doctor may prescribe:
  Medication to reduce pain, nausea or anxiety.
  Anticancer drugs.

ACTIVITY—After surgery, resume your normal activities gradually.

DIET—No special diet.

 CALL YOUR DOCTOR IF

- You have symptoms of lung cancer.
- The following occurs after surgery or during drug treatment:
  Intolerable pain.
  Nausea or vomiting.
  Sleeplessness.
- New, unexplained symptoms develop. Drugs used in treatment may produce side effects.

LUPUS ERYTHEMATOSUS, DISCOID

GENERAL INFORMATION

DEFINITION—A skin disorder. This is different from systemic lupus erythematosus, a connective-tissue disease that affects many different organs. About 1 in 20 persons with discoid lupus progresses to systemic lupus.

BODY PARTS INVOLVED—Skin only of the face, scalp, ears, neck and arms.

SEX OR AGE MOST AFFECTED—Adults of both sexes. The peak incidence occurs in women in their late 20s.

SIGNS & SYMPTOMS—Plaques (red, raised skin lesions) with the following characteristics:
- Plaques are 1cm to 4cm in diameter and have clearly defined borders.
- They may appear anywhere on the face, but the cheeks and jawline are the most common sites. Some people describe them as "butterfly" lesions when two lesions of unequal size appear on both sides of the nose.
- Lesions sometimes appear on the scalp with localized patches of hair loss.
- Lesions scar as they heal.

CAUSES—Unknown, but probably an autoimmune disorder.

RISK INCREASES WITH—Exposure to sunlight.

HOW TO PREVENT—No specific preventive measures. Protection from sunlight decreases the severity.

WHAT TO EXPECT

APPROPRIATE HEALTH CARE
- Self-care after diagnosis.
- Doctor's treatment.

DIAGNOSTIC MEASURES
- Your own observation of symptoms.
- Medical history and physical exam by a doctor.
- Laboratory blood studies and biopsy of skin lesions to rule out systemic lupus erythematosus.

POSSIBLE COMPLICATIONS
- Extensive scarring of the face.
- Systemic lupus erythematosus.

PROBABLE OUTCOME—This disorder is characterized by remissions and flare-ups. It runs its course in 10 to 20 years. 95% of patients (those who don't progress to systemic lupus) live a normal lifespan.

HOW TO TREAT

NOTE—Follow your doctor's instructions. These instructions are supplemental.

GENERAL MEASURES
- Don't go outdoors between 10 a.m. and 2 p.m., when the sun's ultraviolet light is strongest. If you can't avoid exposure to bright sunlight, wear protective clothing and maximum-protection sun-screen products. Avoid fluorescent lighting, if possible.
- See your doctor for regular checkups, even when in remission.

MEDICATION—Your doctor may prescribe:
- Injections of triamcinolone into lesions or hydroxychloroquine by mouth to shrink lesions.
- Topical steroids (occasionally) to decrease redness of lesions.

ACTIVITY—No restrictions.

DIET—No special diet.

CALL YOUR DOCTOR IF

- You have symptoms of discoid lupus erythematosus.
- The following occurs during treatment:
  Lesions on the hands.
  Swelling, redness, pain in joints.

ILLNESSES & DISORDERS

LUPUS ERYTHEMATOSUS, SYSTEMIC

GENERAL INFORMATION

DEFINITION—An inflammatory disease of connective tissue. Lupus is not inherited or cancerous.

BODY PARTS INVOLVED—Connective tissue (collagen). Many body systems are affected, including joints, skin, kidneys, brain, heart and lungs.

SEX OR AGE MOST AFFECTED—All ages and both sexes, but 90% of cases occur in women between ages 30 and 50.

SIGNS & SYMPTOMS—Lupus symptoms frequently flare up and then subside. Episodes generally include fever and fatigue, plus any 4 of the following:
- Rash, usually on the cheeks.
- Ulcers in the mouth.
- Red palms and hands.
- Joint pain with redness, swelling and tenderness—but no deformity.
- Swelling of the face and legs.
- Shortness of breath.
- Rapid or irregular heartbeat.
- Chest pain.
- Hair loss.
- Swelling of the lymph glands.
- Protein in the urine.
- Increased sensitivity to the sun.
- Anemia.
- Mental changes, including psychosis.

CAUSES—Unknown, but lupus is probably an autoimmune disorder. In an autoimmune disorder, the body's immune system functions abnormally and attacks its own normal tissue—usually connective tissue.

RISK INCREASES WITH
- Stress.
- Use of drugs, such as hydralazine, procainamide, methyldopa and chlorpromazine.
- Genetic factors. The incidence is higher among blacks.

HOW TO PREVENT—Cannot be prevented at present.

WHAT TO EXPECT

APPROPRIATE HEALTH CARE
- Self-care after diagnosis.
- Doctor's treatment.

DIAGNOSTIC MEASURES
- Your own observation of symptoms.
- Medical history and physical exam by a doctor. Patients with vague, recurrent symptoms may require long-term observation before a final diagnosis can be made.

- Laboratory studies of antinuclear antibodies, blood count and sedimentation rate (see Glossary).

POSSIBLE COMPLICATIONS
- Bacterial or viral pneumonia.
- Impaired kidney function.
- Pericarditis.
- Seizures.
- Hypertension.

PROBABLE OUTCOME—Lupus is currently considered incurable. The disease is characterized by remissions and relapses. Life expectancy is reduced, but symptoms can be relieved or controlled for many years.

Medical literature cites instances of unexplained recovery. Scientific research into causes and treatment continues, so there is hope for increasingly effective treatment and cure.

HOW TO TREAT

NOTE—Follow your doctor's instructions. These instructions are supplemental.

GENERAL MEASURES
- Obtain prompt medical treatment for any infection.
- Don't take any immunizations or drugs without consulting your doctor. Immunizations and some drugs may cause relapses or worsen current symptoms.
- Don't become pregnant without consulting your doctor. Pregnancy may overload the kidneys and cause death.

MEDICATION—Your doctor may prescribe immunosuppressive, steroid and non-steroidal anti-inflammatory drugs. These relieve symptoms but don't cure the disease.

ACTIVITY—Remain as active as possible.

DIET—If your kidneys or heart are affected, restrict your salt intake. Otherwise, no special diet is necessary.

CALL YOUR DOCTOR IF

- You have symptoms of systemic lupus erythematosus.
- Any of the following occurs after diagnosis:
  Fever of 101F (38.3C) or higher.
  Blood in the urine.
  Shortness of breath.
  Chest pain.
  Bloody stool.
  Severe abdominal pain.
  Any illness with fever.
- New, unexplained symptoms develop. Drugs used in treatment may produce side effects.

LYME DISEASE
(LD; Lyme Arthritis)

GENERAL INFORMATION

DEFINITION—An inflammatory disorder characterized by a skin rash, followed in weeks to months by symptoms in the central nervous system, cardiovascular system and joints. This is named for Lyme, Connecticut, where it was first described.

BODY PARTS INVOLVED—Skin of the thighs, buttocks or underarms; central nervous system; heart and blood vessels; any joint, especially in the neck and back.

SEX OR AGE MOST AFFECTED—Both sexes; all ages.

SIGNS & SYMPTOMS—First stage:
- A red papule (small, raised bump) on the skin of the thighs, buttocks or armpits that grows as large as 5cm.

Later stages—any or some of the following:
- Muscle aches and pains.
- Fatigue.
- Chills and fever.
- Stiff neck with headache.
- Backache.
- Nausea and vomiting.
- Sore throat.
- Enlargement of the spleen and lymph glands.
- Migrating joint pain, eventually accompanied by redness and warmth.
- Enlarged heart and heart-rhythm disturbances.

CAUSES—Unknown, but evidence suggests it is transmitted by the bite of a tiny tick, ixodes dammini. Many patients report a tick bite at the site of the skin lesion 3 days to 3 weeks prior to the skin rash.

RISK INCREASES WITH—Areas where ticks are numerous.

HOW TO PREVENT—Wear protective clothing and use insect repellents in areas with ticks.

WHAT TO EXPECT

APPROPRIATE HEALTH CARE
- Self-care after diagnosis during treatment and convalescence.
- Doctor's treatment.

DIAGNOSTIC MEASURES
- Your own observation of symptoms.
- Medical history and physical exam by a doctor.
- Laboratory blood studies.

POSSIBLE COMPLICATIONS
- Congestive heart failure.
- Permanent joint deformity.
- Permanent brain damage.

PROBABLE OUTCOME—The skin rash is curable in some patients in 10 days with treatment, and this may prevent development of other symptoms. If not, symptoms in the joints, central nervous system and cardiovascular system usually subside slowly over 2 to 3 years. Symptoms often recur after several years—without another tick bite.

HOW TO TREAT

NOTE—Follow your doctor's instructions. These instructions are supplemental.

GENERAL MEASURES
- Use crutches to keep weight off affected joints, if necessary.
- Heat relieves joint pain. Take hot baths or use heating pads, heat lamps or whirlpool treatments.

MEDICATION—Your doctor may prescribe:
- Penicillin or another antibiotic for at least 10 days, if a secondary bacterial infection develops in the affected skin.
- Non-steroidal anti-inflammatory drugs.
- Cortisone drugs to reduce the inflammatory response in the heart or central nervous system.

ACTIVITY—Rest in bed until symptoms of active inflammation subside. You may read or watch TV. Then resume normal activities gradually.

DIET—No special diet.

CALL YOUR DOCTOR IF

- You have symptoms of Lyme disease.
- New, unexplained symptoms develop.

Drugs used in treatment may produce side effects.

LYMPHOGRANULOMA VENEREUM
(LGV; Lymphogranuloma Inguinale)

GENERAL INFORMATION

DEFINITION—A contagious venereal disease. This disease is found mostly in tropical and subtropical areas. It is rare in North America.

BODY PARTS INVOLVED—Genitals; lymph glands.

SEX OR AGE MOST AFFECTED—Both sexes of adults, but most common in men aged 20 to 40.

SIGNS & SYMPTOMS—The following begin 1 to 4 weeks after exposure and progress in order:
- A painless blister on the genitals which ulcerates and heals quickly.
- Enlarged lymph glands in the groin that form large, red, tender masses.
- Multiple areas of deep infection that discharge thick pus and blood-stained material.

Other symptoms include:
- Fever.
- Muscle aches and pain, including backache.
- Headaches.
- Joint pain.
- Appetite loss.
- Vomiting.

CAUSES—The germ chlamydia, which is transmitted by sexual activity.

RISK INCREASES WITH
- Travel and sexual activity with new partners in a country with a tropical or subtropical climate.
- Crowded or unsanitary living conditions.

HOW TO PREVENT
- Use condoms during sexual intercourse with new partners.
- Don't engage in sexual activity with an infected person.

WHAT TO EXPECT

APPROPRIATE HEALTH CARE
- Doctor's treatment.
- Surgery to drain affected lymph glands or remove abscesses and fistulas.

DIAGNOSTIC MEASURES
- Your own observation of symptoms.
- Medical history and physical exam by a doctor.
- Laboratory studies, such as a blood study to rule out syphilis, culture of the discharge from lesions and Frei test (see Glossary).

POSSIBLE COMPLICATIONS
- Chronic infection.
- Interference with bowel and bladder function.
- Impotence (sometimes).

PROBABLE OUTCOME—Usually curable in 6 months if treatment is successful. If not, the disorder is incurable, although it does not reduce life expectancy.

HOW TO TREAT

NOTE—Follow your doctor's instructions. These instructions are supplemental.

GENERAL MEASURES—No specific instructions except those listed under other headings.

MEDICATION
- For minor discomfort, you may use non-prescription drugs such as acetaminophen.
- Your doctor may prescribe:
  Antibiotics or sulfa drugs to fight infection.
  Pain relievers.

ACTIVITY—After treatment, resume normal activity as soon as symptoms improve. Don't resume sexual relations until completely healed.

DIET—No special diet.

CALL YOUR DOCTOR IF

- You have symptoms of lymphogranuloma venereum.
- The following occurs during treatment:
  Fever spikes to 101F (38.3C) or higher.
  Pain cannot be relieved with simple pain medicine.
  You develop symptoms of malabsorption (see Malabsorption in Illness section).
- New, unexplained symptoms develop.

Drugs used in treatment may produce side effects.

LYMPHOMA, NON-HODGKIN'S
(Lymphosarcoma; Reticulum Cell Sarcoma)

GENERAL INFORMATION

DEFINITION—Malignant tumor of the lymph glands. This is more common than Hodgkin's disease.

BODY PARTS INVOLVED
- Lymphocytes (white blood cells).
- Lymph glands (glands which check infection and produce immune substances).
- Spleen (a large lymph gland).

SEX OR AGE MOST AFFECTED—All ages, but most common in men in their 40s.

SIGNS & SYMPTOMS
- Swollen, non-tender, rubbery, distinct lymph glands anywhere in the body—but most commonly in the armpit, neck or groin.
- Weight loss.
- General ill feeling.
- Anemia.
- Bleeding from the gastrointestinal tract.
- Jaundice (yellow skin and eyes).

CAUSES—Unknown, but research suggests a virus infection may be a factor.

RISK INCREASES WITH—Adults over 40.

HOW TO PREVENT—No specific preventive measures.

WHAT TO EXPECT

APPROPRIATE HEALTH CARE
- Doctor's treatment.
- Hospitalization for short periods of treatment.
- Surgery to discover the extent of disease.
- Radiation therapy.

DIAGNOSTIC MEASURES
- Your own observation of symptoms.
- Medical history and physical exam by a doctor.
- Laboratory studies of blood and bone marrow.
- Lymphangiogram (see Glossary).
- Biopsy (see Glossary) of lymph node.
- X-rays of various body parts that may be involved.
- CAT scan (see Glossary).

POSSIBLE COMPLICATIONS—Spread of cancer to other parts of the body.

PROBABLE OUTCOME—Usually curable with radiation therapy and anticancer drugs. If cured, life expectancy is normal. The potential for cure varies according to the cell type discovered from biopsy of the lymph node. Consult your doctor.

HOW TO TREAT

NOTE—Follow your doctor's instructions. These instructions are supplemental.

GENERAL MEASURES—Try to remain optimistic about your treatment and chances for cure. A good mental attitude is a powerful ally.

MEDICATION—Your doctor may prescribe anticancer drugs. Medication may cause side effects or adverse reactions in some people. New symptoms may be caused by the medicine, original disorder or a new illness. Side effects caused by medicine usually disappear when your body adjusts to the drug or when the drug is discontinued.

ACTIVITY—Remain as active as your strength allows.

DIET—No special diet.

CALL YOUR DOCTOR IF

- You have symptoms of lymphoma.
- The following occurs during treatment:
  Fever.
  Signs of infection (redness, swelling, pain or tenderness) anywhere in the body.
  Swelling of the feet and ankles.
  Discomfort when urinating or decreased urination in 1 day.
- You think your medicine is causing symptoms.

ILLNESSES & DISORDERS

MALABSORPTION
(Malabsorptive Syndrome)

 ## GENERAL INFORMATION

DEFINITION—Poor absorption of nutrients from the intestinal tract into the bloodstream.

BODY PARTS INVOLVED—Intestinal tract; liver; pancreas.

SEX OR AGE MOST AFFECTED—Both sexes; all ages.

SIGNS & SYMPTOMS
- Diarrhea.
- Weakness.
- Weight loss.
- Gas and vague abdominal discomfort.
- Bad-smelling, copious stools.
- Mild anemia (sometimes).

CAUSES
- Deficiency of intestinal enzymes.
- Inadequate digestion caused by disease of the pancreas (such as cystic fibrosis), gallbladder or liver.
- Change in bacteria that normally live in the intestinal tract.
- Disease of the intestinal walls, including worms or parasites, tropical sprue and celiac disease.
- Surgery that reduces the intestinal tract, decreasing the area for absorption.

RISK INCREASES WITH
- Family history of malabsorption or cystic fibrosis.
- Excess alcohol consumption.
- Use of drugs, such as mineral oil and other laxatives.
- Travel to foreign countries.
- Intestinal surgery.

HOW TO PREVENT
- Avoid prolonged dependence on mineral oil and other laxatives.
- Avoid excess alcohol consumption.

 ## WHAT TO EXPECT

APPROPRIATE HEALTH CARE
- Self-care after diagnosis.
- Doctor's treatment.

DIAGNOSTIC MEASURES
- Your own observation of symptoms.
- Medical history and physical exam by a doctor.
- Laboratory studies of stool, chromosomes and blood.
- X-rays of the intestinal tract.

POSSIBLE COMPLICATIONS
- Prolonged illness.
- Failure to thrive in infants.
- Additional illness caused by nutritional, vitamin or mineral deficiency.

PROBABLE OUTCOME—The degree to which symptoms can be controlled depends on the cause, but many things are common to all malabsorptive disorders. The onset is usually slow and difficult to diagnose. Disorders may be present for months or years before being recognized. Treatment is long, complicated and may need to be changed often. Patience and a positive attitude are important in cure.

 ## HOW TO TREAT

NOTE—Follow your doctor's instructions. These instructions are supplemental.

GENERAL MEASURES—You may need injections of vitamin B-12 and iron because neither is absorbed well with any malabsorptive disorder.

MEDICATION—Your doctor may prescribe:
- Enzymes to replace missing intestinal enzymes.
- Antispasmodics to reduce discomfort.

ACTIVITY—No restrictions. Resume normal activities as soon as symptoms improve.

DIET
- Don't drink alcohol.
- You will need a special diet, depending on the cause of your illness. Your doctor or nutritionist will provide specific information. For a gluten-free diet for sprue and celiac disease, see Appendix 5. For a milk-free diet for lactase deficiency, see Appendix 4.

 ## CALL YOUR DOCTOR IF

- You have symptoms of malabsorption.
- You have black, tarry bowel movements.
- You have fever of 101F (38.3C) or higher.
- You have severe abdominal pain.
- You have muscle cramps.

MALARIA

GENERAL INFORMATION

DEFINITION—An infection caused by a single-cell parasite, which is transmitted by the bite of an anopheles mosquito.

BODY PARTS INVOLVED—Blood cells; blood vessels; liver; central nervous system.

SEX OR AGE MOST AFFECTED—Both sexes; all ages.

SIGNS & SYMPTOMS—The first episode of the following symptoms usually occurs about 8 to 30 days after the mosquito bite:
- Headache.
- Fatigue.
- Nausea.
- Hard, shaking chills with fever for 12 to 24 hours.
- Rapid breathing.
- Heavy sweating, accompanied by a drop in temperature.

Episodes may recur every 2 or 3 days until the disease is treated. Without treatment, the disease can continue for years.

CAUSES—There are 4 types of malarial parasites; they are transferred from person to person by a mosquito bite. The mosquito becomes infected with malaria after biting a person with the disease. The organisms multiply in the mosquito, then enter the bloodstream of the next person the mosquito bites.

Once in a person's bloodstream, the parasites travel to the liver, where they thrive and multiply rapidly. After several days, thousands re-enter the bloodstream and destroy red-blood cells. Some parasites remain in the liver, continue to multiply and are released again at intervals into the bloodstream.

RISK INCREASES WITH
- Crowded or unsanitary living conditions.
- Hot, humid climates.
- Geographic locations, such as Latin America, Asia and Africa. Malaria is uncommon in the U.S., but it often affects travelers or military personnel stationed in foreign countries.

HOW TO PREVENT
- Take antimalaria drugs before visiting an area where malaria is prevalent. Continue to take the drugs after you return. The public health department or your doctor can give you instructions.
- If you are in a mosquito-infested area, destroy mosquito breeding areas, install window screens and mosquito nets over beds, and use insect repellants.

WHAT TO EXPECT

APPROPRIATE HEALTH CARE
- Self-care after diagnosis.
- Doctor's treatment.
- Hospitalization (severe cases).

DIAGNOSTIC MEASURES
- Your own observation of symptoms.
- Medical history and physical exam by a doctor. Tell your doctor of recent travel.
- Laboratory studies, such as studies of blood smears to identify the parasite.

POSSIBLE COMPLICATIONS
- Anemia caused by blood-cell destruction.
- Clumping of blood cells, which may cause brain or kidney damage.

PROBABLE OUTCOME—Usually curable in 2 weeks with treatment. Malaria can be fatal without treatment in persons who don't receive adequate nourishment or have low resistance to disease.

HOW TO TREAT

NOTE—Follow your doctor's instructions. These instructions are supplemental.

GENERAL MEASURES
- Protect yourself from secondary bacterial infection while you are ill with malaria. Wash your hands and bathe often.
- Make your environment mosquito-free so your infection cannot be transmitted to others. See How to Prevent.

MEDICATION—Your doctor may prescribe antimalaria drugs to kill the parasite.

ACTIVITY—Rest in bed until fever and chills subside. Resume your normal activities gradually as symptoms improve.

DIET—No special diet. Take vitamin and mineral supplements until you recover.

CALL YOUR DOCTOR IF

- You have symptoms of malaria.
- You are weak for a prolonged time after an attack. This may indicate anemia.
- Symptoms of malaria recur after treatment.
- New, unexplained symptoms develop. Drugs used in treatment may produce side effects.

MALIGNANT MELANOMA

 GENERAL INFORMATION

DEFINITION—A skin cancer that spreads to other areas of the body, primarily the lymph nodes, liver, lungs and central nervous system. Most melanomas begin in a mole or other pre-existing skin lesion.

BODY PARTS INVOLVED—Usually in skin of the head, neck, legs or back. It appears rarely in the eye, mouth, vagina or anus.

SEX OR AGE MOST AFFECTED—Adults.

SIGNS & SYMPTOMS—A flat or slightly raised skin lesion that can be black, brown, blue, red, white or a mixture of all colors. Its borders are often irregular and may bleed.

CAUSES—Uncontrolled growth of cells that give skin its brownish color (melanocytes). When the cells grow down into deep skin layers, they invade blood vessels and lymph vessels and are spread to other body areas.

RISK INCREASES WITH
- Moles on the skin.
- Occupations or activities involving excessive sun exposure, such as farming, construction work, athletics or sunbathing.
- Pregnancy.
- Genetic factors. This is most common in light-complexioned, blonde people. It is rare in black people.
- Radiation treatment or excessive exposure to ultraviolet light, as with sun lamps.

HOW TO PREVENT
- Protect yourself from excessive sun exposure. Wear broad-rimmed hats and protective clothing. Use maximum protection sun-block preparations on exposed skin.
- Examine your skin, including soles of the feet, regularly for changes in pigmented areas. Ask a family member to examine your back. See your doctor about any skin area (especially brown or black) that becomes multicolored, develops irregular edges or surfaces, bleeds or changes in any way.

 WHAT TO EXPECT

APPROPRIATE HEALTH CARE
- Doctor's treatment.
- Surgery to remove suspicious skin lesions or to remove nearby lymph glands, if the tumor has spread.
- Hospitalization for radiation treatment, if the tumor has spread.

DIAGNOSTIC MEASURES
- Your own observation of suspicious growths.
- Medical history and physical exam by a doctor.
- Biopsy (see Glossary) of suspicious lesions. The melanoma's depth must be established to determine appropriate treatment.

POSSIBLE COMPLICATIONS—Fatal spread to lungs, liver, brain or other internal organs.

PROBABLE OUTCOME—Varies greatly. Early melanomas that have not grown downward are curable with surgical removal. Once the tumor has spread to distant organs, this condition is currently considered incurable and fatal in a short time. However, symptoms can be relieved or controlled.

Scientific research into causes and treatment continues, so there is hope for increasingly effective treatment and cure.

 HOW TO TREAT

NOTE—Follow your doctor's instructions. These instructions are supplemental.

GENERAL MEASURES—No specific instructions except those listed under other headings.

MEDICATION—Your doctor may prescribe anticancer drugs.

ACTIVITY—No restrictions.

DIET—No special diet.

 CALL YOUR DOCTOR IF

- You have symptoms of malignant melanoma.
- During treatment, changes occur in another skin area.
- New, unexplained symptoms develop. Drugs used in treatment may produce side effects.

MARCH FRACTURE

GENERAL INFORMATION

DEFINITION—A fracture of a bone in the foot that develops after repeated stress, such as prolonged standing, marching or running.

BODY PARTS INVOLVED—Bones in the feet (metatarsal bones).

SEX OR AGE MOST AFFECTED—Adolescents and young adults.

SIGNS & SYMPTOMS
- Severe, unexplained foot pain when standing or walking. Pain disappears when the load is taken off the feet.
- Swelling and increased warmth and tenderness over the painful area.

CAUSES—Fatigue of the foot bone(s) caused by repeated overload, as with marching, dancing, walking, running or jogging.

RISK INCREASES WITH—Fatigue or overwork, especially standing or walking on a hard surface (such as concrete) for prolonged periods.

HOW TO PREVENT—Heed early warnings of impending fracture, such as foot pain after extended standing or walking. Adjust activities *before* a fracture occurs.

WHAT TO EXPECT

APPROPRIATE HEALTH CARE
- Doctor's treatment.
- Self-care after diagnosis.

DIAGNOSTIC MEASURES
- Your own observation of symptoms.
- Medical history and physical exam by a doctor.
- X-rays of both feet. X-rays are often normal for 10 to 24 days after symptoms begin. Then they show a fracture line across one or more metatarsal bones.
- Radioactive technetium 99 scan (see Glossary), if symptoms are typical but X-rays are negative.

POSSIBLE COMPLICATIONS—Complete fracture from continued foot abuse after symptoms begin.

PROBABLE OUTCOME—Complete healing in 6 to 8 weeks with treatment.

HOW TO TREAT

NOTE—Follow your doctor's instructions. These instructions are supplemental.

GENERAL MEASURES—Your doctor will probably apply a short, weight-bearing leg cast. For care of casts, see Appendix 17.

MEDICATION
- You may use non-prescription drugs, such as aspirin or other non-steroidal anti-inflammatory drugs, to relieve minor pain.
- Your doctor may prescribe stronger pain relievers, if necessary.

ACTIVITY—Don't bear weight on the injured foot. Learn to walk with crutches, and prop your foot up whenever possible. Resume your normal activities when the cast is removed.

DIET—No special diet.

CALL YOUR DOCTOR IF

- You have symptoms of a march fracture.
- Toes become dark, blue, cold or numb while the cast is on.

MASTITIS
(Breast Infection)

 GENERAL INFORMATION

DEFINITION—Inflammation and infection in the breast of a woman who has recently given birth. It occurs in about 1% of new mothers and is more likely in women who are breast-feeding.

BODY PARTS INVOLVED—Breasts.

SEX OR AGE MOST AFFECTED—Females of childbearing age.

SIGNS & SYMPTOMS—Symptoms may occur anytime while nursing, but usually begin 3 to 4 weeks after delivery. Common symptoms include:
- Temperature of 101F (38.3C) or higher.
- Tender, swollen, hard, hot breast(s).

CAUSES—Infection from bacteria that enter the mother's breast from the nursing baby's nose or throat. The most-common germs are staphylococcus aureus and beta-hemolytic streptococcus.

RISK INCREASES WITH
- Abrasion of the nipple.
- Blocked milk ducts from wearing too-tight bras, sleeping on the stomach or waiting too long between feedings.
- Use of an electric or manual breast pump.

HOW TO PREVENT
- Wash nipples before nursing. Wash hands before touching breasts.
- Wear a comfortable bra that is not too tight.
- If a nipple cracks or fissures, apply lanolin cream or other topical medication recommended by your doctor.
- Don't sleep on your stomach.

 WHAT TO EXPECT

APPROPRIATE HEALTH CARE
- Self-care after diagnosis.
- Doctor's treatment.

DIAGNOSTIC MEASURES
- Your own observation of symptoms.
- Medical history and physical exam by a doctor.
- Laboratory blood studies and a culture of breast milk.

POSSIBLE COMPLICATIONS—Without treatment, may lead to breast abscess.

PROBABLE OUTCOME—Usually curable in 10 days with treatment.

 HOW TO TREAT

NOTE—Follow your doctor's instructions. These instructions are supplemental.

GENERAL MEASURES
- Apply an ice pack (ice in a plastic bag, covered with a thin towel) to the engorged breast 3 to 6 times a day. Use for 15 to 20 minutes at a time. Don't use ice packs within 1 hour of nursing—use warm compresses instead.
- Wear an uplift bra during treatment.
- Continue to breast-feed, even though breasts are infected. Offer the affected breast first to promote complete emptying.
- If an abscess develops, stop breast-feeding on the affected side. Use a breast pump to empty the infected breast regularly, and continue breast-feeding on the unaffected side.

MEDICATION—Your doctor may prescribe:
- Antibiotics to fight infection. Finish the prescription, even if symptoms subside quickly.
- Pain relievers. For minor discomfort, you may use non-prescription drugs such as acetaminophen.

ACTIVITY—Rest in bed until fever and pain diminish. You may read or watch TV.

DIET—No special diet. Drink extra fluids while you have fever.

 CALL YOUR DOCTOR IF

- You have symptoms of mastitis.
- The following occurs during treatment: Fever spikes to over 101F (38.3C). You have signs of a developing abscess: a localized area with increasing redness, pain, tenderness and fluctuance (feels like pushing on an inflated inner tube).

MEASLES
(Red Measles; Rubeola)

 GENERAL INFORMATION

DEFINITION—A serious virus illness that infects the respiratory tract and skin. This is one of the most contagious diseases known.

BODY PARTS INVOLVED—Skin; eyes; upper-respiratory tract.

SEX OR AGE MOST AFFECTED—All ages, but most common in children.

SIGNS & SYMPTOMS—Measles symptoms usually occur in the following sequence:
- Temperature of 102F (38.9C) or higher.
- Fatigue.
- Appetite loss.
- Sneezing and runny nose.
- Harsh, hacking cough.
- Red eyes and sensitivity to light.
- Koplik spots (tiny white spots) in the mouth and throat.
- Reddish rash on the forehead and around ears that spreads to the body.

CAUSES—Measles is caused by a rubeola-virus infection that chiefly affects the skin and respiratory tract. The incubation period after exposure is 7 to 14 days.

RISK INCREASES WITH
- Crowded or unsanitary living conditions.
- Population groups that are not immunized.
- Measles epidemics. The disease becomes more virulent as it spreads.

HOW TO PREVENT
- Immunize children against measles. See Appendix 16 for the recommended schedule.
- If a person has not been immunized against measles and is exposed to it, a gamma globulin (antibodies) injection may prevent or reduce the severity of the disease.

 WHAT TO EXPECT

APPROPRIATE HEALTH CARE
- Home care after diagnosis.
- Doctor's treatment.

DIAGNOSTIC MEASURES
- Your own observation of symptoms.
- Medical history and physical exam by a doctor.

POSSIBLE COMPLICATIONS
- Pneumonia.
- Encephalitis or meningitis.

PROBABLE OUTCOME—A child who has been immunized against measles or has had the disease will probably never develop it.

A person who has been passively immunized with gamma globulin is protected against measles for about 3 months.

 HOW TO TREAT

NOTE—Follow your doctor's instructions. These instructions are supplemental.

GENERAL MEASURES
- Don't read books or watch TV during the first days when the eyes are sensitive to light.
- Use a cool-mist humidifier to soothe the cough and thin lung secretions so they can be coughed up more easily.
- Take morning and evening temperatures; keep a record. If the fever is 103F (39.4C) or higher, reduce it. See Appendix 19, How to Reduce Fever.

MEDICATION
- Your doctor will not prescribe antibiotics for measles, which is a virus. However, if complications arise, such as pneumonia or a middle-ear infection, antibiotics may be necessary.
- Don't give aspirin to a person younger than 16. Use acetaminophen instead to relieve discomfort and reduce fever. Some research shows a link between the use of aspirin in children during a virus illness and the development of Reye's syndrome.

ACTIVITY—Rest until the fever and rash disappear. Encourage a child to rest, but don't force it. Light activities are acceptable once eyes are not painful. Children should not return to school until 7 to 10 days after the fever and rash disappear.

DIET—No special diet. Drink extra fluids, including water, tea, lemonade, cola and fruit juice. Maintaining an adequate fluid intake is very important in keeping lung secretions thin and preventing lung complications.

 CALL YOUR DOCTOR IF

- You or your child have symptoms of measles.
- The following occurs during treatment:
  Temperature above 103F (39.4C), accompanied by a sore throat.
  Severe headache.
  Earache.
  Convulsion.
  Excessive lethargy or drowsiness.
  Breathing rate above 35 breaths-per-minute or breathing difficulty.
  Blue, gray or purple lips or nails.
  Thick, discolored nasal discharge or sputum.
  Cough that persists longer than 4 or 5 days.

ILLNESSES & DISORDERS

MEASLES, GERMAN
(Rubella)

GENERAL INFORMATION

DEFINITION—A mild, contagious virus illness. German measles is likely to cause serious birth defects to the unborn baby of a pregnant woman who develops the disease in the first 3 or 4 months of pregnancy.

BODY PARTS INVOLVED—Skin; lymph glands behind the ears and in the neck.

SEX OR AGE MOST AFFECTED—All ages, but most common in children.

SIGNS & SYMPTOMS
● Fever.
● Muscle aches and stiffness, especially in the neck.
● Fatigue.
● Headache.
● Reddish rash on the head and body after the 2nd or 3rd day. The rash lasts 1 or 2 days.
● Swollen lymph glands, especially behind the ears and at the back and sides of the neck.
● Joint pain (adults).

CAUSES—RNA virus spread by person-to-person contact. Patients are contagious from 1 week before the rash appears until 1 week after it fades.

RISK INCREASES WITH—Springtime weather when epidemics are common.

HOW TO PREVENT
● Children should be immunized against German measles at approximately 15 months of age.
● Non-pregnant women of childbearing age should be immunized if they have not had German measles or been immunized. Pregnancy should be prevented for 3 months following immunization. (If you don't know whether or not you have had German measles, your doctor or local health department can determine it from a blood test.)
● A person—especially a pregnant woman—who is exposed to German measles, who has not had it or been immunized, should receive a gamma globulin (antibodies) injection. If taken soon after exposure, this may prevent or reduce the severity of the disease.

OTHER—A person should not be immunized if he or she: has an altered autoimmune system, as with cancer; currently takes cortisone or anticancer drugs; is receiving radiation therapy; or has an illness with fever.

WHAT TO EXPECT

APPROPRIATE HEALTH CARE
● Self-care.
● Doctor's treatment.

DIAGNOSTIC MEASURES
● Your own observation of symptoms.
● Medical history and physical exam by a doctor.
● Laboratory blood studies.

POSSIBLE COMPLICATIONS
● Miscarriage or catastrophic birth defects.
● Encephalitis.
● Thrombocytopenia.
● Agranulocytosis.

PROBABLE OUTCOME—Spontaneous recovery in 1 week in children, longer in adults. Symptoms are usually quite mild.

HOW TO TREAT

NOTE—Follow your doctor's instructions. These instructions are supplemental.

GENERAL MEASURES—Contact any pregnant woman who has been exposed. Exposure includes contact with the infected person 1 week prior to, during, or 1 week after the infection. This woman should consult her obstetrician immediately.

MEDICATION—For minor discomfort, you may use non-prescription drugs such as acetaminophen. Don't give aspirin to a person younger than 16. Some research shows a link between the use of aspirin in children during a virus illness and the development of Reye's syndrome (a type of encephalitis).

ACTIVITY—Stay in bed until the fever disappears. Then limit activities until the day after the rash disappears. Resume normal activity gradually as your strength allows. Don't expose yourself to others until 1 week after the rash disappears.

DIET—No special diet.

CALL YOUR DOCTOR IF

● You have symptoms of German measles.
● The following occurs during treatment:
  Fever of 103F (39.4C) or higher.
  Red eyes.
  Cough or shortness of breath.
  Severe headache, drowsiness, lethargy or convulsion.
● Unusual bleeding occurs 1 to 4 weeks after the illness (bleeding gums, nose, uterus or scattered blood specks on the skin).

MENIERE'S DISEASE

GENERAL INFORMATION

DEFINITION—Increased fluid in the inner ear's semicircular canals, which help maintain balance. Excess fluid produces pressure in the inner ear, disturbing balance and sometimes reducing hearing.

BODY PARTS INVOLVED—Semicircular canals of the inner ear, usually on one side only.

SEX OR AGE MOST AFFECTED
- Both sexes, but slightly more common in women.
- Adults between ages 30 and 60.

SIGNS & SYMPTOMS—The following occur with every acute attack:
- Severe dizziness.
- Noises in the affected ear, such as ringing or buzzing.
- Hearing loss that increases with each attack.
Possible accompanying symptoms:
- Vomiting.
- Sweating.
- Jerky eye movements.
- Loss of balance.

CAUSES—Unknown. Theories include:
- Spasms of blood vessels to the inner ear.
- Fluid retention in the inner ear, especially during the premenstrual period in women.
- Allergic reactions.

RISK INCREASES WITH—Unknown.

HOW TO PREVENT—No specific preventive measures.

WHAT TO EXPECT

APPROPRIATE HEALTH CARE
- Self-care after diagnosis.
- Doctor's treatment.
- Surgical destruction of the affected inner ear (rare).

DIAGNOSTIC MEASURES
- Your own observation of symptoms.
- Medical history and physical exam by a doctor.
- Laboratory studies, such as audiometry and ice-water tests (see Glossary for both).
- X-rays of the head.

POSSIBLE COMPLICATIONS
- Permanent hearing loss.
- Chronic noises in the ear.

PROBABLE OUTCOME—Attacks of Meniere's disease usually recur over many years. Some symptoms can be controlled. The condition is frustrating but not life-threatening.

HOW TO TREAT

NOTE—Follow your doctor's instructions. These instructions are supplemental.

GENERAL MEASURES—Avoid glaring light and don't read during attacks.

MEDICATION—Your doctor may prescribe:
- Antinausea drugs.
- Tranquilizers to reduce dizziness.
- Antihistamines, which lessen symptoms in some persons.
- Diuretics to decrease fluid in the inner ear.

ACTIVITY
- Rest quietly in bed until dizziness and nausea disappear.
- Don't walk without assistance.
- Avoid sudden changes in position.
- Don't drive, climb ladders or work around dangerous machinery.

DIET—No special diet, but decrease salt and fluid intake.

CALL YOUR DOCTOR IF

- You have symptoms of Meniere's disease.
- The following occurs during treatment:
  Decreased hearing in either ear.
  Persistent vomiting.
  Convulsions.
  Fainting.
  Fever of 101F (38.3C) or higher.
- New, unexplained symptoms develop. Drugs used in treatment may produce side effects.

MENINGITIS, ASEPTIC
(Non-Bacterial Meningitis)

 GENERAL INFORMATION

DEFINITION—Inflammation of the meninges (thin membranes that cover the brain and spinal cord). This is contagious.

BODY PARTS INVOLVED—Brain; spinal cord.

SEX OR AGE MOST AFFECTED—Both sexes; all ages.

SIGNS & SYMPTOMS
- Fever.
- Headache.
- Irritability.
- Eyes that are sensitive to light.
- Stiff neck.
- Vomiting.
- Confusion, lethargy and drowsiness.

CAUSES
- Viruses of several types, including the polio virus.
- Fungi, including yeasts.
- A reaction—probably an autoimmune response—following various viral illnesses, such as measles.

RISK INCREASES WITH
- Recent measles, German measles or various types of flu.
- Immunosuppressive treatment, such as for cancer or following an organ transplant.
- Poor nutrition.
- Recent illness that has lowered resistance.
- Meningitis epidemics. The disease becomes more virulent as it spreads from person to person.

HOW TO PREVENT—Keep immunizations up to date against all viruses for which vaccines are available. See Appendix 16 for an immunization schedule.

 WHAT TO EXPECT

APPROPRIATE HEALTH CARE
- Doctor's treatment.
- Hospitalization, except in mild cases.

DIAGNOSTIC MEASURES
- Your own observation of symptoms.
- Medical history and physical exam by a doctor.
- Laboratory studies, such as blood-cell counts and examination of the cerebrospinal fluid.

POSSIBLE COMPLICATIONS
- Permanent brain damage (rare).
- Muscle impairment or paralysis (if caused by poliomyelitis).

PROBABLE OUTCOME—Most patients recover fully from viral meningitis without specific therapy—unlike bacterial meningitis, in which antibiotics may be life-saving.

 HOW TO TREAT

NOTE—Follow your doctor's instructions. These instructions are supplemental.

GENERAL MEASURES—No special instructions except those listed under other headings.

MEDICATION—If aseptic meningitis is caused by a virus, there is no medication for it. The body defenses will usually cure it (although a polio virus may leave permanent damage).

   If meningitis is caused by a fungus, your doctor may prescribe antifungal drugs, such as amphoterecin B.

ACTIVITY—Rest in bed in a darkened room. Resume your normal activities as soon as symptoms improve.

DIET—No special diet. Drink 6 to 8 glasses of fluid daily, even if you don't feel like it.

 CALL YOUR DOCTOR IF

- You have symptoms of aseptic meningitis.
- New, unexplained symptoms develop. Drugs used in treatment may produce side effects.

MENINGITIS, BACTERIAL
(Spinal Meningitis)

GENERAL INFORMATION

DEFINITION—Bacterial infection or inflammation of the meninges (thin membranes that cover the brain and spinal cord).

BODY PARTS INVOLVED—Central nervous system.

SEX OR AGE MOST AFFECTED—All ages, but more severe in persons under age 2 or over age 60.

SIGNS & SYMPTOMS
- Fever, chills and sweating (may be absent in critically ill persons).
- Headache.
- Irritability.
- Eyes sensitive to light; pupils may be of different size.
- Stiff neck.
- Vomiting.
- Red or purple skin rash.
- Confusion, lethargy, drowsiness or unconsciousness.
- Sore throat or other signs of respiratory illness may precede other symptoms.

CAUSES—Infection caused by bacteria, from the following sources:
- Infection in another body part, such as the lung, ear or sinus, that spreads to the meninges.
- Head injury, such as a fractured skull, that allows infection to enter.

RISK INCREASES WITH
- Newborns and infants.
- Adults over 60.
- Illness that has lowered resistance.
- Poor nutrition.
- Use of drugs that decrease the body's immune responses, such as anticancer drugs.

HOW TO PREVENT
- Consult your doctor for treatment of any infection in your body to prevent its spread.
- Avoid contact with anyone who has meningitis. Those who have had close contact with a person with meningitis may need preventive antibiotic treatment even if they have no symptoms.

WHAT TO EXPECT

APPROPRIATE HEALTH CARE
- Doctor's care.
- Hospitalization.
- Self-treatment after hospitalization.

DIAGNOSTIC MEASURES
- Your own observation of symptoms.
- Medical history and physical exam by a doctor.
- Laboratory studies, such as blood-sugar tests and cultures of throat, blood, nose or other infection sites.
- Lumbar puncture (see Glossary).

POSSIBLE COMPLICATIONS—Death or permanent brain damage—including paralysis, hearing loss, speech difficulty and intellectual impairment—if not treated quickly.

PROBABLE OUTCOME—Full recovery is likely in 2 to 3 weeks with treatment, if no complications arise.

HOW TO TREAT

NOTE—Follow your doctor's instructions. These instructions are supplemental.

GENERAL MEASURES—Restrict visitors until the doctor determines the disease is no longer contagious.

MEDICATION—Your doctor may prescribe antibiotics, depending on what bacteria is causing meningitis.

ACTIVITY—While in the hospital, you will need bed rest in a darkened room. After a 2- to 3-week recovery, you should be as active as your strength allows.

DIET—You may be given intravenous nutrients in the hospital. At home, eat a normal, well-balanced diet. Vitamin and mineral supplements should not be necessary unless you have a deficiency or cannot eat normally.

CALL YOUR DOCTOR IF

- You have symptoms of bacterial meningitis.
- Temperature rises to 101F (38.3C) or higher during treatment.
- New, unexplained symptoms develop. Drugs used in treatment may produce side effects.
- You have had contact with someone who has meningitis.

MENOPAUSE

GENERAL INFORMATION

DEFINITION—The permanent cessation of menstruation. This occurs as early as age 35 or as late as age 55 and usually spans 1 to 2 years. Menopause is only one event in the "climacteric," a biological change in all body tissue and body systems that occurs in both sexes between the mid-40s and mid-60s.

BODY PARTS INVOLVED—Female reproductive system, with secondary effects in other body parts.

SEX OR AGE MOST AFFECTED—Women, especially between ages 45 and 50.

SIGNS & SYMPTOMS—Physical changes (directly associated with decreased blood levels of female hormones):
- Menstrual irregularity.
- Hot flashes or flushes—sensations of heat spreading from the waist or chest toward the neck, face and upper arms.
- Headaches.
- Dizziness.
- Rapid or irregular heartbeat.
- Vaginal itching, burning or discomfort during intercourse, beginning a few years after menopause.
- Bloating in the upper abdomen.
- Bladder irritability.
- Breast tenderness.

Emotional changes (associated with lower hormone levels *and* conflicting feelings about aging and loss of fertility):
- Mood changes.
- Pronounced tension and anxiety.
- Sleeping difficulty.
- Depression or melancholy and fatigue.

CAUSES
- A normal decline in ovary function, resulting in decreased levels of the female hormones, estrogen and progesterone.
- Surgical removal of both ovaries.

RISK INCREASES WITH—Menopause is a natural part of the aging process for women.

HOW TO PREVENT—Take estrogen replacement therapy, beginning before menopause and extending throughout life.

WHAT TO EXPECT

APPROPRIATE HEALTH CARE
- Doctor's diagnosis to rule out other causes of menstrual changes.
- Self-care after diagnosis.
- Psychotherapy or counseling, if emotional changes interfere with personal relationships or work.

DIAGNOSTIC MEASURES
- Your own observation of symptoms.
- Medical history and physical exam by a doctor.
- Laboratory blood studies of hormone levels.

POSSIBLE COMPLICATIONS
- Increased irritability and susceptibility to infection in the urinary tract.
- Diminished breast size.
- Decreased skin elasticity.
- Accentuation of neurotic tendencies.
- Increased risk of hardening of the arteries, heart disease, stroke and osteoporosis after menopause.

PROBABLE OUTCOME—Menopause is a normal process—not an illness. Most women make an easy transition without crisis.

HOW TO TREAT

NOTE—Follow your doctor's instructions. These instructions are supplemental.

GENERAL MEASURES
- Continue to use birth-control measures for 12 months after your last menstrual period.
- Reduce stress as much as possible. See Appendix 13.
- If you take estrogen-replacement therapy, have a Pap smear every 6 months.

MEDICATION—Most women require no medication. If symptoms are severe, your doctor may prescribe female hormones. Because hormone treatment has some risks, learn all you can about hormone-replacement therapy before deciding on treatment.

Don't take hormones if you have diabetes mellitus or high blood pressure and are obese. Hormones may aggravate the underlying condition and complicate treatment.

ACTIVITY—No restrictions.

DIET—No special diet.

CALL YOUR DOCTOR IF

- You have symptoms of menopause. Other causes should be ruled out.
- You experience excessive bleeding, prolonged periods or spotting between your expected periods. These may be signs of other disorders.
- Bleeding appears 6 months or more after your last period.
- New, unexplained symptoms develop. Hormones used in treatment may produce side effects.
- Symptoms of menopause return while taking estrogen-replacement therapy.

MISCARRIAGE
(Spontaneous Abortion)

 GENERAL INFORMATION

DEFINITION—Premature termination of a pregnancy before the fetus can survive outside the uterus.

BODY PARTS INVOLVED—Reproductive system.

SEX OR AGE MOST AFFECTED—Women of childbearing age.

SIGNS & SYMPTOMS
- Uterine cramps.
- Vaginal bleeding—from slight to heavy. Most miscarriages are only "threatened," and the pregnancy continues to term. Symptoms may be the same for threatened miscarriages as for those in progress.

CAUSES—During the first 3 months (trimester):
- An abnormal or defective fetus.
- Uterine abnormalities that prevent the fertilized egg from growing normally.
During the second trimester:
- Uterine abnormalities that cause detachment of the fetus and placenta.
- Severe psychological stress (maybe).
Anytime:
- Use of drugs that harm the fetus.
- Infections, especially virus infections, such as German measles or influenza.

RISK INCREASES WITH
- Stress.
- Poor nutrition.
- Illness that has lowered resistance.
- Recent serious infection.
- Medical history of endocrine diseases, such as diabetes mellitus or hypothyroidism.

HOW TO PREVENT—During pregnancy:
- Obtain regular medical checkups.
- Eat a normal, well-balanced diet. See Appendix 3.
- Don't drink alcohol, smoke cigarettes or use recreational drugs.
- Don't use any medications, including non-prescription drugs, without consulting your doctor.

 WHAT TO EXPECT

APPROPRIATE HEALTH CARE
- Self-care.
- Doctor's treatment.
- Surgery to remove any remaining tissue or a dead fetus (sometimes).
- Hospitalization (sometimes).
- Psychotherapy or counseling.

DIAGNOSTIC MEASURES
- Your own observation of symptoms.

- Medical history and physical exam by a doctor.

POSSIBLE COMPLICATIONS
- Uterine infection, signaled by fever, chills and aching.
- Hemorrhaging from other body parts.
- "Incomplete" abortion, in which some placenta or fetal tissue remains in the uterus, or missed abortion, in which the fetus dies but remains in the uterus.

PROBABLE OUTCOME—With treatment, a miscarriage is not a life-threatening condition. It does not affect a woman's ability to carry a healthy baby to term in the future.

 HOW TO TREAT

NOTE—Follow your doctor's instructions. These instructions are supplemental.

GENERAL MEASURES
- For a threatened miscarriage, follow your doctor's orders. Bed rest is often enough to stabilize the pregnancy.
- After a miscarriage:
  Expect a small amount of vaginal bleeding or spotting for 8 to 10 days.
  Don't use tampons for 2 to 4 weeks.
  Wait through 2 or 3 normal menstrual cycles before attempting to become pregnant.

MEDICATION
- For a threatened miscarriage: Medicine usually is not necessary. Don't take *any* medication without consulting your doctor.
- After a miscarriage, your doctor may prescribe:
  Antibiotics to fight infection.
  Blood transfusions for severe blood loss.

ACTIVITY
- For a threatened miscarriage: Rest in bed until symptoms disappear. Avoid sexual intercourse until the outcome is known.
- After a miscarriage: Reduce activity and rest often for 48 hours.

DIET
- For a threatened miscarriage: Drink fluids only, if bleeding and cramping are severe.
- After a miscarriage: No special diet.

 CALL YOUR DOCTOR IF

- Vaginal bleeding occurs during pregnancy.
- Bleeding and cramps worsen during a threatened miscarriage or you pass tissue.
- Fever and chills occur during a threatened miscarriage or following miscarriage.
- Bleeding (other than vaginal) or unexplained bruising occurs after a miscarriage.
- Infection develops while you are pregnant.

MOLLUSCUM CONTAGIOSUM

 GENERAL INFORMATION

DEFINITION—A contagious virus infection of the skin.

BODY PARTS INVOLVED—Skin anywhere on the body. The virus usually occurs on the face in children. In adults, it usually occurs on the inner thighs, abdomen and genitals.

SEX OR AGE MOST AFFECTED—Both sexes; all ages.

SIGNS & SYMPTOMS—Papules (small, raised bumps on the skin) with the following characteristics:
- Bumps are firm, smooth, domed, and skin-colored or white. The overlying skin is transparent and thin.
- Bumps are usually 2mm to 3mm in diameter. A few may be as large as 10mm.
- Bumps cause eye irritation if they are on the eyelids.
- Bumps don't hurt or itch.

CAUSES—DNA virus of the pox group. This virus may be transmitted sexually. The incubation is 2 weeks to 6 months.

RISK INCREASES WITH
- Previous allergies or family history of allergy.
- Use of immunosuppressive drugs.

HOW TO PREVENT—To prevent spread to other parts of the body or to other people, don't scratch bumps.

 WHAT TO EXPECT

APPROPRIATE HEALTH CARE
- Doctor's treatment to remove the papules with liquid nitrogen.
- Self-care after removal.

DIAGNOSTIC MEASURES
- Your own observation of symptoms.
- Medical history and physical exam by a doctor.

POSSIBLE COMPLICATIONS—Scarring or disfigurement.

PROBABLE OUTCOME—If untreated, a few papules may increase to 20 to 50 lesions in several weeks. They will disappear spontaneously in 10 to 24 months. However, they should be treated to prevent their spread to other persons.

 HOW TO TREAT

NOTE—Follow your doctor's instructions. These instructions are supplemental.

GENERAL MEASURES
- After treatment with liquid nitrogen, leave the blisters alone. The tops will come off spontaneously in 7 to 14 days.
- Keep blisters dry. Cover with small adhesive bandages any that may be irritated by clothing.

MEDICATION—Medicine usually is not necessary for this disorder. In some cases, your doctor may prescribe cantharidin (Cantherone) to apply topically to kill the virus.

ACTIVITY—No restrictions, except to avoid sexual relations until bumps disappear.

DIET—No special diet.

 CALL YOUR DOCTOR IF

- You have symptoms of molluscum contagiosum.
- The following occurs after treatment:
  Fever.
  Signs of infection (swelling, redness, pain, tenderness or warmth) at the treatment site.

MONONUCLEOSIS, INFECTIOUS
(Mono; "Kissing Disease")

 GENERAL INFORMATION

DEFINITION—An infectious viral disease that affects the respiratory system, liver and lymphatic system.

BODY PARTS INVOLVED—Lymph nodes; liver; spleen; throat; bronchial tubes.

SEX OR AGE MOST AFFECTED—Adolescents and young adults (12 to 40 years).

SIGNS & SYMPTOMS
- Fever.
- Sore throat (sometimes severe).
- Appetite loss.
- Fatigue.
- Swollen lymph glands, usually in the neck, underarms or groin.
- Enlarged spleen.
- Enlarged liver.
- Jaundice with yellow skin and eyes (sometimes).
- Headache.
- General aching.

CAUSES—A contagious virus (Epstein-Barr virus) transmitted from person to person by close contact, such as kissing, shared food or coughing.

RISK INCREASES WITH
- Stress.
- Illness that has lowered resistance.
- Fatigue or overwork. The high incidence among college students and military recruits may result from inadequate rest and crowded living conditions.

HOW TO PREVENT
- Avoid contact with persons having infectious mononucleosis.
- Vaccine (possibly). This is still in the experimental stages.

 WHAT TO EXPECT

APPROPRIATE HEALTH CARE
- Self-care after diagnosis.
- Doctor's treatment.
- Hospitalization (rare).

DIAGNOSTIC MEASURES
- Your own observation of symptoms.
- Medical history and physical exam by a doctor.
- Laboratory blood tests.

POSSIBLE COMPLICATIONS
- Meningitis or encephalitis (rare).
- Misdiagnosis as a streptococcal sore throat, resulting in useless, unnecessary treatment with antibiotics.
- Ruptured spleen, resulting in surgery.

PROBABLE OUTCOME—Spontaneous recovery in 10 days to 6 months. Fatigue frequently persists for 3 to 6 weeks after other symptoms disappear.

 HOW TO TREAT

NOTE—Follow your doctor's instructions. These instructions are supplemental.

GENERAL MEASURES
- To relieve the sore throat, gargle frequently with double-strength tea or warm salt water (1 teaspoon of salt to 8 oz. of water).
- Don't strain hard for bowel movements. This may injure an enlarged spleen.

MEDICATION
- For minor discomfort, you may use non-prescription drugs such as acetaminophen. Don't take aspirin because of its suspected association with Reye's syndrome.
- If symptoms are severe, your doctor may prescribe a short course of cortisone drugs. It is not safe to use cortisone drugs if you have: a positive tuberculin skin test or history of tuberculosis; viral eye infection; chronic bacterial infection; diabetes; high blood pressure; diverticulitis; thrombophlebitis; chronic kidney disease; or if you are pregnant.

ACTIVITY
- Rest in bed, especially when you have fever. Resume activity gradually. Rest when you are fatigued.
- Don't participate in contact sports until at least 1 month after complete recovery.

DIET—No special diet. You may not feel like eating while you are ill. Maintain an adequate fluid intake. Drink at least 8 glasses of water or juice a day—more during periods of high fever.

 CALL YOUR DOCTOR IF

- You have symptoms of infectious mononucleosis.
- The following occurs during treatment:
  Fever over 102F (38.9C).
  Constipation, which may cause straining.
  Severe pain in the upper left abdomen that lasts for 5 minutes or more.
  Swallowing or breathing difficulty from severe throat inflammation.

ILLNESSES & DISORDERS

MORNING SICKNESS DURING PREGNANCY

 GENERAL INFORMATION

DEFINITION—Nausea during pregnancy. This usually occurs in the morning.

BODY PARTS INVOLVED—Muscles of the intestinal tract; vomiting center in the hypothalamus gland.

SEX OR AGE MOST AFFECTED—Pregnant women, most of whom experience at least mild morning sickness.

SIGNS & SYMPTOMS—Mild to severe nausea—with or without vomiting—usually during the first 12 to 14 weeks of pregnancy.

CAUSES—Major hormone changes that take place to permit normal growth of the fetus. Progesterone and other hormones cause involuntary muscles to relax, probably slowing movement of food through the stomach and intestines. They may also affect the vomiting center in the brain.

In addition, blood sugar is lower during early pregnancy in many women, contributing to gastrointestinal upsets.

RISK INCREASES WITH—Unknown.

HOW TO PREVENT—No specific preventive measures.

 WHAT TO EXPECT

APPROPRIATE HEALTH CARE
• Self-care after diagnosis.
• Doctor's treatment, if morning sickness becomes disabling.

DIAGNOSTIC MEASURES
• Your own observation of symptoms.
• Medical history and physical exam by a doctor.

POSSIBLE COMPLICATIONS—Hyperemesis gravidarum, a condition of pregnancy characterized by severe nausea, vomiting, weight loss and electrolyte disturbance (rare).

PROBABLE OUTCOME—Usually stops after the first 3 to 4 months of pregnancy.

 HOW TO TREAT

NOTE—Follow your doctor's instructions. These instructions are supplemental.

GENERAL MEASURES
• Keep rooms well-ventilated to prevent accumulation of cooking odors or cigarette smoke.
• Don't smoke cigarettes, and ask your family and friends not to smoke while you are experiencing morning sickness.
• Keep a positive attitude. If you have conflicts that you cannot resolve, ask for help from family, friends or professional counselors.

MEDICATION—Medicine is usually not necessary for this disorder. Don't take *any* medications during pregnancy without consulting your doctor. Your doctor may prescribe a trial of vitamin B-6, which appears safe at the present.

ACTIVITY—No restrictions.

DIET—The following may help minimize nausea:
• Place a small, quick-energy snack, such as soda crackers, at your bedside. Eat it before getting up in the morning.
• Eat a small snack at bedtime and when you get up to go to the bathroom during the night.
• Eat a snack as often as every hour or two during the day. Avoid large meals. Snacks should consist of high-protein foods, such as: peanut butter on apple slices or celery; nuts; a quarter-sandwich; cheese and crackers; milk; cottage cheese; yogurt sprinkled with granola; and turkey or chicken slices. Avoid foods that are high in fat and salt but low in nutrition.

 CALL YOUR DOCTOR IF

• You have morning sickness that does not improve, despite the above measures.
• You vomit blood or material that resembles coffee grounds.
• You lose more than 1 or 2 pounds.

MOTION SICKNESS

GENERAL INFORMATION

DEFINITION—An unpleasant, temporary disturbance that occurs while traveling, characterized by dizziness and stomach upset.

BODY PARTS INVOLVED—Semicircular canals in the inner ear. These fluid-filled canals maintain balance.

SEX OR AGE MOST AFFECTED—Both sexes; all ages.

SIGNS & SYMPTOMS
- Loss of appetite.
- Nausea and vomiting.
- Spinning sensation.
- Weakness and unsteadiness.

CAUSES—Travel by any means, especially airplane, boat or car. Irregular motion causes fluid changes in the semicircular canals of the inner ear, which transmit signals to the brain's vomiting center.

RISK INCREASES WITH
- Stress.
- Ear disorders.
- Smoky environment or poor ventilation.
- Excess alcohol consumption.

HOW TO PREVENT
- Don't eat large meals or drink alcohol before and during travel.
- Sit in areas of the airplane or boat with the least motion.
- Recline in your seat, if possible.
- Breathe slowly and deeply.
- Avoid areas where others are smoking, if possible.
- On an airplane or bus, turn on the overhead air vent to improve air circulation.
- Take medication to prevent motion sickness before you travel.

OTHER—Some airlines have developed behavior-modification techniques for those who are afraid to fly or have motion sickness. Contact the airline or your travel agent for information.

WHAT TO EXPECT

APPROPRIATE HEALTH CARE
- Self-care.
- Doctor's treatment, if you have a chronic illness that may be worsened by vomiting.
- Psychotherapy or counseling, if your occupation or lifestyle requires travel, and you usually develop motion sickness.

DIAGNOSTIC MEASURES
- Your own observation of symptoms.
- Medical history and physical exam by a doctor, if motion sickness is recurrent and interferes with your life.

POSSIBLE COMPLICATIONS
- Dehydration from vomiting.
- Falls and injuries from unsteadiness.

PROBABLE OUTCOME—Spontaneous recovery when the trip is over.

HOW TO TREAT

NOTE—Follow your doctor's instructions. These instructions are supplemental.

GENERAL MEASURES—Psychological factors contribute to motion sickness. Try to resolve concerns about travel before leaving home. Maintain a positive attitude.

MEDICATION
- For minor discomfort, you may use non-prescription drugs, such as dimenhydrinate (Dramamine), before and during travel.
- Your doctor may prescribe scopolamine to control symptoms.

ACTIVITY—To minimize symptoms during travel, rest in a reclining position and fix your gaze on a distant object.

DIET—Eat lightly or not at all before and during brief trips. For longer trips, sip frequently on beverages—don't take large drinks—to maintain your fluid intake.

CALL YOUR DOCTOR IF

You plan to travel and have had disabling motion sickness in the past.

ILLNESSES & DISORDERS

MOUTH OR TONGUE TUMOR, BENIGN

 GENERAL INFORMATION

DEFINITION—Abnormal new growth in the mouth or tongue that is unlikely to spread to other body parts. Benign mouth and tongue tumors usually occur singly and grow very slowly over 2 to 6 years.

BODY PARTS INVOLVED—Lips; gums; palate; tongue; membrane covering the lips and cheeks; floor of the mouth.

SEX OR AGE MOST AFFECTED—Adults over 60.

SIGNS & SYMPTOMS—A lump in any part of the mouth or tongue with the following characteristics:
- It may ulcerate and bleed.
- It may interfere with the way dentures fit.
- It may interfere with speech or swallowing.

CAUSES—Unknown, although it is most common in people who smoke cigarettes, cigars or pipes, or use chewing tobacco or snuff.

RISK INCREASES WITH
- Use of tobacco.
- Poorly fitting dentures.

HOW TO PREVENT
- Don't smoke or use tobacco.
- See your dentist for annual dental exams and for problems with denture fit.

 WHAT TO EXPECT

APPROPRIATE HEALTH CARE
- Doctor's or dentist's treatment.
- Self-care after diagnosis.
- Surgery to remove the tumor.

DIAGNOSTIC MEASURES
- Your own observation of symptoms.
- Medical history and physical exam by a doctor.
- Biopsy (see Glossary) of the tumor.

POSSIBLE COMPLICATIONS
- Cancerous change in the tumor (rare).
- Bleeding from the tumor.
- Infection in the tumor.

PROBABLE OUTCOME—Curable with surgical removal. Normal facial appearance can usually be restored by plastic surgery.

 HOW TO TREAT

NOTE—Follow your doctor's instructions. These instructions are supplemental.

GENERAL MEASURES—After surgery, cleanse the mouth 3 to 4 times a day with a soothing salt-water solution (1 teaspoon salt in 8 oz. warm water).

MEDICATION
- For minor discomfort, you may use non-prescription drugs such as acetaminophen.
- Your doctor may prescribe antibiotics, if infection exists.

ACTIVITY—No restrictions.

DIET—No special diet after recovery. A liquid diet may be necessary for several days after surgery.

 CALL YOUR DOCTOR IF

- You have symptoms of a mouth or tongue tumor.
- The following occurs after surgery:
  Fever.
  Bleeding at the surgical site.
  Unbearable pain.
- New, unexplained symptoms develop. Drugs used in treatment may produce side effects.

MULTIPLE MYELOMA
(Primary Bone-Marrow Cancer)

GENERAL INFORMATION

DEFINITION—A malignancy beginning in the plasma cells of the bone marrow.

Plasma cells normally produce antibodies to help destroy germs and protect against infection. With myeloma, this function becomes impaired, and the body cannot deal effectively with infection.

BODY PARTS INVOLVED—Bone marrow of all bones, but most common in the thigh, back, pelvis or upper arms.

SEX OR AGE MOST AFFECTED—Both sexes, but most common in men between ages 50 and 70.

SIGNS & SYMPTOMS
- Pain in the affected bone. The pain is severe, boring and deep. If the bone collapses, pain spreads to other parts of the body.
- Weight loss.
- Symptoms of anemia, such as weakness, paleness, tiredness and breathlessness.

CAUSES—Unknown. The bone pain is caused by the cancerous abnormal plasma cells. The anemia is caused by damaged red blood cells and decreased platelets.

RISK INCREASES WITH—Unknown.

HOW TO PREVENT—No specific preventive measures.

WHAT TO EXPECT

APPROPRIATE HEALTH CARE
- Self-care after diagnosis.
- Doctor's treatment.
- Radiation therapy to relieve bone pain.
- Hospitalization in late stages.

DIAGNOSTIC MEASURES
- Your own observation of symptoms.
- Medical history and physical exam by a doctor.
- Laboratory blood studies.
- Biopsy (see Glossary) of bone marrow.
- X-rays of painful bones.

POSSIBLE COMPLICATIONS
- Recurrent infections.
- Kidney failure.
- Spontaneous bleeding.

PROBABLE OUTCOME—This condition is currently considered incurable. However, pain can be relieved or controlled. Some persons live up to 5 years after symptoms appear, and medical literature cites a few instances of unexplained recovery.

Scientific research into causes and treatment continues, so there is hope for increasingly effective treatment and cure.

HOW TO TREAT

NOTE—Follow your doctor's instructions. These instructions are supplemental.

GENERAL MEASURES—No specific instructions except those listed under other headings.

MEDICATION—Your doctor may prescribe:
- Anticancer and cortisone drugs (chemotherapy).
- Pain relievers.
- Antibiotics to fight infections.

ACTIVITY—Stay as active as pain or bone complications allow.

DIET—No special diet.

CALL YOUR DOCTOR IF

- You have symptoms of multiple myeloma.
- The following occurs during treatment:
  Fever.
  Any sign of infection (pain, swelling, redness, tenderness or warmth) anywhere in the body.
  Swelling of the feet and ankles.
  Urination discomfort or decreased urine output in 1 day.
  Unexplained bleeding from any part of the body.
- New, unexplained symptoms develop. Drugs used in treatment may produce side effects.

ILLNESSES & DISORDERS

MULTIPLE SCLEROSIS

GENERAL INFORMATION

DEFINITION—A chronic disorder affecting many nervous-system functions. One-third of patients have mild, non-progressive disease. Another third worsen slowly. The rest worsen rapidly.

BODY PARTS INVOLVED—Central nervous system (brain and spinal cord).

SEX OR AGE MOST AFFECTED—Younger adults (ages 20 to 40) of both sexes, but more common in women.

SIGNS & SYMPTOMS—Early stages:
● Vague eye problems, such as intermittent blurred or double vision.
● Weakness; difficulty with walking or balance.
● Vague loss of sensation or numbness and tingling.
Late stages:
● Marked weakness; tremor.
● Speaking difficulty.
● Loss of bladder or bowel control.
● Extreme mood swings.
● Sexual impotence in men.
Signs and symptoms vary widely between persons. Sometimes they are mistakenly attributed to emotions or "nerves."

CAUSES—Unknown. Research suggests multiple sclerosis may be caused by an autoimmune disorder or slow-acting virus. Patches of white matter in the brain and spinal cord break down and cannot conduct normal nerve impulses.

RISK INCREASES WITH—Children and adolescents raised in cool climates. Moving to a warmer climate later does not help.

HOW TO PREVENT—Cannot be prevented at present, but relapses can be shortened by therapy. Avoid infections, which trigger relapses.

WHAT TO EXPECT

APPROPRIATE HEALTH CARE
● Self-care after diagnosis.
● Doctor's treatment.
● Hospitalization or nursing-home care, depending on the severity of the disease.

DIAGNOSTIC MEASURES
● Your own observation of symptoms.
● Medical history and physical exam by a doctor. Consultation with a neurologist is often valuable.
● EEG (see Glossary).
● CAT scan (see Glossary).
● Laboratory studies of spinal fluid.

POSSIBLE COMPLICATIONS
● Urinary-tract infections caused by bowel and bladder disorders.
● Pressure sores from prolonged bed rest.
● Constipation caused by inactivity.

PROBABLE OUTCOME—Spontaneous recovery sometimes occurs. In most cases, however, multiple sclerosis is incurable. Symptoms can be relieved or controlled, and the condition often remains stable for months or years. Survival of 20 to 30 years is common.
    Scientific research into causes and treatment continues, so there is hope for increasingly effective treatment and cure.

HOW TO TREAT

NOTE—Follow your doctor's instructions. These instructions are supplemental.

GENERAL MEASURES
● Try to lead as normal a life as possible, but avoid fatigue.
● Avoid warm surroundings—even a hot shower. Heat can temporarily worsen symptoms.
● Have frequent massages, which help prevent contractures (shortening of muscles).
● Avoid stress, which may aggravate symptoms. See Appendix 13.
● Some unethical medical practitioners offer unproven treatments of no value. Discuss any unconventional treatment with your doctor before investing your money.

MEDICATION—Your doctor may prescribe:
● Cortisone drugs during periods of relapse or when symptoms worsen.
● Muscle relaxants to control muscle spasms.

ACTIVITY
● A regular program of physical exercise and mental activity is essential. Obtain physical therapy and muscle retraining with mechanical devices to overcome physical handicaps.
● Take regular rest periods.
● Remain sexually active, if possible. Sexual counseling may be helpful.

DIET—Eat a normal, well-balanced diet that is high in fiber to prevent constipation.

CALL YOUR DOCTOR IF

● You have symptoms of multiple sclerosis.
● The following occurs during treatment:
  Breathing or swallowing difficulty.
  Sudden increased weakness.
  Chills and fever, or other signs of infection.

MUMPS

GENERAL INFORMATION

DEFINITION—A mild, contagious viral disease that causes painful swelling of the salivary glands.

BODY PARTS INVOLVED—Parotid glands (salivary glands that lie between the ear and jaw). Other organs, including the testicles, ovaries, pancreas, breasts, brain and meninges (membranes that cover the brain) sometimes become involved.

SEX OR AGE MOST AFFECTED—All ages, but most common in children (2 to 12 years). Approximately 10% of adults are susceptible to mumps.

SIGNS & SYMPTOMS—Mumps without complications:
- Inflammation, swelling and pain of the parotid glands. The glands feel firm, and pain increases with chewing or swallowing.
- Fever.
- Headache.
- Sore throat.
Additional symptoms with complications:
- Painful, swollen testicles.
- Abdominal pain, if the ovaries or pancreas are involved.
- Severe headache, if the brain or meninges are involved.

CAUSES—Person-to-person transmission of the mumps virus. The virus can be transmitted anytime from 48 hours before symptoms begin to 6 days after symptoms appear. Virus incubation is 14 to 24 days after contact; the average is 18 days.

RISK INCREASES WITH—Crowded living conditions.

HOW TO PREVENT
- Obtain mumps immunizations for children at the appropriate age. For an immunization schedule, see Appendix 16.
- If you have not had mumps or been vaccinated and a close family member has mumps, your doctor may suggest an antimumps globulin. The injection *may* prevent the disease—it is not guaranteed—and it is expensive.

WHAT TO EXPECT

APPROPRIATE HEALTH CARE
- Home care after diagnosis.
- Doctor's treatment to confirm the diagnosis and treat complications, if any occur.

DIAGNOSTIC MEASURES
- Your own observation of symptoms.
- Medical history and physical exam by a doctor.

POSSIBLE COMPLICATIONS—Infections of the brain or meninges (meningo-encephalitis), pancreas, ovaries, breasts or testicles. Sterility may occur if both testicles become infected (rare).

PROBABLE OUTCOME—Spontaneous recovery in about 10 days if no complications occur. After having the disease, a person has lifetime immunity to mumps.

HOW TO TREAT

NOTE—Follow your doctor's instructions. These instructions are supplemental.

GENERAL MEASURES
- It is not necessary to isolate the infected person from the family. By the time symptoms appear, the disease has usually already spread.
- Apply heat or ice—whichever feels better—intermittently to the swollen, painful glands (parotid or testicles). Use a hot-water bottle, hot towel or ice pack.

MEDICATION—Once the disease begins, it must run its natural course. There is no safe, readily available medicine that can kill the virus or keep it from multiplying.
- For minor pain, you may use non-prescription drugs such as acetaminophen. Don't use aspirin.
- Your doctor may prescribe:
  Stronger pain relievers.
  Cortisone drugs, if testicles are involved.

ACTIVITY—Bed rest is not essential and does not reduce the possibility of complications. Allow as much activity as strength and feeling of well-being allow. Patients are no longer contagious when swelling disappears.

DIET—No special diet, but increase daily fluid intake to at least 6 to 8 glasses of liquid, including ginger ale, cola, tea or water. Fruit juices or tart beverages may increase pain.

CALL YOUR DOCTOR IF

- Fever (oral) rises above 101F (38.3C).
- The following occurs during the illness:
  Vomiting or abdominal pain.
  Severe headache which is not relieved by acetaminophen.
  Drowsiness or inability to stay awake.
  Swelling or pain in the testicle.
  Twitching of the face muscles.
  Convulsion.
  Discomfort or redness in the eyes.

ILLNESSES & DISORDERS

MUSCLE, PULLED OR TORN

GENERAL INFORMATION

DEFINITION—Stretched or torn muscle fibers.

BODY PARTS INVOLVED—Muscles attached to bones anywhere in the body.

SEX OR AGE MOST AFFECTED—Both sexes; all ages.

SIGNS & SYMPTOMS
- Pain or tenderness in the injury area.
- Gradual stiffening or contraction of the injured muscle.
- Swelling, redness or bruising at the injury site.

CAUSES—Injury caused by overuse or stress of a muscle group.

RISK INCREASES WITH
- Poor nutrition, especially an electrolyte imbalance or vitamin deficiencies.
- Poor physical condition.
- Strenuous activity following excess alcohol consumption.
- Obesity.
- Fatigue or overwork.
- Lifting heavy weights improperly.

HOW TO PREVENT—Avoid vigorous exercise if you are not accustomed to it. If you are out of condition, begin an exercise program to strengthen your muscles gradually and prevent future injury. See Appendix 20.

WHAT TO EXPECT

APPROPRIATE HEALTH CARE
- Self-care after diagnosis.
- Doctor's treatment for severe injuries, or if self-care is not successful.
- Rehabilitation and treatment by a physical therapist or athletic trainer.

DIAGNOSTIC MEASURES
- Your own observation of symptoms.
- Medical history and physical exam by a doctor.
- X-rays of the painful area.

POSSIBLE COMPLICATIONS—Permanent weakness in the affected muscle.

PROBABLE OUTCOME—Healing time for a pulled muscle depends on your age, general physical condition, previous injuries and severity of the injury. Most partial tears or pulls heal with treatment within 1 month. Muscle function will be poor until the torn fibers heal.
  If the muscle is ruptured (torn in two), surgery may be necessary.

HOW TO TREAT

NOTE—Follow your doctor's instructions. These instructions are supplemental.

GENERAL MEASURES
- Apply ice to the injured area during the first 24 hours. Place ice in a plastic bag and separate it from the skin with a thin towel. Hold it against the muscle with your hand or an elastic bandage. Keep the ice pack on the area as long as you can tolerate the cold.
- Wrap the area with a support bandage. Don't wrap it too tightly. If it swells *below* the bandage, loosen it. Elevate the injured part whenever possible.
- After 24 hours, apply heat in any form or continue ice packs, whichever feels better. For heat, use a heating pad, heat lamp, whirlpool, ultrasound, hot baths or hot compresses.

MEDICATION—You may take non-prescription pain relievers such as aspirin. If your pain is severe or the affected area becomes badly swollen, your doctor may prescribe stronger pain relievers or muscle relaxants.

ACTIVITY
- Don't use the pulled muscle as long as it is painful. However, keep uninjured parts of the body active. Severe leg injuries may require crutches, and severe arm injuries may require slings.
- Physical therapy, with a graduated exercise program, may be necessary to restore normal use and strength.

DIET—Eat a normal, well-balanced diet. Increase protein intake (meat, poultry, fish, eggs, beans and dairy products) during healing.

CALL YOUR DOCTOR IF

You have symptoms of a pulled or torn muscle, especially if the following occur:
- You become unable to use the affected muscle.
- Pain becomes intolerable.
- Swelling or bruising increase after 24 hours.
- You think medicine is causing symptoms.

MUSCULAR DYSTROPHY

GENERAL INFORMATION

DEFINITION—A gradual deterioration of the body's muscles, leading to increasing difficulty in walking and moving.

BODY PARTS INVOLVED—Muscular system, especially of the extremities, pelvis and hips.

SEX OR AGE MOST AFFECTED—Male children, usually between ages 5 and 12.

SIGNS & SYMPTOMS—Early symptoms:
- Weakness.
- Ducklike gait.
- Falling, with difficulty getting up.
- Muscles that appear larger and stronger—but are weaker—than normal.

Late symptoms:
- Muscle deterioration severe enough to require confinement to a wheelchair by age 9 to 12.
- Severe distortion of the body.
- Recurrent respiratory infections.

CAUSES—Inherited. Muscular dystrophy is a genetic abnormality. It is carried by a female who does not have the disease; she passes it to male children. When a woman carrier marries a normal male, half the male children will inherit the condition.

RISK INCREASES WITH—Family history of muscular dystrophy.

HOW TO PREVENT—If you have a family history of muscular dystrophy:
- Obtain genetic counseling prior to starting a family.
- If you are pregnant, consider amniocentesis (see Glossary) to determine whether the fetus is male and the disorder is present.

OTHER—Different types of muscular dystrophy exist, depending on the exact genes involved. They affect different areas of the body, such as shoulders, hips or face.

WHAT TO EXPECT

APPROPRIATE HEALTH CARE
- Home care.
- Doctor's treatment.
- Psychotherapy or counseling to learn ways to cope with disability and to adjust socially.
- Physical therapy.
- Nursing-home care, if the patient's needs exceed the resources available at home.

DIAGNOSTIC MEASURES
- Parent's observation of symptoms.
- Medical history and physical exam by a doctor.
- Laboratory studies of muscle enzymes in the blood.
- Muscle biopsy (see Glossary).

POSSIBLE COMPLICATIONS
- Frequent fractures or injuries from falls.
- Spinal curvature caused by weakened muscles of the spine.
- Pneumonia caused by weakened chest muscles and a diminished cough response.
- Muscle shortening (contractures).
- Pressure sores.

PROBABLE OUTCOME—This condition is currently considered incurable. Persons with this condition rarely reach adulthood.

Scientific research into causes and treatment continues, so there is hope for better treatment and increased life expectancy.

HOW TO TREAT

NOTE—Follow your doctor's instructions. These instructions are supplemental.

GENERAL MEASURES
- Contact your local chapter of the Muscular Dystrophy Association for help.
- The child should learn deep-breathing techniques. Your doctor can provide instructions.
- The child should stay active in school as long as possible.

MEDICATION—No medicine can cure this condition. Your doctor may prescribe:
- Stool softeners to prevent constipation.
- Medications appropriate for complications.

ACTIVITY—The child should be as physically and mentally active as possible. Many devices can help overcome handicaps caused by weakness. Your doctor will tell you if braces will help.

If the child cannot voluntarily move muscle groups, family members or a visiting nurse should massage and passively exercise them to prevent contractures. Long periods of inactivity or bed rest should be avoided.

DIET—No special diet. Overweight should be avoided, because it adds stress to weakened muscles.

CALL YOUR DOCTOR IF

- You detect symptoms of muscular dystrophy in your child.
- Infection, especially of the lung, occurs after diagnosis. Symptoms include fever, cough and chest pain.

MYASTHENIA GRAVIS

GENERAL INFORMATION

DEFINITION—Disorder of muscles, especially of the face and head, with increasing fatigue and weakness as muscles are used.

BODY PARTS INVOLVED—Muscles, especially around the eyes, mouth and throat, and the extremities.

SEX OR AGE MOST AFFECTED—Adolescents and young adults of both sexes, but more common in females.

SIGNS & SYMPTOMS
- Drooping eyelids.
- Double vision.
- Loss of normal facial expression.
- Swallowing difficulty.
- Weakness of the arms and legs.
- Difficulty speaking clearly.
- Breathing difficulty.

Most flare-ups appear after a brief period of normal muscle function, and worsen as the muscle is used.

CAUSES
- Autoimmune disorder (probably).
- Tumor of the thymus (newborns only).

RISK INCREASES WITH
- Medical history of other autoimmune diseases.
- Some cancers, especially thymus and lung cancer.
- Newborns and infants of mothers with myasthenia gravis. They show symptoms in 2 to 3 weeks.

HOW TO PREVENT—Cannot be prevented at present.

OTHER—Pregnancy often results in temporary improvement.

WHAT TO EXPECT

APPROPRIATE HEALTH CARE
- Doctor's treatment.
- Surgery to remove a thymus tumor, if present.

DIAGNOSTIC MEASURES
- Your own observation of symptoms.
- Medical history and physical exam by a doctor.
- Laboratory studies of antibodies in the blood and electrical muscle tests.
- X-rays of the chest.
- Therapeutic trial of anticholinesterase drugs.

POSSIBLE COMPLICATIONS
- Choking from swallowing difficulty.
- Respiratory paralysis.

PROBABLE OUTCOME—This condition is currently considered incurable. However, symptoms can be relieved or controlled. Worsening may be followed by improvement. Life expectancy is reduced but patients usually live many years with the disease.

Scientific research into causes and treatment continues, so there is hope for increasingly effective treatment and cure.

HOW TO TREAT

NOTE—Follow your doctor's instructions. These instructions are supplemental.

GENERAL MEASURES—Maintain as normal a life as possible. See Appendix 13.

MEDICATION—Your doctor may prescribe:
- Anticholinesterase drugs to restore normal muscle function. Excessive doses may cause weakness.
- Cortisone drugs at times when symptoms worsen.

ACTIVITY—No restrictions. Remain as active as possible.

DIET—No special diet.

CALL YOUR DOCTOR IF

- You have symptoms of myasthenia gravis.
- You develop swallowing or breathing difficulty. (You should have emergency medications—anticholinesterase drugs—available at all times to use if these symptoms develop.)

MYOCARDITIS

GENERAL INFORMATION

DEFINITION—Inflammation of the heart muscle (myocardium) that usually occurs as a complication of underlying illness, hypersensitive immune reactions, injury or radiation therapy.

BODY PARTS INVOLVED—Heart muscle.

SEX OR AGE MOST AFFECTED—Both sexes; all ages.

SIGNS & SYMPTOMS
- Fatigue.
- Shortness of breath.
- Irregular heartbeat.
- Fever.
- Other symptoms caused by the underlying disorder.

If myocarditis causes congestive heart failure, the following symptoms will also occur:
- Swollen feet and ankles.
- Distended neck veins.
- Rapid heartbeat, even when at rest.
- Breathing difficulty, even when sleeping or at rest.

CAUSES
- Viral infections, such as measles, influenza or adenovirus.
- Bacterial infections, such as tetanus, gonorrhea, typhoid fever, tuberculosis or diphtheria.
- Surgery on the heart.
- Rheumatic fever.
- Parasite infections.
- Radiation therapy for cancers in the chest, such as lung or breast cancer.

RISK INCREASES WITH
- Excess alcohol consumption.
- Geographic location. Parasite infections are common in underdeveloped countries.

HOW TO PREVENT
- Don't drink more than 1 or 2 alcoholic drinks—if any—a day.
- Keep immunizations current against diphtheria, tetanus, measles, German measles and polio. See Appendix 16.

WHAT TO EXPECT

APPROPRIATE HEALTH CARE
- Self-care after diagnosis.
- Doctor's treatment.
- Hospitalization for the underlying disorder (frequently).

DIAGNOSTIC MEASURES
- Your own observation of symptoms.
- Medical history and physical exam by a doctor.
- Laboratory blood studies.
- EKG (see Glossary).
- Other studies appropriate for the underlying disorder.

POSSIBLE COMPLICATIONS—Even with excellent treatment of the underlying disorder, a few patients develop:
- Congestive heart failure.
- Permanent damage to the heart muscle or valves.
- A blood clot inside the heart muscle that can break away and lodge elsewhere in the body. This may be life-threatening.

PROBABLE OUTCOME—Usually curable with detection and treatment of the underlying cause.

HOW TO TREAT

NOTE—Follow your doctor's instructions. These instructions are supplemental.

GENERAL MEASURES—Obtain complete nursing care, including help with bathing and eating.

MEDICATION—Your doctor may prescribe:
- Antibiotics to fight infection, if myocarditis is caused by a bacterial infection.
- Cortisone drugs to reduce inflammation.
- Appropriate medications, if myocarditis develops into congestive heart failure. These include:
  Diuretics to reduce fluid retention.
  Digitalis to stimulate a stronger heartbeat.
  Anticoagulants to prevent clot formation.

ACTIVITY—Rest in bed until symptoms disappear. Recovery time varies, depending on the underlying cause. You may read or watch TV.
  Use a bedside commode for bowel movements while at complete bed rest. This causes less stress than a bedpan.
  After recovery, resume your normal activities gradually.

DIET—Eat a low-salt diet (see Appendix 9).

CALL YOUR DOCTOR IF

- You have symptoms of myocarditis.
- The following occurs during treatment:
  Recurrence of fever or chills.
  Increased shortness of breath.
- New, unexplained symptoms develop. Drugs used in treatment may produce side effects.

ILLNESSES & DISORDERS

NAIL SPLITTING

GENERAL INFORMATION

DEFINITION—Splitting of fingernails and toenails.

BODY PARTS INVOLVED—Toenails and fingernails.

SEX OR AGE MOST AFFECTED—Both sexes; all ages.

SIGNS & SYMPTOMS—Painless splitting of the nail. Cracks may be parallel to the length of the finger, or flakes of nail may chip off the end.

CAUSES
- Scar formation from injury to the nail bed (sometimes).
- Family history of nail-splitting.
- Unknown (usually).

RISK INCREASES WITH—Aging.

HOW TO PREVENT—Protect fingernails from trauma, especially excessive irritation from soap and water.

WHAT TO EXPECT

APPROPRIATE HEALTH CARE
- Self-care after diagnosis.
- Doctor's treatment for diagnosis, if splitting becomes severe.

DIAGNOSTIC MEASURES
- Your own observation of symptoms.
- Medical history and physical exam by a doctor.

POSSIBLE COMPLICATIONS—None expected.

PROBABLE OUTCOME—Splitting may never disappear completely, but it may improve from time to time.

HOW TO TREAT

NOTE—Follow your doctor's instructions. These instructions are supplemental.

GENERAL MEASURES
- Apply multiple layers of clear fingernail polish so cracks, fissures and flakes are cemented together. This can provide a splint or shield to protect nails. Nail polishes that contain nylon fibers will thicken and strengthen nails.
- Don't remove nail polish too often. Polish remover has a drying effect and may increase splitting. Instead, patch chips in the nail polish as they occur.
- Cement false fingernails over the split nail.
- Wear rubber gloves with cotton lining for housework that involves water.
- Use a hand cream often. Massage it into the skin around the nails.

MEDICATION—Medicine usually is not necessary for this disorder.

ACTIVITY—No restrictions.

DIET—No special diet. Many people say the condition improves if they drink large quantities of plain gelatin each day. Evidence does not support this theory.

CALL YOUR DOCTOR IF

- You have severe nail splitting that has become a problem.
- Self-care produces no improvement in 6 months.

NAILS, RINGWORM INFECTION OF
(Onychomycosis; Tinea Unguium)

 GENERAL INFORMATION

DEFINITION—A fungus infection of the toenails or fingernails in which nails become pliable, opaque, white and thickened. This is contagious.

BODY PARTS INVOLVED—Toenails (usually) or fingernails.

SEX OR AGE MOST AFFECTED—All ages, but most common in older adolescents and adults.

SIGNS & SYMPTOMS
- Begins with a small separation between the end of the nail and the nail bed.
- Soft yellow material gradually builds up in the separation.
- The condition usually doesn't itch and is painless, unless the area is extensive and becomes infected.
- Eventually the entire nail is separated, resulting in a partially destroyed, misshapen, yellow nail.

CAUSES—Infection with the trichophyton fungus. Fingernail infection occurs only if the nail has been injured or the nail is affected by another skin disease on the hand. Toenail infections can occur without injury.

RISK INCREASES WITH
- Exposure to occupational heat, wetness and humidity, such as with cooks, dishwashers and housewives.
- Hot, humid weather.

HOW TO PREVENT
- Keep feet cool, dry and exposed to sunlight as much as possible.
- Wear cotton or wool socks. Avoid footwear made from synthetic fibers.

 WHAT TO EXPECT

APPROPRIATE HEALTH CARE
- Self-care.
- Doctor's treatment.
- Surgical removal of the nail.

DIAGNOSTIC MEASURES
- Your own observation of symptoms.
- Medical history and physical exam by a doctor.
- Laboratory fungal cultures of the material under nails.

POSSIBLE COMPLICATIONS—Permanent nail loss or deformity.

PROBABLE OUTCOME—Most fingernail infections are curable with 6 months of continuous treatment. Toenails require 12 to 24 months of treatment because of their slower growth rate. Most fingernail infections respond well to treatment, but toenail infections are more resistant to treatment. Recurrence is likely.

 HOW TO TREAT

NOTE—Follow your doctor's instructions. These instructions are supplemental.

GENERAL MEASURES
- Dry feet and hands with extra care after bathing—even after the infection clears.
- Wear light footwear, such as sandals, to allow free air circulation. Don't wear socks or shoes made of synthetic materials. During acute phases, go barefoot as much as possible. Keep feet and hands cool, dry and exposed to sunlight.
- For fingernail infections, wear cotton-lined latex or rubber gloves for dishwashing or other cleaning that requires immersion in water or chemicals.

MEDICATION—Non-prescription antifungal ointments, creams and powders are available, but they are ineffective in curing these infections. Your doctor may prescribe oral antifungal drugs, such as griseofulvin or ketoconazole, to cure the infection.

ACTIVITY—No restrictions, but avoid heat and excess sweating.

DIET—No special diet.

 CALL YOUR DOCTOR IF

- You have a minor nail infection that becomes a problem.
- After 2 weeks of medication, symptoms fall to improve.
- New, unexplained symptoms develop. Drugs used in treatment may produce side effects.

NARCOLEPSY

 GENERAL INFORMATION

DEFINITION—Rare sleep disorder characterized by uncontrollable episodes of falling asleep at any place or time.

BODY PARTS INVOLVED—Central nervous system.

SEX OR AGE MOST AFFECTED
- Both sexes.
- Begins in adolescence or young adulthood and continues throughout life.

SIGNS & SYMPTOMS—Any of the following (10% of people with narcolepsy have all 4 signs):
- Sleep attacks that may occur up to 10 times a day. These can occur during conversations or other activities. An attack leaves the person feeling refreshed, but another may occur again quickly.
- Vivid dreams, sounds or hallucinations at the beginning of a sleep attack.
- Temporary paralysis when falling asleep or just before complete awakening.
- Momentary paralysis not related to sleep when feeling sudden emotion, such as anger, fear or joy.

CAUSES—Unknown.

RISK INCREASES WITH—Either of the following may trigger an attack:
- Monotonous activity.
- Prolonged laughter.

HOW TO PREVENT—Reduce frequency of attacks by avoiding risks listed above, if possible.

 WHAT TO EXPECT

APPROPRIATE HEALTH CARE
- Self-care after diagnosis.
- Doctor's treatment.

DIAGNOSTIC MEASURES
- Your own observation of symptoms.
- Medical history and physical exam by a doctor.
- EEG (see Glossary).
- Studies in a sleep laboratory.

POSSIBLE COMPLICATIONS—Accidental injury during a sudden sleep attack.

PROBABLE OUTCOME—This disorder lasts throughout life, but it has no effect on life expectancy. Medication can decrease the frequency of sleep attacks.

 HOW TO TREAT

NOTE—Follow your doctor's instructions. These instructions are supplemental.

GENERAL MEASURES—Wear a Medic-Alert bracelet or pendant (see Glossary).

MEDICATION—Your doctor may prescribe stimulants, such as dextroamphetamine, ephedrine or methylphenidate.

ACTIVITY—Don't engage in any activity that carries the risk of injury from a sudden sleep attack. These include activities such as driving long distances, climbing ladders or working around dangerous machinery.

DIET—No special diet.

 CALL YOUR DOCTOR IF

- You have symptoms of narcolepsy.
- New, unexplained symptoms develop. Drugs used in treatment may produce side effects.

NASAL POLYPS

GENERAL INFORMATION

DEFINITION—Non-malignant growths in the nasal cavities, usually in both sides of the nose.

BODY PARTS INVOLVED—Nasal mucous membranes.

SEX OR AGE MOST AFFECTED—All ages, but most common in adults.

SIGNS & SYMPTOMS
- Obstruction of air through the nose (chronic "stuffy-nose" feeling).
- Impaired sense of smell.
- Feelings of fullness in the face.
- Nasal discharge.
- Facial pain (sometimes).
- Headaches (sometimes).

CAUSES—Chronic infection or allergy in the nose (allergic rhinitis) that causes the nasal mucous membranes to swell and produce excess fluid in the nasal cells.

RISK INCREASES WITH—Sinusitis or chronic nasal infection.

HOW TO PREVENT—Obtain medical treatment for the underlying allergy. Consult your doctor about allergy testing and desensitizing procedures.

WHAT TO EXPECT

APPROPRIATE HEALTH CARE
- Self-care (only if surgery cannot be performed).
- Doctor's treatment.
- Surgery to remove polyps under local anesthesia—a minor surgical procedure.

DIAGNOSTIC MEASURES
- Your own observation of symptoms.
- Medical history and physical exam by a doctor.
- Laboratory skin tests to identify allergies.

POSSIBLE COMPLICATIONS
- Repeated infections.
- Nosebleeds.

PROBABLE OUTCOME—Symptoms can be controlled with treatment (usually surgery). Recurrence is common, even with surgical treatment.

HOW TO TREAT

NOTE—Follow your doctor's instructions. These instructions are supplemental.

GENERAL MEASURES—If nosebleeds occur, see treatment described under Nosebleed (in Illness section).

MEDICATION
- For minor pain, you may use acetaminophen. Avoid aspirin, which may increase the tendency to bleed.
- Your doctor may prescribe cortisone drugs in nasal spray or oral form for a short while before surgery to shrink the polyps.

ACTIVITY—Resume your normal activities gradually after surgery.

DIET—No special diet.

CALL YOUR DOCTOR IF

- You have symptoms of nasal polyps.
- The following occurs during treatment: Nosebleeds that cannot be stopped. Fever. Pain that persists despite the use of acetaminophen.

ILLNESSES & DISORDERS

NASAL SEPTUM, DEVIATED

 GENERAL INFORMATION

DEFINITION—Crookedness or other abnormality of the septum, the structure dividing the nose in 2 equal parts.

BODY PARTS INVOLVED—Septum, which is made of cartilage (closer to the tip) and bone (closer to the forehead).

SEX OR AGE MOST AFFECTED—Both sexes of adults.

SIGNS & SYMPTOMS
- An apparently crooked nose.
- Obstruction of air through the nostrils.
- Nasal discharge.

CAUSES
- Rapid growth, especially at puberty.
- Injury.
- Nose surgery.

RISK INCREASES WITH—Unknown.

HOW TO PREVENT—Protect yourself from nose injury. Wear protective headgear for contact sports or cycling. Buckle your auto seat belt or shoulder harness.

 WHAT TO EXPECT

APPROPRIATE HEALTH CARE
- Self-care after diagnosis.
- Doctor's treatment, if symptoms warrant it.
- Surgery to correct the deviation (sometimes). The procedures are:
  Submucosal removal, which relieves obstruction.
  Rhinoplasty, which corrects anatomical deformity.
  Septoplasty, which relieves nasal obstruction and improves appearance.

DIAGNOSTIC MEASURES
- Your own observation of symptoms.
- Medical history and physical exam by a doctor, including inspection of the nose with a bright light and nasal speculum.

POSSIBLE COMPLICATIONS
- Recurrent nosebleeds.
- Recurrent nasal or sinus infections.

PROBABLE OUTCOME—Usually curable with surgery. If symptoms are not troublesome, surgery is probably not necessary.

 HOW TO TREAT

NOTE—Follow your doctor's instructions. These instructions are supplemental.

GENERAL MEASURES—For an explanation of one type of corrective surgery and postoperative care, see Rhinoplasty & Submucosal Removal (in Surgery section).

MEDICATION
- For minor discomfort, you may use non-prescription drugs, such as decongestants, to decrease nasal secretions.
- Your doctor may prescribe antibiotics to fight infection, if necessary.

ACTIVITY—No restrictions unless surgery is necessary. If so, resume your normal activities gradually.

DIET—No special diet.

 CALL YOUR DOCTOR IF

You have symptoms of a deviated nasal septum, especially recurrent nosebleeds or nasal and sinus infections, and you want to consider corrective surgery.

NEPHROSIS
(Nephrotic Syndrome)

GENERAL INFORMATION

DEFINITION—A form of chronic kidney disease beginning in childhood. Nephrosis is characterized by protein in the urine, swelling of the skin and organs, and low protein and high cholesterol in the blood.

BODY PARTS INVOLVED—Kidneys. Late or complicated stages involve all body cells.

SEX OR AGE MOST AFFECTED—Children between ages 1 and 6—especially ages 2 and 3. It affects more boys than girls.

SIGNS & SYMPTOMS
● Fluid retention that appears first as puffy eyes and ankles, then as general puffiness of the skin, and eventually as a swollen abdomen.
● Reduced urine production, sometimes to 20% of normal.
● Appetite loss.
● Weakness.
● General ill feeling.

CAUSES—Unknown. May be primary (of unknown cause) or may occur as a complication of other problems which affect kidney function, such as: diabetes; lupus erythematosus; glomerulonephritis; autoimmune disorders; serum sickness and other severe allergic disorders; blood clot in the kidney; infections, especially of the skin; or congenital heart disease.

RISK INCREASES WITH—Family history of nephrosis (primary form only). The following may reactivate a childhood case:
● Pregnancy.
● Exposure to chemical toxins.
● Congestive heart failure.

HOW TO PREVENT—Obtain prompt medical treatment for any causes listed, especially skin and throat infections.

WHAT TO EXPECT

APPROPRIATE HEALTH CARE
● Home care after diagnosis.
● Doctor's treatment.

DIAGNOSTIC MEASURES
● Your own observation of symptoms.
● Medical history and physical exam by a doctor.
● Laboratory studies, such as urinalysis and blood studies of protein and cholesterol.

POSSIBLE COMPLICATIONS
● Kidney disease that resembles chronic glomerulonephritis.
● Kidney failure.
● Increased susceptibility to infections.

PROBABLE OUTCOME—Nephrosis can't be cured or prevented. However, medication and diet can control swelling and reverse kidney abnormalities in many children.
  Although symptoms usually disappear in 2 weeks with treatment, medication is continued for 6 to 8 weeks. Nephrosis can be arrested with treatment, but relapses are common and the treatment must be repeated. If kidney failure develops, dialysis or a kidney transplant can prolong life.

HOW TO TREAT

NOTE—Follow your doctor's instructions. These instructions are supplemental.

GENERAL MEASURES—During the acute phase:
● Keep a record of the child's temperature each morning and evening.
● Collect all urine the child passes during each 24 hours and record every amount. Record all fluids consumed also. Portions of the urine will be analyzed in the doctor's office.

MEDICATION—Your doctor may prescribe:
● Cortisone or immunosuppressive drugs to reduce kidney inflammation.
● Diuretics, including potassium-saving diuretics, to reduce fluid retention.
● Antibiotics to control infection.

ACTIVITY—Keep the child in bed (except for trips to the bathroom) until the edema (fluid retention) improves. After the swelling decreases, the child may be as mildly active as his or her strength allows.

DIET
● Cook and serve the child's food without salt. Avoid prepared foods that contain salt. Include more protein than usual, such as fish, meat, eggs and low-salt cheese.
● You may need to restrict the child's fluid intake. Ask your doctor.

CALL YOUR DOCTOR IF

● Your child has symptoms of nephrosis.
● The following occurs during treatment:
  Severe headache.
  Convulsion.
  Extreme weakness.
  Signs of infection, such as fever, sores on the skin, cough or burning on urination.
  Failure to pass 1 quart of urine in a 24-hour period.
  Increased fluid retention.
  Vomiting, diarrhea or nausea.

NLD
(Necrobiosis Lipoidica Diabeticorum)

 GENERAL INFORMATION

DEFINITION—An inflammatory disease of the skin which occurs primarily in patients with diabetes. It is not contagious.

BODY PARTS INVOLVED—Skin of the shins.

SEX OR AGE MOST AFFECTED—Adults of both sexes.

SIGNS & SYMPTOMS—One or more plaques (raised, flat-topped skin lesions) with the following characteristics:
● The center of the plaque appears yellow and waxy. The borders are darker and may be violet.
● Plaques measure 2cm to 10cm in diameter.
● Veins under the plaques can be seen easily because the skin is atrophied.
● Plaques don't itch or hurt.
● Plaques may have ulcers in the center.

CAUSES—Unknown. 60% occur in patients with diabetes mellitus; however, less than 0.5% of diabetic persons develop NLD.

RISK INCREASES WITH—Diabetes.

HOW TO PREVENT—Cannot be prevented at present—even with good control of diabetes.

 WHAT TO EXPECT

APPROPRIATE HEALTH CARE
● Self-care.
● Doctor's treatment.
● Biopsy (see Glossary).

DIAGNOSTIC MEASURES
● Your own observation of symptoms.
● Medical history and physical exam by a doctor.

POSSIBLE COMPLICATIONS—Lesions may ulcerate or become infected, delaying or preventing healing.

PROBABLE OUTCOME—The lesions of NLD are slow to heal; they sometimes remain for several years. In rare cases, they are incurable, but life expectancy is not affected.

 HOW TO TREAT

NOTE—Follow your doctor's instructions. These instructions are supplemental.

MEDICATION—Your doctor may prescribe:
● Topical steroids under occlusion to reduce inflammation. Medicine under an occlusive dressing may sting, burn, itch or cause dryness. It can also cause infection of the hair follicles, acnelike eruptions, secondary infection, changes in skin color, softening of the skin or colored stripes on the skin.
● Steroids injected directly into lesions.
● Aspirin or dipyridamole to interfere with blood clotting. The effectiveness of these drugs for this disorder has not been proved.

GENERAL MEASURES—If topical steroids with occlusion have been prescribed:
● Gently rub a small amount of steroid medicine into the affected area.
● Reapply a small amount.
● Cover the area with clear, pliable, non-porous plastic wrap. To provide additional moisture, if needed: cover the area with a damp, clean cloth before applying the plastic, or briefly soak the affected area in water after applying the medicine.
● Change the dressing as often as your doctor instructs.
● Reapply medicine every time you change the plastic-film dressing.

ACTIVITY—No restrictions.

DIET—No special diet.

 CALL YOUR DOCTOR IF

● You have symptoms of NLD.
● Lesions don't improve in 2 months, despite treatment.
● Lesions ulcerate in the center.
● Signs of infection, such as swelling, pain, redness, tenderness or fever, appear around lesions.
● New, unexplained symptoms develop. Drugs used in treatment may produce side effects.

NOSE FRACTURE

GENERAL INFORMATION

DEFINITION—Fracture or damage to the bones and cartilage of the nose. This often happens when other facial bones are also fractured.

BODY PARTS INVOLVED—Nose.

SEX OR AGE MOST AFFECTED—Older children (over age 8) and adults. Young children's noses have only cartilage.

SIGNS & SYMPTOMS
- Pain in the nose.
- Nosebleed.
- Swollen, discolored nose.
- Inability to breathe through the nose.
- Crooked or misshapen nose (sometimes).

CAUSES—Injury to the nose.

RISK INCREASES WITH—Previous nose injury.

HOW TO PREVENT—Protect your nose from injury, whenever possible. Wear protective headgear for contact sports or when riding motorcycles or bicycles. Wear auto seat belts.

WHAT TO EXPECT

APPROPRIATE HEALTH CARE
- Self-care after diagnosis of minor injuries.
- Doctor's treatment.
- Emergency-room treatment for heavy bleeding.
- Surgery, if the nose is crooked or breathing is impaired.

DIAGNOSTIC MEASURES
- Your own observation of symptoms.
- Medical history and physical exam by a doctor.
- Laboratory blood tests, if bleeding is heavy.
- X-ray of the nose.

POSSIBLE COMPLICATIONS
- Infection of the nose and sinuses.
- Shock from loss of blood (rare).
- Permanent breathing difficulty.
- Permanent change in appearance.

PROBABLE OUTCOME—Minor fractures with no deformity usually heal in 4 weeks. Major fractures can be repaired with surgery. If surgery is necessary, it should be done within 2 weeks or not until 6 months after injury.

HOW TO TREAT

NOTE—Follow your doctor's instructions. These instructions are supplemental.

GENERAL MEASURES
- Apply ice packs to the nose immediately after injury to minimize swelling.
- If the nosebleed is heavy or cannot be stopped, obtain emergency medical treatment.

MEDICATION
- For minor discomfort, you may use non-prescription drugs such as acetaminophen.
- Your doctor may prescribe:
  Stronger pain relievers, if needed.
  Antibiotics, if infection develops.

ACTIVITY—Rest until bleeding stops.

DIET—No special diet.

CALL YOUR DOCTOR IF

- You have symptoms of a fractured nose, especially bleeding that is heavy or cannot be stopped.
- You have had a fractured nose and think surgery is needed.

NOSEBLEED
(Epistaxis)

 GENERAL INFORMATION

DEFINITION—Bleeding from the nose.

BODY PARTS INVOLVED—Blood vessels (arteries and veins) in the nose. In children, nosebleeds occur close to the nose opening. In adults, they usually occur deeper in the nose.

SEX OR AGE MOST AFFECTED—All ages, but twice as common in children as adults.

SIGNS & SYMPTOMS
- Blood oozing from the nostril. If the nosebleed is close to the nostril, the blood is bright red. If the nosebleed is deeper in the nose, the blood may be bright or dark.
- Lightheadedness from blood loss.
- Rapid heartbeat, shortness of breath and pallor (with significant blood loss only).

CAUSES
- Injury to the nose or nasal polyps—even simple injury caused by picking the nose.
- Nasal or sinus infection.
- A foreign body in the nose.
- Scarlet fever.
- Malaria or typhoid fever.
- Dry mucous membranes in the nose from any cause.
- Atherosclerosis.
- High blood pressure.
- Bleeding tendencies associated with aplastic anemia, leukemia, thrombocytopenia or liver disease.

RISK INCREASES WITH
- Any disorder listed as a cause.
- Hodgkin's disease.
- Scurvy.
- Rheumatic fever.
- Blood disorders, including leukemia and hemophilia.
- Use of certain drugs, such as anticoagulants, aspirin, or prolonged use of nose drops.
- Exposure to irritating chemicals.
- High altitude or dry climate.

HOW TO PREVENT
- Avoid injury if possible.
- Obtain medical treatment for the underlying cause.
- Humidify the air if you live in a dry climate or at high altitude.

 WHAT TO EXPECT

APPROPRIATE HEALTH CARE
- Self-care (see General Measures).
- Doctor's treatment or emergency-room treatment if self-care is unsuccessful. Gauze packing may be inserted to absorb blood, stop dripping and exert pressure on the ruptured blood vessels. Continued bleeding may require cauterization (see Glossary).
- Surgery (for severe bleeding only) to tie off the artery feeding the bleeding area.

DIAGNOSTIC MEASURES
- Your own observation of symptoms.
- Medical history and physical exam by a doctor.
- Laboratory blood studies.

POSSIBLE COMPLICATIONS—Bleeding severe enough to require transfusion.

PROBABLE OUTCOME—Symptoms can be controlled with treatment. Severe bleeding requires hospitalization and usually is caused by an underlying disorder, such as liver disease, blood disease or hypertension. In these cases, the underlying disorder should be treated also.

 HOW TO TREAT

NOTE—Follow your doctor's instructions. These instructions are supplemental.

GENERAL MEASURES
- Sit up with your head bent forward.
- Clamp your nose closed with your fingers for 5 uninterrupted minutes. During this time, breathe through your mouth.
- If bleeding stops and recurs, repeat—but pinch your nose firmly on both sides for 8 to 10 minutes. Holding your nose tightly closed allows the blood to clot and seal the damaged blood vessels.
- You may apply cold compresses at the same time.
- Don't blow your nose for 12 hours after bleeding stops to avoid dislodging the blood clot.
- Don't swallow blood. It may upset your stomach or make you "gag," causing you to inhale blood.
- Don't talk (also to avoid gagging).

MEDICATION—Your doctor may prescribe drugs to treat any underlying serious disorder.

ACTIVITY—Resume your normal activities as soon as symptoms improve.

DIET—No special diet.

 CALL YOUR DOCTOR IF

- You have a nosebleed that won't stop with self-care described above.
- After the nosebleed, you become nauseous or vomit.
- After the nose has been packed, your temperature rises to 101F (38.3C) or higher.

OBESITY

GENERAL INFORMATION

DEFINITION—Excess fat stored in the body.

BODY PARTS INVOLVED—Total body.

SEX OR AGE MOST AFFECTED—Both sexes; all ages.

SIGNS & SYMPTOMS—Weight of 20% or more than ideal for height and body frame. Most obese persons have no symptoms except associated emotional problems and poor exercise tolerance. Excess weight increases the heart's work.

CAUSES
- Eating more food than the body can use (most common cause). The body cannot store protein and carbohydrates, so excess is converted to fat and stored. 1 pound of fat represents about 3,500 excess calories, depending on individual metabolism.
- Diseases of the central nervous system, such as brain tumor or stroke (rare).
- Disorders of the endocrine glands (rare).

RISK INCREASES WITH
- Excess alcohol consumption.
- Genetic factors. Some people remain thin despite a large food intake, and vice versa.
- A decrease in exercise with no corresponding decrease in food intake.
- Stress, depression, nervous tension, boredom, frustration or dissatisfaction.
- Poor eating habits learned in childhood.

HOW TO PREVENT
- Avoid a sedentary lifestyle. Exercise daily, or at least 3 times a week.
- Eat less food high in fat and sugar. Concentrate on not gaining weight, rather than on gaining and then reducing.
- Limit alcohol consumption to 1 or 2 drinks a day, if any.

OTHER—Surgical procedures to reduce weight, such as bypassing part of the intestine or stomach, cutting away fat, fat suctioning, or wiring the jaw shut, are desperate measures. They are used only in extreme circumstances.

WHAT TO EXPECT

APPROPRIATE HEALTH CARE
- Self-care.
- Doctor's treatment (sometimes).
- Psychotherapy or counseling.

DIAGNOSTIC MEASURES
- Your own observation of symptoms.
- Medical history and physical exam by a doctor.
- Laboratory blood studies of endocrine function.

POSSIBLE COMPLICATIONS—Obesity may contribute to the development of diabetes, high blood pressure, heart disease and gallbladder disease. It complicates treatment and decreases survival chances of patients with stroke, kidney disease and other disorders.

PROBABLE OUTCOME—Obesity can be controlled if motivation stays high for life.

HOW TO TREAT

NOTE—Follow your doctor's instructions. These instructions are supplemental.

GENERAL MEASURES—Join a support group for overweight persons. Many people find it easier to follow a reduction diet and exercise program if they join a group of people with similar problems.

MEDICATION—Most doctors don't recommend medication to aid weight loss. Medications often cause harmful side effects or adverse reactions. At best, they control appetite only for short time periods and don't help you change eating habits.

ACTIVITY—Increase your current level of activity. Daily exercise (bicycle riding, walking, swimming and others) helps you lose weight, feel better and control appetite.

DIET—See Appendix 1 for a reducing diet. The diet is varied and balanced. Choose foods you like so you can establish eating patterns you can maintain indefinitely.

Some nutritionists suggest 4 or 5 small meals a day rather than 3. Skipping meals does not help in losing weight in the long term.

Diets that are not nutritionally balanced can cause more problems than the obesity. Crash diets and fad diets don't produce long-term results.

During your diet and exercise program, there may be periods when you don't lose weight. This is normal; don't stop the program. Weight loss will begin again in a week or two.

A realistic weight loss is 1 to 2-1/2 pounds a week. This may seem slow, but 1 pound of fat lost per week totals 52 pounds in 1 year!

CALL YOUR DOCTOR IF

Obesity increases, despite your self-help measures.

ILLNESSES & DISORDERS

ORAL CANCER

GENERAL INFORMATION

DEFINITION—Growth of malignant cells in the mouth or tongue. These are rare but dangerous.

BODY PARTS INVOLVED—Lips; gums; palate; tongue; membranes inside the lip or cheek; floor of the mouth.

SEX OR AGE MOST AFFECTED—Adults over 40.

SIGNS & SYMPTOMS—A pale lump—usually painless—with a hard rim that appears in any part of the mouth or tongue. It has the following characteristics:
- It enlarges, ulcerates and bleeds easily.
- It may prevent dentures from fitting properly.
- It may make the tongue stiff and difficult to control, causing speaking and swallowing difficulty.

CAUSES—Unknown.

RISK INCREASES WITH
- Use of tobacco in any form.
- Family history of oral cancer.

HOW TO PREVENT—Don't use tobacco.

WHAT TO EXPECT

APPROPRIATE HEALTH CARE
- Self-care after diagnosis.
- Doctor's treatment.
- Surgery to remove the cancerous area.
- Radiation therapy.
- Speech therapy, if surgery impairs speech.

DIAGNOSTIC MEASURES
- Your own observation of symptoms.
- Medical history and physical exam by a doctor.
- Laboratory blood studies.
- Biopsy (see Glossary) of the lump.
- X-rays of the head.

POSSIBLE COMPLICATIONS
- Slow healing after surgery.
- Spread to lymph nodes in the neck, requiring radical head and neck surgery.
- Permanent disfigurement.
- Permanent speech impairment.

PROBABLE OUTCOME—Usually curable with early detection and treatment. Normal facial appearance can often be restored by plastic surgery.

HOW TO TREAT

NOTE—Follow your doctor's instructions. These instructions are supplemental.

GENERAL MEASURES—After surgery, cleanse the mouth 3 to 4 times a day with a soothing salt-water solution (1 teaspoon salt to 8 oz. warm water).

MEDICATION—Your doctor may prescribe:
- Anticancer drugs.
- Pain relievers after surgery.
- Antibiotics, if infection coexists.

ACTIVITY—Resume your normal activities gradually after surgery.

DIET—No special diet after recovery. A liquid diet may be necessary for several days after surgery.

CALL YOUR DOCTOR IF

- You have signs of a mouth or tongue tumor.
- The following occurs after surgery:
  Increasing pain.
  Fever.
  New lumps.
  Excessive bleeding.

OSGOOD-SCHLATTER DISEASE
(Osteochondrosis)

GENERAL INFORMATION

DEFINITION—A temporary condition of the leg at the knee, characterized by swelling, tenderness and pain.

BODY PARTS INVOLVED—Tibial tubercle, a prominence just below the knee cap attached to a large thigh muscle connecting the bone of the upper leg (femur) to the large bone in the lower leg (tibia). This disorder often affects both knees.

SEX OR AGE MOST AFFECTED—Adolescents of both sexes. It is uncommon after age 16.

SIGNS & SYMPTOMS
- A slightly swollen, warm and tender bump below the knee.
- Pain with activity, especially straightening the leg against force, as in stair-climbing, jumping or weight-lifting.

CAUSES—Stress or injury of the tibial tubercle, which is still developing during adolescence. Repeated stress or injury interferes with development, causing inflammation.

RISK INCREASES WITH
- Overzealous conditioning routines, such as running, jumping or jogging.
- Overweight.

HOW TO PREVENT
- Help an overweight child lose weight. A reducing diet appears in Appendix 1.
- Encourage your child to exercise moderately, avoiding extremes.

WHAT TO EXPECT

APPROPRIATE HEALTH CARE
- Home care after diagnosis.
- Doctor's treatment.

DIAGNOSTIC MEASURES
- Your own observation of symptoms.
- Medical history and physical exam by a doctor.
- X-ray of the knee.

POSSIBLE COMPLICATIONS
- Bone infection.
- Recurrence of the condition in adulthood.

PROBABLE OUTCOME—Usually curable with treatment in 4 to 8 months.

HOW TO TREAT

NOTE—Follow your doctor's instructions. These instructions are supplemental.

GENERAL MEASURES—Use heat to relieve pain. Warm compresses, heating pads, warm whirlpool baths, heat lamps, diathermy or ultrasound are effective.

MEDICATION
- For minor discomfort, you may use non-prescription drugs such as aspirin.
- Your doctor may prescribe cortisone injections, if other treatment fails. Cortisone injections may weaken tendons, so it is better to give the condition more time to heal than to use them.

ACTIVITY—Resting the affected leg is the most important treatment. This is done with:
- Crutches.
- A leg cast or splint.
- An elastic knee brace that prevents the knee from bending fully.
The child should not participate in sports during treatment. This is temporary, and normal activity can be resumed when inflammation subsides.

DIET—No special diet, unless the child is overweight. See Appendix 10 for a reducing diet.

CALL YOUR DOCTOR IF

- Your child has symptoms of Osgood-Schlatter disease.
- The following occurs during treatment:
  Symptoms don't improve in 4 weeks, despite treatment.
  Pain increases.
  Temperature rises to 101F (38.3C).

OSTEOARTHRITIS
(Degenerative Joint Disease; Hypertrophic Arthritis)

 GENERAL INFORMATION

DEFINITION—Degeneration of cartilage at a joint and growth of bone "spurs" that inflame surrounding tissue.

BODY PARTS INVOLVED—All joints, but most common in fingers, feet, knees, hips and spine.

SEX OR AGE MOST AFFECTED—Adults over 45.

SIGNS & SYMPTOMS
- Joint stiffness and pain, including backache. Weather changes, especially cold, damp weather, may increase aching.
- Limited movement and loss of dexterity in affected joints.
- No redness, heat or fever in affected joints (usually).
- Swelling of affected joints (sometimes), especially finger joints.
- Cracking or grating sounds with joint movement (sometimes).

CAUSES
- Stress on the joints caused by activity and aging. Almost all people over age 50 have some osteoarthritis.
- Injury to the joint lining.

RISK INCREASES WITH
- Poor posture.
- Obesity.
- Persons with occupations that stress joints, such as dancers, football players, instrumental musicians or carpet layers.

HOW TO PREVENT
- Maintain a normal weight.
- Be physically active, but avoid activities that lead to joint injury, especially after age 40.

 WHAT TO EXPECT

APPROPRIATE HEALTH CARE
- Self-care after diagnosis.
- Doctor's treatment.
- Acupuncture (sometimes).
- Physical therapy for muscle and joint rehabilitation (severe cases only).

DIAGNOSTIC MEASURES
- Your own observation of symptoms.
- Medical history and physical exam by a doctor.
- Laboratory blood studies to rule out inflammatory forms of arthritis.
- X-rays of painful joints.

POSSIBLE COMPLICATIONS
- Crippling (sometimes). This is preventable with treatment.

- Muscles around affected joints may become smaller and weaker because of decreased use due to pain.

PROBABLE OUTCOME—Symptoms can usually be relieved, but joint changes are permanent. Pain may begin as a minor irritant, but it can become severe enough to interfere with daily activities and sleep. As degeneration occurs, pain may decrease.

 HOW TO TREAT

NOTE—Follow your doctor's instructions. These instructions are supplemental.

GENERAL MEASURES
- To relieve pain, apply heat to painful and stiff joints for 20 minutes 2 or 3 times a day. Use hot towels, hot tubs, infrared heat lamps, electric heating pads or deep-heating ointments or lotions. Swim often in a heated pool or move around in a whirlpool spa.
- If osteoarthritis of the neck causes pain in the arms, wear a soft, immobilizing collar (Thomas collar). If this isn't helpful, buy or rent a neck-traction device for home use.
- Massage the muscles around painful joints. Massaging the joint itself is not helpful.
- If osteoarthritis affects the spine, sleep on your back on a very firm mattress or place 3/4-inch plywood between your box springs and mattress. Waterbeds help some people.
- Avoid chilling. Wear thermal underwear or avoid outdoor activity in cold weather.
- Consider moving to a warm, dry climate, such as southwest desert areas of the U.S.
- Keep a positive outlook on life. Don't think of yourself as an invalid. Remain active to prevent wasting of muscles.

MEDICATION—Your doctor may prescribe:
- Aspirin or other non-steroidal anti-inflammatory drugs.
- Cortisone injections into painful, stiff joints. These may provide temporary relief.
  Don't take oral cortisone drugs. They are not effective for long-term relief and have many harmful side effects.

ACTIVITY—Rest is important only during acute phases of the disease when joints are very painful. Resume normal activity as soon as symptoms improve.

DIET—If you are overweight, lose weight. A reducing diet appears in Appendix 1.

 CALL YOUR DOCTOR IF

- You have joint pain or stiffness.
- New, unexplained symptoms develop. Drugs used in treatment may produce side effects.

OSTEOMYELITIS

GENERAL INFORMATION

DEFINITION—Infection of the bone and bone marrow.

BODY PARTS INVOLVED—Any bone in the body. In a child, the femur (upper-leg bone), tibia (lower-leg bone) or humerus or radius (bones in the arm) is usually affected. In an adult, the pelvis or spine is usually affected.

SEX OR AGE MOST AFFECTED
- Both sexes, but more common in males.
- All ages, but most common in rapidly growing children (5 to 14 years).

SIGNS & SYMPTOMS
- Fever. Sometimes this is the only symptom.
- Pain, swelling, redness, warmth and tenderness in the area over the infected bone, especially when moving a nearby joint. Nearby joints—especially the knee—may also be red, warm and swollen.
  If a child is too young to talk, signs of pain are: reluctance to move an arm or leg or refusal to walk; limping; or screaming when the limb is touched or moved.
- Pus drainage through a skin abscess, without fever or severe pain (chronic osteomyelitis only).
- General ill feeling.

CAUSES—Usually staphylococcal infection, but many other bacteria may be responsible. The bacteria may spread to the bone through the bloodstream from the following sources:
- Compound fracture or other injury.
- Boil, carbuncle or any break in the skin.
- Middle-ear infection.
- Pneumonia.

RISK INCREASES WITH
- Illness that has lowered resistance.
- Rapid growth during childhood.

HOW TO PREVENT—Obtain prompt medical treatment of any bacterial infection to prevent its spread to bone or other body parts.

WHAT TO EXPECT

APPROPRIATE HEALTH CARE
- Doctor's treatment.
- Hospitalization for surgery to drain abscesses or to remove pockets of infected bone, and to administer high doses of antibiotics—sometimes intravenously.

DIAGNOSTIC MEASURES
- Your own observation of symptoms.
- Medical history and physical exam by a doctor.
- Laboratory blood studies and blood cultures to identify the bacteria.
- X-rays of the bone. X-rays often don't show changes until 2 to 3 weeks after the infection begins.
- CAT scan (see Glossary).

POSSIBLE COMPLICATIONS
- Abscess that breaks through the skin and won't heal until the underlying bone heals.
- Permanent stiffness in a nearby joint (rare).
- Blood poisoning that makes amputation necessary (rare).

PROBABLE OUTCOME—Usually curable with prompt and aggressive treatment.

HOW TO TREAT

NOTE—Follow your doctor's instructions. These instructions apply to home care after hospitalization for treatment of the infection.

GENERAL MEASURES
- Wear sterile gloves to change dressings.
- Keep the involved limb level or slightly elevated and immobilized with pillows. Don't let it dangle.
- Keep unaffected parts of the body as active as possible to prevent pressure sores during required, prolonged bed rest.

MEDICATION—Your doctor may prescribe:
- Large doses of antibiotics, usually intravenously. Antibiotics may be necessary—either orally or by injection—for 8 to 10 weeks.
- Pain relievers.
- Laxatives, if constipation develops during prolonged bed rest.

ACTIVITY—Rest in bed until 2 to 3 weeks after symptoms disappear. Resume your normal activities gradually.

DIET—No special diet. Eat heartily. Take vitamin and mineral supplements.

CALL YOUR DOCTOR IF

- You or your child have symptoms of osteomyelitis.
- The following occurs during treatment:
  An abscess forms over the infected bone, or drainage from an existing abscess increases.
  Fever rises to 101F (38.3C) or higher.
  Pain becomes intolerable.
- New, unexplained symptoms develop. Drugs used in treatment may produce side effects.

OSTEOPOROSIS

GENERAL INFORMATION

DEFINITION—Loss of normal bone density, mass and strength, leading to increased porousness and vulnerability to fracture.

BODY PARTS INVOLVED—Bones.

SEX OR AGE MOST AFFECTED—Women after menopause.

SIGNS & SYMPTOMS—Early symptoms:
- Backache.
- No symptoms (often).
Late symptoms:
- Sudden back pain with a cracking sound indicating fracture.
- Deformed spinal column with humps.
- Loss of height.
- Fractures occurring with minor injury, especially of the hip or arm.

CAUSES—Loss of bony structure and strength. Factors include:
- Prolonged lack of adequate calcium and protein in the diet.
- Low estrogen levels after menopause.
- Decreased activity with increased age.
- Smoking (possibly).
- Use of cortisone drugs.
- Prolonged disease, including alcoholism.
- Vitamin deficiency (especially of vitamin D).
- Hyperthyroidism.
- Cancer.

RISK INCREASES WITH
- Surgery to remove the ovaries.
- Radiation treatment for ovarian cancer.
- Chronic or recurrent urinary-tract or other pelvic infections.
- Poor nutrition, especially inadequate calcium and protein.
- Body type. Thin women with a small frame are more susceptible.

HOW TO PREVENT
- Ensure an adequate calcium intake—up to 1500mg a day—with milk and milk products or calcium supplements.
- Exercise regularly.
- Protect yourself against falls, especially in the home.
- Consult your doctor about taking estrogen, calcium and fluoride after menopause begins or the ovaries have been removed.

OTHER—Older persons may need assistance in maintaining a good diet, remaining physically active, and creating an accident-proof home environment.

WHAT TO EXPECT

APPROPRIATE HEALTH CARE
- Self-care.
- Doctor's treatment.

DIAGNOSTIC MEASURES
- Your own observation of symptoms.
- Medical history and physical exam by a doctor.
- X-rays of bones.

POSSIBLE COMPLICATIONS—Bone fracture, especially of the hip or spine, after a fall. Sometimes a bone will break or collapse without injury or a fall.

PROBABLE OUTCOME—Diet, calcium and fluoride supplements, vitamin D, exercise and estrogen can halt—and may reverse—bone deterioration. Fractures will heal with standard treatment.

HOW TO TREAT

NOTE—Follow your doctor's instructions. These instructions are supplemental.

MEDICATION
- For minor pain, you may use non-prescription drugs such as acetaminophen.
- Your doctor may prescribe calcium and vitamin-D supplements or estrogen.

GENERAL MEASURES
- Avoid all circumstances which may lead to injury. Stay off icy streets and wet or waxed floors. Hold banisters when using stairs, and make sure banisters are sturdy.
- If estrogen is prescribed, visit your doctor for regular pelvic exams and Pap smears. Examine your breasts for lumps once a month. Report any vaginal bleeding or discharge.
- Use heat or ice in any form to ease pain.
- Sleep on a firm mattress.
- Use a back brace, if prescribed by your doctor.
- Use correct posture when lifting.
- See Back Care (Appendix 14).

ACTIVITY—Stay active, but avoid the risk of falls. Exercise—especially weight-bearing exercise, such as walking or running—helps maintain bone strength.

DIET—Eat a normal, well-balanced diet high in protein, calcium and vitamin D.

CALL YOUR DOCTOR IF

- You have symptoms of osteoporosis.
- Pain develops, especially after injury.
- New, unexplained symptoms develop, such as vaginal bleeding. Drugs used in treatment may produce side effects.

OTOSCLEROSIS

GENERAL INFORMATION

DEFINITION—Slow formation of abnormal spongy bone growth in the middle ear. The growth prevents one of the small bones in the middle ear from vibrating sound waves, leading to hearing loss.

BODY PARTS INVOLVED—Middle-ear bones and nerves in the ear that allow us to hear. Otosclerosis usually affects both ears.

SEX OR AGE MOST AFFECTED
- Both sexes, but twice as likely in females.
- All ages, but most common from ages 15 to 30.

SIGNS & SYMPTOMS
- Slow, progressive hearing loss.
- Ringing in the ears.
- Hearing that is better in noisy environments than quiet ones.

CAUSES—Inherited. This is a dominant genetic trait.

RISK INCREASES WITH
- Family history of hearing loss.
- Caucasian heritage. Otosclerosis affects to some degree about 10% of all white people.
- Pregnancy, which may trigger the onset.

HOW TO PREVENT—Cannot be prevented at present. Obtain genetic counseling before starting a family if you or your spouse have otosclerosis.

WHAT TO EXPECT

APPROPRIATE HEALTH CARE
- Doctor's treatment.
- Surgery to remove the stapes (a bone in the middle ear).

DIAGNOSTIC MEASURES
- Your own observation of symptoms.
- Medical history and physical exam by a doctor.
- Laboratory studies such as audiogram and Rinne test (see Glossary).

POSSIBLE COMPLICATIONS—Total deafness in 10 to 15 years without treatment. The younger the patient, the more rapid the hearing loss.

PROBABLE OUTCOME—In most cases, hearing is at least partially restored with surgery.

HOW TO TREAT

NOTE—Follow your doctor's instructions. These instructions are supplemental.

GENERAL MEASURES—To prevent complications after surgery:
- Don't blow your nose for 1 week.
- Avoid unnecessary contact with persons who have a respiratory infection, such as a cold, flu or bronchitis.
- Protect ears against cold.
- Avoid activities that might cause dizziness, such as bending, lifting or straining.
- Avoid loud noises and sudden pressure changes (flying or scuba diving) for 6 months or until healing is complete.

MEDICATION—Your doctor may prescribe antibiotics after surgery.

ACTIVITY—After surgery, resume your normal activities gradually.

DIET—No special diet.

CALL YOUR DOCTOR IF

- You have symptoms of otosclerosis.
- Signs of infection, such as fever, pain or excessive dizziness, develop after treatment.

OVARIAN CANCER

 GENERAL INFORMATION

DEFINITION—A malignant growth in the ovary that is likely to spread to other body parts and threaten life.

BODY PARTS INVOLVED—One or both ovaries. It may spread to the lungs and bone.

SEX OR AGE MOST AFFECTED—Females of all ages, but most common between ages 40 and 65.

SIGNS & SYMPTOMS—Frequently no symptoms occur until the tumor becomes large. The earliest symptoms include:
- Vague discomfort in the lower abdomen.
- Gastrointestinal upsets.
- Irregular menstrual periods.
Later symptoms:
- Deep voice.
- Excessive hair growth.
- Unexplained weight loss.
- An enlarged, hard and sometimes tender mass in the lower abdomen.
- Pain with intercourse.
- Anemia.

CAUSES—Unknown.

RISK INCREASES WITH—Unknown.

HOW TO PREVENT—Have yearly pelvic examinations, which offer the best chance of early detection and cure.

 WHAT TO EXPECT

APPROPRIATE HEALTH CARE
- Doctor's treatment.
- Surgery to remove the cancerous ovary and other affected areas, including Fallopian tubes, uterus and the other ovary (sometimes).
- Radiation treatment.
- Psychotherapy or counseling to learn to accept and cope with cancer.

DIAGNOSTIC MEASURES
- Your own observation of symptoms.
- Medical history and physical exam by a doctor.
- Laboratory blood studies.
- Sonogram (see Glossary) of the abdomen.
- X-rays of the abdomen.
- Surgical diagnostic procedures, such as culdoscopy and laparoscopy (see Glossary).

POSSIBLE COMPLICATIONS—Death from spread of cancer to other body parts.

PROBABLE OUTCOME—25% to 50% of women with ovarian cancer survive at least 5 years after treatment.

 HOW TO TREAT

NOTE—Follow your doctor's instructions. These instructions are supplemental.

GENERAL MEASURES—For an explanation of surgery and postoperative care, see Hysterectomy (in Surgery section).

MEDICATION—Your doctor may prescribe:
- Anticancer drugs.
- Pain relievers.
- Female hormones until menopause.

ACTIVITY—No restrictions after recovery from surgery.

DIET—Eat a normal, well-balanced diet that is high in protein to promote repair of body tissues.

 CALL YOUR DOCTOR IF

- You have symptoms of an ovarian tumor.
- The following occurs after surgery:
  Increased pain, swelling, redness or drainage from the surgical wound.
  Pain or swelling in the leg.
  Signs of infection, such as fever, chills, headache or muscle aches.

OVARIAN CYST

 ## GENERAL INFORMATION

DEFINITION—A closed cavity or sac containing liquid or semisolid material which develops in the ovary. Ovarian cysts are rarely cancerous.

BODY PARTS INVOLVED—Ovary; fallopian tubes; peritoneum; colon.

SEX OR AGE MOST AFFECTED—Women of all ages.

SIGNS & SYMPTOMS—Some produce no symptoms. Others produce any of the following:
- Swelling without pain in the lower abdomen.
- Painful sexual intercourse.
- Stinging or burning on urination (if the cyst presses on the bladder).
- Difficulty emptying the bladder completely.
- Brownish vaginal discharge.
- Irregular menstruation or increased hairiness (if the cyst produces excess hormones).

The following may occur if the cyst twists, bleeds or breaks:
- Severe abdominal pain.
- Fever.
- Vomiting.

CAUSES—Hormone disturbance. Ovarian cysts sometimes develop during pregnancy.

RISK INCREASES WITH
- Pregnancy.
- Use of hormones.

HOW TO PREVENT—Cannot be prevented at present.

 ## WHAT TO EXPECT

APPROPRIATE HEALTH CARE
- Doctor's treatment.
- Surgery to drain the cyst through a laparoscope (see Glossary) or surgery to remove the ovary.

DIAGNOSTIC MEASURES
- Your own observation of symptoms.
- Medical history and physical exam—including a complete pelvic examination—by a doctor.
- X-ray of the abdomen.
- Pelvic ultrasonography (see Glossary).

POSSIBLE COMPLICATIONS
- Rupture of the cyst or twisting of the cyst's stalk. This requires emergency surgery.
- Urinary obstruction.
- Increased risk of ovarian cancer.

PROBABLE OUTCOME—Ovarian cysts are curable with surgery. Without surgery, they often recur.

 ## HOW TO TREAT

NOTE—Follow your doctor's instructions. These instructions are supplemental.

GENERAL MEASURES—For an explanation of surgery and postoperative care, see Ovarian-Cyst or Tumor Removal (in Surgery section).

MEDICATION—Medicine is usually not necessary for this disorder. For minor discomfort, you may use non-prescription drugs such as acetaminophen.

ACTIVITY—No restrictions. If surgery is necessary, resume activities gradually.

DIET—No special diet.

 ## CALL YOUR DOCTOR IF

- You have symptoms of an ovarian cyst.
- Any of the following develops after diagnosis:
  You lose weight for no apparent reason.
  You feel generally ill.
  You have pain in the lower abdomen.
  You have severe abdominal pain, nausea, and fever that comes on suddenly. This may indicate rupture of a cyst.

OVARIAN TUMOR, BENIGN

GENERAL INFORMATION

DEFINITION—A benign, cystic (saclike) tumor on the ovary that contains fluid or semisolid material. These are usually small, but in some cases they may grow large enough to make a woman appear pregnant. Ovarian tumors are usually benign, but a few undergo malignant change.

BODY PARTS INVOLVED—One or both ovaries.

SEX OR AGE MOST AFFECTED—Females between puberty and menopause.

SIGNS & SYMPTOMS—May not cause symptoms. If symptoms occur, they may include:
- Mild pelvic pain.
- Pain in the lower back.
- Discomfort with sexual intercourse.
- Abnormal menstruation, including changes in menstrual flow, length of periods and intervals between periods.
- Excessive hair growth, deep voice and weight gain (sometimes).

If a large ovarian tumor twists or ruptures, the following will occur in the lower abdomen:
- Severe pain.
- Rigid muscles.
- Swelling.

CAUSES—Unknown, but it is probably related to abnormalities of female hormone production and secretion.

RISK INCREASES WITH—Unknown.

HOW TO PREVENT—No specific preventive measures.

WHAT TO EXPECT

APPROPRIATE HEALTH CARE
- Doctor's treatment.
- Surgery to remove the tumor or diseased ovary (sometimes).

DIAGNOSTIC MEASURES
- Your own observation of symptoms.
- Medical history and physical exam by a doctor.
- Laboratory blood studies.
- Laparoscopy, a surgical diagnostic procedure. A small tube is inserted in the abdomen under local anesthesia. The tube allows the doctor to see the organs and biopsy or drain the tumor, if necessary.

POSSIBLE COMPLICATIONS—Emergency abdominal surgery caused by twisting, rupture or bleeding of a tumor.

PROBABLE OUTCOME—Most ovarian tumors require no treatment and disappear spontaneously within 2 months.

Some tumors require surgery to diagnose accurately, ruling out malignancy, or to treat. If one ovary must be removed, normal conception and childbirth is possible as long as a normal ovary remains on the other side.

HOW TO TREAT

NOTE—Follow your doctor's instructions. These instructions are supplemental.

GENERAL MEASURES
- Have yearly medical checkups and pelvic exams to detect tumors early. Treatment may not be necessary, except to have regular pelvic examinations so the tumor's growth can be monitored.
- If surgery is required, see Laparotomy (in Surgery section) for an explanation of surgery and postoperative care.

MEDICATION—Your doctor may prescribe female hormones or clomiphene. These help shrink or destroy some tumors.

ACTIVITY—No restrictions if surgery is not necessary.

DIET—No special diet.

CALL YOUR DOCTOR IF

- You have symptoms of an ovarian tumor, especially severe pain, rigidity and abdominal distention.
- New, unexplained symptoms develop. Drugs used in treatment may produce side effects.

PAGET'S DISEASE
(Osteitis Deformans)

 GENERAL INFORMATION

DEFINITION—A gradual, progressive bone disease, characterized by bones breaking down and regenerating excessively. New bone is fragile and weak. This affects 2.5 million people in the U.S., and it occurs worldwide. It is not cancerous.

BODY PARTS INVOLVED—Bones of the skull, spine, legs, collar bone and pelvis.

SEX OR AGE MOST AFFECTED—Both sexes, but most common in men over age 40.

SIGNS & SYMPTOMS—Early stages:
• Mild bone pain.
Later stages:
• Affected bones are chronically painful—especially at night—enlarged, misshapen, tender and warm.
• Movement is impaired.
• Spinal curvature compresses sensory nerves.
• Fractures occur from minor trauma and heal slowly with deformity.

CAUSES—Unknown.

RISK INCREASES WITH—Family history of Paget's disease.

HOW TO PREVENT—No specific preventive measures.

 WHAT TO EXPECT

APPROPRIATE HEALTH CARE
• Self-care after diagnosis.
• Doctor's treatment.

DIAGNOSTIC MEASURES
• Your own observation of symptoms.
• Medical history and physical exam by a doctor.
• X-rays of affected bones.
• Laboratory blood and urine studies to determine levels of serum alkaline phosphatase and urinary calcium.

POSSIBLE COMPLICATIONS
• Blindness or hearing loss caused by the skull pressing on the brain.
• High blood pressure.
• Kidney stones.
• Gout.
• Bone cancer.
• Congestive heart failure. The heart is strained by the greatly increased blood flow through diseased bones.
• Misdiagnosis of Paget's disease as an overactive parathyroid gland or spread of cancer from the prostate gland, breast or bone marrow.

PROBABLE OUTCOME—This condition is currently considered incurable. However, symptoms can be relieved or controlled. The disease has a pattern of remissions and flare-ups that become progressively worse. Sometimes adjacent joints become involved. Life expectancy is reduced, but most persons live with the disease for at least 10 to 15 years.

Scientific research into causes and treatment continues, so there is hope for increasingly effective treatment and cure.

 HOW TO TREAT

NOTE—Follow your doctor's instructions. These instructions are supplemental.

GENERAL MEASURES
• Use heat to relieve pain, including hot compresses, hot soaks (see Glossary) or heat lamps.
• If you don't have a firm bed, place 3/4-inch plywood under your mattress.
• Accident-proof your home as much as possible. Avoid throw rugs and slippery floors. Install hand rails next to the tub.

MEDICATION—Your doctor may prescribe: male and female hormones; fluoride; radiation treatment; pain relievers; calcitonin injections; or cytotoxic drugs, such as mithromycin. All relieve pain, but none cure the disease.

ACTIVITY—Rest in bed during active phases. Move or turn often to prevent pressure sores. Resume your normal activities during remissions.

DIET—No special diet.

 CALL YOUR DOCTOR IF

• You have symptoms of Paget's disease.
• The following occurs during treatment:
Fever of 101F (38.3C) or higher.
Unbearable pain.
Weight loss.
Worsening symptoms.
• New, unexplained symptoms develop. Drugs used in treatment may produce side effects.

ILLNESSES & DISORDERS

PANCREAS, CANCER OF

GENERAL INFORMATION

DEFINITION—Uncontrolled growth of malignant cells in the pancreas. This is the 4th leading cause of cancer deaths in the U.S.

BODY PARTS INVOLVED—Pancreas, an organ in the back of the upper abdomen. The pancreas produces intestinal enzymes to help digest food, and insulin to control blood sugar.

SEX OR AGE MOST AFFECTED—Men between ages 35 and 70. It is rare in women.

SIGNS & SYMPTOMS
- Depression.
- Rapid, unexplained weight loss.
- Pain in the back or upper abdomen that is often relieved by bending forward.
- Blood clots in veins anywhere, especially the arms and legs. This is often an early sign.
- Jaundice (yellow skin and eyes) from blockage of the nearby bile duct. Jaundice is usually accompanied by intense itching.

CAUSES—Unknown.

RISK INCREASES WITH
- Chronic pancreatitis.
- Diabetes mellitus.
- Genetic factors. This is more common in blacks than Caucasians.
- Smoking.
- Excess alcohol consumption.
- Geographic location. The incidence is higher in Israel, the U. S., Sweden and Canada than in other parts of the world.
- Poor nutrition, especially a diet high in fat, protein and processed foods containing many food additives.
- Exposure to industrial chemicals, such as urea, naphthalene or benzidine.

HOW TO PREVENT—Cannot be prevented. To reduce the risk:
- Don't smoke.
- Don't drink more than 1 or 2 alcoholic drinks—if any—a day.
- Eat more poultry, fish, fresh fruits and vegetables, and eat less red meat, processed foods and fat in any form.
- Avoid exposure to harmful chemicals.

WHAT TO EXPECT

APPROPRIATE HEALTH CARE
- Doctor's treatment.
- Psychotherapy or counseling to help adjust to incurable illness.
- Surgery to:
  Remove the tumor, if it is small.
  Relieve any bile-duct blockage.
  Relieve or prevent bowel obstruction.

DIAGNOSTIC MEASURES
- Your own observation of symptoms.
- Medical history and physical exam by a doctor.
- Laboratory blood-chemistry studies of the pancreas, liver and gallbladder, and blood-sugar tests.
- Needle biopsy (see Glossary) of the liver.
- Exploratory abdominal surgery (laparotomy).
- X-rays of the abdomen, liver, gallbladder and blood vessels (angiography).
- Ultrasonography (see Glossary) of the pancreas.
- CAT scan (see Glossary) of the pancreas.

POSSIBLE COMPLICATIONS
- Hemorrhage into the intestinal tract.
- Pancreas infections.
- Spread of cancer to liver, other abdominal organs and lungs.

PROBABLE OUTCOME—This condition is currently considered incurable. Survival chances for more than 1 or 2 years are unlikely. However, symptoms can be relieved or controlled.

Scientific research into causes and treatment continues, so there is hope for increasingly effective treatment and cure.

HOW TO TREAT

NOTE—Follow your doctor's instructions. These instructions are supplemental.

GENERAL MEASURES—No specific instructions except those listed under other headings.

MEDICATION—Your doctor may prescribe:
- Antibiotics for coexisting infections.
- Pain relievers.
- Anticancer drugs.
- Pancreatic enzymes to replace those the pancreas cannot manufacture.
- Sedatives for sleep.

ACTIVITY—Remain as active as your strength allows.

DIET—No special diet.

CALL YOUR DOCTOR IF

- You have symptoms of pancreatic cancer.
- The following occurs during treatment:
  Fever and headache.
  Muscle aches and fatigue.
  Nausea and vomiting.
  Severe abdominal pain and swelling.
  Black, tarry stools.
- New, unexplained symptoms develop. Drugs used in treatment may produce side effects.

PANCREATITIS

GENERAL INFORMATION

DEFINITION—Inflammation of the pancreas. Chronic pancreatitis usually follows recurrent attacks of acute pancreatitis, because the pancreas does not recover completely between attacks. It gradually becomes unable to supply digestive juices and hormones necessary for good health.

BODY PARTS INVOLVED—Pancreas.

SEX OR AGE MOST AFFECTED—Adults.

SIGNS & SYMPTOMS—Severe acute pancreatitis:
- Extreme abdominal pain.
- Vomiting.
- Abdominal swelling and gas.
- Fever.
- Muscle aches.
- Drop in blood pressure.
Chronic pancreatitis:
- Persistent, mild or severe pain in the upper abdomen, sometimes radiating to the back or generalized. Pain is aching, burning, gnawing or stabbing. Pain episodes may last days or weeks, but rarely less than 1 day.
- Mild jaundice (yellow skin and eyes).
- Rapid weight loss.

CAUSES
- Alcoholism.
- Disease of the gallbladder or bile ducts.
- Obstruction of the pancreatic duct by stones, scarring or slow-growing cancer (rare).
- Abdominal injury.
- Virus infection.

RISK INCREASES WITH
- Poor nutrition.
- Obesity.
- Excess alcohol consumption.
- Use of drugs, such as sulfa drugs, azothioprene, chlorothiazide or cortisone drugs.

HOW TO PREVENT—Don't drink more than 1 or 2 alcoholic drinks—if any—a day.

WHAT TO EXPECT

APPROPRIATE HEALTH CARE
- Doctor's treatment.
- Hospitalization (severe cases).

DIAGNOSTIC MEASURES
- Your own observation of symptoms.
- Medical history and physical exam by a doctor. This may be difficult to diagnose.
- Laboratory studies, such as blood and urine tests and radioisotope scans (see Glossary).
- X-rays of the pancreas.
- CAT scan (see Glossary) of the pancreas.

POSSIBLE COMPLICATIONS
- Diabetes mellitus.
- Chronic calcium deficiency.
- Secondary bacterial infection in the pancreas.
- Massive hemorrhage and destruction of the pancreas.

PROBABLE OUTCOME—Acute pancreatitis is usually curable in 5 to 7 days with intensive care. Treatment includes resting the gastrointestinal tract completely and providing intravenous fluids and nourishment. About 5% of cases don't respond to treatment and are fatal.

Chronic pancreatitis may cause recurrent attacks for many years.

HOW TO TREAT

NOTE—Follow your doctor's instructions. These instructions are supplemental.

GENERAL MEASURES—Use heat from a heating pad, heat lamp or hot compresses to relieve pain.

MEDICATION—Your doctor may prescribe:
- Pain relievers.
- Digestive enzymes that the damaged pancreas cannot manufacture.
- Antibiotics, if bacterial infection develops.

ACTIVITY—No restrictions.

DIET—No special diet. Abstain totally from drinking alcohol.

CALL YOUR DOCTOR IF

- You have symptoms of acute pancreatitis.
- The following occurs during or after treatment:
  Jaundice.
  Fever of 101F (38.3C) or higher.
  Continued weight loss.
  Signs of calcium deficiency, such as muscle cramps or seizures.

ILLNESSES & DISORDERS

PARAPLEGIA OR QUADRIPLEGIA

 ## GENERAL INFORMATION

DEFINITION
- Paraplegia is partial or complete paralysis of both legs.
- Quadriplegia is partial or complete paralysis of both arms *and* legs.

BODY PARTS INVOLVED—Spinal cord and all body parts below the spinal-cord damage.

SEX OR AGE MOST AFFECTED—Both sexes; all ages.

SIGNS & SYMPTOMS—The following vary, depending on the site and extent of spinal-cord damage:
- Loss of movement and sensation in affected arms or legs.
- Loss of urinary and bowel control.
- Impaired sexual function.
- Loss of normal blood pressure.
- Loss of body-temperature control.
- Constipation.

CAUSES—Paraplegia is caused by spinal-cord damage in the back. Quadriplegia is caused by spinal-cord damage in the neck. Spinal-cord damage results from accidents, spinal-cord tumors or birth defects.

RISK INCREASES WITH
- Occupations, sports or other activities with a high risk of injury.
- Excess alcohol consumption or drug use. These increase the risk of accidents—especially vehicle accidents.

HOW TO PREVENT
- Observe safety precautions and don't take risks.
- Don't dive into shallow swimming pools or into water of unknown depth.
- Don't drink alcohol or use mind-altering drugs and drive.
- Use seat belts in cars.
- Wear protective headgear during contact sports, or while riding a bicycle or motorcycle.

 ## WHAT TO EXPECT

APPROPRIATE HEALTH CARE
- Doctor's treatment.
- Surgery to limit further spinal-cord damage, or to remove bones or a tumor.
- Time in an extended-care facility or nursing home (sometimes).
- Occupational rehabilitation.
- Psychotherapy or counseling for depression or for sexual problems.

DIAGNOSTIC MEASURES
- Your own observation of symptoms.
- Medical history and physical exam by a doctor.

- Laboratory studies of blood and urine.
- X-rays of the injured area.

POSSIBLE COMPLICATIONS
- Kidney infections, especially if a urinary catheter is needed.
- Lung infections.
- Fecal impaction.
- Pressure sores.
- Deep-vein blood clot.
- Depression.

PROBABLE OUTCOME—Depends on the extent of injury. A damaged spinal cord is limited in its ability to recover from injury. With rehabilitation, uninjured areas can take over some lost functions.

 ## HOW TO TREAT

NOTE—Follow your doctor's instructions. These instructions are supplemental.

GENERAL MEASURES
- If someone is in an accident and has neck pain or possible spinal-cord injury, *don't move the person unless absolutely necessary.* Splint the neck to avoid movement and additional damage.
- If you have a spinal-cord injury, you will need emotional support from family and friends. Don't be afraid to ask for help.
- Wear thigh-length elastic stockings during convalescence—and knee-length stockings later—to reduce the chance of deep-vein blood clots.
- Sleep on a waterbed or egg-crate foam mattress to reduce the chance of pressure sores.

MEDICATION—No medication can heal a damaged spinal cord. Your doctor may prescribe:
- Antibiotics to fight infection. Urinary-tract infections are most common.
- Stool softeners and laxatives to prevent constipation.

ACTIVITY—Stay as active as your strength and condition allow. The body can be retrained to compensate for or restore some lost functions, including sexual abilities.

DIET
- Eat a high-fiber diet to prevent constipation.
- If you have a urinary catheter, drink up to 16 glasses of water a day to prevent bladder stones and urinary-tract infections.

 ## CALL YOUR DOCTOR IF

- You observe signs of a neck or spine injury in someone.
- Signs of infection occur during treatment. These include fever, chills, cloudy urine, muscle aches and headache.

PARKINSON'S DISEASE

GENERAL INFORMATION

DEFINITION—A disease of the central nervous system in older adults characterized by gradual, progressive muscle rigidity, tremors and clumsiness.

BODY PARTS INVOLVED—Area of the brain that regulates movement; muscles.

SEX OR AGE MOST AFFECTED—Adults over 60.

SIGNS & SYMPTOMS

- Tremors, especially when not moving.
- General muscle stiffness and slowness.
- Awkward or shuffling walk.
- Stooped posture.
- Loss of facial expression.
- Voice changes. The voice becomes weak and high pitched.
- Swallowing difficulty.
- Intellectual ability is unchanged until advanced stages, when it deteriorates slowly.

CAUSES—Usually unknown. Some cases may be caused by: medications, such as phenothiazine tranquilizers; brain injury; tumors; post-influenza encephalitis; slow-virus infection; or carbon-monoxide poisoning (possibly).

RISK INCREASES WITH—Stress.

HOW TO PREVENT—No specific preventive measures.

WHAT TO EXPECT

APPROPRIATE HEALTH CARE

- Doctor's treatment.
- Psychotherapy or counseling to help relieve depression.
- Physical therapy, if muscle rigidity is severe.
- Surgery using heat, cold or radiation to destroy areas of the brain that cause Parkinson's disease (rare).

DIAGNOSTIC MEASURES

- Your own observation of symptoms.
- Medical history and physical exam by a doctor.
- Laboratory blood studies.
- EEG (see Glossary).

POSSIBLE COMPLICATIONS

- Depression, sometimes severe.
- Pneumonia.
- Severe constipation.
- Urine retention caused by medication.
- Falls and fractures.

PROBABLE OUTCOME—This condition is currently considered incurable. However, symptoms can be relieved or controlled. Life expectancy is not significantly reduced.

Scientific research into causes and treatment continues, so there is hope for increasingly effective treatment and cure.

HOW TO TREAT

NOTE—Follow your doctor's instructions. These instructions are supplemental.

GENERAL MEASURES

- Take frequent, warm baths and have massages to forestall muscle rigidity.
- Shave with an electric razor.
- Wear shoes without laces, such as loafers or those with zipper or Velcro fasteners.
- Accidentproof your home to prevent falls and injuries.
- Gradual restrictions of the disease may frustrate you. Seek professional help and ask your family for support in finding ways to remain active and useful.

MEDICATION—Your doctor may prescribe: anticholinergics; antihistamines; antiviral drugs, such as amantadine; or antiparkinson medications, including bromocriptine, levodopa and carbidopa. All these decrease tremors and reduce muscle rigidity, but they often have significant side effects.

ACTIVITY—Remain as active as possible, and rest often. Physical abilities vary greatly between persons with this disease. The only restrictions are those imposed by muscle rigidity. Physical therapy helps reduce this.

DIET—No special diet, but soft foods may be necessary if swallowing becomes difficult. Add bulk or fiber to the diet and increase fluid intake to prevent constipation.

CALL YOUR DOCTOR IF

- You have symptoms of Parkinson's disease or symptoms worsen during treatment.
- New, unexplained symptoms develop, especially urination difficulty, confusion or blurred vision. Drugs used in treatment may produce side effects.

PARONYCHIA

GENERAL INFORMATION

DEFINITION—Inflammation of tissue folds that surround the fingernail. The inflammation can be bacterial or fungal and is not contagious.

BODY PARTS INVOLVED—Fingernails.

SEX OR AGE MOST AFFECTED—Both sexes; all ages.

SIGNS & SYMPTOMS—Bacterial paronychia:
- Pain or tenderness, redness, warmth and swelling in the affected finger.
- Drops of pus that can be squeezed out of swollen tissue.
Fungal paronychia:
- Redness and swelling around the fingernail.
- No pain, warmth, itching or pus.

CAUSES
- Bacterial paronychia is preceded by injury, such as a torn hangnail. The infecting germ is usually staphylococcus.
- Fungal paronychia is caused by a fungus or yeast infection.

RISK INCREASES WITH
- Injury around the fingernail.
- Occupational exposure to constant wetness (dishwashers, bartenders, housewives).

HOW TO PREVENT
- Protect hands from wetness.
- Leave hangnails alone.
- Avoid fingertip injury.

WHAT TO EXPECT

APPROPRIATE HEALTH CARE
- Self-care after diagnosis.
- Doctor's treatment.

DIAGNOSTIC MEASURES
- Your own observation of symptoms.
- Medical history and physical exam by a doctor.
- Laboratory studies, such as culture of the discharge, to identify the germ.

POSSIBLE COMPLICATIONS—If untreated, may permanently damage the fingernail and nail bed.

PROBABLE OUTCOME
- Bacterial paronychia is curable with treatment in 2 weeks.
- Fungal paronychia is chronic and may require 6 months to heal.
- Recurrence is common with both forms.

HOW TO TREAT

NOTE—Follow your doctor's instructions. These instructions are supplemental.

GENERAL MEASURES
- Wear heavy-duty vinyl gloves to prevent contact with irritating substances, such as water, soap, detergent, metal scrubbing pads, scouring pads, scouring powder and other chemicals.
- Dry the insides of gloves after use. Discard gloves if they develop a hole. A glove with a hole harms the hand more than not wearing a glove.
- Wear gloves when you peel or squeeze lemons, oranges, grapefruit, tomatoes or potatoes.
- Wear leather or heavy-duty fabric gloves for housework or gardening.
- Use a dishwashing machine or ask someone else to wash dishes.
- Avoid contact with irritating chemicals, such as paint, paint thinner, turpentine, and polish for cars, floors, shoes, furniture or metal.
- Use lukewarm water and very little mild soap to shower or bathe. All soaps are irritating. Expensive soaps offer no more protection against irritation than less-expensive ones.
- For bacterial paronychia, apply warm soaks.

MEDICATION
- For minor pain, you may use non-prescription drugs, such as aspirin or acetaminophen.
- Your doctor may prescribe antibiotics or antifungal medicine (depending on the type of infection).

ACTIVITY—No restrictions.

DIET—No special diet.

CALL YOUR DOCTOR IF

- You have symptoms of paronychia.
- Fever develops.
- Pain is not relieved by treatment.

PELVIC INFLAMMATORY DISEASE (PID)

GENERAL INFORMATION

DEFINITION—Infection of the female internal reproductive organs. This is contagious if it is caused by a sexually transmitted organism.

BODY PARTS INVOLVED—Fallopian tubes; cervix; uterus; ovaries; urinary bladder.

SEX OR AGE MOST AFFECTED—Sexually active females after puberty. The peak incidence occurs in late teens and early 20s.

SIGNS & SYMPTOMS—Early symptoms (up to 1 week):
● Pain in the lower pelvis on one or both sides, especially during menstrual periods. Menstrual flow may be heavy.
● Bad-smelling vaginal discharge.
● General ill feeling.
● Low fever (up to 101F or 38.3C).
● Frequent, painful urination.
Later symptoms (1 to 3 weeks later):
● Severe pain and tenderness in the lower abdomen.
● Temperature over 101F (38.3C).
● Increased bad-smelling, vaginal discharge.

CAUSES
● Bacterial infection (chlamydia, gonorrhea or mycoplasma) or a virus. This may be transmitted by an infected sexual partner.
● Childbirth.
● Abortion.
● Pelvic surgery.

RISK INCREASES WITH
● Many sexual partners.
● Use of an intrauterine contraceptive device (IUD).

HOW TO PREVENT—Use rubber condoms to prevent sexually transmitted infections.

OTHER—Your sexual partner may also need examination and treatment.

WHAT TO EXPECT

APPROPRIATE HEALTH CARE
● Doctor's treatment.
● Self-care after diagnosis.
● Hospitalization (usually).
● Surgery to drain a pelvic abscess (sometimes).
● Psychotherapy or counseling, if infertility occurs.

DIAGNOSTIC MEASURES
● Your own observation of symptoms.
● Medical history and physical exam by a doctor.
● Laboratory blood studies and culture of the vaginal discharge.
● Surgical diagnostic procedures, such as laparoscopy or culdocentesis (see Glossary).

POSSIBLE COMPLICATIONS
● Pelvic abscess and rupture. This can be life-threatening.
● Adhesions (bands of scar tissue) inside the pelvis.
● Infertility.
● Blood poisoning.
● Thrombophlebitis (blood clots that break off and travel to the lungs).

PROBABLE OUTCOME—Usually curable with early treatment. Complications may be fatal. The illness lasts from 1 to 6 weeks, depending on its severity.

HOW TO TREAT

NOTE—Follow your doctor's instructions. These instructions are supplemental.

GENERAL MEASURES
● Use heat to relieve pain:
Place a heating pad or hot water bottle on the abdomen or back.
Take frequent hot baths. This may reduce the bad odor of the vaginal discharge, as well as relax muscles and relieve discomfort. Sit in a tub of hot water for 10 to 15 minutes as often as needed.
● Use sanitary pads to absorb the discharge or menstrual flow.
● Don't douche during treatment.

MEDICATION—Your doctor may prescribe:
● Intravenous antibiotics to fight infection during hospitalization. Oral antibiotics may be necessary for about 1 month following hospitalization.
● Pain relievers.

ACTIVITY—Avoid sexual intercourse until you are well. Rest in bed until the fever subsides. Sit and lie in different positions until you find one that is comfortable for you. Allow 6 weeks for recovery.

DIET—No special diet.

CALL YOUR DOCTOR IF

● You have symptoms of pelvic inflammatory disease.
● Symptoms recur after treatment.
● New, unexplained symptoms develop. Drugs used in treatment may produce side effects.

PENIS, CANCER OF

GENERAL INFORMATION

DEFINITION—Malignant tumor of the penis.

BODY PARTS INVOLVED—Penis, including the glans (tip), corona (rounded border of the glans) or prepuce (foreskin covering the glans).

SEX OR AGE MOST AFFECTED—Men over age 50.

SIGNS & SYMPTOMS—Early stages:
- A small circular lesion (resembles a pimple) or persistent, painless sore on the penis. The lesion is easily visible in a circumcised male, but it may go unnoticed in an uncircumcised male.
Later stages:
- Pain, bleeding or discharge from the tumor.
- Discomfort with urination.
- Enlarged lymph nodes in the groin.

CAUSES—Unknown, but penile cancer is rare in men circumcised at birth or shortly thereafter. This may explain why it is rare among Jews, Muslims, and other cultures where early circumcision is customary.

RISK INCREASES WITH
- Previous leukoplakia of the penis, balanitis or epithelial horn on the penis.
- Personal uncleanliness, especially of the genitals in uncircumcised males.

HOW TO PREVENT
- Have male children circumcised soon after birth. Circumcision 2 to 3 months after birth or later offers no protection against penile cancer.
- Examine the penis and testicles monthly to detect possible cancers early, when treatment is most successful. Seek medical treatment for any sign of infection or sore on the penis.

WHAT TO EXPECT

APPROPRIATE HEALTH CARE
- Self-care after diagnosis.
- Doctor's treatment.
- Hospitalization and surgery to remove the tumor. Local tumors of the foreskin may require circumcision only. Invasive tumors require total removal of the penis and regional lymph nodes.
- Radiation treatment after surgery.
- Psychotherapy or counseling after surgery to learn to cope with an altered self-image.

DIAGNOSTIC MEASURES
- Your own observation of symptoms.
- Medical history and physical exam by a doctor.

- Laboratory studies, such as culture of the tumor discharge, urinalysis and blood tests.
- Biopsy (see Glossary).

POSSIBLE COMPLICATIONS—This spreads quickly to nearby lymph nodes, but slowly to distant sites or organs. Many men delay treatment due to denial or fear of disfigurement and loss of sexual function. This increases the likelihood the cancer will spread and cause death.

PROBABLE OUTCOME—Often curable with early diagnosis, surgery and radiation treatment. Without treatment, this condition is incurable, and the 5-year survival rate is less than 40%.

HOW TO TREAT

NOTE—Follow your doctor's instructions. These instructions are supplemental.

GENERAL MEASURES—A bladder catheter will be necessary for a prolonged period—sometimes permanently—after surgery and irradiation treatment.

MEDICATION—Your doctor may prescribe:
- Pain relievers, if necessary.
- Anticancer drugs for widespread cancer. However, the effectiveness of presently available drugs is only temporary.

ACTIVITY—Resume your normal activities as soon as possible after treatment. Sexual relations are possible if enough penile tissue remains following surgery.

DIET—No special diet.

CALL YOUR DOCTOR IF

- You have any lump or sore on the penis.
- Excessive bleeding occurs at the surgical site.
- New, unexplained symptoms develop. Drugs used in treatment may produce side effects.

PERICARDITIS, ACUTE

GENERAL INFORMATION

DEFINITION—Inflammation of the pericardium (thin membrane around the heart). This is not contagious or cancerous, unless caused by the spread of cancer elsewhere.

BODY PARTS INVOLVED—Pericardium.

SEX OR AGE MOST AFFECTED—Both sexes; all ages.

SIGNS & SYMPTOMS
● Dull or sharp pain in the front of the chest, radiating to the neck and shoulder. The pain worsens with movement and eases when sitting up or leaning forward.
● Rapid breathing.
● Cough.
● Fever and chills.
● Weakness.
● Anxiety.
● The most important signs are apparent only with medical examination: friction rub heard through a stethoscope; elevated white-blood-cell count; rapid sedimentation rate (see Glossary); abnormal EKG (see Glossary).

CAUSES—Sometimes unknown. The most common known causes are:
● Viral infection.
● Rheumatic fever and other diseases of connective tissue, such as lupus erythematosus.
● Chronic kidney failure.
● Complication of a heart attack.
● Complication following heart surgery.
● Complication of a chest injury, including use of a cardiac catheter.
● Spread of cancer to the pericardium.

RISK INCREASES WITH
● Recent illness, such as a heart attack, viral illness or rheumatic fever.
● Medical history of tuberculosis.

HOW TO PREVENT—No specific preventive measures except medical treatment of the disorders that cause pericarditis.

WHAT TO EXPECT

APPROPRIATE HEALTH CARE
● Doctor's treatment.
● Surgery (sometimes) to remove fluid through a needle if fluid collects in the pericardium.
● Self-care.

DIAGNOSTIC MEASURES
● Your own observation of symptoms.
● Medical history and physical exam by a doctor.
● EKG.
● Chest X-ray.
● Thoracentesis (fluid removal with a needle). This procedure may be diagnostic or therapeutic.

POSSIBLE COMPLICATIONS—Fluid in the pericardium may cause pressure on the heart. This can be fatal unless fluid is removed quickly.

PROBABLE OUTCOME—Usually curable in 6 months unless pericarditis is caused by cancer. After cure, there should be no functional disability.

HOW TO TREAT

NOTE—Follow your doctor's instructions. These instructions are supplemental.

GENERAL MEASURES—Apply a heating pad or warm compresses to the chest to relieve pain.

MEDICATION
● Your doctor may prescribe steroid drugs if pericarditis is a complication of heart attack, connective-tissue disease or metabolic disorder. No medication is needed if pericarditis is caused by a virus.
● You may use non-prescription drugs, such as acetaminophen, for minor pain.

ACTIVITY
● Rest in bed until fever and pain subside. You may read or watch TV.
● Resume your normal activities gradually.
● Resume sexual relations when fever and pain disappear.

DIET—No special diet.

CALL YOUR DOCTOR IF

● You have symptoms of pericarditis.
● The following occurs during treatment:
  Fever above 102F (38.9C).
  Shortness of breath and rapid heartbeat.
  Cough with blood.
  Unexplained weight loss.
  Pain not controlled by acetaminophen.
● New, unexplained symptoms develop. Steroids used in treatment may produce side effects, especially restlessness.

ILLNESSES & DISORDERS

PERIODONTITIS
(Gum Inflammation)

 GENERAL INFORMATION

DEFINITION—Inflammation and infection of the gums, causing loss of supporting bone. Periodontitis is responsible for more tooth loss than tooth decay. It is not contagious.

BODY PARTS INVOLVED—Gums; jaw bones.

SEX OR AGE MOST AFFECTED—Adults over age 20.

SIGNS & SYMPTOMS
- Unpleasant taste in the mouth.
- Bad breath.
- Loosening of teeth in the sockets.
- Aching teeth and gums when eating hot, cold or sweet food.
- If an abscess develops, tenderness, swelling, pain and fever will also occur.

CAUSES—Plaque (a sticky deposit of food, bacteria and mucus) destroys bone that surrounds and supports teeth. Poor dental hygiene causes the accumulation of plaque.

RISK INCREASES WITH—Illness that has lowered resistance.

HOW TO PREVENT
- Practice good oral hygiene (see General Measures).
- Avoid sweet snacks, which contribute to plaque formation.
- Visit your dentist regularly to have teeth cleaned. Ask your dentist about the level of fluoride in local drinking water. Fluoride supplements may provide added protection.

 WHAT TO EXPECT

APPROPRIATE HEALTH CARE
- Self-care after diagnosis.
- Dentist's care.
- Surgery to remove unhealthy gum tissue and reshape underlying bone to eliminate pockets.

DIAGNOSTIC MEASURES
- Your own observation of symptoms.
- Medical history and physical exam by a dentist.
- X-rays of the mouth.

POSSIBLE COMPLICATIONS—Without treatment, teeth loosen so much in their bony sockets that they must be extracted.

PROBABLE OUTCOME—Usually curable with a combination of dental treatment and strict adherence to a good oral-hygiene program (see General Measures).

 HOW TO TREAT

NOTE—Follow your dentist's instructions. These instructions are supplemental.

GENERAL MEASURES
- To brush teeth: Scrub the clear, sticky plaque off teeth daily with a soft toothbrush. A soft brush is less likely to damage teeth and gums than a hard brush. Place the brush at the gum line and gently rotate it, pointing the bristles toward the gum. Brush one section of teeth at a time.
- To floss teeth: Wind waxed or unwaxed dental floss around one finger on each hand. Force the dental floss between teeth. Gently clean the tooth surfaces with a back-and-forth, sawing motion at the gum line. Floss between all lower teeth, using your fingers as guides. Next, loosen the floss and place it on the tops of your thumbs. Floss between all upper teeth, using your thumbs as guides.

MEDICATION—For minor pain, you may use non-prescription drugs such as acetaminophen.

ACTIVITY—No restrictions.

DIET—No special diet, except to avoid sweets.

 CALL YOUR DENTIST IF

You have symptoms of periodontitis.

PERIPHERAL NEUROPATHY
(Peripheral Neuritis)

 GENERAL INFORMATION

DEFINITION—A group of symptoms caused by abnormalities in sensory or motor nerves.

BODY PARTS INVOLVED—Many nerves that end in muscles, blood vessels and skin. This usually affects fingers, toes, hands, feet, lower arms and legs, and may affect bladder or bowel control.

SEX OR AGE MOST AFFECTED—Adults of both sexes.

SIGNS & SYMPTOMS—Symptoms usually appear gradually over many months:
- Tingling and numbness that begins in the hands and feet, and spreads gradually.
- Gradual muscle weakness throughout the body—generally in same place on both sides.
- Shooting pains that are often worse at night. Pains are aggravated by touch or temperature changes.
- Painless ulcers on the toes or fingers.
- Pale, dry skin that becomes sensitive to touch.
- Weight loss.
- Severe back pain or loss of bladder or bowel control, if caused by intervertebral disk disease.

CAUSES
- Reactions to drugs or chemicals, including: emetine; hexobarbitol; chlorbutanol; sulfonamides; phenytoin; nitrofurantoin; heavy metals; carbon monoxide; solvents; or industrial poisons. Interactions of drugs required by people with cardiovascular disease sometimes cause symptoms.
- Complication of an underlying disorder, such as: diabetes mellitus; alcoholism; vitamin deficiency; vitamin B-12 deficiency anemia; or thyroid disorder.
- Poor nutrition.
- Malabsorption disorders.
- Excessive vomiting, including vomiting of early pregnancy.
- Decreased thyroid function.
- Acute porphyria.
- Complication of dialysis treatment.
- Cancer.
- Ruptured intervertebral disc.

RISK INCREASES WITH
- Adults over 60.
- Use of drugs listed in Causes, especially multiple medications.
- Exposure to chemicals listed in Causes.
- Poor nutrition, such as in alcoholism.
- Poor control of diabetes.

HOW TO PREVENT
- Avoid as many causes and risks as possible.
- If an underlying disorder is causing peripheral neuropathy, follow your doctor's instructions rigidly to control the disorder.

 WHAT TO EXPECT

APPROPRIATE HEALTH CARE
- Doctor's care.
- Hospitalization (sometimes).
- Surgery to relieve pressure, if nerves are compressed.

DIAGNOSTIC MEASURES
- Your own observation of symptoms.
- Medical history and physical exam by a doctor.
- Laboratory studies of blood, urine, vitamin B-12 levels, thyroid function and spinal fluid.
- Electromyography (see Glossary).

POSSIBLE COMPLICATIONS—Chronic pain and disability.

PROBABLE OUTCOME—Mild cases can be cured if the underlying cause is diagnosed and treated. Serious cases may be incurable, but symptoms can improve.

 HOW TO TREAT

NOTE—Follow your doctor's instructions. These instructions are supplemental.

GENERAL MEASURES
- If peripheral neuropathy is caused by an incurable disorder, obtain biofeedback training to learn relaxation techniques that relieve pain.
- If peripheral neuropathy is interfering with normal activities, consult a physical therapist.
- If you have difficulty maintaining balance, walk with a cane or other support.
- Install rails next to the bathtub.
- Inspect hands and feet daily for unnoticed wounds.
- Keep feet clean and toenails trimmed properly; wear shoes that fit well.

MEDICATION—For minor pain, you may use non-prescription drugs such as aspirin or acetaminophen.

ACTIVITY—Stay as active as possible.

DIET—No special diet. Vitamin and mineral supplements probably will be necessary.

 CALL YOUR DOCTOR IF

- You have symptoms of peripheral neuropathy.
- Symptoms (especially muscle weakness) persist or worsen, despite treatment.
- You develop a severe bruise or open sore.

ILLNESSES & DISORDERS

PERITONITIS

GENERAL INFORMATION

DEFINITION—A serious infection or inflammation of part or all of the peritoneum, the covering of the intestinal tract.

BODY PARTS INVOLVED—Abdomen, including intestines and peritoneum (a thin membrane that covers all the organs and walls of the abdomen).

SEX OR AGE MOST AFFECTED—Both sexes; all ages.

SIGNS & SYMPTOMS
- Pain in one area or throughout the abdomen. Pain usually starts suddenly and becomes increasingly severe. Pain may be crampy at first, and then steady. The patient often prefers to lie quietly on the back because movement or pressure on the abdomen increases pain.
- Shoulder pain (sometimes).
- Chills and fever (often high).
- Dizziness and weakness.
- Rapid heartbeat.
- Low blood pressure.

CAUSES—Intense inflammation of the peritoneum lining that occurs when foreign material enters the abdominal cavity. Foreign material includes bacteria or gastrointestinal contents, such as digestive juices, blood, partly digested food or feces. These materials enter the abdomen following:
- Rupture or perforation of any organ in the abdomen, such as an inflamed appendix, peptic ulcer, or infected diverticulum or gallbladder.
- Injury to the abdominal wall, such as from a knife or bullet wound.
- Pelvic inflammatory disease.
- Rupture of an ectopic pregnancy.

RISK INCREASES WITH
- Delay in treatment of causes listed above.
- Recent abdominal surgery.

HOW TO PREVENT—Obtain prompt medical treatment for underlying disorders.

WHAT TO EXPECT

APPROPRIATE HEALTH CARE
- Doctor's treatment.
- Hospitalization.
- Surgery to repair the organ damage or injury that allowed foreign material into the abdomen.
- Self-care after treatment.

DIAGNOSTIC MEASURES
- Your own observation of symptoms.
- Medical history and physical exam by a doctor.
- Laboratory white-blood-cell count to detect inflammation, red-blood-cell count to detect bleeding and measurement of fluid and electrolyte levels.
- Surgical diagnostic procedures, such as passing a small needle into the abdomen to obtain fluid, blood or other material.
- X-rays of the abdomen.

POSSIBLE COMPLICATIONS
- Shock.
- Blood poisoning (septicemia).
- Intestinal obstruction caused by later adhesions (bands of scar tissue).

PROBABLE OUTCOME—Usually curable with early diagnosis and treatment. Treatment delay and complications can be fatal.

HOW TO TREAT

NOTE—Follow your doctor's instructions. These instructions are supplemental.

GENERAL MEASURES—Early diagnosis and treatment of the underlying disorder, such as appendicitis, ulcer or ectopic pregnancy, are essential. If abdominal pain develops, don't waste valuable time with home treatments—especially laxative use. Laxatives may cause inflamed abdominal organs to rupture.

MEDICATION—Your doctor may prescribe:
- Antibiotics to fight infection.
- Pain relievers (sometimes) after diagnosis or surgery.

ACTIVITY—Rest in bed after treatment until symptoms disappear. You may read or watch TV. If surgery is necessary, resume your activities gradually after surgery.

DIET—Don't eat or drink anything so the intestinal tract can rest until the acute infection subsides. You will be given intravenous nourishment and fluids.

CALL YOUR DOCTOR IF

- You have symptoms of peritonitis. This is an emergency!
- The following occurs during treatment:
  Constipation.
  Signs of new infection, including fever, chills, muscle aches, dizziness, headache and increasing abdominal pain.
- New, unexplained symptoms develop. Drugs used in treatment may produce side effects.

PHARYNGITIS

GENERAL INFORMATION

DEFINITION—Throat inflammation and infection from a variety of germs.

BODY PARTS INVOLVED—Throat area, including tonsils.

SEX OR AGE MOST AFFECTED
- Both sexes.
- All ages except infancy.

SIGNS & SYMPTOMS
- Sore throat.
- Swallowing difficulty.
- Tickle or "lump" in the throat.
- Fever.
- Swollen glands in the neck (sometimes).
- Throat may be red or covered with a grayish membrane (sometimes).
- Generalized aching.

CAUSES—Infection from bacteria, viruses or fungi. Following are the most common germs.
- Bacteria—streptococci, diphtheria, gonococci, hemophilus, pneumococci or staphylococci.
- Viruses—Epstein-Barr and many types of respiratory viruses.
- Fungi—Monilial.

RISK INCREASES WITH
- Illness that has lowered resistance.
- Fatigue or overwork.
- Diabetes mellitus.
- Immune deficiencies.
- Smoking.
- Excess alcohol consumption.
- Oral sex.
- Epidemics, during which all persons are at increased risk.

HOW TO PREVENT
- Avoid contact with anyone with a sore throat.
- Keep immunizations, including diphtheria, up to date. An immunization schedule appears in Appendix 16.

WHAT TO EXPECT

APPROPRIATE HEALTH CARE
- Self-care after diagnosis.
- Doctor's treatment.
- Hospitalization for pharyngitis caused by diphtheria or hemophilus bacteria.

DIAGNOSTIC MEASURES
- Your own observation of symptoms.
- Medical history and physical exam by a doctor.
- Laboratory throat culture and blood count.

POSSIBLE COMPLICATIONS
- Epiglottitis, leading to complete breathing obstruction.
- Pneumonia.

- Rheumatic fever, scarlet fever or glomerulonephritis, if pharyngitis is caused by strep bacteria and does not receive adequate antibiotic treatment.

PROBABLE OUTCOME—Spontaneous recovery for most cases of viral pharyngitis. Other cases are curable with antibiotic or antifungal drugs.

HOW TO TREAT

NOTE—Follow your doctor's instructions. These instructions are supplemental.

GENERAL MEASURES
- Use gargles to relieve throat pain. Prepare double-strength tea, hot or cold, or a salt-water solution (1 teaspoon salt in 8 oz. warm water). Use to gargle as often as you wish.
- Use a cool-mist humidifier to increase air moisture. This will relieve the dry, tight feeling in the throat.
- To reduce a high fever, or for fever in a child who has had a convulsion, see Appendix 19, How to Reduce Fever.
- If the glands are large and tender, apply moist, warm soaks (see Appendix 18) at least 4 times a day for 30 to 60 minutes. The compresses will be more effective if they are kept warm. Be careful not to burn the skin.

MEDICATION
- For minor discomfort, you may use non-prescription drugs such as acetaminopohen. Don't give aspirin to a child for any viral illness. Studies link its use with the development of Reye's syndrome.
- Your doctor may prescribe antibiotics or antifungal agents to fight bacterial or fungal infections.

ACTIVITY—Bed rest is necessary until symptoms disappear. Reading or watching TV is acceptable.

DIET—Extra fluids are necessary—at least 8 glasses of water daily, more for high fevers. If swallowing solid food is painful, a liquid diet may be necessary. See Appendix 7.

CALL YOUR DOCTOR IF

- You have symptoms of pharyngitis.
- The following occurs during treatment:
  Breathing or swallowing difficulty.
  Fever (oral) over 102F (38.9C).
  Severe headache.
  Thick mucus drainage from the nose.
  Cough that produces green, yellow, brown or bloody sputum.
  Skin rash.

ILLNESSES & DISORDERS

PHEOCHROMOCYTOMA

GENERAL INFORMATION

DEFINITION—A tumor of the core (medulla) of the adrenal glands. The tumor is usually benign and does not spread to other organs.

BODY PARTS INVOLVED—Adrenal medulla.

SEX OR AGE MOST AFFECTED—Adults of both sexes between ages 30 and 50.

SIGNS & SYMPTOMS
- Rapid heartbeat following exercise, emotional upset or exposure to cold.
- Tremors and nervousness.
- Feelings of impending doom.
- Sweating.
- Paleness.
- Weakness and fatigue.
- Very high blood-pressure spikes, accompanied by headaches.
- Unexplained weight loss.

Episodes of at least some of these symptoms may occur several times a day or only occasionally (up to 2 months apart).

CAUSES—The hormones adrenalin and noradrenalin, produced by the core of each adrenal gland, work with the central nervous system to control heart rate, blood pressure and other vital body functions. When a tumor (the pheochromocytoma) exists—even though it is benign—excess hormones are produced. The excess hormones cause symptoms. Cause of the tumor is unknown.

RISK INCREASES WITH
- Pregnancy.
- Family history of pheochromocytoma.

HOW TO PREVENT—No specific preventive measures.

WHAT TO EXPECT

APPROPRIATE HEALTH CARE
- Doctor's treatment.
- Surgery to remove the tumor. The tumor is usually removed through an abdominal incision after several days of study and preparation with medications that block release of hormones during surgery.

DIAGNOSTIC MEASURES
- Your own observation of symptoms.
- Medical history and physical exam by a doctor.
- Laboratory studies of urine and blood to measure catecholamine levels. Catecholamines are breakdown products of hormone production.
- Angiography (see Glossary).
- CAT scan (see Glossary).

POSSIBLE COMPLICATIONS
- Stroke caused by very high blood pressure during an episode.
- Kidney, brain, heart damage and death caused by unrecognized and untreated pheochromocytoma.

PROBABLE OUTCOME—Usually curable with surgery.

HOW TO TREAT

NOTE—Follow your doctor's instructions. These instructions are supplemental.

GENERAL MEASURES—For a description of abdominal surgery and postoperative care, see Laparotomy.

MEDICATION—Your doctor my prescribe alpha- and beta-adrenergic blockers before surgery to suppress the effect of hormones.

ACTIVITY—No restrictions after recovery from surgery.

DIET—No special diet.

CALL YOUR DOCTOR IF

- You have symptoms of pheochromocytoma.
- New, unexplained symptoms develop.

Drugs used in treatment may produce side effects.

PICA

GENERAL INFORMATION

DEFINITION—Eating bizarre substances that have no food value.

BODY PARTS INVOLVED—Brain; gastrointestinal tract.

SEX OR AGE MOST AFFECTED—Children between ages 1 and 6, and pregnant women. Pica does not apply to infants and children up to about 18 months old who "put everything" in the mouth. That is normal.

SIGNS & SYMPTOMS
- Eating non-food substances, such as starch, clay, ice, plaster, paint, hair or gravel.
- Abdominal pain (sometimes).

CAUSES
- Instinctive need to replace minerals absent in the diet. This is especially true of eating clay for iron content.
- Psychological factors that are not well-understood, related to substandard housing, low income or emotional deprivation.

RISK INCREASES WITH
- Family history of pica.
- Poor nutrition.
- Poverty.
- Mental retardation.

HOW TO PREVENT
- Remove substances from the reach of children.
- Repaint homes in which lead-base paints have been used. Don't use older baby cribs painted with lead-base paint.
- Provide a well-balanced diet for yourself and your children.
- Provide a loving, supportive home environment for your children.

WHAT TO EXPECT

APPROPRIATE HEALTH CARE
- Self-care after diagnosis.
- Doctor's treatment.
- Psychotherapy or counseling.

DIAGNOSTIC MEASURES
- Your own observation of symptoms.
- Medical history and physical exam by a doctor.
- Laboratory blood studies to detect anemia and measure fluids and electrolytes.
- X-rays of the abdomen.

POSSIBLE COMPLICATIONS
- Lead poisoning from paint or plaster.
- Intestinal infections or parasites from soil.
- Anemia.
- Malnutrition.
- Intestinal obstruction.

PROBABLE OUTCOME—Pica during pregnancy usually ends with childbirth. Other forms can be controlled with treatment.

HOW TO TREAT

NOTE—Follow your doctor's instructions. These instructions are supplemental.

GENERAL MEASURES
- Childproof your home by removing substances the child is eating.
- Examine your home environment and family interactions. If you feel they are not what they should be, seek ways to create a healthier atmosphere. Consult a counselor, if necessary.

MEDICATION—Medicine usually is not necessary for this disorder.

ACTIVITY—No restrictions.

DIET—Provide a well-balanced diet. Vitamin and mineral supplements may be necessary. If you need help planning meals, consult the home-extension service, a dietitian or a visiting nurse.

CALL YOUR DOCTOR IF

- Your child has symptoms of pica.
- You are pregnant and have symptoms of pica.
- Pica does not improve in 2 weeks, despite treatment.

ILLNESSES & DISORDERS

PILONIDAL CYST

GENERAL INFORMATION

DEFINITION—A small, hair-containing skin sac at the base of the spine. The cyst looks like a small opening—sometimes no more than a dimple—with a few hairs protruding (sometimes). It is prone to infection. Pilonidal cysts are uncommon in black people.

BODY PARTS INVOLVED—Skin.

SEX OR AGE MOST AFFECTED—Both sexes, but more common in men. Cyst infections usually begin in young adulthood (ages 18 to 40).

SIGNS & SYMPTOMS—No symptoms when not infected. When infected, it causes:
- Pain, redness, tenderness and swelling in the area.
- Fever and chills.
- Discharge of pus.

CAUSES—The cyst is a minor abnormality that occurs during fetal development. Infection is usually caused by staphylococcal bacteria.

RISK INCREASES WITH
- Heavy perspiration. Obesity increases perspiration.
- Tight clothing.

HOW TO PREVENT
- Bathe or shower daily to keep the area clean. Hot tub baths seem more effective in preventing infection of the cyst.
- Wear light, loose-fitting clothing.
- Avoid overweight.

WHAT TO EXPECT

APPROPRIATE HEALTH CARE
- Self-care after diagnosis.
- Doctor's treatment.
- Surgery to remove the cyst, if it repeatedly becomes infected.

DIAGNOSTIC MEASURES
- Your own observation of symptoms.
- Medical history and physical exam by a doctor.
- Laboratory culture of the discharge.

POSSIBLE COMPLICATIONS—Spread of infection (rare).

PROBABLE OUTCOME—Curable with antibiotic treatment.

HOW TO TREAT

NOTE—Follow your doctor's instructions. These instructions are supplemental.

GENERAL MEASURES
- If the cyst is infected, take warm baths to relieve pain. Sit in a tub of warm water for 10 to 15 minutes as often as it feels good.
- If surgery is necessary, see Pilonidal Cyst Removal (in Surgery section) for an explanation of the surgery and postoperative care.

MEDICATION—Your doctor may prescribe antibiotics to fight infection.

ACTIVITY—No restrictions, unless the cyst becomes infected. Then, limit activities until the infection is cured.

DIET—Lose weight if you are overweight. A reducing diet appears in Appendix 1.

CALL YOUR DOCTOR IF

- You have symptoms of a pilonidal cyst. It should be diagnosed.
- After diagnosis, a cyst shows signs of infection.

PINWORMS
(Enterobiasis; Seatworm; Threadworm; Oxyuriasis)

GENERAL INFORMATION

DEFINITION—Infestation with intestinal parasites, a common occurrence in children. Pinworm infestations are more a nuisance than a major health problem.

BODY PARTS INVOLVED—Cecum (pouchlike beginning of the large intestine on the right side to which the appendix is attached); large intestine; anus; skin around the anus.

SEX OR AGE MOST AFFECTED—All ages, but most common in children.

SIGNS & SYMPTOMS
- Skin irritation and painful itching around the anus.
- Restless sleep.
- Vaginal discharge, itching and discomfort, if pinworms migrate into the vaginal opening.
- Poor appetite and stomach pain (sometimes).
- Paleness (sometimes).

CAUSES—Infestation of the cecum by a very small worm (oxyuria) that measures only 10mm in its adult form.

Pinworms travel from the cecum to the rectum to lay eggs around the anus and buttocks. The tiny eggs are picked up on the fingers by scratching.

Eggs are transferred to others on toilet seats or by hand-to-hand or hand-to-mouth contact. They also drift in the air, where they are inhaled or swallowed.

Eggs hatch in the small intestine. The larvae travel to the cecum, where they mature, mate and repeat the cycle.

RISK INCREASES WITH
- Groups of children, as in schools or large families.
- Poor personal hygiene.
- Dishwashing water that is not hot enough to kill eggs.

HOW TO PREVENT
- Wash hands carefully after using the toilet and before meals.
- Keep the nails short and clean.
- Wash the anus and genitals at least once a day. Rinse well, preferably under a shower.
- Have children wear snug cotton underpants day and night, and change them daily.
- Don't scratch the anus or put fingers near the nose or mouth.
- Use very hot water to wash dishes.

WHAT TO EXPECT

APPROPRIATE HEALTH CARE
- Home care after diagnosis.
- Doctor's treatment.

DIAGNOSTIC MEASURES
- Your own observation of symptoms.
- Medical history and physical exam by a doctor.
- Microscopic study of the worms or eggs.

POSSIBLE COMPLICATIONS—No serious complications expected.

PROBABLE OUTCOME—Usually curable in one treatment—two treatments at the most. Treatment should include all family members at once. Recurrence is common.

If worms reappear soon after treatment, they usually represent a new infection—not treatment failure.

HOW TO TREAT

NOTE—Follow your doctor's instructions. These instructions are supplemental.

GENERAL MEASURES—The following should be done on the day the family is treated with medicine:
- Clean the house with extra care. Wash the sheets and clothing with extra bleach or ammonia, or boil them.
- Scrub washable toys. Sterilize metal toys and similar objects in a hot oven.
- Cut and clean fingernails.
- Change towels.
- Scrub toilet bowls.
- Take extra-long showers.

About 2 weeks after treatment, your doctor will probably check to be sure all parasites have been destroyed.

MEDICATION—Your doctor may prescribe antiworm medicine. Follow directions carefully. Take the medicine on an empty stomach. The medicine may cause nausea, vomiting and diarrhea. It is not absorbed by the stomach or intestines, so the bowel movement following treatment will probably be the color of the medicine.

ACTIVITY—No restrictions.

DIET—No special diet.

CALL YOUR DOCTOR IF

- Anyone in your family has symptoms of pinworms.
- Pinworms reappear after treatment.
- You think medicine is causing side effects that don't disappear quickly.

PITUITARY GLAND, UNDERACTIVE
(Hypopituitarism)

 GENERAL INFORMATION

DEFINITION—Underactivity of the pituitary gland, resulting in inadequate amounts of hormones produced by the pituitary. The anterior lobe of the pituitary produces the following hormones:
- Growth hormone.
- Prolactin, which stimulates breasts to produce milk.
- Thyroid-stimulating hormone.
- Adrenal-stimulating hormone.
- Ovarian- or testicular-stimulating hormones.

The posterior lobe of the pituitary gland produces two hormones:
- Antidiuretic hormone, which affects the kidneys in regulating concentration and quantity of urine.
- Oxytocin, which stimulates contractions of the uterus during childbirth and releases milk during breast-feeding.

BODY PARTS INVOLVED—Pituitary gland and body parts mentioned above.

SEX OR AGE MOST AFFECTED—Both sexes; all ages.

SIGNS & SYMPTOMS
- Menstrual irregularities.
- Impotence.
- Infertility.
- Low blood sugar and weakness.
- Retarded growth in children (evident after 6 months of age).
- Lack of secondary sexual features that develop in puberty, such as voice changes, breast development and growth of pubic hair.
- Mental changes, including psychosis.
- Extreme lethargy.
- Persistent headaches.

CAUSES
- Unknown (sometimes).
- Serious head injury with pressure (usually from bleeding) on the pituitary gland.
- Reduced blood supply to the pituitary gland in a mother following severe hemorrhage and shock during childbirth.
- Tumor of the pituitary gland.
- Infection in the brain.
- Aneurysm of blood vessels in the base of the brain.

RISK INCREASES WITH
- Family history of pituitary disorders.
- Pregnancy.

HOW TO PREVENT—Obtain medical treatment for the underlying injury, infection or tumor, if possible.

 WHAT TO EXPECT

APPROPRIATE HEALTH CARE
- Doctor's treatment. This requires close supervision and continuing treatment.
- Surgery to remove underlying tumors or blood clots, if necessary.

DIAGNOSTIC MEASURES
- Your own observation of symptoms.
- Medical history and physical exam by a doctor.
- Laboratory blood studies of hormone levels and function.
- CAT scan (see Glossary) of the head.

POSSIBLE COMPLICATIONS—Hormonal failure and death without treatment.

PROBABLE OUTCOME—Usually curable with surgery or replacement therapy of pituitary, thyroid, adrenal and sex hormones.

 HOW TO TREAT

NOTE—Follow your doctor's instructions. These instructions are supplemental.

GENERAL MEASURES—No specific instructions except those listed under other headings.

MEDICATION—Your doctor may prescribe:
- Hormones to replace those the pituitary is not producing.
- Pain relievers after surgery.
- Antibiotics or antiviral medications, if infection is causing the disorder.

ACTIVITY—Stay as active as your condition allows.

DIET—No special diet.

 CALL YOUR DOCTOR IF

- You have symptoms of an underactive pituitary gland.
- After surgery, you develop signs of infection, such as fever, lethargy and muscle aches.
- New, unexplained symptoms develop. Drugs used in treatment may produce side effects.

PITUITARY TUMOR

 ## GENERAL INFORMATION

DEFINITION—Abnormal growth in the pituitary gland. Pituitary tumors may be benign or malignant—but even malignant pituitary tumors rarely spread to other body parts.

BODY PARTS INVOLVED—Pituitary gland, located at the base of the brain.

SEX OR AGE MOST AFFECTED—Both sexes and all ages, but most common between ages 30 and 50.

SIGNS & SYMPTOMS
- Blurred vision, double vision, dizziness or a drooping eyelid caused by tumor pressure on nerves to the eye.
- Headache in the forehead.
- Nausea and vomiting.
- Seizures.
- Runny nose.
- Excessive thirst.
- Menstrual changes.
- Unexplained weight gain.
- Retarded or excessive growth in children.
- Low blood sugar.
- Low blood pressure.
- Symptoms of abnormalities in other endocrine glands. See Hyperthyroidism, Hyperparathyroidism, Cushing's Disease and Ovarian Tumor (all in Illness section).

CAUSES—Unknown, but it may be caused by a dominant genetic trait.

RISK INCREASES WITH—Unknown.

HOW TO PREVENT—No specific preventive measures.

 ## WHAT TO EXPECT

APPROPRIATE HEALTH CARE
- Doctor's treatment.
- Surgery to remove the tumor (see Craniotomy), cryohypophysectomy (freezing the tumor with liquid nitrogen) or surgery to implant tiny radioactive pellets in the tumor.
- Postoperative radiation therapy.
- Self-care after surgery and radiation.

DIAGNOSTIC MEASURES
- Your own observation of symptoms.
- Medical history and physical exam by a doctor.
- Laboratory studies of cerebrospinal fluid and blood.
- X-rays of the skull.
- CAT scan (see Glossary).
- Angiogram (see Glossary).

POSSIBLE COMPLICATIONS—The following complications may diminish or be reversed after surgery:
- Blindness.
- Loss of sense of smell.
- Extreme hormone imbalance.

PROBABLE OUTCOME—Curable with surgery if the tumor has not spread from the pituitary gland. If it has, fatal complications usually develop.

 ## HOW TO TREAT

NOTE—Follow your doctor's instructions. These instructions are supplemental.

GENERAL MEASURES—No specific instructions except those listed under other headings.

MEDICATION—Your doctor may prescribe:
- Pain relievers.
- Hormone replacement medication for life. This may require frequent dosage adjustments.
- Anticancer drugs.

ACTIVITY—Resume your normal activities gradually after surgery.

DIET—No special diet.

 ## CALL YOUR DOCTOR IF

- You have symptoms of a pituitary tumor.
- The following occurs after surgery:
  Bleeding at the surgical site.
  Signs of general infection, such as fever, chills, muscle aches and headache.
  Clear discharge from the nose.

PITYRIASIS ALBA

 GENERAL INFORMATION

DEFINITION—A benign disorder of the skin in which skin temporarily loses pigmentation in patches.

BODY PARTS INVOLVED—Skin of the cheeks and arms.

SEX OR AGE MOST AFFECTED—Occurs most in children, but may occur up to age 25.

SIGNS & SYMPTOMS—Skin lesions with the following characteristics:
- Lesions are small white patches with vague borders. They sometimes have pinpoint-sized white papules (small, raised bumps).
- Patches are most apparent in summer because the lesions cannot tan, and tanning heightens the contrast between the areas.
- One person may have 1 to 12 patches at a time.
- Patches feel smooth.
- Patches may itch occasionally, but they are not painful.

CAUSES—Unknown. The tendency may be inherited.

RISK INCREASES WITH—Family history of allergies of any kind.

HOW TO PREVENT—No specific preventive measures.

 WHAT TO EXPECT

APPROPRIATE HEALTH CARE
- Self-care after diagnosis.
- Doctor's treatment.

DIAGNOSTIC MEASURES
- Your own observation of symptoms.
- Medical history and physical exam by a doctor.

POSSIBLE COMPLICATIONS—None expected.

PROBABLE OUTCOME—Patches may come and go for years. Between ages 20 and 30, they disappear completely.

 HOW TO TREAT

NOTE—Follow your doctor's instructions. These instructions are supplemental.

MEDICATION—Your doctor may prescribe prescription or non-prescription topical steroid medicine to control itching and prevent papules.

GENERAL MEASURES
- Apply prescribed topical steroids only once or twice a day unless directed otherwise. Apply immediately after bathing for better spreading and penetration. For the face, use only low-potency steroid products without fluorine. Apply a thin layer; a heavy layer wastes medicine and is no more beneficial than a thin layer. Rub in gently for several minutes until the cream disappears.
- Use sunscreen or protective clothing to prevent sunburn in affected areas.

ACTIVITY—No restrictions.

DIET—No special diet.

 CALL YOUR DOCTOR IF

- You have symptoms of pityriasis alba.
- New, unexplained symptoms develop. Drugs used in treatment may produce side effects.

PITYRIASIS ROSEA

GENERAL INFORMATION

DEFINITION—A non-contagious, inflammatory skin disorder with a faint rash that lasts 3 to 4 weeks.

BODY PARTS INVOLVED—Skin, especially of the chest and abdomen.

SEX OR AGE MOST AFFECTED—All ages, but most common in adolescents and young adults.

SIGNS & SYMPTOMS
- A faint rash—often found in skin creases—of oval or round, pale-pink or brown areas. One larger patch (the "herald patch") may appear first.
- Mild fatigue.
- Itching, usually mild.
- Occasional slight fever and headache.

CAUSES—Unknown, but may be caused by a virus or autoimmune disorder.

RISK INCREASES WITH—Fall and spring seasons.

HOW TO PREVENT—Cannot be prevented at present.

WHAT TO EXPECT

APPROPRIATE HEALTH CARE
- Self-care after diagnosis.
- Doctor's treatment, if severe itching occurs.

DIAGNOSTIC MEASURES
- Your own observation of symptoms.
- Medical history and physical exam by a doctor to rule out other disorders.

POSSIBLE COMPLICATIONS—Secondary bacterial infection of the rash area.

PROBABLE OUTCOME—Pityriasis rosea usually runs its natural course in 5 weeks to 4 months. No medication or treatment is available to shorten its course, but itching and discomfort can be relieved.

The skin eruptions won't leave scars unless complicated by a secondary infection. New rash areas continue to break out for several weeks. Once over, one episode seems to confer lifelong immunity.

Although pityriasis is probably caused by an infectious agent, it is not contagious. Even close family contacts are unlikely to develop the disease.

HOW TO TREAT

NOTE—Follow your doctor's instructions. These instructions are supplemental.

GENERAL MEASURES
- Bathe as usual with a mild soap. You don't need to sterilize the tub or shower after bathing.
- Expose the skin to moderate amounts of sunlight. This may decrease the rash.

MEDICATION—For minor discomfort, you may use non-prescription drugs, such as:
- Calamine lotion to decrease itching.
- Acetaminophen to reduce fever.

ACTIVITY—Usually no restrictions. Be as active as your strength allows.

DIET—No special diet.

CALL YOUR DOCTOR IF

- You have symptoms of pityriasis rosea.
- The following occurs during treatment: Fever over 101F (38.3C). Signs of infection (warmth, redness, tenderness, pain and swelling) in the rash area.

PITYRIASIS VERSICOLOR
(Tinea Versicolor)

 GENERAL INFORMATION

DEFINITION—A yeast infection of the skin that changes the color of skin it affects.

BODY PARTS INVOLVED—Skin of the chest, back, shoulders, upper arms, trunk or groin. This rarely affects the face.

SEX OR AGE MOST AFFECTED—Adolescents and adults.

SIGNS & SYMPTOMS—Lesions with the following characteristics:
• Lesions on exposed skin are white; on covered areas, they are brown or brownish red.
• Lesions are flat with clearly defined borders. They don't scale unless scraped.
• Lesions begin at 3 to 4mm in diameter and spread. They often join together to form large patches.

CAUSES—A developing stage of the yeast, pityrosborum orbiculare. High heat and high humidity favor the growth of this yeast. The infection is contagious, but how it spreads is unknown.

RISK INCREASES WITH—Environmental exposure to heat and high humidity.

HOW TO PREVENT—No specific preventive measures.

 WHAT TO EXPECT

APPROPRIATE HEALTH CARE
• Doctor's treatment.
• Self-care after diagnosis.

DIAGNOSTIC MEASURES
• Your own observation of symptoms.
• Medical history and physical exam by a doctor.
• Laboratory culture of scrapings for positive diagnosis.

POSSIBLE COMPLICATIONS—Unlimited recurrence without treatment.

PROBABLE OUTCOME—Untreated pityriasis versicolor persists indefinitely but seems to come and go at times. It frequently recurs, even with treatment. Following treatment, the white patches will remain for months after the yeast infection has been cured.

 HOW TO TREAT

NOTE—Follow your doctor's instructions. These instructions are supplemental.

GENERAL MEASURES
• Apply prescribed medicine with cotton balls to affected parts once a day for 3 weeks. Rinse off in 30 minutes if you wish.
• Expose affected skin to air as much as possible.
• Repeat treatment prior to tanning season each year.

MEDICATION—Your doctor may prescribe selenium sulfide shampoo (Exgel and Selsun) or other antifungal medication to apply to affected areas.

ACTIVITY—No restrictions.

DIET—No special diet.

 CALL YOUR DOCTOR IF

• You have symptoms of pityriasis versicolor.
• Infection doesn't improve despite treatment.

PLACENTA PREVIA

GENERAL INFORMATION

DEFINITION—Bleeding late in pregnancy caused by placenta attachment too low in the uterus, covering the cervix. This can be life-threatening to the unborn child. It occurs to some degree in 1 of 200 pregnancies.

BODY PARTS INVOLVED—Uterus; placenta (the organ that transfers nourishment and oxygen from mother to fetus); cervix (opening to the uterus).

SEX OR AGE MOST AFFECTED—Pregnant women.

SIGNS & SYMPTOMS
- Sudden, painless bleeding during the second or third trimester of pregnancy—especially the last 13 weeks. Bleeding may begin moderately and become severe.
- Abnormal fetal position in the uterus.

CAUSES—Normally, placenta attaches high on the uterus wall, away from the cervix. In placenta previa, the placenta covers the cervix partially or completely. Any change in the cervix, such as the softening and dilating that occurs close to delivery, can cause the placenta to separate from the uterus and bleed.

RISK INCREASES WITH
- Fibroid tumors of the uterus.
- Diabetes mellitus.
- Previous uterine surgery.
- Smoking.
- Multiple previous pregnancies and deliveries.
- Mothers over age 35.

HOW TO PREVENT—Don't smoke during pregnancy.

WHAT TO EXPECT

APPROPRIATE HEALTH CARE
- Doctor's treatment.
- Hospitalization.
- Surgery to deliver the fetus by Cesarean section (sometimes). Vaginal delivery is possible if the placenta separation is small or the cervix is covered only partially.

DIAGNOSTIC MEASURES
- Your own observation of symptoms, especially of vaginal bleeding during pregnancy.
- Medical history and physical exam by a doctor.
- Laboratory blood tests to determine the amount of blood loss.
- Ultrasonography to determine the exact location of the placenta.

POSSIBLE COMPLICATIONS
- Premature delivery or fetal death, if extensive placenta previa develops before the expected delivery date.
- Hazardous blood loss, requiring blood transfusions for the mother.

PROBABLE OUTCOME—With prompt care, mothers and most infants survive without complications. In some cases, delivery is necessary before the fetus is mature enough to survive.

HOW TO TREAT

NOTE—Follow your doctor's instructions. These instructions are supplemental.

GENERAL MEASURES—Have regular checkups during pregnancy. If signs of placenta previa appear, be prepared to go to the hospital early for observation and possible delivery. Arrange for fast transportation to the hospital in case of emergency, especially massive bleeding.

A marginal placenta previa requires bed rest in the hospital until bleeding stops. If bleeding stops, you may get up—but you should stay in the hospital until delivery. If you leave the hospital, your life and that of your child will be at risk. Massive bleeding can occur before you can get back to the hospital.

If you are near the expected delivery date and studies reveal more than a marginal or low-lying placenta, immediate Cesarean section is necessary—even though the child is below optimal size and development.

MEDICATION—Only minimal analgesic medications—if any—will be used in delivery to increase the child's survival chances. Blood transfusions may be necessary.

Don't use aspirin during pregnancy—it increases the risk of bleeding.

ACTIVITY—Rest in bed until bleeding stops or you deliver your child.

DIET—While you are bleeding and as long as surgery is being considered, drink liquids only. Eating solid food before surgery can cause anesthesia problems.

CALL YOUR DOCTOR IF

You have symptoms of placenta previa. Report any bleeding immediately. This is an emergency!

PLEURISY

GENERAL INFORMATION

DEFINITION—Inflammation and irritation of the pleura, a thin, two-layered membrane that encloses the lung and lines the inside of the chest.

BODY PARTS INVOLVED—Pleura.

SEX OR AGE MOST AFFECTED—Both sexes; all ages.

SIGNS & SYMPTOMS
- Sudden chest pain that worsens with breathing and coughing. The pain varies from vague discomfort that occurs only with deep breathing or coughing to intense, stabbing pain. Pain is usually over the area of pleura inflammation, but it may also occur in the lower chest or abdomen.
- Fever.
- Discomfort on moving the affected side.
- Rapid, shallow breathing.

If fluid develops at the site of inflammation between the two membrane layers, the liquid is called pleural effusion. When this happens, the pleurisy pain usually subsides, but breathlessness worsens.

CAUSES—Complication of:
- Lung or chest infections, such as pneumonia or tuberculosis.
- Bronchiectasis.
- Collapse of part of the lung.
- Blood clot in the lung.
- Injury to the chest or rib fracture.
- Cancer in other parts of the body.
- Collagen vascular disease, such as systemic lupus erythematosus or rheumatoid arthritis.
- Congestive heart failure.
- Kidney disorders.
- Liver disorders.

RISK INCREASES WITH
- Obesity.
- Smoking.
- Use of immunosuppressive drugs.

HOW TO PREVENT—Obtain medical treatment for the underlying disorder.

WHAT TO EXPECT

APPROPRIATE HEALTH CARE
- Self-care after diagnosis.
- Doctor's treatment.

DIAGNOSTIC MEASURES
- Your own observation of symptoms.
- Medical history and physical exam by a doctor.
- Laboratory blood studies to detect infection or autoimmune disease.
- X-rays of the chest.

POSSIBLE COMPLICATIONS
- Pneumonia.
- Lung compression and impaired breathing from leakage of pleural effusion.
- Scarring and adhesions at the site of inflammation, restricting lung expansion.

PROBABLE OUTCOME—Successful treatment of pleurisy depends on successful treatment of the disorder causing it. Often, symptoms without complications clear completely and spontaneously in 2 weeks.

HOW TO TREAT

NOTE—Follow your doctor's instructions. These instructions are supplemental.

GENERAL MEASURES
- For chest pain, wrap the entire chest loosely with 2 or 3 non-adhesive, 6-inch-wide elastic bandages.
- For coughing, use a cool-mist humidifier to help loosen bronchial secretions so they can be coughed up easily.

MEDICATION—Your doctor may prescribe antibiotics or pain relievers after diagnosis of the underlying disorder. You may take simple pain relievers, such as acetaminophen or aspirin, to relieve pain if no complicating disorders exist.

ACTIVITY—Reduce activity until pain and fever disappear. Then resume normal activities gradually.

DIET—No special diet.

CALL YOUR DOCTOR IF

- You have symptoms of pleurisy.
- The following occurs during treatment:
  Temperature spikes over 101F (38.3C).
  Increased pain.
  Increased breathlessness.
  Cough that is dry and non-productive.
  Blue or dark fingernails, toenails or lips.
  Blood in the sputum.

PNEUMOCONIOSIS

 GENERAL INFORMATION

DEFINITION—Inflammation of the lung caused by breathing industrial dusts. This is not contagious. It may lead to lung cancer.

BODY PARTS INVOLVED—Lungs.

SEX OR AGE MOST AFFECTED—Men over age 40.

SIGNS & SYMPTOMS—Early symptoms:
- Shortness of breath.
- Cough that produces little or no sputum.
- General ill feeling.

Late symptoms:
- Fitful sleep.
- Appetite and weight loss.
- Chest pain.
- Hoarseness.
- Coughing blood.
- Symptoms of congestive heart failure.
- Bluish nails.
- Shadows on the lungs (visible with chest X-rays).

CAUSES—At least 20 years of exposure to small particles of industrial dusts cause the following forms of pneumoconiosis:
- Coal dust causes black-lung disease (coal miner's pneumoconiosis, anthracosis).
- Beryllium and its compounds—once used in manufacturing fluorescent lamp bulbs, ceramics and chemicals—cause berylliosis.
- Talc, iron, cotton, synthetic fiber and aluminum dusts cause a rare form of pneumoconiosis.
- Asbestos and silica cause asbestosis and silicosis. These are described separately in the Illness section.

RISK INCREASES WITH
- Poor nutrition.
- Smoking.
- Excess alcohol consumption.

HOW TO PREVENT
- During exposure to industrial dusts, wear a protective mask or external-air-supplied hood.
- Don't smoke.
- Participate in a regular physical exercise program to maintain good cardio-pulmonary fitness.

 WHAT TO EXPECT

APPROPRIATE HEALTH CARE
- Self-care after diagnosis.
- Doctor's treatment.

DIAGNOSTIC MEASURES
- Your own observation of symptoms.
- Medical history and physical exam by a doctor.
- X-ray of chest.

POSSIBLE COMPLICATIONS
- Congestive heart failure.
- Lung collapse.
- Pleurisy.
- Tuberculosis in the late stages.

PROBABLE OUTCOME—This condition is currently considered incurable. However, symptoms can be relieved or controlled. It reduces life expectancy, but many patients live into their 60s and 70s. Scientific research into causes and treatment continues, so there is hope for increasingly effective treatment and cure.

 HOW TO TREAT

NOTE—Follow your doctor's instructions. These instructions are supplemental.

GENERAL MEASURES—The following measures may relieve symptoms and protect against recurrent lung infections:
- Obtain medical treatment for any respiratory infection, including the common cold.
- Consider moving to a warm, dry climate if your disease is advanced.
- Practice bronchial drainage. Your doctor will provide instructions.
- Use a cool-mist humidifier to loosen bronchial secretions so they may be coughed up easily.

MEDICATION
- Your doctor may prescribe:
  Antibiotics for infections.
  Bronchodilators (inhaled or oral) with inhalation therapy (supervised at first by an inhalation therapist) to open bronchial tubes to the maximum.
- For minor discomfort, you may use non-prescription drugs, such as acetaminophen or aspirin.

ACTIVITY
- Rest in bed with infections. You may read or watch TV.
- After treatment, resume normal activity as soon as symptoms improve.

DIET—No special diet.

 CALL YOUR DOCTOR IF

- You have symptoms of pneumoconiosis.
- The following occurs during treatment:
  Temperature spike of 101F (38.3C) or more.
  Increased chest pain or breathlessness.
  Blood in sputum.
  Continuing weight loss.
- New, unexplained symptoms develop.
Drugs used in treatment may produce side effects.

PNEUMONIA, BACTERIAL

 GENERAL INFORMATION

DEFINITION—Infection and inflammation of the lungs with bacterial germs. This is not usually contagious.

BODY PARTS INVOLVED—Lungs; bronchial tubes.

SEX OR AGE MOST AFFECTED—All ages, but most severe in young children and adults over age 60.

SIGNS & SYMPTOMS
- High fever (over 102F or 38.9C) and chills.
- Shortness of breath.
- Cough with sputum that may contain blood or blood streaks.
- Rapid breathing.
- Chest pain that worsens with inhalations.
- Abdominal pain.
- Fatigue.
- Bluish lips and nails (rare).

CAUSES—Infection with bacteria, such as pneumococci, hemophilus, streptococci or staphylococci.

RISK INCREASES WITH
- Newborns and infants.
- Adults over 60.
- Use of anticancer drugs.
- Smoking.
- Illness that has lowered resistance, such as: heart disease; recent surgery; cancer; tuberculosis; congestive heart failure; diabetes; alcoholism; or chronic lung disease.
- Poor general health from any cause.
- Crowded or unsanitary living conditions.

HOW TO PREVENT
- Obtain prompt medical treatment for respiratory infections.
- Arrange for pneumococcal and influenza immunizations of persons at risk.

 WHAT TO EXPECT

APPROPRIATE HEALTH CARE
- Self-care after diagnosis.
- Doctor's treatment.
- Hospitalization (severe cases only).

DIAGNOSTIC MEASURES
- Your own observation of symptoms.
- Medical history and physical exam by a doctor.
- Laboratory studies, such as a sputum culture, blood culture and blood count.
- X-rays of lungs.

POSSIBLE COMPLICATIONS
- Pleurisy.
- Pleural effusion (fluid between the membranes that cover the lung).
- Spread of infection to the brain or meninges (meningitis).

PROBABLE OUTCOME—Usually curable in 1 to 2 weeks with treatment, but may take longer for the very young or elderly.

 HOW TO TREAT

NOTE—Follow your doctor's instructions. These instructions are supplemental.

GENERAL MEASURES
- Use a cool-mist humidifier to increase air moisture. Putting medicine in the humidifier probably will not help.
- Don't suppress the cough with medicine if the cough produces sputum or mucus. It is useful in ridding the body of lung secretions.
- Suppress the cough with medicine if it is dry, non-productive and painful. Consult your doctor about a cough suppressant.
- Use a heating pad or hot compresses to relieve chest pain.

MEDICATION
- Your doctor may prescribe antibiotics to fight infection.
- You may use non-prescription drugs, such as acetaminophen, to relieve minor discomfort.

ACTIVITY—Rest in bed until fever declines and pain and shortness of breath disappear. You may read or watch TV. After treatment, resume normal activity as soon as possible.

DIET—No special diet. Increase fluid intake; drink at least 1 glass of water or other beverage every hour. Extra fluid helps thin lung secretions so they are easier to cough up.

 CALL YOUR DOCTOR IF

- You have symptoms of pneumonia.
- The following occurs during treatment: Fever higher than 102F (38.9C).
  Pain not relieved by heat or prescribed medication.
  Increased shortness of breath.
  Dark or bluish fingernails, skin or toenails.
  Blood in the sputum.
  Nausea, vomiting or diarrhea.
- New, unexplained symptoms develop.
Drugs used in treatment may produce side effects.

PNEUMONIA, MYCOPLASMA
(Primary Atypical Pneumonia; Eaton-Agent Pneumonia)

GENERAL INFORMATION

DEFINITION—Contagious lung inflammation caused by mycoplasma bacteria. This germ can cause infection in other body parts.

BODY PARTS INVOLVED—Upper-respiratory system.

SEX OR AGE MOST AFFECTED—All ages, but most common in children (1 to 12 years).

SIGNS & SYMPTOMS
- Cough (with or without sputum).
- Fever.
- Labored breathing.
- Chest pain.
- Abdominal pain.
- Bluish skin (severe cases).

CAUSES—Preceding mycoplasma infection in the nose, throat or bronchial tubes.

RISK INCREASES WITH
- Stress.
- Illness that has lowered resistance.
- Exposure to cold, harsh weather.
- Crowded or unsanitary living conditions.

HOW TO PREVENT
- Avoid exposure to persons who are ill with respiratory infections.
- Don't get chilled or wet in cold weather.

WHAT TO EXPECT

APPROPRIATE HEALTH CARE
- Home care after diagnosis.
- Doctor's treatment.
- Hospitalization of seriously ill children.

DIAGNOSTIC MEASURES
- Your own observation of symptoms.
- Medical history and physical exam by a doctor.
- Laboratory culture of sputum and blood studies.
- Chest X-rays.

POSSIBLE COMPLICATIONS—Prolonged illness.

PROBABLE OUTCOME—This form of pneumonia is characteristically slow to heal. It is usually curable in 4 to 6 weeks with treatment. Lungs should not have residual scars.

HOW TO TREAT

NOTE—Follow your doctor's instructions. These instructions are supplemental.

GENERAL MEASURES
- Use a cool-mist humidifier to increase air moisture. Putting medicine in the humidifier probably will not help.
- Don't suppress the cough with medicine if it produces sputum or mucus. Coughing is useful in ridding the body of lung secretions.
- Suppress the cough with medicine if it is dry, non-productive and painful. Consult your doctor about a cough suppressant.
- Use a heating pad on low heat or hot compresses to relieve chest pain.
- Catch sneezes and coughs with disposable tissue.

MEDICATION—Your doctor may prescribe:
- Antibiotics, such as erythromycin, to fight infection.
- Cough medicine to make the cough more tolerable.
- Nose drops, sprays or oral decongestants to reduce congestion in the upper-respiratory system.

ACTIVITY—Bed rest is necessary until fever subsides. Normal activities should be resumed gradually.

DIET—No special diet. Increase fluids to at least 1 glass of water or other beverage every hour. Extra fluid helps thin lung secretions so they can be coughed up more easily .

CALL YOUR DOCTOR IF

- You or your child have symptoms of mycoplasma pneumonia.
- The following occurs during treatment:
  Fever higher than 102F (38.9C).
  Pain that is not relieved by heat or prescribed medication.
  Increased shortness of breath.
  Dark or bluish fingernails, skin or toenails.
  Blood in the sputum.
  Nausea, vomiting or diarrhea.
- New, unexplained symptoms develop.
Drugs used in treatment may produce side effects.

PNEUMONIA, VIRAL

GENERAL INFORMATION

DEFINITION—Lung infection caused by a virus. It is unlikely that others will develop pneumonia from exposure to a person with viral pneumonia.

BODY PARTS INVOLVED
- Lower respiratory tract (bronchial tubes, bronchioles and lungs).
- Upper respiratory tract (nose, throat, tonsils, sinuses, trachea and larynx).

SEX OR AGE MOST AFFECTED—Both sexes; all ages.

SIGNS & SYMPTOMS
- Fever and chills.
- Muscle aches and fatigue.
- Cough, with or without sputum or "croup."
- Rapid, labored (sometimes) breathing.
- Chest pain.
- Sore throat.
- Loss of appetite.
- Enlarged lymph glands in the neck.
- Bluish nails.

CAUSES—Virus infections, including influenza, chickenpox (especially in adults), respiratory viruses, measles and cytomegalovirus (especially in infants).

RISK INCREASES WITH
- Newborns and infants.
- Adults over 60.
- Asthma.
- Cystic fibrosis.
- Inhalation of a foreign body into the lung.
- Smoking.
- Crowded or unsanitary living conditions.

HOW TO PREVENT—No specific preventive measures.

WHAT TO EXPECT

APPROPRIATE HEALTH CARE
- Self-care after diagnosis.
- Doctor's treatment.
- Hospitalization (rare).

DIAGNOSTIC MEASURES
- Your own observation of symptoms.
- Medical history and physical exam by a doctor.
- Laboratory blood studies.
- X-rays of the chest.

POSSIBLE COMPLICATIONS
- Secondary bacterial infections of the lungs.
- Post-infectious depression.

PROBABLE OUTCOME—Usually curable in 4 weeks.

HOW TO TREAT

NOTE—Follow your doctor's instructions. These instructions are supplemental.

GENERAL MEASURES
- Use a cool-mist humidifier to increase air moisture. Putting medicine in the vaporizer probably will not help.
- Use a heating pad on the chest to relieve chest pain.

MEDICATION
- If the cough produces sputum, it is ridding the lungs of secretions and should not be suppressed with medicine. If the cough is dry, non-productive and painful, you may suppress it with non-prescription cough medicine that contains dextromethorphan.
- For minor pain and fever, you may use non-prescription drugs, such as acetaminophen or decongestant nose drops, nasal sprays or tablets.
- Your doctor may prescribe antibiotics to fight secondary bacterial infections.

ACTIVITY—Bed rest is necessary until fever, pain and shortness of breath have been gone at least 48 hours. Then normal activity may be resumed slowly. Many people are fatigued and weak for up to 6 weeks after recovery, so don't expect a quick return to normal strength.

DIET—No special diet, but do everything possible to maintain a normal intake of nutritious foods and drinks. Drink at least 1 full glass of fluid each hour. This helps thin lung secretions so they are easier to cough up.

CALL YOUR DOCTOR IF

- You have symptoms of pneumonia.
- The following occurs during treatment:
  Temperature spikes over 102F (38.9C).
  Intolerable pain, despite medication and heat treatment.
  Increasing shortness of breath.
  Increasing blueness of nails and skin.
  Blood in the sputum.
  Nausea, vomiting, or diarrhea.

PNEUMOTHORAX

GENERAL INFORMATION

DEFINITION—Collapse of part or all of a lung caused by pressure from free air in the chest between the two layers of the pleura (thin membranes that cover the lung).

BODY PARTS INVOLVED—Lung; pleura.

SEX OR AGE MOST AFFECTED—All ages, but most common in active young men (20 to 40 years).

SIGNS & SYMPTOMS—The following symptoms vary according to the degree of lung collapse and extent of underlying lung disease. Symptoms may be less acute if the pneumothorax develops slowly:
- Sharp chest pain. Pain may extend to a shoulder or across the chest or abdomen.
- Shortness of breath.
- Dry, hacking cough (occasionally).

CAUSES—Spontaneous pneumothorax:
- Rupture of a small air sac in the lung resulting from asthma, lung abcess or empyema, or physical exertion, such as diving, high-altitude flying or stretching. Causes related to activity occur most often in healthy persons.
Pneumothorax due to trauma:
- Penetrating wounds to the chest, which permit outside air to rush into the pleural space and cause the lung to collapse.
- Complication of removing fluid from the lung (thoracentesis).

RISK INCREASES WITH
- Chest injury.
- Chronic lung disease.
- Smoking.

HOW TO PREVENT
- Obtain medical treatment for lung disorders, such as asthma or emphysema.
- Don't smoke.

WHAT TO EXPECT

APPROPRIATE HEALTH CARE
- Self-care after diagnosis.
- Doctor's treatment.
- Hospitalization, if the extent of lung collapse is disabling.

DIAGNOSTIC MEASURES
- Your own observation of symptoms.
- Medical history and physical exam by a doctor.
- X-rays of the chest to confirm the diagnosis.

POSSIBLE COMPLICATIONS
- Respiratory failure.
- Lung infection.

PROBABLE OUTCOME—A small pneumothorax is inconsequential and heals itself. However, if the collapse is extensive and it occurs in middle-aged or older adults whose lungs are damaged by asthma, chronic bronchitis or emphysema, it can lead to respiratory failure and critical illness.

Treatment depends on the size of the pneumothorax and the condition of the lungs. The disorder may heal itself, but hospitalization and treatment may be necessary to remove the air.

HOW TO TREAT

NOTE—Follow your doctor's instructions. These instructions are supplemental.

GENERAL MEASURES
- Don't smoke.
- Try not to cough.
- Avoid loud talking, laughing or singing.
- You may be more comfortable if you rest in a sitting position.

MEDICATION—Medication usually is not necessary. However, you may use non-prescription drugs, such as acetaminophen, for minor pain. For severe pain, your doctor may prescribe stronger pain relievers.

ACTIVITY—Stay as active as your strength allows. Rest often. Resume your normal activities as soon as possible. Allow about 2 weeks for recovery.

DIET—No special diet.

CALL YOUR DOCTOR IF

- You have symptoms of pneumothorax.
- The following occurs during treatment:
Temperature rises to 101F (38.3C).
Chest pain or shortness of breath increases.
Painful, debilitating coughing or sputum production begins.

POLYARTERITIS
(Polyarteritis Nodosa; Periarteritis Nodosa; Necrotizing Angiitis)

 GENERAL INFORMATION

DEFINITION—A disorder of connective tissue that is one of several related diseases of collagen tissue. Collagen is a protein molecule that forms the major part of all connective tissue.

Polyarteritis causes inflammation of small and medium arteries, decreasing the blood supply to tissues supplied by the affected blood vessels. It is not contagious.

BODY PARTS INVOLVED—All body parts.

SEX OR AGE MOST AFFECTED
- Both sexes, but more common in men.
- All ages, but most common in adults under age 50.

SIGNS & SYMPTOMS—Varies, depending on which organ is affected by the decreased blood supply. The most common include:
- Chest pain (heart involvement).
- Shortness of breath (lung involvement).
- Abdominal pain (intestinal and liver involvement).
- Blood in the urine (kidney involvement).
- Numbness and tingling of the hands and feet (nerve involvement).
The course may be acute, with fever, weight loss and rapid deterioration. If the course is chronic, body tissues will waste away over several years.

CAUSES—This is considered a disease of autoimmunity or hypersensitivity, although the cause is uncertain. In many persons, no predisposing factors can be found. Following are the most common preceding factors:
- Bacterial infections.
- Viral infections.
- Use of certain drugs, including sulfa drugs, penicillin, antithyroid drugs, gold and thiazide diuretics.
- Vaccines.

RISK INCREASES WITH
- Family history of collagen or hypersensitivity disease.
- Smoking.

HOW TO PREVENT—No specific preventive measures.

 WHAT TO EXPECT

APPROPRIATE HEALTH CARE
- Self-care after diagnosis.
- Doctor's treatment.
- Surgery to remove part of the intestines, if they are involved.
- Hospitalization for intensive treatment (severe cases).

DIAGNOSTIC MEASURES
- Your own observation of symptoms.
- Medical history and physical exam by a doctor.
- Laboratory studies of kidneys and blood, including sedimentation rate (see Glossary).

POSSIBLE COMPLICATIONS—Kidney failure and death, despite treatment.

PROBABLE OUTCOME—This condition is currently considered incurable. However, symptoms can be relieved or controlled. Many patients live many years with the disease, and medical literature cites a few instances of unexplained recovery.

Scientific research into causes and treatment continues, so there is hope for increasingly effective treatment and cure.

 HOW TO TREAT

NOTE—Follow your doctor's instructions. These instructions are supplemental.

GENERAL MEASURES—No specific instructions except those listed under other headings.

MEDICATION—Your doctor may prescribe:
- Cortisone drugs in high doses until acute symptoms diminish. Then symptoms may be controlled by a schedule of 1 cortisone dose every other day. Take only as long as necessary. Long-term use of cortisone produces serious adverse effects.
- Drugs to treat disorders of organs involved with this serious disease, such as heart medications for heart involvement or antihypertensives for high blood pressure.
- Immunosuppressive drugs—either alone or with steroids—if other drugs fail. These drugs pose additional risks, including severe generalized septic bacterial infections.

ACTIVITY—Resume your normal activities gradually as symptoms improve.

DIET—Low-salt diet (see Appendix 9).

 CALL YOUR DOCTOR IF

- You have symptoms of polyarteritis.
- New, unexplained symptoms develop. Drugs used in treatment may produce side effects.

POLYCYTHEMIA

GENERAL INFORMATION

DEFINITION—An increase in red blood cells in the body. The disease has 3 forms:
● Polycythemia vera, which involves overproduction of red blood cells, white blood cells and platelets.
● Secondary polycythemia (pseudo-polycythemia), which is a complication of diseases or factors other than blood-cell disorders.
● Stress polycythemia (pseudo-polycythemia), which involves decreased blood plasma.

BODY PARTS INVOLVED—Blood-forming organs: bone marrow; spleen; lymph glands; lymph channels.

SEX OR AGE MOST AFFECTED—Adults of both sexes over age 60, but more common in men.

SIGNS & SYMPTOMS—Some patients have no symptoms. Others have any of the following:
● Fatigue; headache; drowsiness; dizziness.
● Itching or flushed skin.
● Enlarged spleen.
● Unexplained bleeding.

CAUSES
● Polycythemia vera: unknown.
● Secondary polycythemia: congenital heart disease; chronic lung disease; cigarette or cigar smoking; living at high altitude.
● Stress polycythemia: use of diuretic drugs; smoking; dehydration.

RISK INCREASES WITH
● Smoking.
● Heart or lung disease.
● Stress.
● Family history of polycythemia.

HOW TO PREVENT
● Polycythemia vera cannot be prevented at present.
● To prevent secondary polycythemia or stress polycythemia:
  Don't smoke.
  Avoid dehydration.
  Obtain medical treatment for heart or lung disease.

WHAT TO EXPECT

APPROPRIATE HEALTH CARE
Your doctor may use 1 of 3 forms of treatment available to keep the hematocrit range (see Glossary) near normal and prevent clotting or hemorrhage:
● Phlebotomy (withdrawal of blood).
● Radioisotope therapy (see Glossary).
● Drug therapy.

The treatment chosen will depend upon symptoms and response to treatment. More than one form of treatment may be needed.

DIAGNOSTIC MEASURES
● Your own observation of symptoms.
● Medical history and physical exam by a doctor.
● Laboratory studies of bone marrow and blood (red-blood-cell count, measurement of hematocrit).
● X-ray of the kidneys.
● Radioactive chromium studies.

POSSIBLE COMPLICATIONS
● Clots in veins or arteries.
● Gout.
● Stroke.
● Heart attack.
● Peptic ulcer.
● Kidney stones.
● Chronic leukemia from radioisotope therapy (rare).

PROBABLE OUTCOME
● Polycythemia vera is incurable, but symptoms can be controlled and it does not affect life expectancy.
● Other forms of polycythemia can be cured if the causes can be eliminated.

HOW TO TREAT

NOTE—Follow your doctor's instructions. These instructions are supplemental.

GENERAL MEASURES—No specific instructions except those under other headings.

MEDICATION—Your doctor may prescribe:
● Aspirin to decrease clotting and reduce the chance of stroke or heart attack.
● Radioactive phosphorus, or cytotoxic drugs, such as chlorambucil or cyclophosphamide, to decrease production of red blood cells.

ACTIVITY—After treatment, resume normal activity as soon as possible.

DIET—No special diet. Drink 6 to 8 oz. of fluid every 2 hours to maintain adequate body fluid.

CALL YOUR DOCTOR IF

● You have symptoms of polycythemia.
● You have symptoms of complications (refer to specific disorder in this book).
● New, unexplained symptoms develop. Drugs used in treatment may produce side effects.

ILLNESSES & DISORDERS

POLYMYALGIA RHEUMATICA OR TEMPORAL ARTERITIS
(Giant-Cell Arteritis; Cranial Arteritis)

 GENERAL INFORMATION

DEFINITION—Inflammatory disease of the large arteries, especially those in the head and neck. Symptoms of polymyalgia rheumatica and temporal arteritis are the same, so the two diseases may be identical.

BODY PARTS INVOLVED—Muscles; temporal arteries; eyes; connective tissue.

SEX OR AGE MOST AFFECTED—Adults over 50. The disease occurs 4 times more often in women than men.

SIGNS & SYMPTOMS—The following symptoms may resemble those of an infection such as influenza.
- Low fever.
- Muscle stiffness, aches and pains—especially in the morning. The muscles involved are usually those of the trunk, upper arms and legs.
- Severe, throbbing headache (usually in one temple).
- Redness, swelling, tenderness and pulsating nodules along the temporal artery on one side of the head.
- Appetite loss.

CAUSES—An autoimmune disorder in which the body's immune system attacks and destroys its own tissues (especially connective tissue). The underlying cause is unknown.

RISK INCREASES WITH—Adults over 60, especially women.

HOW TO PREVENT—No specific preventive measures.

 WHAT TO EXPECT

APPROPRIATE HEALTH CARE
- Self-care after diagnosis.
- Doctor's treatment for this disorder or problems associated with it. These may include heart disease, high blood pressure or decreased blood supply to the bowel.
- Surgery, if the bowel develops intestinal gangrene.

DIAGNOSTIC MEASURES
- Your own observation of symptoms.
- Medical history and physical exam by a doctor.
- Laboratory studies, such as sedimentation rate (see Glossary), white-blood-cell count and blood tests for anemia.
- Biopsy (see Glossary) of the temporal artery.

POSSIBLE COMPLICATIONS
- Without treatment:
  Loss of vision.
  Coronary-artery disease.
  Stroke.
  Poor blood circulation to the arms and legs.
- With treatment: Cortisone drugs may be necessary for 2 years. Complications of long-term cortisone use are significant, including osteoporosis and peptic-ulcer disease.

PROBABLE OUTCOME—Usually curable in 2 years with cortisone treatment.

 HOW TO TREAT

NOTE—Follow your doctor's instructions. These instructions are supplemental.

GENERAL MEASURES
- Apply heat to the painful side of the head. You may use warm compresses or a heat lamp.
- Gently massage the back of the neck and sore muscles.

MEDICATION—Your doctor may prescribe:
- Cortisone drugs in high doses until the acute phase ends. These dramatically relieve symptoms by altering the inflammation causing them.
  For continuing treatment with cortisone, the lowest possible single dose taken every other day may keep symptoms under control.
- Immunosuppressive drugs—either alone or with cortisone—if other treatment is not successful. These drugs impose additional risks, including severe generalized bacterial infections.
- Heart medications (if the heart is involved).
- Antihypertensive drugs (if high blood pressure is part of the problem).

ACTIVITY—No restrictions.

DIET—No special diet.

 CALL YOUR DOCTOR IF

- You have symptoms of polymyalgia rheumatica and temporal arteritis.
- The following occurs during treatment:
- Temperature of 101F (38.3C).
  Blood in the urine.
  Shortness of breath.
  Chest pain.
  Bloody bowel movements.
  Severe abdominal pain.
  Any illness with fever.
- New, unexplained symptoms develop. Drugs used in treatment may produce side effects.

POLYMYOSITIS & DERMATOMYOSITIS

GENERAL INFORMATION

DEFINITION—Inflammation of connective tissue, with degenerative changes in the muscles (polymyositis) and skin (dermatomyositis). This causes weakness and muscle wasting, especially in the arms and legs. This disease has many similarities to rheumatoid arthritis and lupus erythematosus.

BODY PARTS INVOLVED—Muscles, including large muscles of the skeleton and tiny muscles that control small arteries; skin; connective tissue.

SEX OR AGE MOST AFFECTED
- Twice as common in women as men.
- All ages, but most likely to begin between ages 30 and 50.

SIGNS & SYMPTOMS—Sudden or slow onset of the following:
- Weakness in the pelvic-girdle and shoulder-girdle muscles.
- Skin rash that may itch on the face, shoulders, arms and over joints.
- Cold hands and feet.
- Frequent falls and difficulty in getting up.
- Speaking or swallowing difficulty.
- Infection with fever, muscle weakness, weight loss and joint pain (sometimes) preceding other symptoms.

CAUSES—Probably a disease of hypersensitivity or autoimmunity, although the cause is uncertain. This disease has been associated with the use of certain drugs and preceding bacterial infections, viral infections and vaccines.

RISK INCREASES WITH
- Allergies.
- Use of sulfa drugs, penicillin, antithyroid drugs, gold and thiazide diuretics.
- Family history of hypersensitivity diseases from illness or drugs, such as lupus.
- Cancer of the lung, colon or breast.

HOW TO PREVENT—No specific preventive measures.

WHAT TO EXPECT

APPROPRIATE HEALTH CARE
- Self-care after diagnosis.
- Doctor's treatment.
- Hospitalization during early, active phases.
- Surgery, if intestinal obstruction occurs.
- Time in an extended-care facility for physical therapy and rehabilitation.

DIAGNOSTIC MEASURES
- Your own observation of symptoms.
- Medical history and physical exam by a doctor.

- Laboratory blood studies to measure antinuclear antibodies (ANA).
- Surgical diagnostic procedures, such as biopsy of muscle and electromyography (see Glossary for both).

POSSIBLE COMPLICATIONS
- Muscle and body wasting.
- Congestive heart failure.
- High blood pressure.
- Intestinal obstruction.
- Kidney damage.

PROBABLE OUTCOME—The disease may begin suddenly or gradually. Most patients become wheelchair-bound or bedridden because of muscle weakness. Some symptoms can be controlled briefly with treatment, but the disease is often fatal in a short time. However, remissions or spontaneous recovery can occur—especially in children.
   Scientific research into causes and treatment continues, so there is hope for increasingly effective treatment and cure.

HOW TO TREAT

NOTE—Follow your doctor's instructions. These instructions are supplemental.

GENERAL MEASURES
- The patient may need a wheelchair and attendants to help with the daily routine.
- If confined to bed, the patient should be moved frequently to prevent pressure sores.
- Passive exercise should be provided to prevent contractures (muscle shortening).
- Cool-water compresses may relieve itching.

MEDICATION—Your doctor may prescribe:
- Cortisone drugs in high doses until acute symptoms diminish, then in lower doses.
- Immunosuppressive drugs, if other treatment is not effective. These drugs impose additional risks, including life-threatening septic bacterial infections.

ACTIVITY—No restrictions, except those imposed by muscle weakness.

DIET—No special diet.

CALL YOUR DOCTOR IF

- You have symptoms or polymyositis and dermatomyositis.
- The following occurs during treatment:
   Blood in the urine.
   Shortness of breath.
   Chest pain.
   Bloody bowel movements.
   Severe abdominal pain.
   Fever.

PORPHYRIA

 GENERAL INFORMATION

DEFINITION—A rare inherited disorder characterized by excessive formation and excretion of porphyrins (chemicals in all living things).

BODY PARTS INVOLVED—Central nervous system; skin; liver; digestive system.

SEX OR AGE MOST AFFECTED
- Both sexes, but more common and severe in females.
- All ages, but less likely in older adults.

SIGNS & SYMPTOMS
- Increased sensitivity to light.
- Mental changes, including depression and mania.
- Skin changes, including itching and blistering.
- Dark urine that darkens more if left standing in a specimen jar.
- Abdominal pain and vomiting.
- Muscle cramps and weakness.
- Numbness and tingling in the feet and hands.

CAUSES—An inherited disturbance in the metabolism of porphyrins.

RISK INCREASES WITH
- Family history of porphyria.
- Use of drugs, such as birth-control pills, alcohol, barbiturates. These don't cause the disease, but they may trigger attacks.
- Exposure to sunlight. This may trigger attacks.

HOW TO PREVENT—Cannot be prevented at present. To reduce the frequency and severity of attacks:
- Avoid all drugs, including non-prescription medicines, until you talk with your doctor.
- Don't take birth-control pills.
- Avoid bright sunlight.

OTHER—If you are a woman and your disease is severe, pregnancy may not be advisable. Any person with a family history of porphyria should seek genetic counseling before starting a family.

 WHAT TO EXPECT

APPROPRIATE HEALTH CARE
- Doctor's treatment.
- Psychotherapy or counseling.
- Hospitalization during attacks for supportive care.

DIAGNOSTIC MEASURES
- Your own observation of symptoms.
- Medical history and physical exam by a doctor.
- Laboratory studies to measure porphyrins in the urine, blood and stool.

POSSIBLE COMPLICATIONS
- A fatal porphyria crisis may occur during pregnancy. Special medical care is necessary in prenatal and postnatal stages.
- Misdiagnosis as a psychological or emotional problem may delay recognition and appropriate treatment.

PROBABLE OUTCOME—This condition is currently considered incurable, but many patients live several years with the disorder. Symptoms can be relieved or controlled.

Scientific research into causes and treatment continues, so there is hope for increasingly effective treatment and cure.

 HOW TO TREAT

NOTE—Follow your doctor's instructions. These instructions are supplemental.

GENERAL MEASURES—Avoid bright sunlight. If you must be in bright sun, use a hat and protective clothing.

MEDICATION—Medicine usually is not necessary for this disorder, and some drugs may trigger attacks. Don't take any medicine until you ask your doctor. Your doctor may prescribe tranquilizers to decrease anxiety.

ACTIVITY—No restrictions.

DIET—No special diet.

 CALL YOUR DOCTOR IF

- You have symptoms of porphyria.
- Dark urine or other symptoms of an attack recur.

POSTPARTUM DEPRESSION
(Postnatal Depression)

GENERAL INFORMATION

DEFINITION—Depression beginning up to 6 weeks following childbirth.

BODY PARTS INVOLVED—Brain.

SEX OR AGE MOST AFFECTED—Females of childbearing age.

SIGNS & SYMPTOMS
- Feelings of sadness, hopelessness or gloom.
- Appetite and weight loss.
- Sleep disturbances or frightening dreams.
- Loss of energy; fatigue.
- Slow speech and thought.
- Frequent headaches and other physical discomfort.
- Confusion about one's ability to improve life.

CAUSES—Most people consider it almost normal for a mother to be depressed during the first weeks after birth. Pregnancy and birth are accompanied by sudden hormonal changes that affect emotions.

Additionally, the 24-hour responsibility for a newborn infant represents a major psychological and lifestyle adjustment for most mothers—even if it is not the first child.

These physical and emotional stresses are usually accompanied by inadequate rest until the baby's routine stabilizes, so fatigue and depression are not unusual.

RISK INCREASES WITH
- Stress.
- Lack of sleep.
- Poor nutrition.
- Lack of support from one's partner, family or friends.
- Pre-existing neurosis or psychosis.

HOW TO PREVENT—Cannot be prevented, but can be minimized with rest, an adequate diet and a strong emotional support system.

WHAT TO EXPECT

APPROPRIATE HEALTH CARE
- Self-care after diagnosis.
- Doctor's treatment.
- Psychotherapy or counseling, if depression persists.
- Hospitalization (severe cases only).

DIAGNOSTIC MEASURES
- Your own observation of symptoms.
- Medical history and physical exam by a doctor.

POSSIBLE COMPLICATIONS
- Lack of bonding between mother and infant, which is harmful to both.

- Serious depression that may be accompanied by aggressive feelings toward the baby, a loss of pride in appearance and home, loss of appetite or compulsive eating, withdrawal from others or suicidal tendencies.

PROBABLE OUTCOME—With support from friends and family, mild postpartum depression usually disappears quickly.

If depression becomes severe, a mother may not be able to care for herself and the baby, and hospitalization may be necessary. Medication, counseling and support from others usually cure even severe depression in 3 to 6 months.

HOW TO TREAT

NOTE—Follow your doctor's instructions. These instructions are supplemental.

GENERAL MEASURES
- Don't feel guilty if you have mixed feelings about motherhood. Adjustment and bonding take time.
- Schedule frequent outings, such as walks and short visits with friends or family. These help prevent feelings of isolation.
- Have your baby sleep in a separate room. You will sleep more restfully.
- Ask for daytime help from family or friends who will shop for you or care for the baby while you rest.
- If you feel depressed, share your feelings with your partner or a friend who is a good listener. Talking with other mothers can help you keep problems in perspective.
- If depression becomes severe and hospitalization is necessary, choose a facility close enough to home so you can continue a close relationship with your baby.

MEDICATION—Your doctor may prescribe antidepressant drugs. These are often effective when used for 3 to 4 weeks.

ACTIVITY—No restrictions. Resume your normal activities as soon as possible. Resume sexual relations within 3 to 4 weeks after delivery. Ask your doctor for specific instructions.

DIET—No special diet.

CALL YOUR DOCTOR IF

- You have postpartum depression and additional life changes occur, such as divorce, career change or moving.
- Postpartum depression does not improve in 4 to 6 weeks.
- You seriously consider suicide. This is an emergency!

POTASSIUM IMBALANCE

 GENERAL INFORMATION

DEFINITION—Above- or below-normal levels of potassium in the blood, body fluids and body cells.

BODY PARTS INVOLVED—Blood, which affects all body cells and body fluids.

SEX OR AGE MOST AFFECTED—Both sexes; all ages.

SIGNS & SYMPTOMS—For above-normal levels (hyperkalemia):
- Weakness and paralysis.
- Dangerously rapid, irregular heartbeat or slow heartbeat (sometimes).
- Nausea and diarrhea.
For below-normal levels (hypokalemia):
- Weakness and paralysis.
- Low blood pressure.
- Life-threatening rapid, irregular heartbeat. This is more severe than with hyperkalemia.

CAUSES—Hyperkalemia:
- Chronic kidney disease with kidney failure. Failing kidneys eliminate potassium too slowly, causing an excess in the body.
- Use of oral potassium supplements.
- Burns or crushing injuries. These may release potassium from body tissues into body fluids.
- Addison's disease.
Hypokalemia:
- The use of diuretics drugs for hypertension or heart failure.
- Prolonged loss of body fluids from vomiting or diarrhea.
- Chronic kidney disease with kidney failure. At certain stages, this may cause the body to lose potassium.

RISK INCREASES WITH
- Diabetes mellitus.
- Adrenal disease.
- Use of drugs, such as diuretics, potassium supplements and digitalis. Low potassium levels—especially in persons who take digitalis—often lead to serious heartbeat disturbances.

HOW TO PREVENT
- If you have a disorder or take drugs that affect potassium levels (see Causes and Risks), learn as much as you can about your condition, your drugs and how you can prevent a potassium imbalance.
- If you take digitalis *and* diuretics, have frequent blood studies to monitor potassium levels.
- Obtain medical care for prolonged vomiting or diarrhea.

OTHER—A normal medium to high blood level of potassium may help protect against coronary-artery disease.

 WHAT TO EXPECT

APPROPRIATE HEALTH CARE
- Self-care after diagnosis.
- Doctor's treatment.
- Hospitalization (severe cases).

DIAGNOSTIC MEASURES
- Your own observation of symptoms, especially muscle weakness and heart-rhythm changes.
- Medical history and physical exam by a doctor.
- Laboratory blood and urine studies of potassium and other electrolytes.
- EKG (see Glossary).

POSSIBLE COMPLICATIONS—Cardiac arrest and death.

PROBABLE OUTCOME—Usually can be corrected with intravenous fluids and treatment of the underlying disorder.

 HOW TO TREAT

NOTE—Follow your doctor's instructions. These instructions are supplemental.

GENERAL MEASURES—If you take diuretics and digitalis, your friends and family members should learn cardiopulmonary resuscitation (CPR). Learn to count your own pulse at the wrist or neck.

MEDICATION—Your doctor may prescribe:
- Oral potassium supplements to raise low levels.
- Diuretics to increase urination and decrease high potassium levels.
- Intravenous fluids to correct a serious imbalance.
- Medications appropriate for the underlying disease.

ACTIVITY—Resume your normal activities as soon as symptoms improve.

DIET—Depends on the condition. Mild hypokalemia can be corrected by increasing consumption of potassium-containing foods, such as orange juice and bananas.

 CALL YOUR DOCTOR IF

You have symptoms of a potassium imbalance or are having problems with a disorder that affects potassium levels.

PREMATURE EJACULATION

GENERAL INFORMATION

DEFINITION—Male orgasm and ejaculation following brief sexual stimulation, and prior to satisfactory arousal and orgasm in the sexual partner.

BODY PARTS INVOLVED—Brain and central nervous system; reproductive system.

SEX OR AGE MOST AFFECTED—Male adolescents and adults.

SIGNS & SYMPTOMS
- Repeated episodes of premature ejaculation.
- Feelings of self-doubt, inadequacy and guilt.

CAUSES—Usually psychological, including:
- Poor relationship or communication with the sexual partner.
- Fear of impregnating the partner.
- Fear of contracting a sexually transmitted disease.
- Anxiety about sexual performance.
- Cultural or religious conflicts.
- Belief that sex is sinful or dirty.

RISK INCREASES WITH—Recent illness such as prostatitis.

HOW TO PREVENT—No specific preventive measures.

WHAT TO EXPECT

APPROPRIATE HEALTH CARE
- Self-care after diagnosis.
- Doctor's treatment, if self-help measures fail.
- Counseling from a qualified sex therapist.

DIAGNOSTIC MEASURES
- Your own observation of signs.
- Medical history and physical exam by a doctor.

POSSIBLE COMPLICATIONS
- Low self-esteem.
- Damage to marital or interpersonal relationships.

PROBABLE OUTCOME—Usually curable in most people within 6 months after recognition and treatment.

HOW TO TREAT

NOTE—Follow your doctor's instructions. These instructions are supplemental.

GENERAL MEASURES—The following methods are recommended by sex researchers and therapists Masters and Johnson. These measures usually lead to ejaculatory control for 5 to 10 minutes or longer:
- Sensate-focus exercises, in which each partner caresses the other's body without intercourse to learn relaxed, pleasurable aspects of touching.
- Mutual physical examination of each other's bodies to acquaint both partners thoroughly with anatomy. This helps reduce shameful feelings about sex.
- Stop-and-start technique, in which the man is stimulated through controlled intercourse or masturbation until he feels an impending ejaculation. Stimulation is stopped, then resumed in 20 to 30 seconds.
- Squeeze technique, in which the woman squeezes her partner's penis with her thumb and forefinger when he feels an impending ejaculation. When ejaculatory feelings pass, intercourse is resumed. This is repeated as often as necessary until the man can control ejaculation to the satisfaction of both partners.

MEDICATION—Medicine usually is not necessary for this disorder.

ACTIVITY—No restrictions.

DIET—No special diet.

CALL YOUR DOCTOR IF

You have had repeated episodes of premature ejaculation and want professional guidance to solve the problem.

ILLNESSES & DISORDERS

PREMATURE INFANTS

GENERAL INFORMATION

DEFINITION—Infants born before 37 weeks of pregnancy.

BODY PARTS INVOLVED—All body systems.

SEX OR AGE MOST AFFECTED—Both sexes of newborns.

SIGNS & SYMPTOMS
- Birth weight of less than 5-1/2 pounds (2.5 kg).
- Low body temperature.
- Breathing difficulty.
- Weak sucking and swallowing reflexes.
- Susceptibility to infection.
- Fluid and electrolyte imbalance (sometimes).
- Jaundice caused by poor elimination of bilirubin, a byproduct of breakdown of red blood cells.

CAUSES
- Premature labor.
- Induced (artificially-started) labor or Cesarean section because of serious injury or illness in the mother.

RISK INCREASES WITH
- Poor nutrition.
- Smoking.
- Injury to the uterus.
- Excess alcohol consumption.
- Use of mind-altering drugs.
- Inadequate prenatal care.
- Damage to cervix in previous deliveries.
- Vaginal infections that spread to the uterus.
- Urinary-tract infection.
- More than one fetus (twins or more).
- Previous premature delivery.
- Adolescent mothers.

HOW TO PREVENT
- Obtain good prenatal care throughout pregnancy.
- Don't smoke, use mind-altering drugs or drink alcohol during pregnancy.
- Eat a normal, well-balanced diet during pregnancy (see Appendix 3). Take prenatal vitamin and mineral supplements, if your doctor prescribes them.
- Don't use medications of any kind, including non-prescription drugs, without consulting your doctor.
- If you have a weak cervix, which is sometimes evident before pregnancy, ask your doctor about a minor operation to strengthen the cervix.
- Rest more and decrease activity in the 3rd trimester, especially if you have blood spotting or other warning signs.

WHAT TO EXPECT

APPROPRIATE HEALTH CARE
- Doctor's treatment.
- Hospitalization in a nursery for premature infants. This provides temperature-controlled bassinets, mechanical breathing machines and continuous nursing care.

DIAGNOSTIC MEASURES
- Medical history and physical exam by a doctor.
- Laboratory blood studies to detect anemia or infection and determine the degree of jaundice.

POSSIBLE COMPLICATIONS
- Anemia.
- Serious infections, such as meningitis or colitis.
- Hyaline-membrane disease (see Glossary).
- Blindness, if excessive oxygen is necessary to maintain life.

PROBABLE OUTCOME—The infant's survival chances depend on its maturity. With good care, most premature infants "catch up" developmentally with other children and lead normal lives.

HOW TO TREAT

NOTE—Follow your doctor's instructions. These instructions are supplemental.

GENERAL MEASURES—Premature infants require special care once they are mature enough to leave the hospital. Ask for assistance from a visiting-nurse service or your local health department.

MEDICATION—Medicine usually is not necessary for prematurity, but your doctor may prescribe drugs for complications.

ACTIVITY—No restrictions.

DIET—Feeding by stomach tube may be necessary if the infant's sucking reflex is too weak. When normal feeding is possible, most premature infants tolerate mother's milk best. You may return to the hospital as often as possible to feed the baby. Use a breast pump to express and store milk for feedings when you cannot be present. Hold the baby often. Bonding is important.

CALL YOUR DOCTOR IF

After returning home, your baby has any of the following:
- Fever.
- Poor appetite or poor weight gain.
- Excessive crying that persists even when the child is picked up.

PREMATURE LABOR

GENERAL INFORMATION

DEFINITION—Labor that begins before the 37th week of pregnancy.

BODY PARTS INVOLVED—Female reproductive system.

SEX OR AGE MOST AFFECTED—Pregnant females.

SIGNS & SYMPTOMS
- Uterine contractions at regular intervals that begin before the fetus is mature, usually before the due date of delivery.
- Passage of bloody mucus (sometimes).
- Flow of fluid (amniotic fluid) from the uterus (sometimes). This may occur with a gush or may be only a continuous watery discharge.

CAUSES
- Premature rupture of the membranes (the "water breaks").
- Illness of the mother, including toxemia, high blood pressure or diabetes.
- Abnormal shape or size of the uterus.
- Weak cervix.
- Hormone imbalance.
- Vaginal infection that spreads to the uterus.
- Large fetus or more than one fetus.
- Abnormalities of the placenta, such as placenta previa.
- Excessive amniotic fluid.

RISK INCREASES WITH
- Poor nutrition, especially when associated with weight loss.
- Previous premature labor.
- Smoking.
- Injury to the uterus.
- Excess alcohol consumption.
- Urinary-tract infection.
- Use of mind-altering drugs, such as narcotics, psychedelics, hallucinogens, marijuana, sedatives, hypnotics or cocaine.
- Adolescent mothers.

HOW TO PREVENT
- Obtain good prenatal care throughout pregnancy.
- Don't smoke, use mind-altering drugs or drink alcohol during pregnancy.
- Eat a normal, well-balanced diet during pregnancy (see Appendix 3). Take prenatal vitamin and mineral supplements, if your doctor prescribes them.
- Don't use medications of any kind, including non-prescription drugs, without consulting your doctor.
- If you have a weak cervix, which is sometimes evident before pregnancy, ask your doctor about a minor operation to strengthen the cervix.
- Rest more and decrease activity in the 3rd trimester, especially if you have blood spotting or irregular contractions.

WHAT TO EXPECT

APPROPRIATE HEALTH CARE
- Doctor's treatment.
- Hospitalization.

DIAGNOSTIC MEASURES
- Your own observation of watery vaginal drainage or regular uterine contractions.
- Medical history and physical exam by a doctor.
- Laboratory blood studies.
- Amniocentesis (in Surgery section) to determine fetal maturity.
- Ultrasound (see Glossary) to determine fetal maturity and position.

POSSIBLE COMPLICATIONS
- Premature infant.
- Uterine infection after delivery.
- Fetal death.

PROBABLE OUTCOME—Labor can often be stopped with treatment to allow more time for the fetus to mature. However, if the membranes have ruptured or the placenta has separated from the uterus, labor must proceed—sometimes by Cesarean section. The outcome depends on fetal maturity.

HOW TO TREAT

NOTE—Follow your doctor's instructions. These instructions are supplemental.

GENERAL MEASURES—Don't douche or use tampons to absorb fluid or blood. This increases the risk of infection.

MEDICATION—Your doctor may prescribe:
- Medication to stop labor.
- Antibiotics to fight infection, if it develops.
- *No* sedatives and pain relievers. These are withheld to give the fetus the greatest chance for survival.

ACTIVITY—Complete bed rest is necessary once signs of premature labor begin. Avoid sexual activity.

DIET—Once labor begins, drink only clear liquids until after delivery.

CALL YOUR DOCTOR IF

- You have symptoms of premature labor. Call immediately. This is an emergency!
- During pregnancy, you think you have a urinary-tract infection.
- After delivery, you have abdominal pain, chills and fever, headache, muscle aches or a bad-smelling vaginal discharge.
- New, unexplained symptoms develop. Drugs used in treatment may produce side effects.

ILLNESSES & DISORDERS

PREMENSTRUAL SYNDROME
(Premenstrual Tension; PMS)

 GENERAL INFORMATION

DEFINITION—Symptoms that begin 7 to 14 days prior to a menstrual period and usually stop when menstruation begins.

BODY PARTS INVOLVED—Gastrointestinal system; central nervous system; skin; reproductive system; breasts.

SEX OR AGE MOST AFFECTED—About half of all women experience PMS at some time—some very frequently. The peak incidence occurs between ages 25 and 40.

SIGNS & SYMPTOMS
- Nervousness and irritability.
- Dizziness or fainting.
- Emotional instability.
- Increased or decreased sex drive.
- Headaches.
- Tender, swollen breasts.
- Bloating, constipation, diarrhea or other digestive disturbances.
- Fluid retention that causes puffiness in the ankles, hands and face.
- Higher incidence of minor infections such as colds.
- Acne outbreaks.
- Decreased urination.

CAUSES
- Fluctuations in the circulating level of hormones (especially estrogen and progesterone). These fluctuations cause retention of sodium in the bloodstream, resulting in edema in body tissues—including the brain.
- Increased levels of prostaglandin (a chemical) in the bloodstream.

RISK INCREASES WITH—The older a woman is and the more children she has, the more likely she is to have PMS.

HOW TO PREVENT—No specific preventive measures.

 WHAT TO EXPECT

APPROPRIATE HEALTH CARE
- Self-care.
- Doctor's treatment.

DIAGNOSTIC MEASURES
- Your own observation of symptoms.
- Medical history and physical exam by a doctor.

POSSIBLE COMPLICATIONS—Emotional stress caused by symptoms severe enough to disrupt a woman's life.

PROBABLE OUTCOME—Present treatments may or may not be effective. Medication can relieve some symptoms. However, many new treatments are in the experimental stage, offering hope for the future.

 HOW TO TREAT

NOTE—Follow your doctor's instructions. These instructions are supplemental.

GENERAL MEASURES—Reduce stress whenever possible. See Appendix 13.

MEDICATION—Your doctor may prescribe:
- Tranquilizers or sedatives to relieve tension.
- Non-steroidal anti-inflammatory drugs to decrease prostaglandin levels.
- Diuretics to reduce fluid retention.

ACTIVITY—No restrictions.

DIET
- Decrease salt intake during the premenstrual phase.
- Your doctor may prescribe vitamin B-6 (50mg to 100mg daily) and extra calcium (either in tablets or in milk or milk products). These supplements decrease symptoms in some women.

 CALL YOUR DOCTOR IF

- You have symptoms of PMS that interfere with normal activities or relationships, and self-care is not sufficient.
- Symptoms don't improve, despite treatment.
- New, unexplained symptoms develop. Drugs used in treatment may produce side effects.

PRICKLY HEAT
(Miliaria Rubra; Sweat Retention)

GENERAL INFORMATION

DEFINITION—A skin disorder characterized by a non-inflammatory, itchy rash caused by obstructed sweat-gland ducts.

BODY PARTS INVOLVED—Skin.

SEX OR AGE MOST AFFECTED—All ages, but most common in infants.

SIGNS & SYMPTOMS—Clusters of vesicles (small, fluid-filled skin blisters) or red rash without vesicles in areas of heavy perspiration.

CAUSES—Obstruction of sweat-gland ducts for unknown reasons.

RISK INCREASES WITH
- Obesity
- Stress.
- Hot, humid weather.
- Genetic factors, such as fair, sensitive skin.

HOW TO PREVENT—Stay indoors in refrigerated air-conditioned buildings during hot, humid weather.

WHAT TO EXPECT

APPROPRIATE HEALTH CARE
- Home care.
- Doctor's treatment, if home care fails.

DIAGNOSTIC MEASURES
- Your own observation of symptoms.
- Medical history and physical exam by a doctor (severe cases only).

POSSIBLE COMPLICATIONS—Secondary skin infection.

PROBABLE OUTCOME—Usually curable with treatment in 6 weeks to 6 months. Recurrence is common.

HOW TO TREAT

NOTE—Follow your doctor's instructions. These instructions are supplemental.

GENERAL MEASURES
- Take frequent cool showers or tub baths.
- Apply lubricating ointment or cream to skin 6 or 7 times a day.
- Use cool-water soaks (see Appendix 18) to relieve itching and hasten healing. Pat skin dry, and dust with cornstarch after and between soaks.
- Wear cotton socks and leather-soled footwear rather than shoes made of man-made materials.
- Expose the affected skin to air as much as possible.
- Don't use binding materials, such as adhesive tape, or wear tight girdles.
- Change diapers on infants as soon as they are wet.
- Avoid sunburn once you have had prickly heat. The body's inflammatory reaction to sunburn may trigger a new outbreak of prickly heat.

MEDICATION—Your doctor may suggest non-prescription steroid cream to apply 2 or 3 times a day.

ACTIVITY—Decrease activity during hot, humid weather or until skin heals.

DIET—No special diet.

CALL YOUR DOCTOR IF

Prickly heat doesn't improve in 10 days, despite home care.

ILLNESSES & DISORDERS

PROCTITIS

GENERAL INFORMATION

DEFINITION—Inflammation of the rectum and tissues around the anus.

BODY PARTS INVOLVED—Anus; rectum.

SEX OR AGE MOST AFFECTED—Adolescents and adults of both sexes, but more common in males around age 30.

SIGNS & SYMPTOMS
- Rectal pain.
- Constant urge to have a bowel movement, often when little or no stool is present.
- Blood or mucus discharge from the rectum.
- Cramping pain in the left lower abdomen.

CAUSES
- Sexually transmitted infections of gonorrhea, syphilis and herpes.
- Chronic constipation.
- Ulcerative colitis (early stages).
- Cancer of the rectum.
- Rectal injury.
- Aftereffects of radiation therapy for cancer of the cervix and uterus.
- Endocrine disorders.
- Bacterial infections, including food poisoning.
- Food allergies.

RISK INCREASES WITH
- Homosexual males.
- Use of laxatives.

HOW TO PREVENT
- Avoid anal intercourse.
- To prevent constipation, establish a regular pattern for bowel movements. Eat a diet high in fiber and drink many fluids.
- Don't use laxatives regularly.
- Don't eat foods to which you are sensitive.

OTHER—Sexually transmitted diseases, such as gonorrhea and syphilis, must be reported to the local health department to prevent their spread. Information is kept confidential.

WHAT TO EXPECT

APPROPRIATE HEALTH CARE
- Self-care after diagnosis.
- Doctor's treatment.
- Surgery to remove any underlying tumor.

DIAGNOSTIC MEASURES
- Your own observation of symptoms.
- Medical history and physical exam by a doctor.
- Laboratory studies, such as: blood counts; tests for gonorrhea, syphilis, and other sexually transmitted diseases; and stool cultures.
- Surgical diagnostic procedures such as proctoscopy (see Glossary).

POSSIBLE COMPLICATIONS—Anal scarring and stricture (permanent narrowing of the anus).

PROBABLE OUTCOME—The outcome of proctitis depends on the outcome of the underlying cause:
- Infections can usually be cured with antibiotics.
- Cancer is often curable with surgery.
- Food allergies can be minimized if the offending foods are avoided.
- Symptoms of other disorders can be relieved or controlled with treatment.

HOW TO TREAT

NOTE—Follow your doctor's instructions. These instructions are supplemental.

GENERAL MEASURES
- Keep the anal area clean with frequent bathing.
- Take sitz baths often to relieve pain. Sit in a tub of hot water for 10 to 15 minutes as often as necessary.

MEDICATION
- You may use non-prescription topical anesthetics to relieve discomfort.
- Your doctor may prescribe:
  Antibiotics for sexually transmitted infections.
  Steroid suppositories to reduce inflammation from other causes.

ACTIVITY—No restrictions.

DIET
- Eat a high-fiber diet.
- Drink at least 8 glasses of water a day.
- Don't eat foods to which you are sensitive.

CALL YOUR DOCTOR IF

- You have symptoms of proctitis, or symptoms recur after treatment.
- New, unexplained symptoms develop. Drugs used in treatment may produce side effects.

PROSTATE CANCER

GENERAL INFORMATION

DEFINITION—Growth of malignant cells in the prostate gland, the gland at the base of the urinary bladder in men that helps form semen. Many prostate cancers grow very slowly and never cause symptoms or spread.

BODY PARTS INVOLVED—Prostate.

SEX OR AGE MOST AFFECTED—Men over age 50.

SIGNS & SYMPTOMS—Early stages:
- No symptoms (usually). Most prostate cancers are discovered during a routine rectal examination.
Later stages:
- Urinary obstruction.
- Pain in the low back or pelvis from spread of cancer.

CAUSES—Unknown. Prostate cancer does *not* seem related to an enlarged prostate, a common condition in older men.

RISK INCREASES WITH—Unknown.

HOW TO PREVENT—No specific preventive measures.

WHAT TO EXPECT

APPROPRIATE HEALTH CARE
- Doctor's treatment.
- Psychotherapy or counseling, if sexual difficulties occur after treatment.
- Surgery to remove the prostate gland and testes (sometimes), if the cancer has not spread.
- Hospitalization for radiation or hormone treatment, if the cancer has spread.

DIAGNOSTIC MEASURES
- Your own observation of symptoms, especially urinary obstruction.
- Medical history and physical exam by a doctor, including rectal examination.
- Laboratory blood tests for enzymes (acid phosphatase), which appear in higher quantities in the blood if cancer has spread to bone.
- Needle biopsy (see Glossary) of the prostate.
- X-rays of bone.

POSSIBLE COMPLICATIONS
- Fatal spread to bone, bladder and other organs.
- Urinary incontinence.
- Sexual impotence after surgery (sometimes).

PROBABLE OUTCOME—Often curable with surgery if treated before cancer spreads. Even after spread, therapy can relieve symptoms and prolong life.

HOW TO TREAT

NOTE—Follow your doctor's instructions. These instructions are supplemental.

GENERAL MEASURES—No appropriate self-care. Surgery is the usual treatment, unless pre-existing medical conditions, such as chronic heart, lung, kidney or liver disease, prohibit it. A yearly rectal examination after age 40 is the best way to detect early prostate cancer.

MEDICATION—Your doctor may prescribe:
- Hormones (usually estrogens) to slow malignant growth in bones.
- Analgesics to control pain.

ACTIVITY—Resume your normal activities gradually after surgery. Resume sexual relations when able.

DIET—No special diet.

CALL YOUR DOCTOR IF

- You have symptoms of prostate cancer.
- During treatment, any sign of urinary-tract infection occurs, such as: frequent, difficult or painful urination; fever and chills; aching around the genitals or rectum; or backache.
- New, unexplained symptoms develop. Drugs used in treatment may produce side effects.

ILLNESSES & DISORDERS

PROSTATE, ENLARGED
(Prostate Hypertrophy; Benign Prostatic Hypertrophy; BPH)

 GENERAL INFORMATION

DEFINITION—Enlargement of the prostate (a gland surrounding the neck of the bladder and urethra in the male). The enlargement may obstruct the flow of urine from the bladder, but it is not cancerous.

BODY PARTS INVOLVED—Prostate gland; bladder; urethra.

SEX OR AGE MOST AFFECTED—Men over age 50.

SIGNS & SYMPTOMS
- Increased urinary urgency and frequency, especially at night.
- Burning on urination.
- Weak urinary stream.
- Straining and dribbling on urination.
- Feeling that the bladder cannot be emptied completely.
- Urine of abnormal color.
- Impotence (sometimes).

CAUSES
- Overgrowth of the prostate due to hormonal changes that accompany aging.
- Diminishing sex life with few or no ejaculations.

RISK OF OBSTRUCTION INCREASES WITH
- Stress.
- Smoking.
- Excess alcohol consumption.
- Cold, moist weather.
- Use of many drugs, including atropine, antihistamines, muscle relaxers, beta-adrenergic blockers and calcium-channel blockers.

HOW TO PREVENT
- Maintain physical fitness.
- Continue an active sex life or masturbation into the aging years.
- Drink alcohol in moderation—1 to 2 drinks a day—if at all.
- Take only medication that is essential for your health.

 WHAT TO EXPECT

APPROPRIATE HEALTH CARE
- Doctor's treatment.
- Hospitalization for surgery to remove the prostate. Surgery is recommended for these conditions:
  Inability to empty the bladder completely, leading to chronic infection of the urinary tract.

One or more episodes of urinary retention (complete inability to empty the bladder).
Kidney failure caused by the obstruction.
Swelling or destruction of the kidney as revealed by X-ray.
Persistent bleeding from the prostate.
Recurrent prostate infection.

DIAGNOSTIC MEASURES
- Your own observation of symptoms.
- Medical history and physical exam by a doctor.
- Laboratory studies, such as urinalysis and blood-enzyme studies.

POSSIBLE COMPLICATIONS—Any of the conditions listed above requiring surgery.

PROBABLE OUTCOME—Curable with surgery.

 HOW TO TREAT

NOTE—Follow your doctor's instructions. These instructions are supplemental.

GENERAL MEASURES
- Urinate as soon as you feel the urge. Don't let the bladder become too full before emptying it.
- Sit on hard chairs rather than soft ones whenever possible.
- Avoid exposure to dampness or cold temperatures.
- For an explanation of surgery and postoperative care, see Prostate-Gland Removal in Surgery section.

MEDICATION—Your doctor may prescribe antibiotics if you develop a urinary-tract infection.

ACTIVITY
- Engage in frequent sexual intercourse. Avoid sexual stimulation and arousal without ejaculation.
- Avoid long bus, train or plane rides unless restrooms are available so you can urinate at any time.

DIET—No special diet. Avoid spicy foods and pepper, which irritate the urethra.

 CALL YOUR DOCTOR IF

- You cannot urinate.
- Your temperature rises to 101F (38.3C).
- You have an enlarged prostate and the symptoms are worsening.

PROSTATITIS

GENERAL INFORMATION

DEFINITION—Inflammation or infection of the prostate (the gland surrounding the neck of the bladder and urethra). Prostatitis is not contagious. It may rarely accompany cancer of the prostate.

BODY PARTS INVOLVED—Prostate gland.

SEX OR AGE MOST AFFECTED—Male adolescents and adults.

SIGNS & SYMPTOMS
- Urgency to urinate.
- Burning with urination.
- Frequent urination; waking to urinate at night.
- Difficulty starting urination and emptying the bladder completely.
- Fever; chills.
- Pain between the scrotum and anus.
- Joint and muscle aches.
- Blood in the urine (sometimes).
- Low back pain.
- Pain with a doctor's rectal examination.

CAUSES
- Bacterial infection, usually from gram-negative germs such as those found in feces. These may reach the prostate through the bloodstream, the lymphatic system or directly from the urethra.
- Infection caused by prostate cancer (rare).

RISK INCREASES WITH
- Recent urinary-tract infection.
- Smoking.
- Excess alcohol consumption.

HOW TO PREVENT—Men who have never had prostatitis are less likely to develop it if they are sexually active. Men who have prostatitis at least once may decrease the likelihood of recurrence by increasing sexual activity.

WHAT TO EXPECT

APPROPRIATE HEALTH CARE
- Self-care after diagnosis.
- Doctor's treatment. This may include prostate massage for chronic forms, after acute symptoms subside.
- Hospitalization for 3 to 4 days in serious cases if blood poisoning is suspected.
- Surgery to drain an abscess of the prostate (rare).

DIAGNOSTIC MEASURES
- Your own observation of symptoms.
- Medical history and physical exam by a doctor.
- Laboratory studies, such as urinalysis and culture of secretions obtained at the time of the doctor's prostate exam.

POSSIBLE COMPLICATIONS—If untreated, may lead to:
- Blood poisoning.
- Chronic bacterial or non-bacterial prostate infections. These have similar symptoms, but they are more likely to recur and respond less readily to treatment.

PROBABLE OUTCOME—Usually curable with treatment, but recurrence is common.

HOW TO TREAT

NOTE—Follow your doctor's instructions. These instructions are supplemental.

GENERAL MEASURES—Sit in a tub with 6 or 8 inches of warm water (106F or 41.1C) for 15 minutes at least 3 times a day. Use a whirlpool bath, if possible.

MEDICATION—Your doctor may prescribe:
- Antibiotics to fight infection (usually for at least 30 days).
- Pain relievers.

ACTIVITY—Rest in bed until fever and pain subside. Then resume your normal activities gradually. The ability to be sexually active during acute prostatitis depends on the degree of disability. Symptoms are usually relieved in 1 to 10 days, so during convalescence, let your sense of well-being be your guide.

DIET—No special diet, but don't drink alcohol or eat spicy foods. These irritate the urethra. Drink 8 to 10 glasses of water a day to ensure an adequate urine flow.

CALL YOUR DOCTOR IF

- You have symptoms of prostatitis.
- Symptoms worsen or you have fever during treatment.
- Symptoms don't improve after 3 days of treatment.
- Symptoms recur after treatment.

ILLNESSES & DISORDERS

PRURITIS ANI

GENERAL INFORMATION

DEFINITION—Itching around the anus and genitals.

BODY PARTS INVOLVED—Anus; vulva (vaginal lips) in women, scrotum in men.

SEX OR AGE MOST AFFECTED—Both sexes; all ages.

SIGNS & SYMPTOMS—Itching, often intense and worse at night.

CAUSES
- Yeast infection.
- Pinworms.
- Scabies.
- Contact dermatitis caused by soaps, contraceptive foams or jellies, perfumed toilet paper, deodorant sprays, douches or underwear made of synthetic fabric.
- Various skin disorders, including psoriasis or seborrheic dermatitis.
- Vaginal discharge or skin atrophy in women caused by low estrogen levels.
- Chronic diarrhea.
- Unknown (often).

RISK INCREASES WITH
- Stress.
- Diabetes mellitus.
- Excessive sweating.

HOW TO PREVENT
- Keep the body clean with regular showers or baths.
- Cleanse carefully after bowel movements with moistened tissue.
- Avoid contact with substances to which you are sensitive (see Causes).

WHAT TO EXPECT

APPROPRIATE HEALTH CARE
- Self-care after diagnosis.
- Doctor's treatment, if self-care is not successful.

DIAGNOSTIC MEASURES
- Your own observation of symptoms.
- Medical history and physical exam by a doctor.
- Laboratory studies, such as cultures for fungi, or microscopic examinations for pinworm eggs or scabies in skin burrows.

POSSIBLE COMPLICATIONS
- Skin damage, allowing secondary bacterial infection to develop.
- Skin thickening and chronic inflammation.
- Fatigue from chronic sleep disturbance.

PROBABLE OUTCOME—Symptoms can be controlled with treatment, even if the cause cannot be determined.

HOW TO TREAT

NOTE—Follow your doctor's instructions. These instructions are supplemental.

GENERAL MEASURES
- Keep showers or baths brief to minimize dryness and soap irritation. Use plain, unscented soap—if any.
- Keep the rectal area clean, dry and cool. Wear loose clothing and underclothing. Clean carefully after bowel movements, using moist tufts of cotton or plain soap and water.
- Don't use irritants listed as causes.
- Wear underwear with a cotton crotch or underwear made of cotton, rather than nylon or other synthetics.
- Women may be more comfortable using tampons for menstrual periods, rather than sanitary napkins.

MEDICATION
- You may use non-prescription cortisone ointment or cream. Apply 3 times a day, and rub in gently until it disappears.
- Your doctor may prescribe:
  More potent topical cortisone drugs.
  Zinc oxide.

ACTIVITY—Avoid activities that cause excessive perspiration.

DIET—Avoid spicy or highly seasoned foods. These irritate mucous membranes of the anus.

CALL YOUR DOCTOR IF

- You have symptoms of pruritis ani that persist, despite self-care.
- You develop a fever.
- The irritated area seems infected.

PRURITIS VULVAE

GENERAL INFORMATION

DEFINITION—An acute or chronic disorder of the skin around the vulva (the vaginal lips) and anus. This disorder is characterized by severe itching. It is not contagious.

BODY PARTS INVOLVED—Vulva and skin surrounding the vulva and anus.

SEX OR AGE MOST AFFECTED—Female adolescents and adults, especially after menopause.

SIGNS & SYMPTOMS
- Intense itching, sensitivity and irritation in the genital area. The skin may be dry.
- Thin, white vaginal discharge (sometimes).
- Discomfort during sexual intercourse.

CAUSES
- Skin disease, such as psoriasis or lichen planus.
- Systemic disease, such as diabetes.
- Atrophy and dryness caused by estrogen deficiency.
- Skin reaction to irritants, such as: toilet tissue; sanitary pads; soap; douches; deodorants; powders; perfume; and fabric.
- Systemic allergies, including food allergies.
- Disorder of the vagina or rectum, such as vaginitis or hemorrhoids.

RISK INCREASES WITH
- Stress.
- Days prior to menstruation.
- Hot, humid weather.
- Diabetes mellitus.
- Lack of urinary control.

HOW TO PREVENT
- Wear cotton panties rather than nylon.
- Avoid contact with irritants listed above.
- Obtain medical treatment for underlying causes.

WHAT TO EXPECT

APPROPRIATE HEALTH CARE
- Self-care.
- Doctor's treatment.

DIAGNOSTIC MEASURES
- Your own observation of symptoms.
- Medical history and physical exam by a doctor.

POSSIBLE COMPLICATIONS—Secondary bacterial infection of the inflamed skin.

PROBABLE OUTCOME—Home treatment usually provides relief in 4 to 7 days. If medical treatment becomes necessary, allow 2 weeks for recovery.

HOW TO TREAT

NOTE—Follow your doctor's instructions. These instructions are supplemental.

GENERAL MEASURES
- Follow suggestions under How to Prevent.
- Keep the area as dry and cool as possible. Wear loose clothing.
- Don't scratch the itchy area. Scratching will aggravate soreness and irritation.
- Wash the genital area with water and unscented soap only once a day.
- Use a lubricant, such as K-Y Lubricating Jelly or baby oil, during intercourse.
- After urinating or having a bowel movement, clean the genital area gently with absorbent cotton or antiseptic wipes. Wipe from front to back (vagina to anus).
- During menstruation, use tampons rather than sanitary napkins until the disorder heals.

MEDICATION—You may use low-potency, non-prescription steroid creams or ointments. If these are not effective, your doctor may prescribe:
- More potent steroid creams or lotions to reduce inflammation. These require 24 to 36 hours to provide relief.
- Ointments that contain hormones.
- Benzodiazepines or antihistamines at night to ensure rest.

ACTIVITY—Avoid overexertion, heat and excessive sweating.

DIET—No special diet, except to avoid foods to which you may be allergic.

CALL YOUR DOCTOR IF

- You have symptoms of pruritis vulvae.
- Symptoms don't improve in 2 weeks, despite treatment.
- Scratching leads to skin infection.
- New, unexplained symptoms develop. Drugs used in treatment may produce side effects.

ILLNESSES & DISORDERS

PSEUDOMEMBRANOUS ENTEROCOLITIS

 GENERAL INFORMATION

DEFINITION—A rare, severe illness in the small and large intestines. It usually follows 5 to 7 days after extensive gastrointestinal surgery and antibiotic treatment in a person who was debilitated before surgery. It is characterized by inflammation and tissue death of the lining membrane and deeper layers of the intestine.

BODY PARTS INVOLVED—Large and small intestines.

SEX OR AGE MOST AFFECTED—Adults, especially those over age 60.

SIGNS & SYMPTOMS
- Watery diarrhea (sometimes bloody) with abdominal cramps.
- Fever.
- High white-blood-cell count.
- Drop in blood pressure, sometimes to shock levels, with weak pulse and rapid heartbeat.
- Nausea and vomiting.
- Disorientation.

CAUSES—Infection from bacteria, usually the germ clostridium difficile, which manufactures a toxin that causes the symptoms, or from the staphylococcus germ. These germs normally inhabit the intestinal tract. They cause enterocolitis when other normal bacterial of the intestinal tract have been killed by heavy use of broad-spectrum antibiotics. This upsets the bacterial balance of the intestinal tract. The illness usually occurs as a complication of surgery.

RISK INCREASES WITH
- Adults over 60.
- Recent surgery with a drop in blood pressure during surgery.
- Kidney failure.
- Obesity.
- Poor nutrition.
- Use of antibiotics, especially lincomycin, clindamycin, ampicillin, chloramphenicol, cephalosporins, penicillin or sulfa drugs.

HOW TO PREVENT—No specific preventive measures.

 WHAT TO EXPECT

APPROPRIATE HEALTH CARE
- Doctor's treatment.
- Hospitalization for intravenous nutrition and intensive care.
- Self-care during convalescence after hospitalization.

DIAGNOSTIC MEASURES
- Your own observation of symptoms.

- Medical history and physical exam by a doctor.
- Biopsy (see Glossary) of the membrane lining of the large intestine through a colonoscope (see Glossary).
Note: A barium emema should *not* be administered. It may cause intestinal perforation.

POSSIBLE COMPLICATIONS—The following occur only if the problem is not recognized and treated:
- Shock and severe dehydration.
- Peritonitis caused by perforation of the intestine.

PROBABLE OUTCOME—Symptoms will usually disappear in 1 to 2 weeks after the offending antibiotic is discontinued. A substitute antibiotic is usually not prescribed; the body's defense mechanisms must take over for the withdrawn antibiotic. The worst cases are fatal.

 HOW TO TREAT

NOTE—Follow your doctor's instructions. These instructions are supplemental.

GENERAL MEASURES—The most important treatment is to discontinue use of the antibiotic causing the illness.

MEDICATION
- Your doctor may prescribe: Cholestyramine, vancomycin or metronidazole to prevent secondary, non-bacterial infections that occur when the balance of intestinal organisms is upset.
High doses of cortisone for a short time to decrease inflammation.
- Don't take antidiarrheal drugs unless prescribed by your doctor. They may contribute to intestinal perforation.

ACTIVITY—Rest in bed until all symptoms of the illness disappear. Flex legs often while in bed to decrease the likelihood of deep-vein blood clots. Resume normal activities gradually.

DIET—Intravenous nourishment will be necessary at first, progressing to a liquid diet, a soft diet and finally to a normal diet.

 CALL YOUR DOCTOR IF

- You have symptoms of pseudomembranous enterocolitis following intestinal surgery.
- Symptoms return after treatment.
- New, unexplained symptoms develop. Drugs used in treatment may produce side effects.

PSITTACOSIS
(Parrot Fever; Ornithosis)

 GENERAL INFORMATION

DEFINITION—An infectious form of pneumonia transmitted by birds.

BODY PARTS INVOLVED—Lungs.

SEX OR AGE MOST AFFECTED—Both sexes; all ages.

SIGNS & SYMPTOMS
- Fever and chills.
- General ill feeling.
- Appetite loss.
- Cough without sputum that progresses to cough with occasional discolored sputum.
- Shortness of breath.

CAUSES—Infection by the germ, chlamydia. Microscopic chlamydia organisms are not bacteria, viruses or fungi. However, they can be destroyed with antibiotics.

Psittacosis is found in psittacine birds (parrots, parakeets, lovebirds), poultry, pigeons, canaries and some sea birds. Germs enter the human body by inhalation of air that contains the germ, or by a bite from an infected bird. Incubation is 1 to 3 weeks after exposure.

RISK INCREASES WITH—Exposure to birds, especially in zoos, pet shops or on farms.

HOW TO PREVENT
- Avoid dust from bird feathers and cage contents.
- Don't handle any sick bird. Imported psittacine birds must be treated for 45 days with feed that contains chlortetracycline. This eliminates the organisms from the birds' blood and feces.

 WHAT TO EXPECT

APPROPRIATE HEALTH CARE
- Self-care after diagnosis.
- Doctor's treatment.

DIAGNOSTIC MEASURES
- Your own observation of symptoms.
- Medical history and physical exam by a doctor.
- Laboratory blood studies and sputum culture.
- X-rays of the lungs.

POSSIBLE COMPLICATIONS—Severe or fatal pneumonia.

PROBABLE OUTCOME—Usually curable in 7 to 14 days with early diagnosis and treatment. Fever may remain for 2 or 3 weeks before falling slowly, unless antibiotics are used.

 HOW TO TREAT

NOTE—Follow your doctor's instructions. These instructions are supplemental.

GENERAL MEASURES
- Keep the patient isolated to avoid transmitting the disease through cough droplets and sputum.
- Use a cool-mist humidifier to increase air moisture and loosen lung secretions. Use pure water; don't put medication in the humidifier.
- Use a heating pad on the chest to relieve pain.
- The patient should not smoke.

MEDICATION
- Your doctor may prescribe tetracycline (an antibiotic) for at least 10 days to control fever and other symptoms.
- Don't suppress the cough if it produces sputum. It is performing a useful function in ridding the lungs of mucus. If the cough is non-productive and painful, you may suppress it with prescribed medication.
- For minor pain, take non-prescription drugs such as aspirin or acetaminophen.

ACTIVITY—Bed rest is necessary until the fever, pain and shortness of breath have been gone at least 48 hours. Then normal activities may be resumed gradually. Fatigue and weakness may persist for a long time, so don't expect a quick return to normal strength.

DIET—No special diet. Increase fluid intake to at least 1 glass of fluid every hour. This helps to thin lung secretions so they can be coughed up more easily.

 CALL YOUR DOCTOR IF

- You have symptoms of psittacosis.
- The following occurs during treatment:
  Fever rises to 102F (38.9C) or higher.
  Pain is not relieved by heat or prescribed medication.
  Shortness of breath increases.
  Fingernails become dark or bluish.
  Blood appears in the sputum.
  Nausea, vomiting or diarrhea occur.

ILLNESSES & DISORDERS

PSORIASIS

GENERAL INFORMATION

DEFINITION—A chronic, scaly skin disorder characterized by frequent remissions and recurrences.

BODY PARTS INVOLVED—Skin, especially of the scalp, elbows, knees, chest, back, arms, legs, toenails, fingernails and fold between the buttocks.

SEX OR AGE MOST AFFECTED—Begins in late childhood or young adulthood and continues throughout life.

SIGNS & SYMPTOMS
- Skin areas that are slightly raised, have red borders and are covered with large white or silver-white scales. The areas crack and become painful.
- Itching (sometimes).
- Joint pain.

CAUSES—Unknown, but probably caused by autoimmune disorder.

RISK INCREASES WITH
- Rheumatoid arthritis.
- Local injury.
- Infections (viral and bacterial) elsewhere in the body.
- Family history of psoriasis.
- Stress.
- Cold climates.
- Genetic factors. Persons with psoriasis have HLA antigens, and the incidence is highest among Caucasians.

HOW TO PREVENT—Cannot be prevented at present.

WHAT TO EXPECT

APPROPRIATE HEALTH CARE
- Self-care after diagnosis.
- Doctor's treatment.
- Psychotherapy or counseling (sometimes) to help in adapting to the disorder.

DIAGNOSTIC MEASURES
- Your own observation of symptoms.
- Medical history and physical exam by a doctor.
- Laboratory blood tests.

POSSIBLE COMPLICATIONS
- Secondary bacterial infection in the affected area.
- Generalized secondary bacterial infection—sometimes fatal—characterized by the eruption of many pustules, fever and joint pain.

PROBABLE OUTCOME—Symptoms can be controlled but not cured. The disease may have long periods of inactivity. In women, severity decreases during pregnancy.

HOW TO TREAT

NOTE—Follow your doctor's instructions. These instructions are supplemental.

GENERAL MEASURES
- Move to a warm climate, if possible. Severity increases during cold weather.
- Maintain good skin hygiene with daily baths or showers.
- Avoid skin injury, including harsh scrubbing, which can trigger new outbreaks.
- Avoid skin dryness to decrease the frequency of recurrences. To reduce scaling, use non-prescription waterless cleansers and hair preparations containing coal tar or cortisone.
- Expose skin to moderate amounts of sunlight as often as possible.
- Oatmeal baths may loosen scales. Use 1 cup of oatmeal to a tub of warm water.

MEDICATION—Your doctor may prescribe the following to decrease inflammation and scaling:
- Ointments containing coal tar.
- Topical cortisone drugs to use under plastic dressings.
- Ultraviolet light.
- Immunosuppressive drugs (severest cases).

ACTIVITY—No restrictions.

DIET—No special diet.

CALL YOUR DOCTOR IF

- You have symptoms of psoriasis, or symptoms recur after treatment.
- During an outbreak, pustules erupt on the skin, accompanied by fever, muscle aches and fatigue.
- New, unexplained symptoms develop. Drugs used in treatment may produce side effects.

PSORIATIC ARTHRITIS

GENERAL INFORMATION

DEFINITION—Joint inflammation that accompanies psoriasis lesions in nearby nails and skin.

BODY PARTS INVOLVED
- Joints in any part of the body, but most likely in finger joints and low-back and neck joints in the spine.
- Skin or nails that have psoriasis lesions and are close to the affected joint. Sometimes additional skin sites include the scalp, navel, underarm and groin.

SEX OR AGE MOST AFFECTED—Usually begins between ages 30 and 35, and continues intermittently throughout life.

SIGNS & SYMPTOMS
- Pain, swelling, restricted movement, tenderness and warmth in the affected joint.
- Scaling skin.
- Pitted, ridged, yellow nails.

CAUSES
- Physical or emotional trauma.
- Immunological response to a streptococcal infection.
- Unknown (usually).

RISK INCREASES WITH
- Strep infections.
- Family history of rheumatoid arthritis or psoriasis.

HOW TO PREVENT—Obtain prompt antibiotic treatment for strep infections.

WHAT TO EXPECT

APPROPRIATE HEALTH CARE
- Self-care after diagnosis.
- Doctor's treatment.

DIAGNOSTIC MEASURES
- Your own observation of symptoms.
- Medical history and physical exam by a doctor.
- Laboratory blood studies to detect a rheumatic factor and measure antinuclear antibodies (ANA).

POSSIBLE COMPLICATIONS—Permanent joint deformity and crippling—although this is less likely than with rheumatoid arthritis.

PROBABLE OUTCOME—This condition is currently considered incurable. It is characterized by acute flare-ups and remissions. However, symptoms can be relieved or controlled, and medical literature cites a few instances of unexplained recovery.

Scientific research into causes and treatment continues, so there is hope for increasingly effective treatment and cure.

HOW TO TREAT

NOTE—Follow your doctor's instructions. These instructions are supplemental.

GENERAL MEASURES
- Immobilize inflamed joints with splints.
- Use heat to relieve joint pain. Hot soaks (see Glossary), whirlpool treatments, heat lamps, ultrasound or diathermy (see Glossary) are all effective.
- Schedule periods for regular, moderate exposure to sunlight.
- See Psoriasis for treatment of the skin and nails.

MEDICATION
- For minor discomfort, you may use non-prescription drugs such as aspirin.
- To reduce joint inflammation, your doctor may prescribe:
  Non-steroidal anti-inflammatory drugs.
  Cortisone injections into inflamed joints (occasionally).
  Immunosuppressive drugs (sometimes) such as methotrexate.

ACTIVITY—Rest inflamed joints during flare-ups, then resume your normal activities gradually. Try to increase outdoor activity in sunshine.

DIET—No special diet.

CALL YOUR DOCTOR IF

- You have symptoms of psoriatic arthritis.
- New, unexplained symptoms develop. Drugs used in treatment may produce side effects.

ILLNESSES & DISORDERS

PTOSIS

 GENERAL INFORMATION

DEFINITION—Drooping of the upper eyelid, partially or completely covering the eye.

BODY PARTS INVOLVED—Upper eyelid; eye.

SEX OR AGE MOST AFFECTED—Both sexes; all ages.

SIGNS & SYMPTOMS—Drooping of one or both eyelids, accompanied by poor blinking reflexes. The extent of droop may vary at different times of the day.

CAUSES—May be present at birth or may accompany other problems, including:
- Paralysis of nerve fibers to the eyelids.
- Myasthenia gravis.
- Muscular dystrophy.
- Diabetes.
- Brain tumor.
- Birth injury.
- Head or eyelid injury.
- Tumor in the upper lobe of a lung.

RISK INCREASES WITH
- Adults over 60.
- Family history of ptosis.

HOW TO PREVENT—No specific preventive measures.

 WHAT TO EXPECT

APPROPRIATE HEALTH CARE
- Self-care after diagnosis.
- Doctor's treatment. Some ophthalmologists recommend keeping the lid raised with a support that is part of eyeglasses.
- Surgery to strengthen the muscles of the eyelid (sometimes).

DIAGNOSTIC MEASURES
- Medical history and physical exam by a doctor.
- Your own observation of symptoms.
- X-rays of various body regions to look for the underlying cause.

POSSIBLE COMPLICATIONS
- Permanent disfigurement.
- Irritation and infection in the eye caused by poor blinking reflexes and continuous contact between the eyelid and eye surface.
- Visual disturbance.

PROBABLE OUTCOME—Sometimes curable if the underlying cause can be corrected by surgery or medication.

 HOW TO TREAT

NOTE—Follow your doctor's instructions. These instructions are supplemental.

GENERAL MEASURES
- Keep the eye moist with non-prescription, artificial tears.
- Wear safety goggles to protect the eye from injury when exposed to dust or flying debris.

MEDICATION—Medicine usually is not necessary for ptosis, but it may be necessary for the underlying disorder.

ACTIVITY—No restrictions.

DIET—No special diet.

 CALL YOUR DOCTOR IF

- You have symptoms of ptosis.
- Ptosis worsens or vision is affected.

PUERPERAL INFECTION
(Puerperal Fever)

GENERAL INFORMATION

DEFINITION—Infection of the birth canal after the first 24 hours following delivery of a baby.

BODY PARTS INVOLVED—Any or all: vagina; vulva; perineum (area between the vagina and rectum); cervix, uterus; peritoneum (membrane that covers abdominal organs).

SEX OR AGE MOST AFFECTED—Females of childbearing age.

SIGNS & SYMPTOMS
- Unexplained fever and chills for 2 or more days after the first postpartum day (first day after delivery).
- Headache.
- Muscle aches.
- Appetite loss.
- Rapid heartbeat.
- Soft, large, tender uterus.
- Vaginal discharge with an unpleasant odor.
- Abdominal pain.

CAUSES—Infection by bacteria normally found in a healthy vagina. These bacteria can infect the uterus, vagina, adjacent tissues and kidney, especially in conjunction with risk factors.

RISK INCREASES WITH
- Insertion of a fetal scalp electrode during labor.
- Anemia, either pre-existing or from loss of blood during delivery.
- Toxemia during pregnancy.
- Long delay between rupture of the placental membranes and delivery.
- Prolonged labor.
- Traumatic delivery.
- Repeated vaginal examinations with unsterile equipment during labor.
- Retained fragments of placenta in the uterus.
- Excessive bleeding after delivery.

HOW TO PREVENT
- Avoid anyone with an active infection for the last 2 weeks of pregnancy.
- Notify your doctor as soon as placental membranes rupture (your "water breaks"). Don't have sexual intercourse after membranes rupture.
- Wash the perineal area often during the first week after delivery.

WHAT TO EXPECT

APPROPRIATE HEALTH CARE
- Doctor's treatment.
- Surgery to remove fragments of placenta (sometimes).
- Hospitalization for intensive treatment.

DIAGNOSTIC MEASURES
- Medical history and physical exam by a doctor.
- Laboratory blood studies, blood culture and culture of the vaginal discharge.

POSSIBLE COMPLICATIONS
- Deep-vein blood clot in the pelvis.
- Blood poisoning.
- Shock.

PROBABLE OUTCOME—Usually curable in 7 to 10 days with intensive treatment. Without treatment, complications can be fatal.

HOW TO TREAT

NOTE—Follow your doctor's instructions. These instructions are supplemental.

GENERAL MEASURES
- To relieve pain, place a heating pad or hot-water bottle on the abdomen or back.
- Take frequent hot baths to relax muscles and relieve pain.
- Use sanitary pads rather than tampons for the vaginal discharge.
- If you plan to breast-feed, use a breast pump to express milk until the infection heals.

MEDICATION—Your doctor may prescribe:
- Antibiotics in high doses—intravenously, if necessary.
- Codeine and acetaminophen to reduce fever and pain.
- Anticoagulants to prevent blood-clot formation.

ACTIVITY
- Rest in bed, except to use the bathroom, until fever and other signs of infection subside. You will probably be more comfortable if you lie on your left side.
- Abstain from sexual relations until signs of infection have been gone at least 7 days.

DIET—Drink lots of fluids to prevent dehydration from high fever. Vitamin and mineral supplements should not be necessary unless you are anemic.

CALL YOUR DOCTOR IF

- You have symptoms of a puerperal infection.
- You faint.
- You develop a skin rash.
- New, unexplained symptoms develop. Drugs used in treatment may produce side effects.
- Symptoms of infection recur after treatment.

ILLNESSES & DISORDERS

PULMONARY EDEMA

 GENERAL INFORMATION

DEFINITION—A set of dramatic, life-threatening symptoms caused by congestive heart failure.

BODY PARTS INVOLVED—Lungs and heart.

SEX OR AGE MOST AFFECTED—Adults over 40.

SIGNS & SYMPTOMS—The following symptoms often begin suddenly in the middle of the night and worsen rapidly:
- Extreme shortness of breath, sometimes with wheezing.
- Rapid breathing.
- Restlessness and anxiety.
- Paleness.
- Sweating.
- Bluish nails and lips.
- Low blood pressure.
- Cough. This may be unproductive at first, but later it can produce a frothy, blood-stained sputum.

CAUSES—Failure of the heart's left ventricle to pump well enough to supply all body cells with oxygen. The underlying cause of heart failure includes many forms of heart disease, especially heart-rhythm disturbances or hypertension with atherosclerosis or narrowing of the aortic valve.

RISK INCREASES WITH
- Adults over 60.
- Stress.
- Recent heart attack.
- High blood pressure or any form of heart disease.
- Obesity.
- Smoking.
- Fatigue or overwork.

HOW TO PREVENT—If you have any form of heart disease, obtain prompt treatment for less dramatic signs of congestive heart failure. The treatment will include a low-salt diet, smoking cessation, maintenance of an ideal weight, adequate rest and prescription drugs.

 WHAT TO EXPECT

APPROPRIATE HEALTH CARE
- Doctor's treatment.
- Hospitalization for oxygen and medication.

DIAGNOSTIC MEASURES
- Your own observation of symptoms.
- Medical history and physical exam by a doctor.
- Laboratory blood studies and EKG (see Glossary).

POSSIBLE COMPLICATIONS
- Death (if treatment is delayed or unsuccessful).
- Misdiagnosis as asthma, resulting in inappropriate treatment.

PROBABLE OUTCOME—In most cases, symptoms can be controlled with treatment. The treatment for pulmonary edema usually brings dramatic and effective relief. However, the underlying heart disease causing pulmonary edema will require lifelong treatment.

 HOW TO TREAT

NOTE—Follow your doctor's instructions. These instructions are supplemental.

GENERAL MEASURES—Self-care is not appropriate for pulmonary edema. This is a medical emergency requiring intensive medical care. Delay can lead to death.

MEDICATION—Your doctor may prescribe:
- Narcotics to relieve anxiety, decreasing the breathing rate.
- Diuretics to decrease excess fluid circulating in the bloodstream and lessen fluid accumulated in the lungs.
- Digitalis to stimulate a stronger heartbeat.
- Antibiotics (if pulmonary edema has been triggered by infection).

ACTIVITY—Rest in bed until your condition stabilizes. You may read or watch TV. After treatment, resume your normal activities gradually. Resume sexual relations when symptoms disappear and strength returns.

DIET—Low-salt, low-fat diet (see Appendices 8 and 9).

 CALL YOUR DOCTOR IF

You have symptoms of pulmonary edema. This is an emergency!

PULMONARY EMBOLISM

GENERAL INFORMATION

DEFINITION—A blood clot or fat cells (rarely) in one of the arteries carrying blood to the lungs. The blood clot begins in a deep vein of the leg or pelvis. A fat embolus usually begins at a fracture site. The embolus moves through the bloodstream, passing through the heart and lodging in the branch of an artery that nourishes the lungs. This blockage decreases breathing ability and sometimes destroys lung tissue.

BODY PARTS INVOLVED—Veins, especially veins in the legs; pulmonary artery and smaller artery branches that nourish the lungs; broken bone.

SEX OR AGE MOST AFFECTED—All ages, but most common in adults.

SIGNS & SYMPTOMS
- Sudden shortness of breath.
- Faintness or fainting.
- Pain in the chest.
- Cough (sometimes with bloody sputum).
- Rapid heartbeat.
- Low fever.
These symptoms are often preceded by swelling and pain in the leg.

CAUSES—Deep-vein thrombosis, which can occur anytime that blood pools in a vein.

RISK INCREASES WITH
- Adults over 60.
- Any injury or illness that requires prolonged bed rest.
- Sitting in one position for prolonged periods, as on airplane flights.
- Recent surgery.
- Congestive heart failure.
- Heart-rhythm disturbances.
- Polycythemia.
- Hemolytic anemia.
- Bone fractures.
- Obesity.
- Smoking.
- Pregnancy.
- Use of oral contraceptives, especially in women over age 35.

HOW TO PREVENT
- Avoid prolonged bed rest during illnesses. Wear elastic stockings during recuperation—in or out of bed.
- Start moving lower limbs and walking as soon as possible after surgery.
- Don't smoke, especially if you are a woman 35 or older who takes birth-control pills.
- Avoid needless surgery. Get a second opinion.
- When traveling, stand and walk every 1 to 2 hours.

WHAT TO EXPECT

APPROPRIATE HEALTH CARE
- Doctor's treatment.
- Hospitalization for anticoagulation and oxygen.
- Surgery to tie off the big vein leading to the heart and lungs (vena cava) or insertion of a filter to trap recurrent clots (rare).

DIAGNOSTIC MEASURES
- Your own observation of symptoms.
- Medical history and physical exam by a doctor.
- Laboratory blood studies to measure coagulation factors and prothrombin time.
- X-rays of the chest.
- CAT scan (see Glossary) of the lungs.

POSSIBLE COMPLICATIONS
- Rapid death from a large clot that obstructs more than 50% of the blood to the lungs.
- Massive bleeding in the lungs caused by smaller clots.

PROBABLE OUTCOME—Usually curable in 10 to 14 days with intensive care.

HOW TO TREAT

NOTE—Follow your doctor's instructions. These instructions are supplemental.

GENERAL MEASURES
- Wear elastic stockings or leg wraps with elastic bandages.
- Don't sit with your legs or ankles crossed.
- Elevate your feet higher than your hips when sitting for long periods.
- Elevate the foot of your bed.

MEDICATION—Your doctor may prescribe anticoagulant drugs to dissolve and prevent clots. The anticoagulant level must be monitored to keep it in a safe range.

ACTIVITY—Rest in bed until all symptoms and signs of clot inflammation disappear. While in bed, move your legs often to stimulate circulation.

DIET—No special diet.

CALL YOUR DOCTOR IF

- You have symptoms of pulmonary embolism. This is an emergency!
- The following occurs during treatment:
  Chest pain.
  Coughing up blood.
  Shortness of breath.
  Increased swelling and pain in the leg, despite treatment.
- You take anticoagulants and develop any signs of bleeding.

PULMONARY-VALVE STENOSIS

GENERAL INFORMATION

DEFINITION—Narrowing of the pulmonary valve. The pulmonary valve separates the right ventricle (major chamber) of the heart from the pulmonary artery (the large artery that goes from the heart to the lungs). When this valve becomes narrowed, heart function is impaired.

BODY PARTS INVOLVED—Heart.

SEX OR AGE MOST AFFECTED—Both sexes; all ages.

SIGNS & SYMPTOMS—Early stages:
- No symptoms.

Later stages:
- Chest pain.
- Dizziness.
- Faintness upon exertion.
- Congestive heart failure, with the following symptoms:
  Fatigue.
  Swelling in the lower parts of the body—the feet if standing or sitting and the back if lying down.
  Breathlessness with exertion—walking, climbing stairs or sexual intercourse.
  Later, breathlessness appears without exertion—sometimes even after going to sleep.
  Cough, sometimes with frothy or bloody sputum.
  Nausea and loss of appetite.
  Loss of sex drive.

CAUSES
- Congenital (present at birth).
- Complication of rheumatic fever (rare).

RISK INCREASES WITH—Prior streptococcal infection.

HOW TO PREVENT
- Obtain a throat culture and prompt medical treatment for strep infections to prevent rheumatic fever.
- If you have had rheumatic fever, take antibiotics before any surgery, even dental procedures.

WHAT TO EXPECT

APPROPRIATE HEALTH CARE
- Self-care after diagnosis.
- Doctor's treatment.
- Surgery (only if the defective valve must be repaired).

DIAGNOSTIC MEASURES
- Your own observation of symptoms.
- Medical history and physical exam by a doctor.
- Laboratory studies such as EKG, cardiac catheterization and echocardiography (see Glossary for all).
- X-rays of the heart and lungs.

POSSIBLE COMPLICATIONS—Congestive heart failure.

PROBABLE OUTCOME—Mild pulmonary-valve stenosis may cause little if any disability. Severe impairment is usually curable with surgery to stretch the defective pulmonary heart valve.

HOW TO TREAT

NOTE—Follow your doctor's instructions. These instructions are supplemental.

GENERAL MEASURES
- Weigh yourself daily and keep a record.
- Advise any doctor or dentist who treats you that you have a disease of heart valves.

MEDICATION—Your doctor may prescribe diuretics to reduce the fluid retention of congestive heart failure.

ACTIVITY—If surgery is not advised and your condition allows, continue normal activity. Avoid strenuous activity, but don't treat yourself as an invalid—even if you have some disability. Walks, golf, sexual intercourse and other exercises may be possible.

DIET—Low-salt diet (see Appendix 9).

CALL YOUR DOCTOR IF

- You have symptoms of pulmonary-valve stenosis.
- The following occurs during treatment:
  Unexplained weight gain of 3 to 4 pounds in 2 to 3 days, indicating fluid retention.
  Increased breathlessness.
  Wheezing at night.
  Fever.
  Rapid heartbeat.
  Cough.

PURPURA, ALLERGIC
(Anaphylactoid Purpura; Henoch-Schönlein Purpura)

 GENERAL INFORMATION

DEFINITION—An allergic disorder.

BODY PARTS INVOLVED
- Joints (usually knees, ankles, hips, wrists and elbows).
- Skin of the legs, thighs and abdomen.
- Gastrointestinal tract.
- Kidneys.

SEX OR AGE MOST AFFECTED—Boys (2 to 8 years).

SIGNS & SYMPTOMS
- Sore throat about 2 weeks prior to other symptoms.
- Itching skin rash that seems to be just beneath the skin surface. The rash usually consists of large hives with small bruises or blood spots in the centers. The rash is most often on the legs, thighs and lower abdomen, but it may be scattered over the body.
- Joint inflammation at the knees, ankles, hips, wrists or elbows.
- Cramping abdominal pain and vomiting.
- Protein and blood in the urine.
- Low fever.

CAUSES—Purpura is probably an allergic reaction in the inflamed small blood vessels throughout the body. The allergic trigger is not known, but attacks often follow an upper-respiratory infection or the use of some drugs, especially sulfa drugs.

RISK INCREASES WITH
- Recent illness, especially a bacterial sore throat.
- Use of sulfa drugs.

HOW TO PREVENT
- Don't allow your child to be exposed to respiratory infections, if possible.
- Obtain prompt medical treatment of any bacterial throat infection.
- Avoid the use of any drug that has triggered allergic purpura in your child. Consult the doctor before giving any medication to a child.

 WHAT TO EXPECT

APPROPRIATE HEALTH CARE
- Home care after diagnosis.
- Doctor's treatment.
- Hospitalization (for complications).

DIAGNOSTIC MEASURES
- Your own observation of symptoms.
- Medical history and physical exam by a doctor.
- Laboratory blood studies and a urinalysis.

POSSIBLE COMPLICATIONS
- Kidney failure, resulting from kidney inflammation and damage.
- Permanent joint deformity.

PROBABLE OUTCOME—Allergic purpura usually lasts 1 to 3 weeks. Some children only have a few spots and fever. Others require hospitalization for severe abdominal pain and kidney inflammation.

Most children with allergic purpura recover completely. In some, however, allergic purpura recurs or persists for years.

 HOW TO TREAT

NOTE—Follow your doctor's instructions. These instructions are supplemental.

GENERAL MEASURES—Use warm soaks (see Appendix 18) to relieve joint pain.

MEDICATION—Your doctor may prescribe cortisone drugs or immunosuppressive drugs, such as cyclophosphamide, to suppress inflammation. Effectiveness of treatment varies.

ACTIVITY—If the child has fever or pain, encourage bed rest. The child may sit up for meals and walk to the bathroom. When fever and pain are gone, the child may gradually resume normal activities as strength and well-being allow.

DIET—The child should eat a normal, well-balanced diet. Vitamin and mineral supplements should not be necessary unless the child shows evidence of deficiency.

 CALL YOUR DOCTOR IF

- Your child has symptoms of allergic purpura.
- The following symptoms occur during treatment:
  Unrelenting abdominal pain.
  Blood in the stool.
  Black, tarry bowel movements.
  New bleeding under the skin.
  Blood in the urine.

PYLORIC STENOSIS, CONGENITAL
(Hypertrophic Pyloric Stenosis)

 GENERAL INFORMATION

DEFINITION—A condition of infancy in which encircling muscles at the end of the stomach enlarge and cause obstruction.

BODY PARTS INVOLVED—Pylorus (a muscular tube that carries food from the stomach to the small intestine).

SEX OR AGE MOST AFFECTED
- Both sexes, but more common in firstborn males.
- Usually begins between 2 and 5 weeks of age, but can occur as late as 4 months.

SIGNS & SYMPTOMS
- Recurrent vomiting after feedings that becomes increasingly forceful.
- Muscular mass in the upper abdomen (sometimes).
- No pain or fever. Infant seems happy but hungry after vomiting.
- Constipation.
- Gradual weight loss and dehydration.

CAUSES—The muscular band that encircles the pylorus thickens and eventually closes off the outlet from the stomach.

RISK INCREASES WITH—Family history of pyloric stenosis.

HOW TO PREVENT—Cannot be prevented at present.

 WHAT TO EXPECT

APPROPRIATE HEALTH CARE
- Doctor's treatment.
- Surgery to cut the thickened muscle (pyloromyotomy)
- Hospitalization for about 3 days after surgery.

DIAGNOSTIC MEASURES
- Your own observation of symptoms.
- Medical history and physical exam by a doctor.
- Laboratory blood counts and studies of fluids and electrolytes.
- X-rays of the stomach (sometimes).

POSSIBLE COMPLICATIONS—Weight loss, dehydration, shock and death without treatment.

PROBABLE OUTCOME—Curable with surgery. The child usually recovers quickly.

 HOW TO TREAT

NOTE—Follow your doctor's instructions. These instructions are supplemental.

GENERAL MEASURES—After surgery:
- A firm ridge will appear at the incision site. This is a healthy sign and requires no treatment.
- Wash the incision site gently several times a day.
- If the baby seems uncomfortable, apply warm compresses to the incision site.

MEDICATION—Intravenous fluids and electrolytes until the baby is ready for surgery. Medication is usually not necessary after surgery.

ACTIVITY—No restrictions.

DIET—The baby may tolerate small feedings of half-strength formula while awaiting surgery—check with your doctor. If not, formula will be given by stomach tube.

 CALL YOUR DOCTOR IF

- Your baby vomits repeatedly.
- The following occurs after surgery: Pain, swelling, redness, bleeding or drainage at the surgical site. Temperature spike to 101F (38.3C).

RABIES
(Hydrophobia)

GENERAL INFORMATION

DEFINITION—A serious virus infection of the central nervous system, transmitted by the bite of infected animals.

BODY PARTS INVOLVED—Brain and central nervous system; body parts bitten by the rabid animal.

SEX OR AGE MOST AFFECTED—Both sexes; all ages.

SIGNS & SYMPTOMS—Symptoms may appear 3 to 7 weeks after the bite. Early symptoms are:
- Restlessness and irritability.
- Fatigue.
- Slight fever.
- Cough.
- Sore throat.
- Increased saliva and tears.

2 to 10 days later:
- Violent spasms of throat muscles that make swallowing impossible.
- Hyperactivity and violent behavior.
- Confusion.
- High fever.
- Irregular heartbeat.
- Irregular breathing.

CAUSES—A virus in the saliva of infected animals passes to humans through broken skin or a mucous membrane. The virus travels slowly from the bite area to the brain.

Animals that are commonly infected include dogs (especially wild dogs), bats, skunks, foxes, coyotes and raccoons. Other animals can also be infected, so consult your local health department after *any* animal bite.

RISK INCREASES WITH
- Multiple bites or bites on the face, head, neck or upper body.
- Outdoor activities that involve exposure to wild animals, especially cave exploration and hunting (in which animals are handled).

HOW TO PREVENT
- Vaccinate your dog or cat against rabies.
- Report stray animals in the neighborhood, and teach children to avoid them.
- Have a rabies immunization, if your work involves animals.
- Keep tetanus immunizations up-to-date. See Appendix 16 for an immunization schedule.

WHAT TO EXPECT

APPROPRIATE HEALTH CARE
- Doctor's treatment.
- Surgery to clean and repair the bite wound (sometimes).
- Hospitalization, if symptoms develop.

DIAGNOSTIC MEASURES
- Your own observation of the animal's behavior. Determine if the animal was provoked. Attacking animals are more likely to be infected.
- Medical history and physical exam by a doctor.
- Laboratory blood tests and fluid and electrolyte measurements.
- Pathological exam of the animal's tissue.

POSSIBLE COMPLICATIONS
- Dehydration and shock.
- Coma.
- Paralysis and death.

PROBABLE OUTCOME—Rabies can be prevented with early treatment following animal bites. Once symptoms begin, survival is unlikely. The mortality rate is 80%..

HOW TO TREAT

NOTE—Follow your doctor's instructions. These instructions are supplemental.

GENERAL MEASURES
- Wash the bite area for 10 minutes with soap and water to remove all saliva.
- Cover the wound with a clean bandage.
- Call your doctor or local emergency room for advice.
- Call your local animal-control center to catch the animal, if possible.
- If the animal is killed, remove the head and refrigerate or freeze it until it can be examined by pathologists.
- Don't panic. The incubation period allows time for diagnosis and treatment.

MEDICATION—Your doctor may prescribe one of the following:
- Injections of rabies-immune globulin.
- Injections of human diploid-cell-strain vaccine, if the animal is proven rabid.
- Tetanus booster.

Painful injections in the abdomen are no longer necessary.

ACTIVITY—No restrictions unless symptoms begin. If they do, bed rest in a hospital is necessary.

DIET—No special diet during outpatient treatment before symptoms begin. Intravenous fluids and nutrients are necessary during hospitalization.

CALL YOUR DOCTOR IF

Anyone is bitten by an animal.

RADIATION SICKNESS

GENERAL INFORMATION

DEFINITION—Side effects that accompany radiation treatment for cancer or aftereffects of accidental exposure to radiation.

BODY PARTS INVOLVED—Depends on the location of treatment or exposure. See Signs & Symptoms below.

SEX OR AGE MOST AFFECTED—Both sexes; all ages.

SIGNS & SYMPTOMS—The following vary widely, and are often temporary, depending on the radiation dosage and area radiated:
- Nausea, vomiting and diarrhea.
- Headache.
- Fatigue and shortness of breath.
- Rapid heartbeat.
- Yeast infection in the mouth.
- Dry mouth and loss of taste.
- Swallowing difficulty.
- Worsening of tooth or gum disease.
- Hair loss.
- Dry cough.
- Heart inflammation with chest pain.
- Burning, inflammation or scarring of skin.
- Permanent skin darkening.
- Bleeding spots anywhere under the skin.
- Anemia.
- Sexual impotence.

CAUSES—Radiation damage to the immune system and to healthy tissues.

RISK INCREASES WITH—For radiation treatment:
- Poor nutrition.
- Illness that has lowered resistance.

HOW TO PREVENT
- Have a thorough dental checkup to detect tooth or gum disease before head or neck radiation.
- Eat well before radiation treatment to be in optimal nutritional condition.
- If you work around radiation, learn and observe safety regulations.

WHAT TO EXPECT

APPROPRIATE HEALTH CARE
- Doctor's treatment.
- Psychotherapy or counseling to reduce the stress of radiation treatment.
- Hospitalization for radiation treatment or complications.

DIAGNOSTIC MEASURES
- Laboratory blood studies of hemoglobin, platelet counts and white-blood-cell counts.
- X-rays of treated areas.

POSSIBLE COMPLICATIONS
- Susceptibility to infections due to decreased resistance.
- Sterility or birth defects may occur.
- Increased susceptibility to cancer—especially bone-marrow cancer or leukemia.
- With radiation treatment, other complications depend on the area involved. Your doctor will explain possible complications. Modern radiation equipment makes serious complications unlikely.

PROBABLE OUTCOME
- With radiation treatment, most side effects or complications disappear gradually afterward.
- With radiation accidents not severe enough to cause immediate death, side effects may not appear for years.

HOW TO TREAT

NOTE—Follow your doctor's instructions. These instructions are supplemental.

GENERAL MEASURES
- Join a support group of people with similar experiences.
- During radiation treatment, keep your doctor informed of how you are feeling. Treatments can sometimes be interrupted until you feel better.
- If you lose your hair, wear a wig until hair growth resumes.
- Use effective birth-control measures to prevent pregnancy until your doctor determines it is safe to have children.

MEDICATION—Your doctor may prescribe:
- Antinausea drugs.
- Pain relievers.
- Blood transfusions for anemia.
- Antibiotics to fight infections.

ACTIVITY—Be as active as your strength allows. Rest often.

DIET—Eat a balanced diet. You may temporarily need a liquid diet (see Appendix 7) or want to prepare food in a blender if you have trouble swallowing. Intravenous feeding or use of a small stomach tube is also possible until you resume normal eating. A dietitian can help.

CALL YOUR DOCTOR IF

- You are accidentally exposed to radiation.
- You feel very ill during radiation treatment, especially if you have unexpected symptoms.
- You develop signs of infection, such as fever and chills, muscle aches, headache and dizziness, during or after exposure or treatment.
- New, unexplained symptoms develop. Drugs in treatment may produce side effects.

RAPE CRISIS SYNDROME

GENERAL INFORMATION

DEFINITION—The physical and emotional aftereffects of rape (forced sexual entry into the body).

BODY PARTS INVOLVED—Genitals; rectum; mouth; brain.

SEX OR AGE MOST AFFECTED—All ages and both sexes, but more common in females.

SIGNS & SYMPTOMS
- Cuts, bruises or other injuries, including vaginal and rectal tears.
- Effects of exposure to the elements, if the attack occurred outdoors or in a remote place.
- Fear, anger, crying, or unusual behavior such as laughter.
- Unwarranted self-blame and guilt.
- Depression and withdrawal, even from family and friends.
- No outward signs (sometimes).

CAUSES—Rape is not a sexual act for pleasure. It is a show of power and an attempt to degrade or humiliate the victim. Some rapists have been victims of sexual abuse. Many know their victims—at least casually—and their attacks may be planned, not impulsive.

RISK INCREASES WITH
- Economically depressed areas.
- Excess alcohol consumption or drug abuse by the potential rapist.

HOW TO PREVENT—At home:
- Keep doors and windows locked.
- Install security devices.
Away from home:
- Avoid dark, quiet or isolated places. Stay within sight of others.
- Never hitchhike.
- Always lock your car.
- Check the back seat of your car before getting in.
- Take a self-defense course.
- If you are threatened with rape, remain calm. Panic may worsen the situation. Sometimes a rapist can be stopped by unexpected behavior, such as asking for help with a task.
- Carry a rape siren or whistle. Most authorities don't recommend that you carry a weapon.

WHAT TO EXPECT

APPROPRIATE HEALTH CARE
- Doctor's treatment *always*—regardless of whether there are physical injuries.
- Surgery to repair any wounds.
- Hospitalization (rare).

- Psychotherapy or counseling to learn to cope with fear, sexual trauma and unrealistic feelings of guilt or worthlessness.

DIAGNOSTIC MEASURES
- Your own observation of symptoms.
- Medical history and physical exam by a doctor.
- Laboratory studies, such as:
  Cultures and blood tests for gonorrhea or other venereal disease.
  Detailed examination of the body for evidence from the rapist, such as hair, sperm or bits of clothing.
- X-rays, if fractures are suspected.

POSSIBLE COMPLICATIONS
- Prolonged psychological trauma.
- Pregnancy.
- Venereal disease.

PROBABLE OUTCOME—Complete physical and psychological recovery is often possible with professional treatment.

HOW TO TREAT

NOTE—Follow your doctor's instructions. These instructions are supplemental.

GENERAL MEASURES—If you are raped:
- Report the rape to police or a rape crisis center. If you don't, the rapist will probably attack others.
- Call your doctor or go to the nearest emergency room. Many cities have rape-crisis teams to help you through the stress of the medical examination.
- Don't bathe, douche or change clothes.
- Talk over your feelings with trusted friends and family. Suppressing your feelings increases distress.

MEDICATION—Your doctor may prescribe:
- Antibiotics, if venereal infection is suspected or diagnosed.
- Hormones to prevent pregnancy ("day-after pill").
- Sedatives or tranquilizers for a short time to reduce anxiety.

ACTIVITY—Resume your normal life as quickly as possible.

DIET—No special diet.

CALL YOUR DOCTOR IF

You or someone you know has been raped.

RAYNAUD'S DISEASE

 ## GENERAL INFORMATION

DEFINITION—A primary disorder of the circulatory system that affects blood circulation to fingers and occasionally toes. This is different from Raynaud's phenomenon, which is a circulatory-system disorder that occurs as a complication of other diseases.

BODY PARTS INVOLVED—Small arteries to the hands and feet.

SEX OR AGE MOST AFFECTED—Both sexes, but most common in females between ages 12 and 40.

SIGNS & SYMPTOMS—Early symptoms:
● Fingers that turn pale when exposed to cold or stress. Paleness is followed by a bluish tinge, then redness. Pain, numbness and tingling accompany the color changes. Warmth relieves these symptoms.
Late symptoms:
● Chronic infections around fingernails and toenails.
● Ulcers on the fingertips caused by inadequate blood circulation in the fingers. Symptoms develop gradually over a period of years. With Raynaud's phenomenon, symptoms may begin suddenly.

CAUSES—Spasms of arteries that supply blood to the fingers and toes caused by extreme sensitivity to cold. The sensitivity may be due to poor function of the autoimmune system.

RISK INCREASES WITH
● Stress.
● Smoking, which impairs circulation to the extremities.
● Cold, wet weather.

HOW TO PREVENT—Don't start smoking. Tobacco triggers the problem. This disease is rare among non-smokers.

OTHER—There are many similarities between Raynaud's disease and Raynaud's phenomenon. Diagnosis between the two may require years of observation.

 ## WHAT TO EXPECT

APPROPRIATE HEALTH CARE
● Self-care after diagnosis.
● Doctor's treatment.
● Biofeedback training (see Glossary).
● Surgery to sever sympathetic nerves to the involved extremities. Surgery usually relieves symptoms for 1 to 2 years before they recur.

DIAGNOSTIC MEASURES
● Your own observation of symptoms.
● Medical history and physical exam by a doctor.
● Laboratory blood studies.
● X-rays of the hands and feet.

POSSIBLE COMPLICATIONS
● Permanent weakness and numbness in the toes and fingers.
● Gangrene and amputation (worst cases only).

PROBABLE OUTCOME—This condition is currently considered incurable. The disease worsens gradually over many years. However, symptoms can be relieved or controlled. Most persons cope well with Raynaud's disease and live a normal life span if complications don't arise.

Scientific research into causes and treatment continues, so there is hope for increasingly effective treatment and cure.

 ## HOW TO TREAT

NOTE—Follow your doctor's instructions. These instructions are supplemental.

GENERAL MEASURES
● Stop smoking. Symptoms will improve if you do.
● Avoid exposure to cold in any form. Wear mittens and gloves outdoors and when handling ice or frozen foods.
● Wear comfortable, roomy shoes and wool socks.
● Avoid stressful situations. See Appendix 13.
● Move to a warm climate, if possible.

MEDICATION—Your doctor may prescribe:
● Vasodilator drugs to dilate the small arteries and improve circulation.
● Sedatives to reduce stress.

ACTIVITY—No restrictions, except to keep warm. Avoid chilling while participating in active sports.

DIET
● No special diet.
● Because alcohol dilates blood vessels and may temporarily improve circulation slightly, you may have an occasional alcoholic drink.

 ## CALL YOUR DOCTOR IF

● You have symptoms of Raynaud's disease.
● Discomfort worsens, despite treatment.
● Ulcers that do not heal appear on fingers or toes.

RAYNAUD'S PHENOMENON

GENERAL INFORMATION

DEFINITION—A circulatory-system disorder affecting fingers and toes that is a complication of an underlying disease or emotional disturbance. This is different from Raynaud's disease, a primary disease. Symptoms arise suddenly with Raynaud's phenomenon. With Raynaud's disease, they appear slowly over several years.

BODY PARTS INVOLVED—Small arteries to the hands and feet.

SEX OR AGE MOST AFFECTED—Both sexes and all ages, but most common in young adult women (20 to 45 years).

SIGNS & SYMPTOMS—Early symptoms:
- Fingers that turn pale when exposed to cold or stress. Paleness is followed by a bluish tinge and then redness. Numbness and tingling accompany the color changes, and symptoms are relieved by warmth.
Late symptoms:
- Ulcers on the fingertips caused by lack of normal blood flow to the fingers.
- Chronic infections under and around fingernails and toenails.

CAUSES—Spasms of arteries that supply blood to fingers and toes. Spasms may be caused by:
- Scleroderma or other connective-tissue disorders.
- Buerger's disease.
- Cor pulmonale.
- Certain medications, including ergot preparations, antihypertensives, alpha- and beta-adrenergic blockers, and calcium-channel blockers.

RISK INCREASES WITH
- Stress.
- Smoking.
- Cold, wet weather.
- Occupations that involve work with heavy equipment that vibrates forcefully, such as a chain saw or pneumatic drill.

HOW TO PREVENT
- Don't smoke.
- Avoid exposure to the cold.
- Obtain medical treatment for diseases listed as causes.

OTHER—Because of the similarities between Raynaud's disease and Raynaud's phenomenon, an accurate diagnosis between the two may require years of observation.

WHAT TO EXPECT

APPROPRIATE HEALTH CARE
- Self-care after diagnosis.
- Doctor's treatment.
- Surgery to sever sympathetic nerves to the affected extremities. Surgery sometimes relieves symptoms for 1 or 2 years before they recur.

DIAGNOSTIC MEASURES
- Your own observation of symptoms.
- Medical history and physical exam by a doctor.
- Laboratory blood studies.
- X-rays of the hands and feet.

POSSIBLE COMPLICATIONS
- Permanent weakness and numbness in the toes and fingers caused by blockage of the blood supply.
- Gangrene that necessitates amputation, caused by loss of blood supply (worst cases only).

PROBABLE OUTCOME—Curable if the underlying cause can be cured.

HOW TO TREAT

NOTE—Follow your doctor's instructions. These instructions are supplemental.

GENERAL MEASURES
- Don't smoke.
- Avoid exposure to cold in any form. Wear mittens and gloves outdoors and when handling ice or frozen food.
- Wear comfortable, roomy shoes and wool socks. Don't go barefoot outdoors.
- Avoid stressful situations whenever possible. See Appendix 13.
- Move to a warm climate, if possible.

MEDICATION—Your doctor may prescribe:
- Vasodilator drugs to dilate small arteries and improve circulation.
- Sedatives to relieve tension and anxiety.

ACTIVITY—No restrictions, except to keep warm. Avoid chilling, which may happen following any active recreational sport.

DIET—No special diet. Alcohol dilates blood vessels and may temporarily improve circulation slightly. An occasional alcoholic beverage may be helpful.

CALL YOUR DOCTOR IF

- You have symptoms of Raynaud's phenomenon.
- Discomfort worsens, despite treatment.
- Ulcers appear on fingers or toes and do not heal.

ILLNESSES & DISORDERS

RECTAL PROLAPSE

GENERAL INFORMATION

DEFINITION—Protrusion of rectal tissues outside the anus.

BODY PARTS INVOLVED—Anus and rectum.

SEX OR AGE MOST AFFECTED—Adults over 60, usually women.

SIGNS & SYMPTOMS
- A vague sense of fullness in the lower abdomen or rectal area.
- A mucus discharge—sometimes tinged with blood—from the rectum.
- A firm mass of tissue that can be felt at the anus after a bowel movement.

CAUSES
- Weak pelvic muscles.
- Abdominal pressure caused by:
  Chronic cough.
  Prolonged constipation and straining to have bowel movements.
  Standing or walking for long periods.

RISK INCREASES WITH
- Aging.
- Previous surgery on the rectum or vagina.

HOW TO PREVENT—Women can practice pelvic-strengthening exercises (Kegel exercises) to prevent recurrences.

OTHER—Rectal prolapse in infants can be a sign of cystic fibrosis.

WHAT TO EXPECT

APPROPRIATE HEALTH CARE
- Self-care.
- Doctor's treatment.
- Surgery to strengthen tissues that support the rectum (sometimes).

DIAGNOSTIC MEASURES
- Your own observation of symptoms.
- Medical history and physical exam by a doctor.
- Examination of the rectal area by anoscope or sigmoidoscope (see Glossary for both).

POSSIBLE COMPLICATIONS
- Ulceration and bleeding in tissue that protrudes permanently.
- Bowel incontinence.

PROBABLE OUTCOME—Minor degrees of prolapse can be managed by general measures listed below. Surgery cures major prolapse.

HOW TO TREAT

NOTE—Follow your doctor's instructions. These instructions are supplemental.

GENERAL MEASURES
- Occasional minor prolapse can often be reversed by gently pushing the protruding tissue back into the rectum.
- Use sanitary napkins or absorbent pads to absorb the mucus discharge.
- Women can learn to recognize, control and develop the muscles of the pelvic floor. These are the ones you use to interrupt urination in mid-stream. The following exercises (Kegel exercises) strengthen these muscles so you can control or relax them completely:

To identify which muscles are involved, alternately start and stop urinating when using the toilet.

Practice tightening and releasing these muscles while sitting, standing, walking, driving, watching TV or listening to music.

Tighten the muscles a small amount at a time—"like an elevator going up to the 10th floor." Then release very slowly—"one floor at a time."

Tighten the muscles from front to back, including the anus, as in the previous exercise.

Practice exercises every morning, afternoon and evening. Start with 5 times each, and gradually work up to 20 or 30 each time.

MEDICATION—Your doctor may prescribe stool softeners to prevent constipation.

ACTIVITY
- Avoid standing or walking for long periods; this increases abdominal pressure.
- Practice pelvic-strengthening exercises to prevent a recurrence.

DIET—No special diet. Drink at least 8 glasses of water a day and eat a diet high in fiber to prevent constipation.

CALL YOUR DOCTOR IF

- Rectal tissue remains outside the anus.
- Rectal pain or bleeding occur.
- Fever or chills develop, indicating infection.

REITER'S SYNDROME

GENERAL INFORMATION

DEFINITION—An inflammatory disease characterized by a complex of symptoms resembling those of arthritis, urethritis, conjunctivitis and psoriasis. This is probably a sexually transmitted disease.

BODY PARTS INVOLVED—Joints; eyes, including white eye covering; urethra and head of the penis; skin.

SEX OR AGE MOST AFFECTED—Male adolescents and young adults (12 to 40 years). This is rare in women and children.

SIGNS & SYMPTOMS
- Inflammation of the urethra and discharge within 7 to 14 days after sexual intercourse.
- Frequent urinary urgency.
- Small ulcers inside the mouth, tongue and on the penis tip.
- Low fever.
- Red eyes.
- Painful joints, especially toes, legs, hip and back.
- Aching in the pelvis.
- Skin lesions similar to psoriasis on the soles, palms, and around fingernails and toenails.

CAUSES—Unknown. The predisposition is inherited, and the disease usually follows sexual contact. It probably represents an unusual response to a sexually-transmitted infection.

RISK INCREASES WITH
- Recent gastrointestinal illness with diarrhea.
- Previous sexually-transmitted infections.
- Family history of Reiter's syndrome.
- Genetic factors. Most persons with this disease carry antigen HLA-B27.

HOW TO PREVENT—Use rubber condoms for sexual intercourse.

WHAT TO EXPECT

APPROPRIATE HEALTH CARE
- Doctor's treatment for diagnosis and supervision of treatment.
- Self-care after diagnosis.

DIAGNOSTIC MEASURES
- Your own observation of symptoms.
- Medical history and physical exam by a doctor.
- Laboratory blood studies and culture of the urethral discharge.

POSSIBLE COMPLICATIONS—Osteoporosis.

PROBABLE OUTCOME—Arthritis symptoms may continue up to 4 months, others disappear sooner. Most patients recover in 2 to 16 weeks with no residual signs of the disease, but some persons have recurrent flare-ups and remissions.

HOW TO TREAT

NOTE—Follow your doctor's instructions. These instructions are supplemental.

GENERAL MEASURES—To relieve foot pain, wear cushion pads and arch supports in your shoes.

MEDICATION—Your doctor may prescribe:
- Non-steroidal anti-inflammatory drugs.
- Antibiotics, such as tetracyclines, for urethritis.

ACTIVITY
- Stay as active as your condition allows, but avoid sexual excitement and activity during the illness.
- Exercise the affected joints according to instructions from your doctor or physical therapist. Don't immobilize affected joints.

DIET—No special diet.

CALL YOUR DOCTOR IF

- You have symptoms of Reiter's syndrome.
- Symptoms recur after recovery.
- New, unexplained symptoms develop. Drugs used in treatment may produce side effects.

ILLNESSES & DISORDERS

RETINAL DETACHMENT

 GENERAL INFORMATION

DEFINITION—A separation or tear of the retina (the light-sensitive tissue at the back of the eye) from the remainder of the eye.

BODY PARTS INVOLVED—Eye.

SEX OR AGE MOST AFFECTED—All ages and both sexes, but more common in men.

SIGNS & SYMPTOMS—The following usually affect one eye, but sometimes both are affected:
- Light flashes in the field of vision.
- Floating spots in the field of vision.
- Blurred vision.
- Wavy visual images (sometimes).
- Gradual loss of vision. This may not be noticed because it is so gradual.
- No pain.

CAUSES
- Extreme nearsightedness (myopia).
- Complications of eye surgery.
- Eye injury.
- Inherited tendency (possibly).

RISK INCREASES WITH
- Age.
- Diabetes mellitus.
- Vascular disease.
- Previous retinal detachment.
- Family history of retinal detachment.

HOW TO PREVENT
- Wear protective eye shields when participating in sports.
- If you have diabetes mellitus or vascular disease, obtain medical treatment to control the disorder. See an opthalmologist at least once a year.

 WHAT TO EXPECT

APPROPRIATE HEALTH CARE
- Doctor's (ophthalmologist's) treatment.
- Surgery to reattach the retina using special lasers or cryotherapy (see Glossary), or by changing the shape of the eye (sometimes).

DIAGNOSTIC MEASURES
- Your own observation of symptoms.
- Medical history and physical exam by a doctor.

POSSIBLE COMPLICATIONS
- Without treatment: Partial or complete blindness in the affected eye.
- With delayed treatment: Detachment which extends to the macula (the area of most detailed vision). This causes permanent loss of detailed (central) vision.

PROBABLE OUTCOME—Often curable with early surgical treatment.

 HOW TO TREAT

NOTE—Follow your doctor's instructions. These instructions are supplemental.

GENERAL MEASURES—The following instructions apply after surgery:
- Both eyes will be patched for a time. Your family and friends can help overcome this stress by providing companionship and assistance.
- Use dark glasses after the patches are removed.
- Don't rub your eyes.
- Don't bend over.
- Avoid straining, such as from constipation, heavy lifting or harsh coughing. This may increase pressure in the eyes.

MEDICATION—Your doctor may prescribe:
- Mydriatic eye drops to dilate the pupil. Dilation reduces eye activity during healing. If you cannot instill the drops, ask someone to be available to help at the appropriate times.
- Sedatives or tranquilizers to reduce anxiety during convalescence.

ACTIVITY—After surgery, lie on your back in bed with your head elevated. Move your legs frequently to prevent blood clots from forming in deep veins. Resume your normal activities when your ophthalmologist considers it safe.

DIET—No special diet.

 CALL YOUR DOCTOR IF

- You have flashes or floating spots in your field of vision.
- Any sign of infection (bleeding, redness, pain, swelling or fever) occurs after surgery.
- Your vision worsens after full recovery from surgery.

REYE'S SYNDROME

GENERAL INFORMATION

DEFINITION—A disease in children and adolescents that involves the brain and other major organs.

BODY PARTS INVOLVED—Brain; liver; kidneys; heart.

SEX OR AGE MOST AFFECTED—Children from infancy through adolescence.

SIGNS & SYMPTOMS
- Confusion.
- Lethargy.
- Personality changes.
- Seizures.
- Weakness and paralysis in an arm or leg.
- Double vision.
- Speech impairment.
- Hearing loss.
- Drowsiness that progresses to coma.

CAUSES—Unknown. Reye's syndrome usually follows a virus infection. Some studies link it to the use of aspirin during a viral illness, especially chickenpox and influenza.

RISK INCREASES WITH
- Recent illness, such as chickenpox, influenza or other respiratory illness.
- Use of aspirin.
- Genetic factors. This is more common in Caucasians than in blacks.

HOW TO PREVENT—Don't give a child aspirin for any illness with fever until the doctor has diagnosed it. If the illness is diagnosed as viral, *don't use aspirin.*

WHAT TO EXPECT

APPROPRIATE HEALTH CARE
- Doctor's treatment.
- Hospitalization for intensive care to monitor pressure on the brain.
- Home care during convalescence.

DIAGNOSTIC MEASURES
- Your own observation of symptoms.
- Medical history and physical exam by a doctor.
- Laboratory studies, such as blood studies of liver function and an analysis of cerebrospinal fluid.

POSSIBLE COMPLICATIONS—Permanent brain damage, coma or death caused by pressure on the brain.

PROBABLE OUTCOME—With treatment, 80% of patients survive. Most recover completely, but some have varying degrees of brain damage.

HOW TO TREAT

NOTE—Follow your doctor's instructions. These instructions are supplemental.

GENERAL MEASURES—No specific instructions except those listed under other headings.

MEDICATION—Your doctor may prescribe:
- Intravenous fluids.
- Anticoagulant drugs to prevent blood-clot formation during prolonged bed rest.
- Drugs, such as dexamethasone, to reduce cerebral swelling.
- Antibiotics to fight secondary bacterial infections, if they develop.

ACTIVITY—Bed rest is necessary until the acute stage is over. Reading or watching TV is acceptable. Normal activities may then be resumed gradually.

DIET—No special diet.

CALL YOUR DOCTOR IF

- Your child has symptoms of Reye's syndrome. Call at the first sign of confusion, lethargy or other mental changes!
- After hospitalization, any symptoms of Reye's syndrome recur or the child develops fever of 100F (37.8C) or higher.
- New, unexplained symptoms develop. Drugs used in treatment may produce side effects.

ILLNESSES & DISORDERS

RH INCOMPATIBILITY
(Erythroblastosis Fetalis)

 GENERAL INFORMATION

DEFINITION—Incompatibility between an infant's blood type and that of its mother, resulting in destruction of the infant's red blood cells (hemolytic anemia) after birth by antibodies from its mother's blood.

BODY PARTS INVOLVED—Blood of pregnant mother and fetus.

SEX OR AGE MOST AFFECTED—Newborn infants only.

SIGNS & SYMPTOMS—Signs in a newborn:
- Paleness.
- Jaundice (yellow skin and eyes) that begins within 24 hours after delivery.
- Unexplained bruising or blood spots under the skin.
- Tissue swelling (edema).
- Breathing difficulty.
- Seizures.
- Lack of normal movement.
- Poor reflex response.

CAUSES—The fetus of an Rh-negative (blood type) mother and an Rh-positive father may be Rh-positive. During delivery, a small amount of the infant's blood is absorbed by the mother through the placenta, stimulating her body to produce antibodies against Rh-positive blood. The antibodies are produced after delivery, so the first infant is not affected. With succeeding pregnancies, the antibodies in the mother's blood destroy fetal blood cells. The fetus is unharmed in the uterus, because the mother's blood is supplying the infant's oxygen needs. After birth, however, the antibodies in the infant's blood destroy its blood cells, causing jaundice and other symptoms.

RISK INCREASES WITH
- Each pregnancy after the first involving different blood types.
- Previous blood transfusions. These might have contained unidentified, incompatible blood types.

HOW TO PREVENT
- Obtain prenatal care throughout pregnancy. Medical supervision early in pregnancy is essential to determine the risk of Rh incompatibility.
- Special anti-Rh gamma globulin is given to the mother at 28 weeks gestation and within 72 hours after delivery, miscarriage, ectopic pregnancy or abortion. This prevents formation of antibodies that might affect future infants.

 WHAT TO EXPECT

APPROPRIATE HEALTH CARE
- Doctor's treatment.
- Transfusion to exchange completely the infant's blood.
- Hospitalization. The newborn child will remain in the hospital up to 2 weeks after an exchange transfusion.

DIAGNOSTIC MEASURES
- Medical history and physical exam by a doctor. Tell your doctor if you have had a miscarriage or abortion.
- Blood tests to: type mother's, father's and infant's blood; measure the mother's Rh-positive antibodies; and detect hemolytic anemia in the infant's blood.
- Amniocentesis (in Surgery section).

POSSIBLE COMPLICATIONS
- Permanent neurological damage, such as cerebral palsy or hearing loss (rare).
- Blood-transfusion reaction.

PROBABLE OUTCOME—With prompt recognition of the disorder, damage to the infant can be prevented with exchange transfusions.

 HOW TO TREAT

NOTE—Follow your doctor's instructions. These instructions are supplemental.

GENERAL MEASURES—If you have an Rh-negative blood type:
- Tell any doctor or medical professional who treats you. Make sure this information is in your medical records.
- Wear a Medic-Alert bracelet or pendant (see Glossary).

MEDICATION—If you are pregnant and have Rh-negative blood type, your doctor will prescribe an anti-Rh gamma globulin injection at 28 weeks and again within 72 hours after delivery or termination of a pregnancy for any reason.

ACTIVITY—No restrictions after treatment.

DIET—The infant may be breast-fed or bottle-fed normally.

📞 **CALL YOUR DOCTOR IF**

Your baby has any of the following after returning home:
- Fever.
- Jaundice.
- Poor appetite or poor weight gain.
- Excessive crying that does not stop when the baby is held.

RHEUMATIC FEVER

GENERAL INFORMATION

DEFINITION—An inflammatory complication of Group A streptococcal infections that affects many parts of the body, especially the joints and heart. Strep infections are contagious, but rheumatic fever is not.

BODY PARTS INVOLVED—Joints; heart and heart valves; skin and brain (sometimes).

SEX OR AGE MOST AFFECTED—Both sexes of children between ages 4 and 18.

SIGNS & SYMPTOMS
- Joint inflammation, characterized by pain, redness, swelling and warmth. Wrists, elbows, knees or ankles are most often affected. Joint inflammation usually subsides in 10 to 14 days, but without treatment, other joints may become inflamed.
- Fever.
- Appetite loss.
- Abdominal pain.
- General ill feeling.
- Mild skin rash on the chest, back and abdomen.
- Small, painless bumps just under the skin in bony areas such as the elbows or knees.
- Fatigue.
- Paleness.

If the heart is involved:
- Shortness of breath.
- Fluid retention that causes swelling of the legs and back.
- Rapid heartbeat, especially when lying down.

CAUSES—Rheumatic fever is caused by a preceding strep infection, usually in the throat, that occurs 1 to 6 weeks prior to the onset of symptoms. It is probably an autoimmune disorder in which antibodies produced to attack the strep bacteria also attack tissues of the joints or heart.

RISK INCREASES WITH
- Poor nutrition.
- Family history of rheumatic fever.
- Crowded or unsanitary living conditions.

HOW TO PREVENT
- Request a throat culture for strep from your doctor's office for any throat infection, especially in a child.
- Obtain prompt antibiotic treatment of any strep infection, including those of the skin. Strep infections must be treated with antibiotics, usually penicillin, for a *minimum of 10 days orally or by long-lasting injection.*

WHAT TO EXPECT

APPROPRIATE HEALTH CARE
- Doctor's treatment.
- Home care after diagnosis (mild cases).
- Hospitalization (severe cases).

DIAGNOSTIC MEASURES
- Your own observation of symptoms.
- Medical history and physical exam by a doctor.
- Laboratory studies, such as blood studies, a throat culture and EKG (see Glossary).
- X-rays of the chest and heart.

POSSIBLE COMPLICATIONS—Permanently damaged heart valves, leading to congestive heart failure.

PROBABLE OUTCOME—Usually curable with treatment. In some cases, rheumatic fever may damage the heart valves. A damaged valve can be replaced with surgery.

In rare cases, rheumatic fever is fatal—even with treatment.

HOW TO TREAT

NOTE—Follow your doctor's instructions. These instructions are supplemental.

GENERAL MEASURES
- Take the patient's temperature and count the pulse; keep a record for your doctor.
- Use a cool-mist humidifier if the patient has a sore throat or cough.

MEDICATION—Your doctor may prescribe:
- Steroids (anti-inflammatory drugs) or aspirin to reduce inflammation.
- Diuretics to reduce fluid retention.
- Antibiotics to fight any remaining strep bacteria. Once rheumatic fever reaches the inactive stage, low-dose antibiotics may be continued indefinitely to prevent recurrence.

ACTIVITY—The patient should stay in bed until studies show the disease has subsided. Bed rest for 2 to 5 weeks is usually required, but some cases require months. Provide a bed pan or bedside commode so the patient won't have to get up to use the bathroom.

DIET—A liquid or soft diet in the early stages (see Appendices 7 and 11), progressing to a normal diet high in protein, calories and vitamins.

CALL YOUR DOCTOR IF

- Your child has symptoms of rheumatic fever.
- The following symptoms occur during treatment:
  Swelling of the legs or back.
  Shortness of breath.
  Vomiting or diarrhea.
  Cough.
  Severe abdominal pain.
  Fever of 101F (38.3C) or higher.
- New, unexplained symptoms develop.
Drugs in treatment may produce side effects.

RINGWORM

GENERAL INFORMATION

DEFINITION—Fungus (tinea) infection of the skin. This is transmitted by person-to-person contact or by contact with infected surfaces, such as towels, shoes or shower stalls.

BODY PARTS INVOLVED—Scalp (tinea capitis); skin (tinea corporis); groin skin (tinea cruris); nails (tinea unguium); feet (tinea pedis); skin with beard (tinea barbae).

SEX OR AGE MOST AFFECTED—Adolescents and adults. It is more common in males than females.

SIGNS & SYMPTOMS—Lesions that itch (sometimes) and have the following characteristics:
- On the scalp, lesions cause patchy hair loss and scaling scalp.
- On body skin, lesions are red, circular, flat, scaling and have well-defined borders.
- On the bearded area of the face, lesions cause an itchy, scaling rash under the beard.
- On the feet: see Athlete's Foot in the Illness section.
- Of the nails: see Paronychia in the Illness section.

CAUSES—Fungus infection with one or more of 5 different fungi.

RISK INCREASES WITH
- Diabetes mellitus.
- Exposure to darkness, moisture and warmth.
- Crowded or unsanitary living conditions.

HOW TO PREVENT—The fungi are so prevalent that total prevention is impossible. To minimize risk:
- Avoid continuous exposure to overheated humid environments.
- Avoid contact with pets that have skin problems.

WHAT TO EXPECT

APPROPRIATE HEALTH CARE
- Self-care after diagnosis.
- Doctor's treatment.

DIAGNOSTIC MEASURES
- Your own observation of symptoms.
- Medical history and physical exam by a doctor.
- Microscopic exam of skin scrapings in potassium hydroxide solution.
- Laboratory culture of skin scrapings.
- Examination with ultraviolet light (Wood's lamp) for ringworm on the scalp.

POSSIBLE COMPLICATIONS—Secondary bacterial infection of ringworm lesions.

PROBABLE OUTCOME—Usually curable in 6 weeks with treatment, but recurrence is common. Ringworm becomes chronic in 20% of cases.

HOW TO TREAT

NOTE—Follow your doctor's instructions. These instructions are supplemental.

GENERAL MEASURES—For ringworm on the body:
- Boil or chemically sterilize all clothing, towels or bed linens that have touched the lesions.
- Keep the skin dry. Moist areas favor fungus growth.
- Wear cotton underwear. Change more than once a day. Avoid tight clothes.
- If the area is red, swollen and weeping, use compresses made of 1 teaspoon salt to 1 pint water. Apply 4 times a day for 2 to 3 days before starting the local antifungal medication.

For ringworm of the scalp:
- Shampoo the hair every day.
- Have the hair cut short, but don't shave the scalp. Place large sheets of paper under and around the hair and chair to catch all the clippings. Place a cloth drape around the shoulders, chest and back. Don't wear street clothes for a haircut. Wear something that can be sterilized, such as pajamas, a house coat or smock. Repeat this procedure every 2 weeks, or whenever the hair grows back.

MEDICATION—Your doctor may prescribe oral or topical antifungal drugs.

ACTIVITY—No restrictions.

DIET—No special diet.

CALL YOUR DOCTOR IF

- You have symptoms of ringworm.
- Ringworm lesions become redder, painful and ooze pus.
- Symptoms don't improve in 3 or 4 weeks, despite treatment.
- New, unexplained symptoms develop. Drugs used in treatment may produce side effects.

ROCKY MOUNTAIN SPOTTED FEVER
(Tick Fever; Tick Typhus; Spotted Fever)

 GENERAL INFORMATION

DEFINITION—An acute illness with fever caused by a germ transmitted by infected ticks. This is not contagious from person to person.

BODY PARTS INVOLVED—Skin; central nervous system; gastrointestinal tract; muscles.

SEX OR AGE MOST AFFECTED—Both sexes; all ages.

SIGNS & SYMPTOMS—The following occur 2 to 5 days after a tick bite:
● Fever up to 105F (40.6C) with chills.
● Red skin rash that begins on hands and feet and spreads to ankles, wrists, legs, trunk and abdomen.
● Headache.
● Muscle aches and weakness; stiff back.
● Nausea and vomiting.
● Mental confusion; coma.

CAUSES—Rickettsia germs that live inside ticks. People are infected through tick bites, usually in the spring or summer. Rickettsia also infect rodents, squirrels and chipmunks.

The disease occurs in all states of the U.S., especially on the Eastern seaboard from Georgia to Maryland, and in heavy brushy areas, such as Long Island.

RISK INCREASES WITH—Outdoor activities in tick-infested areas.

HOW TO PREVENT
● Wear protective clothing in tick-infested areas, and use insect repellant.
● During outdoor activity, carefully inspect the body frequently to remove ticks. Don't crush them during removal—the whole tick must be removed. Hold a lighted cigarette near the tick, or apply gasoline, kerosene or oil to the tick's body. Pull it off with tweezers.

 WHAT TO EXPECT

APPROPRIATE HEALTH CARE
● Doctor's treatment. This may be a medical emergency.
● Home care during convalescence.

DIAGNOSTIC MEASURES
● Your own observation of symptoms.
● Medical history and physical exam by a doctor.
● Laboratory studies, such as blood counts and serological tests (see Glossary).

POSSIBLE COMPLICATIONS—Rocky Mountain spotted fever is often fatal if untreated.

PROBABLE OUTCOME—Curable if antibiotic treatment is begun in the early stages.

 HOW TO TREAT

NOTE—Follow your doctor's instructions. These instructions are supplemental.

GENERAL MEASURES—No specific instructions except those listed under other headings.

MEDICATION—Your doctor may prescribe antibiotics, such as tetracycline or chloramphenicol.

ACTIVITY—Rest in bed until fever and other symptoms disappear. You may read or watch TV.

DIET—No special diet.

 CALL YOUR DOCTOR IF

● You have symptoms of Rocky Mountain spotted fever.
● New, unexplained symptoms develop. Drugs used in treatment may produce side effects.

ILLNESSES & DISORDERS

ROSEOLA INFANTUM
(Exanthem Subitum; Pseudorubella)

 GENERAL INFORMATION

DEFINITION—A common, contagious childhood disease characterized by high fever and skin rash.

BODY PARTS INVOLVED—Skin; central nervous system.

SEX OR AGE MOST AFFECTED—Infants and young children (1 to 3 years).

SIGNS & SYMPTOMS
● Fever of 103F (39.4C) to 105F (40.6C) for 3 to 4 days.
● Irritability.
● Drowsiness.
● Flat, reddish skin rash after 3 or 4 days of high fever. When the rash appears, fever and other symptoms disappear.

CAUSES—Unknown. Because roseola has many features of viral illness, it is commonly believed to be caused by a virus—but the organism has not been identified. Incubation is 5 to 15 days.

RISK INCREASES WITH
● Spring and autumn seasons.
● Exposure to others in public places.

HOW TO PREVENT—Avoid exposure if possible.

 WHAT TO EXPECT

APPROPRIATE HEALTH CARE
● Home care after diagnosis.
● Doctor's treatment. Middle-ear infection, meningitis, pneumonia or urinary-tract infection should be ruled out as possible causes for the high fever.

DIAGNOSTIC MEASURES
● Your own observation of symptoms.
● Medical history and physical exam by a doctor.
● Laboratory studies, such as urinalysis and blood counts, to rule out other reasons for high fever.

POSSIBLE COMPLICATIONS
● Convulsions caused by high fever.
● Dehydration.

PROBABLE OUTCOME—Spontaneous recovery in 1 week.

 HOW TO TREAT

NOTE—Follow your doctor's instructions. These instructions are supplemental.

GENERAL MEASURES—Try to reduce fever if it reaches 102F (38.9C) or higher. See How to Reduce Fever, Appendix 19.

MEDICATION—For minor discomfort and to reduce fever, you may use non-prescription drugs such as acetaminophen.

ACTIVITY—The child should rest in bed until fever disappears.

DIET—The child should eat a normal, well-balanced diet. Continue baby-vitamin supplements if the child is accustomed to taking them.

 CALL YOUR DOCTOR IF

● Fever exceeds 103F (39.4C) rectally.
● Twitching or other signs of a convulsion begin.
● The child refuses liquids.
● The child cries loudly and persistently, and does not stop when picked up.
● The child is listless and has a stiff neck.

ROUNDWORMS
(Ascariasis)

GENERAL INFORMATION

DEFINITION—Intestinal parasites shaped like earthworms that can be seen easily without a microscope. Roundworms thrive in the gastrointestinal tract. They are contagious.

BODY PARTS INVOLVED—Gastrointestinal tract; lungs (sometimes).

SEX OR AGE MOST AFFECTED—All ages, but most common in children.

SIGNS & SYMPTOMS
- Irritability.
- Restlessness at night.
- Erratic or poor appetite.
- Frequent fatigue.
- Weight loss or lack of weight gain.
- Colicky abdominal discomfort.
- Diarrhea (sometimes).
- Cough and wheezing (rare).

CAUSES—A parasite called ascaris whose eggs enter the human body through contaminated water, food or soil-contaminated hands.

RISK INCREASES WITH—Crowded or unsanitary living conditions.

HOW TO PREVENT
- Wash hands frequently—*always* before eating.
- Keep fingers away from the mouth.
- Have pets treated for worms. Avoid strange animals.

OTHER—Worms may sometimes be seen in bowel movements or in the child's bed. Rarely, one may be vomited.

WHAT TO EXPECT

APPROPRIATE HEALTH CARE
- Home care after diagnosis.
- Doctor's treatment.

DIAGNOSTIC MEASURES
- Your own observation of symptoms.
- Medical history and physical exam by a doctor.
- Laboratory studies to identify the worm.

POSSIBLE COMPLICATIONS—If untreated:
- Anemia or malnutrition. May cause failure to thrive and abnormal physical and mental development in children.
- Intestinal obstruction (rare).

PROBABLE OUTCOME—Usually curable in 1 week with treatment.

HOW TO TREAT

NOTE—Follow your doctor's instructions. These instructions are supplemental.

GENERAL MEASURES
- Wash hands carefully after using the toilet or before meals. Keep fingers away from the mouth. Keep nails short and clean.
- Wash the anus and genitals with warm soap and water at least twice a day. Rinse well, preferably under a shower. Don't take tub baths.
- If possible, boil all soiled linen, nightclothes, underwear, towels and washcloths that have been used by anyone with roundworms. Fabrics that cannot be boiled can be soaked in an ammonia solution (1 cup of household ammonia to 5 gallons of cold water).
- After treatment, scrub all toilet seats, bathroom floors and fixtures. Vacuum rugs, table tops, curtains, sofa and chairs carefully. Sterilize metal toys or similar objects in a hot oven.

MEDICATION—Your doctor may prescribe drugs to kill roundworms, such as:
- Pyrantel pamoate or piperazine.
- Mebendazole. This medication may cause fetal abnormalities. Don't use it if you are pregnant.

ACTIVITY—Patient may resume normal activities as soon as symptoms improve.

DIET—No special diet.

CALL YOUR DOCTOR IF

- You or your child have symptoms of roundworms.
- Roundworms reappear after treatment.
- New, unexplained symptoms develop. Drugs used in treatment may produce side effects.

ST. VITUS' DANCE
(Sydenham's Chorea; Rheumatic Chorea)

 GENERAL INFORMATION

DEFINITION—A temporary disorder of parts of the brain that control movement and coordination. St. Vitus' dance is not contagious.

BODY PARTS INVOLVED—Central nervous system.

SEX OR AGE MOST AFFECTED—Children of both sexes, but more common in girls.

SIGNS & SYMPTOMS
- Uncontrollable, purposeless and non-repetitive movements that are wandering or jerky. The eyes are not involved.
- Facial grimacing that disappears during sleep.

Symptoms are similar to those of cerebral palsy, except these last for a limited time, while cerebral palsy lasts a lifetime.

CAUSES—A delayed (up to 6 months) complication of inadequately treated Group A streptococcal infections, usually of the throat or skin. St. Vitus' dance is more likely to occur in summer and early autumn.

RISK INCREASES WITH—Prior strep infection.

HOW TO PREVENT
- Obtain prompt antibiotic treatment for strep infections of the throat, tonsils or skin. Take medication at least 10 days.
- A child who has had St. Vitus' dance should take daily antibiotics (usually penicillin or erythromycin) until adulthood to prevent strep infections.

OTHER—Use of phenothiazine drugs and other tranquilizers may produce symptoms identical to those of St. Vitus' dance, leading to misdiagnosis. If you have these symptoms and take these drugs, consult your doctor.

 WHAT TO EXPECT

APPROPRIATE HEALTH CARE
- Home care after diagnosis.
- Doctor's treatment.
- Psychotherapy or counseling for the patient and family. Parents and teachers should understand that the unusual movements are temporary, and the condition is not contagious.

DIAGNOSTIC MEASURES
- Your own observation of symptoms. Sometimes the symptoms are so mild that you may think only that the child seems unusually clumsy.
- Medical history and physical exam by a doctor.
- Laboratory throat culture and tests of spinal fluid (to rule out other causes of symptoms).
- EEG (see Glossary).

POSSIBLE COMPLICATIONS
- Injury from involuntary movements.
- Psychosocial problems.

PROBABLE OUTCOME—Spontaneous recovery in 3 to 6 months without lasting effects on personality, intelligence, emotions or muscle control.

 HOW TO TREAT

NOTE—Follow your doctor's instructions. These instructions are supplemental.

GENERAL MEASURES
- Keep the child away from dangerous implements, such as knives. Use plastic tableware with dull edges to prevent mouth injury.
- Help the child dress and eat, if necessary.
- Provide the child with love, support and reassurance.

MEDICATION—Your doctor may prescribe:
- Mild sedatives, tranquilizers or muscle relaxants to control abnormal, unintentional movements and help prevent self-injury.
- Cortisone drugs to control movements if the above drugs fail.
- Penicillin or other antibiotics until adulthood to prevent strep infections.

ACTIVITY—The child should resume normal activities as soon as possible. Try to educate teachers and classmates so the child can return to school—even before all involuntary movements cease. Avoid bed rest.

DIET—No special diet.

 CALL YOUR DOCTOR IF

- Your child has symptoms of St. Vitus' dance.
- Injury occurs from uncontrolled movements.

SALIVARY-DUCT STONE

GENERAL INFORMATION

DEFINITION—A tiny hard particle which forms in a salivary-gland duct (usually a salivary gland under the tongue). Chemicals in the saliva cause crusting in the duct. The disorder is not contagious or cancerous but symptoms of stones and tumors may be identical.

BODY PARTS INVOLVED—Salivary ducts or glands under the tongue or in the cheeks.

SEX OR AGE MOST AFFECTED—Both sexes, but more common in men.

SIGNS & SYMPTOMS
● Pain and swelling in the salivary gland (between ear and jaw).
● Redness and tenderness in the floor of the mouth and under the jaw.
● Swollen, tender lymph glands in the neck or under the jaw.
● Fever (if infection is present).

CAUSES—Chemical change of unknown cause in salivary-gland secretions. Infections and injuries sometimes precede stone formation.

RISK INCREASES WITH
● Smoking.
● Recent infection in the salivary gland.

HOW TO PREVENT
● Brush and floss teeth regularly to prevent infection in the mouth.
● Visit your dentist regularly for checkups.

WHAT TO EXPECT

APPROPRIATE HEALTH CARE
● Doctor's treatment.
● Surgery to remove the stone—generally under local anesthesia.
● Self-care after surgery.

DIAGNOSTIC MEASURES
● Your own observation of symptoms.
● Medical history and physical exam by a doctor.
● X-rays of the salivary duct (sialogram).

POSSIBLE COMPLICATIONS—Recurrence of the stone. If it recurs, a surgeon can permanently open the duct so saliva drains from the gland directly into the mouth.

PROBABLE OUTCOME—Many stones pass spontaneously. Others are usually curable with surgery.

HOW TO TREAT

NOTE—Follow your doctor's instructions. These instructions are supplemental.

GENERAL MEASURES—Use warm-water or cool-water soaks (see Appendix 18)—whichever feels better—to relieve pain and hasten healing.

MEDICATION
● Your doctor may prescribe antibiotics if infection is present with the stone.
● For minor pain, you may use non-prescription drugs, such as acetaminophen.

ACTIVITY—After surgery, resume normal activities as soon as possible.

DIET—No special diet.

CALL YOUR DOCTOR IF

● You have symptoms of a salivary-duct stone.
● Symptoms worsen or don't improve in 4 days despite treatment.
● Temperature rises to 101F (38.3C) or higher.

ILLNESSES & DISORDERS

SALIVARY-GLAND INFECTION

GENERAL INFORMATION

DEFINITION—An infection of a salivary gland caused by an infectious organism other than the virus that causes mumps.

BODY PARTS INVOLVED—Salivary glands and ducts.

SEX OR AGE MOST AFFECTED—Both sexes, but most common in men.

SIGNS & SYMPTOMS
- Pain and swelling of parotid (behind ear) or sublingual (under tongue) salivary glands.
- Pain and swelling of lymph glands in the neck (below jaw).
- Bitter pus in the mouth from the infected gland.
- Fever.

CAUSES—Bacterial infection caused by staphylococci or another of many strains of bacteria.

RISK INCREASES WITH
- Adults over 60.
- Smoking.
- Dehydration.
- Poor nutrition, especially vitamin deficiency.
- Recent or chronic illness that has lowered resistance, especially mouth infection.
- Use of drugs that cause a dry mouth.

HOW TO PREVENT
- Brush and floss teeth often and use antiseptic mouthwash, especially when ill.
- Visit your dentist regularly for checkups.

WHAT TO EXPECT

APPROPRIATE HEALTH CARE
- Self-care after diagnosis.
- Doctor's treatment.

DIAGNOSTIC MEASURES
- Your own observation of symptoms.
- Medical history and physical exam by a doctor.
- Laboratory studies, such as culture of pus from the infected gland.

POSSIBLE COMPLICATIONS—Complete, permanent blockage of the salivary-gland duct, which requires surgery.

PROBABLE OUTCOME—Usually curable in 2 weeks with treatment. If the gland becomes blocked with a stone or scar tissue, surgery is necessary before the infection can clear.

HOW TO TREAT

NOTE—Follow your doctor's instructions. These instructions are supplemental.

GENERAL MEASURES—Apply warm soaks (see Appendix 18) or a heating pad on low setting to ease pain and hasten healing.

MEDICATION
- Your doctor may prescribe antibiotics to fight bacterial infection.
- For minor pain, you may use non-prescription drugs such as acetaminophen.

ACTIVITY—No restrictions. Resume normal activities when fever disappears.

DIET—No special diet. Drink at least 6 to 8 glasses of fluid a day.

CALL YOUR DOCTOR IF

- You have symptoms of a salivary-gland infection.
- The infection does not improve in 4 days or symptoms worsen despite treatment.
- Fever persists, despite treatment, or recurs after treatment.

SALIVARY-GLAND TUMOR

GENERAL INFORMATION

DEFINITION—An abnormal growth in the salivary-gland. Most salivary-gland tumors are benign and require several years to develop. Even malignant tumors rarely spread to distant body parts.

BODY PARTS INVOLVED—Parotid glands (salivary glands in the jaw); submaxiliary and sublingual glands (salivary glands in the floor of the mouth).

SEX OR AGE MOST AFFECTED—Adults.

SIGNS & SYMPTOMS—A soft, painful swelling or firm mass above the angle of either jaw or in the floor of the mouth.

CAUSES—Unknown.

RISK INCREASES WITH
- Dehydration.
- Poor oral hygiene.
- Smoking.
- Salivary-duct stone.
- Dentures.

HOW TO PREVENT—Some can't be prevented, but the risk can be minimized by:
- Not smoking.
- Brushing and flossing the teeth at least twice a day to keep the mouth healthy.

WHAT TO EXPECT

APPROPRIATE HEALTH CARE
- Doctor's treatment.
- Surgery to remove the tumor and lymph glands in the neck, if malignant cells have spread.
- Self-care after surgery.

DIAGNOSTIC MEASURES
- Your own observation of symptoms.
- Medical history and physical exam by a doctor.
- X-rays of the salivary glands.

POSSIBLE COMPLICATIONS
- Infection at the surgical site.
- Disfigurement after surgery.
- Fatal spread to other organs.

PROBABLE OUTCOME
- Malignant tumors are usually curable with surgery, radiation treatment and anticancer drugs.
- Benign tumors are usually curable with surgery alone.

HOW TO TREAT

NOTE—Follow your doctor's instructions. These instructions are supplemental.

GENERAL MEASURES—After surgery, keep the mouth clean with salt-water mouthwashes. At least 3 or 4 times a day, rinse the mouth with a solution of 1 teaspoon salt in 8 oz. of warm water.

MEDICATION—Your doctor may prescribe:
- Pain relievers.
- Antibiotics, if infection is present.
- Anticancer drugs, if surgery and radiation treatment don't destroy a malignant tumor.

ACTIVITY—Resume your normal activities as soon as possible after surgery.

DIET—After surgery, a liquid diet (see Appendix 7) will be necessary until your mouth heals so you can eat normally.

CALL YOUR DOCTOR IF

- You have symptoms of a salivary-gland tumor.
- After surgery, signs of infection develop in your mouth, including increased warmth, redness, pain or tenderness and swelling.
- New, unexplained symptoms develop. Drugs used in treatment may produce side effects.

SALMONELLA INFECTIONS

GENERAL INFORMATION

DEFINITION—A general infection caused by one of the 12,000 or more germs in the salmonella family.

BODY PARTS INVOLVED—Gastrointestinal tract; lymphatic system.

SEX OR AGE MOST AFFECTED—Both sexes; all ages.

SIGNS & SYMPTOMS
- Diarrhea, often accompanied by abdominal cramps. In mild cases, diarrhea may be only 2 or 3 loose bowel movements a day. In severe cases, it may be watery diarrhea as often as every 10 or 15 minutes.
- Vomiting.
- Fever.
- Blood in the stool (sometimes).

A relatively mild salmonella infection may be mistaken for simple gastroenteritis.

CAUSES—Infection with salmonella bacteria after eating meat that contains the bacteria. Salmonella bacteria survive freezing, but thorough cooking kills them. Pet turtles can also carry salmonella bacteria.

Salmonella epidemics often occur when many people eat the same contaminated food at a picnic, social gathering or restaurant. The infection can be transmitted from person to person.

RISK INCREASES WITH
- Recent gastrointestinal illness.
- Crowded or unsanitary living conditions.

HOW TO PREVENT
- Follow these recommendations in any area with a substandard water supply:
  Drink purified water, boil water or add 2 to 4 drops of 4% to 6% chlorine bleach to each quart of water 30 minutes before use. If in a hotel, draw hot water from the faucet, let it cool and use it as drinking water. Don't use ice.
  Don't eat raw fruits and vegetables unless you can peel them.
- Drink only pasteurized milk.
- Wash your hands after bowel movements and before handling food.
- Isolate anyone in the family who has the infection.
- Ask your doctor about preventive antibiotics before traveling in countries with unsanitary water and food supplies.

WHAT TO EXPECT

APPROPRIATE HEALTH CARE
- Self-care.
- Doctor's treatment, if symptoms continue longer than 48 hours or for complications.
- Hospitalization (rare).

DIAGNOSTIC MEASURES
- Your own observation of symptoms.
- Medical history and physical exam by a doctor.
- Laboratory stool studies.

POSSIBLE COMPLICATIONS
- Dehydration from excessive diarrhea and vomiting. Severe dehydration can be fatal, especially in infants and persons over 60.
- Infection of other organs, such as the kidneys, gallbladder, spleen and lungs, from salmonella bacteria in the bloodstream (rare).

PROBABLE OUTCOME—Most salmonella infections are mild and curable with treatment in 24 to 48 hours. Patients with severe infections require hospitalization and isolation. The infection may last 2 to 3 weeks.

HOW TO TREAT

NOTE—Follow your doctor's instructions. These instructions are supplemental.

GENERAL MEASURES
- Isolate the ill person, if possible.
- Use a heating pad or hot-water bottle to relieve abdominal cramps.
- If diarrhea is severe, use a bedside commode.

MEDICATION—Medicine is usually not necessary for mild cases. Antidiarrhea medications may retard recovery. For severe cases, your doctor may prescribe antidiarrhea medication, antibiotics to fight infection and intravenous fluids for severe dehydration.

ACTIVITY—Stay in bed, except for trips to the bathroom, until at least 3 days after diarrhea, fever and other symptoms disappear. Then resume normal activities gradually. Flex the legs regularly in bed to prevent formation of blood clots.

DIET—Drink clear liquids until diarrhea stops. Then eat a high-calorie, well-balanced diet. Vitamin and mineral supplements may be helpful after prolonged illness.

CALL YOUR DOCTOR IF

- An infant has symptoms of a salmonella infection and shows signs of dehydration, such as dry, wrinkled skin, decreased urination or dark urine.
- You have symptoms of a salmonella infection that persist longer than 48 hours.
- The following occurs during the illness:
  Fever of 102F (38.9C) or higher.
  Jaundice.
  Cough with blood.
  Worsening diarrhea.

SCABIES

GENERAL INFORMATION

DEFINITION—A disease of the skin caused by a mite (the "itch" mite) with a characteristic pattern of distribution. Scabies is contagious from person to person (by shared clothing or bed linen) and from one site to another in the same person.

BODY PARTS INVOLVED—Skin of the finger webs, and folds under the arms, breasts, elbows, genitals and buttocks.

SEX OR AGE MOST AFFECTED—Both sexes; all ages.

SIGNS & SYMPTOMS
- Small, itchy blisters in several parts of the body. The blisters break easily when scratched.
- Broken blisters leave scratch marks and thickened skin, crisscrossed by grooves and scaling.

CAUSES—A mite that burrows into deep skin layers, where the female mite deposits eggs. Eggs mature into adult mites in 3 weeks. Mites are 0.1mm in diameter and can only be seen under a microscope. Scratching collects mites and eggs under the fingernails, so they spread to other parts of the body.

RISK INCREASES WITH—Crowded or unsanitary living conditions.

HOW TO PREVENT
- Avoid contact with persons or linen and clothing that you suspect may be infected with scabies.
- Maintain personal cleanliness:
  Bathe daily, or at least 2 to 3 times a week.
  Wash hands before eating.
  Launder clothes often.

WHAT TO EXPECT

APPROPRIATE HEALTH CARE
- Self-care after diagnosis.
- Doctor's treatment.

DIAGNOSTIC MEASURES
- Your own observation of symptoms.
- Medical history and physical exam by a doctor. The diagnosis is confirmed by discovering the mite, lifting it from its burrow and identifying it under a microscope.

POSSIBLE COMPLICATIONS—Secondary bacterial infection of mite-infested areas of inflammation.

PROBABLE OUTCOME—Itching usually disappears quickly, and evidence of the disease is gone in 1 to 2 weeks with treatment.

In 20% of cases, re-treatment is necessary in 20 days. If skin irritation persists longer than this, oral antihistamines or topical steroids may be necessary to break the itch-scratch cycle.

Scabies may last for years if left untreated. This accounts for the term, "seven-year itch."

HOW TO TREAT

NOTE—Follow your doctor's instructions. These instructions are supplemental.

MEDICATION—Your doctor may prescribe a pediculicide, such as gamma benzene hexachloride or crotamiton cream.

Infants and pregnant women may need a pediculicide that is less toxic, such as a 6% solution of sulfur.

GENERAL MEASURES
- Bathe thoroughly before applying the prescribed medicine.
- Apply from the neck down, and cover the entire body.
- Wait 15 minutes before dressing.
- Carefully wash all clothes and toys used prior to or during treatment. You don't need to clean furniture or floors with special care.
- Leave medicine on the skin for 2 hours before bathing.
- You may need to repeat in 1 week. Ask your doctor.

ACTIVITY—No restrictions.

DIET—No special diet.

CALL YOUR DOCTOR IF

- You have symptoms of scabies.
- After treatment, the lesions show signs of infection (redness, pus, swelling or pain).
- New, unexplained symptoms develop. Drugs used in treatment may produce side effects.

SCARLET FEVER

GENERAL INFORMATION

DEFINITION—A childhood disorder characterized by a bright red rash. Scarlet fever is preceded by a streptococcal throat infection. Both are very contagious.

BODY PARTS INVOLVED—Throat; tonsils; skin.

SEX OR AGE MOST AFFECTED—Children and adolescents, especially between ages 2 and 10.

SIGNS & SYMPTOMS—Symptoms may vary from person to person. Following is the usual course of the disease:
- Day 1—Fever as high as 104F (40C); a red sore throat; swollen tonsils (tonsils may have a whitish coating); enlarged lymph glands in the neck; cough; vomiting.
- Day 2—Bright red rash on the face, except around the mouth.
- Day 3—Reddened tongue and rash in body creases, spreading to the neck, chest, back, then the entire body. The rash resembles a sunburn with bumps.
- Day 6—Faded rash and skin that begins peeling, continuing for 10 to 14 days.

CAUSES—Strep infection caused by a specific type of strep germ that manufactures a scarlet-fever toxin (poison). All strep infections don't cause scarlet fever, because everyone is not susceptible to the rash-producing toxin. In one family, one child may contract scarlet fever, another may have a strep throat only, and a third may carry the germ and transmit it to others without being sick.

RISK INCREASES WITH
- Family history of recurrent strep infections.
- Recent impetigo.
- Crowded or unsanitary living conditions.
- Exposure to others in public places.

HOW TO PREVENT—Cannot be prevented completely, because some healthy persons are carriers of the strep germ without being ill. However, partial preventive measures include:
- Antibiotic treatment for at least 10 days for any strep infection.
- Avoidance of persons with sore throats.

WHAT TO EXPECT

APPROPRIATE HEALTH CARE
- Home care after diagnosis.
- Doctor's treatment.

DIAGNOSTIC MEASURES
- Your own observation of symptoms.
- Medical history and physical exam by a doctor.
- Laboratory throat culture.

POSSIBLE COMPLICATIONS—Without treatment:
- Rheumatic fever.
- Impaired hearing.
- Glomerulonephritis.
- Meningitis.
- Pneumonia.
- Encephalitis.

PROBABLE OUTCOME—Usually curable in 10 days or more with treatment. Scarlet fever is not as prevalent as it once was, and it is rarely fatal. With antibiotic treatment, the severity and likelihood of complications decrease.

HOW TO TREAT

NOTE—Follow your doctor's instructions. These instructions are supplemental.

GENERAL MEASURES
- Prepare a soothing tea gargle for adults or children old enough to gargle. Double the usual strength of tea. This may be gargled warm or cold as often as is soothing.
- Use a cool-mist humidifier to relieve the dry, tight feeling in the throat.
- Use moist, warm soaks (see Appendix 18) to relieve tender, enlarged glands in the neck.
- Isolate the ill person from other people, including family members.

MEDICATION—Your doctor may prescribe penicillin to shorten the course of scarlet fever and prevent complications. If the patient is allergic to penicillin, other antibiotics, such as erythromycin, are also effective.

ACTIVITY—Bed rest is necessary until all signs of illness have disappeared. The patient may read or watch TV.

DIET—No special diet.

CALL YOUR DOCTOR IF

- You or your child have symptoms of strep throat or scarlet fever.
- The following occurs during treatment: Temperature becomes normal for 2 days, then rises over 101F (38.3C).
  New symptoms begin, such as: nausea; vomiting; earache; cough; headache; thick, colored, nasal drainage; chest pain; or labored breathing.

SCLERITIS

GENERAL INFORMATION

DEFINITION—Deep, localized inflammation of the sclera, the outermost white layer of tissue covering the eyeball. Scleritis is not contagious.

BODY PARTS INVOLVED—Sclera, which includes the conjunctiva and cornea. Scleritis may affect one or both eyes.

SEX OR AGE MOST AFFECTED—All ages, but most common in adults from ages 30 to 60.

SIGNS & SYMPTOMS
- Eye pain (usually dull).
- Purple-red, inflamed areas in one or more areas of the white of the eye.
- Partial vision loss (sometimes).

CAUSES—Unknown, but scleritis frequently occurs with rheumatoid arthritis, Crohn's disease and other connective-tissue disorders. It is probably an autoimmune disorder.

RISK INCREASES WITH
- Rheumatoid arthritis.
- Crohn's disease (regional ileitis).
- Chronic gastrointestinal disorder.

HOW TO PREVENT—No specific preventive measures.

WHAT TO EXPECT

APPROPRIATE HEALTH CARE
- Self-care after diagnosis.
- Doctor's treatment.
- Surgery to close a perforation, if perforation occurs as a complication.

DIAGNOSTIC MEASURES
- Your own observation of symptoms.
- Medical history and physical exam by a doctor.

POSSIBLE COMPLICATIONS—Rupture of the scleral tissue, perforating the eyeball and causing loss of the eye. The eye can sometimes be saved with surgery after perforation.

PROBABLE OUTCOME—Usually curable with treatment. If partial vision loss occurs, it is usually permanent.

HOW TO TREAT

NOTE—Follow your doctor's instructions. These instructions are supplemental.

GENERAL MEASURES—Use warm-water soaks (see Appendix 18) to relieve pain.

MEDICATION
- Your doctor may prescribe immunosuppressive drugs, oral cortisone drugs or cortisone eye drops to reduce inflammation.
- For minor pain, you may use non-prescription drugs, such as acetaminophen.

ACTIVITY—Reduce normal activity until inflammation subsides.

DIET—No special diet.

CALL YOUR DOCTOR IF

- You have symptoms of scleritis.
- The following occurs during treatment:
  Symptoms don't improve in 48 hours.
  Temperature rises to 100F (37.8C) or higher.
  Pain becomes worse.
  Vision is affected.

ILLNESSES & DISORDERS

SCLERODERMA
(Progressive System Sclerosis)

GENERAL INFORMATION

DEFINITION—A widespread connective tissue disease in which the skin and other body parts gradually degenerate, thicken and become stiff.

BODY PARTS INVOLVED—Skin; joints; digestive system, especially the esophagus; heart; kidneys; lungs; blood vessels; fingers; toes.

SEX OR AGE MOST AFFECTED—Adults of both sexes, but more common in women between ages 30 and 50.

SIGNS & SYMPTOMS
- Fingers—hardening and thickening of the skin, stiffness, poor circulation, numbness and fingertip ulceration.
- Digestive system—swallowing difficulty, poor food absorption, bloating after eating, weight loss, heartburn and a feeling that food sticks in the chest.
- Skin—hardening and thickening, especially in the face, which becomes tight and loses its elasticity.
- Muscle aches.
- Weakness and fatigue.
- Joint pain, stiffness and swelling.
- Anemia.

CAUSES—Unknown, but may be an autoimmune disorder. The connective tissue (the framework for all body tissues and blood vessels) thickens, becoming stiff and inflexible.

RISK INCREASES WITH—Unknown.

HOW TO PREVENT—Cannot be prevented at present.

WHAT TO EXPECT

APPROPRIATE HEALTH CARE
- Self-care during treatment.
- Doctor's treatment.
- Psychotherapy or counseling to adjust to living with an incurable disease.
- Hospitalization for heart, lung or kidney complications.

DIAGNOSTIC MEASURES
- Your own observation of symptoms.
- Medical history and physical exam by a doctor.
- Laboratory blood tests to detect anemia and measure antibodies.
- Urinalysis to detect red cells in the urine.
- EKG (see Glossary).
- X-rays of the hands, esophagus and chest.

POSSIBLE COMPLICATIONS
- Poor wound healing and gangrene.
- Bleeding tendencies.
- Heart-rhythm disturbances.
- Congestive heart failure.
- Kidney failure.
- High blood pressure.
- Lung destruction.

PROBABLE OUTCOME—This condition is currently considered incurable, but symptoms can be controlled for a while with treatment. With treatment, most patients live at least 5 years.

HOW TO TREAT

NOTE—Follow your doctor's instructions. These instructions are supplemental.

GENERAL MEASURES
- Because of poor circulation, wear warm clothing—especially socks and gloves. Avoid exposure to extreme cold.
- Protect yourself from burns and cuts.
- Sleep on 2 or 3 pillows, or raise the head of your bed 5 to 8 inches to prevent stomach acid from rolling back into the esophagus.
- Learn biofeedback techniques to increase circulation to the extremities.

MEDICATION
- You may take non-prescription antacids to relieve heartburn or indigestion, and aspirin or ibuprofen to relieve muscle aches and joint pain.
- Use skin lotions, lubricants and bath oil to soften skin.
- Your doctor may prescribe cortisone drugs to relieve inflammatory symptoms and antibiotics to fight infections.

ACTIVITY—Be as active as your strength permits. Poor circulation in the legs may restrict exercise.

DIET—Eat frequent, small meals to minimize bloating, heartburn and gastrointestinal discomfort. Use additional fluids to help with swallowing. A dietitian can help plan a nutritious diet. Consult your doctor about taking vitamin and mineral supplements.

CALL YOUR DOCTOR IF

- You have symptoms of scleroderma.
- The following occurs during treatment:
  Unexplained bruising or bleeding under the skin.
  Slow healing of a wound.
  Fever.
  General ill felling.

SCOLIOSIS
(Curvature of the Spine)

GENERAL INFORMATION

DEFINITION—A painless, progressive bending and twisting of the upper spinal column, which eventually distorts the chest and back.

BODY PARTS INVOLVED—Spinal vertebrae (bones).

SEX OR AGE MOST AFFECTED
- Adolescents between ages 12 and 15.
- Both sexes, but more common in girls.

SIGNS & SYMPTOMS
- Early stages: No obvious symptoms or signs, but scoliosis can be detected by your doctor or school nurse with a simple screening test.
- Later stages: Visible curving of the upper body. The spine becomes S-shaped and shoulders become uneven.

CAUSES—Usually unknown. Scoliosis is sometimes a result of:
- Diseases of the central nervous system, such as polio or muscular dystrophy.
- Congenital defects of the spine.

RISK INCREASES WITH—Family history of scoliosis.

HOW TO PREVENT—Cannot be prevented at present.

WHAT TO EXPECT

APPROPRIATE HEALTH CARE
- Doctor's treatment.
- Exercises to strengthen back muscles.
- Orthopedic back brace.
- Surgery to correct the deformity (severe cases only).

DIAGNOSTIC MEASURES
- Your own observation of symptoms.
- Medical history and physical exam by a doctor.

POSSIBLE COMPLICATIONS
- Severe distortion of the spine and ribs.
- Breathing difficulty.
- Lung infection.
- Congestive heart failure.

PROBABLE OUTCOME—When diagnosed early, scoliosis can usually be corrected completely. A back brace is usually worn daily for several years.

HOW TO TREAT

NOTE—Follow your doctor's instructions. These instructions are supplemental.

GENERAL MEASURES—A teenager may be embarrassed to wear a brace. Be sure your teenager understands that the brace is temporary. Explain the eventual consequences of not wearing the brace. Insist on keeping doctor appointments for follow-up evaluation.

MEDICATION—Medicine usually is not necessary for this disorder. For minor discomfort from muscle imbalance or complications, you may use non-prescription drugs, such as aspirin or acetaminophen.

ACTIVITY—Consult your doctor. Special exercises may be part of therapy. If a brace is necessary, sports participation will be restricted.

DIET—No special diet.

CALL YOUR DOCTOR IF

You suspect your child is developing scoliosis.

SEBACEOUS CYST
(Epidermoid Cyst; Wens)

 GENERAL INFORMATION

DEFINITION—A dome-shaped cyst filled with semisolid material (keratin, the same material that forms skin, hair and nails). The name *sebaceous cyst* is in error, because a real sebaceous cyst would be filled with material called sebum and manufactured in hair follicles.

BODY PARTS INVOLVED—Skin of the trunk, face, neck and scalp.

SEX OR AGE MOST AFFECTED—All ages, but most common in adolescents and adults.

SIGNS & SYMPTOMS—A cyst with the following characteristics:
- The cyst has sloped shoulders or a dome-shaped, nodular appearance and a smooth surface.
- The cyst is whitish or skin-colored.
- Cysts range from 1cm to 4cm in diameter.
- If the cyst becomes injured or infected, it may become bright red and painful.

CAUSES—Sebaceous cysts are caused by plugged ducts in malformed hair follicles. They may enlarge from hormonal stimulation or injury.

RISK INCREASES WITH
- Skin injury.
- Hormonal stimulation at puberty.

HOW TO PREVENT—Cannot be prevented at present.

 WHAT TO EXPECT

APPROPRIATE HEALTH CARE
- Self-care.
- Doctor's treatment.
- Surgery to remove the cyst (sometimes).
  Small cysts can be removed through a simple incision, but rupture of the cyst—and corresponding incomplete removal—frequently results in recurrence.
  Large cysts do better if incised and drained in an initial procedure, with removal of the complete cyst at another time.

DIAGNOSTIC MEASURES
- Your own observation of symptoms.
- Medical history and physical exam by a doctor.

POSSIBLE COMPLICATIONS
- Infection of a cyst.
- Injury to a cyst, causing rupture or inflammation.

PROBABLE OUTCOME—Cysts which cause no symptoms require no medical treatment. Those that are unsightly or are repeatedly injured can be removed.
  Infected cysts may require incision, drainage and packing with gauze.

 HOW TO TREAT

NOTE—Follow your doctor's instructions. These instructions are supplemental.

GENERAL MEASURES—Before surgery, apply warm compresses to the cyst to reduce inflammation and size.

MEDICATION—Medicine usually is not necessary for this disorder. If a cyst becomes infected, your doctor may prescribe antibiotics.

ACTIVITY—Resume your normal activities as soon as symptoms improve.

DIET—No special diet.

 CALL YOUR DOCTOR IF

- After removal, signs of infection (pain, redness, warmth and increased tenderness) occur at the surgical site.
- Fever of 101F (38.3C) or higher develops.
- The treated area does not appear to be healing well within 1 week.
- You are taking antibiotics, and new, unexplained symptoms develop. Antibiotics may produce side effects.

SEXUAL DYSFUNCTION, FEMALE

GENERAL INFORMATION

DEFINITION—Difficulty in becoming sexually aroused or achieving orgasm in a woman.

BODY PARTS INVOLVED—Brain and central nervous system; autonomic nervous system.

SEX OR AGE MOST AFFECTED—Sexually active women.

SIGNS & SYMPTOMS
- Lack of sexual desire.
- Inability to enjoy sex.
- Failure to achieve orgasm, even when sexually aroused.

CAUSES
- Inadequate foreplay.
- Anxiety, preoccupation and worry about other important areas of life.
- Psychological problems, including depression and poor self-esteem.
- Feelings of shame or guilt about sex.
- Fear of pregnancy.
- Exhaustion.
- Acute illness.
- Chronic illness, especially of the central nervous system or endocrine system, as with multiple sclerosis or hypothyroidism.
- Inexperience or inadequate information about sexuality on the part of either partner.
- Repressed anger toward the sexual partner that may result from: feelings of being used as a sexual object; physical or emotional abuse; jealousy or fears of disloyalty; or lack of true intimacy.

RISK INCREASES WITH
- Previous sexual abuse or sexual trauma.
- Use of some drugs, such as:
  Female hormones, including oral contraceptives (although these heighten sexual pleasure in some women).
  Antihypertensives.
  Antihistamines.
  Beta-adrenergic blockers.
  Calcium-channel blockers.
- Withdrawal from long-term use of mind-altering drugs, including narcotics, psychedelics, hallucinogens, marijuana, sedatives, hypnotics or cocaine.

HOW TO PREVENT
- Talk with your partner about your sexual needs and feelings.
- Seek counseling to resolve feelings about past sexual trauma or abuse.

WHAT TO EXPECT

APPROPRIATE HEALTH CARE
- Self-care after diagnosis.
- Doctor's treatment.
- Counseling with a professional trained in sex therapy.

DIAGNOSTIC MEASURES
- Your own observation of symptoms.
- Medical history and physical exam by a doctor.

POSSIBLE COMPLICATIONS
- Permanent inability to enjoy sex.
- Damage to interpersonal relationships.

PROBABLE OUTCOME—With open communication between partners and professional counseling, when necessary, most sexual problems can be resolved.

HOW TO TREAT

NOTE—Follow your doctor's instructions. These instructions are supplemental.

GENERAL MEASURES
- Admit the problem and try to establish open communication with your partner. Pretending that you are aroused or have orgasms leaves the problem unsolved.
- See Appendix 13 for recommendations to reduce stress in your life.

MEDICATION—Medication is not necessary unless the sexual problem is due to some underlying medical condition. There is no known aphrodisiac that is effective and safe.

ACTIVITY—No restrictions. Exercise regularly (see Appendix 20) to reduce stress and improve your self-image. A healthy body and mind make enjoyable sex more likely.

DIET—Eat a well-balanced diet. Vitamin and mineral supplements may be helpful. Consult your doctor.

CALL YOUR DOCTOR IF

You have sexual problems and you want help in resolving them.

ILLNESSES & DISORDERS

SHINGLES
(Herpes Zoster; Zona;
Acute Posterior Ganglionitis)

 GENERAL INFORMATION

DEFINITION—A viral infection of the central nervous system. Shingles is contagious to persons who have not had chickenpox.

BODY PARTS INVOLVED—Sensory nerves of the skin on one side of the body only.

SEX OR AGE MOST AFFECTED—All ages, but most common in adults over age 50.

SIGNS & SYMPTOMS
- Mild chills and fever.
- General ill feeling.
- Mild nausea, abdominal cramps or diarrhea.
- Painful red blisters anywhere on the body. Blisters appear 4 to 5 days after early symptoms begin. The blisters appear on a broad streak of reddened skin along sensory-nerve routes to a particular area of skin. They occur most often on the chest, and spread only on one side of the body.
- Chest pain, face pain, or burning pain in the skin of the abdomen, depending on the affected area.

CAUSES—Shingles is caused by the varicella-zoster virus, the same virus that causes chickenpox. It may lie dormant in the spinal cord until triggered by risk factors.

RISK INCREASES WITH
- Adults over 60.
- Stress.
- Hodgkin's disease.
- Illness that has lowered resistance.
- Use of immunosuppressive or anticancer drugs.

HOW TO PREVENT—Cannot be prevented at present.

 WHAT TO EXPECT

APPROPRIATE HEALTH CARE
- Self-care after diagnosis.
- Doctor's treatment.

DIAGNOSTIC MEASURES
- Your own observation of symptoms.
- Medical history and physical exam by a doctor.

POSSIBLE COMPLICATIONS
- Secondary infection in the shingles blisters.
- Chronic pain—especially in the elderly—that persists for months or years in the sensory nerves where the blisters have been.

PROBABLE OUTCOME—Most patients recover spontaneously without lasting complications, except for mild scarring. One attack usually provides immunity against shingles, but a few persons have had more than one attack.

 HOW TO TREAT

NOTE—Follow your doctor's instructions. These instructions are supplemental.

GENERAL MEASURES
- Avoid chilling drafts.
- When bathing, wash blisters gently.
- Don't bandage the sores.
- Apply heat or moist compresses if this decreases the pain.

MEDICATION
- For minor discomfort, you may use non-prescription drugs such as acetaminophen.
- Your doctor may prescribe:
  Pain relievers.
  Tranquilizers for a short time.
  Cortisone drugs to relieve pain in severe cases.
  Antiviral drugs. These may be useful, but they are still experimental.

ACTIVITY—No restrictions.

DIET—No special diet.

 CALL YOUR DOCTOR IF

- You have symptoms of shingles.
- Pain is intolerable, despite treatment.
- New, unexplained symptoms develop. Drugs used in treatment may produce side effects.

SHOCK

GENERAL INFORMATION

DEFINITION—Low blood pressure that is extensive enough so the body cannot maintain normal functions. Shock does not include a person's reaction to emotional trauma.

BODY PARTS INVOLVED—Heart; blood vessels; blood.

SEX OR AGE MOST AFFECTED—Both sexes; all ages.

SIGNS & SYMPTOMS
- Cold hands and feet.
- Fast, weak pulse.
- Disorientation or confusion.
- Anxiety with feelings of impending doom.
- Skin that is pale, moist and sweaty.
- Shortness of breath and rapid breathing.
- Lack of urination.
- Low blood pressure. This may be so low that it cannot be measured by usual means.

CAUSES
- Sudden loss of blood from injury or disorders, such as bleeding peptic ulcer, ruptured aneurysm or ruptured ectopic pregnancy.
- Fluid loss, such as occurs with severe burns, fluid and electrolyte imbalance, or peritonitis.
- Impaired heart-pumping function from heart attack, heart-rhythm irregularities, pericarditis or pulmonary embolism.
- Blood poisoning, which causes blood vessels to greatly expand, such as occurs with toxic shock syndrome or major infections.
- Some endocrine diseases, such as Addison's disease or diabetes mellitus.

RISK INCREASES WITH
- Recent serious injury.
- Recent surgery.
- Infection.
- Childbirth.
- Anemia.
- Cancer.
- Use of drugs that cause anaphylactic (allergic) shock as an adverse reaction, such as penicillin, local anesthetics and many others.
- Overdose of mind-altering drugs.
- Excess alcohol consumption.

HOW TO PREVENT—Avoid causes and risk factors when possible.

WHAT TO EXPECT

APPROPRIATE HEALTH CARE
- Doctor's treatment.
- Surgery to stop hemorrhaging.

- Hospitalization for intravenous fluids and medications to raise blood pressure and treat the underlying cause.

DIAGNOSTIC MEASURES
- Medical history and physical exam by a doctor.
- Laboratory blood studies to measure the amount of blood in circulation and to measure fluids and electrolytes.

POSSIBLE COMPLICATIONS
- Cardiac arrest.
- Permanent brain damage.

PROBABLE OUTCOME—Usually curable with early diagnosis and treatment. Without treatment, shock can be fatal.

HOW TO TREAT

NOTE—Follow your doctor's instructions. These instructions are supplemental.

GENERAL MEASURES—If you observe signs of shock in someone, do the following until medical help arrives:
- Stop external bleeding by applying pressure.
- Keep the victim lying down with legs elevated. Cover the victim for warmth.
- Make sure the victim's airway is open to allow breathing. If breathing stops, give mouth-to-mouth resuscitation. If breathing *and* pulse stop, give cardiopulmonary resuscitation.

MEDICATION—Depends on the underlying disorder:
- If shock is from blood or fluid loss, treatment includes blood transfusion or intravenous fluids.
- If blood pressure is at a life-threatening low level, hypertensive drugs to raise blood pressure may be given.
- If infection is present, antibiotics will be used.

ACTIVITY—Rest in bed until completely recovered. Move legs actively while in bed to decrease the likelihood of deep-vein blood clots.

DIET—No special diet.

CALL YOUR DOCTOR IF

- You have symptoms of shock or observe them in someone else. Call immediately. This is a life-threatening emergency!
- New, unexplained symptoms develop. Drugs used in treatment may produce side effects.

SHOULDER, FROZEN
(Adhesive Capsulitis)

GENERAL INFORMATION

DEFINITION—Pain and stiffness in the shoulder joint that progresses to inability to use the shoulder. In this case, "frozen" does not relate to freezing temperatures.

BODY PARTS INVOLVED—Shoulder tendons, bursa, joint capsule, muscles, blood vessels and nerves.

SEX OR AGE MOST AFFECTED—All ages, but most common in athletic adolescents and young adults.

SIGNS & SYMPTOMS—Early stages:
- Pain in the shoulder, often slight, that progresses to severe pain that interferes with sleep and normal activities. Pain worsens with shoulder movement.
- Stiffness in the shoulder that prevents normal movement. Reduced movement increases stiffness.
Later stages:
- Pain in the arm or neck.
- Inability to move the shoulder.
- Intolerable shoulder pain.

CAUSES—Minor shoulder injury or inflammation, such as bursitis or tendinitis, that worsens from lack of use. Adhesions (constricting bands of tissue) form with disuse in 7 to 10 days. Adhesions increase disuse. After 3 weeks of disuse, adhesions grow so severe that the joint cannot move.

RISK INCREASES WITH
- Neglect of minor injuries, including bursitis or tendinitis.
- Poor nutrition, especially lack of adequate protein.
- Poor physical conditioning and occasional athletic activity.

HOW TO PREVENT—Obtain medical treatment for bursitis and tendinitis, including exercises to prevent formation of adhesions.

WHAT TO EXPECT

APPROPRIATE HEALTH CARE
- Self-care after diagnosis.
- Doctor's treatment, including manipulation of the shoulder to break up adhesions. This is done in a hospital or outpatient surgical facility under general anesthesia.
- Physical therapy and exercises.

DIAGNOSTIC MEASURES
- Your own observation of symptoms.
- Medical history and physical exam by a doctor.
- X-rays of the shoulder.

POSSIBLE COMPLICATIONS—Permanent shoulder disability and pain without treatment or with delayed treatment.

PROBABLE OUTCOME—Usually curable with treatment and rehabilitation.

HOW TO TREAT

NOTE—Follow your doctor's instructions. These instructions are supplemental.

GENERAL MEASURES—After treatment and rehabilitation begin, your doctor will prescribe ice treatment and exercises.

MEDICATION
- Your doctor may prescribe:
  Pain relievers.
  Non-steroidal anti-inflammatory drugs.
  Injections of cortisone and local anesthesia into joints to reduce pain and inflammation.
- For minor pain, you may use non-prescription drugs such as aspirin.

ACTIVITY—Resume your normal activities as soon as symptoms improve.

DIET—No special diet. Vitamins and mineral supplements don't help unless you can't eat a normal, well-balanced diet.

CALL YOUR DOCTOR IF

- You have symptoms of a frozen shoulder.
- You have persistent shoulder pain, indicating possible bursitis or tendinitis.
- New, unexplained symptoms develop. Drugs used in treatment may produce side effects.

SICKLE-CELL ANEMIA

GENERAL INFORMATION

DEFINITION—An inherited blood disorder that causes anemia, episodes of severe pain, low resistance to infection and chronic poor health. It is not cancerous.

BODY PARTS INVOLVED—Bone marrow; lymph glands; spleen; liver; thymus.

SEX OR AGE MOST AFFECTED—Usually begins around 6 months of age and lasts a lifetime.

SIGNS & SYMPTOMS
- Anemia with shortness of breath, rapid heartbeat, fatigue and jaundice.
- Episodes of pain in joints, chest, abdomen and back.
- Frequent infections, especially pneumonia.
- Nerve impairment.
- Delayed growth and development.
- Skin ulcers, especially on the legs.

CAUSES—This disease is hereditary. Persons with the gene may pass it on to their children. Red blood cells change from round to sickle shapes, which causes blockage in the capillaries. Low oxygen in the tissues is partly responsible for the changed shape. The change occurs in attacks that cause pain and disability. The disease occurs mostly in black people.

RISK INCREASES WITH—Family history of sickle-cell anemia. The following may aggravate symptoms:
- Ascending to high altitude, as in driving up a mountain or flying.
- Pregnancy.
- Surgery.
- Injury.

HOW TO PREVENT—If you have a family history of sickle-cell anemia, ask your doctor to test you. If the condition is present, obtain genetic counseling before starting a family. A less serious condition, sickle-cell trait, may be present. It will not cause the disease, but genetic counseling is still desirable.

WHAT TO EXPECT

APPROPRIATE HEALTH CARE
- Doctor's treatment. If a child has the condition, seek special treatment from a pediatrician with special knowledge of this condition.
- Psychotherapy or counseling may be helpful in adapting to this condition, especially for children.
- Hospitalization at times of severe attacks.

DIAGNOSTIC MEASURES
- Your own observation of symptoms.
- Medical history and physical exam by a doctor.
- Laboratory blood studies. Simple screening tests are also available. They may be done at birth if there is a family history of sickle-cell anemia.
- X-rays of bones and lungs.

POSSIBLE COMPLICATIONS
- Infections of lungs and bones.
- Kidney failure.
- Eye disease.
- Stroke.

PROBABLE OUTCOME—Sickle-cell anemia is incurable and life expectancy is reduced. A few patients reach adulthood. Most patients die prematurely of infection or stroke.

HOW TO TREAT

NOTE—Follow your doctor's instructions. These instructions are supplemental.

GENERAL MEASURES
- During an attack, stay warm. Apply warm compresses to painful areas.
- Maintain your immunization schedule, including a pneumonia vaccine.
- Don't fly, even in pressurized planes, without oxygen. Check with your airline.
- Wear a Medic-Alert bracelet or pendant (see Glossary).

MEDICATION—No medications are yet available to control this condition. For severe attacks, intravenous fluids, blood transfusions and pain relievers are helpful.

ACTIVITY—Avoid strenuous exercise and exposure to cold temperatures. Rest in bed during acute attacks.

DIET—Drink at least 8 glasses of water a day—more if you have a fever. This helps keep blood cells from collecting and blocking capillaries.

CALL YOUR DOCTOR IF

- Your child has signs and symptoms of sickle-cell anemia.
- You want to know if you have the sickle-cell gene.
- You have the disease, and symptoms recur after a period of remission or you develop fever or other signs of infection.

ILLNESSES & DISORDERS

SILICOSIS

GENERAL INFORMATION

DEFINITION—Inflammation of the lung due to breathing silica (quartz) dust. Silicosis may lead to lung cancer.

BODY PARTS INVOLVED—Lungs.

SEX OR AGE MOST AFFECTED—Men over age 40.

SIGNS & SYMPTOMS—Early symptoms:
- Shortness of breath.
- Cough that produces little or no sputum.
- General ill feeling.

Late symptoms:
- Fitful sleep.
- Appetite loss.
- Chest pain.
- Hoarseness.
- Coughing blood.
- Symptoms of heart failure.
- Bluish nails.

CAUSES—20 to 30 years of exposure to small particles of silica in work such as mining, granite-cutting, manufacturing pottery or metal-grinding.

RISK INCREASES WITH
- Poor nutrition.
- Smoking.
- Excess alcohol consumption.

HOW TO PREVENT
- During exposure to silica, wear a protective mask or external-air-supplied hood.
- Don't smoke.
- Participate in a regular physical exercise program to maintain good cardiopulmonary fitness.

WHAT TO EXPECT

APPROPRIATE HEALTH CARE
- Self-care after diagnosis.
- Doctor's treatment.

DIAGNOSTIC MEASURES
- Your own observation of symptoms.
- Medical history and physical exam by a doctor.
- X-ray of the chest.

POSSIBLE COMPLICATIONS
- Tuberculosis (late stages of silicosis).
- Heart failure due to lung disease.
- Lung collapse.
- Pleurisy.
- Lung cancer.

PROBABLE OUTCOME—This condition is currently considered incurable. Life expectancy is reduced, and it causes increasing respiratory disability. However, symptoms can be relieved or controlled. Scientific research into causes and treatment continues, so there is hope for increasingly effective treatment and cure.

HOW TO TREAT

NOTE—Follow your doctor's instructions. These instructions are supplemental.

GENERAL MEASURES—The following measures may relieve symptoms and protect against recurrent lung infections:
- Obtain medical treatment for any respiratory infection, including the common cold.
- Consider moving to a warm, dry climate if you have advanced disease.
- Practice bronchial drainage. Your physician will provide instructions.
- Use a cool-mist humidifier to loosen bronchial secretions so they may be coughed up easily.

MEDICATION
- Your doctor may prescribe:
  Antibiotics for infections.
  Bronchodilators (inhaled or oral) with inhalation therapy (supervised at first by an inhalation therapist) to open bronchial tubes to the maximum.
- For minor discomfort, you may use non-prescription drugs, such as acetaminophen or aspirin.

ACTIVITY
- Rest in bed with infections. You may read or watch TV.
- After treatment, resume normal activity as soon as symptoms improve.

DIET—No special diet.

CALL YOUR DOCTOR IF

- You have symptoms of silicosis.
- The following occurs during treatment:
  Temperature spike of 101F (38.3C) or more.
  Increased chest pain or breathlessness.
  Blood in the sputum.
  Continuing weight loss.
  Confusion or lethargy.
- New, unexplained symptoms develop. Drugs used in treatment may produce side effects.

SINUS INFECTION
(Sinusitis)

 GENERAL INFORMATION

DEFINITION—Inflammation of the sinuses adjacent to the nose. Germs that cause sinusitis are contagious.

BODY PARTS INVOLVED—Sinuses.

SEX OR AGE MOST AFFECTED—Both sexes; all ages.

SIGNS & SYMPTOMS—Early stages:
- Nasal congestion with green-yellow (sometimes blood-tinged) discharge.
- Feeling of pressure inside the head.
- Eye pain.
- Headache that is worse in the morning or when bending forward.
- Cheek pain that may resemble a toothache.
- Post-nasal drip.
- Cough (sometimes) that is usually non-productive.
- Disturbed sleep (sometimes).
- Fever (sometimes).
Late stages:
- Complete blockage of the sinus openings, blocking the discharge and increasing pain.

CAUSES
- Infection (usually initiated by a cold or other upper-respiratory infection). The infection may be complicated by a bacterial invasion of organisms that normally inhabit the nose and throat.
- Irritation of the nasal passages from: allergies; smoking; harsh sneezes with the mouth closed; chilling; swimming, especially jumping into the water without holding the nose; and fatigue.

RISK INCREASES WITH
- Illness that has lowered resistance.
- Smoking.
- Exposure to cold, damp weather outdoors and dry heat indoors.
- Exposure to others in public places.
- Excessive nose-blowing during an upper-respiratory infection.

HOW TO PREVENT
- Keep the humidity level at 45% to 50% in heated buildings during the winter.
- Don't stifle sneezes.

 WHAT TO EXPECT

APPROPRIATE HEALTH CARE
- Self-care.
- Doctor's treatment.
- Surgery to drain blocked sinuses (rare).

DIAGNOSTIC MEASURES
- Your own observation of symptoms.
- Medical history and physical exam by a doctor.
- X-rays of the sinuses.

POSSIBLE COMPLICATIONS—Meningitis or brain abscess (rare).

PROBABLE OUTCOME—Usually curable with intense treatment. Recurrence is common.

 HOW TO TREAT

NOTE—Follow your doctor's instructions. These instructions are supplemental.

MEDICATION
- Your doctor may prescribe:
  Nasal sprays, nose drops or decongestant medicine to reduce congestion. Antibiotics to fight infection.
- For minor pain, you may use non-prescription drugs such as acetaminophen.

GENERAL MEASURES
- Use a cool-mist humidifier to help thin secretions so they will drain more easily.
- For infants and young children who cannot blow the nose, use a nasal aspirator to suction each nostril gently before applying nose drops. Suction again 10 minutes after using nose drops.
- Apply heat to relieve pain in the sinuses and nose. Use an electric heating pad or warm compresses.
- Don't allow other persons to use your nose drops. They will be contaminated by the infection. Discard them after treatment.
- Don't use nose drops after the prescribed time. They can interfere with normal nasal and sinus function and become addictive, causing a rebound phenomenon (see Glossary).

ACTIVITY—Resume your normal activities gradually.

DIET—No special diet, but drink extra fluids to help thin secretions.

 CALL YOUR DOCTOR IF

- You have symptoms of sinusitis.
- The following occurs during treatment:
  Fever of 101F (38.3C) or higher.
  Bleeding from the nose.
  Severe headache.
  Swelling of the face (forehead, eyes, side of the nose or cheek).
  Blurred vision.

SKIN CANCER, BASAL-CELL

GENERAL INFORMATION

DEFINITION—Skin cancer affecting skin's basal layer (the 5th layer). Basal-cell skin cancer invades areas under skin, but it does not spread to distant areas.

BODY PARTS INVOLVED—Skin of face, ears, backs of hands, shoulders and arms.

SEX OR AGE MOST AFFECTED
- Both sexes.
- Adults 40 and older.

SIGNS & SYMPTOMS—A small skin lesion that does not heal in 3 weeks with the following characteristics:
- The lesion appears flat and "pearly." Its edges are translucent and rounded or rolled. The edges may have small, curvy, new blood vessels. The ulcer in the center is dimpled. Lesion size varies from 4mm to 6mm, but it may grow larger if untreated.
- The lesion occurs on skin that is exposed to the sun and shows evidence of sun damage.
- The lesion grows slowly. It does not hurt or itch.

CAUSES—Skin damage from sun that occurs many years prior to the cancer's appearance.

RISK INCREASES WITH
- Adults over 60.
- Exposure to excess sunlight.
- Fair skin complexion.

HOW TO PREVENT—Limit exposure to sun. Protect skin from sun exposure with a hat, clothing and sunscreen.

WHAT TO EXPECT

APPROPRIATE HEALTH CARE
- Removal of cancer by one of the following methods. The treatment method is chosen in a doctor-patient conference:
  Surgery in the doctor's office or an out-patient surgical unit of the hospital.
  Electrosurgery (see Glossary).
  Cryosurgery (see Glossary).
  Radiation treatment.
- Self-care after removal.

DIAGNOSTIC MEASURES
- Your own observation of symptoms.
- Medical history and physical exam by a doctor.
- Pathological exam of tissue after removal to confirm diagnosis.

POSSIBLE COMPLICATIONS—Without treatment, cancers may enlarge, ulcerate and disfigure. Less than 1% spread to other sites, but they should be removed to prevent local damage.

PROBABLE OUTCOME—Curable in 2 weeks if cancer is removed. This does not become life-threatening unless it is ignored completely.

HOW TO TREAT

NOTE—Follow your doctor's instructions. These instructions are supplemental.

GENERAL MEASURES—After surgery:
- Apply rubbing alcohol to the scab twice a day.
- Apply an adhesive bandage to the scab during the day. Leave it uncovered at night.
- Wash the wound as usual. Dry gently and completely after bathing or swimming.

MEDICATION
- For minor pain, you may use non-prescription drugs, such as acetaminophen or aspirin.
- If the scab cracks or oozes, apply a non-prescription antibiotic ointment several times a day.
- Your doctor may prescribe an antibiotic ointment to prevent wound infection.

ACTIVITY—No restrictions.

DIET—No special diet.

CALL YOUR DOCTOR IF

- You have symptoms of basal-cell skin cancer.
- The wound bleeds after surgery, and the bleeding cannot be stopped by applying pressure for 10 minutes.
- The wound shows signs of infection, such as pain, redness, swelling or increased tenderness.

SKIN CANCER, SQUAMOUS-CELL

GENERAL INFORMATION

DEFINITION—A malignant growth of the epithelial layer (external surface) of the skin.

BODY PARTS INVOLVED—Skin in areas exposed to the sun, such as the face, ears, hands or arms.

SEX OR AGE MOST AFFECTED—Adults over 40.

SIGNS & SYMPTOMS—A small, disfiguring, scaling, raised bump on the skin with a crusting ulcer in the center. The bump doesn't hurt or itch.

CAUSES
- Excessive exposure to sunlight.
- Overexposure to X-rays.

RISK INCREASES WITH
- Adults over 60.
- Light complexion.
- Recent illness with chronic skin ulcers from any cause.
- Outdoor occupation.
- Occupation or treatment requiring exposure to X-rays.

HOW TO PREVENT—Wear sunscreen or hat and protective clothing to protect skin from sun damage.

WHAT TO EXPECT

APPROPRIATE HEALTH CARE
- Doctor's treatment.
- Treatment with any of the following methods:
  Surgical removal.
  Scraping and electrocautery (see Glossary).
  Radiation therapy.

DIAGNOSTIC MEASURES
- Your own observation of symptoms.
- Medical history and physical exam by a doctor.
- Biopsy (see Glossary).

POSSIBLE COMPLICATIONS
- Cancer must be treated again in 10% of cases.
- Cancer will spread to other tissue if untreated.

PROBABLE OUTCOME—This type of skin cancer responds well to treatment. It is usually curable in 2 weeks with treatment.

HOW TO TREAT

NOTE—Follow your doctor's instructions. These instructions are supplemental.

GENERAL MEASURES—After removal of the tumor, keep the area clean, dry and protected from clothing until healed. Your doctor will provide additional instructions, depending on the treatment used.

MEDICATION
- For minor discomfort, you may use non-prescription drugs such as acetaminophen.
- Your doctor may prescribe topical antibiotic ointment or cream to prevent infection after surgery.

ACTIVITY—After treatment, resume normal activity as soon as possible.

DIET—No special diet.

CALL YOUR DOCTOR IF

- You have symptoms of squamous-cell skin cancer.
- The following occurs after treatment:
  Redness, swelling, bleeding or tenderness at the treatment site.
  Pain that is not controlled by non-prescription pain relievers.
- The sore has not healed 3 weeks after treatment.

ILLNESSES & DISORDERS

SKIN LESIONS, BENIGN

 GENERAL INFORMATION

DEFINITION—Non-cancerous growths or areas of pigment or color change on the skin.

BODY PARTS INVOLVED—Skin.

SEX OR AGE MOST AFFECTED—Both sexes; all ages.

SIGNS & SYMPTOMS—Benign skin lesions fall into the following categories:
- Tags—Soft, flesh-colored buds, often on stalks, found on the neck, armpits or groin.
- Moles—Flat or raised lesions with clearly defined borders. Moles may be black, blue, red, yellow or brown.
- Cherry spots—Pinhead-sized, bright-red lesions on the chest or back.
- Strawberry marks—Bright-red raised areas in infants that grow until they are removed.
- Keloids—Thick, pale, irregular growths that begin at the site of a scar and gradually increase in size.
- Dermatofibromas—Rounded nodules, usually brownish and usually on the legs.
- Freckles—Flat, brownish spots of pinhead-size or larger.

CAUSES—Unknown, but most people have a few benign skin lesions.

RISK INCREASES WITH
- Family history of benign skin lesions.
- Pregnancy or use of oral contraceptives (brownish, frecklelike patches only).

HOW TO PREVENT—To decrease freckles, avoid excessive sun exposure. Other forms cannot be prevented.

 WHAT TO EXPECT

APPROPRIATE HEALTH CARE
- Self-care after diagnosis.
- Doctor's treatment.
- Surgery to remove lesions that enlarge, bleed, change color, are slow to heal or are unsightly.
- Radiation treatment following removal of keloids to prevent their recurrence.

DIAGNOSTIC MEASURES
- Your own observation of symptoms.
- Medical history and physical exam by a doctor.
- Skin biopsy (see Glossary).

POSSIBLE COMPLICATIONS
- Malignant change in moles.
- Bleeding in strawberry marks.

PROBABLE OUTCOME—Treatment is usually unnecessary because most skin lesions are harmless. Suspicious or unsightly lesions can be removed surgically. If the affected area is large or in a prominent place, plastic surgery may be necessary after removal.

 HOW TO TREAT

NOTE—Follow your doctor's instructions. These instructions are supplemental.

GENERAL MEASURES
- Examine skin lesions—especially those that are constantly rubbed or irritated by clothing—regularly for signs of growth, color change, pain, infection or bleeding.
- If a lesion is removed, cover the area with a clean dressing and protect against injury. Ointments are rarely needed.

MEDICATION—Medicine usually is not necessary for this disorder. Makeup may be helpful in covering unsightly blemishes.

ACTIVITY—No restrictions.

DIET—No special diet.

 CALL YOUR DOCTOR IF

You have a skin lesion that enlarges, bleeds, changes color, is painful or doesn't heal.

SLEEP APNEA IN ADULTS

GENERAL INFORMATION

DEFINITION—Temporary cessation of breathing while in deep sleep.

BODY PARTS INVOLVED—Central nervous system.

SEX OR AGE MOST AFFECTED—All ages, but most common in adults over 60.

SIGNS & SYMPTOMS
- Long periods (up to 1 or 2 minutes) of not breathing while asleep. Sleep apnea must be observed by others—it is most reliably recorded in a sleep laboratory.
- Choking while asleep caused by obstruction in the back of the throat from the uvula and other loose tissue. This causes cycles of sleep, choking, startled awakening, drowsiness and sleep. The cycles often continue throughout the day because poor sleep causes chronic sleepiness.

CAUSES
- Unknown (often).
- Airway obstruction, especially in obese patients.
- Chronic respiratory-system disease.
- Central-nervous-system disorder, such as a brain tumor, viral brain infection or stroke.

RISK INCREASES WITH
- Stress, including anxiety and depression.
- Recent stroke.
- Senility.
- Obesity.
- Smoking.
- Excess alcohol consumption.
- Use of mind-altering drugs.

HOW TO PREVENT—If you have an underlying disease listed as a cause of sleep apnea, avoid as many risk factors as possible to decrease the chance of triggering the disorder.

WHAT TO EXPECT

APPROPRIATE HEALTH CARE
- Doctor's treatment.
- Self-care after diagnosis.
- Surgery to perform a tracheostomy (sometimes).

DIAGNOSTIC MEASURES
- Observation of symptoms by someone close to you.
- Medical history and physical exam by a doctor.
- Laboratory studies to measure oxygen in blood, chest-wall movement and air flow through nose.
- EEG (see Glossary).
- Studies in a sleep laboratory.

POSSIBLE COMPLICATIONS
- Impaired productivity and depression caused by sleep deprivation.
- Permanent brain damage caused by recurrent episodes of inadequate oxygen to the brain.
- Heartbeat irregularities and congestive heart failure.

PROBABLE OUTCOME—If sleep laboratory studies reveal significant sleep disturbance, surgery (tracheostomy) is usually necessary to cure the sleep apnea—no matter what the underlying cause. No other effective treatment is currently available.

HOW TO TREAT

NOTE—Follow your doctor's instructions. These instructions are supplemental.

GENERAL MEASURES
- If sleep apnea occurs only when you sleep on your back, sew a ping-pong ball to the back of your pajamas. This forces you to sleep on your side.
- For a description of surgery and postoperative care, see Tracheostomy (in Surgery section).

MEDICATION—Medicine usually is not necessary for this disorder. Consult your doctor about withdrawing medications that may be causing sleep apnea.

ACTIVITY—No restrictions. Engage in regular physical exercise to become physically fit, but don't exercise vigorously before bedtime.

DIET—Lose weight if you are obese. A reducing diet appears in Appendix 10.

CALL YOUR DOCTOR IF

- You suspect you have sleep apnea.
- You observe signs of sleep apnea in another family member.

SLEEP APNEA IN INFANTS

 GENERAL INFORMATION

DEFINITION—Unexplained lapses in breathing during sleep, leading to lack of oxygen to the brain and heart with life-threatening heartbeat irregularity. This can cause sudden infant death syndrome (SIDS), a mysterious tragedy that kills apparently healthy infants.

BODY PARTS INVOLVED—Central nervous system.

SEX OR AGE MOST AFFECTED—Infants of both sexes.

SIGNS & SYMPTOMS—Episodes when breathing stops and skin color changes. Episodes may last several minutes. Breathing usually resumes spontaneously. Unless death occurs, these episodes are apparent only with careful observation by hospital nurses or parents during the first weeks after birth.

CAUSES—Unknown.

RISK INCREASES WITH
- Prematurity or low birth weight.
- Young mothers (under 20 years old). Older mothers (over age 35) do *not* have a higher incidence of infants with sleep apnea, as has been theorized.
- Lower socioeconomic groups.

HOW TO PREVENT—Special equipment (respiration monitor) is used continuously to monitor breathing in infants that experience sleep apnea or in those suspected of being at risk for SIDS.

 WHAT TO EXPECT

APPROPRIATE HEALTH CARE
- Home care that includes monitoring equipment and close, constant observation.
- Doctor's supervision.

DIAGNOSTIC MEASURES—None, except the observations of breathing lapses by persons caring for the infant.

POSSIBLE COMPLICATIONS—Sudden infant death syndrome. When this occurs, infants die in their sleep without signs of struggle or injury. Autopsies show no apparent cause of death. There are approximately 6,000 to 7,000 such deaths each year in the U.S. Autopsies must be performed on all SIDS victims.

PROBABLE OUTCOME—As long as SIDS can be averted, infants with sleep apnea grow and develop normally. Most children are considered out of danger and can be taken off the monitor between 6 months and 1 year of age.

 HOW TO TREAT

NOTE—Follow your doctor's instructions. These instructions are supplemental.

GENERAL MEASURES
- If your baby suffers from sleep apnea, obtain and use a respiration monitor. The manufacturer and your doctor or nurse will demonstrate and provide full instructions.
- If your baby has a monitor, obtain detailed cardiopulmonary resuscitation training (CPR). In many cases, CPR can revive an infant who has stopped breathing, and the child experiences no serious aftereffects.

MEDICATION—No medication is currently available to prevent sleep apnea in infants.

ACTIVITY—No restrictions.

DIET—No special diet. Bottle-feeding has *no* association with SIDS, as was once theorized.

 CALL YOUR DOCTOR IF

Your baby has lapses in breathing (apnea). Call immediately!

SMALL-INTESTINE TUMOR

GENERAL INFORMATION

DEFINITION—Abnormal new growth in the small intestine. Only 10% of small-intestine tumors are cancerous.

BODY PARTS INVOLVED—Small intestine.

SEX OR AGE MOST AFFECTED—All ages, but most likely in adults.

SIGNS & SYMPTOMS
- No symptoms (sometimes).
- Tiredness.
- Paleness.
- Blood in stools or black, tarry stools.
- Unexplained weight loss.

CAUSES—Unknown.

RISK INCREASES WITH
- Regional ileitis (Crohn's disease).
- Celiac disease.

HOW TO PREVENT—No specific preventive measures.

WHAT TO EXPECT

APPROPRIATE HEALTH CARE
- Doctor's treatment.
- Surgery to remove the tumor (sometimes).
- Radiation treatment (sometimes).
- Self-care after surgery or during treatment.

DIAGNOSTIC MEASURES
- Your own observation of symptoms.
- Medical history and physical exam by a doctor.
- Laboratory blood studies for anemia.
- X-rays of the intestinal tract (upper and lower GI series).

POSSIBLE COMPLICATIONS—Intestinal obstruction. Symptoms are: distended abdomen; severe colicky pain; nausea, vomiting; fever.

PROBABLE OUTCOME—Most tumors are removed surgically, regardless of whether they are malignant. With surgery or other treatment, the disorder is curable and a normal life span is expected.

HOW TO TREAT

NOTE—Follow your doctor's instructions. These instructions are supplemental.

GENERAL MEASURES—No specific instructions except those under other headings.

MEDICATION—Your doctor may prescribe:
- Anticancer drugs.
- Cortisone drugs to reduce bowel inflammation that may cause obstruction.

ACTIVITY—No restrictions. Resume normal activities as soon as possible after surgery.

DIET—Your doctor may prescribe a special diet following surgery or during treatment with radiation or anticancer drugs.

CALL YOUR DOCTOR IF

- You have symptoms of a tumor of the small intestine.
- You have symptoms of intestinal obstruction (see Possible Complications).
- New, unexplained symptoms develop during treatment. Drugs used in treatment may produce side effects.

SNAKEBITE

GENERAL INFORMATION

DEFINITION—Bite from a poisonous snake. Bites on the extremities are most common, but bites on the head and trunk are most dangerous.

BODY PARTS INVOLVED—Exposed skin; blood; lymphatic system.

SEX OR AGE MOST AFFECTED—Both sexes; all ages.

SIGNS & SYMPTOMS—Early symptoms:
- Severe pain and swelling around the bite.
Late symptoms:
- Fever.
- Skin discoloration that resembles bruising around the bite.
- Bleeding spots under the skin all over the body.
- Numbness and tingling around the mouth and in the hands and feet.
- Excessive sweating.
- Low blood pressure and shock.
- Breathing difficulty.
- Blurred vision.
- Headache.
- Seizures.
- Coma.
Signs:
- Multiple fang marks and small cuts, if the bite is from a coral snake. Symptoms may not appear for 3 to 4 hours.
- Deep single or double fang marks, if the bite is from another snake. Symptoms begin quickly.

CAUSES—Bite from a poisonous snake, including rattlesnake, copperhead, water moccasin or coral snake.

RISK INCREASES WITH—Outdoor activities during warm months in areas where poisonous snakes are abundant.

HOW TO PREVENT—Wear protective shoes, boots and clothing for hiking, camping, fishing and hunting. Prevent complications by carrying a snakebite kit and instructions.

WHAT TO EXPECT

APPROPRIATE HEALTH CARE
- Immediate self-care.
- Doctor's treatment as soon as possible.
- Surgery (sometimes) to remove injured or gangrenous tissue 2 to 3 days after bite.

DIAGNOSTIC MEASURES
- Your own observation of symptoms.
- Medical history and physical exam by a doctor.
- Laboratory blood studies.

POSSIBLE COMPLICATIONS
- Gangrene, requiring amputation of the affected part.
- DIC (disseminated intravascular coagulation).
- Severe immunological response, if the victim has had a previous venomous snakebite.

PROBABLE OUTCOME—Usually curable with rapid medical care. Severe bites involving a large amount of poisonous venom may be fatal—even with treatment. After one snakebite, succeeding snakebites may produce more severe reaction.

HOW TO TREAT

NOTE—Follow your doctor's instructions. These instructions are supplemental.

GENERAL MEASURES
- Don't panic! Venom will spread more quickly through the body if the victim runs or becomes excited.
- Before giving first aid, identify the snake.
- Don't pack the affected part in ice.
- If the bite is from a coral snake, elevate and immobilize the bitten part and go to the nearest emergency facility.
- If it is from another poisonous snake:
  Put a *light* tourniquet (constricting band of any sort) 3 or 4 inches above the bite, toward the body. Don't use a tourniquet if 30 minutes or more have passed since the bite.
  Wash the bite with soap and water.
  Immobilize the bitten area.
  Go to the nearest emergency facility.

MEDICATION—Your doctor may prescribe:
- Antivenin to neutralize snake poison.
- Tetanus booster injection.
- Antibiotics to prevent infection.
- Pain relievers. (Narcotics cannot be used for coral-snake bites. They may cause shock.)

ACTIVITY—Resume normal activities as soon as symptoms improve.

DIET—No special diet.

CALL YOUR DOCTOR IF

- You or someone you are with receives a snakebite.
- New, unexplained symptoms develop. Drugs used in treatment may produce side effects.

SODIUM IMBALANCE

GENERAL INFORMATION

DEFINITION—Above- or below-normal levels of sodium in the blood.

BODY PARTS INVOLVED—All body cells.

SEX OR AGE MOST AFFECTED—Both sexes; all ages.

SIGNS & SYMPTOMS
- Confusion.
- Restlessness and anxiety.
- Weakness.
- Muscle cramps (usually in the legs).
- Changes in pulse rate and blood pressure.
- Tissue swelling (edema).
- Stupor or coma.

Sodium imbalance may be part of a disease with other symptoms that predominate, such as fever, vomiting, diarrhea or excessive sweating.

CAUSES—Hyponatremia (below-normal sodium):
- Prolonged loss of body fluids from vomiting or diarrhea.
- Addison's disease.
- Congestive heart failure.
- Prolonged, excessive drinking of water. (This is usually a psychiatric condition.)
- Some cancers of the adrenal glands.
- Infections with high fever.

Hypernatremia (above-normal sodium):
- Inability to drink water, as with stroke or gastrointestinal diseases.
- Use of cortisone drugs.
- Excessive intake of salty food or liquid, as in near-drowning in salt water.

RISK INCREASES WITH
- Diabetes mellitus.
- Congestive heart failure.
- Use of diuretics.
- Kidney diseases. Healthy kidneys can usually control sodium levels.

HOW TO PREVENT—Because sodium disturbance is the result of underlying disease, obtain early medical treatment to prevent a sodium imbalance.

WHAT TO EXPECT

APPROPRIATE HEALTH CARE
- Self-care after diagnosis and treatment.
- Doctor's treatment.
- Hospitalization (sometimes).

DIAGNOSTIC MEASURES
- Your own observation of symptoms.
- Medical history and physical exam by a doctor.
- Laboratory blood and urine studies of sodium and other electrolytes.

POSSIBLE COMPLICATIONS—Shock and death.

PROBABLE OUTCOME—Usually can be corrected with intravenous fluids and treatment of the underlying disorder.

HOW TO TREAT

NOTE—Follow your doctor's instructions. These instructions are supplemental.

GENERAL MEASURES—If you have a disorder or take drugs that affect sodium balance, learn as much as possible about your drugs, your condition and how to prevent a sodium imbalance.

MEDICATION—Your doctor may prescribe:
- Intravenous sodium if sodium levels are low.
- Diuretics to decrease high sodium levels.
- Medications to correct underlying disorders.

ACTIVITY—Resume your normal activities after recovery.

DIET—No special diet for low sodium levels. Most persons with high sodium levels benefit from a low-salt diet (see Appendix 9). Low-salt diets contain enough sodium to prevent hyponatremia. However, sodium levels are not influenced by diet alone.

CALL YOUR DOCTOR IF

- You have symptoms of a sodium imbalance.
- You are having problems with a disorder that affects sodium levels.

ILLNESSES & DISORDERS

SORES, PRESSURE
(Bed Sores; Decubitus Ulcers)

 GENERAL INFORMATION

DEFINITION—Skin ulcerations, usually in an area of pressure over a bony prominence. Pressure sores are not contagious or cancerous.

BODY PARTS INVOLVED—Skin over pressure points in the lower back, buttocks, elbows, knees, shoulders, heels, ankles and other areas with bony prominences.

SEX OR AGE MOST AFFECTED—All ages, but most likely in the elderly.

SIGNS & SYMPTOMS—Spots of skin that are red and shiny. Spots progress to blisters, then ulcers, leading to a breakdown of tissue under the ulcer. Ulcers are usually painless.

CAUSES—Constant pressure on the skin, especially over bony areas. Pressure reduces the blood supply, causing death in the tissue layers. Pressure sores usually develop in persons who cannot move because of chronic illness or disability that confines them to bed.

RISK INCREASES WITH
- Adults over 60.
- Poor circulation.
- Decreased or absent sensation.
- Malnutrition.
- Obesity.
- Illness or accident requiring prolonged bed confinement, especially with unsanitary living conditions and wrinkled or wet bed linen.

HOW TO PREVENT—Provide good nursing care for the disabled, including the following:
- Frequent changes of position in bed.
- Protective, soft padding, such as gel flotation pads or sheepskin, over bony areas.
- A water mattress, egg-crate rubber mattress or alternating-pressure mattress.
- Dry, clean, smooth bed linen.
- Frequent inspection of skin areas at risk.

 WHAT TO EXPECT

APPROPRIATE HEALTH CARE
- Home care.
- Doctor's treatment.
- Surgery to remove dead tissue (sometimes).

DIAGNOSTIC MEASURES
- Your own observation of symptoms.
- Medical history and physical exam by a doctor.

POSSIBLE COMPLICATIONS
- Local or general infection.
- Infection of bone (osteomyelitis) adjacent to the ulcer.

PROBABLE OUTCOME—Usually curable with treatment. Sores may heal very slowly. Healing time varies with the site and size of the ulcer and the patient's general health.

 HOW TO TREAT

NOTE—Follow your doctor's instructions. These instructions are supplemental.

GENERAL MEASURES
- Provide good nursing care for the patient (see How to Prevent).
- Provide warm whirlpool treatments, if a pressure sore is on an arm, hand, foot or leg.
- Apply lotions or ointment if prescribed by your doctor. Apply a thin layer of the cream, ointment or lotion 3 or 4 times daily. A heavy layer wastes medicine and is no more beneficial than a thin layer. Rub in gently for several minutes until it disappears.

MEDICATION
- Your doctor may prescribe:
  Antibiotics to fight infection.
  Ointments, dressings and drying agents, such as zinc oxide, granulated sugar, povidone-iodine packs or 3% hydrogen peroxide.
- Avoid harsh soaps, tincture of benzoin or hexachlorophene.

ACTIVITY—The patient may resume normal activities as soon as symptoms improve.

DIET—Normal, well-balanced diet that includes extra protein. Vitamin and mineral supplements may be necessary.

 CALL YOUR DOCTOR IF

- You have symptoms of pressure sores or observe them in someone else.
- The following occurs during treatment:
  Skin inflammation or breakdown.
  Signs of infection, such as: pain, redness, tenderness, swelling or increased warmth of the affected area.
  Fever.

SPINAL-CORD TUMOR

GENERAL INFORMATION

DEFINITION—An abnormal growth that compresses the spinal cord or its nerve roots. The growth may be benign or malignant—but a non-malignant tumor may be as disabling as a malignant tumor unless treated appropriately.

BODY PARTS INVOLVED—Spinal cord; nerves below the level of the spinal-cord tumor.

SEX OR AGE MOST AFFECTED—All ages, but most common in adults.

SIGNS & SYMPTOMS
- Progressive weakness, numbness and wasting of muscles whose nerve supply comes from the affected area of the spinal cord.
- Difficult urination or bowel movements; incontinence.
- Chronic back pain.

CAUSES—Tumors originating in the spinal cord (primary tumors) are rare—especially in childhood or old age—and their cause is unknown.

A spinal-cord tumor usually results from cancer that has spread from another part of the body, such as: lung; breast; intestinal tract; prostate; kidney; thyroid; or lymphatic system.

RISK INCREASES WITH—Cancer in any of the body parts listed above.

HOW TO PREVENT
- Because spinal-cord tumors frequently result from the spread of cancer, be alert to early symptoms of cancer in other organs.
- Don't smoke.
- Eat a high-fiber diet to reduce the likelihood of intestinal cancer.
- Be alert to enlargement of the thyroid gland.
- For men over 45, request a prostate exam with your annual physical.
- For women, practice breast self-exam (see Appendix 14).

WHAT TO EXPECT

APPROPRIATE HEALTH CARE
- Self-care after diagnosis and treatment.
- Doctor's treatment.
- Surgery to remove tumors and surrounding bone that compress the spinal cord.
- Radiation therapy following surgery.
- Physical therapy.

DIAGNOSTIC MEASURES
- Your own observation of symptoms.
- Medical history and physical exam by a doctor.
- Laboratory studies of blood and spinal fluid.
- X-rays of the spine.

POSSIBLE COMPLICATIONS—Total paralysis caused by a blockage of blood vessels that nourish spinal-cord cells.

PROBABLE OUTCOME—The success of treatment depends on the type, size, and location of the growth.

Surgery to remove bone surrounding the cord can relieve pressure on spinal nerves and nerve pathways. This operation generally relieves pain and other symptoms immediately, but may impair motor functions. Physical therapy and rehabilitation may restore lost function.

If the tumor originated on the exterior of the spinal cord and has not spread, surgery restores a normal life expectancy.

HOW TO TREAT

NOTE—Follow your doctor's instructions. These instructions are supplemental.

GENERAL MEASURES—No specific instructions except those listed under other headings.

MEDICATION—Your doctor may prescribe:
- Pain relievers.
- Cortisone drugs to decrease swelling around the tumor and reduce pressure on the spinal cord.
- Anticancer drugs, if the tumor is malignant.

ACTIVITY—Stay as active as your strength allows. Work and exercise moderately. Rest when you tire.

DIET—Eat a normal, well-balanced diet. Vitamin and mineral supplements should not be necessary unless you show evidence of deficiency or cannot eat normally.

CALL YOUR DOCTOR IF

You have any symptoms of a spinal-cord tumor.

SPOROTRICHOSIS

GENERAL INFORMATION

DEFINITION—An infectious fungal disease that causes ulcers and abscesses of the skin, lymph nodes and lymph channels. Farm laborers and gardeners, especially those handling barberry bushes, are most often infected. Sporotrichosis is not contagious from person to person.

BODY PARTS INVOLVED—Skin; lymph system; lungs; joints; bones (rare).

SEX OR AGE MOST AFFECTED—Adults of both sexes, but more common in men.

SIGNS & SYMPTOMS—Early stages:
● A small, movable, non-tender nodule appears under the skin of the fingers. The nodule enlarges slowly, becomes pink and ulcerates.
In a few days or weeks:
● Dark nodules appear along the lymphatic channel that drains the area.
● Cough with sputum begins, if the organism reaches the lungs (rare).
● Usually no other symptoms—unlike other fungal diseases, which cause fever, chills, a general ill feeling and appetite loss.

CAUSES—Infection by a fungus, sporotricum schenckii, that lives in soil, sphagnum moss, weeds and decaying organic vegetation.

RISK INCREASES WITH
● Medical history of sarcoidosis or tuberculosis.
● Occupations that involve work with plants and soil, such as farming, nursery work and horticulture.

HOW TO PREVENT—Wear gloves when working with soil.

WHAT TO EXPECT

APPROPRIATE HEALTH CARE
● Self-care after diagnosis.
● Doctor's treatment.
● Hospitalization, if complications occur.

DIAGNOSTIC MEASURES
● Your own observation of symptoms.
● Medical history and physical exam by a doctor.
● Laboratory culture of pus from the lesions.

POSSIBLE COMPLICATIONS—Spread of the fungi throughout the body, causing widespread, life-threatening infection.

PROBABLE OUTCOME—With treatment, usually curable within 1 to 2 months after lesions heal—but recovery may require 6 or 7 months. The fatality rate is high if infection spreads throughout the body.

HOW TO TREAT

NOTE—Follow your doctor's instructions. These instructions are supplemental.

GENERAL MEASURES
● Because sporotrichosis is not contagious, the patient does not need to be isolated.
● Cover lesions with loose-fitting bandages to prevent secondary infection with bacteria.
● Weigh daily and keep a record.

MEDICATION—Your doctor may prescribe:
● Saturated solution of potassium iodide. Dilute this in water, fruit juice or other beverages and take 3 times a day after meals. Drink this with a straw to prevent discoloration of the teeth.
● Antifungal medicine, such as amphotericin B. This medication is potent and may cause severe adverse reactions. It is reserved for serious cases. Hospitalization is necessary so the drug can be administered intravenously.

ACTIVITY—No restrictions unless you develop signs of widespread infection.

DIET—No special diet.

CALL YOUR DOCTOR IF

● You have symptoms of sporotrichosis.
● The following occurs during treatment:
   Unexplained weight loss.
   Fever of 101F (38.3C) orally.
● New, unexplained symptoms develop. Antifungal drugs used in treatment may produce side effects, including skin rash, tongue and mouth irritation, and cough.

SPRAINS & STRAINS

GENERAL INFORMATION

DEFINITION—Injury to ligaments that hold a joint together and in position. A strain is a stretched ligament. A sprain is a stretched and torn ligament. Sprains occur most often in ankles, knees or fingers, although any joint can be sprained. Sprained joints can function—but only with pain.

BODY PARTS INVOLVED—Any ligament (tendon) attached to any joint.

SEX OR AGE MOST AFFECTED—Both sexes; all ages.

SIGNS & SYMPTOMS
● Pain or tenderness in the area of injury; severity varies with the extent of injury.
● Swelling of the affected joint.
● Redness or bruising in the area of injury, either immediately or several hours after injury.
● Loss of normal mobility in the injured joint.

CAUSES—Overuse or stress of a ligament or membrane around a joint. A sprain usually occurs when the body weight is placed abnormally on ligaments, causing them to stretch and tear. The ankle is injured most often because of its anatomical weakness, its exposed position and the stress it sustains in athletic and recreational activities.

RISK INCREASES WITH—Obesity.

HOW TO PREVENT—Avoid injury:
● Wrap weak joints with support bandages before strenuous activity.
● Strengthen weak joints with rehabilitative exercises to prevent a recurrence. Consult your doctor or a physical therapist for exercises.
● Accident-proof your home.

WHAT TO EXPECT

APPROPRIATE HEALTH CARE
● Self-care if the injury is not severe.
● Doctor's treatment if the joint cannot move or bear weight normally.
● Cast for a severely sprained joint.
● Surgery to repair badly torn ligaments.
● Physical therapy to regain strength and normal use of the joint.

DIAGNOSTIC MEASURES
● Your own observation of symptoms.
● Medical history and physical exam by a doctor.
● X-rays of the injured area.

POSSIBLE COMPLICATIONS—Permanent weakness if the sprain is severe or if a joint is sprained repeatedly.

PROBABLE OUTCOME—Strains usually heal in 1 to 2 weeks. Sprains generally heal in 2 weeks without complications.

HOW TO TREAT

NOTE—Follow your doctor's instructions. These instructions are supplemental.

GENERAL MEASURES
● Apply ice to the injured joint during the first 24 hours. Place ice in a plastic bag and separate it from the skin with a thin towel. Hold it against the joint with your hand or an elastic bandage. Keep the ice pack on the joint up to 2 hours at a time—either constantly or intermittently—depending on your ability to tolerate the cold. Continue the ice treatment at 2-hour intervals for 24 hours.
● After 24 hours, some doctors recommend continued ice treatment. Others recommend heat.
● To use heat, soak the joint in hot water or apply heat for 15 minutes every 2 hours or whenever possible. Don't apply heat during the first 24 hours. It may increase bleeding and swelling and prolong healing time.
● Whenever possible, elevate the joint so fluid can drain and diminish swelling.
● A cast may be necessary for severe sprains or following surgery. See Care of Casts, Appendix 17. Following cast removal, you will wear support bandages for a while.
● Learn how to use crutches, if needed.

MEDICATION—You may use non-prescription pain relievers such as aspirin. If the sprain is severe, your doctor may prescribe a stronger pain reliever.

ACTIVITY—Allow the joint to rest 1 or 2 days. Then begin exercising the joint gently, without putting weight on it.

DIET—No special diet.

CALL YOUR DOCTOR IF

● You have a sprained joint that won't bear weight or move normally.
● Pain becomes intolerable.
● Swelling or bruising increases, despite treatment.

STEIN-LEVENTHAL SYNDROME
(Polycystic Ovarian Syndrome)

GENERAL INFORMATION

DEFINITION—Ovary enlargement from many small cysts. The surface of the ovaries becomes too thick to allow ovulation (the monthly release of the egg from the ovary). Women with this problem cannot become pregnant without treatment.

BODY PARTS INVOLVED—Either or both ovaries.

SEX OR AGE MOST AFFECTED—Young adult women.

SIGNS & SYMPTOMS
- Irregular menstrual bleeding, usually a lighter flow.
- Increased time between periods, often up to several months.
- Increased hair growth on the face, arms, legs and from pubic area to navel.
- Enlarged clitoris.
- Increased sex drive.
- Higher energy level.
- Obesity.
- Acne.

CAUSES—Unknown, but probably hereditary.

RISK INCREASES WITH—Unknown.

HOW TO PREVENT—Cannot be prevented at present.

WHAT TO EXPECT

APPROPRIATE HEALTH CARE
- Doctor's treatment.
- Surgery to remove a small section from each ovary (usually). This often permits ovulation.

DIAGNOSTIC MEASURES
- Your own observation of symptoms.
- Medical history and physical exam by a doctor.
- Laboratory studies of blood hormone levels.
- Surgical diagnostic procedures, such as laparoscopy or culdoscopy (see Glossary for both).

POSSIBLE COMPLICATIONS
- Permanent hormone imbalance.
- Infertility.
- Increased likelihood of uterine cancer and breast cancer.

PROBABLE OUTCOME—Hormone therapy and surgery usually decrease masculine characteristics and often restore fertility. Some signs and symptoms may never disappear completely.

HOW TO TREAT

NOTE—Follow your doctor's instructions. These instructions are supplemental.

GENERAL MEASURES—You may need professional help if you want to remove excess hair from your face, arms and legs.

MEDICATION—Your doctor may prescribe clomiphene citrate. This occasionally lessens symptoms without surgery.

ACTIVITY—No restrictions on activity, including sexual intercourse.

DIET—No special diet.

CALL YOUR DOCTOR IF

- You have symptoms of Stein-Leventhal syndrome.
- Your periods become profuse or more frequent than usual.
- You develop a lump or swelling in the breast.
- Symptoms recur after treatment or surgery.
- You want a referral to remove excess body hair.
- New, unexplained symptoms develop. Drugs used in treatment may produce side effects.

STOMACH CANCER
(Gastric Carcinoma)

 GENERAL INFORMATION

DEFINITION—Uncontrolled growth of malignant cells in the stomach. In the past 30 years, the incidence of stomach cancer has decreased by 50% in the U.S. Incidence and mortality rates still remain high for unknown reasons in Japan, Iceland and Austria.

BODY PARTS INVOLVED—Stomach.

SEX OR AGE MOST AFFECTED—Men over age 40.

SIGNS & SYMPTOMS—Early stages:
• Vague symptoms of indigestion, such as fullness, burping, nausea and poor appetite. Later stages:
• Unexplained weight loss.
• Vomiting blood.
• Black stools.
• Fullness after eating small amounts.
• Anemia.
• Pain in the upper abdomen.
• Mass in the upper abdomen that can be felt (sometimes).

CAUSES—Unknown.

RISK INCREASES WITH
• Persons over age 65.
• Family history of stomach cancer.
• Blood type. This is most common in people with type-A blood.
• Pernicious anemia.
• Excess alcohol consumption.
• Absence of normal stomach acid, previous stomach surgery or partial stomach removal.
• Diet that includes many smoked, pickled and salted meats.

HOW TO PREVENT
• Don't ignore symptoms of indigestion that last more than a few days.
• Avoid eating processed or smoked meats, such as bacon, prepared ham and lunch meats.
• Decrease alcohol consumption if you drink more than 1 or 2 drinks a day.

 WHAT TO EXPECT

APPROPRIATE HEALTH CARE
• Doctor's treatment.
• Surgery to remove part or all of the stomach.
• Radiation treatment.

DIAGNOSTIC MEASURES
• Your own observation of symptoms.
• Medical history and physical exam by a doctor.
• Laboratory blood studies for anemia, stomach tests for acid and stool tests for bleeding.
• Surgical diagnostic procedures such as biopsy through a gastroscope (see Glossary).
• X-rays of the stomach, esophagus and small intestine.

POSSIBLE COMPLICATIONS
• Internal bleeding.
• Misdiagnosis as a stomach ulcer.
• Fatal spread to liver, bones and lungs.

PROBABLE OUTCOME—This condition is currently considered incurable. With early diagnosis and treatment, the 5-year survival rate is 65%. Scientific research into causes and treatment continues, so there is hope for increasingly effective treatment and cure.

 HOW TO TREAT

NOTE—Follow your doctor's instructions. These instructions are supplemental.

GENERAL MEASURES—No specific instructions except those listed under other headings.

MEDICATION—Your doctor may prescribe:
• Anticancer drugs (sometimes).
• Pain relievers.

ACTIVITY—Resume your normal activities as soon as symptoms improve after surgery or chemotherapy.

DIET—Eat frequent, small meals of soft foods. Consult a dietician for menu planning.

 CALL YOUR DOCTOR IF

• You have symptoms of stomach cancer.
• Indigestion occurs after surgery and does not respond to medication in a few days.
• New, unexplained symptoms develop. Drugs used in treatment may produce side effects.

ILLNESSES & DISORDERS

STRABISMUS

GENERAL INFORMATION

DEFINITION—Lack of coordinated muscle movement or focusing ability between the eyes, causing the eyes to point in different directions. One or both eyes may turn inward (crossed eyes) or outward ("walleye").

BODY PARTS INVOLVED—Eyes; brain area that controls vision.

SEX OR AGE MOST AFFECTED—Both sexes; all ages.

SIGNS & SYMPTOMS
- Uncoordinated eye movements. This is sometimes evident only when looking in certain directions.
- Double vision (sometimes).
- Vision in one eye only, with loss of depth perception.

CAUSES—Eye movement is controlled by brain signals to four muscles around each eye. Loss of coordinated movement results from:
- Muscle imbalance between the eyes.
- Lack of equal focusing ability in the eyes. The brain cannot tolerate differing focused images, so it ignores signals from one field of vision. The weaker eye eventually becomes useless from disuse, and a "lazy" or wandering eye results.
- Brain damage or head injury.

RISK INCREASES WITH—Family history of strabismus.

HOW TO PREVENT—No specific preventive measures.

WHAT TO EXPECT

APPROPRIATE HEALTH CARE
- Home care after diagnosis.
- Doctor's (opthalmologist's) treatment.
- Surgery to correct the condition of the eye muscles (sometimes).

DIAGNOSTIC MEASURES
- Your own observation of symptoms. Note particularly if a young child covers one eye—this may indicate the eyes are not focusing together.
- Medical history and physical exam by a doctor, including tests of visual acuity, retina examination, total neurological exam and muscle tests.

POSSIBLE COMPLICATIONS
- Loss of normal vision in one eye.
- Psychological distress from an unattractive facial appearance.

PROBABLE OUTCOME—With early diagnosis, strabismus can be corrected with glasses, an eye patch, eye exercises or surgery. Without prompt treatment, vision loss in one eye may become permanent.

Many persons adapt well to single-eye vision and learn to drive a car or fly an airplane.

If vision is lost in one eye, take extra precautions against injury in the other eye. Wear goggles for sports and other activities, such as carpentry or welding, that carry the risk of injury.

HOW TO TREAT

NOTE—Follow your doctor's instructions. These instructions are supplemental.

GENERAL MEASURES—Your doctor may recommend:
- Glasses or an eye patch over the stronger eye to correct focusing imbalance. These force the weak eye to work.
- Eye-muscle exercises.

MEDICATION—Medicine usually is not necessary for this disorder.

ACTIVITY—No restrictions. Protect your child against falls or injury while he or she adjusts to an eye patch.

DIET—No special diet.

CALL YOUR DOCTOR IF

Your child has symptoms of strabismus.

STREP THROAT
(Streptococcal Sore Throat)

 GENERAL INFORMATION

DEFINITION—Infection and inflammation of the pharynx by streptococcal bacteria. Strep throat is contagious. One out of 4 family members usually catches it within 2 to 7 days after exposure.

BODY PARTS INVOLVED—Throat; tonsils.

SEX OR AGE MOST AFFECTED—Both sexes; all ages.

SIGNS & SYMPTOMS
- Fever.
- Throat pain that is worse when swallowing.
- Appetite loss.
- Headache.
- General ill feeling.
- Ear pain when swallowing (sometimes).
- Swollen glands in the neck.
- Bright-red tonsils that may have specks of pus.

CAUSES—Streptococcal bacteria.

RISK INCREASES WITH
- Recent strep infection in the household.
- Smoking.
- Fatigue.
- Cold, wet weather.
- Crowded living conditions.

HOW TO PREVENT—Avoid contact with infected people.

 WHAT TO EXPECT

APPROPRIATE HEALTH CARE
- Self-care after diagnosis.
- Doctor's treatment.

DIAGNOSTIC MEASURES
- Your own observation of symptoms.
- Medical history and physical exam by a doctor.
- Laboratory studies, such as a throat culture and blood count. A throat culture is the only way to diagnose a strep-throat infection. This is an inexpensive, quick, painless procedure in a doctor's office.

POSSIBLE COMPLICATIONS
- Dehydration (if throat is too sore to swallow liquid).
- The following complications can be prevented with at least 10 days of treatment with penicillin or other effective antibiotics:
  - Abscess next to the tonsil.
  - Rheumatic fever.
  - Glomerulonephritis.

PROBABLE OUTCOME—Usually curable in 10 to 12 days with antibiotic treatment.

 HOW TO TREAT

NOTE—Follow your doctor's instructions. These instructions are supplemental.

GENERAL MEASURES
- For adults or children old enough to gargle, prepare a soothing tea gargle. Double the usual strength of tea, and gargle warm or cold as often as it feels good.
- Use a cool-mist humidifier to provide moisture. This relieves the dry, tight feeling in the throat.
- Use warm soaks (see Glossary) to relieve pain in swollen glands.

MEDICATION—Your doctor may prescribe penicillin or another antibiotic to take orally or by injection.

ACTIVITY
- Rest in bed until fever drops below 100F (37.8C). You may read or watch TV.
- After treatment, resume normal activity as symptoms improve. Children may return to school 5 days after beginning antibiotics, if symptoms have improved.

DIET—A liquid diet may be necessary while the throat is sore. Drink as many fluids as possible, including milk shakes, soups, tea, carbonated drinks and iced coffee. Any type and amount of solid food is acceptable as long as it can be swallowed without too much pain.

 CALL YOUR DOCTOR IF

- You have symptoms of a strep throat.
- The following occurs during treatment: Temperature is normal for 1 or 2 days, then rises to 101F (38.3C).
  New symptoms appear, such as: nausea; vomiting; earache; cough; swollen glands; skin rash; severe headache; nasal drainage; chest pain; or shortness of breath.
  Convulsions occur.
  Joints become red or painful.
  Cough begins that produces green, yellow-brown or bloody sputum.

ILLNESSES & DISORDERS

STROKE
(Cerebrovascular Accident; CVA)

 GENERAL INFORMATION

DEFINITION—A sudden decrease in the blood supply to part of the brain, damaging the area so it cannot function normally.

BODY PARTS INVOLVED—Central nervous system; musculo-skeletal system.

SEX OR AGE MOST AFFECTED—Adults over 60.

SIGNS & SYMPTOMS—The following symptoms may vary according to the site of brain damage:
- Inability to speak.
- Inability to move part of the body.
- Loss of consciousness.
- Sudden heaviness in an arm or leg, or numbness and inability to control muscles.
- Headache.
- Vision disturbances.
- Confusion.
- Dizziness.
- Loss of bowel and bladder control.

CAUSES—Usually hardening of the arteries (atherosclerosis) or high blood pressure. These may result in the following:
- Thrombosis, in which blood flow is blocked by a narrow or closed artery.
- Embolism, in which a small part of an artery wall or a small blood clot from a diseased artery or heart travels to the brain.
- Cerebral hemorrhage, in which a blood vessel to the brain ruptures and bleeds into surrounding brain tissue.
- Rupture of an aneurysm of a small artery to the brain.

RISK INCREASES WITH
- Smoking.
- Obesity.
- Diet that is high in fat or salt.
- High blood pressure.
- Diabetes mellitus.
- Coronary-artery disease.
- Previous transient ischemic attacks.
- Family history of stroke.
- Excess alcohol consumption.

HOW TO PREVENT
- Exercise regularly. See Appendix 20.
- Eat a diet that is low in fat. See Appendix 8.
- Don't smoke.
- Have your blood pressure checked regularly. If it is high, consult your doctor.
- Ask your doctor about taking 1 aspirin tablet daily. Recent studies indicate this may affect blood clotting enough to decrease the chance of cerebral thrombosis or embolism.

 WHAT TO EXPECT

APPROPRIATE HEALTH CARE
- Doctor's treatment.
- Self-care after diagnosis.
- Hospitalization.
- Surgery (sometimes) to remove a clot in an artery (carotid) to the brain.
- Nursing-home care (sometimes).
- Physical therapy and speech therapy.

DIAGNOSTIC MEASURES
- Your own observation of symptoms.
- Medical history and physical exam by a doctor.
- Laboratory studies of spinal fluid and blood.
- CAT scan (see Glossary).
- X-rays of the head.

POSSIBLE COMPLICATIONS
- Pneumonia.
- Depression.
- Pressure sores from prolonged bed rest.
- Permanent paralysis or disability.

PROBABLE OUTCOME—Stroke causes death, permanent damage or disability in 2/3 of all cases. In the rest, complete recovery without long-term disability is possible.

A mild stroke may be the forerunner of more severe attacks. For stroke survivors, partial paralysis may last for months.

 HOW TO TREAT

NOTE—Follow your doctor's instructions. These instructions are supplemental.

GENERAL MEASURES—Following a stroke, consider installing ramps at entries to the house and hand bars next to tubs and toilets.

MEDICATION—Your doctor may prescribe:
- Anticoagulant drugs to reduce the chance of clot formation.
- Antihypertensive drugs, if you have high blood pressure.

ACTIVITY—If you have lost muscle control, therapy will help you learn to use affected limbs to regain basic skills, such as eating, dressing and toilet functions.

DIET—Eat a diet that is low in salt (see Appendix 9) and low in fat (see Appendix 8).

 CALL YOUR DOCTOR IF

- You have symptoms of a stroke or observe them in someone else. This is an emergency!
- The following occurs during treatment:
  Fever.
  Pressure sores.
  Worsening symptoms.

STY
(Hordeolum)

GENERAL INFORMATION

DEFINITION—A small abscess of hair-follicle glands in the eyelid.

BODY PARTS INVOLVED—Eyelid; eyelashes; conjunctiva (white of the eye).

SEX OR AGE MOST AFFECTED—Both sexes; all ages.

SIGNS & SYMPTOMS
- Redness, swelling, warmth, tenderness or pain on the edge of the top or bottom eyelid. The head of the sty is usually on the outside, but it may be on the underside of the lid.
- Increased tear production.
- Sensitivity to bright light.
- A gritty feeling in the eye.

CAUSES—Bacterial infection (usually staphylococcal). The infection may be limited to the eyelid or may have spread from somewhere else in the body. A sty may result from general poor health or may occasionally indicate a need for glasses.

RISK INCREASES WITH
- Stress.
- Illness that has lowered resistance.
- Eye irritation from smoking.
- Exposure to chemical or environmental irritants.
- Crowded or unsanitary living conditions.
- Poor nutrition.

HOW TO PREVENT
- Wash hands frequently, and dry with clean towels.
- Avoid environments with excessive dust or other irritating substances.
- Eat a normal, well-balanced diet.

WHAT TO EXPECT

APPROPRIATE HEALTH CARE
- Self-care.
- Doctor's treatment.
- Surgery to drain the abscess.

DIAGNOSTIC MEASURES
- Your own observation of symptoms.
- Medical history and physical exam by a doctor.
- Laboratory culture of the discharge from the sty.

POSSIBLE COMPLICATIONS—Spread of infection to other glands in the eyelid.

PROBABLE OUTCOME—Usually curable within 1 week after the sty discharges its pus. Sties frequently recur, even with treatment.

HOW TO TREAT

NOTE—Follow your doctor's instructions. These instructions are supplemental.

GENERAL MEASURES—Use warm-water soaks (see Appendix 18) to relieve pain and inflammation and hasten healing. Apply soaks for 20 minutes, then rest at least 1 hour. Repeat as often as needed.

MEDICATION—Your doctor may prescribe:
- Antibiotic eye drops to prevent the spread of infection to other parts of the eye. Oral antibiotics or antibiotic injections are usually not needed.
- Topical antibiotic ointments or creams, such as erythromycin or bacitracin. Apply a thin layer of medication to the eyelid edge 3 or 4 times daily. A heavy layer wastes medicine and is no more beneficial than a thin layer.

ACTIVITY—No restrictions.

DIET—No special diet.

CALL YOUR DOCTOR IF

- A ripened sty does not drain spontaneously or after gentle removal of the affected eyelash.
- Pain occurs in the *eye.*
- Vision changes.

SUBARACHNOID HEMORRHAGE

GENERAL INFORMATION

DEFINITION—Sudden bleeding into the subarachnoid space (the area between 2 of the membranes that cover the brain). The space is normally filled with cerebrospinal fluid.

BODY PARTS INVOLVED—Brain; meninges (membranes that cover the brain); blood vessels to the brain.

SEX OR AGE MOST AFFECTED—All ages, but most common in adults aged 25 to 50.

SIGNS & SYMPTOMS
- Acute, severe headache, often followed by unconsciousness.
- Drowsiness, dizziness, convulsions or coma.
- Eye pain with extreme sensitivity to light.
- Vomiting.
- Rapid heartbeat and breathing.
- Stiff neck with pain on movement.
- Fever.
- Numbness, weakness or inability to move an arm or leg.

CAUSES
- Head injury (the most common cause).
- Hardening of the arteries.
- Infection in any part of the central nervous system.
- Rupture of an aneurysm (weakened part of an artery) that has been present since birth. Rupture is often preceded by high blood pressure or hardening of the arteries.
- Bleeding disorder, such as sickle-cell anemia, leukemia or any that is a side effect of prescription drugs.

RISK INCREASES WITH
- Atherosclerosis (hardening of the arteries) or high blood pressure.
- Family history of bleeding disorders.
- Family history of subarachnoid hemorrhage. Cerebral aneurysms run in families.

HOW TO PREVENT
- Avoid head injury. Use seat belts in cars and protective head gear in contact sports.
- Have your blood pressure checked regularly. If it is high, consult your doctor for treatment to reduce it.

WHAT TO EXPECT

APPROPRIATE HEALTH CARE
- Doctor's treatment. This is an emergency.
- Surgery to stop bleeding and remove collected blood.
- Long-term rehabilitation.
- Self-care after treatment.

DIAGNOSTIC MEASURES
- Your own observation of symptoms.
- Medical history and physical exam by a doctor.
- Laboratory studies of blood and cerebrospinal fluid.
- X-rays of the skull.
- CAT scan (see Glossary).

POSSIBLE COMPLICATIONS—Death or permanent disability if treatment does not begin soon enough.

PROBABLE OUTCOME—If surgery is possible, recovery chances are good. Partial paralysis, weakness or numbness, and speech and visual difficulties may remain in some cases.

The damaged area of the brain cannot be restored. However, undamaged areas of the brain often can be taught the lost functions. This usually requires rehabilitation, including physical therapy or speech therapy. Determination and a positive attitude greatly affect the success of the rehabilitation process.

HOW TO TREAT

NOTE—Follow your doctor's instructions. These instructions are supplemental.

GENERAL MEASURES—At home, consider installing hand bars at the tub and toilet, and ramps at each entry to the house.

MEDICATION—Your doctor may prescribe cortisone drugs to reduce brain swelling and pressure.

ACTIVITY—If you have lost some motor functions, occupational and physical therapists will help you use the affected limbs to regain basic skills, such as eating, dressing and toilet functions.

After recovery, resume as many of your former activities as your strength and sense of well-being allow. Allow 6 to 12 months for recovery.

DIET—No special diet. Vitamin and mineral supplements should not be necessary unless you cannot eat normally.

CALL YOUR DOCTOR IF

- You have any symptoms of a subarachnoid hemorrhage. This is an emergency!
- Symptoms recur after surgery.

SUBCONJUNCTIVAL HEMORRHAGE

 GENERAL INFORMATION

DEFINITION—Sudden appearance of blood in the white area of the eye. Although the bleeding may appear frightening, it is not painful or serious.

BODY PARTS INVOLVED—Conjunctiva (white of the eye).

SEX OR AGE MOST AFFECTED—Both sexes; all ages.

SIGNS & SYMPTOMS—A small, painless collection of bright red blood over the white of the eye. Swelling may occur in the affected area of the conjunctiva. The blood changes color gradually to brown or green before disappearing. The condition doesn't interfere with vision.

CAUSES—Usually spontaneous bleeding with no known cause. It may follow coughing, sneezing or vomiting.

RISK INCREASES WITH
- Use of mind-altering drugs.
- Use of anticoagulant drugs.

HOW TO PREVENT—No specific preventive measures.

 WHAT TO EXPECT

APPROPRIATE HEALTH CARE
- Self-care after diagnosis.
- Doctor's treatment, if there has been injury or a change in vision.

DIAGNOSTIC MEASURES
- Your own observation of symptoms.
- Medical history and physical exam by a doctor (sometimes).

POSSIBLE COMPLICATIONS—None expected.

PROBABLE OUTCOME—The blood should be absorbed in 2 or 3 weeks. It is very unlikely that any scarring will occur.

 HOW TO TREAT

NOTE—Follow your doctor's instructions. These instructions are supplemental.

GENERAL MEASURES
- Use cold compresses for several days to prevent additional bleeding. Fold a clean cloth in several layers, dip it in ice water and wring it out a little. Apply it to the eye for 10 minutes every hour.
- Use warm compresses when signs of bleeding have stopped for 2 days. This will hasten blood absorption. Dip the compress in warm water instead of cold water. Apply to the eye for 10 minutes 3 times a day.

MEDICATION—Medicine is usually not necessary for this disorder.

ACTIVITY—No restrictions.

DIET—No special diet.

 CALL YOUR DOCTOR IF

You have symptoms of subconjunctival hemorrhage, especially if you have eye pain or your vision changes.

SUBDURAL HEMORRHAGE & HEMATOMA

 GENERAL INFORMATION

DEFINITION—Bleeding (hemorrhage) that causes blood to collect and clot (hematoma) beneath the outermost of 3 membranes that cover the brain (meninges).

There are 2 types of subdural hematomas. An acute subdural hematoma occurs soon after a severe head injury. A chronic subdural hematoma is a complication that may develop weeks after a head injury. The injury may have been so minor that the patient does not remember it.

BODY PARTS INVOLVED—Brain; meninges; blood vessels to the brain.

SEX OR AGE MOST AFFECTED—Both sexes; all ages.

SIGNS & SYMPTOMS
- Recurrent headaches that worsen each day.
- Fluctuating drowsiness, dizziness, mental changes or confusion.
- Weakness or numbness on one side of the body.
- Vision disturbances.
- Vomiting without nausea.
- Pupils of different size (sometimes).

CAUSES—Head injury.

RISK INCREASES WITH—Injuries occur more often after:
- Excess alcohol consumption.
- Use of mind-altering drugs.

HOW TO PREVENT—Avoid head injury in the following ways:
- Use seat belts in cars.
- Wear protective head gear during contact sports, or while riding a bicycle or motorcycle.
- Don't drink alcohol or use mind-altering drugs and drive.

 WHAT TO EXPECT

APPROPRIATE HEALTH CARE
- Doctor's treatment.
- Surgical exploration and removal of the clot.

DIAGNOSTIC MEASURES
- Your own observation of symptoms.
- Medical history and physical exam by a doctor.
- Laboratory studies of blood and cerebrospinal fluid.
- Hospital diagnostic tests, such as X-ray, arteriography, radioscopic scan and CAT scan (see Glossary for all).

POSSIBLE COMPLICATIONS—Death or permanent brain damage, including partial or complete paralysis, behavioral and personality changes, and speech problems.

PROBABLE OUTCOME—The degree of recovery depends upon general health, age, severity of the injury, rapidity of the treatment, and extensiveness of the bleeding or clot. After the clot is removed, brain tissue that has been compressed usually expands slowly to fill its original space. The outlook is good under the best circumstances.

 HOW TO TREAT

NOTE—Follow your doctor's instructions. These instructions are supplemental.

GENERAL MEASURES—There is no self-treatment. These suggestions apply to care at home following surgery.

MEDICATION—Your doctor may prescribe cortisone drugs to reduce swelling inside the skull.

ACTIVITY—Stay as active as your strength allows. Work and exercise moderately. Rest when you tire.

If your speech or muscle control has been damaged, you may need physical therapy or speech therapy.

DIET—Eat a normal, well-balanced diet. Vitamin and mineral supplements should not be necessary unless you cannot eat normally.

 CALL YOUR DOCTOR IF

- You have had a head injury—even if it seems minor—and you develop any symptoms of subdural hemorrhage. This is an emergency!
- The following occurs during or after treatment:
  Temperature rises to 101F (38.3C) or higher.
  Surgical wound becomes red, swollen or tender.
  Headache worsens.

SUN POISONING

GENERAL INFORMATION

DEFINITION—Reaction to overexposure to the sun.

BODY PARTS INVOLVED—Skin in areas most exposed to sunlight.

SEX OR AGE MOST AFFECTED—Both sexes; all ages.

SIGNS & SYMPTOMS
- Red skin rash, sometimes with small blisters, in areas exposed to sunlight.
- Fever.
- Fatigue or dizziness.

CAUSES—Sun poisoning is most likely to occur during hot seasons when ultraviolet light is strongest. It is triggered by exposure to the sun, usually in conjunction with sunburn. It is especially likely in persons who take medications that cause photosensitivity (increased sensitivity to ultraviolet light). The most common drugs include tetracycline antibiotics, thiazide diuretics, sulfa drugs and oral contraceptives. Some cosmetics, including lipstick, perfume and soaps, can also cause a photosensitive reaction.

RISK INCREASES WITH
- Underlying infection.
- Previous episodes of sun poisoning.
- Metabolic disorders, such as diabetes mellitus or thyroid disease.
- Use of immunosuppressive drugs or any drugs listed under Causes.

HOW TO PREVENT—Stay out of the sun when possible if you have a history of sun poisoning.

WHAT TO EXPECT

APPROPRIATE HEALTH CARE
- Self care after diagnosis.
- Doctor's treatment.

DIAGNOSTIC MEASURES
- Your own observation of symptoms.
- Medical history and physical exam by a doctor.

POSSIBLE COMPLICATIONS—Recurrence of the rash and other symptoms when exposed to the sun—even for short periods—especially in spring and summer.

PROBABLE OUTCOME—Symptoms can be controlled with treatment if you stay out of the sun. Allow up to 1 week for recovery.

HOW TO TREAT

NOTE—Follow your doctor's instructions. These instructions are supplemental.

GENERAL MEASURES
- Stay out of the sun during the hours of strongest ultraviolet light (10 a.m. to 2 p.m.).
- If you must go out in the sun, wear protective clothing and the most protective sun-screen preparation available.

MEDICATION—Your doctor may prescribe:
- Beta-carotene to reduce discomfort.
- Chloroquine prior to sun exposure to prevent a recurrence of symptoms.

ACTIVITY—No restrictions, except to avoid prolonged sun exposure.

DIET—No special diet. Drink extra fluids to prevent dehydration.

CALL YOUR DOCTOR IF

- You have symptoms of sun poisoning.
- New, unexplained symptoms develop. Drugs used in treatment may produce side effects.

SUNBURN

GENERAL INFORMATION

DEFINITION—Inflammation of the skin that follows overexposure to the sun, sun lamps or occupational light sources.

BODY PARTS INVOLVED—Exposed skin.

SEX OR AGE MOST AFFECTED—Both sexes; all ages.

SIGNS & SYMPTOMS
- Red, swollen, painful and sometimes blistered skin.
- Chills and fever.
- Nausea and vomiting (severe burns).
- Delirium (severe, extensive burns).
- Tanning or peeling of the skin after recovery, depending on severity of the burn.

CAUSES—Excess exposure to ultraviolet (UV) light. This is not screened out by thin clouds on overcast days, but it is partially screened by smoke and smog. A great deal of ultraviolet light reflects from snow, water, sand and sidewalks.

RISK INCREASES WITH
- Genetic factors, especially fair skin, blue eyes, and red or blonde hair.
- Exposure to industrial light sources, such as welding arcs.
- Use of drugs, including sulfa, tetracyclines, amoxicillin or oral contraceptives.

HOW TO PREVENT
- Avoid the sun from noon to 3 p.m.
- Use a sun-block preparation for outdoor activity. Products with a sun-protective value of 10 or more protect almost totally. Those with lower values offer partial protection and allow minimal tanning. Some of these resist water and perspiration, but reapply them after swimming or after prolonged exposure. Baby oil, mineral oil or cocoa butter offer no protection from the sun.
- For maximum protection, use a physical-barrier agent such as zinc-oxide ointment. Reapply after swimming and at frequent intervals during exposure. Barrier agents are especially helpful on skin areas that are most susceptible to burns, such as the nose, ears, backs of the legs and back of the neck.
- If you rarely burn, use a sun-screen product that permits tanning and provides minimal protection.
- Wear muted colors such as tan. Avoid brilliant colors and whites, which reflect the sun into your face.
- If you insist on tanning, limit your sun exposure on the 1st day to 5 to 10 minutes on each side. Add 5 minutes per side each day.

WHAT TO EXPECT

APPROPRIATE HEALTH CARE
- Self-care for minor sunburn.
- Doctor's treatment for severe sunburn.

DIAGNOSTIC MEASURES
- Your own observation of symptoms.
- Medical history and physical exam by a doctor.

POSSIBLE COMPLICATIONS
- Skin changes leading to skin cancer, including life-threatening malignant melanoma.
- Keratoses, premalignant skin lesions.
- Premature wrinkling and loss of skin elasticity.
- Temporary delirium in worst cases.

PROBABLE OUTCOME—Spontaneous recovery in 3 days to 3 weeks, depending on the severity of the sunburn.

HOW TO TREAT

NOTE—Follow your doctor's instructions. These instructions are supplemental.

GENERAL MEASURES
- To reduce heat and pain, dip gauze or towels in cool water and lay these on the burned areas.
- After skin swelling subsides, apply cold cream or baby lotion.
- For badly blistered skin, apply a light coating of petroleum jelly. This prevents anything from sticking to the blisters.

MEDICATION
- Use non-prescription drugs, such as aspirin or acetaminophen, to relieve pain and reduce fever. Non-prescription burn remedies that contain local anesthetics, such as benzocaine or lidocaine, may be useful, but they produce allergic reactions in some.
- Your doctor may prescribe pain relievers or cortisone drugs to use briefly.

ACTIVITY—Rest in any comfortable position until fever and discomfort diminish. Cover yourself with an upside-down "cradle" or tent of cardboard or other material to keep bed linens off the burned skin.

DIET—No special diet. Increase fluid intake.

CALL YOUR DOCTOR IF

The following occurs after sunburn:
- Oral temperature spikes to 101F (38.3C).
- Vomiting or diarrhea.
- Delirium.
- Pain and fever that persist longer than 48 hours.

SURGICAL-WOUND INFECTION

GENERAL INFORMATION

DEFINITION—Infection from bacterial contamination during or after a surgical procedure. Infections occur following surgery in 1.5% to 30% of cases, depending on the type of procedure.

BODY PARTS INVOLVED—Any body part with a surgical incision.

SEX OR AGE MOST AFFECTED—Both sexes; all ages.

SIGNS & SYMPTOMS—The following usually begin within 5 to 10 days after surgery, but in some cases, they begin months later:
- Fever.
- Pain and redness around the surgical wound.
- Edema (collection of fluid) around the incision, making the sutures tighter.

CAUSES
- Infection with bacteria, including streptococcal, staphylococcal or other germs. These sometimes cause infection, in spite of elaborate precautions against them and scrupulous surgical technique. They occur most often in people who must have emergency surgery on the gastrointestinal tract, such as for perforation of an ulcer or intestinal bleeding.
- Infection from any material left in the surgical area, including instruments or gauze.

RISK INCREASES WITH
- Adults over 60.
- Poor nutrition.
- Any chronic illness, especially diabetes mellitus.
- Gastrointestinal surgery.
- Use of immunosuppressive drugs.

HOW TO PREVENT—Skillful surgical techniques and presurgical procedures that include the following:
- Use of certain antibiotics, such as neomycin, before gastrointestinal surgery to sterilize the intestinal tract.
- Meticulous cleansing of the skin before surgery.
- Use of as few sutures as possible.

WHAT TO EXPECT

APPROPRIATE HEALTH CARE
- Doctor's treatment.
- Surgery to incise and drain a wound abscess.
- Self-care during convalescence.

DIAGNOSTIC MEASURES
- Your own observation of symptoms.
- Medical history and physical exam by a doctor.
- Laboratory culture of pus from the infection site.

POSSIBLE COMPLICATIONS
- Peritonitis.
- Blood poisoning.
- Interference with normal incision healing after surgery, sometimes necessitating further surgery and repairs.

PROBABLE OUTCOME—Usually curable in most patients with drainage of pus and antibiotic treatment. Allow about 2 weeks for the surgical-wound infection to heal.

HOW TO TREAT

NOTE—Follow your doctor's instructions. These instructions are supplemental.

GENERAL MEASURES
- Relieve pain with heat. Use a heat lamp or apply a heating pad or warm compress 3 or 4 times a day for 30 to 40 minutes.
- Change dressings frequently if the wound oozes.

MEDICATION—Your doctor may prescribe:
- Antibiotics to fight infection.
- Vitamin and mineral supplements to hasten healing.
- Pain relievers. You may use non-prescription drugs, such as acetaminophen, to relieve minor pain.

ACTIVITY—Rest in bed until all signs of infection disappear. You may read or watch TV.

DIET—Your surgeon will prescribe a diet.

CALL YOUR DOCTOR IF

- You have symptoms of a surgical-wound infection.
- You develop high fever and a general ill feeling, or infection seems to worsen after treatment.
- New, unexplained symptoms develop. Drugs used in treatment may produce side effects.

ILLNESSES & DISORDERS

SYPHILIS

GENERAL INFORMATION

DEFINITION—A contagious, sexually-transmitted disease that causes widespread tissue destruction. Syphilis is known as the "great mimic," because its symptoms resemble those of many other diseases.

BODY PARTS INVOLVED—Genitals; skin; central nervous system.

SEX OR AGE MOST AFFECTED
- Newborns (0 to 2 weeks) born to mothers with syphilis (congenital form).
- Persons of all ages and both sexes who have sexual contact (contagious form).

SIGNS & SYMPTOMS
First stage (contagious; appears 3 to 6 days after contact):
- A painless, red sore (chancre) on the genitals, mouth or rectum. The sore affects the penis in males and vagina or cervix in females.
Second stage (contagious; begins 6 or more weeks after the chancre appears):
- Fever (sometimes).
- Enlarged lymph glands in the neck, armpit or groin.
- Headache.
- Rash on skin and mucous membranes of the penis, vagina or mouth. The rash has small, red, scaly bumps.
Third stage (non-contagious; may appear years after the first and second stages):
- Mental deterioration.
- Sexual impotence.
- Loss of balance.
- Loss of feeling or shooting pains in the legs.
- Heart disease.

CAUSES—The infecting germ for both forms is treponema pallidum.
- The congenital form is spread to the fetus through the bloodstream.
- The contagious form is spread by intimate sexual contact with someone who has syphilis in the first or second stages.

RISK INCREASES WITH—Many sexual partners.

HOW TO PREVENT
- Obtain blood serum test for syphilis early in pregnancy. If infected, consult your doctor immediately for treatment.
- Use rubber condoms during intercourse.
- Avoid any sexual contact if you suspect a partner is infectious.

WHAT TO EXPECT

APPROPRIATE HEALTH CARE—Doctor's treatment.

DIAGNOSTIC MEASURES
- Your own observation of symptoms.
- Medical history and physical exam by a doctor.
- Laboratory studies, such as a blood serum test for syphilis, a microscopic exam of discharge from the chancre, and a study of spinal fluid. Tests are repeated after treatment.

POSSIBLE COMPLICATIONS—Widespread tissue destruction and death without treatment.

PROBABLE OUTCOME—Usually curable in 3 months with treatment. In spite of treatment, syphilis returns within 1 year in 10% of patients. If this happens, re-treatment is necessary.

HOW TO TREAT

NOTE—Follow your doctor's instructions. These instructions are supplemental.

GENERAL MEASURES
- Ensure that all your sexual partners obtain treatment. The public health department will work with you to notify contacts confidentially and help them obtain treatment.
- After treatment, have blood studies done each month for 6 months to check for recurrence. Then repeat blood studies every 3 months for 2 years.

MEDICATION—Your doctor will probably prescribe penicillin unless you are allergic to it. If penicillin cannot be used, other antibiotics can be equally as effective.

ACTIVITY—Avoid sexual intercourse for at least 2 months after treatment begins. Then use rubber condoms during sexual intercourse.

DIET—No special diet.

CALL YOUR DOCTOR IF

- You have symptoms of syphilis.
- The following occurs during or after treatment:
    Fever over 101F (38.3C).
    Skin rash, sore throat or swelling in any joint, such as the ankle or knee.
- New, unexplained symptoms develop. Drugs used in treatment may produce side effects.
- You once had syphilis and have not had a medical checkup in the past year.
- You have had sexual contact with someone who has syphilis.

TAPEWORM
(Taenia Saginata)

 GENERAL INFORMATION

DEFINITION—An infestation of the intestinal tract by the tapeworm, a parasite. This is not contagious from person to person.

BODY PARTS INVOLVED—Intestinal tract.

SEX OR AGE MOST AFFECTED—Both sexes; all ages.

SIGNS & SYMPTOMS—Most people with this problem have no symptoms. However, some experience the following:
- Pain in the upper abdomen.
- Diarrhea.
- Unexplained weight loss.
- Symptoms of anemia (weakness, fatigue and shortness of breath).
- Bowel movements containing worm eggs and worm body parts.

CAUSES—An intestinal parasite called taenia saginata. People become infected by eating improperly cooked or raw beef muscle infected with the parasite.

RISK INCREASES WITH—Travel to Africa, the Middle East, Eastern Europe, Mexico and South America. This is uncommon in the U.S., except in California and New England.

HOW TO PREVENT
- Cook beef long enough for all parts to reach at least 133F (56.1C), and hold it at that temperature at least 5 minutes.
- Buy only meat that has been inspected.

 WHAT TO EXPECT

APPROPRIATE HEALTH CARE—Doctor's treatment.

DIAGNOSTIC MEASURES
- Your own observation of symptoms.
- Medical history and physical exam by a doctor.
- Laboratory stool studies to identify the worm.

POSSIBLE COMPLICATIONS—Anemia.

PROBABLE OUTCOME—Usually curable in 1 day with treatment.

 HOW TO TREAT

NOTE—Follow your doctor's instructions. These instructions are supplemental.

GENERAL MEASURES
- Wash your hands before eating.
- Have all family members examined by a doctor for possible infection.

MEDICATION—Your doctor may prescribe an antihelminthic drug, such as niclosamide or paromomycin, to kill the parasite. Either drug cures with a single dose.

ACTIVITY—No restrictions.

DIET—No special diet.

 CALL YOUR DOCTOR IF

- You have symptoms of a tapeworm.
- New, unexplained symptoms develop. Drugs used in treatment may produce side effects.

ILLNESSES & DISORDERS

TAY-SACHS DISEASE

GENERAL INFORMATION

DEFINITION—An inherited, rare disorder of the central nervous system in infants and young children. It causes progressive impairment and early death. Less than 100 children are born with the disease each year in the U.S.

BODY PARTS INVOLVED—Brain and central nervous system.

SEX OR AGE MOST AFFECTED—Infants and young children (up to age 5).

SIGNS & SYMPTOMS—The child seems normal at birth. Between 3 and 6 months, the following symptoms begin to appear:
- Loss of alertness and retarded mental development.
- Loss of muscle strength, such as difficulty sitting up or turning over.
- Deafness.
- Blindness.
- Severe constipation caused by an impaired nerve supply to the colon.
- Seizures.

CAUSES—An inherited disease resulting from a recessive gene that causes enzyme deficiency. If both parents have the gene, they have a 25% chance of having a child with Tay-Sachs disease. If only one parent is a carrier, the children will not have the disease.

RISK INCREASES WITH—Genetic factors. Most parents who carry the recessive gene are of Eastern European Jewish origin (Ashkenazi).

HOW TO PREVENT
- Obtain genetic screening for children in families with Tay-Sachs.
- Obtain genetic counseling if you or your spouse have a family history of Tay-Sachs or are of Ashkenazi background.
- If you are expecting a child and have a family history of Tay-Sachs, consider amniocentesis (see Glossary) to detect if the fetus has the disease.

WHAT TO EXPECT

APPROPRIATE HEALTH CARE
- Doctor's treatment.
- Time in an extended-care facility for basic care if parents are unable to provide it at home.
- Psychotherapy or counseling for parents and siblings to learn to cope with the distress produced by this condition.

DIAGNOSTIC MEASURES
- Your own observation of symptoms.
- Medical history and physical exam by a doctor.
- Laboratory blood tests to detect the hexosaminidase A enzyme deficiency.

POSSIBLE COMPLICATIONS
- Pneumonia.
- Pressure sores.

PROBABLE OUTCOME—Death usually occurs before age 5.

HOW TO TREAT

NOTE—Follow your doctor's instructions. These instructions are supplemental.

GENERAL MEASURES—Seek out support groups for families of Tay-Sachs victims.

MEDICATION—Your doctor may prescribe:
- Anticonvulsants to control seizures.
- Stool softeners and laxatives to relieve constipation.
- Other medicines to control complicating disorders as they arise.

ACTIVITY—In the early stages, encourage the child to be as active as possible. Increasing mental, nervous and muscular deficiencies will eventually confine the child to bed much of the time.

DIET—Provide adequate fluids and a normal, high-fiber diet to minimize constipation. Feeding by tube usually becomes necessary as the disease progresses.

CALL YOUR DOCTOR IF

- You are concerned about your infant's mental and physical development.
- You think you or any member of your family carries the abnormal gene. A genetic counselor can advise you on how to prevent having children with this disease.

TEAR DUCT, INFECTION OR BLOCKAGE OF
(Dacryocystitis or Dacryostenosis)

 GENERAL INFORMATION

DEFINITION—Infection of the tear duct, sac or gland is called dacryocystitis. The germs that cause the infection can be spread to other people.

Scarring or blockage of the tear duct—usually from inherited abnormality or prior infection—is called dacryostenosis.

BODY PARTS INVOLVED—Eye; tear (nasolacrimal) gland, sac or duct.

SEX OR AGE MOST AFFECTED
- Infection of the tear duct or sac occurs in all ages, but it is most common in children.
- Inherited blockage of the tear duct usually appears in infants at 3 to 12 weeks.
- Blockage caused by infection can occur at any age following an infection.

SIGNS & SYMPTOMS—The following symptoms may apply to either blockage or infection:
- Persistent tearing of one or both eyes.
- Drainage of mucus and pus instead of water from the tear duct. The drainage may flow spontaneously or with pressure on the area.
- Pain below the eye.
- Redness and swelling of the tear duct.
- Redness of the white of the eye surrounding the tear duct.

CAUSES—Obstruction of the tear duct resulting from the following:
- Inherited abnormality.
- Bacterial infection of the duct.
- Sinus or nasal infection, especially chronic nasal infection.
- Nasal polyps.
- Eye injury.
- Eye infection, including severe pink eye (conjunctivitis).
- Fracture of the nose or facial bones.

RISK INCREASES WITH
- Newborns and infants, especially those with a family history of blocked tear ducts.
- Recent infection, such as those listed above.

HOW TO PREVENT—Obtain prompt medical treatment for eye, nose or sinus infections.

 WHAT TO EXPECT

APPROPRIATE HEALTH CARE
- Home care after diagnosis.
- Doctor's treatment.
- Surgery to dilate and probe the tear-duct canal. In infants, this usually requires a brief general anesthesia in an out-patient surgical facility. In adults, it is often done in the doctor's office with local anesthesia.

After dilation, the tear-duct system is irrigated with saline.

Complete obstruction may require a surgical opening from the eye into the nasal passage.

DIAGNOSTIC MEASURES
- Your own observation of symptoms.
- Medical history and physical exam by a doctor.

POSSIBLE COMPLICATIONS
- Without treatment, an obstruction may cause chronic infection.
- Without treatment, infection may spread to the cornea and other parts of the eye or permanently scar the tear duct.

PROBABLE OUTCOME
- Infection is usually curable with antibiotics.
- Obstruction is usually curable with dilation of the duct or surgery. Allow 3 weeks for recovery.

 HOW TO TREAT

NOTE—Follow your doctor's instructions. These instructions are supplemental.

GENERAL MEASURES
- For obstruction (if surgery is not necessary): Massage the tear duct twice a day with fingertips to milk the contents.
- For infection: Relieve pain by applying warm soaks (see Appendix 18).

MEDICATION—Your doctor may prescribe oral or topical antibiotics for infection.

ACTIVITY—Reduce activity during treatment for the infection. Avoid swimming and contact sports.

DIET—No special diet.

 CALL YOUR DOCTOR IF

- You have symptoms of a tear-duct infection or blockage.
- You have a temperature of 101F (38.3C) or more.
- Symptoms don't improve, despite treatment.
- Your vision is affected.

ILLNESSES & DISORDERS

TEETHING
(Cutting Teeth; Tooth Eruption)

GENERAL INFORMATION

DEFINITION—Sequential appearance of baby teeth and adult teeth. New teeth erupt continually from age 6 months to 3 years. Between ages 6 and 12, children lose baby teeth, which are replaced with adult teeth.

BODY PARTS INVOLVED—Mouth; teeth.

SEX OR AGE MOST AFFECTED—Both sexes of children from ages 6 months to 3 years and 6 to 12 years.

SIGNS & SYMPTOMS
- Excess saliva production and drooling.
- Pain. (This symptom cannot be proved, but probably does occur.)
- Blood or blood blisters at the site of tooth eruption (rarely). This usually requires no treatment.

Signs & symptoms *not* related to teething:
- Fever.
- Infection.
- Personality or sleep disturbance. These problems are most likely occurring concurrently; there is no cause-and-effect relationship.

CAUSES—Normal physiological development.

RISK INCREASES WITH—Teething problems are not related to any known risk factor.

HOW TO PREVENT—Teething problems cannot be prevented, but symptoms can be relieved.

OTHER—The sequence of normal tooth eruption in children is:
- First teeth (lower front teeth) at about 6 months, sooner in girls than boys.
- First adult teeth at about age 6.
- Bicuspids (side teeth) between ages 10 and 12.
- Permanent molars at about age 12.

WHAT TO EXPECT

APPROPRIATE HEALTH CARE
- Home care for teething discomfort.
- Dentist's treatment (complications only).

DIAGNOSTIC MEASURES—Your own observation of teething symptoms.

POSSIBLE COMPLICATIONS
- If not cared for properly, baby teeth may decay and need filling.
- Teething may be misdiagnosed as a fever-causing illness.

PROBABLE OUTCOME—Teething discomfort can be partially relieved.

HOW TO TREAT

NOTE—Follow your doctor's instructions. These instructions are supplemental.

GENERAL MEASURES
- Rub the child's gums with your finger; this is very comforting.
- Freeze a coarse washcloth and allow the child to chew it.
- Offer the child a teething biscuit or teething ring (you may chill it).
- Don't use any *imported,* fluid-filled teething rings—even if they are less expensive. The liquid inside may be contaminated.
- Clean new teeth with a cotton swab and water if you notice any collection of tartar. Otherwise, wait until the child is 2 or 3 years old before brushing teeth regularly. By this age, children want to imitate parents by brushing teeth.
- Begin regular dental visits at age 2 or 3.
- At age 5, explain to the child that losing baby teeth is normal. This prevents the child from becoming concerned when tooth loss begins.

MEDICATION—Medicine usually is not necessary for teething discomfort. Don't use tooth powder, ointment or cream to relieve discomfort.

ACTIVITY—No restrictions.

DIET—No special diet.

📞 CALL YOUR DOCTOR IF

- The child's temperature rises above normal.
- Signs of infection, such as pain, pus, excessive swelling, or very red gums, occur at the site of the erupting tooth.

TELOGEN EFFLUVIUM

GENERAL INFORMATION

DEFINITION—Generalized hair loss in which numerous, scattered hair follicles simultaneously change from the growing phase to the resting stage of the hair-growth cycle. Persons with telogen effluvium rarely progress to significant baldness, and it is not contagious.

BODY PARTS INVOLVED—Hair; scalp.

SEX OR AGE MOST AFFECTED—Both sexes and all ages but most common in young females (age 8 through adolescence).

SIGNS & SYMPTOMS
● Hair loss of 4 to 5 times the normal rate. Normal hair loss is approximately 400 hairs a day, mostly during washing or brushing.
● No itching or pain.

CAUSES
● Hormonal changes, such as those that occur during adolescence, following childbirth or after discontinuing use of oral contraceptives.
● Severe psychological stress—including that of serious illness, such as high fever, heart attack or stroke.

RISK INCREASES WITH
● Stress.
● Pregnancy.
● Menopause.

HOW TO PREVENT—No specific preventive measures.

WHAT TO EXPECT

APPROPRIATE HEALTH CARE—Self-care.

DIAGNOSTIC MEASURES
● Your own observation of symptoms.
● Medical history and physical exam by a doctor (severe, prolonged cases only).

POSSIBLE COMPLICATIONS—None expected.

PROBABLE OUTCOME—Spontaneous recovery in 6 to 12 months.

HOW TO TREAT

NOTE—Follow your doctor's instructions. These instructions are supplemental.

GENERAL MEASURES
● Continue to wash and brush your hair as usual.
● Confront and define areas of conflict in your family life, occupational and leisure-time activities. If you cannot resolve conflicts, ask for help from family, friends or competent counselors.
● Aim for a balance of work, recreation, reflection and rest.
● Concentrate on feeling positive. A good attitude toward yourself and others is a powerful asset.

MEDICATION—Medicine usually is not necessary for this disorder.

ACTIVITY—No restrictions. Engage in a regular exercise program at least 3 times a week to reduce stress and maintain good overall fitness.

DIET—No special diet or supplements. Eat a normal, well-balanced diet to provide the nutrients necessary for healthy hair growth.

CALL YOUR DOCTOR IF

● Hair loss doesn't improve in 4 months.
● Signs of infection (pain, redness, tenderness, swelling) begin at the site of hair loss.

ILLNESSES & DISORDERS

TEMPORO-MANDIBULAR JOINT SYNDROME (TMJ)
(Myofascial Pain-Dysfunction Syndrome; MPD)

 GENERAL INFORMATION

DEFINITION—Pain and inflammation in the temporo-mandibular joint (the joint on either side of the jaw that opens and closes the mouth) and adjoining muscles.

BODY PARTS INVOLVED—Temporo-mandibular joint; facial muscles; sensory nerves.

SEX OR AGE MOST AFFECTED—Adults of both sexes, but more common in women.

SIGNS & SYMPTOMS
- Dull, aching pain on one side of the jaw (below the ear) that radiates to the temples, back of the head and along the jaw line.
- Tenderness of the muscles used to chew.
- "Clicking" or "popping" sounds when opening the mouth.
- Inability to open the jaw completely.

CAUSES—Grinding teeth and contracting jaw muscles in an unconscious attempt to:
- Relieve muscle tension caused by stress.
- Correct a faulty alignment ("bite") between the upper and lower jaws.

RISK INCREASES WITH
- Stress.
- Osteoarthritis.

HOW TO PREVENT—Don't grind your teeth. Learn techniques for relaxing muscles and relieving tension, such as biofeedback, meditation and exercise.

 WHAT TO EXPECT

APPROPRIATE HEALTH CARE
- Self-care after diagnosis.
- Doctor's or dentist's treatment. Your dentist may manufacture, fit and install a night-guard prosthesis to prevent tooth-grinding while asleep. A night-guard prosthesis consists of removable splints that fit over the tops of the teeth to eliminate incorrect biting pressure.
- Psychotherapy or counseling, including biofeedback training, to learn new ways to cope with stress.

DIAGNOSTIC MEASURES
- Your own observation of symptoms.
- Medical history and physical exam by a doctor or dentist.
- X-rays of the temporo-mandibular joint.

POSSIBLE COMPLICATIONS—Without treatment, bone in the temporo-mandibular joint may erode and deteriorate.

PROBABLE OUTCOME—With treatment, symptoms can be controlled, and behavior that produces symptoms can be modified. A jaw misalignment can also be corrected.

 HOW TO TREAT

NOTE—Follow your doctor's instructions. These instructions are supplemental.

GENERAL MEASURES—No specific instructions except those listed under other headings.

MEDICATION
- Your doctor may prescribe:
  Tranquilizers or muscle relaxants for a short time.
  Non-steroidal anti-inflammatory drugs.
- For minor pain, you may use non-prescription drugs, such as aspirin or acetaminophen.

ACTIVITY—No restrictions.

DIET—Eat a soft diet (see Appendix 11) until symptoms subside.

 CALL YOUR DOCTOR OR DENTIST IF

- You have symptoms of temporo-mandibular joint syndrome.
- New, unexplained symptoms develop. Drugs used in treatment may produce side effects.

TENDINITIS

GENERAL INFORMATION

DEFINITION—Painful inflammation of a tendon (ligament). Tendon fibers merge into muscle fibers. A typical skeletal muscle has a tendon on each end that attaches to bone. The force of a muscle contraction is transmitted through the tendon to produce movement.

BODY PARTS INVOLVED—Tendons; bones; joints.

SEX OR AGE MOST AFFECTED—Adolescents and adults.

SIGNS & SYMPTOMS
● Restricted movement, tenderness and swelling around the inflamed tendon. Common sites are the shoulder, elbow, Achilles' tendon or hamstring.
● Weakness in the tendon caused by calcium deposits that often accompany tendinitis.

CAUSES
● Injury, usually from strenuous athletic activity.
● Musculo-skeletal disorders, including congenital defects and rheumatism.
● Poor posture.

RISK INCREASES WITH
● Overuse of certain tendons and joints from participation in active, competitive sports.
● Incorrect movement and strain during activity. For example, repeatedly holding and swinging a tennis racket incorrectly may cause tendinitis at the elbow (tennis elbow).

HOW TO PREVENT
● Precondition your body and build up strength gradually for a sport before beginning it on a regular, competitive basis.
● Warm up before each workout.
● Learn the proper techniques for any sport you intend to play regularly.

WHAT TO EXPECT

APPROPRIATE HEALTH CARE
● Self-care for mild cases.
● Doctor's treatment, if self-care is not successful.

DIAGNOSTIC MEASURES
● Your own observation of symptoms.
● Medical history and physical exam by a doctor.
● X-rays of the involved area.

POSSIBLE COMPLICATIONS—Large deposits of calcium in the inflamed tendon, leading to permanent impairment ("frozen joint").

PROBABLE OUTCOME—Usually curable with treatment and rest of the tendon. Allow 6 weeks for healing.

HOW TO TREAT

NOTE—Follow your doctor's instructions. These instructions are supplemental.

GENERAL MEASURES—Treatment varies with the cause, severity and duration of the condition:
● With severe pain, stiffness and tenderness, relax completely with the injured area resting in a splint or on a pillow until pain becomes more bearable.
● Apply ice packs to the affected area during the acute stage or after receiving injections.
● When pain diminishes, wear a sling or use crutches until pain becomes bearable.
● After the acute phase, apply heat. Take hot showers, apply hot compresses, use a heat lamp or heating pad, or rub in deep-heating ointment.
● If you have a shoulder injury, perform shoulder exercises that your doctor or physical therapist will give you. If done conscientiously, these exercises help prevent stiffness and increase strength.

MEDICATION—Your doctor may prescribe:
● Anti-inflammatory drugs.
● Pain relievers.
● Injections of local anesthetics.
● Injections of cortisone into painful and calcified tendons. This reduces pain and inflammation and allows movement, preventing a frozen joint.

ACTIVITY—Resume your normal activities as soon as symptoms improve.

DIET—No special diet.

CALL YOUR DOCTOR IF

● You have symptoms of tendinitis.
● Pain and swelling increases, despite treatment.
● New, unexplained symptoms develop. Drugs used in treatment may produce side effects.

ILLNESSES & DISORDERS

TENNIS ELBOW
(Epicondylitis)

GENERAL INFORMATION

DEFINITION—Inflammation of bony areas of the elbow.

BODY PARTS INVOLVED—Elbow muscles, tendons and epicondyle (a bony prominence on the outside of the elbow where muscles of the forearm attach to the bone of the upper arm).

SEX OR AGE MOST AFFECTED—Adults (20 to 40 years).

SIGNS & SYMPTOMS
- Pain and tenderness over the epicondyle.
- Weak grip.
- Pain when twisting the hand and arm, as in using a screwdriver or playing tennis.

CAUSES—Partial tear of the tendon and attached covering of the bone caused by:
- Chronic stress on the tissues that attach the forearm muscles to the elbow area.
- Sudden strain on the forearm.

RISK INCREASES WITH
- Occupations that require strenuous forearm movement, such as mechanics or carpentry.
- Participation in sports that require strenuous forearm movement, such as tennis.
- Poor physical conditioning.

HOW TO PREVENT
- Don't play sports, such as tennis, for long periods until you are in excellent condition. Take frequent rest periods.
- Do forearm conditioning exercises to build your strength gradually.
- Warm up slowly and completely before participating in sports—especially before competition.
- Use a tennis-elbow strap when you resume normal activity after treatment.

WHAT TO EXPECT

APPROPRIATE HEALTH CARE
- Self-care after diagnosis.
- Doctor's treatment.
- Physical therapy.
- Surgery (rare).

DIAGNOSTIC MEASURES
- Your own observation of symptoms.
- Medical history and physical exam by a doctor.
- X-rays of the elbow.

POSSIBLE COMPLICATIONS—Complete ligament tear, requiring surgery to repair.

PROBABLE OUTCOME—Usually curable, but treatment may require 3 to 6 months.

HOW TO TREAT

NOTE—Follow your doctor's instructions. These instructions are supplemental.

GENERAL MEASURES
- Use heat to relieve pain. Use warm soaks (see Appendix 18), a heat lamp or soak in a whirlpool.
- You may receive diathermy (see Glossary), ultrasound (see Glossary) or massage treatments in your doctor's office or a physical-therapy facility. These may bring quicker symptom relief and healing.
- You may need to wear a forearm splint to immobilize the elbow.
  Do the following exercise 3 or 4 times a day while wearing the splint: Stretch your arm, flex your wrist, then press the back of your hand against a wall. Hold for 1 minute.

MEDICATIONS—Your doctor may prescribe:
- Non-steroidal anti-inflammatory drugs to reduce inflammation.
- Injections of anesthetics or cortisone drugs. Cortisone reduces inflammation, and anesthetics temporarily relieve pain. Caution: Repeated injections may weaken the muscle ligament.

ACTIVITY—Don't repeat the activity that caused tennis elbow until symptoms disappear. Then resume your normal activities gradually after proper conditioning.

DIET—No special diet.

CALL YOUR DOCTOR IF

- You have symptoms of tennis elbow.
- Symptoms don't improve in 2 weeks, despite treatment.

TESTES, UNDESCENDED
(Cryptorchidism)

 GENERAL INFORMATION

DEFINITION—A disorder present at birth in which one or both testicles have not descended from the pelvis into their normal position in the scrotum. 3% of full-term newborn males and 30% of premature newborn males have undescended testes. Most descend spontaneously without treatment by age 1.

BODY PARTS INVOLVED—One or both testes (testicles); scrotum; spermatic cord.

SEX OR AGE MOST AFFECTED—Male infants and children.

SIGNS & SYMPTOMS
● Scrotum appears undeveloped on one or both sides.
● Testicle can't be felt in its normal position in the scrotum.

CAUSES—Unknown, but probably related to hormone deficiency in the mother or fetus.

RISK INCREASES WITH—Unknown.

HOW TO PREVENT—No specific preventive measures.

 WHAT TO EXPECT

APPROPRIATE HEALTH CARE
● Doctor's treatment.
● Surgery to move the testes into the scrotum.

DIAGNOSTIC MEASURES
● Your own observation of symptoms.
● Medical history and physical exam by a doctor.
● Laboratory blood studies of gonadotrophin (hormone) levels. Normal levels indicate normally functioning testes which are undescended. Abnormal levels indicate a congenital absence of testes.

POSSIBLE COMPLICATIONS
● Increased likehood of testicular cancer.
● Sterility, if testes are not repositioned before puberty.
● Psychological problems associated with an altered male self-image, if the problem is not corrected.
● Lack of normal sexual development, if testes are not present.

PROBABLE OUTCOME—Usually curable if treated before puberty with surgery or hormones.

 HOW TO TREAT

NOTE—Follow your doctor's instructions. These instructions are supplemental.

GENERAL MEASURES—Surgery is the only treatment for those who don't respond to hormone treatment. Surgery ideally should be performed at about age 5 and *must* be performed prior to puberty to preserve reproductive function.

MEDICATION—Your doctor may prescribe human chorionic gonadotrophins by injection. These are usually given 3 times a week for 4 to 6 weeks. This treatment causes testes to descend normally in about 25% of cases.

ACTIVITY—No restrictions.

DIET—No special diet.

 CALL YOUR DOCTOR IF

Your child has undescended testes. Call as soon as you identify this abnormality.

TESTICLE, CANCER OF
(Testicular Cancer)

GENERAL INFORMATION

DEFINITION—Uncontrolled growth of malignant cells in the testicle. There are several types of testicular cancer, some more dangerous than others.

This is the most common form of cancer in young men.

BODY PARTS INVOLVED—Testicles (usually one only).

SEX OR AGE MOST AFFECTED—Older adolescent and young adult males.

SIGNS & SYMPTOMS
● A firm swelling in one testicle discovered by accident or by self-examination.
● No pain (usually).

CAUSES—Unknown.

RISK INCREASES WITH—Undescended testicle(s) in infancy—even if the testicle was surgically moved into the scrotum.

HOW TO PREVENT—Males should examine testicles routinely at least once a month.

WHAT TO EXPECT

APPROPRIATE HEALTH CARE
● Doctor's treatment.
● Surgery to remove the cancerous testicle.
● Radiation therapy or chemotherapy for some types of tumors.
● Hospitalization for treatment.

DIAGNOSTIC MEASURES
● Your own observation of symptoms. Testicular self-examination is the most important diagnostic measure.
● Medical history and physical exam by a doctor.
● Laboratory and radioactive studies of hormone levels.
● Biopsy (see Glossary).
● X-rays of the chest or kidneys to determine if cancer has spread.

POSSIBLE COMPLICATIONS—Without treatment, some tumors may spread to other parts of the body.

PROBABLE OUTCOME—Most types of testicular tumors are curable with surgery and other treatment. A few types are extremely malignant and have a high death rate unless discovered and treated early.

Removal of one testicle does not interfere with normal sexual function or the ability to have normal children.

HOW TO TREAT

NOTE—Follow your doctor's instructions. These instructions are supplemental.

GENERAL MEASURES—No special instructions except those listed under other headings.

MEDICATION—Your doctor may prescribe anticancer drugs for some types of tumors.

ACTIVITY
● Resume your normal activities as soon as possible. Radiation and chemotherapy may cause temporary fatigue requiring extra rest.
● Resume sexual relations when you are able. Contraception may be necessary for 12 to 18 months because some forms of treatment cause temporary genetic damage to sperm in the remaining testicle.

DIET—No special diet.

CALL YOUR DOCTOR IF

● You have a firm swelling or mass in the scrotum.
● New, unexplained symptoms develop. Drugs used in treatment may produce side effects.

TESTICLE TORSION

GENERAL INFORMATION

DEFINITION—Twisting of the spermatic cord of the testicle, damaging the testicle—sometimes irreversibly. Testicle torsion usually occurs on one side only. Prompt treatment is necessary to salvage the affected testicle.

BODY PARTS INVOLVED—Testicle; spermatic cord; blood supply to each.

SEX OR AGE MOST AFFECTED—Males of all ages, but most common in adolescents (12 to 20 years).

SIGNS & SYMPTOMS
- Sudden pain in one testicle.
- Swelling, redness and tenderness of the scrotum.
- Nausea and vomiting.
- Sweating.
- Rapid heartbeat, if pain is severe.

CAUSES—Usually unknown. It is occasionally present at birth, or may rarely be caused by an injury or sudden, forceful contraction of muscles attached to the testicle and spermatic cord.

RISK INCREASES WITH—Unknown.

HOW TO PREVENT—Wear an athletic supporter or cup when participating in contact sports to prevent genital injury.

WHAT TO EXPECT

APPROPRIATE HEALTH CARE
- Doctor's treatment.
- Surgery to untangle the twisted spermatic cord, and to attach the affected testicle to the inside scrotal wall, which prevents recurrence. The surgeon will probably operate on the unaffected testicle also to prevent torsion.

DIAGNOSTIC MEASURES
- Your own observation of symptoms.
- Medical history and physical exam by a doctor.

POSSIBLE COMPLICATIONS—Death of cells in the testicle caused by a diminished or blocked blood supply. This strangulation requires removal of the affected testicle and spermatic cord.

PROBABLE OUTCOME—Sometimes the torsion will correct itself, symptoms will disappear and no treatment will be needed. However, the testicle is usually injured beyond repair unless surgery is done within 3 to 4 hours after symptoms begin.

If one testicle must be removed, the remaining healthy testicle should provide enough hormones for normal male maturation, sex life and reproduction.

HOW TO TREAT

NOTE—Follow your doctor's instructions. These instructions are supplemental.

GENERAL MEASURES
- After surgery, use ice packs to relieve pain and swelling. Wrap the ice in plastic. Apply it to the affected side, separating the ice from the skin with a cloth towel. Apply ice 5 to 10 minutes at a time. Repeat as often as necessary.
- Return to your doctor for suture removal in about 7 days.

MEDICATION—After surgery, your doctor may prescribe pain relievers.

ACTIVITY—Resume your normal activities gradually after surgery.

DIET—No special diet.

CALL YOUR DOCTOR IF

- You have symptoms of testicular torsion. This is an emergency!
- Signs of infection begin after surgery. These include fever, chills, muscle aches, headache, dizziness and a general ill feeling.
- Excessive bleeding occurs at the surgical site.

TETANUS
(Lockjaw)

GENERAL INFORMATION

DEFINITION—An infection in a wound or injury that causes severe muscle spasms. Tetanus is not contagious from person to person.

BODY PARTS INVOLVED—Injured tissue; muscles throughout the body, especially the jaw, neck, back and abdomen.

SEX OR AGE MOST AFFECTED—Both sexes; all ages.

SIGNS & SYMPTOMS
- Muscle pain, irritability and frequent, severe spasms.
- Severe swallowing difficulty.
- Fever.
- Difficulty using chest muscles to breathe.

CAUSES—Bacteria (clostridium tetani) that are present almost everywhere—especially in soil, manure or dust. They enter the body through a puncture caused by a nail or other object. Toxins produced by the bacteria travel to nerves that control muscle contraction, producing muscle spasms and seizures.

RISK INCREASES WITH
- Diabetes mellitus.
- Adults over 60.
- Lack of up-to-date tetanus immunizations.
- Warm, humid weather.
- Crowded or unsanitary living conditions, especially for newborn infants born to non-immunized mothers.
- Use of street drugs administered with unclean needles and syringes.

HOW TO PREVENT—Obtain tetanus immunizations. These consist of 3 immunization shots, with a booster shot every 10 years. An additional booster shot may be necessary at the time of injury. Private doctors or local health departments may provide immunizations at little or no cost.

WHAT TO EXPECT

APPROPRIATE HEALTH CARE
- Doctor's treatment.
- Surgery to remove infected tissue.
- Hospitalization in a quiet, dark room. Treatment may include the use of breathing tubes, a respirator and 24-hour nursing care.

DIAGNOSTIC MEASURES
- Your own observation of symptoms.
- Medical history and physical exam by a doctor.

POSSIBLE COMPLICATIONS
- Pneumonia.
- Pressure sores.
- Irregular heartbeat.
- Respiratory paralysis and death.

PROBABLE OUTCOME—The death rate from tetanus is 50%. With early diagnosis and treatment, however, full recovery is likely. Allow 4 weeks for recovery.

HOW TO TREAT

NOTE—Follow your doctor's instructions. These instructions are supplemental.

GENERAL MEASURES—Provide the patient with reassurance and psychological support. Despite the seriousness of tetanus, patients are usually conscious.

MEDICATION—Your doctor may prescribe:
- Antitoxins to neutralize the nerve toxin.
- Muscle relaxants to control spasms.
- Sedatives to relieve anxiety.

ACTIVITY—During hospitalization, bed rest is necessary with as little disturbance as possible. During recovery, activities should be resumed gradually.

DIET—During hospitalization, intravenous fluids will be necessary because of swallowing difficulty.

CALL YOUR DOCTOR IF

- You have symptoms of tetanus or observe them in someone else. Call immediately. This is an emergency!.
- You or someone in your family needs basic or booster tetanus immunizations.
- You have a puncture wound or injury that breaks the skin, and you have not had an immunization or booster in 5 years.

THALASSEMIA
(Mediterranean Anemia; Hereditary Leptocytosis)

 GENERAL INFORMATION

DEFINITION—An inherited form of anemia in which red blood cells contain less hemoglobin than normal.

BODY PARTS INVOLVED—Blood.

SEX OR AGE MOST AFFECTED—Both sexes; all ages.

SIGNS & SYMPTOMS
- Fatigue.
- Paleness.
- Breathlessness.
- Irregular heartbeat, especially with exertion.
- Bloody or dark urine.
- Jaundice (yellow skin and eyes).
- Leg ulcers.
- Enlarged spleen.

CAUSES
- Destruction of abnormal blood cells in the spleen and other sites.
- Inadequate manufacture of normal amounts of hemoglobin-A.

RISK INCREASES WITH
- Poor nutrition, especially a diet likely to produce other anemias.
- Obesity.
- Family history of thalassemia.
- Genetic factors, including absence of the gene necessary to manufacture hemoglobin-A. The disorder first appeared in persons of Mediterranean heritage; it also affects people from the Middle East and Far East.

HOW TO PREVENT—Cannot be prevented at present, especially if the mother *and* father have thalassemia or the thalassemia genetic trait. If you have a family history of thalassemia, obtain genetic counseling before having children.

 WHAT TO EXPECT

APPROPRIATE HEALTH CARE
- Self-care.
- Doctor's treatment.
- Hospitalization for repeated transfusions as needed.

DIAGNOSTIC MEASURES
- Your own observation of symptoms.
- Medical history and physical exam by a doctor.
- Laboratory blood tests and bone-marrow examinations.

POSSIBLE COMPLICATIONS
- Many years of thalassemia produce gallstones.
- Repeated transfusions increase the risk of transfusion reaction or kidney damage.

PROBABLE OUTCOME—This condition is currently considered incurable. However, symptoms can be relieved or controlled. It usually causes death by early adulthood or middle age, depending on the severity of the symptoms.

Scientific research into causes and treatment continues, so there is hope for increasingly effective treatment and cure.

 HOW TO TREAT

NOTE—Follow your doctor's instructions. These instructions are supplemental.

GENERAL MEASURES—The only treatment for thalassemia is periodic hospitalization for blood transfusions when symptoms become disabling.

MEDICATION—Medicine usually is not necessary for this disorder. For minor pain, you may use non-prescription drugs such as acetaminophen.

ACTIVITY—After treatment, resume normal activity as soon as possible.

DIET—No special diet. Don't take iron supplements; they make symptoms worse.

 CALL YOUR DOCTOR IF

You have symptoms of anemia (fatigue, paleness, irregular heartbeat, breathlessness).

ILLNESSES & DISORDERS

THORACIC-OUTLET-OBSTRUCTION SYNDROME
(Cervical-Rib Syndrome)

 GENERAL INFORMATION

DEFINITION—Pain and weakness from compression of nerves in the neck that affect the shoulders, arms and hands.

BODY PARTS INVOLVED—Nerves and blood vessels that supply the neck, shoulders, arms and hands.

SEX OR AGE MOST AFFECTED—Adults between ages 35 and 55, usually women.

SIGNS & SYMPTOMS
- Pain, numbness and tingling in the neck, shoulders, arms and hands.
- Weakness in the arms and hands.
- Poor blood circulation, characterized by coldness, swelling and blueness in the hands and fingers.
- Absent pulse in the wrist when raising the arm and turning the head toward the opposite shoulder.

CAUSES—The nerves and blood vessels that supply the shoulder, arms and hands start in the neck and pass as a bundle near the cervical ribs and collarbone. Pressure on this nerve and blood-vessel bundle creates symptoms. Pressure may be caused by:
- An extra rib in the lower neck or overdeveloped neck muscles.
- Muscle weakness and drooping in the shoulder.
- Prolonged, abnormal position of the neck or arm, as during surgery with general anesthesia.
- Injury from overextending the arm or shoulder.
- Tumor that has spread to the head and neck area from another part of the body.

RISK INCREASES WITH
- Recent unconsciousness from illness, injury, or alcohol or drug use.
- Recent surgery with general anesthesia.

HOW TO PREVENT
- Avoid shoulder and neck injury whenever possible. Wear seat belts and use padded headrests in cars.
- Don't use mind-altering drugs or drink excessive amounts of alcohol.

 WHAT TO EXPECT

APPROPRIATE HEALTH CARE
- Doctor's treatment.
- Surgery to relieve pressure on the nerves and blood vessels (rare).
- Exercise and physical therapy.

DIAGNOSTIC MEASURES
- Your own observation of symptoms.
- Medical history and physical exam by a doctor.
- X-rays of the neck and shoulder area to look for an extra cervical rib or tumor.

POSSIBLE COMPLICATIONS—If the disorder is caused by a tumor or an extra cervical rib, treatment may be unsuccessful. These can cause permanent numbness or loss of full arm or hand strength, or gangrene in the fingers (rare).

PROBABLE OUTCOME—Usually curable in most patients with physical therapy or surgery.

 HOW TO TREAT

NOTE—Follow your doctor's instructions. These instructions are supplemental.

GENERAL MEASURES—Use heat to relieve pain. Use a heating pad, heat lamp, hot showers or warm compresses.

MEDICATION—You may use non-prescription drugs, such as acetaminophen or aspirin, to relieve pain. Medication cannot correct the underlying condition.

ACTIVITY—Your doctor will prescribe physical therapy and exercises.

DIET—No special diet.

 CALL YOUR DOCTOR IF

- You have symptoms of thoracic-outlet-obstruction syndrome.
- Symptoms don't improve in 2 weeks, despite treatment.

THROMBOCYTOPENIA

GENERAL INFORMATION

DEFINITION—Reduction of platelets in the blood, which reduces blood clotting and increases the risk of bleeding.

BODY PARTS INVOLVED—Blood, which affects all body parts.

SEX OR AGE MOST AFFECTED—Both sexes; all ages.

SIGNS & SYMPTOMS
- Abnormal bleeding in the mouth.
- A rash of pinpoint-size dots that doesn't fade when the skin is pressed.
- Unexplained bruising.
- Spontaneous nosebleeds.
- Blood in the urine.
- Unexplained vaginal bleeding.
- Black, tarry stools.
- Signs of anemia: weakness, fatigue, paleness (if bleeding is prolonged).

CAUSES—Frequently unknown. The following often precede the disorder:
- Allergies.
- Virus infections.
- Use of drugs, such as: non-steroidal anti-inflammatory drugs including ibuprofen, aspirin, indomethacin, phenylbutazone; tricyclic antidepressants; antihistamines; phenothiazines.
- Collagen disorders, such as lupus erythematosus.
- Blood transfusions and surgery.
- Blood poisoning.
- Liver disease.
- Radiation treatment for cancer.
- Enlarged spleen from any cause.
- Uremia.
- Scurvy.
- Pernicious anemia.
- Leukemia.

RISK INCREASES WITH
- Family history of bleeding disorders.
- Use of any drug.
- Poor nutrition.

HOW TO PREVENT
- Avoid any drug which has lowered your platelet count in the past.
- Take only drugs that are necessary.
- Eat a well-balanced diet.

WHAT TO EXPECT

APPROPRIATE HEALTH CARE
- Doctor's treatment.
- Hospitalization to transfuse platelets.
- Self-care after diagnosis.

DIAGNOSTIC MEASURES
- Your own observation of symptoms.
- Medical history and physical exam by a doctor.
- Laboratory blood studies.

POSSIBLE COMPLICATIONS—The spleen may enlarge and require surgical removal.

PROBABLE OUTCOME—Usually curable in 2 to 3 weeks if the cause can be treated.

HOW TO TREAT

NOTE—Follow your doctor's instructions. These instructions are supplemental.

GENERAL MEASURES
- To stop bleeding at any accessible site, apply cold compresses or ice packs and pressure until bleeding stops.
- Inform any doctor or dentist who treats you that you have thrombocytopenia.
- Avoid surgery, including dental surgery, unless it is essential.
- Avoid injections. If a shot is necessary, apply pressure continuously to the injection site for 5 minutes.
- Avoid injury whenever possible.

MEDICATION
- Stop taking all drugs, including non-prescription drugs (especially aspirin) and vitamins.
- Your doctor may prescribe cortisone drugs to reduce the body's autoimmune response.

ACTIVITY
- Don't engage in contact sports.
- Avoid overexertion or dehydration.
- If your occupation involves a risk of injury, don't go to work until you are cured.

DIET—No special diet.

CALL YOUR DOCTOR IF

- You have symptoms of thrombocytopenia.
- The following occurs during treatment:
  Bleeding that can't be stopped.
  Enlargement of the abdomen.
  Black, tarry stools or vomit that looks like coffee grounds.
  A rash (described under Signs & Symptoms)—especially if fever is present.
- New, unexplained symptoms develop. Drugs used in treatment may produce side effects.

ILLNESSES & DISORDERS

THROMBOPHLEBITIS, SUPERFICIAL
(Phlebitis; Phlebothrombosis)

GENERAL INFORMATION

DEFINITION—Inflammation and small blood clots in a superficial vein, usually caused by infection or injury. This type of inflammation seldom causes clots to break loose and flow in the bloodstream, as does deep-vein thrombosis.

BODY PARTS INVOLVED—Superficial veins, usually in the legs.

SEX OR AGE MOST AFFECTED
- Both sexes, but more common in females.
- All ages, but most common in adults.

SIGNS & SYMPTOMS
- Hardness of a superficial vein (feels like a cord).
- Redness, tenderness and pain in the affected area.
- Fever (sometimes).

CAUSES—Increased fibrin and clotting of red blood cells in a vein due to:
- Injury to the vein's membrane lining from injections. This allows bacteria to enter.
- Spread of malignant blood cancer.
- Pooling of blood following surgery or prolonged bed rest.

RISK INCREASES WITH
- Illness with prolonged bed confinement.
- Smoking.
- Use of birth-control pills. The combination of birth-control pills and smoking greatly increases the risk.

HOW TO PREVENT
- Don't smoke if you take birth-control pills.
- If confined to bed for any reason, move the legs as much as possible to prevent pooling of blood in the veins.
- Don't use any drug intravenously, if you can avoid it.

OTHER—Repeated episodes may indicate pancreatic cancer.

WHAT TO EXPECT

APPROPRIATE HEALTH CARE
- Doctor's treatment.
- Self-care after diagnosis.

DIAGNOSTIC MEASURES
- Your own observation of symptoms.
- Medical history and physical exam by a doctor.
- Laboratory blood studies, if the cause is not immediately apparent.

POSSIBLE COMPLICATIONS—Embolism, in which part of the clot breaks off and travels through the bloodstream, lodging in the lung or elsewhere (extremely rare).

PROBABLE OUTCOME—Usually curable in 2 weeks.

HOW TO TREAT

NOTE—Follow your doctor's instructions. These instructions are supplemental.

GENERAL MEASURES
- Stop smoking and stop taking birth-control pills. If you continue both, the next episode of vein clots may be a dangerous, deep-vein clot.
- Wear elastic stockings or wrapped elastic bandages to hasten the blood flow through the veins, relieving discomfort and helping prevent further clot formation. Don't wear garters or knee-high hosiery.
- To relieve pain, use wrapped soaks (see Appendix 18).

MEDICATION—Your doctor may prescribe:
- Non-steroidal anti-inflammatory drugs to decrease inflammation and pain.
- Antibiotics, if bacterial infection is suspected (rare).

ACTIVITY—Bed rest with the affected limb elevated may be helpful for 1 or 2 days. Move the feet, ankles and legs often. When the inflammation begins to subside, resume normal activity slowly. Rest often. Don't sit or stand for prolonged periods, and don't cross legs.

DIET—No special diet.

CALL YOUR DOCTOR IF

- You have symptoms of superficial thrombophlebitis.
- The following occurs during treatment:
  Fever of 102F (38.9C) or higher.
  Intolerable pain.
  Coughing blood.
  Shortness of breath.
  Chest pain.
- New, unexplained symptoms develop. Drugs used in treatment may produce side effects.

THROMBOSIS, DEEP-VEIN

GENERAL INFORMATION

DEFINITION—A blood clot that forms inside a vein. It may partially or completely block blood flow, or break off and travel to the lung. This is different from clots in superficial veins, where clots rarely break off.

BODY PARTS INVOLVED—Usually lower legs (calves) or lower abdomen, but occasionally affects other veins in the body.

SEX OR AGE MOST AFFECTED—All ages, but most common in persons over age 60.

SIGNS & SYMPTOMS
- Swelling and pain in the area drained by the vein, usually the ankle, calf or thigh. Swelling in the leg includes everything below the clot, extending to the toes.
- Tenderness and redness of the affected parts.
- Soreness or pain when walking. The soreness does not disappear with rest.
- Pain when raising the leg and flexing the foot (sometimes).
- Fever (sometimes).
- Increased heartbeat (sometimes).

CAUSES—Pooling of blood in the vein, which triggers blood-clotting mechanisms. The pooling may occur after prolonged bed rest following surgery, or from debilitating illness, such as heart attack, stroke or bone fracture.

RISK INCREASES WITH
- Persons over 60.
- Obesity.
- Smoking.
- Use of estrogen in oral contraceptives or for replacement after menopause. This is especially hazardous if estrogen use is combined with smoking.

HOW TO PREVENT
- Avoid prolonged bed rest during illnesses. Start moving the lower limbs as soon as possible after any surgical procedure or during any bed-confining illness.
- On long auto or airplane trips, exercise your legs at least every 1 or 2 hours.
- Stop smoking, especially if you take estrogen for any purpose.

WHAT TO EXPECT

APPROPRIATE HEALTH CARE
- Doctor's treatment.
- Hospitalization for anticoagulant injections.
- Self-care after hospitalization.

DIAGNOSTIC MEASURES
- Your own observation of symptoms.
- Medical history and physical exam by a doctor.
- Laboratory studies, such as ultrasound, radioactive fibrinogen and prothrombin time (see Glossary for all).
- X-rays of veins after dye is injected into a foot vein.

POSSIBLE COMPLICATIONS—Pulmonary embolism, in which the clot breaks away and travels to the lung. The lung's blood supply is blocked, causing affected lung tissue to die.

PROBABLE OUTCOME—Usually curable with anticoagulant treatment, if pulmonary embolism can be avoided.

HOW TO TREAT

NOTE—Follow your doctor's instructions. These instructions are supplemental.

GENERAL MEASURES—The following suggestions apply after hospitalization or if the condition can be treated safely at home:
- Wear fitted elastic stockings or wrapped elastic bandages, but don't wear garters or knee-high hosiery.
- Don't cross your legs or ankles while sitting, lying in bed or traveling.
- Elevate the feet higher than the hips when sitting for long periods.
- Elevate the foot of the bed.

MEDICATION—After hospitalization, your doctor may prescribe oral anticoagulant drugs, such as coumarin. To minimize the danger of pulmonary embolism, blood tests to monitor the anticoagulant level are mandatory. Oral anticoagulants may be necessary up to 6 months.

ACTIVITY—Rest in bed until all signs of inflammation have disappeared. While resting, make it a habit to move leg muscles, bend ankles and wiggle toes.

DIET—No special diet.

CALL YOUR DOCTOR IF

- You have symptoms of deep-vein thrombosis.
- The following occurs during treatment:
  Unexpected bleeding anywhere.
  Chest pain.
  Coughing up blood.
  Shortness of breath.
  Continued or increased swelling and pain, despite treatment.
- New, unexplained symptoms develop. Drugs used in treatment may produce side effects.

ILLNESSES & DISORDERS

THROMBOSIS & EMBOLUS, ARTERIAL

 GENERAL INFORMATION

DEFINITION—Blood-clot formation in an artery (thrombosis) that may travel to distant organs (embolus).

BODY PARTS INVOLVED—Large or medium arteries anywhere in the body, especially arteries in the neck or arteries to the brain, intestine, legs, arms or kidney.

SEX OR AGE MOST AFFECTED—Adults of both sexes.

SIGNS & SYMPTOMS—The following depend on where the embolus lodges:
● Brain: temporary blindness, speaking difficulty, partial paralysis, hearing loss, headache and dizziness.
● Extremities: pain in the arm or calf after exercise (subsides with rest); weakness, numbness, burning and tingling sensations; weak or absent pulse beyond the blocked blood flow. These symptoms subside with rest.
● Intestine: abdominal pain; nausea; vomiting; and shock.

CAUSES—Clots may form with any condition that damages the smooth lining of a blood vessel. As the clot grows, small or large portions break away and are carried by the bloodstream to the brain, abdomen, extremities or other areas. Conditions that damage the blood-vessel lining include:
● Atherosclerosis (hardening of the arteries).
● Injury to a blood vessel from accident or surgery.

RISK INCREASES WITH
● Adults over 60.
● Smoking.
● High blood pressure.
● Diabetes mellitus.
● Previous transient ischemic attacks.

HOW TO PREVENT
● Follow suggestions to prevent atherosclerosis (in Illness section).
● If you have high blood pressure or diabetes mellitus, adhere to your treatment program to control the disease.
● Take anticoagulant drugs for a short time after injury or surgery to prevent blood clots.
● Exercise regularly (see Appendix 20) to keep blood vessels healthy.

 WHAT TO EXPECT

APPROPRIATE HEALTH CARE
● Self-care after diagnosis.
● Doctor's treatment.
● Surgery to repair or replace damaged blood vessels, or to remove an embolus by suction or bypass.

DIAGNOSTIC MEASURES
● Your own observation of symptoms.
● Medical history and physical exam by a doctor.
● Laboratory studies of blood clotting and blood flow.
● X-rays of arteries (angiography).

POSSIBLE COMPLICATIONS—Tissue death or gangrene in cells deprived of oxygen by a clot.

PROBABLE OUTCOME—Depends on the organs affected, size of the affected blood vessel and size of the embolus. Clots in the extremities can be removed with surgery, relieving symptoms. Clots to the brain, kidney and intestines often cause death or permanent disability before they can be removed.

 HOW TO TREAT

NOTE—Follow your doctor's instructions. These instructions are supplemental.

GENERAL MEASURES—Follow suggestions under Diet and Activity to maintain a healthy lifestyle.

MEDICATION—Your doctor may prescribe:
● Anticoagulants to thin the blood and reduce the chance of embolus.
● Aspirin (1 tablet a day). This reduces the chance of small clots to brain in men over 45.
● Vasodilators to widen blood vessels.

ACTIVITY—Complete rest is necessary until circulation is re-established by surgery or other treatment.

DIET—No special diet during recovery. However, atherosclerosis and diabetes require dietary control.

 CALL YOUR DOCTOR IF

● You have symptoms of arterial thrombosis or embolus.
● Symptoms return after surgery.
● New, unexplained symptoms develop. Drugs used in treatment may produce side effects.

THRUSH
(Oral Thrush)

GENERAL INFORMATION

DEFINITION—A common fungus infection of the mouth.

BODY PARTS INVOLVED—Mouth; gums; tongue; soft palate; cheeks; lips.

SEX OR AGE MOST AFFECTED—Newborns and infants, but may also affect older children and adults.

SIGNS & SYMPTOMS—Patches appear in the mouth with the following characteristics:
- Patches are white to creamy yellow and slightly raised. They are similar to milk curds, but they don't wipe off.
- Patches are not painful unless they are rubbed off. Then they leave small, painful ulcers.
- The mouth is dry.

CAUSES—A fungus called candida albicans, which may develop under the following circumstances:
- Treatment with antibiotics. This may upset the natural balance of organisms in the mouth and allow thrush to develop.
- Birth. Newborns may acquire the infection during passage through the birth canal—especially if the mother has a vaginal yeast infection. Thrush appears within hours or up to 7 days after birth.
- Aging. Older persons develop thrush because of lower natural resistance.

RISK INCREASES WITH
- Poor nutrition.
- Illness that has lowered resistance.
- Diabetes.
- Irritation from dentures.
- Use of immunosuppressive drugs.

HOW TO PREVENT—If you have had thrush and must take antibiotics, drink buttermilk or eat yogurt during treatment to replenish helpful bacteria in the digestive tract.

WHAT TO EXPECT

APPROPRIATE HEALTH CARE
- Self-care.
- Doctor's treatment if self-care is not successful.

DIAGNOSTIC MEASURES
- Your own observation of symptoms.
- Medical history and physical exam by a doctor.

POSSIBLE COMPLICATIONS—Can spread to vagina, skin, larynx, gastrointestinal tract or respiratory system.

PROBABLE OUTCOME—Treatment usually clears this infection in 3 days. It is not dangerous or serious, but it has a tendency to recur.

HOW TO TREAT

NOTE—Follow your doctor's instructions. These instructions are supplemental.

GENERAL MEASURES
- To avoid transmitting thrush to others, boil eating utensils or use disposable items. Boil anything that touches the mouth or saliva.
- Rinse the mouth with a salt solution (1/2 teaspoon salt to 8 ounces water) 3 times a day or more after eating.
- If an infant has the infection, boil bottle nipples separately for 20 minutes before the final sterilization.

MEDICATION
- Gently swab patches of thrush in the mouth with antiseptic mouthwash or non-prescription 1% gentian-violet solution.
- If these simple medicines don't cure the infection, your doctor may prescribe an antifungal drug, nystatin, to apply to the patches.

ACTIVITY—No restrictions.

DIET—No changes in infants. Older children and adults should maintain an adequate fluid intake with milk, liquid gelatin, ice cream, custard, water, tea or other beverages and foods that are easy to swallow. Use a straw for drinking if the patches are painful.

CALL YOUR DOCTOR IF

- Signs of dehydration (sunken eyes, poor elasticity of the skin and lethargy) appear in a child.
- An infant fails to gain weight or an unexplained weight loss occurs in an older person.
- Fever develops.
- Lesions on the skin or vagina appear.
- Signs of secondary bacterial infection (pain, redness, tenderness, swelling, sometimes fever) appear in the mouth.

ILLNESSES & DISORDERS

THUMB-SUCKING

GENERAL INFORMATION

DEFINITION—Placing the finger or thumb on the roof of the mouth behind the teeth and sucking with lips and teeth closed. Thumb-sucking is a behavior—not a disorder.

BODY PARTS INVOLVED—Mouth; teeth; tongue; pharynx; finger or thumb.

SEX OR AGE MOST AFFECTED—Children of both sexes up to age 12, but most common in young children.

SIGNS & SYMPTOMS—Protruding front teeth. Thumb-sucking may put enough pressure on front teeth to move them forward eventually.

CAUSES—Some psychiatrists believe thumb-sucking provides a mother substitute and is caused by a need to cling to the mother. Others believe it is an instinctive behavior that becomes habitual.

RISK INCREASES WITH—Lack of love and attention during infancy and childhood.

HOW TO PREVENT
- Provide a loving and secure environment for the child.
- Provide other comfort mechanisms early in infancy, such as orthodontic pacifiers designed to minimize tooth misalignment.

OTHER—Thumb-sucking does not cause serious damage until the permanent teeth begin cutting through gums at age 6 or 7. Most children have outgrown the habit by this age. If not, parents should work with the child to change the habit for the sake of appearance and dental health.

WHAT TO EXPECT

APPROPRIATE HEALTH CARE
- Home care.
- Doctor's or dentist's treatment.
- Psychotherapy or counseling (prolonged or excessive thumb-sucking only).

DIAGNOSTIC MEASURES
- Your own observation of symptoms.
- Medical history and physical exam by a doctor or dentist.

POSSIBLE COMPLICATIONS—Unsightly facial appearance without treatment.

PROBABLE OUTCOME—Protruding front teeth should improve in 6 months to 2 years with dental treatment.

HOW TO TREAT

NOTE—Follow your doctor's or dentist's instructions. These instructions are supplemental.

GENERAL MEASURES—For a child over 6 or 7 who sucks the fingers or thumb:
- Give the child extra attention. Observe if conflicts or anxiety-producing situations provoke sucking. Help the child explore other solutions to stress.
- If the child decides to try to stop sucking, help the child set goals. Give rewards for *any* progress toward the goal. Reward is not a bribe, but something earned through effort.

MEDICATION—Medicine usually is not necessary for this disorder.

ACTIVITY—No restrictions.

DIET—No special diet.

CALL YOUR DOCTOR OR DENTIST IF

- Your child wishes to stop and behavior-modification efforts (rewards for progress) have not solved the problem. The dentist may fit a training device in the child's mouth to prevent the thumb from touching the roof of the mouth.
- The child becomes intolerant of the training device or it loosens.
- The sucking behavior does not diminish in 6 months, despite treatment. Referral for psychological counseling may be necessary at this point.

THYROID TUMOR

GENERAL INFORMATION

DEFINITION—A benign or malignant thyroid nodule. Benign tumors are unlikely to spread to other body parts. These growths may be cystic or solid (thyroid adenoma). Malignant thyroid nodules can spread and threaten life. Early symptoms of both types are the same.

BODY PARTS INVOLVED—Thyroid gland in the front of the neck.

SEX OR AGE MOST AFFECTED
- Both sexes, but benign nodules are more common in women than men.
- All ages, but malignant nodules are more likely in children between ages 4 and 7.

SIGNS & SYMPTOMS
- Swelling or lump in the thyroid gland.
- Pain and tenderness in the thyroid gland.
- Swallowing difficulty.
- Hoarseness.
- Breathing difficulty (rare).
- Symptoms of hypothyroidism or hyperthyroidism (both in Illness section).

CAUSES—Unknown.

RISK INCREASES WITH
- Radiation treatment during childhood—even in small doses—to the head, neck and upper chest.
- Family history of thyroid tumors.

HOW TO PREVENT—Avoid radiation treatments to the neck for acne, tonsillitis, enlarged thymus gland or other minor conditions.

WHAT TO EXPECT

APPROPRIATE HEALTH CARE
- Home care after diagnosis.
- Doctor's treatment.
- Surgery to aspirate a cystic tumor or to remove a solid tumor and the affected lobe of the thyroid.
- Radioactive iodine treatment (see Glossary).
- Speech therapy, if the voice is affected after surgery.

DIAGNOSTIC MEASURES
- Your own observation of symptoms.
- Medical history and physical exam by a doctor.
- Laboratory tests, such as radioactive-iodine uptake studies, CAT scan (see Glossary for both) and blood studies of thyroid function.
- Biopsy (see Glossary).

POSSIBLE COMPLICATIONS
- Spread of a malignant tumor to adjacent parts, requiring radical surgery to remove lymph nodes and muscles of one side of the neck.
- Hypothyroidism or hypoparathyroidism, caused by inadvertent injury to the thyroid or parathyroid glands during surgery.
- Permanent hoarseness and loss of voice following surgery for some thyroid cancers.

PROBABLE OUTCOME—Usually curable with surgery or a combination of surgery and radioactive-iodine treatment.

HOW TO TREAT

NOTE—Follow your doctor's instructions. These instructions are supplemental.

GENERAL MEASURES
- For an explanation of surgery and postoperative care, see Thyroidectomy (in Surgery section).
- If you lose your voice, special equipment is available from the telephone company and other agencies to assist you with speech.
- After thyroid surgery, when rising from a lying to a sitting position, put a pillow under your head and support it with your hands to prevent neck-muscle strain.

MEDICATION—Your doctor may prescribe:
- Antithyroid medications or replacement thyroid hormone.
- Radioactive iodine to treat cancer (I-131).
- Pain relievers.

ACTIVITY—Resume your normal activities as soon as symptoms improve after surgery.

DIET—No special diet.

CALL YOUR DOCTOR IF

- You have symptoms of thyroid nodules or thyroid enlargement.
- The following occurs after surgery:
  Symptoms of hypothyroidism (fatigue, puffy face, rapid weight gain, coarse hair and decreased sex drive).
  Bleeding, pain or swelling at the surgical site.
  Fever.
  Twitching muscles.
  Breathing difficulty.
- New, unexplained symptoms develop. Drugs used in treatment may produce side effects.

THYROIDITIS

GENERAL INFORMATION

DEFINITION—Inflammation of the thyroid gland.

BODY PARTS INVOLVED—Thyroid gland, a hormone-producing organ at the base of the neck, next to the trachea (windpipe).

SEX OR AGE MOST AFFECTED—Middle-aged persons of both sexes between ages 30 and 50, but more common in women.

SIGNS & SYMPTOMS
- Enlarged, painful, tender thyroid gland.
- Fever.
- Pain in the jaw or ears (sometimes).
- Hyperthyroidism (rapid heartbeat, nervousness, tremor and rapid weight loss).

CAUSES—Disorder of the autoimmune system, accompanied by one of the following:
- Various viruses, such as mumps or influenza.
- Rheumatoid arthritis.
- Bacterial infection of the thyroid gland (rare).

RISK INCREASES WITH
- Recent illness, such as tuberculosis or any infection.
- Pregnancy.
- Family history of thyroiditis.
- Previous thyroid disorders.

HOW TO PREVENT—No specific preventive measures.

WHAT TO EXPECT

APPROPRIATE HEALTH CARE
- Self-care after diagnosis.
- Doctor's treatment. Consultation with an endocrinologist may be valuable.
- Hospitalization (rare).
- Surgery to relieve pressure on adjacent areas of the neck or to drain an abscess (rare).

DIAGNOSTIC MEASURES
- Your own observation of symptoms.
- Medical history and physical exam by a doctor.
- Laboratory blood counts and tests of thyroid function.

POSSIBLE COMPLICATIONS—Permanent loss of thyroid function, requiring lifelong thyroid-hormone replacement.

PROBABLE OUTCOME—Usually curable with treatment. Some persons recover spontaneously. Regular medical follow-up is recommended after the condition is apparently cured.

HOW TO TREAT

NOTE—Follow your doctor's instructions. These instructions are supplemental.

GENERAL MEASURES—No specific instructions except those listed under other headings.

MEDICATION—Your doctor may prescribe:
- Antithyroid medication or thyroid replacement hormones, depending on the activity of your thyroid hormones.
- Beta-adrenergic blockers to suppress symptoms of an overactive thyroid.
- Antibiotics to fight infection, if necessary.
- Cortisone drugs to decrease inflammation (rare).

ACTIVITY—Resume your normal activities as soon as symptoms improve.

DIET—No special diet.

CALL YOUR DOCTOR IF

- You have symptoms of thyroiditis.
- The following occurs during treatment: Fever and redness of the thyroid gland. Lethargy.
- New, unexplained symptoms develop. Drugs used in treatment may produce side effects.

TIC DOULOUREUX
(Trigeminal Neuralgia)

 GENERAL INFORMATION

DEFINITION—A nerve condition that causes brief, but often severe, face pain.

BODY PARTS INVOLVED—Nerve branches from the trigeminal or 5th cranial nerve (nerve from the brain that supplies sensation to the face, scalp, teeth, mouth and nose).

SEX OR AGE MOST AFFECTED—Adults over 40, usually men.

SIGNS & SYMPTOMS—Severe face pain, described as "jabbing" or "searing." Pain is often triggered by touching or stroking the face, brushing teeth, shaving, exposure to wind or chewing. Bouts of pain usually last 1 to 15 minutes. Attacks may occur several times a day, or may disappear for weeks or months. Between bouts, there is little or no discomfort.

CAUSES
- Pressure on the nerve from adjacent blood vessels (sometimes).
- Unknown (often).

RISK INCREASES WITH—Multiple sclerosis.

HOW TO PREVENT—No specific preventive measures.

 WHAT TO EXPECT

APPROPRIATE HEALTH CARE
- Self-care after diagnosis.
- Doctor's treatment.
- Surgery to relieve pressure on the nerve. This is a major operation.
- Nerve destruction by injections of alcohol or ultrasound treatment (high-frequency sound waves).

DIAGNOSTIC MEASURES
- Your own observation of symptoms.
- Medical history and physical exam by a doctor.
- X-rays of the head to rule out other conditions, such as brain tumor.

POSSIBLE COMPLICATIONS—Interference with normal activities from frequent, severe pain episodes.

PROBABLE OUTCOME—Most patients obtain pain relief with anticonvulsant medication. If the problem persists, injecting the involved nerve with alcohol usually relieves pain but leaves the face numb. Major surgery will relieve pain, but pain often returns within 5 to 10 years when nerves regenerate.

 HOW TO TREAT

NOTE—Follow your doctor's instructions. These instructions are supplemental.

GENERAL MEASURES
- Following are suggestions for ways to prevent sudden pain:
  Avoid blasts of hot or cold air.
  Chew on the unaffected side of the mouth.
  Grow a beard.
- Assure good oral health with dental checkups at least twice a year.

MEDICATION—Your doctor may prescribe anticonvulsant medication to prevent painful attacks.

ACTIVITY—No restrictions.

DIET—No special diet.

 CALL YOUR DOCTOR IF

- You have symptoms of tic douloureux.
- New, unexplained symptoms develop. Drugs used in treatment may produce side effects.

TOENAIL, INGROWN

GENERAL INFORMATION

DEFINITION—A condition in which the sharp edge of a nail grows into the flesh of a toe, usually the great (big) toe.

BODY PARTS INVOLVED—Toes.

SEX OR AGE MOST AFFECTED—All ages, but most common in adolescents and adults.

SIGNS & SYMPTOMS—Pain, tenderness, redness, swelling and heat in the toe where the sharp nail edge pierces the surrounding fold of tissue. Once tissue surrounding the nail becomes inflamed, infection usually develops in the injured area.

CAUSES—An ingrown toenail is likely to accompany one of the following conditions:
● The nail formation is more curved than normal.
● The toenail is clipped back too far, allowing tissue to grow up over it.
● Shoes fit poorly, forcing the toe of the shoe against the nail and surrounding tissue.
● The person participates in activities that require sudden stops ("toe jamming").

RISK INCREASES WITH—Any of the circumstances listed as causes.

HOW TO PREVENT
● Wear roomy, well-fitting shoes.
● Cut toenails carefully. Persons with diabetes mellitus or peripheral vascular disease should be especially careful in trimming toenails. Foot injury is dangerous with these disorders because of impaired blood circulation to the feet.

WHAT TO EXPECT

APPROPRIATE HEALTH CARE
● Self-care.
● Doctor's treatment.
● Surgery to remove the nail.

DIAGNOSTIC MEASURES
● Your own observation of symptoms.
● Medical history and physical exam by a doctor.

POSSIBLE COMPLICATIONS—Chronic infection that cannot be cured without surgery.

PROBABLE OUTCOME—Curable with treatment. Oral antibiotics usually relieve symptoms of infection within 1 week. Then part or all of the toenail is removed surgically and the nail bed is scraped so the problem will not recur. The nail should grow back, but it probably won't look the same.

HOW TO TREAT

NOTE—Follow your doctor's instructions. These instructions are supplemental.

GENERAL MEASURES—The following home treatment is appropriate either before or after surgery:
● Use immersion soaks (see Appendix 18).
● Lift the nail corners free of surrounding inflamed tissue by wedging a small piece of cotton under the nail around the edges. Protect the inflamed tissue from further injury.

MEDICATION—Your doctor may prescribe antibiotics to fight infection.

ACTIVITY—Resume your normal activities as soon as symptoms improve. You may need to wear a shoe with the toe cut out until the toe heals.

DIET—No special diet.

CALL YOUR DOCTOR IF

● You have symptoms of an ingrown toenail.
● The following occurs during treatment or after surgery:
Fever.
Increased pain.
Signs of infection (pain, redness, tenderness, swelling or heat) in the toe.

TONGUE INFLAMMATION
(Glossitis)

GENERAL INFORMATION

DEFINITION—Acute or chronic inflammation of the tongue from a variety of causes. This is sometimes contagious, but not cancerous.

BODY PARTS INVOLVED—Tongue and adjacent parts of the mouth.

SEX OR AGE MOST AFFECTED—Both sexes; all ages.

SIGNS & SYMPTOMS—Any of the following:
- Bright red, swollen tongue.
- Ulcers on the tongue.
- Hairy-looking tongue.
- A tongue with red tip and edges.

CAUSES
- Infections, including herpes.
- Burns.
- Injury from jagged teeth, ill-fitting dentures, mouth-breathing or repeated biting during convulsive seizures.
- Excessive consumption of alcohol, tobacco, hot food or spices.
- Poor dental health.
- Allergy to toothpaste, mouthwash (especially mouthwash containing peroxide), candy, dye or material used in dental work.
- Lack of B-vitamins, resulting in pellagra, B-12-deficiency anemia or iron-deficiency anemia.
- Adverse reaction to antibiotic drugs.

RISK INCREASES WITH
- Poor nutrition, especially vitamin deficiencies.
- Smoking.
- Chemical or environmental exposure to irritating or corrosive chemicals.

HOW TO PREVENT
- Practice good oral hygiene. Brush teeth and tongue at least twice a day, and floss teeth daily. Get regular dental checkups.
- Don't smoke.
- Prevent tongue injury by wearing protective headgear for contact sports or cycling.

WHAT TO EXPECT

APPROPRIATE HEALTH CARE
- Self-care.
- Doctor's treatment if self-care doesn't relieve symptoms.

DIAGNOSTIC MEASURES
- Your own observation of symptoms.
- Medical history and physical exam by a doctor.

POSSIBLE COMPLICATIONS—Tongue inflammation can become chronic if not adequately treated.

PROBABLE OUTCOME—Usually curable in 2 weeks with treatment.

HOW TO TREAT

GENERAL MEASURES
- Observe if there is an association between eating specific foods and tongue inflammation. Irritating foods may include chocolate, citrus, acid foods (vinegar, pickles), salted nuts or potato chips.
- Rinse mouth 3 or more times a day with a salt solution (1/2 teaspoon salt to 8 oz. water).
- If tongue inflammation is caused by a rough tooth or denture, consult your dentist. Inflammation won't heal until the cause is eliminated.

MEDICATION
- For minor pain, you may use non-prescription drugs, such as anesthetic mouthwashes or acetaminophen.
- For infection and pain, your doctor may prescribe antibiotics or topical anesthetics.

ACTIVITY—No restrictions.

DIET—No special diet, except to avoid foods that aggravate inflammation. Drink as many fluids and eat as well-balanced a diet as possible while healing. To minimize pain, sip liquids through straws. Foods that cause the least pain are milk, liquid gelatin, yogurt, ice cream and custard.

CALL YOUR DOCTOR IF

- Fever develops.
- Symptoms don't improve in 3 days despite treatment.
- Pain is unbearable and isn't relieved by treatment.
- Skin rash appears.
- Weight loss occurs.

ILLNESSES & DISORDERS

TONSILLITIS
(Pharyngitis)

GENERAL INFORMATION

DEFINITION—Inflammation of the tonsils (clumps of lymphoid tissue at the back of the throat).

Tonsils are small at birth, enlarge during childhood, and become smaller at puberty. When not infected, tonsils help prevent infection in the sinuses, mouth and throat from spreading to other body parts. Tonsillitis is contagious.

BODY PARTS INVOLVED—Tonsils; pharynx.

SEX OR AGE MOST AFFECTED—All ages, but most common in children between ages 5 and 10.

SIGNS & SYMPTOMS
● Throat pain, either mild or severe.
● Swallowing difficulty.
● Chills and fever as high as 104F (40C) or more.
● Swollen lymph glands on either side of the jaw.
● Headache.
● Ear pain.
● Cough (sometimes).
● Vomiting (sometimes).

CAUSES—Viral or bacterial infection of the tonsils.

RISK INCREASES WITH
● Crowded or unsanitary living conditions.
● Exposure to others in public places.

HOW TO PREVENT—Avoid exposure to people with upper-respiratory infections.

WHAT TO EXPECT

APPROPRIATE HEALTH CARE
● Home care.
● Doctor's treatment.
● Surgery to remove the tonsils (occasionally).

DIAGNOSTIC MEASURES
● Your own observation of symptoms.
● Medical history and physical exam by a doctor.
● Laboratory throat culture.

POSSIBLE COMPLICATIONS
● Abscess of the tonsils and nearby throat area, requiring surgery to drain.
● Chronic tonsillitis, with a recurrent sore throat and greatly enlarged tonsils, caused by repeated attacks.
● Rheumatic fever, if the bacterial infection is streptococcal and it is not treated with antibiotics.

PROBABLE OUTCOME—Usually spontaneous recovery. Symptoms generally begin to improve in 2 to 3 days, but treatment may last longer.

If attacks of tonsillitis are so severe and frequent that they affect one's general health or interfere with schooling, hearing or breathing, your doctor may recommend surgery to remove the tonsils.

A tonsillectomy involves small risk, but the risk increases with age.

HOW TO TREAT

NOTE—Follow your doctor's instructions. These instructions are supplemental.

GENERAL MEASURES
● Use a cool-mist humidifier to relieve throat irritation and cough.
● Prepare a soothing tea or other gargle. Double the usual strength of tea. This may be gargled warm or cold as often as is soothing.

MEDICATION
● If the tonsillitis is caused by a streptococcal infection, your doctor will prescribe penicillin or other antibiotics for at least 10 days.
● To relieve pain, you may use acetaminophen.

ACTIVITY
● Keep the patient away from others until fever, pain and other symptoms disappear.
● Bed rest, except to use the bathroom, is necessary until fever subsides. Normal activity may be resumed when temperature has been normal for 2 or 3 days.

DIET—Increase all fluid intake. While the throat is very sore, use liquid nourishment, such as milk shakes, soups, and high-protein fluids (diet or instant-breakfast milk drinks).

CALL YOUR DOCTOR IF

● You have symptoms of tonsillitis. If tonsils cover the opening of the throat (hold down the tongue with a spoon and look with a flashlight), call your doctor immediately.
● Symptoms worsen or the following occurs during treatment:
  Temperature is normal for 1 or 2 days, then rises above 101F (38.3C) orally or 102F (38.9C) rectally.
  New symptoms begin, such as: nausea; vomiting; skin rash; thick nasal drainage; chest pain; or shortness of breath.
  There is a convulsion.
  Joints become red or painful.
  Cough produces a discolored (green, yellow, brown or bloody) sputum.

TOOTH ABSCESS
(Periapical Abscess; Periodontal Abscess)

 GENERAL INFORMATION

DEFINITION—An abscess around a tooth root, which is imbedded in bone of the upper or lower jaw.

BODY PARTS INVOLVED—Gums; jawbone.

SEX OR AGE MOST AFFECTED—Both sexes; all ages.

SIGNS & SYMPTOMS
- Persistent toothache or throbbing, extreme pain upon biting or chewing.
- Swelling and tenderness in the neck glands and on the side of the face.
- Earache.
- Fever.
- General ill feeling.
- Foul taste and bad breath (if the abscess opens spontaneously).

CAUSES
- Tartar beneath the gum.
- Deep decay which has entered the tooth nerve. The infection spreads down the nerve and into surrounding bone and gum tissue, but does not affect adjacent teeth.

RISK INCREASES WITH
- Poor nutrition.
- Improper diet.
- Inadequate fluoride in drinking water.

HOW TO PREVENT
- Prevent decay with good brushing and flossing:
  Use a soft-bristle toothbrush to remove plaque from the teeth's front and back surfaces, especially at the gum line.
  Learn to use dental floss correctly. Ask your dentist or hygienist to demonstrate the technique.
- Use fluoride mouthwash, toothpaste, tablets or liquid supplements if your dentist recommends them.
- Reduce sugar consumption. Tooth decay increases as sugar consumption increases.

 WHAT TO EXPECT

APPROPRIATE HEALTH CARE—Tooth abscesses can be drained in one of 3 ways:
- If the tooth has poor bone and gum support, the tooth can be extracted, allowing the abscess to drain through the socket and heal.
- A hole can be drilled through the top of the tooth, and a tiny metal or plastic wick inserted into the narrow nerve canal through the center of the tooth. This allows the abscess to drain.

- An incision can be made in the gum at the site of infection, which dramatically relieves pain and pressure. Your dentist may place a small rubber wick in the incision for a few days. When the infection improves, your dentist can perform root-canal therapy.

DIAGNOSTIC MEASURES
- Your own observation of symptoms.
- Medical history and physical exam by a dentist.
- X-rays of the mouth.

POSSIBLE COMPLICATIONS
- Rupture into the sinus of an abscess in the upper jaw.
- Loss of the tooth.
- Spread of infection through the bloodstream to other body parts.

PROBABLE OUTCOME—Usually curable with oral surgery.

 HOW TO TREAT

NOTE—Follow your dentist's instructions. These instructions are supplemental.

GENERAL MEASURES
- Rinse your mouth with warm water to draw infection from the abscess. Repeat each hour or as often as feels good.
- Don't chew on the affected side of your mouth for at least 2 days.
- If a tube has been used to drain the abscess, keep the small hole free of infection. Carefully remove impacted food.
- If a drain has been placed in gum tissue, return to your dentist in several days to have it removed.

MEDICATION
- For minor pain, you may use non-prescription drugs such as acetaminophen.
- Your doctor or dentist may prescribe:
  Antibiotics to control infection.
  Pain relievers.

ACTIVITY—Resume your normal activities as soon as possible.

DIET—A liquid diet may be necessary for 1 or 2 days until pain subsides.

 CALL YOUR DOCTOR OR DENTIST IF

- You have symptoms of a tooth abscess.
- The following occurs during treatment:
  Fever spikes to 101F (38.3C) or higher.
  Pain becomes unbearable.
- New, unexplained symptoms develop. Drugs used in treatment may produce side effects.

ILLNESSES & DISORDERS

TOOTH DECAY
(Caries; Dental Decay; Cavities)

 GENERAL INFORMATION

DEFINITION—Disintegration of tooth enamel, allowing injury to the dentin (layer below the enamel) and eventual involvement of the pulp (the layer below the dentin), which contains nerves and blood vessels. Tooth decay and the common cold are the most common human disorders.

BODY PARTS INVOLVED—Teeth.

SEX OR AGE MOST AFFECTED—Both sexes; all ages.

SIGNS & SYMPTOMS
- Tooth sensitivity to heat and cold.
- Tooth discomfort after eating sugar.
- Darkening on or between the teeth (cavity) when the decay has progressed enough to be seen. The most common tooth-cavity sites are the gum line, biting surfaces and surfaces between adjacent teeth.
- Unpleasant taste in the mouth and bad breath because of stagnant food and bacteria trapped in the cavity.
- Persistent tooth pain (in the final stages of decay when the pulp becomes inflamed).

CAUSES—Cavities are caused by acid destruction of tooth material. Acid is produced by bacteria in the mouth. The bacteria feed on food debris—usually sugar—and produce the acid that dissolves tooth material.

The combination of sugars from food debris, bacteria and chemicals in the saliva form a substance called plaque. Plaque becomes a localized site of acid production, which forms continuously at the neck of each tooth. This plaque must be thoroughly cleaned away at the gum line daily or it fosters tooth decay.

RISK INCREASES WITH
- Poor nutrition and improper diet.
- Poor dental hygiene.

HOW TO PREVENT
- Brush and floss teeth regulary.
- Consult your dentist about using fluoride mouthwash, liquid, tablets or having fluoride treatments once or twice a year.
- Drinking fluoridated water or taking fluoride supplements during pregnancy has not proven to protect the unborn child's teeth.

 WHAT TO EXPECT

APPROPRIATE HEALTH CARE
- Self-care.
- Dentist's treatment to remove all decay in the tooth and replace it with a restorative material (filling). The filling prevents further decay.

DIAGNOSTIC MEASURES
- Your own observation of symptoms.
- Examination by a dentist. The decayed area feels soft when the dentist probes it with a sharp instrument.
- X-rays of the teeth and mouth.

POSSIBLE COMPLICATIONS
- Abscess around a decayed tooth.
- Death of the tooth, caused by destruction of the tooth pulp that contains the tooth's nerve and blood supply.

PROBABLE OUTCOME—Usually curable with dental treatment.

 HOW TO TREAT

NOTE—Follow your dentist's instructions. These instructions are supplemental.

GENERAL MEASURES—No specific instructions except those listed under other headings.

MEDICATION
- For minor pain, you may use non-prescription drugs such as acetaminophen.
- Your dentist may prescribe stronger pain relievers or fluoride supplements.

ACTIVITY—No restrictions.

DIET—For 48 hours after your dentist fills the decayed tooth, don't put pressure on the tooth, as by eating apples, hard candy, raw vegetables or chewing on ice. Avoid very hot or cold foods. The tooth remains sensitive for 48 hours to 10 days after a cavity has been filled.

 CALL YOUR DENTIST IF

- You have symptoms of tooth decay.
- The following occurs after treatment:
  Fever.
  Increased pain that is not relieved by non-prescription medication.
  Discomfort with hot or cold food that persists longer than 2 weeks after the filling procedure.
  Brown spots on the tops of any other teeth.

TOOTH-GRINDING
(Bruxism)

 GENERAL INFORMATION

DEFINITION—The habit of grinding teeth. Tooth-grinding is often done while asleep, but grinding or tapping teeth during the day is also common. Continual tooth-grinding may erode gums and supporting bones in the mouth.

BODY PARTS INVOLVED—Teeth; gums; tempero-mandibular joints.

SEX OR AGE MOST AFFECTED—Both sexes; all ages.

SIGNS & SYMPTOMS
- Frequent contraction of muscles on the side of the face.
- Annoying, tooth-grinding noises at night. These may be loud enough to awaken others.
- Damaged teeth, supporting gums and bone (apparent in a dental exam).
- Headaches.

CAUSES
- Anxiety.
- Unconscious attempts to correct a faulty "bite" (contact between upper and lower teeth when jaws are closed).

RISK INCREASES WITH—Stress or anxiety.

HOW TO PREVENT—Avoid stressful situations if possible. See Appendix 13.

 WHAT TO EXPECT

APPROPRIATE HEALTH CARE
- Self-care after diagnosis.
- Dentist's care. Your dentist may manufacture, fit and install a night-guard prosthesis to prevent tooth-grinding while asleep. A night-guard prosthesis consists of removable splints which fit over the tops of the teeth to eliminate incorrect biting pressure.
- Biofeedback training or counseling to learn ways to cope more effectively with stress.

DIAGNOSTIC MEASURES
- Your own observation of symptoms.
- Medical history and physical exam by a dentist.
- X-rays of the mouth.

POSSIBLE COMPLICATIONS—Without treatment, teeth, bones and gums may erode from the pressure of grinding.

PROBABLE OUTCOME—Usually curable in 6 months with treatment.

 HOW TO TREAT

GENERAL MEASURES—No specific instructions except those listed under other headings.

MEDICATION—Medicine usually is not necessary for this disorder.

ACTIVITY—No restrictions.

DIET—No special diet.

 CALL YOUR DOCTOR OR DENTIST IF

- You grind your teeth at night.
- You develop pain around the ears, dizziness or ringing in the ears.
- You develop pain or clicking in the jaw.
- You lose or break your night-guard prosthesis.

ILLNESSES & DISORDERS

TORTICOLLIS
(Wryneck)

 GENERAL INFORMATION

DEFINITION—Shortened neck muscles or chronic neck-muscle spasm that causes the head to turn and bend.

BODY PARTS INVOLVED—Brain and central nervous system; muscular system.

SEX OR AGE MOST AFFECTED—Both sexes, but more common in females of all ages.

SIGNS & SYMPTOMS—The following may be permanent or intermittent:
- Head that turns sideways and bends down.
- Neck-muscle spasm that is sometimes painful.

CAUSES—For constant torticollis:
- Birth defect.
- Injury to neck muscles or vertebrae at birth or later.
- Neck-muscle inflammation.
For intermittent torticollis:
- Stress and psychological conflict.

RISK INCREASES WITH
- Sleeping in an awkward position.
- Emotional disturbances, such as neurosis or hypochondriasis.

HOW TO PREVENT—Stress-related forms can be prevented with stress-reduction techniques, including biofeedback.

 WHAT TO EXPECT

APPROPRIATE HEALTH CARE
- Self-care after diagnosis.
- Doctor's treatment.
- Psychotherapy or counseling, if the cause is stress-related.
- Surgery to lengthen neck muscles, if the cause is congenital.
- Physical therapy (sometimes), including gentle massage.

DIAGNOSTIC MEASURES
- Your own observation of symptoms.
- Medical history and physical exam by a doctor.
- Laboratory blood tests for infection and inflammation.
- X-rays of the spinal column in the neck.

POSSIBLE COMPLICATIONS—Without treatment, the congenital form becomes permanent, causing an unattractive, abnormal appearance of the head and neck.

PROBABLE OUTCOME
- Congenital torticollis can usually be corrected with muscle-stretching exercises or surgery.
- Other forms will improve or heal with treatment. Healing time varies. Some cases require treatment for several years.

 HOW TO TREAT

NOTE—Follow your doctor's instructions. These instructions are supplemental.

GENERAL MEASURES—If your infant has signs of torticollis:
- Ask your doctor or physical therapist for muscle-stretching exercises to do with the child twice a day.
- Place attention-getting objects in the crib opposite the side that the head turns.
For non-congenital forms of torticollis:
- Your doctor may recommend that you wear a neck brace.
- Relieve pain from neck spasms with heat. Take hot showers or use hot compresses, deep-heating ointments or heat lamps.

MEDICATION—If the condition is caused by injury or inflammation, your doctor may prescribe muscle relaxants and pain relievers.

ACTIVITY—Normal activities may be resumed as soon as symptoms improve.

DIET—No special diet.

 CALL YOUR DOCTOR IF

- Your infant has symptoms of torticollis.
- You have neck pain or spasms that persist longer than 1 week.

TOXEMIA OF PREGNANCY
(Pre-eclampsia & Eclampsia)

 GENERAL INFORMATION

DEFINITION—A serious disturbance in blood pressure, kidney function and the central nervous system that may occur from the 20th week of pregnancy until 7 days after delivery.

BODY PARTS INVOLVED—Female reproductive system; kidneys; brain and central nervous system; blood and blood vessels.

SEX OR AGE MOST AFFECTED—Pregnant females.

SIGNS & SYMPTOMS—Mild pre-eclampsia:
- Significant blood-pressure rise, even if still in the normal range.
- Puffiness in the face, hands and feet that is worse in the morning.
- Excessive weight gain (more than a pound a week during the last trimester).
- Protein in the urine.
Severe pre-eclampsia:
- Continued blood-pressure rise.
- Continued swelling and puffiness.
- Blurred vision.
- Headache.
- Irritability.
- Abdominal pain.
Eclampsia:
- Worsening of above symptoms.
- Muscle twitching.
- Seizures.
- Coma.

CAUSES—Unknown.

RISK INCREASES WITH
- Poor nutrition.
- Diabetes mellitus.
- Previous high blood pressure.
- Chronic kidney disease.
- First pregnancy. Toxemia during one pregnancy does not mean it will recur with subsequent pregnancies.
- Smoking.
- Excess alcohol consumption.
- Use of mind-altering drugs.

HOW TO PREVENT
- Obtain good prenatal care throughout pregnancy.
- Don't smoke, use mind-altering drugs or drink alcohol during pregnancy.
- Eat a normal, well-balanced diet during pregnancy (see Appendix 3). Take prenatal vitamin and mineral supplements, if your doctor prescribes them.
- Don't use medications of any kind, including non-prescription drugs, without consulting your doctor.

 WHAT TO EXPECT

APPROPRIATE HEALTH CARE
- Doctor's treatment.
- Hospitalization.

DIAGNOSTIC MEASURES
- Your own observation of symptoms.
- Medical history and physical exam by a doctor.
- Laboratory blood studies of kidney, liver and blood-clotting functions.
- Urinalysis to detect protein in the urine.

POSSIBLE COMPLICATIONS
- Premature labor.
- Stroke.
- DIC (in Illness section).
- Increased risk of high blood pressure unrelated to pregnancy after age 30.

PROBABLE OUTCOME—If diagnosed and treated throughout pregnancy, toxemia usually disappears without complications within 7 days after delivery. It is fatal in rare cases. If toxemia causes premature labor, the newborn's survival chances depend on its maturity. Fetal death is common.

 HOW TO TREAT

NOTE—Follow your doctor's instructions. These instructions are supplemental.

GENERAL MEASURES
- Weigh yourself daily and keep a record.
- Ask your doctor about testing for urine protein at home.

MEDICATION—Your doctor may prescribe:
- Antihypertensive drugs to lower blood pressure.
- Anticonvulsants or sedatives to prevent seizures.
- Diuretics to decrease fluid accumulation.

ACTIVITY—Rest often—this is important in controlling toxemia. Rest on your left side, if possible, to help circulation.

DIET—A special diet will be necessary. Consult a dietitian.

 CALL YOUR DOCTOR IF

- You have symptoms of mild toxemia at any stage of pregnancy.
- The following occurs during treatment:
  Severe headache or vision disturbance.
  Weight gain of 3 or more pounds in 24 hours.
  Nausea, vomiting and diarrhea.
  Cramping abdominal pains.
  Excessive irritability.

TOXIC SHOCK SYNDROME

GENERAL INFORMATION

DEFINITION—A form of blood poisoning caused by poisons (toxins) released by staphylococcal bacteria.

BODY PARTS INVOLVED—Female reproductive system; respiratory system.

SEX OR AGE MOST AFFECTED—All ages and both sexes, but most common in women of childbearing age.

SIGNS & SYMPTOMS
- Sudden, high fever (at least 101F or 38.3C) in a previously healthy person.
- Vomiting and watery diarrhea.
- Rash that resembles sunburn.
- Low blood pressure.
- Thirst.
- Rapid pulse.
- Feeling of impending doom.
- Mental changes, such as confusion.
- Extreme fatigue and weakness.
- Headache.
- Sore throat.

CAUSES—Some strains of staphylococcal bacteria produce toxins that enter the bloodstream, causing sudden symptoms. Most serious cases have come from staphylococci in the vagina of women using tampons. Toxic shock syndrome can also arise from wounds or infections in the throat, skin, lungs or bone.

RISK INCREASES WITH
- Continuous use of tampons during menstrual periods.
- Any infection.

HOW TO PREVENT
- Change tampons frequently, and alternate them at night with sanitary napkins.
- Don't use superabsorbent tampons. Use those made of cotton.
- Don't use tampons if you have a skin infection, especially near the genitals.
- Wash hands thoroughly before inserting tampons. Staphylococci are commonly found on hands.

WHAT TO EXPECT

APPROPRIATE HEALTH CARE
- Doctor's treatment.
- Immediate hospitalization for intravenous fluids to administer antibiotics and correct fluid and electrolyte loss and dehydration.

DIAGNOSTIC MEASURES
- Your own observation of symptoms.
- Medical history and physical exam by a doctor.
- Laboratory studies, such as blood counts, blood cultures and cultures from the vagina or other areas of infection.

POSSIBLE COMPLICATIONS
- Severe shock.
- Kidney failure.
- Congestive heart failure.

PROBABLE OUTCOME—Most patients recover with early diagnosis and prompt hospital treatment, but some cases are fatal. Skin of the palms and soles often peels during recovery.

HOW TO TREAT

NOTE—Follow your doctor's instructions. These instructions are supplemental.

GENERAL MEASURES—No specific instructions except those listed under other headings.

MEDICATION—Your doctor may prescribe:
- Antibiotics, usually intravenous, for infection.
- Intravenous fluids and electrolytes.

ACTIVITY—Resume your normal activities as soon as symptoms improve.

DIET—No special diet after recovery. Intravenous nourishment is usually necessary during hospitalization.

CALL YOUR DOCTOR IF

- You have symptoms of toxic shock syndrome. Call immediately! Shock develops rapidly.
- New, unexplained symptoms develop. Drugs used in treatment may produce side effects.

TRANSIENT ISCHEMIC ATTACK (T.I.A.)

GENERAL INFORMATION

DEFINITION—A temporary decrease in the blood supply to part of the brain. The affected part of the brain is temporarily unable to function normally.

BODY PARTS INVOLVED—Blood vessels to the brain and the part of the brain supplied by the affected blood vessels.

SEX OR AGE MOST AFFECTED—Adults over age 40.

SIGNS & SYMPTOMS—The following symptoms are brief, lasting from several minutes to a few hours.
- Loss of muscle function on one side of the body.
- Headache.
- Dizziness.
- Tingling in the arms and legs.
- Numbness.
- Vision disturbance or temporary blindness in one eye.
- Confusion.
- Faintness without loss of consciousness.
- Slurred speech or inability to speak.

CAUSES—T.I.A.s are caused by a partial blockage in a small artery in the brain or a larger artery (usually the carotid artery in the neck) that supplies blood to brain arteries. The blockage is often caused by a small clot or piece of an artery wall or heart valve that breaks away and is carried into the brain. This temporarily decreases blood flow to an area of the brain and causes strokelike symptoms.

RISK INCREASES WITH
- Smoking.
- Personal or family medical history of high blood pressure and atherosclerosis.

HOW TO PREVENT
- Exercise at least 3 times a week to maintain good cardiovascular fitness.
- Follow recommendations under Diet.
- Don't smoke.
- Have your blood pressure checked regularly. If it is high, consult your doctor for treatment to reduce it.

WHAT TO EXPECT

APPROPRIATE HEALTH CARE
- Self-care after diagnosis.
- Doctor's treatment.
- Surgery to remove plaques (fatty deposits) from carotid arteries in the neck (sometimes).

DIAGNOSTIC MEASURES
- Your own observation of symptoms.
- Medical history and physical exam by a doctor.
- Laboratory blood studies to analyze cholesterol and other fats.
- X-rays and sonograms (see Glossary) of blood vessels in the neck or brain.

POSSIBLE COMPLICATIONS—Stroke. Without treatment, about 50% of persons who have T.I.A.s have strokes within 5 years.

PROBABLE OUTCOME—Transient ischemic attacks are often signals of an impending stroke. They should be treated to attempt to prevent a stroke, which may cause serious brain damage.

T.I.A.s are likely to recur. A person may have several attacks daily or only 2 or 3 over several years. The symptoms of each attack may be similar or quite different from others. In some patients symptoms appear repeatedly without leaving permanent damage.

HOW TO TREAT

NOTE—Follow your doctor's instructions. These instructions are supplemental.

GENERAL MEASURES—No specific instructions except those listed under other headings.

MEDICATION—Your doctor may prescribe:
- Anticoagulants, such as warfarin, to decrease the formation of blood clots. These drugs must be monitored with laboratory studies of prothrombin time (see Glossary).
- 1 or 2 aspirin tablets a day. Recent medical experiments indicate aspirin can decrease blood-clotting enough to reduce the likelihood of T.I.A.s developing into stroke. The aspirin seems more effective in men than women.

ACTIVITY—If you have frequent T.I.A.s, don't drive, work in high places or operate machinery.

DIET—Eat a normal, well-balanced diet that is low in salt and fat, especially saturated fat. (See Appendices 8 and 9).

CALL YOUR DOCTOR IF

- You have your first symptoms of a T.I.A.
- Symptoms of a T.I.A. recur after diagnosis and persist longer than 2 hours.

ILLNESSES & DISORDERS

TRENCH MOUTH
(Necrotizing Ulcerative Gingivitis; Vincent's Disease; Fusospirochetosis)

 GENERAL INFORMATION

DEFINITION—Infection of tissue between the teeth. This is not contagious or cancerous.

BODY PARTS INVOLVED—Gums. If untreated, trench mouth can spread to: lymph glands in the neck; tonsils; vocal cords; bronchial tubes; rectum; or vagina.

SEX OR AGE MOST AFFECTED—Both sexes and all ages, but most common in young adults (20 to 40 years).

SIGNS & SYMPTOMS
- Painful gums.
- Gums that bleed when pressed.
- Excess salivation.
- Bad breath.
- Ulcers covered with gray membrane on the gums.
- Swallowing difficulty.
- Speaking difficulty.

CAUSES
- Spirochetes, a fusiform bacteria.
- Tartar, plaque or food debris between teeth.

RISK INCREASES WITH
- Poor nutrition.
- Illness that has lowered resistance.
- Smoking.
- Stress.

HOW TO PREVENT
- Maintain good oral hygiene.
  To brush teeth: Scrub clear, sticky plaque off teeth daily with a soft toothbrush. Place the brush at the gum line and gently rotate, pointing bristles toward the gum. Brush one section of teeth at a time. Then brush tongue. A soft brush is less likely to damage teeth and gums than a hard brush.
  To floss: Use waxed or unwaxed dental floss according to instructions on the package label or your dentist's instructions.
- Eat a well-balanced diet.
- Don't smoke.

 WHAT TO EXPECT

APPROPRIATE HEALTH CARE
- Self-care after diagnosis.
- Doctor's treatment.
- Scaling of teeth by a dentist to remove plaque.
- Frequent dental checkups—up to once a month—after treatment.

DIAGNOSTIC MEASURES
- Your own observation of symptoms.
- Medical history and physical exam by a doctor.
- Laboratory culture to identify the infecting germs.

POSSIBLE COMPLICATIONS—Surgery may be necessary to trim rough, infected gums.

PROBABLE OUTCOME—Usually curable in 2 weeks with treatment.

 HOW TO TREAT

NOTE—Follow your doctor's or dentist's instructions. These instructions are supplemental.

GENERAL MEASURES
- Rinse your mouth every 2 hours, alternating the following rinses:
  Mixture of 1 teaspoon salt in large glass of very warm water.
  Mixture of equal parts 2% hydrogen peroxide and warm water.
- Don't smoke.
- Avoid any gum irritation until gums heal completely.

MEDICATION
- Your doctor may prescribe penicillin or another antibiotic to fight infection.
- You may use non-prescription drugs, such as acetaminophen, for minor pain.

ACTIVITY—Rest at home for the first 2 days of treatment, then resume normal activities.

DIET—A liquid diet (see Appendix 7) may be necessary for 2 or 3 days because of gum tenderness. When pain subsides, eat many fresh fruits and vegetables. Don't eat spicy or hot (temperature) food.
- Drink juices and 4 to 6 glasses of water each day. Don't drink carbonated beverages or alcohol.

 CALL YOUR DOCTOR OR DENTIST IF

- You have symptoms of trench mouth.
- The following occurs during treatment:
  Fever of 101F (38.3C) or higher.
  Swelling of neck or face.
  Swallowing difficulty.
  Inability to eat.

TRICHINOSIS

GENERAL INFORMATION

DEFINITION—Infection caused by larvae of parasites that live in the intestines of pigs and bears.

BODY PARTS INVOLVED—Gastrointestinal tract (where larvae enter); lymphatic system and bloodstream (through which they are transported); large muscles of the body, especially diaphragm large muscle used in breathing that separates the chest from the abdomen, arms and legs (in which they become embedded).

SEX OR AGE MOST AFFECTED—Both sexes; all ages.

SIGNS & SYMPTOMS—Early stages (usually begin in 7 to 10 days):
● Appetite loss, nausea, vomiting, diarrhea and abdominal cramps.
Later stages:
● Puffy eyelids and face.
● Muscle pain.
● Itching, burning skin.
● Sweating.
● High fever (102F to 104F or 38.9C to 40C).
Late stages:
● Symptoms subside, but some muscle tissues remain permanently infected with microscopic cysts. In rare cases, these cause heart and central-nervous-system disorders.

CAUSES—Infection with a parasite, trichina spiralis, which is transmitted to people when they eat infected animals. Thorough cooking kills the parasite and makes infected meat safe to eat. The parasites pass from animal to animal in contaminated food—usually raw garbage.

RISK INCREASES WITH
● Eating improperly cooked or raw pork or bear meat.
● Use of immunosuppressive drugs.

HOW TO PREVENT—Don't eat raw or undercooked pork (including sausage) or bear meat.

WHAT TO EXPECT

APPROPRIATE HEALTH CARE
● Self-care after diagnosis.
● Doctor's treatment.
● Hospitalization (worst cases).

DIAGNOSTIC MEASURES
● Your own observation of symptoms.
● Medical history and physical exam by a doctor.
● Laboratory blood studies.
● Muscle biopsy.

POSSIBLE COMPLICATIONS—Overwhelming infection, which can lead to:
● Congestive heart failure.
● Respiratory failure.
● Permanent damage to central nervous system.

PROBABLE OUTCOME—Usually curable in most persons with antiparasite drugs and, in severe cases, expert supportive care. Some deaths have been reported. Allow up to 6 months for recovery.

HOW TO TREAT

NOTE—Follow your doctor's instructions. These instructions are supplemental.

GENERAL MEASURES—Reduce fever if it goes over 103F (39.4C). See Appendix 19, How to Reduce Fever.

MEDICATION
● Your doctor may prescribe antihelminthic drugs (usually thiabendazole) to kill the parasites.
● You may take non-prescription drugs, such as acetaminophen, to reduce fever and discomfort.

ACTIVITY—Rest in bed until symptoms subside. While confined to bed, move legs frequently to reduce the likelihood of deep-vein blood clots. Resume normal activities gradually.

DIET—Special high-protein diet to help rebuild damaged muscle tissue. The diet will be prescribed by your doctor and explained by a dietitian. Usually, you may progress to an unrestricted, well-balanced diet within 6 months.

CALL YOUR DOCTOR IF

● You have symptoms of trichinosis.
● The following occurs during treatment:
  Fever spike to over 104F (40C).
  Irregular heartbeat.
  Shortness of breath.
  Puffy ankles.
  Clumsy finger or thumb movement.
● New, unexplained symptoms develop. Drugs used in treatment may produce side effects, especially nausea, vomiting, skin rash or fever.

ILLNESSES & DISORDERS

TUBERCULOSIS (TB)

GENERAL INFORMATION

DEFINITION—An acute or chronic, contagious, bacterial infection.

BODY PARTS INVOLVED—Lungs primarily, but may spread to other organs. Childhood tuberculosis is usually confined to the middle of the lungs, but it may spread to cause meningitis. Tuberculosis in adults usually affects the top of the lungs.

SEX OR AGE MOST AFFECTED—Both sexes; all ages.

SIGNS & SYMPTOMS
Early stages:
- No symptoms (often).
- Symptoms that resemble those of influenza.

Second stages:
- Low fever.
- Weight loss.
- Chronic fatigue.
- Heavy sweating, especially at night.

Later stages:
- Cough with sputum that becomes progressively bloody, yellow, thick or gray.
- Chest pain.
- Shortness of breath.
- Reddish or cloudy urine (sometimes).

CAUSES—Infection by the germ, mycobacterium tuberculosis. The germ is transmitted in the air from one person to another. Cattle are also susceptible, and can transmit TB through non-pasteurized milk.

RISK INCREASES WITH
- Adults over 60.
- Newborns and infants.
- Chronic illness that has lowered resistance.
- Use of cortisone or immunosuppressive drugs. These may reactivate inactive TB.
- Crowded or unsanitary living conditions.

HOW TO PREVENT
- Vaccination with BCG, a strain of the tuberculosis bacteria. This may prevent infection, or shorten and diminish the severity of the infection.
- Preventive treatment for several months with isonicotinic acid if a tuberculin skin test is positive.

OTHER—Health authorities recommend vaccination and preventive treatment for the following groups:
- Persons who have positive reactions to TB tests, but show no symptoms of disease—especially children under age 5.
- Children with negative reactions to TB tests in areas where 20% or more of classmates have positive reactions.
- Persons traveling to countries where TB is prevalent.
- Persons who must take immuno-sup-pressive or cortisone drugs for a long time.
- Post-gastrectomy patients whose X-rays show evidence of inactive TB.
- Persons with silicosis.

WHAT TO EXPECT

APPROPRIATE HEALTH CARE
- Self-care after diagnosis.
- Doctor's treatment.

DIAGNOSTIC MEASURES
- Your own observation of symptoms.
- Medical history and physical exam by a doctor.
- Tuberculin skin test.
- Laboratory cultures of sputum and urine.
- X-rays of the chest.

POSSIBLE COMPLICATIONS
- Lung abscess.
- Bronchiectasis.
- COPD (see Glossary).
- Spread of infection to other organs (brain, bone, spine and kidneys).
- Respiratory failure.

PROBABLE OUTCOME—Usually curable with treatment. Without treatment, it can be fatal.

HOW TO TREAT

NOTE—Follow your doctor's instructions. These instructions are supplemental.

GENERAL MEASURES
- It may not be necessary to isolate or hospitalize a person with TB. The disease is usually spread before diagnosis. Patients are probably not infectious after 10 days to 2 weeks of treatment.
- Occasionally you will need to collect a 24-hour sputum specimen for laboratory analysis to see if TB is still active.

MEDICATION—Your doctor may prescribe antitubercular drugs, including: INH (isonicotinic acid hydrizide); ethambutol; para-aminosalicylic acid; or rifampin.

ACTIVITY—Rest in bed until symptoms disappear and tests show TB germs are gone. You may need to restrict activities for 6 months.

DIET—No special diet.

CALL YOUR DOCTOR IF

- You have symptoms of TB.
- Symptoms persist or worsen, despite treatment.
- New, unexplained symptoms develop. Drugs used in treatment may produce side effects.

TYPHOID FEVER

GENERAL INFORMATION

DEFINITION—A bacterial infection of the gastrointestinal tract.

BODY PARTS INVOLVED—Gastrointestinal tract; skin; central nervous system.

SEX OR AGE MOST AFFECTED—Both sexes; all ages. Infants and persons over 60 usually have the severest cases.

SIGNS & SYMPTOMS
- Diarrhea. In mild cases, this may be only 2 or 3 loose bowel movements a day. In severe cases, it may be watery diarrhea as often as every 10 or 15 minutes.
- Vomiting.
- Fever.
- Headache.
- Muscle aches.
- Skin rash on the abdomen.
- Abdominal cramps (sometimes).
- Blood in the stool (sometimes).

A relatively mild attack may be mistaken for simple gastroenteritis.

CAUSES—Infection with the salmonella typhi bacteria. The bacteria is found in infected animals and transmitted to persons in contaminated meat or milk. Thorough cooking kills the germ.

The infection can also be transmitted by ill persons or non-ill carriers who handle food without careful hand-washing after bowel movements.

RISK INCREASES WITH
- Illness that has lowered resistance.
- Crowded or unsanitary living conditions.

HOW TO PREVENT
- Follow these recommendations in any area with a substandard water supply:
  Drink purified water, boil water or add 2 to 4 drops of 4% to 6% chlorine bleach to each quart of water 30 minutes before use. If in a hotel, draw hot water from the faucet, let it cool and use it as drinking water. Don't use ice.
  Don't eat raw fruits and vegetables unless you can peel them.
- Drink only pasteurized milk.
- Wash your hands after bowel movements and before handling food.
- Obtain a vaccination for anyone exposed to typhoid.

WHAT TO EXPECT

APPROPRIATE HEALTH CARE
- Doctor's treatment.
- Self-care during the convalescent stage.
- Hospitalization for severe cases.

DIAGNOSTIC MEASURES
- Your own observation of symptoms.
- Medical history and physical exam by a doctor.
- Laboratory studies, such as stool studies and a blood culture.
- X-rays of the gastrointestinal tract.
- Sigmoidoscopy (see Glossary).

POSSIBLE COMPLICATIONS
- Dehydration.
- Perforation of the intestines.
- Gastrointestinal hemorrhage or abscess.
- Deep-vein blood clot.
- Pneumonia.
- Bone infection.
- Congestive heart failure.

PROBABLE OUTCOME—Usually curable in 2 to 3 weeks with treatment. Without treatment, it can be fatal.

HOW TO TREAT

NOTE—Follow your doctor's instructions. These instructions are supplemental and apply if hospitalization is not necessary.

GENERAL MEASURES
- Isolate ill persons and have them use bedside commodes or a separate bathroom.
- Use a heating pad or hot-water bottle to relieve abdominal cramps.
- Wash hands carefully and often.
- Turn patients frequently in bed.
- Apply lukewarm wet towels to the groin and underarms to reduce fever. *Don't* use aspirin or acetaminophen; both irritate the gastrointestinal tract.

MEDICATION—Your doctor may prescribe antibiotics, such as ampicillin or sulfa drugs.

ACTIVITY—Bed rest is necessary until all symptoms have been gone at least 3 days. The legs should be flexed often in bed to prevent formation of deep-vein blood clots.

DIET—A clear-liquid diet is necessary during the diarrhea phase. Later, a high-calorie, well-balanced diet is necessary. Vitamin and mineral supplements may be helpful.

CALL YOUR DOCTOR IF

- You have symptoms of typhoid fever.
- The following occurs during treatment:
  Fever of 102F (38.9C) or higher.
  Sore throat.
  Severe cough or coughing up blood.
  Shortness of breath.
  Severe abdominal pain or swelling.
  Rectal bleeding.
  Pain in the calf or leg.
  Headache, earache or swollen joints.

ILLNESSES & DISORDERS

ULCER, DUODENAL
(Peptic Ulcer)

 GENERAL INFORMATION

DEFINITION—An ulcer (or "sore") in the duodenum which causes symptoms similar to those of a stomach ulcer. An ulcer is not contagious or cancerous.

BODY PARTS INVOLVED—Duodenum (first 12 inches of small intestine beyond the stomach).

SEX OR AGE MOST AFFECTED
- Both sexes, but more common in males.
- All ages, but most common in adults.

SIGNS & SYMPTOMS
- Pain that has the following characteristics:
  A burning, boring or gnawing feeling that lasts 30 minutes to 3 hours. The pain is often interpreted as heartburn, indigestion or hunger.
  Pain is usually in the upper abdomen, but occasionally below the breastbone.
  Pain occurs in some persons immediately after eating; in others, it may not occur until hours later. It frequently awakens one at night.
  Pain comes and goes. Weeks of intermittent pain may alternate with short pain-free periods.
  Pain may be relieved by drinking milk, eating, resting or taking antacids.
- Appetite and weight loss.
- Recurrent vomiting.
- Blood in the stool.
- Anemia.

CAUSES—Unknown. An ulcer can develop wherever stomach acid comes in contact with the gastrointestinal lining—especially the lower end of the esophagus, the stomach and the duodenum.

An ulcer is most likely to develop in an anxious, tense or worried person. A person with an ulcer usually has an overactive stomach that manufactures too much hydrochloric acid.

In addition, persons with ulcers often have irregular living habits (see risks below).

RISK INCREASES WITH
- Family history of ulcers.
- Stress.
- Improper diet, irregular mealtimes and skipped meals.
- Smoking.
- Excess alcohol consumption.
- Use of drugs, including caffeine, which irritate the stomach.
- Fatigue or overwork.

HOW TO PREVENT—Avoid as many risk factors as possible.

 WHAT TO EXPECT

APPROPRIATE HEALTH CARE
- Self-care after diagnosis.
- Doctor's treatment.
- Hospitalization (complications).

DIAGNOSTIC MEASURES
- Your own observation of symptoms.
- Medical history and physical exam by a doctor.
- Gastroscopy (see Glossary) to determine the ulcer size and location.

POSSIBLE COMPLICATIONS—The following complications are most likely in adults over 60:
- Perforation (erosion of the ulcer through the intestinal wall) or dangerous bleeding.
- Unrelenting pain, failure to heal and scarring.
- Extensive peptic-ulcer disease, with increased likelihood of stomach cancer.

PROBABLE OUTCOME—Usually curable with lifestyle changes and medical treatment.

 HOW TO TREAT

NOTE—Follow your doctor's instructions. These instructions are supplemental.

GENERAL MEASURES
- Don't smoke.
- Check your stool daily for bleeding. If the stool is black, remove it from the toilet and take it to your doctor's office for analysis.

MEDICATION—Your doctor may prescribe:
- Antacids to help neutralize excess stomach acid.
- H-2 blockers to reduce stomach acid.

ACTIVITY—Resume your normal activities as soon as symptoms improve.

DIET
- Eat small frequent meals for at least 2 weeks.
- Don't drink alcohol.
- Avoid caffeine and any food that seems to make symptoms worse.

 CALL YOUR DOCTOR IF

- You have symptoms of an ulcer.
- Vomiting begins that is bloody or looks like coffee grounds.
- Stool is bloody, black or tarry-looking.
- Diarrhea begins which may be caused by antacids.
- Pain is severe, despite treatment.
- You are unusually weak or pale.

ULCER, STOMACH
(Peptic Ulcer; Gastric Ulcer)

GENERAL INFORMATION

DEFINITION—A raw spot that develops in the stomach lining.

BODY PARTS INVOLVED—Stomach, including stomach lining.

SEX OR AGE MOST AFFECTED—Both sexes of young adults (20 to 45 years). It is rare in children.

SIGNS & SYMPTOMS—Pain with the following characteristics:
- Burning, gnawing pain in the upper abdomen or the lower chest below the breastbone. The pain is often interpreted as indigestion, heartburn or hunger and may be relieved temporarily with milk, antacids or bland food.
- Pain lasts 30 minutes to 3 hours. It may occur immediately after eating or hours later.
- Pain comes and goes. Weeks of intermittent pain may alternate with short, pain-free periods.

Other symptoms include:
- Loss of appetite.
- Weight loss.
- Anemia
- Occasional vomiting.

Sometimes the symptoms are not typical, and diagnostic procedures are necessary.

CAUSES—Unknown. Persons with ulcers often have irregular living habits (see risks below). Many doctors believe emotional tension causes ulcers.

RISK INCREASES WITH
- Stress.
- Improper diet or irregular meals.
- Smoking.
- Excessive consumption of alcohol or caffeine-containing drinks.
- Use of drugs, such as cortisone, aspirin or other non-steroidal anti-inflammatory drugs.
- Family history of ulcers.
- Type "O" blood.

HOW TO PREVENT—See Appendices 12 and 13 for suggestions for a healthy lifestyle.

WHAT TO EXPECT

APPROPRIATE HEALTH CARE
- Self-care after diagnosis.
- Doctor's treatment.
- Hospitalization (sometimes) during the initial treatment.
- Psychotherapy or counseling.
- Surgery to remove part of the stomach or cut nerves that stimulate acid production, if conservative treatment fails.

DIAGNOSTIC MEASURES
- Your own observation of symptoms.
- Medical history and physical exam by a doctor.
- Laboratory studies to measure stomach acid.
- X-rays of the stomach.
- Gastroscopy (see Glossary).

POSSIBLE COMPLICATIONS
- Bleeding.
- Perforation, in which the ulcer erodes through the stomach wall.
- Scarring and obstruction in the stomach caused by recurrent ulcers.
- Malignant change in an ulcer.
- Anemia.

PROBABLE OUTCOME—Usually curable with 6 to 8 weeks of treatment. If an ulcer doesn't heal in that time, or if recovery is only temporary, surgery may be necessary. For perforation or hemorrhaging, surgery is mandatory. It usually produces complete cure.

HOW TO TREAT

NOTE—Follow your doctor's instructions. These instructions are supplemental.

GENERAL MEASURES
- Don't smoke during convalescence.
- Examine your stool daily for signs of bleeding. If the stool is black, take a specimen to your doctor's office.

MEDICATION
- Don't take aspirin or other non-steroidal anti-inflammatory drugs.
- Your doctor may prescribe:
  Antacids to reduce stomach acid.
  H-2 blockers to decrease the stomach's production of hydrochloric acid.
- Don't medicate yourself with antacids unless your doctor prescribes them and you are under medical supervision.

ACTIVITY—Rest in bed 2 weeks. You may read or watch TV.

DIET
- Eat small, frequent meals for 2 weeks.
- Don't drink alcohol. After recovery, don't drink more than 1 or 2 alcoholic drinks a day.

CALL YOUR DOCTOR IF

- You have symptoms of a stomach ulcer, or symptoms recur after treatment.
- You have signs of bleeding, such as passing a black stool, or vomiting blood or material that looks like coffee grounds.
- Diarrhea begins.
- Pain becomes intolerable.
- You become unusually weak or pale.

URETHRITIS

 GENERAL INFORMATION

DEFINITION—Inflammation or infection of the urethra (the tube through which urine travels from the bladder to the outside), frequently accompanied by bladder infection or inflammation (cystitis). The female urethra is much shorter than the male's.

BODY PARTS INVOLVED—Urethra; bladder (sometimes).

SEX OR AGE MOST AFFECTED—All ages and both sexes, but 10 times more common in females.

SIGNS & SYMPTOMS
- Painful or burning urination with cloudy, yellow-green mucus discharge from the urethra.
- Frequent urge to urinate, even when there is not much urine in the bladder.
- Painful sexual intercourse or temporary impotence in males.
- Dribbling of urine in men over 50.

CAUSES—Bacterial infection. *In women,* the infection is associated with:
- Bacteria that enter the urethra from the skin around the genitals and anal area.
- Bruising during sexual intercourse.
In men, infection is associated with:
- Non-specific urethritis, which may be caused by sexual contact or irritation of the urethra.
- Infections that reach the urethra through the bloodstream from the prostate gland or through the penis.
In both sexes, the infection may be associated with gonorrhea, which is spread by contact with an infected sexual partner.

RISK INCREASES WITH
- Use of a urinary catheter.
- Use of drugs to which bacteria causing infection have become resistant.
- Multiple sexual partners.
- Previous kidney stones, prostatitis, epididymitis or genital injury.

HOW TO PREVENT
- For causes related to sexual activity:
  Drink a glass of water before sexual intercourse, and urinate within 15 minutes afterward.
  Use a rubber condom.
  Use a water-soluble lubricant, such as K-Y Lubricating Jelly.
  Use varying sexual positions to decrease the chance of trauma to the female urethra.
- For causes related only to women:
  After bowel movements, wipe from front to back and wash with soap and water.
  Take showers rather than tub baths.
- For both sexes:
  Drink 8 glasses of water every day.

 WHAT TO EXPECT

APPROPRIATE HEALTH CARE
- Self-care after diagnosis.
- Doctor's treatment.

DIAGNOSTIC MEASURES
- Your own observation of symptoms.
- Medical history and physical exam by a doctor.
- Urinalysis and urine culture.

POSSIBLE COMPLICATIONS
- Chronic urethritis and cystitis, if treatment is inadequate.
- Spread of infection to ureters and kidneys.

PROBABLE OUTCOME—Urethritis is usually "low grade," seldom producing serious, long-term illness. Recurrence is common.

 HOW TO TREAT

NOTE—Follow your doctor's instructions. These instructions are supplemental.

GENERAL MEASURES
- To relieve pain, take sitz baths by sitting in a tub of hot water for 15 minutes at least twice a day.
- Men: Don't irritate the urethra by pulling the penis skin down to open it and see if the discharge is still present. The penis may be inspected, but don't squeeze it.
- Keep the area around the genitals clean. Use unscented, plain soap.

MEDICATION—Your doctor may prescribe antibiotics to fight infection. Be sure to finish the prescribed dose, even if symptoms subside sooner.

ACTIVITY—No restrictions. Avoid sexual excitement and intercourse until you have been free of symptoms for 2 weeks.

DIET
- Drink 8 glasses of water every day.
- Avoid caffeine and alcohol during treatment.
- Drink cranberry juice to acidify urine. Some drugs are more effective with acid urine.

☎ **CALL YOUR DOCTOR IF**

- You have symptoms of urethritis.
- The following occurs during treatment:
  Oral temperature of 101F (38.3C) or higher.
  Bleeding from the urethra or blood in urine.
  No improvement in 1 week, despite treatment.
- New, unexplained symptoms develop.
Drugs used in treatment may produce side effects.

UTERINE BLEEDING, DYSFUNCTIONAL
(Premenopausal Abnormal Uterine Bleeding)

 GENERAL INFORMATION

DEFINITION — Bleeding that is not related to a woman's normal menstrual pattern. Uterine bleeding is a symptom of other disorders.

BODY PARTS INVOLVED — Uterus; vagina.

SEX OR AGE MOST AFFECTED — Female adolescents and premenopausal adults.

SIGNS & SYMPTOMS — Painful, prolonged or irregular bleeding through the vagina.

CAUSES
- Hormone imbalance.
- Cervicitis and cervical erosion.
- Disorders of blood cells, bone marrow or the lymphatic system.
- High blood pressure.
- Congestive heart failure.
- Liver disorders.
- Use of drugs containing hormones, anticoagulants or aspirin.
- Tumors of the uterus and cervix, including polyps and fibroid tumors.
- Infection in the uterus (rare).
- Lacerations of the cervix (rare).
- Psychological factors such as stress.

RISK INCREASES WITH — Use of birth-control pills.

HOW TO PREVENT — Cannot be prevented at present.

 WHAT TO EXPECT

APPROPRIATE HEALTH CARE
- Self-care after diagnosis.
- Doctor's treatment.
- Hospitalization for diagnostic tests (sometimes).
- Surgery to remove tumors, if they are causing the disorder.
- Psychotherapy or counseling, if no underlying physical disorder can be identified.

DIAGNOSTIC MEASURES
- Your own observation of symptoms.
- Medical history and physical exam by a doctor.
- Laboratory studies, such as a Pap smear, pregnancy test and blood studies and chemistries.
- Surgical diagnostic procedures, such as culposcopy, biopsy and dilatation and curettage (D&C) of the uterus (see Glossary for all).

POSSIBLE COMPLICATIONS — Anemia.

PROBABLE OUTCOME — Usually curable in 2 or 3 months, sooner with surgery. Recurrence is common, depending on the underlying cause.

 HOW TO TREAT

NOTE — Follow your doctor's instructions. These instructions are supplemental.

GENERAL MEASURES
- Use heat to relieve pain:
  Place a heating pad or hot-water bottle on the abdomen or back.
  Take a hot bath for 10 to 15 minutes as often as needed.
- Seek professional counseling, if necessary, to resolve any psychological or emotional factors that may complicate your illness and delay recovery.

MEDICATION — Your doctor may prescribe:
- Hormones to correct a hormone imbalance.
- Pain relievers.
- Tranquilizers to reduce anxiety.
- Antihypertensives, if high blood pressure is causing the disorder.
- Diuretics and digitalis medications, if congestive heart failure is the underlying cause.

ACTIVITY — Stay as active as possible, depending on the underlying condition. Consult your doctor about continuing sexual relations.

DIET — No special diet. Iron supplements may be necessary for anemia.

 CALL YOUR DOCTOR IF

- You have abnormal uterine bleeding.
- The following occurs during treatment:
  Bleeding becomes excessive. (You saturate a pad or tampon more often than once an hour).
  You develop signs of infection, such as: fever; a general ill feeling; headache; dizziness; or muscle aches.
- New, unexplained symptoms develop. Drugs used in treatment may produce side effects.

ILLNESSES & DISORDERS

UTERINE BLEEDING, POST-MENOPAUSAL

GENERAL INFORMATION

DEFINITION—Unexpected, menstrual-like bleeding that begins 1 or more years after menopause.

BODY PARTS INVOLVED—Vulva (vaginal lips); vagina; cervix (lower third of the uterus); endometrium (inner uterine lining).

SEX OR AGE MOST AFFECTED—Women after menopause.

SIGNS & SYMPTOMS
- Vaginal bleeding, which may be a light-brown discharge or heavy, red bleeding (with or without clots). Mucus may accompany the bleeding. Bleeding episodes vary in length—there is no expected range.
- Pelvic pain.

CAUSES
- Cancer of the reproductive system.
- Irritation, infection or thinning of the membranes lining the vulva.
- Injury or trauma to the vagina, associated with reduced estrogen levels.
- Polyps or benign tumors of the cervix.
- Polyps on the inner uterine lining, myomas (see Glossary) or fibroid tumors of the uterus.
- Hormone therapy that stimulates the endometrium (uterine lining), causing sloughing similar to normal menstruation. Estrogens (female hormones) taken irregularly are a common cause of this.
- Disorders of the blood cells, lymphatic system or bone marrow.
- High blood pressure.
- Congestive heart failure.
- Liver disorders.
- Anticoagulant or aspirin-containing drugs.

RISK INCREASES WITH
- Recent vaginal infection.
- Adults over 60, due to fragile blood vessels and thin vaginal lining.

HOW TO PREVENT—No specific preventive measures.

WHAT TO EXPECT

APPROPRIATE HEALTH CARE
- Doctor's treatment.
- Surgery (hysterectomy) to remove the uterus (sometimes).
- Psychotherapy or counseling to reduce anxiety about the bleeding.

DIAGNOSTIC MEASURES
- Your own observation of symptoms.
- Medical history and physical exam by a doctor.
- Laboratory studies, such as a Pap smear (see Glossary), blood studies and pregnancy test.
- Surgical diagnostic procedures, such as dilatation and curettage (D & C) and colposcopy (see Glossary).
- Biopsy (see Glossary) of suspicious areas.

POSSIBLE COMPLICATIONS
- Anemia.
- If cancer is the cause, it may spread to other body parts and cause death.

PROBABLE OUTCOME—Depends on the underlying cause and treatment chosen. Hysterectomy cures bleeding immediately. Hormone treatment may require up to 6 months.

HOW TO TREAT

NOTE—Follow your doctor's instructions. These instructions are supplemental.

GENERAL MEASURES
- Use heat to relieve pain. Place a heating pad or hot-water bottle on the abdomen or back.
- Take frequent hot baths to relax muscles and relieve discomfort. Sit in a tub of hot water for 10 to 15 minutes as often as necessary.
- Use sanitary pads instead of tampons.

MEDICATION—Your doctor may prescribe:
- Hormones.
- Medication to treat the underlying disorder, such as antihypertensives for high blood pressure.

ACTIVITY
- Resume your normal activities as soon as symptoms improve.
- Resume sexual relations as soon as possible after diagnosis and treatment.

DIET—No special diet.

CALL YOUR DOCTOR IF

- You have post-menopausal vaginal bleeding.
- Bleeding persists for 1 week, despite treatment.
- Your bleeding becomes excessive (saturates a pad more frequently than once each hour).
- You develop signs of infection: fever, a general feeling of ill health, headache, dizziness and muscle aches.
- New, unexplained symptoms develop. Drugs used in treatment may produce side effects.

UTERINE CANCER

GENERAL INFORMATION

DEFINITION—Cancer of the uterus. Approximately 40,000 new cases are reported each year.

BODY PARTS INVOLVED—Uterus.

SEX OR AGE MOST AFFECTED—Post-menopausal women, usually between ages 50 and 60.

SIGNS & SYMPTOMS—Early stages:
● Bleeding or spotting, especially after sexual intercourse. This often occurs after menstrual activity has ceased for 12 months or more. A watery or blood-streaked vaginal discharge may precede bleeding or spotting.
● Enlarged uterus. It is sometimes a large enough mass to be felt externally.
Later stages:
● Spread to other organs, causing abdominal pain, chest pain and weight loss.

CAUSES—Unknown.

RISK INCREASES WITH
● Diabetes mellitus.
● Obesity.
● High blood pressure.
● Use of estrogen.
● Family history of breast or ovarian cancer.
● History of menstrual cycles without ovulation, uterine polyps or other signs of hormone imbalance.

HOW TO PREVENT
● See your doctor for pelvic examinations every 6 to 12 months.
● Obtain medical care for any uterine bleeding or spotting after menopause.

WHAT TO EXPECT

APPROPRIATE HEALTH CARE
● Doctor's treatment.
● Psychotherapy or counseling for depression.
● Surgery to remove the uterus, and usually, the ovaries and Fallopian tubes.
● Hospitalization.
● Radiation therapy.

DIAGNOSTIC MEASURES
● Your own observation of symptoms, especially abnormal bleeding.
● Medical history and physical exam by a doctor.
● Laboratory blood studies and Pap smear (although this is only 40% accurate in detecting this condition).
● Surgical diagnostic procedures, such as uterine biopsy or dilatation and curettage (see Glossary for both).

POSSIBLE COMPLICATIONS
● Depression.
● Fatal spread of cancer to the bladder, rectum and distant organs.

PROBABLE OUTCOME—With early diagnosis and treatment, 90% of patients survive at least 5 years.

HOW TO TREAT

NOTE—Follow your surgeon's instructions. These instructions are supplemental.

GENERAL MEASURES—During treatment, maintain an optimistic outlook. Counseling may help.

MEDICATION—Your doctor may prescribe:
● Anticancer drugs, including cortisone drugs.
● Hormone replacement therapy.

ACTIVITY—Resume your normal activities as soon as symptoms improve after treatment. Discuss concerns regarding sexual activity with your partner and doctor. In most cases, full sexual activity after therapy should be resumed as soon as possible.

DIET—No special diet, but try to eat a well-balanced diet—even if you lose your appetite from radiation or drug therapy. Vitamin and mineral supplements are helpful. Work with a dietitian to plan nutritious meals.

CALL YOUR DOCTOR IF

● You have symptoms of uterine cancer.
● The following occurs after surgery:
  Excessive bleeding (soaking a pad or tampon at least once an hour).
  Signs of infection, such as fever, muscle aches and headache.
● New, unexplained symptoms develop. Drugs used in treatment may produce side effects.

UTERINE PROLAPSE

GENERAL INFORMATION

DEFINITION—A uterus that has fallen or sunk from its normal location, causing it to bulge into the vagina. In its most pronounced form, it projects outside the vagina.

BODY PARTS INVOLVED—Uterus; ligaments that suspend the uterus; vagina.

SEX OR AGE MOST AFFECTED—Women over age 40.

SIGNS & SYMPTOMS
- Lump in front or back of the vagina, or projecting outside it.
- Vague discomfort in the pelvic region.
- Backache that worsens with lifting.
- Discomfort with urinating.
- Occasional stress incontinence (urine leakage when laughing, sneezing or coughing).
- Difficulty in moving bowels.
- Pain with sexual intercourse.

CAUSES—Prolapse occurs when muscles and ligaments at the base of the abdomen become extremely stretched, usually as a result of childbirth or aging.

RISK INCREASES WITH
- Poor nutrition.
- Poor physical fitness.
- Obesity.
- Repeated childbirth, although one pregnancy and vaginal delivery can weaken the area enough to lead to prolapse eventually.
- Straining to have bowel movements.

HOW TO PREVENT
- Practice Kegel exercises during pregnancy and after childbirth (see General Measures).
- Eat a normal, well-balanced diet.
- Engage in a regular exercise program to maintain good muscle strength.

WHAT TO EXPECT

APPROPRIATE HEALTH CARE
- Self-care (Kegel exercises).
- Doctor's treatment to fit a pessary (see Glossary).
- Surgery to remove the uterus (sometimes).

DIAGNOSTIC MEASURES
- Your own observation of symptoms.
- Medical history and physical exam by a doctor.

POSSIBLE COMPLICATIONS
- Total prolapse, requiring surgery.
- Ulceration of the cervix.
- Increased risk of infection or injury to pelvic organs.

PROBABLE OUTCOME—Aggressive treatment is not always necessary because prolapse is not a health risk. Exercise can often improve muscle function. If the prolapse is severe, it can be cured with surgery.

HOW TO TREAT

NOTE—Follow your doctor's instructions. These instructions are supplemental.

GENERAL MEASURES—Learn to recognize, control and develop the pelvic muscles. These are the ones you use to interrupt urination in mid-stream. The following exercises (Kegel exercises) strengthen these muscles so you can control or relax them completely:
- To identify which muscles are involved, alternately start and stop urinating when using the toilet.
- Practice tightening and releasing these muscles while sitting, standing, walking, driving, watching TV or listening to music.
- Tighten the muscles a small amount at a time, "like an elevator going up to the 10th floor." Then release very slowly, "one floor at a time."
- Tighten the muscles from front to back, including the anus, as in the previous exercise.
- Practice exercises every morning, afternoon and evening. Start with 5 times each, and gradually work up to 20 or 30 each time.

MEDICATION—Medicine is not necessary. Your doctor may prescribe a pessary made of rubber or other material to fit inside the vagina to support the uterus.

ACTIVITY—No restrictions. If surgery is necessary, resume your normal activities gradually.

DIET
- Lose weight if you are obese. A reducing diet appears in Appendix 1.
- Eat a diet high in fiber to prevent constipation.

CALL YOUR DOCTOR IF

- You have symptoms of uterine prolapse.
- Symptoms don't improve in 3 months despite treatment or exercise, or symptoms become intolerable and you wish to consider surgery.
- The following occurs if a pessary is fitted: unusual vaginal bleeding; discomfort; or urination difficulty.

VAGINA OR VULVA, CANCER OF

 GENERAL INFORMATION

DEFINITION—Uncontrolled growth of malignant cells in the vagina or on the vulva (vaginal lips).

BODY PARTS INVOLVED—Vagina; vulva.

SEX OR AGE MOST AFFECTED—Females of all ages, but the peak incidence is from ages 45 to 65. One type (rhabdo-myosarcoma) occurs in children.

SIGNS & SYMPTOMS
- Abnormal vaginal bleeding.
- Discomfort or bleeding with intercourse.
- Small or large, firm, ulcerated, painless lesion of the vulva. Cancers on the vulva have thick, raised edges and bleed easily.
- Uncomfortable urination, if cancer spreads to the bladder.
- Rectal bleeding, if it spreads to the rectum.

CAUSES—Unknown.

RISK INCREASES WITH
- Family history of cancer of reproductive organs.
- Infants born to mothers who take estrogen during pregnancy.

HOW TO PREVENT—No specific preventive measures. Have a yearly pelvic exam to detect the disease during early stages when treatment is most effective.

 WHAT TO EXPECT

APPROPRIATE HEALTH CARE
- Doctor's treatment.
- Surgery (usually) to remove the vaginal lips.
- Radiation treatment (sometimes). External radiation shrinks the primary tumor. Internal radiation (implants) affects cancer that has spread to adjoining tissues. Implants of radium or cesium are used for 48 to 72 hours.
- Self-care after diagnosis, radiation treatment or surgery.

DIAGNOSTIC MEASURES
- Your own observation of symptoms.
- Medical history and physical exam by a doctor.
- Laboratory studies, such as a Pap smear and culposcopy (see Glossary for both).
- Surgical diagnostic procedures such as dilatation and curettage (D & C, see Glossary).

POSSIBLE COMPLICATIONS—Fatal spread to other body parts. Common sites of spread are the lymph nodes in the groin, wall of the pelvis, bladder, rectum, bone, lungs or liver.

PROBABLE OUTCOME—This condition is currently considered incurable, but early detection and treatment offer a good chance for normal life expectancy. Symptoms can be relieved or controlled during treatment.

Scientific research into causes and treatment continues, so there is hope for increasingly effective treatment and cure.

 HOW TO TREAT

NOTE—Follow your doctor's instructions. These instructions are supplemental.

GENERAL MEASURES—No specific instructions except those listed under other headings.

MEDICATION—Your doctor may prescribe:
- Pain relievers.
- Antibiotics, if urinary-tract infection results from use of a bladder catheter during radiation treatment.
- Stool softeners beginning a week after treatment.

ACTIVITY
- A catheter will remain in the bladder for about 2 weeks following surgery or during radiation treatment.
- If you have radiation implants, lie on your back while the radiation source is in place. Move your arms and legs often to prevent formation of deep-vein blood clots.
- After radiation treatment—internal or external—resume your normal activities in about 5 days.
- After surgery, resume your normal activities gradually, allowing 6 weeks for full recovery.
- Resume sexual relations when healing is complete in 8 to 10 weeks.

DIET—No special diet after treatment.

 CALL YOUR DOCTOR IF

- You have symptoms of cancer of the vagina or vulva.
- The following occurs at the treatment site after surgery or radiation treatment:
  Signs of infection, such as increasing pain, fever and swelling.
  Excessive bleeding.

VAGINISMUS

GENERAL INFORMATION

DEFINITION—Spasm of the muscles around the opening to the vagina.

BODY PARTS INVOLVED—Muscles surrounding the vagina and muscles of the lower vagina.

SEX OR AGE MOST AFFECTED—Females of all ages.

SIGNS & SYMPTOMS—Involuntary contraction of the muscles around the vagina and rectum. The vagina closes so tightly that the penis cannot penetrate for sexual intercourse.

CAUSES
● An unconscious desire to prevent penile penetration because of emotional or psychological factors. These may include fear, anxiety, hostility, anger or a distaste for sex.
● An insensitive sexual partner, insufficient or unskillful foreplay, or inadequate vaginal lubrication prior to attempted penetration.
● Physical disorders (rare), such as infections, allergic reactions or a rigid, non-perforated hymen.

RISK INCREASES WITH
● First sexual experiences.
● Previous sexual trauma.
● Stress.

HOW TO PREVENT—Pelvic examination by a doctor and counseling prior to beginning sexual activity.

WHAT TO EXPECT

APPROPRIATE HEALTH CARE
● Self-care after diagnosis.
● Doctor's treatment. Your doctor or nurse will probably teach you how to dilate the vaginal opening gently and gradually with rubber or glass dilators. Office treatments will probably be necessary 3 times a week, and you should practice at home at least twice a day.
● Psychotherapy or counseling, if medical treatment is unsuccessful.

DIAGNOSTIC MEASURES
● Your own observation of symptoms.
● Medical history and physical exam by a doctor.

POSSIBLE COMPLICATIONS
● Psychological trauma caused by guilt, anxiety, loss of self-esteem and feelings of inadequacy, or interpersonal problems resulting from the disorder.
● Painful intercourse for sexual partner.

PROBABLE OUTCOME—Usually curable if the underlying cause can be cured or a coping method can be developed through medical treatment and psychological counseling.

HOW TO TREAT

NOTE—Follow your doctor's instructions. These instructions are supplemental.

GENERAL MEASURES
● Learn dilation techniques and practice twice daily at home.
● Prior to dilation exercises or attempted intercourse, sit in a tub of hot water for 10 to 15 minutes. Baths often relax muscles and relieve discomfort. Repeat baths as often as is helpful.
● Before attempting intercourse, you and your partner should use a lubricant, such as K-Y Lubricating Jelly or baby oil.

MEDICATION—Medicine is usually not necessary for vaginismus, but your doctor may prescribe mild sedatives or tranquilizers for short periods of time.

ACTIVITY—No restrictions.

DIET—No special diet.

CALL YOUR DOCTOR IF

● You have symptoms of vaginismus.
● Symptoms don't improve after 3 weeks, despite treatment
● Symptoms recur after treatment.

VAGINITIS, GARDNERELLA OR NON-SPECIFIC

 GENERAL INFORMATION

DEFINITION—Vaginitis means infection or inflammation of the vagina. Non-specific vaginitis implies that any of several infecting germs, including gardnerella, escherichia coli, mycoplasma, streptococci, staphylococci and viruses, have caused the infection. These infections are contagious.

BODY PARTS INVOLVED—Vagina; urethra; bladder; skin around the genitals.

SEX OR AGE MOST AFFECTED—Female adolescents and adults of all ages.

SIGNS & SYMPTOMS—Severity of the following symptoms varies between women and from time to time in the same woman:
● Vaginal discharge that has an unpleasant odor.
● Genital itching.
● Vaginal discomfort.
● Change in vaginal color from pale pink to red.
● Discomfort during sexual intercourse.

CAUSES—The germs normally present in the vagina can multiply and cause infection when the pH and hormone balance of the vagina and surrounding tissue are disturbed.
  E. coli bacteria normally inhabit the rectum and can cause infection if spread to the vagina. The following conditions increase the likelihood of non-specific and gardnerella infections:
● General poor health.
● Hot weather, non-ventilating clothing—especially underwear—or any other condition that increases genital moisture, warmth and darkness. These foster the growth of germs.

RISK INCREASES WITH
● Diabetes mellitus.
● Menopause.
● Illness that has lowered resistance.

HOW TO PREVENT
● Keep the genital area clean. Use plain unscented soap.
● Take showers rather than tub baths.
● Wear cotton panties or pantyhose with a cotton crotch. Avoid panties made from non-ventilating materials, such as nylon.
● Don't sit around in wet clothing—especially a wet bathing suit.
● After urination or bowel movements, cleanse by wiping or washing from front to back (vagina to anus).
● Lose weight if you are obese.
● Avoid frequent douches.
● If you have diabetes, adhere strictly to your treatment program.

 WHAT TO EXPECT

APPROPRIATE HEALTH CARE
● Self-care after diagnosis.
● Doctor's treatment.

DIAGNOSTIC MEASURES
● Your own observation of symptoms.
● Medical history and physical exam (including pelvic exam) by a doctor.
● Laboratory studies, such as a Pap smear (see Glossary) and culture of the vaginal discharge.

POSSIBLE COMPLICATIONS—Secondary bacterial infection of the vagina.

PROBABLE OUTCOME—Usually curable in 2 weeks with treatment. Your sexual partner will need treatment also.

 HOW TO TREAT

NOTE—Follow your doctor's instructions. These instructions are supplemental.

GENERAL MEASURES
● Follow the first 4 instructions under How to Prevent.
● Don't douche unless your doctor recommends it.
● If urinating causes burning:
  Urinate through a tubular device, such as a toilet-paper roll or plastic cup with the end cut out.
  Urinate while bathing.

MEDICATION—Your doctor may prescribe:
● Antibiotics or antiparasitic drugs for gardnerella vaginitis.
● Soothing vaginal creams or lotions for non-specific forms of vaginitis.
  Use a thin sanitary pad to protect clothing from creams or suppositories, and keep them in the refrigerator. After treatment, you may want to keep a refill of the medication so you can begin treatment quickly if the infection recurs. Follow the prescription directions carefully.

ACTIVITY—Avoid overexertion, heat and excessive sweating. Delay sexual relations until after treatment.

DIET—No special diet.

 CALL YOUR DOCTOR IF

● You have symptoms of vaginitis.
● Symptoms persist longer than 1 week or worsen, despite treatment.
● Unusual vaginal bleeding or swelling develops.

ILLNESSES & DISORDERS

VAGINITIS, MONILIAL
(Vaginal Yeast Infection; Vaginal Candidiasis)

 GENERAL INFORMATION

DEFINITION—Infection or inflammation of the vagina caused by a yeastlike fungus (monilia or candida albicans).

BODY PARTS INVOLVED—Vagina and adjacent skin. Monilial vaginitis causes at least 50% of infections in the vagina.

SEX OR AGE MOST AFFECTED—Females of all ages, especially after puberty.

SIGNS & SYMPTOMS—Severity of the following symptoms varies between women and from time to time in the same woman:
- White, "curdy" vaginal discharge, (resembles lumps of cottage cheese). The odor may be unpleasant, but not foul.
- Swollen, red, tender, itching vaginal lips (labia) and surrounding skin.
- Burning on urination.
- Change in vaginal color from pale-pink to red.

CAUSES—Monilia (or candida) live in a healthy vagina, rectum and mouth. When the vagina's hormone and pH balance is disturbed, the organisms multiply and cause infections. Monilial vaginitis tends to appear before menstrual periods and improves as soon as the period begins. Factors that may disturb the vagina's balance include:
- Pregnancy.
- Diabetes mellitus.
- Antibiotic treatment.
- Oral contraceptives.
- High carbohydrate intake.
- Hot weather or non-ventilating clothing, which increase moisture, warmth and darkness, fostering fungal growth.
- Immunosuppression from drugs or disease.

RISK INCREASES WITH—Factors listed under Causes.

HOW TO PREVENT
- Keep the genital area clean. Use plain unscented soap.
- Take showers rather than tub baths.
- Wear cotton panties or pantyhose with a cotton crotch. Avoid panties made from non-ventilating materials.
- Don't sit around in wet clothing—especially a wet bathing suit.
- Avoid frequent douches.
- Ask your doctor about eating yogurt, sour cream, buttermilk or taking acidophilus tablets when you take antibiotics.
- After urination or bowel movements, cleanse by wiping or washing from front to back (vagina to anus).
- Lose weight if you are obese.
- If you have diabetes, adhere strictly to your treatment program.

 WHAT TO EXPECT

APPROPRIATE HEALTH CARE
- Self-care after diagnosis.
- Doctor's treatment.

DIAGNOSTIC MEASURES
- Your own observation of symptoms.
- Medical history and physical exam (including pelvic exam) by a doctor.
- Laboratory studies, such as a Pap smear (see Glossary), and culture and microscopic exam of the vaginal discharge.

POSSIBLE COMPLICATIONS—Secondary bacterial infections of the vagina and other pelvic organs.

PROBABLE OUTCOME—Usually curable with 2 weeks of treatment. Recurrence is common.

 HOW TO TREAT

NOTE—Follow your doctor's instructions. These instructions are supplemental.

GENERAL MEASURES
- Follow the first 4 instructions under How to Prevent.
- Don't douche unless your doctor recommends it.
- If urination causes burning:
  Urinate through a tubular device, such as a toilet-paper roll or plastic cup with the end cut out.
  Urinate while bathing.

MEDICATION—Your doctor may prescribe antifungal drugs, either in oral form (rare) or in vaginal creams or suppositories (usually). Keep creams or suppositories in the refrigerator.
After treatment, you may keep a refill of the medication so you can begin treatment quickly if the infection recurs. Follow the prescription carefully.

ACTIVITY—Avoid overexertion, heat and excessive sweating. Delay sexual relations until symptoms cease.

DIET—Increase consumption of yogurt, buttermilk or sour cream.

 CALL YOUR DOCTOR IF

- You have symptoms of monilial vaginitis.
- Despite treatment, symptoms worsen or persist longer than 1 week.
- Unusual vaginal bleeding or swelling develops.
- After treatment, symptoms recur.

VAGINITIS, POST-MENOPAUSAL
(Atrophic Vaginitis)

 GENERAL INFORMATION

DEFINITION—Infection or inflammation of the vagina caused by lowered estrogen levels that upset the vagina's normal hormone and pH balance. Post-menopausal vaginitis is not contagious.

BODY PARTS INVOLVED—Vagina.

SEX OR AGE MOST AFFECTED—Women over age 40.

SIGNS & SYMPTOMS—Severity of the following symptoms varies greatly between women and from time to time in the same woman.
- Bad-smelling vaginal discharge. The discharge is usually thin, whitish and sometimes tinged with blood.
- Genital pain and itching.
- Discomfort during sexual intercourse.
- Change in vaginal color from pale-pink to red.

CAUSES—Germs that inhabit the vagina cause infection when the normal physiology of the vagina is disturbed. After menopause, the estrogen level that helped maintain a normal vaginal environment decreases, leaving the vagina more vulnerable to infection. The following conditions increase the likelihood of post-menopausal vaginitis:
- General poor health.
- Hot weather, non-ventilating clothing—especially underwear—or any other condition that increases genital moisture, warmth and darkness. These foster the growth of germs.

RISK INCREASES WITH
- Diabetes.
- Illness that has lowered resistance.
- More frequent sexual intercourse.

HOW TO PREVENT
- Keep the genital area clean. Use plain unscented soap.
- Take showers rather than tub baths.
- Wear cotton panties or pantyhose with a cotton crotch. Avoid panties made from non-ventilating materials, such as nylon.
- Don't sit around in wet clothing—especially a wet bathing suit.
- After urination or bowel movements, cleanse by wiping or washing from front to back (vagina to anus).
- Lose weight if you are obese.
- Avoid frequent douches.
- If you have diabetes, adhere strictly to your treatment program.
- Ask your doctor about replacement estrogen.

 WHAT TO EXPECT

APPROPRIATE HEALTH CARE
- Self-care after diagnosis.
- Doctor's treatment.

DIAGNOSTIC MEASURES
- Your own observation of symptoms.
- Medical history and physical exam (including pelvic exam) by a doctor.
- Laboratory studies, such as a Pap smear (see Glossary), and microscopic exam and culture of the vaginal discharge.

POSSIBLE COMPLICATIONS—Secondary bacterial infection in any pelvic organ.

PROBABLE OUTCOME—Usually curable in 10 days with treatment.

 HOW TO TREAT

NOTE—Follow your doctor's instructions. These instructions are supplemental.

GENERAL MEASURES
- Follow the first 4 instructions under How to Prevent.
- Don't douche unless your doctor recommends it.
- If urinating causes burning:
  Urinate through a tubular device, such as a toilet-paper roll or plastic cup with the end cut out.
  Urinate while bathing.

MEDICATION—Your doctor may prescribe:
- Topical or oral estrogen. If you use a cream or suppository, use a small sanitary pad to protect clothing. Keep creams or suppositories in the refrigerator. After treatment, you may want to keep a refill of the medication so you can begin treatment quickly if the infection recurs. Follow the prescription directions carefully.
- Other creams, ointments or suppositories to suppress the organisms causing the infection.

ACTIVITY—Avoid overexertion, heat and excessive sweating. Delay sexual relations until you are well. Allow about 10 days for recovery.

DIET—No special diet.

 CALL YOUR DOCTOR IF

- You have symptoms of vaginitis.
- Symptoms persist longer than 1 week or worsen, despite treatment.
- Unusual vaginal bleeding or swelling develops.
- After treatment, symptoms recur.

VAGINITIS, TRICHOMONAL
(Trichomoniasis)

 GENERAL INFORMATION

DEFINITION—Infection or inflammation of the vagina caused by a parasite that lives in the lower genitourinary tract of males and females. This is very contagious between sexual partners.

BODY PARTS INVOLVED—Vagina, urethra and bladder in women; prostate gland and urethra in men.

SEX OR AGE MOST AFFECTED—Adolescents and adults.

SIGNS & SYMPTOMS
- Foul-smelling, frothy vaginal discharge that is most noticeable several days after a menstrual period.
- Vaginal itching and pain.
- Redness of the vaginal lips (labia) and vagina.
- Painful urination, if urine touches inflamed tissue.

The severity of discomfort varies greatly from woman to woman and from time to time in the same woman. Infected men may have no symptoms.

CAUSES—Infection from a tiny parasite, trichomonas vaginalis. The parasite passes from person to person during sexual intercourse. It may live in its host for years without producing symptoms. Then, perhaps from altered resistance, it will suddenly multiply rapidly and cause distressing symptoms. Since it thrives in both the male and female, both sexual partners must receive treatment.

RISK INCREASES WITH—Number of sexual partners.

HOW TO PREVENT—Use rubber condoms during sexual intercourse.

 WHAT TO EXPECT

APPROPRIATE HEALTH CARE
- Self-care after diagnosis.
- Doctor's treatment. Both sexual partners require simultaneous treatment.

DIAGNOSTIC MEASURES
- Your own observation of symptoms.
- Medical history and physical exam (including pelvic exam) by a doctor.
- Microscopic exam of the vaginal discharge or prostate secretions.

POSSIBLE COMPLICATIONS—Secondary bacterial infections.

PROBABLE OUTCOME—Usually curable with treatment.

 HOW TO TREAT

NOTE—Follow your doctor's instructions. These instructions are supplemental.

GENERAL MEASURES
- Don't douche unless recommended by your doctor.
- Wear cotton panties or pantyhose with a cotton crotch. Avoid panties made from nylon, silk or other non-ventilating materials.
- Take showers instead of tub baths.
- If urinating causes burning:
  Urinate through a tubular device, such as a toilet-paper roll or plastic cup with the end cut out.
  Urinate while bathing.
- Don't sit around in wet clothing—especially in a wet bathing suit.
- Don't wear tight garments, such as jeans.

MEDICATION—Your doctor may prescribe metronidazole for you and your sexual partner or partners. Follow directions carefully. *Don't drink alcohol or use vinegar when you take metronidazole.* Alcohol or vinegar and metronidazole interact to cause a violent reaction with nausea, vomiting, sweating, weakness and other symptoms.

ACTIVITY—Avoid overexertion, heat and excessive sweating. Delay sexual relations until you are well. Allow about 10 days for recovery.

DIET—No special diet.

 CALL YOUR DOCTOR IF

- You have symptoms of trichomonal vaginitis.
- Symptoms persist longer than 1 week or worsen, despite treatment.
- Unusual vaginal bleeding or swelling develops.
- After treatment, symptoms recur.

VALLEY FEVER
(San Joaquin Valley Fever; Coccidioidomycosis; "Cocci")

 GENERAL INFORMATION

DEFINITION—An infection caused by a fungus whose spores are found in soil. Valley fever is not contagious from person to person.

BODY PARTS INVOLVED—Upper respiratory tract; lymph glands.

SEX OR AGE MOST AFFECTED—Both sexes; all ages.

SIGNS & SYMPTOMS—The infection is usually so mild that it produces no symptoms. In a few cases the symptoms may be quite severe. They include:
- Cough.
- Sore throat.
- Chills and fever.
- Chest pain.
- Headache.
- Muscle aches.
- Shortness of breath.
- Skin rash.
- General ill feeling.
- Depression
- Sweating at night.
- Weight loss.
- Stiff neck (sometimes).

CAUSES—Infection by the fungus, coccidioides immitis, which thrives in soil—especially soil that lines rodent burrows. Susceptible persons become infected when they breathe the dust from such soil, and the fungi lodge in the lungs. Incubation is 1 to 4 weeks after exposure.

RISK INCREASES WITH
- Geographic location. The disease is most common in California's San Joaquin Valley, scattered regions in southern and central Arizona and southwest Texas.
- Occupational or environmental exposure to dust, such as from construction or archeological sites.
- Illness that has lowered resistance, especially uremia, diabetes mellitus, chronic lung disease, tuberculosis, Hodgkin's disease, leukemia or severe burns.
- Use of immunosuppressive drugs, cortisone drugs or antimetabolites.
- Genetic factors. Black people are most likely to have severe complications from valley fever.

HOW TO PREVENT—Cannot be prevented at present.

 WHAT TO EXPECT

APPROPRIATE HEALTH CARE
- Self-care after diagnosis.
- Doctor's treatment.
- Hospitalization (severe cases only).

DIAGNOSTIC MEASURES
- Your own observation of symptoms.
- Medical history and physical exam by a doctor.
- Laboratory skin tests and blood studies.

POSSIBLE COMPLICATIONS—Spread of infection throughout the body and severe illness, especially in the brain or membranes that cover the brain.

PROBABLE OUTCOME—Spontaneous recovery in 3 to 6 weeks. Most persons continue to feel ill for 3 to 6 weeks after signs of infection disappear.

Antifungal drugs are reserved for persons with severe, widespread infection, in which case they are life-saving.

 HOW TO TREAT

NOTE—Follow your doctor's instructions. These instructions are supplemental.

GENERAL MEASURES
- Use a cool-mist humidifier, without medicine added, to increase moisture and help relieve a cough and sore throat.
- Keep a daily weight chart.

MEDICATION—Medicine is usually not necessary. For severe infection, hospitalization may be necessary for treatment with intravenous antifungal drugs, such as amphotericin B or ketoconazole. Both drugs are potent and have potential severe adverse reactions.

ACTIVITY—Stay as active as your strength allows. Rest often.

DIET—No special diet.

 CALL YOUR DOCTOR IF

- You have symptoms of valley fever.
- The following occurs during treatment:
  Continued weight loss.
  Fever of 101F (38.3C) orally.
  Diarrhea that cannot be controlled.
  Stiff neck with severe headache.

ILLNESSES & DISORDERS

VARICOSE VEINS

GENERAL INFORMATION

DEFINITION—Veins, usually in the legs, that become permanently dilated and twisted.

BODY PARTS INVOLVED—Veins in the legs, including superficial veins, deep veins and veins that connect superficial and deep veins. Veins in the vaginal lips during pregnancy and those around the anus (hemorrhoids) also may become varicose.

SEX OR AGE MOST AFFECTED—Adults of both sexes.

SIGNS & SYMPTOMS
- Enlarged, disfiguring, snakelike, bluish veins that are visible under the skin upon standing. They appear most often in the back of the calf or on the inside of the leg from ankle to groin.
- Vague discomfort and aching in the legs, especially after standing.
- Fatigue.

CAUSES—The veins of the legs contain one-way valves every few inches to help blood return against gravity to the heart. If the valves leak, blood pressure in the veins prevents blood from draining properly. Valves may fail because of: previous vein disease, such as thrombophlebitis; prolonged standing; or pressure on veins in the pelvis from pregnancy, tumors or fluid in the abdomen.

RISK INCREASES WITH
- Pregnancy.
- Menstrual cycle. Symptoms worsen before and during menstruation.
- Family history of varicose veins.
- Occupations that require prolonged standing.

HOW TO PREVENT—Exercise regularly, especially by walking, swimming or bicycling, to keep circulation healthy.

WHAT TO EXPECT

APPROPRIATE HEALTH CARE
- Self-care after diagnosis.
- Doctor's treatment.
- Surgery to remove enlarged veins.
- Hospitalization for complications.

DIAGNOSTIC MEASURES
- Your own observation of symptoms.
- Medical history and physical exam by a doctor.
- X-rays of veins (venogram).

POSSIBLE COMPLICATIONS
- Ulcer near the ankle (stasis dermatitis) caused by poor circulation to the skin. This may be slow to heal.
- Deep-vein blood clot.
- Bleeding under the skin or externally.
- Skin problems adjacent to the varicose veins that resemble eczema.

PROBABLE OUTCOME—Symptoms can be controlled with treatment or cured with surgery.

HOW TO TREAT

NOTE—Follow your doctor's instructions. These instructions are supplemental.

GENERAL MEASURES
- Exercise to keep circulation and leg muscles in good condition. Walking is ideal.
- Wear elastic support stockings.
- Rest often with legs slightly elevated to promote good circulation.
- Don't sit with your legs crossed.
- Don't wear girdles, garters or pantyhose with tight elastic tops that obstruct blood flow.
- If the skin over a varicose vein breaks and the vein bleeds, lie down and press on it with your hand in a cloth until bleeding stops.
- Don't stretch skin over varicose veins.
- Elevate the foot of your bed with 2-inch blocks to help circulation in the legs at night.

MEDICATION—Medicine usually is not necessary for this disorder. However, your doctor may inject a chemical into small varicose veins to make them clot and scar (sometimes). Other veins will take over circulation in the area.

ACTIVITY—No restrictions.

DIET—No special diet.

CALL YOUR DOCTOR IF

- You have varicose veins.
- After diagnosis, varicose veins begin causing circulation problems in your feet, especially stasis dermatitis.

VITAMIN-B DEFICIENCIES

GENERAL INFORMATION

DEFINITION—Diseases caused by inadequate or absent B vitamins: B-1 (thiamine); B-2, (riboflavin); niacin; B-6 (pyridoxine); B-12 (cyanocobalamin). Vitamins are organic chemicals that occur in many natural foods. They are necessary for normal body function. B vitamins are water soluble and excess amounts cannot be stored by the body.

BODY PARTS INVOLVED—Central nervous system; heart; skin; eyes; blood.

SEX OR AGE MOST AFFECTED—Both sexes; all ages.

SIGNS & SYMPTOMS—One or several of the following deficiencies may exist at the same time:
- B-1 deficiency (beriberi).
  Tingling or loss of sensation in the legs.
  Weakness.
  Congestive heart failure.
  Mental changes, including poor memory or psychosis.
  Lack of urinary control.
  Abdominal pain.
- B-2 deficiency.
  Cracked lips.
  Pallor.
  Sore tongue.
- Niacin deficiency (pellagra).
  Fatigue and weakness.
  Poor appetite.
  Inflamed skin that may blister, weep and split.
  Sore, burning mouth and tongue.
  Indigestion, nausea, vomiting and diarrhea.
  Mental changes, including confusion and psychosis.
- B-6 deficiency.
  Dermatitis.
  Sore mouth and tongue.
  Abdominal pain, vomiting and diarrhea.
  Convulsions.
- B-12 deficiency (see Pernicious Anemia in Illness section).

CAUSES
- Malnutrition, including malnutrition incurred from fad diets or malnutrition present in infants born to malnourished mothers.
- Alcoholism.
- Gastrointestinal diseases with poor absorption.
- Stomach surgery (B-12 deficiency only).
- Use of some medications, such as isoniazid or oral contraceptives, which inactivate vitamin B-6.

RISK INCREASES WITH
- Adults over 60.
- Improper diet.
- Prolonged illness.
- Pregnancy.
- Smoking (maybe). This decreases absorption of vitamin C and may affect other vitamins.

HOW TO PREVENT
- Eat a well-balanced, nutritious diet.
- Take multiple-vitamin supplements if you cannot eat well.

WHAT TO EXPECT

APPROPRIATE HEALTH CARE
- Self-care after diagnosis.
- Doctor's treatment.
- Hospitalization for severe malnutrition of alcoholism.

DIAGNOSTIC MEASURES
- Your own observation of symptoms.
- Medical history and physical exam by a doctor.
- Laboratory blood studies of vitamin levels.

POSSIBLE COMPLICATIONS
- Permanent brain or nerve damage.
- Severe heart disease.

PROBABLE OUTCOME—Prompt recovery if vitamin-B deficiency is treated with proper nutrition and oral supplements in the early stages. Without treatment, severe malnutrition can cause permanent disability or death.

HOW TO TREAT

NOTE—Follow your doctor's instructions. These instructions are supplemental.

GENERAL MEASURES—No specific instructions except those listed under other headings.

MEDICATION—Your doctor may prescribe vitamin supplements, depending on the type of deficiency. Don't take more than the prescribed amount. Excessive doses of vitamin B-6 can *cause* the same symptoms produced by deficiency.

ACTIVITY—No restrictions.

DIET—No special diet. Prepare well-balanced meals. Don't overcook food or expose it to the air for prolonged periods—these destroy vitamins. Use fresh fruits, vegetables and meats rather than processed foods, if possible.

CALL YOUR DOCTOR IF

You have symptoms of vitamin-B deficiency.

VITAMIN-C DEFICIENCY
(Scurvy)

GENERAL INFORMATION

DEFINITION—Illness caused by an inadequate intake of vitamin C. Vitamin C is essential for the body to manufacture collagen, connective tissue that helps form healthy bones, teeth and capillaries, and promotes wound healing.

BODY PARTS INVOLVED—Bones; teeth; gums; capillaries.

SEX OR AGE MOST AFFECTED—Both sexes; all ages.

SIGNS & SYMPTOMS—Infants and children:
- Tender swollen legs. The child prefers to lie with legs partly bent, and cries if moved.
- Bleeding and bruising under the skin.
- Anemia.
- Tender ribs (sometimes).
- Bleeding gums (if teeth are present).
- Fever.
Adults:
- Swollen bleeding gums.
- Loss of teeth.
- Rough skin.
- Bleeding or bruising under the skin or into joints.
- Weakness and fatigue.
- Mental changes, including hallucinations and bizarre behavior.
Children and adults:
- Increased susceptibility to infection.

CAUSES—Diet that is lacking in adequate vitamin C.

RISK INCREASES WITH
- Improper diet, including following fad diets that don't include fruits and vegetables.
- Loss of vitamin C from foods by overcooking or improper or prolonged storage.
- Maintaining an infant on formula without vitamin supplements.
- Hyperthyroidism.
- Pregnancy.

HOW TO PREVENT—Eat a diet rich in vitamin-C-containing foods. These include citrus fruits, tomatoes and green vegetables, such as green peppers, broccoli and cabbage. 4 to 6 ounces of orange juice a day provides the minimum daily requirement of vitamin C.

WHAT TO EXPECT

APPROPRIATE HEALTH CARE
- Self-care after diagnosis.
- Doctor's treatment.

DIAGNOSTIC MEASURES
- Your own observation of symptoms.
- Medical history and physical exam by a doctor.
- Laboratory blood studies, such as: blood counts for anemia; tests for blood levels of vitamin C; and bleeding and clotting tests.
- X-rays of bones.

POSSIBLE COMPLICATIONS—Fractures or dislocations, especially in children with tender legs or ribs.

PROBABLE OUTCOME—Curable with vitamin-C (ascorbic acid) supplements and a balanced diet that contains foods high in vitamin C. All symptoms and effects, except tooth loss, are reversible. Without treatment, vitamin-C deficiency can be fatal.

HOW TO TREAT

NOTE—Follow your doctor's instructions. These instructions are supplemental.

GENERAL MEASURES—No specific instructions except those listed under other headings.

MEDICATION—Your doctor will prescribe vitamin-C tablets. Don't take more than the prescribed amount. Excessive doses of vitamin C can contribute to kidney-stone formation. If massive doses are suddenly decreased, scurvy can result.

ACTIVITY—Handle infants and children carefully to avoid bone or joint injury until the deficiency is corrected.

DIET
- Eat a well-balanced diet that includes foods rich in vitamin C (see How to Prevent).
- Take prenatal vitamin supplements if you are pregnant.
- Provide your infant with vitamin supplements or vitamin-fortified formula.

CALL YOUR DOCTOR IF

- You have symptoms of vitamin-C deficiency.
- Symptoms don't improve in 3 weeks, despite treatment.

VITAMIN-D DEFICIENCY

GENERAL INFORMATION

DEFINITION—Insufficient intake or absorption of vitamin D, coupled with too little exposure to sunlight. This deficiency causes rickets in children and osteomalacia (softening of the bone) in adults.

BODY PARTS INVOLVED—Total body, but bones are more affected than other tissues.

SEX OR AGE MOST AFFECTED—All ages, but most common in infants and young children up to age 10.

SIGNS & SYMPTOMS—In infants:
- Restlessness.
- Poor sleep habits.
- Profuse sweating.
- Delayed sitting, crawling or walking.
- Delayed closing of the fontanels.
- Poor muscular development, causing a pot belly.
- Bowed legs, "knock knees" and "pigeon breast" after weight-bearing activities begin (standing and walking).

In adults:
- No symptoms until late stages (sometimes).
- Bone pain.
- Muscle weakness.
- Shortening of the vertebral column and flattening of pelvic bones.

CAUSES
- Insufficient dietary intake of vitamin D.
- Poor absorption of vitamin D, causing poor absorption of calcium and phosphorous necessary for healthy bone. Vitamin-D absorption is affected by chronic diseases, such as: pancreatitis; celiac disease; cystic fibrosis; colitis; bile-duct disorders; liver disorders; kidney disease; or surgery on the stomach or small bowel.
- Inadequate exposure to sunlight. This is especially likely in persons confined to bed or home, or those who work at night and sleep during the day.
- Poor function of the parathyroid glands (sometimes).

RISK INCREASES WITH
- Genetic factors, such as black skin, which decreases the absorption of sunlight.
- Use of anticonvulsant drugs.
- Exposure to polluted air. Smog reduces sunlight penetration.
- Improper diet as a result of poverty, food faddism, bulimia or anorexia nervosa.
- Pregnancy, in which the body needs additional vitamin D.

HOW TO PREVENT
- Provide vitamin-D supplements for yourself and your family—including breast-fed babies—unless you are sure your diet supplies a satisfactory amount.
- Exercise outdoors in sunlight.
- Don't follow fad diets, which may be deficient in many nutrients, including vitamin D.

WHAT TO EXPECT

APPROPRIATE HEALTH CARE
- Self-care after diagnosis.
- Doctor's treatment.

DIAGNOSTIC MEASURES
- Your own observation of symptoms.
- Medical history and physical exam by a doctor.
- Laboratory blood studies of calcium, phosphorous and alkaline levels.

POSSIBLE COMPLICATIONS
- Spontaneous fractures in softened bones.
- Difficult or impossible vaginal childbirth in women with flattened pelvic bones. Delivery by Cesarean section is usually necessary.

PROBABLE OUTCOME—Usually curable with an adequate diet, vitamin-D supplements, and treatment for any underlying disease. Bone malformation cannot be reversed.

HOW TO TREAT

NOTE—Follow your doctor's instructions. These instructions are supplemental.

GENERAL MEASURES—Sleep on a firm mattress.

MEDICATION—Your doctor may prescribe vitamin-D tablets or injections.

ACTIVITY
- Exercise whenever possible, especially in sunlight. Weight-bearing exercise, such as walking or running, is especially beneficial.
- Avoid excessive bed rest.
- Stoop—don't bend—to lift heavy objects.

DIET—Increase your intake of foods rich in vitamin D—even if you take vitamin-D supplements. Dietary sources include: fortified milk; liver; eggs; margarine; green vegetables; cauliflower; tomatoes; cheese.

CALL YOUR DOCTOR IF

- You or your child have symptoms of vitamin-D deficiency.
- Your child's symptoms don't improve in 1 month, despite treatment
- Pain or suspected fracture occurs following an injury—even minor injury.

VITAMIN-E DEFICIENCY

 GENERAL INFORMATION

DEFINITION—The effects of inadequate intake of vitamin E. Vitamin E is present in many foods, so deficiency is rare in otherwise healthy persons. Vitamin E promotes normal growth and development. It also enhances enzyme action necessary for body cells to use oxygen efficiently.

BODY PARTS INVOLVED—Blood and body cells.

SEX OR AGE MOST AFFECTED—Both sexes; all ages.

SIGNS & SYMPTOMS
- Muscle weakness or cramps.
- Swelling of the ankles, abdomen and face in infants.
- Anemia in premature infants.

CAUSES
- Malnutrition.
- Malabsorption.

RISK INCREASES WITH—Poor nutrition.

HOW TO PREVENT
- Eat a well-balanced diet.
- Determine if your infant's formula has adequate vitamin E.
- Take vitamin supplements, if your diet is inadequate.

OTHER—No evidence exists that vitamin E has any effect on human sexual reproduction or activity.

 WHAT TO EXPECT

APPROPRIATE HEALTH CARE
- Self-care after diagnosis.
- Doctor's treatment.

DIAGNOSTIC MEASURES
- Your own observation of symptoms.
- Medical history and physical exam by a doctor.
- Laboratory studies to measure blood level of vitamin E.

POSSIBLE COMPLICATIONS—Chronic anemia, resulting in fatigue and underachievement.

PROBABLE OUTCOME—Curable with proper diet and vitamin-E supplements.

 HOW TO TREAT

NOTE—Follow your doctor's instructions. These instructions are supplemental.

GENERAL MEASURES—No specific instructions except those listed under other headings.

MEDICATION—Your doctor may prescribe vitamin-E supplements.

ACTIVITY—No restrictions.

DIET—Eat a well-balanced diet and avoid fad reducing diets. Good sources of vitamin E include salad and cooking oil, margarine, peanuts, beef, eggs and green vegetables.

 CALL YOUR DOCTOR IF

You have symptoms of vitamin-E deficiency.

VITAMIN-K DEFICIENCY

GENERAL INFORMATION

DEFINITION—Inadequate or absent vitamin K, a fat-soluble vitamin necessary for proper blood clotting. Some vitamin K is produced in the gastrointestinal tract.

BODY PARTS INVOLVED—Liver; blood.

SEX OR AGE MOST AFFECTED—Both sexes; all ages. A newborn infant lacks vitamin K until its body begins to produce it.

SIGNS & SYMPTOMS
- Unusual bleeding, such as from the gums, nose or gastrointestinal tract.
- Unexplained bruising.

CAUSES
- Excessive amounts of anticoagulant drugs, such as warfarin or dicumarol.
- Prolonged use of antibiotics. Vitamin K is produced by intestinal bacteria that are destroyed by antibiotics.
- Gallbladder disease.
- Malabsorption disorders, such as celiac disease, pellagra, Crohn's disease, ulcerative colitis or cystic fibrosis.

RISK INCREASES WITH—Poor nutrition, especially an unbalanced diet with inadequate amounts of vitamin K.

HOW TO PREVENT—Injections of vitamin K are given to newborn infants and to persons with gallbladder disease or malabsorption disorders to prevent deficiency. For most people, a well-balanced diet should provide all the vitamin K necessary.

WHAT TO EXPECT

APPROPRIATE HEALTH CARE
- Doctor's treatment.
- Self-care after diagnosis.

DIAGNOSTIC MEASURES
- Your own observation of symptoms.
- Medical history and physical exam by a doctor.
- Laboratory studies of blood clotting.

POSSIBLE COMPLICATIONS—Severe or fatal hemorrhage.

PROBABLE OUTCOME—Curable with vitamin-K supplements by mouth or injection.

HOW TO TREAT

NOTE—Follow your doctor's instructions. These instructions are supplemental.

GENERAL MEASURES—If you take anticoagulants, take only the prescribed amount. Have frequent blood tests to monitor prothrombin time (see Glossary) and prevent unexpected bleeding.

MEDICATION—Your doctor will prescribe vitamin K orally or by injection.

ACTIVITY—No restrictions.

DIET—Eat a well-balanced diet that includes foods high in vitamin K, such as green leafy vegetables, cauliflower, tomatoes, cheese, egg yolks and liver.

CALL YOUR DOCTOR IF

You have unexplained bleeding or bruising, especially if you take anticoagulants, or have gallbladder disease or a malabsorptive disorder.

ILLNESSES & DISORDERS

VITILIGO

 GENERAL INFORMATION

DEFINITION—Loss of skin pigmentation in patches. This can affect persons of any race or ethnic group.

BODY PARTS INVOLVED—Skin on the back of the hands, face and armpits.

SEX OR AGE MOST AFFECTED—Late childhood (9 to 12 years) to mid-adulthood.

SIGNS & SYMPTOMS—Macules (small areas of different skin color) or patches with the following characteristics:
- They are flat, white and can't be felt with fingers.
- They spread to form very large, irregularly-shaped areas without pigmentation.
- They are usually on both sides of the body in approximately the same place.
- Their size varies from 2mm or 3mm to several centimeters in diameter.
- They don't hurt or itch.

CAUSES—Probably autoimmune disease. The pigment-producing cells (melanocytes) don't function normally, allowing destruction of pigment. Once pigment has been destroyed, melanocytes can't produce more pigment.

RISK INCREASES WITH
- Family history of vitiligo.
- Thyroid or adrenal disease.
- Diabetes mellitus.

HOW TO PREVENT—Cannot be prevented at present.

 WHAT TO EXPECT

NOTE—Follow your doctor's instructions. These instructions are supplemental.

APPROPRIATE HEALTH CARE
- Self-care.
- Doctor's treatment.

POSSIBLE COMPLICATIONS—Disorder may never disappear completely, causing permanent disfigurement.

PROBABLE OUTCOME—Treatment is prolonged and often unsatisfactory. Complete and permanent repigmentation is rarely possible. Treatment consists of using an oral medication called psoralens. When discontinued, most of the regained pigmentation is usually lost.

It is impossible to predict how much improvement will occur with treatment. Younger individuals (under 30) and those who obtain treatment early usually respond best. Allow 1 year to evaluate results.

 HOW TO TREAT

GENERAL MEASURES
- If you don't choose to use oral medication (or if it is unsuccessful), cover the lesions with waterproof, opaque makeup such as Lydia O'Leary's Cover Mark.
- If you don't use cosmetic makeup, apply sunscreen to protect areas without pigment from sun damage.

MEDICATION—Your doctor may prescribe psoralens, which stimulates pigmentation from healthy pigment cells bordering damaged cells. Results may be disappointing and adverse effects are frequent.

ACTIVITY—No restrictions.

DIET—No special diet.

 CALL YOUR DOCTOR IF

- You have symptoms of vitiligo.
- New, unexplained symptoms develop. The drug used in treatment may produce side effects.

VOCAL-CORD NODULES
("Singer's Nodes")

 GENERAL INFORMATION

DEFINITION—Non-malignant overgrowths of tissue on the vocal cords.

BODY PARTS INVOLVED—Larynx (voicebox).

SEX OR AGE MOST AFFECTED—Adults of both sexes.

SIGNS & SYMPTOMS—Persistent hoarseness without pain.

CAUSES—Continued overuse of the voice by singing, shouting, yelling, lecturing or other forms of talking too loudly or too much.

RISK INCREASES WITH
- Smoking.
- Vocal performers or public speakers, such as professional singers, teachers, ministers or auctioneers.

HOW TO PREVENT
- Use voice amplification, such as a microphone or megaphone, when performing or speaking.
- Take voice or speech lessons to learn to make your voice carry with less effort.
- Ask others to remind you when you get overexcited, especially in activities such as sporting events, so you can lower your voice.
- Don't smoke.

 WHAT TO EXPECT

APPROPRIATE HEALTH CARE
- Self-care after diagnosis.
- Doctor's treatment.
- Surgery to remove nodules (usually).

DIAGNOSTIC MEASURES
- Your own observation of symptoms.
- Medical history and physical exam by a doctor, usually an ear, nose and throat specialist.

POSSIBLE COMPLICATIONS
- Without treatment, permanent hoarseness or voice alteration.
- Failure to diagnose larynx cancer, which also begins with hoarseness.

PROBABLE OUTCOME—Curable with a simple surgical procedure.

 HOW TO TREAT

NOTE—Follow your doctor's instructions. These instructions are supplemental.

GENERAL MEASURES
- Nodules may disappear if the voice is rested for several months. If you choose this treatment rather than surgery, speak in a whisper or write notes.
- Don't smoke, and avoid smoky environments.

MEDICATION—After surgery:
- Your doctor may prescribe antibiotics to prevent infection.
- You may take mild non-prescription pain relievers, if necessary, such as acetaminophen or aspirin.

ACTIVITY—Don't use your voice after surgery until your doctor determines that healing is complete.

DIET—No special diet.

 CALL YOUR DOCTOR IF

You are hoarse for more than 2 weeks.

ILLNESSES & DISORDERS

VULVOVAGINITIS BEFORE PUBERTY

 GENERAL INFORMATION

DEFINITION—Infection or inflammation of the vagina or vulva before a young girl reaches puberty.

BODY PARTS INVOLVED—Vagina; cervix; vulva (vaginal lips); skin around the genitals.

SEX OR AGE MOST AFFECTED—Female infants and children.

SIGNS & SYMPTOMS
- Redness, pain and itching around the genital area.
- Vaginal discharge, which may or may not smell bad.
- Pain with urination.
- Bleeding from the affected area (sometimes).

CAUSES
- Infections caused by: bacteria; parasites, including pinworms; yeastlike fungi; or viruses. See Vaginitis (several charts in Illness section).
- Allergies to synthetic fabrics, soap or other items in contact with the genitals.
- Scratches, abrasions or genital injury from insertion of foreign bodies in the vagina by the child or a playmate.
- Genital injury from sexual abuse.

RISK INCREASES WITH
- Diabetes mellitus.
- Infrequent bathing or unsanitary living conditions.

HOW TO PREVENT
- Teach the child to wipe after bowel movements from the vagina toward the anus.
- Don't let the child sit around in wet clothing—especially a wet bathing suit.
- Don't use colored or perfumed toilet tissue, scented soap or bubble baths.
- Provide the child with cotton panties or nylon panties with a cotton crotch—not panties made of non-ventilating materials.
- If antibiotics are prescribed for any reason, the child should eat more yogurt and sour cream. This helps prevent vaginal yeast infections.
- Teach your child to resist and report any attempted sexual contact by an older person.

 WHAT TO EXPECT

APPROPRIATE HEALTH CARE
- Doctor's treatment, including removal of any foreign object in the vagina.
- Home care after diagnosis.

DIAGNOSTIC MEASURES
- Your own observation of symptoms.
- Medical history and physical exam by a doctor.
- Laboratory culture and microscopic exam of the discharge.

POSSIBLE COMPLICATIONS—Psychological trauma if the condition is caused by sexual abuse.

PROBABLE OUTCOME—Usually curable in 10 days with treatment.

 HOW TO TREAT

NOTE—Follow your doctor's instructions. These instructions are supplemental.

GENERAL MEASURES
- Follow suggestions under How to Prevent.
- Remove the source of any irritation or allergy, such as soap.
- Don't try to remove a foreign object from the vagina. This may be painful or cause further injury. Take your child to the doctor for removal.
- If urinating causes burning, the child may urinate while bathing or urinate through a toilet-paper roll or plastic cup with the end cut out. This prevents urine from stinging inflamed skin.

MEDICATION—Your doctor may prescribe:
- Medication appropriate for the infection, including antibiotics, antifungal or antiparasitic drugs.
- Topical ointments to relieve pain and itching.

ACTIVITY—No restrictions.

DIET—No special diet.

 CALL YOUR DOCTOR IF

- Your child has symptoms of vulvovaginitis.
- You suspect your child has been sexually abused.
- Symptoms don't improve in 7 to 10 days or symptoms worsen, despite treatment.
- Unusual vaginal bleeding or swelling develops.

WARTS
(Verruca Vulgaris)

GENERAL INFORMATION

DEFINITION—Benign tumors caused by a virus in the outer skin layer. Warts are not cancerous. They are contagious from person to person and from one area to another on the same person.

BODY PARTS INVOLVED—Skin anywhere, but most likely on the fingers, hands and arms.

SEX OR AGE MOST AFFECTED—Most common in children and young adults between ages 1 and 30, but may occur at any age.

SIGNS & SYMPTOMS—A small, raised bump on the skin with the following characteristics:
- Warts begin very small (1mm to 3mm) and grow larger.
- Warts have a rough surface and clearly defined borders.
- They are usually the same color as the skin, but sometimes darker.
- Warts often appear in clusters around a "mother wart."
- If you cut into the wart surface, it contains small black dots or bleeding points.
- Warts are painless and don't itch.

CAUSES—Invasion of the outer skin layer (epidermis) by the papilloma virus. The virus stimulates some cells to grow more rapidly than normal.

Warts are very common. By adulthood, 90% of all people have antibodies to the virus, indicating a history of at least one wart infection.

RISK INCREASES WITH—Unknown.

HOW TO PREVENT—To keep from spreading warts, don't scratch them. Warts spread readily to small cuts and scratches.

WHAT TO EXPECT

APPROPRIATE HEALTH CARE
- Home care after diagnosis and treatment.
- Doctor's treatment.
- Cryotherapy (freezing cells to destroy them). This is an office procedure that doesn't require anesthesia or cause bleeding. Freezing stings or hurts slightly during application, and pain may increase a bit after thawing. 3 to 5 weekly treatments are usually necessary to destroy the wart.
- Electrosurgery (using heat to destroy cells). This treatment can usually be completed in one office visit, but healing takes longer, and secondary bacterial infections and scarring are more common.

DIAGNOSTIC MEASURES
- Your own observation of symptoms.
- Medical history and physical exam by a doctor.

POSSIBLE COMPLICATIONS
- Spread to other body parts.
- Secondary infection of a wart.

PROBABLE OUTCOME—20% of warts disappear spontaneously in 1 month. Without treatment, the remainder disappear in most children in 2 to 3 years.

HOW TO TREAT

NOTE—Follow your doctor's instructions. These instructions are supplemental.

GENERAL MEASURES
- If you have electrosurgery, keep the treatment site clean with soap and water. Cover with an adhesive bandage, if you wish.
- If you have cryotherapy, a blister (sometimes with blood) will develop at the treatment site. The roof of the blister will come off without further treatment in 10 to 14 days. You should have little or no scarring. Wash and use make-up or cosmetics as usual. If clothing irritates the blister, cover with a small adhesive bandage.

MEDICATION—Your doctor may prescribe chemicals, such as mild salicylic acid, to destroy warts. If so, apply twice a day for 4 to 6 weeks.

ACTIVITY—No restrictions.

DIET—No special diet.

CALL YOUR DOCTOR IF

- You or your child have warts and you want them removed.
- After removal by cryosurgery or electrocautery, signs of infection appear at the treatment site.
- After treatment, temperature rises over 101F (38.3C).
- Warts don't disappear completely after treatment.
- Other warts appear after treatment.

WARTS, FLAT

 GENERAL INFORMATION

DEFINITION—Benign, small tumors of the skin caused by a virus. This type of wart is not passed by sexual activity, but it is contagious.

BODY PARTS INVOLVED—Skin along scratch marks or other areas of injury. In children, flat warts occur most often on the face or injured surfaces of the arms and legs. In men, they usually occur on areas of the face that are shaved. In women, they are common on the legs or other areas that are shaved.

SEX OR AGE MOST AFFECTED—Children and young adults (up to age 40).

SIGNS & SYMPTOMS—Flat warts have the following characteristics:
- They are flat-topped, square-shouldered, solid elevations barely raised above the skin surface.
- They appear along scratch marks or other areas of skin injury and accumulate in lines or clusters.
- They don't hurt or itch.

CAUSES—Flat warts are caused by the contagious papilloma virus. The virus is shed from fingers and spaces beneath the fingernails.

RISK INCREASES WITH—Use of immunosuppressive drugs.

HOW TO PREVENT—No specific preventive measures except to protect the skin from injury and wash hands frequently.

 WHAT TO EXPECT

APPROPRIATE HEALTH CARE
- Self-care to apply topical medications.
- Doctor's treatment to remove warts with chemicals, cryotherapy or curettage (see Glossary), with or without electrosurgery (see Glossary).

DIAGNOSTIC MEASURES
- Your own observation of symptoms.
- Medical history and physical exam by a doctor.

POSSIBLE COMPLICATIONS—None expected.

PROBABLE OUTCOME—In children, flat warts spread rapidly, reach a plateau period and disappear soon after. In adults, flat warts are stubborn and may last for years without treatment.

 HOW TO TREAT

NOTE—Follow your doctor's instructions. These instructions are supplemental.

GENERAL MEASURES—Remove the source of trauma, if possible. Men with flat warts on the face should shave with an electric shaver or grow a beard. Women with flat warts on areas that are shaved should use other methods to remove hair, such as depilatory cream or wax.

MEDICATION—Your doctor may prescribe:
- Retinoic acid (Retin-A) or benzoyl peroxide. Either should be applied once or twice a day for 4 to 6 weeks. Apply a small amount to each wart with the tip of a toothpick.
- Duofilm (16% salicylic acid). Follow directions on the medication label.

ACTIVITY—No restrictions.

DIET—No special diet.

 CALL YOUR DOCTOR IF

- You have symptoms of flat warts.
- Warts continue to spread despite treatment.
- Signs of infection (redness, pain or fever) develop in a treated area.

WARTS, PLANTAR

GENERAL INFORMATION

DEFINITION—Warts on the soles of the feet.

BODY PARTS INVOLVED—Skin of the plantar surface (bottom) of the feet.

SEX OR AGE MOST AFFECTED—Children and adults between ages 20 and 50.

SIGNS & SYMPTOMS
- Pinhead-sized bump that grows to 2mm or 3mm. Shaving off the top reveals small black dots, pinpoint bleeding and an underlying translucent core.
- Pain on walking. The wart compresses underlying tender tissue.

CAUSES—Infection with the human papilloma virus, which passes from person to person by direct contact. The virus invades the skin, making infected cells reproduce faster than normal cells.

RISK INCREASES WITH—Unknown.

HOW TO PREVENT
- Don't touch warts on other people.
- Don't wear another person's shoes.
- Wear footwear in public locker rooms or showers.

WHAT TO EXPECT

APPROPRIATE HEALTH CARE
- Self-care after diagnosis.
- Doctor's treatment. Your doctor will probably pare away the overlying calloused skin, and apply chemical cauterants, such as trichloracetic acid, 20% salicylic acid or 20% formalin.

DIAGNOSTIC MEASURES
- Your own observation of symptoms.
- Medical history and physical exam by a doctor.

POSSIBLE COMPLICATIONS—None expected.

PROBABLE OUTCOME—Usually curable in 6 to 10 weeks with treatment, but some cases are resistant to treatment. Recurrence is common.

HOW TO TREAT

NOTE—Follow your doctor's instructions. These instructions are supplemental.

GENERAL MEASURES—Insert pads or cushions in your shoes to make walking more comfortable.

MEDICATION
- For minor discomfort, you may use non-prescription drugs such as acetaminophen.
- Your doctor may prescribe chemically treated plaster for you to apply. Follow instructions carefully.

ACTIVITY—No restrictions. Because walking aggravates the wart, find the most comfortable way to walk without putting weight on the wart, such as walking on the heels.

DIET—No special diet.

CALL YOUR DOCTOR IF

- You have a plantar wart.
- The treated area becomes infected, with redness, heat, increased pain and tenderness.

ILLNESSES & DISORDERS

WARTS, VENEREAL
(Condylomata Acuminata; Genital Warts; Moist Warts)

 GENERAL INFORMATION

DEFINITION—Warts in the genital area. These are more contagious than other warts.

BODY PARTS INVOLVED—Urethra; genitals; rectum.

SEX OR AGE MOST AFFECTED—Both sexes of sexually active adolescents and adults.

SIGNS & SYMPTOMS—Venereal warts have the following characteristics:
- They appear on moist surfaces, especially the penis, entrance to the vagina and entrance to the rectum.
- They are thin, flexible, solid elevations of the skin, growing in stalks or clusters. They are taller than they are wide.
- Each wart measures 1mm to 2mm in diameter, but clusters may be quite large.
- They don't hurt or itch.

CAUSES—Venereal warts are caused by a subtype of the same virus that causes other warts, but they are more contagious. They spread easily on the skin of the infected person and pass easily to other people. They are usually transmitted sexually, often as a result of poor hygiene. They have an incubation of 1 to 6 months.

RISK INCREASES WITH
- Poor nutrition.
- Other venereal disease.
- Crowded or unsanitary living conditions.

HOW TO PREVENT—To prevent spread of warts to other parts of the body or to other persons:
- Don't scratch warts.
- Avoid sexual activity until warts heal completely.
- Use rubber condoms during sexual intercourse.

OTHER—Recent clinical evidence suggests the virus that causes venereal warts may also be associated with genital malignancies.

 WHAT TO EXPECT

APPROPRIATE HEALTH CARE
- Self-care after diagnosis.
- Doctor's treatment, which may include application of liquid nitrogen to warts.

DIAGNOSTIC MEASURES
- Your own observation of symptoms.
- Medical history and physical exam by a doctor.

POSSIBLE COMPLICATIONS—Medication used to treat venereal warts (podophyllin) may damage an unborn child. Systemic toxicity to the fetus has occurred after intravaginal application. Don't use podophyllin if you are pregnant.

PROBABLE OUTCOME—These small warts usually cause no symptoms. If untreated, they probably will disappear eventually. However, because the virus may be associated with genital malignancy, obtain medical treatment.

 HOW TO TREAT

MEDICATION—If your doctor prescribes podophyllin, a topical medication, apply it carefully to avoid damaging surrounding healthy tissue. Use petroleum jelly on surrounding tissue first. Don't apply to large areas at one time. This may cause irritation or absorption of the drug. Keep podophyllin out of eyes.

GENERAL MEASURES—These warts are generally treated with chemicals: podophyllin, trichloracetic acid or liquid nitrogen. After applying any of these, wait 4 hours; then wash the treated area carefully.

ACTIVITY—No restrictions, except to avoid sexual relations until warts are completely gone.

DIET—No special diet.

 CALL YOUR DOCTOR IF

- You have symptoms of venereal warts.
- The following occurs after treatment:
  The treated area becomes infected (red, swollen, painful or tender).
  Temperature rises to 101F (38.3C) or above.
  You feel generally ill.

WHIPLASH
(Acceleration-Deceleration Cervical Injury)

 GENERAL INFORMATION

DEFINITION—Injury to the neck caused when it is whipped backward forcefully—usually in an accident.

BODY PARTS INVOLVED—Muscles, tendons, disks and nerves in the neck.

SEX OR AGE MOST AFFECTED—Both sexes; all ages.

SIGNS & SYMPTOMS
- Pain or stiffness in the front and back of the neck—either immediately following or up to 24 hours after injury.
- Dizziness.
- Headache.
- Nausea and vomiting (sometimes).

CAUSES—Injury, usually from contact sports or motor-vehicle accidents.

RISK INCREASES WITH
- Osteoarthritis of the spine.
- Situations that make accidents more likely, such as:
  Driving in rainy, icy or snowy weather.
  "Tail-gaiting" or other poor driving habits.
  Driving after excess alcohol consumption or use of mind-altering drugs.

HOW TO PREVENT—Use the padded headrests in your auto. These have decreased the frequency and severity of auto whiplash injuries. Drive carefully and defensively. Don't drink or use mind-altering drugs and drive.

 WHAT TO EXPECT

APPROPRIATE HEALTH CARE
- Self-care after diagnosis.
- Doctor's treatment.
- Diathermy or ultrasound treatments (see Glossary).
- Surgery to remove an injured spinal disk (rare).

DIAGNOSTIC MEASURES
- Your own observation of symptoms.
- Medical history and physical exam by a doctor.
- X-rays of the neck.

POSSIBLE COMPLICATIONS—Temporary numbness and weakness in the arms, if nerve roots are injured. This may persist until recovery.

PROBABLE OUTCOME—Usually curable in 1 week to 3 months with treatment.

 HOW TO TREAT

NOTE—Follow your doctor's instructions. These instructions are supplemental.

GENERAL MEASURES
- Apply ice packs to the injured area for 10 to 20 minutes each hour during the first 24 hours.
- After 24 hours, use ice packs or heat to relieve pain. Heat may include hot showers twice a day, in which the water beats on your neck and shoulders for 10 to 20 minutes. Between showers, apply hot soaks (see Appendix 18) to the neck, or use a heat lamp several times a day for 10 to 15 minutes.
- Try to improve your posture. Pull in your chin and abdomen when sitting or standing. Sit in a firm chair and force your buttocks to touch the chair's back.
- If symptoms are severe, buy and wear a soft, padded, fabric collar (Thomas collar) until pain subsides.
- Sleep without a pillow. Instead, roll a small towel to 2 inches in diameter, or use a cervical pillow or a Thomas collar. Poor sleeping positions delay healing.
- If you have nerve-root pressure, with numbness and weakness in the hand or arm, buy or rent a cervical-traction apparatus. This can be hung over a doorway. Ask your doctor for specific instructions.

MEDICATION
- Your doctor may prescribe pain relievers or muscle relaxants (sometimes).
- You may use non-prescription drugs, such as aspirin or acetaminophen, for minor pain.

ACTIVITY—Depends on the severity of symptoms. During the acute or severe stage, rest as much as possible. As symptoms improve, resume normal activity gradually.

DIET—No special diet.

 CALL YOUR DOCTOR IF

- You have a painful neck injury.
- Pain, numbness, tingling or weakness develops in the arm or face.
- New, unexplained symptoms develop. Drugs used in treatment may produce side effects.

WHOOPING COUGH
(Pertussis)

GENERAL INFORMATION

DEFINITION—A serious, contagious, bacterial infection of the bronchial tubes and lungs. Immunization throughout the world has greatly decreased the incidence of whooping cough.

BODY PARTS INVOLVED—Bronchial tubes; larynx; lungs.

SEX OR AGE MOST AFFECTED—All ages, but most common in children.

SIGNS & SYMPTOMS—Early stages:
- Runny nose.
- Dry cough that progresses to a cough with thick sputum.
- Slight fever.

Late stages:
- Severe, continual coughing bouts that last up to 1 minute. The face turns red or blue from lack of oxygen while coughing. At the end of each coughing effort, the child gasps for breath with a "whooping" sound.
- Vomiting and diarrhea.
- Fever.

CAUSES—Infection with bordetella pertussis bacteria.
  The disease is transmitted by direct contact with a contagious person, or by indirect contact, such as breathing air containing infected droplets or handling linen or other contaminated articles. The incubation period is 5 to 7 days.

RISK INCREASES WITH
- Non-immunized populations.
- Epidemics in late winter or early spring. The bacteria become more virulent as they spread.
- Crowded or unsanitary living conditions.

HOW TO PREVENT—Obtain immunizations against whooping cough for all children. Immunizations normally begin at 2 months. See Appendix 16 for an immunization schedule.

WHAT TO EXPECT

APPROPRIATE HEALTH CARE
- Doctor's treatment.
- Hospitalization with intensive care for severely ill infants. Older children can usually be treated at home.

DIAGNOSTIC MEASURES
- Your own observation of symptoms.
- Medical history and physical exam by a doctor.

- Laboratory studies, such as culture of the sputum and fluorescent antibody studies (see Glossary).
- X-rays of the chest.

POSSIBLE COMPLICATIONS
- Nosebleeds.
- Retinal detachment.
- Seizures and encephalitis.
- Pneumonia.
- Apnea (slowed or stopped breathing).
- Middle-ear infection.
- Ruptured blood vessels in the brain.

PROBABLE OUTCOME—Usually curable in about 6 weeks with treatment. The usual course of illness is: 2 weeks with the non-characteristic cough; 2 weeks with bouts of the "whooping" cough; and 2 weeks for convalescence. Some persistent cough may continue for months.

HOW TO TREAT

NOTE—Follow your doctor's instructions. These instructions are supplemental.

GENERAL MEASURES
- Isolate the ill person until fever disappears. Necessary visitors should wear masks.
- During a coughing bout in a baby, raise the foot of the crib. Place the baby face down with the head turned to one side to help drain the lungs. Older children usually prefer to sit up and lean forward during coughing bouts.
- Use a cool-mist humidifier to soothe the cough and help loosen bronchial and lung secretions.

MEDICATION
- Don't use cough medicine unless your doctor prescribes it.
- Your doctor may prescribe antibiotics for complications, such as middle-ear infection or pneumonia.

ACTIVITY—Keep the child in bed until the fever disappears. Normal activity should be resumed slowly, according to strength.

DIET
- Encourage extra fluids, such as fruit juice, tea, carbonated drinks and bouillon.
- No special diet. Small, frequent meals may decrease vomiting.

CALL YOUR DOCTOR IF

- Your child has signs of whooping cough, especially blueness of the face with coughing bouts.
- Fever rises to 103F (39.4C).
- Vomiting persists more than 1 or 2 days.

WILM'S TUMOR
(Congenital Nephroblastoma)

 GENERAL INFORMATION

DEFINITION—A malignant mixed tumor (one that contains several cell types) of the kidney that occurs primarily in children.

BODY PARTS INVOLVED—Kidney (90% affect only one kidney).

SEX OR AGE MOST AFFECTED—Both sexes of children under age 7, with a peak incidence between ages 3 and 4.

SIGNS & SYMPTOMS
- Enlarged abdomen. A large, firm, smooth tumor can be felt easily within the abdominal wall.
- High blood pressure.
- Blood in the urine.
- Abdominal pain (sometimes).
- Repeated vomiting.
- Fever.
- Weight loss.

CAUSES—Unknown. It is probably congenital, but dormant, until it becomes active at some point before age 7.

RISK INCREASES WITH—Genetic factors. Wilm's tumor is most likely in children with other congenital abnormalities.

HOW TO PREVENT—Cannot be prevented at present.

 WHAT TO EXPECT

APPROPRIATE HEALTH CARE
- Doctor's treatment.
- Surgery to remove the affected kidney and adjacent tissue, if the cancer has spread.
- Hospitalization for radiation treatment and anticancer drugs.

DIAGNOSTIC MEASURES
- Your own observation of symptoms.
- Medical history and physical exam by a doctor.
- Laboratory studies, such as 24-hour urine studies.
- X-rays of the abdomen, kidneys and chest.
- Sonogram and CAT scan (see Glossary for both) of the kidneys.

POSSIBLE COMPLICATIONS
- Kidney failure.
- Tumor spread to lungs, bones, liver or brain, if untreated.
- Adverse reactions, including hair loss, from radiation treatment and anticancer drugs.

PROBABLE OUTCOME—With appropriate treatment, the outlook is better than for most malignant tumors in children. In most cases, Wilm's tumor is curable with surgery, radiation treatment and anticancer drugs. If the tumor is detected before it spreads, the 5-year-survival rate is 90%.

 HOW TO TREAT

NOTE—Follow your doctor's instructions. These instructions are supplemental.

GENERAL MEASURES—For an explanation of surgery and postoperative care, see Kidney Removal (in Surgery section).

MEDICATION—Your doctor may prescribe:
- Anticancer drugs.
- Antinausea drugs.
- Pain relievers.
- Antibiotics, if infection occurs during anticancer drug treatment.
- Stool softeners to prevent constipation following surgery.

ACTIVITY—No restrictions. The child may be as active as strength allows.

DIET—No special diet.

 CALL YOUR DOCTOR IF

- Your child has symptoms of Wilm's tumor.
- The following occurs during treatment:
  Vomiting, abdominal pain or constipation.
  Shortness of breath.
  Swelling in feet or ankles.
- New, unexplained symptoms develop. Drugs used in treatment may cause side effects.

WINTER ITCH
(Xerotic Eczema; Asteatocic Eczema)

GENERAL INFORMATION

DEFINITION—Severely chapped skin that becomes cracked, fissured and inflamed. The disorder is most common in winter. It is not contagious.

BODY PARTS INVOLVED—Skin anywhere on the body, but most commonly on the legs.

SEX OR AGE MOST AFFECTED—Both sexes; all ages.

SIGNS & SYMPTOMS—Lesions with the following characteristics:
- The lesions are round plaques (flat-topped patches), 2cm to 5cm in diameter. The plaques are sometimes piled like flat discs on top of each other. They usually have very definite borders.
- The plaques itch, burn and sting.
- Redness is most pronounced within the cracks and fissures which crisscross the plaque surface.
- The plaques usually don't weep or become crusty.

CAUSES—Insufficient oil on the skin's surface, which allows evaporation of water through the skin. Skin cells shrink so much that islands of cells begin to separate, causing cracks and fissures.

Oil in the skin decreases with aging, excessive bathing and excessive rubbing of the skin.

RISK INCREASES WITH—An environment with low humidity, especially in homes heated with hot-air fans in the winter.

HOW TO PREVENT—Reduce water loss from the skin:
- Bathe less frequently and use cool water.
- Use soap sparingly.
- Pat dry skin rather than rubbing it.
- Apply skin lubricants to dry skin before chapped areas become inflamed.
- Use humidifiers in rooms with very dry air.

WHAT TO EXPECT

APPROPRIATE HEALTH CARE
- Self-care after diagnosis.
- Doctor's treatment.

DIAGNOSTIC MEASURES
- Your own observation of symptoms.
- Medical history and physical exam by a doctor.

POSSIBLE COMPLICATIONS—Secondary bacterial infection in the affected area.

PROBABLE OUTCOME—Usually curable with treatment, but recurrence is common unless environmental conditions can be controlled.

HOW TO TREAT

NOTE—Follow your doctor's instructions. These instructions are supplemental.

GENERAL MEASURES
- See instructions under How to Prevent.
- To apply lubricants: Use hand cream 4 to 8 times per day on the hands and twice daily on the trunk and extremities. When possible, apply immediately after bathing—while the skin is wet—to trap additional moisture before evaporation occurs. Bath oils probably don't help.

MEDICATION
- For minor discomfort, you may use non-prescription skin lubricants, such as petroleum jelly, mineral oil or cold cream.
- For serious discomfort, your doctor may prescribe topical cortisone creams or lotions.

ACTIVITY—No restrictions.

DIET—No special diet.

CALL YOUR DOCTOR IF

- You have severely chapped skin, and self-care does not relieve symptoms in 1 week.
- Chapped skin becomes inflamed.

ZINC DEFICIENCY

 GENERAL INFORMATION

DEFINITION—Inadequate amounts of zinc in body cells. This affects function of the testes, liver and muscles, and affects the structure of bones, teeth, hair and skin. Zinc is a vital part of many enzymes that facilitate chemical reactions necessary for normal body function—including immune function and skin healing.

BODY PARTS INVOLVED—All body cells.

SEX OR AGE MOST AFFECTED—All ages, but most common in children during periods of rapid growth (10 to 18 years).

SIGNS & SYMPTOMS—2 or more of the following:
- Poor appetite.
- Sensations of unpleasant tastes and odors, and decreased senses of taste and smell.
- Decreased sex drive.
- Darkening of skin all over the body.
- Sparse hair growth.
- Deformed nails.

CAUSES
- Excessive consumption of substances that bind zinc and prevent its absorption from the gastrointestinal tract. These include calcium, vitamin D and phytate enzyme (found in unleavened bread).
- Surgical removal of any part of the gastrointestinal tract, especially the stomach.
- Parasite infestation in the gastrointestinal tract.

RISK INCREASES WITH
- Alcoholism. Alcohol increases the excretion of zinc.
- Use of cortisone drugs, which increase zinc excretion.

HOW TO PREVENT
- Adults should not drink or eat more than the recommended amounts of milk, other dairy products or unleavened bread. Keep calcium intake at 1500mg or less daily.
- Don't take large doses of vitamin-D supplements.
- Take zinc supplements if you have had gastrointestinal surgery.
- Obtain medical treatment for parasite infections.
- Don't drink more than 1 or 2 alcoholic drinks—if any—a day.

 WHAT TO EXPECT

APPROPRIATE HEALTH CARE
- Home care after diagnosis.
- Doctor's treatment.

DIAGNOSTIC MEASURES
- Your own observation of symptoms.
- Medical history and physical exam by a doctor.
- Laboratory blood studies of zinc levels.

POSSIBLE COMPLICATIONS
- Iron-deficiency anemia. Zinc is necessary for iron absorption.
- Poor wound healing.
- Liver and spleen enlargement.
- Excess zinc replacement or overdose may interfere with body's manufacture of necessary enzymes.

PROBABLE OUTCOME—Usually curable in 2 months with zinc supplements and removal or treatment of the underlying causes.

 HOW TO TREAT

NOTE—Follow your doctor's instructions. These instructions are supplemental.

GENERAL MEASURES—No specific instructions except those listed under other headings.

MEDICATION—Your doctor may prescribe zinc supplements. Take with milk or meals to prevent stomach upset.

ACTIVITY—No restrictions.

DIET—Eat foods high in zinc such as red meat.

 CALL YOUR DOCTOR IF

You or your child have symptoms of zinc deficiency.

ABDOMINAL-AORTIC ANEURYSM, REMOVAL OF

GENERAL INFORMATION

DEFINITION—Removal of an abdominal-aortic aneurysm (swelling or ballooning of a blood vessel).

BODY PARTS INVOLVED—Abdominal aorta.

REASONS FOR SURGERY—Protection of the heart from dangers caused by the aneurysm.

SURGICAL RISK INCREASES WITH
- Obesity.
- Smoking.
- Atherosclerosis; hypertension; coronary-artery disease; peripheral-vascular disease; (see Glossary); or diabetes mellitus.
- Alcoholism or chronic illness.
- Use of drugs such as: antihypertensives; muscle relaxants; tranquilizers; sleep inducers; insulin; sedatives; beta-adrenergic blockers; or cortisone.
- Use of mind-altering drugs, including: narcotics; psychedelics; hallucinogens; marijuana; sedatives; hypnotics; or cocaine.

WHAT TO EXPECT

WHO OPERATES—General surgeon or vascular surgeon.

WHERE PERFORMED—Hospital.

DIAGNOSTIC TESTS
- Before surgery: Blood and urine studies; X-rays of chest; EKG; sonogram; or angiogram (see Glossary for all).
- After surgery: Blood studies.

ANESTHESIA—General anesthesia by inhalation and injection, with an airway tube placed in the windpipe.

DESCRIPTION OF OPERATION
- An incision is made from the breastbone to the lower abdomen.
- The abdominal muscles are separated.
- The aneurysm is located, isolated and clamped at both ends.
- The section of the artery between the clamps is cut free and removed.
- A plastic or polyester graft to fit the removed artery section is fashioned and sewn in place.
- Abdominal organs are replaced, and muscles are closed in layers. The skin is closed with sutures or clips, which usually can be removed about 1 week after surgery.

POSSIBLE COMPLICATIONS
- Excessive bleeding.
- Surgical-wound infection.
- Incisional hernia.

- Inadvertent injury to the ureters, small intestine or branches of the aorta.

AVERAGE HOSPITAL STAY—7 to 10 days.

PROBABLE OUTCOME—Expect complete healing without complications. Allow about 6 weeks for recovery from surgery.

POSTOPERATIVE CARE

NOTE—This information is supplemental and should not replace your doctor's instructions.

GENERAL MEASURES
- Don't smoke.
- Keep feet warm and dry.
- A hard ridge should form along the incision. As it heals, the ridge will recede gradually.
- Use an electric heating pad, a heat lamp or a warm compress to relieve incisional pain.
- Bathe and shower as usual. You may wash the incision gently with mild unscented soap.
- Move legs often while resting in bed to decrease the likelihood of deep-vein blood clots.

MEDICATION—Your doctor may prescribe:
- Pain relievers. Don't take prescription pain medication longer than 4 to 7 days. Use *only* as much as you need.
- Stool softeners to prevent constipation.
- Antibiotics to fight infection.

ACTIVITY
- Resume work and normal activity as soon as possible to reduce postoperative depression, which is common.
- Avoid vigorous exercise for 6 weeks after surgery.
- Resume driving 5 weeks after returning home.
- Resume sexual activity when your doctor determines that healing is complete.

DIET—Clear liquid diet until the gastrointestinal tract begins to function again. Then eat a well-balanced, high-protein diet to promote healing. After recovery, eat a diet low in fat, low in salt and high in fiber. See Appendices 8 and 9.

CALL YOUR DOCTOR IF

Any of the following occurs:
- Pain, swelling, redness, drainage or bleeding increases in the surgical area.
- Signs of infection: headache, muscle aches, dizziness or a general ill feeling and fever.
- New symptoms such as nausea, vomiting, constipation or abdominal swelling.
- Your feet become cold, discolored or numb.

ABDOMINO-PERINEAL RESECTION

GENERAL INFORMATION

DEFINITION—Removal of cancerous cells in the rectum and anus through an incision in the lower abdomen and the perineum. Enough of the anus and rectum are removed so that the intestines cannot be reconnected. A colostomy is performed at the same time so that digestive function is not disrupted.

BODY PARTS INVOLVED—Rectum; anus; sigmoid colon; perineum; abdomen.

REASONS FOR SURGERY—Cancer of the rectum.

SURGICAL RISK INCREASES WITH
- Adults over 60.
- Obesity.
- Smoking.
- Poor nutrition.
- Recent illness.
- Alcoholism or other chronic illness.
- Use of drugs such as: antihypertensives; muscle relaxants; tranquilizers; sleep inducers; insulin; sedatives; beta-adrenergic blockers; or cortisone.
- Use of mind-altering drugs.

WHAT TO EXPECT

WHO OPERATES—Proctologist or general surgeon.

WHERE PERFORMED—Hospital.

DIAGNOSTIC TESTS
- Before surgery: X-rays of lower gastrointestinal tract; blood and urine studies; colonoscopy (see Glossary).
- After surgery: Laboratory examination of removed tissue; blood studies.

ANESTHESIA—General anesthesia by inhalation and injection, with an airway tube placed in the windpipe.

DESCRIPTION OF OPERATION
- An incision is made in the abdomen. The abdominal muscles are divided and the peritoneal cavity is entered. The sigmoid colon is located, isolated and divided. The closer bowel portion is brought to the skin surface for a colostomy.
- The farther bowel portion is closed and placed deep in the pelvis.
- Incisions are made in the perineum.
- The rectum, anus and end of the bowel (intestine) are isolated and cut free of connective tissue.
- Tubes are left in to allow drainage.
- The skin edges of both incisions are closed with sutures or clips, which usually can be removed in 7 to 10 days after surgery.

POSSIBLE COMPLICATIONS
- Excessive bleeding.

- Surgical-wound infection.
- Adhesions leading to intestinal obstruction.

AVERAGE HOSPITAL STAY—7 to 10 days.

PROBABLE OUTCOME—Expect complete healing without complications. Allow about 3 months for recovery from surgery.

POSTOPERATIVE CARE

NOTE—This information is supplemental and should not replace your doctor's instructions.

GENERAL MEASURES
- A hard ridge should form along each incision. The ridges will recede gradually as they heal.
- Use an electric heating pad, a heat lamp or a warm compress to relieve incisional pain.
- Bathe and shower as usual. You may wash the incisions gently with mild soap.
- Move legs often while in bed to decrease the likelihood of deep-vein blood clots.
- An enterostomy specialist (see Glossary) can teach you how to care for your colostomy.

MEDICATION
- Your doctor may prescribe:
  Pain relievers. Don't take prescription pain medication longer than 4 to 7 days. Use *only* as much as you need.
  Stool softeners to prevent constipation.
  Antibiotics to fight infection.
- You may use non-prescription drugs, such as acetaminophen, for minor pain.

ACTIVITY
- Return to work and normal activity as soon as possible. This reduces postoperative depression, which is common.
- Avoid vigorous exercise for 6 weeks after surgery. Resume driving 1 week after returning home.

DIET—Clear liquid diet until the gastrointestinal tract functions again. Then eat a well-balanced, high-protein diet to promote healing. Avoid coffee, tea, cocoa, cola drinks, alcoholic beverages and any food or spice that causes painful or unpleasant digestive symptoms. Your doctor may prescribe a special diet.

CALL YOUR DOCTOR IF

Any of the following occur:
- Nausea, vomiting, constipation or abdominal swelling.
- Increased pain, swelling, redness, drainage or bleeding in the surgical areas.
- Signs of infection: headache, muscle aches, dizziness or a general ill feeling and fever.
- New, unexplained symptoms. Drugs used in treatment may produce side effects.

SURGERIES

ABORTION
(Suction Curettage)

 GENERAL INFORMATION

DEFINITION—Removal of a fetus and accompanying tissue from the uterus.

BODY PARTS INVOLVED—Uterus; placenta; vagina (route for surgery).

REASONS FOR SURGERY
- Elective termination of pregnancy. The patient should receive competent counseling before making this decision.
- Missed or incomplete miscarriages.

SURGICAL RISK INCREASES WITH
- Obesity.
- Smoking.
- Poor nutrition.
- Recent or chronic illness.
- Use of drugs such as: antihypertensives; muscle relaxants; tranquilizers; sleep inducers; insulin; sedatives; narcotics; beta-adrenergic blockers; or cortisone.
- Use of mind-altering drugs, including: narcotics; psychedelics; hallucinogens; marijuana; sedatives; hypnotics; or cocaine.

 WHAT TO EXPECT

WHO OPERATES—General surgeon or obstetrician-gynecologist.

WHERE PERFORMED—Hospital or outpatient surgical facility.

DIAGNOSTIC TESTS
- Before surgery: Pregnancy test; psychological counseling and testing; blood and urine studies.
- After surgery: Laboratory examination of removed tissue.

ANESTHESIA—Local anesthesia by injection.

DESCRIPTION OF OPERATION
- A small plastic tube is passed through the vagina and cervix into the uterus. The tube is connected to a suction apparatus.
- Gentle suction through the tube removes the uterine contents. You may feel cramps in the lower abdomen, nausea, sweating and faintness.
- The tube is removed.

POSSIBLE COMPLICATIONS
- Excessive bleeding.
- Surgical-wound infection.
- Perforation of the uterus.

AVERAGE HOSPITAL STAY—None.

PROBABLE OUTCOME—Expect complete healing without complications. Allow about 1 week for recovery from surgery.

 POSTOPERATIVE CARE

NOTE—This information is supplemental and should not replace your doctor's instructions.

GENERAL MEASURES
- Use sanitary pads for bleeding, which may last for several days. Beginning 3 days after surgery, you may use tampons.
- If you have pain, place a heating pad or hot-water bottle on the abdomen or back. Hot baths frequently aid muscle relaxation and relieve discomfort. Repeat baths as often as they provide comfort.
- Do not have sexual relations for 1 week after surgery.
- If you wish to take birth-control pills, begin taking them either on the night you return from surgery or the next day. If you prefer an IUD, diaphragm or cervical cap, the fitting can be made during your next doctor's appointment.

MEDICATION
- Your doctor may prescribe:
  Pain relievers. Don't take prescription pain medication longer than 4 to 7 days. Use *only* as much as you need.
  Stool softeners to prevent constipation.
  Antibiotics to fight infection.
- You may use non-prescription drugs, such as acetaminophen, for minor pain.

ACTIVITY—Have someone drive you home from surgery. Rest quietly there for the remainder of the day. Resume normal activities slowly the next day, if you feel able. You will probably experience light or moderate vaginal bleeding on and off for 10 to 14 days after surgery. Bed rest will reduce bleeding.

DIET—No special diet.

 CALL YOUR DOCTOR IF

- Pain, swelling, redness or drainage increases in the surgical area.
- You develop signs of infection: headache, muscle aches, dizziness or a general ill feeling and fever.
- You experience new symptoms, such as nausea, vomiting, constipation or abdominal swelling.
- New, unexplained symptoms develop. Drugs used in treatment may produce side effects.

ABSCESS DRAINAGE

 ## GENERAL INFORMATION

DEFINITION—To open and drain an abscess.

BODY PARTS INVOLVED—Abscesses may occur anywhere in the body. The most common areas include: female breast during lactation; armpit; rectum; vaginal lips; face; area around the tonsils; area under the tongue; scrotum; and arms, legs, hands and feet.

REASONS FOR SURGERY—Treatment of infections: If an abscess breaks open and drains spontaneously, surgery is still required to assure complete drainage.

SURGICAL RISK INCREASES WITH
- Obesity.
- Smoking.
- Poor nutrition.
- Recent or chronic illness.
- Use of drugs such as: antihypertensives; muscle relaxants; tranquilizers; sleep inducers; insulin; sedatives; beta-adrenergic blockers; or cortisone.
- Use of mind-altering drugs, including: narcotics; psychedelics; hallucinogens; marijuana; sedatives; hypnotics; or cocaine.

 ## WHAT TO EXPECT

WHO OPERATES—Family doctor or general surgeon.

WHERE PERFORMED—Doctor's office, outpatient surgical facility, hospital or emergency room.

DIAGNOSTIC TESTS
- Before surgery: Blood and urine studies.
- After surgery: Laboratory examination of removed pus (sometimes).

ANESTHESIA
- Local anesthesia by injection.
- General anesthesia by inhalation and injection, with an airway tube placed in the windpipe.

DESCRIPTION OF OPERATION
- An incision is made over the abscess.
- The incision is spread apart, and a sterile-gloved finger is inserted inside the abscess to break up small pockets. The pus is drained.
- Gauze is packed into the space left by the abscess. This provides a drain that allows the cavity to heal from the bottom outwards. The gauze drain is removed in about 48 hours after surgery.
- The skin is left open to hasten healing.
- A gauze dressing is applied over the wound.

POSSIBLE COMPLICATIONS
- Excessive bleeding.
- Surgical-wound infection.

AVERAGE HOSPITAL STAY—0 to 1 day.

PROBABLE OUTCOME—Expect complete healing without complications. Allow about 2 weeks for recovery from surgery.

 ## POSTOPERATIVE CARE

NOTE—This information is supplemental and should not replace your doctor's instructions.

GENERAL MEASURES
- Use an electric heating pad, a heat lamp or a warm compress to relieve pain.
- Bathe and shower as usual. You may wash the wound gently with mild unscented soap, after the gauze drain is removed.
- Change the gauze dressing daily after bathing.

MEDICATION
- Your doctor may prescribe:
  Pain relievers. Don't take prescription pain medication longer than 4 to 7 days. Use *only* as much as you need.
  Antibiotics to fight infection (sometimes).
- You may use non-prescription drugs, such as acetaminophen, for minor pain.

ACTIVITY
- Avoid vigorous exercise for 1 week after surgery.
- Resume driving 3 days after returning home.

DIET—Eat a well-balanced, high-protein diet to promote healing.

 ## CALL YOUR DOCTOR IF

Any of the following occurs:
- Nausea or vomiting.
- Increased pain, swelling, redness, drainage or bleeding in the surgical area.
- Signs of infection: headache, muscle aches, dizziness or a general ill feeling and fever.
- New, unexplained symptoms. Drugs used in treatment may produce side effects.

ADHESIONS, SEPARATION OF

GENERAL INFORMATION

DEFINITION—Separation of adhesions, fibrous bands of tissue that cause parts of the abdomen and pelvis to cling together abnormally.

BODY PARTS INVOLVED—Abdominal or pelvic organs.

REASONS FOR SURGERY—Removal of an intestinal obstruction caused by adhesions. Adhesions usually result from:
- Previous abdominal surgery.
- Congenital defects.
- Pelvic inflammatory disease.
- Endometriosis.
- Ruptured ectopic pregnancy.
- Radiation treatment for cancers in the abdomen or pelvis.
- Any ruptured organ that has caused infection and scarring.

SURGICAL RISK INCREASES WITH
- Adults over 60.
- Obesity.
- Smoking.
- Excess alcohol consumption.
- Poor nutrition.
- Any chronic illness.
- Use of drugs such as: antihypertensives; muscle relaxants; tranquilizers; sleep inducers; insulin; sedatives; beta-adrenergic blockers; or cortisone.
- Use of mind-altering drugs.

WHAT TO EXPECT

WHO OPERATES—General surgeon.

WHERE PERFORMED—Hospital.

DIAGNOSTIC TESTS
- Before surgery: Blood and urine studies.
- After surgery: Blood studies.

ANESTHESIA—General anesthesia by inhalation and injection, with an airway tube placed in the windpipe.

DESCRIPTION OF OPERATION
- An incision is made in the abdomen over the obstruction.
- The obstruction is isolated and the adhesions are divided carefully.
- The bowel is examined for strangulation (lost blood supply). Any strangulated portion is removed, and the normal ends are joined.
- The abdominal contents are then inspected for undetected disease. Other surgeries may be performed at this time.
- The abdominal contents are replaced. Muscle layers are closed with sutures, and skin is closed with sutures or clips, which can usually be removed in 1 week.

POSSIBLE COMPLICATIONS
- Excessive bleeding.
- Surgical-wound infection.
- Incisional hernia.
- Inadvertent bowel injury.
- Recurrence of adhesions.

AVERAGE HOSPITAL STAY—5 to 7 days.

PROBABLE OUTCOME—Expect complete healing without complications. Allow about 6 weeks for recovery from surgery.

POSTOPERATIVE CARE

NOTE—This information is supplemental and should not replace your doctor's instructions.

GENERAL MEASURES
- Wear an abdominal-support binder, available in drugstores, for 4 to 6 weeks.
- A hard ridge should form along the incision. As it heals, the ridge will recede gradually.
- Bathe and shower as usual. You may wash the incision gently with mild unscented soap.
- Use an electric heating pad, a heat lamp or a warm compress to relieve incisional pain.
- Move legs often while resting in bed to decrease the likelihood of deep-vein blood clots.

MEDICATION
- You may use non-prescription drugs, such as acetaminophen, to relieve minor pain.
- Your doctor may prescribe:
  Pain relievers. Don't take prescription pain medication longer than 4 to 7 days. Use *only* as much as you need.
  Stool softeners to prevent constipation.
  Antibiotics to fight infection.

ACTIVITY
- Resume work and normal activity as soon as possible to reduce postoperative depression, which is common.
- Resume driving 5 weeks after returning home.
- Resume sexual relations when your doctor determines healing in complete.

DIET—Clear liquid diet until the gastrointestinal tract begins to function again. Then eat a well-balanced, high-protein diet to promote healing.

CALL YOUR DOCTOR IF

- Pain, swelling, redness, bleeding or drainage increases in the surgical area.
- You develop signs of infection: headache, muscle aches, dizziness or a general ill feeling and fever.
- You experience new symptoms, such as nausea, vomiting, constipation or abdominal swelling.

ADRENAL-GLAND REMOVAL
(Adrenalectomy)

GENERAL INFORMATION

DEFINITION—Removal of the adrenal glands.

BODY PARTS INVOLVED—Adrenal glands.

REASONS FOR SURGERY
- Cushing's syndrome.
- Pheochromocytoma.
- Adrenal-gland tumors.
- Breast cancer (sometimes).

SURGICAL RISK INCREASES WITH
- Adults over 60.
- Obesity.
- Smoking.
- Stress.
- Poor nutrition.
- Recent illness.
- Alcoholism or other chronic illness.
- Use of drugs such as: antihypertensives; muscle relaxants; tranquilizers; sleep inducers; insulin; sedatives; beta-adrenergic blockers; or cortisone.
- Use of mind-altering drugs, including: narcotics; psychedelics; hallucinogens; marijuana; sedatives; hypnotics; or cocaine.

WHAT TO EXPECT

WHO OPERATES—General surgeon.

WHERE PERFORMED—Hospital.

DIAGNOSTIC TESTS
- Before surgery: Blood and urine studies; X-rays of kidneys; CAT scan (see Glossary) of adrenal area.
- After surgery: Blood studies; laboratory examination of removed tissue.

ANESTHESIA—General anesthesia by inhalation and injection, with an airway tube placed in the windpipe.

DESCRIPTION OF OPERATION
- The adrenal glands are usually approached through incisions in the sides.
- The adrenal glands are located, isolated, cut free and removed. Tubes are left in to allow drainage.
- The skin incisions are closed with sutures or clips, which usually can be removed about 1 week after surgery.

POSSIBLE COMPLICATIONS
- Excessive bleeding.
- Surgical-wound infection.
- Adrenal-hormone shortage.
- Fluid retention.
- Increased risk of life-threatening infections.

AVERAGE HOSPITAL STAY—7 to 10 days.

PROBABLE OUTCOME—Expect complete healing without complications. Allow about 6 weeks for recovery from surgery.

POSTOPERATIVE CARE

NOTE—This information is supplemental and should not replace your doctor's instructions.

GENERAL MEASURES
- Hard ridges should form along the incisions. As they heal, the ridges will recede gradually.
- Bathe and shower as usual. You may wash the incisions gently with mild unscented soap.
- Use an electric heating pad, a heat lamp or a warm compress to relieve incisional pain.
- Weigh yourself daily. Report any weight gain of 2 or more pounds in any 24-hour period to your doctor.
- Move legs often while resting in bed to decrease the likelihood of deep-vein blood clots.

MEDICATION
- Your doctor may prescribe:
  Pain relievers. Don't take prescription pain medication longer than 4 to 7 days. Use *only* as much as you need.
  Stool softeners to prevent constipation.
  Antibiotics to fight infection.
  Steroids to replace those formerly manufactured by the adrenal glands.
- You may use non-prescription drugs, such as acetaminophen, for minor pain.

ACTIVITY
- Resume work and normal activity as soon as possible. This reduces postoperative depression and irritability, which are common.
- Avoid vigorous exercise for 3 months after surgery.
- Resume driving 1 week after returning home.
- Resume sexual relations when your doctor determines that healing is complete.

DIET—Your doctor will prescribe a low-salt diet.

CALL YOUR DOCTOR IF

- Pain, swelling, redness, drainage or bleeding increases in the surgical area.
- You develop signs of infection: headache, muscle aches, dizziness or a general ill feeling and fever. If any of these develop—even after recovery—call your doctor.
- You experience new symptoms such as: nausea; vomiting; dizziness; fatigue; weakness; fluid retention; or weight gain.

AMNIOCENTESIS

 ## GENERAL INFORMATION

DEFINITION—Removal of fluid from the amniotic sac during pregnancy.

BODY PARTS INVOLVED—Uterus; amniotic sac.

REASONS FOR SURGERY—Laboratory examination of amniotic fluid helps diagnose abnormalities of the unborn child. The best time for amniocentesis is between the 15th and 18th weeks of pregnancy. There is ample fluid, and enough time exists to terminate the pregnancy if necessary. Amniocentesis is often done for one or more of the following reasons:
- Mother is over 35 years old.
- Either parent has a chromosome abnormality.
- Mother has previously had a child with a chromosome abnormality, such as Down's syndrome.
- Mother carries a sex-linked abnormality, and the unborn child's sex must be determined.
- Unborn child's maturity or other conditions must be determined late in pregnancy.

SURGICAL RISK INCREASES WITH
- Obesity.
- Previous abdominal surgery.
- Previous infection in pelvic organs.

 ## WHAT TO EXPECT

WHO OPERATES—Obstetrician-gynecologist or family doctor.

WHERE PERFORMED—Outpatient surgical facility or hospital.

DIAGNOSTIC TESTS
- Before surgery: Blood and urine studies.
- During surgery: Ultrasonography (see Glossary).
- After surgery: Laboratory examination of the amniotic fluid.

ANESTHESIA—Local anesthesia by injection. To ensure the unborn child's safety, sedatives and pain relievers will not be used.

DESCRIPTION OF OPERATION
- A local anesthetic is injected into the abdomen.
- A hollow needle is inserted through the abdominal wall into the uterus. The needle will cause temporary pain, but should not hurt more than any injection.
- A small amount of amniotic fluid is suctioned through the needle, and the needle removed.

POSSIBLE COMPLICATIONS
- Excessive bleeding.
- Surgical-wound infection.
- Unwanted abortion triggered by procedure in 1 out of 100 to 150 cases.

AVERAGE HOSPITAL STAY—None.

PROBABLE OUTCOME—More than 95 % of amniocentesis tests indicate no abnormalities. Some couples at high risk want the surgery done to reduce their anxiety during pregnancy. However, normal amniocentesis results cannot guarantee a child without defects. At present there are no tests for *all* abnormalities.

 ## POSTOPERATIVE CARE

NOTE—This information is supplemental and should not replace your doctor's instructions.

GENERAL MEASURES—Bathe and shower as usual. You may wash the injection site gently with mild unscented soap.

MEDICATION—Medicine is usually not necessary.

ACTIVITY—No restrictions after 2 or 3 hours following the operation.

DIET—No special diet.

 ## CALL YOUR DOCTOR IF

Any of the following occurs:
- Nausea and vomiting.
- Pain in the lower abdomen or shoulder.
- Vaginal bleeding.
- Signs of infection: headache, muscle aches, dizziness or a general ill feeling and fever.

AMPUTATION

GENERAL INFORMATION

DEFINITION—Removal of a limb or appendage.

BODY PARTS INVOLVED—Arms; legs; hands; feet; fingers; or toes.

REASONS FOR SURGERY—Performed when blood circulation to a part of the body is irreversibly interrupted, usually caused by one of the following:
- Injury to blood vessels that cannot be repaired or reconstructed.
- Hardening of the arteries.
- Impaired blood circulation as a complication of diabetes mellitus.
- Buerger's disease.
- Raynaud's phenomena.
- Severe infection with gangrene.
- Obstructions in the arteries.
- Severe frostbite.

SURGICAL RISK INCREASES WITH
- Adults over 60.
- Smoking.
- Obesity.
- Stress.
- Poor nutrition.
- Excess alcohol consumption.
- Newborns and infants.
- Coronary artery disease.
- Disease that increases coagulability of blood.
- Use of drugs such as: antihypertensives; muscle relaxants; tranquilizers; sleep inducers; insulin; sedatives; narcotics; beta-andrenergic blockers; or cortisone.
- Use of mind-altering drugs.

WHAT TO EXPECT

WHO OPERATES—General surgeon or orthopedic surgeon.

WHERE PERFORMED—Hospital.

DIAGNOSTIC TESTS
- Before surgery: Blood and urine studies; X-rays of part to be amputated.
- After surgery: Blood studies.

ANESTHESIA—General anesthesia by inhalation and injection, with an airway tube placed in the windpipe.

DESCRIPTION OF OPERATION
- An incision is made around the part to be amputated.
- Tissue, muscles, blood vessels, nerves and bone are severed.
- The bone is filed smooth, and the bone end is covered with connective tissue. Frequently tubes are left in the wound to allow drainage.

- Muscles are closed with large sutures. The skin is closed with fine sutures, which are left in place for 3 to 4 weeks after surgery.

POSSIBLE COMPLICATIONS—Excessive bleeding, surgical-wound infection or muscle contractures (shortening of muscles).

AVERAGE HOSPITAL STAY—2 to 7 days.

PROBABLE OUTCOME—Expect complete healing without complications. Allow about 6 weeks for recovery from surgery. A physical rehabilitation program may be frustrating, but it will lead to improved self-esteem and independence.

POSTOPERATIVE CARE

NOTE—This information is supplemental and should not replace your doctor's instructions.

GENERAL MEASURES
- Don't smoke.
- Use an electric heating pad, a heat lamp or a warm compress to relieve surgical-wound pain, if your doctor approves.
- Bathe and shower as usual. You may wash the surgical wound gently with mild unscented soap.
- Move legs often while resting in bed to decrease the likelihood of deep-vein blood clots.

MEDICATION
- Your doctor may prescribe:
  Pain relievers. Don't take prescription pain medication longer than 4 to 7 days. Use *only* as much as you need.
  Stool softeners to prevent constipation.
  Antibiotics to fight infection.
- You may use non-prescription drugs, such as acetaminophen, for minor pain.

ACTIVITY
- Resume work and normal activity as soon as possible to reduce postoperative depression, which is common.
- Avoid vigorous exercise for 3 months after surgery.
- Resume driving 5 weeks after returning home, if able.

DIET—Clear liquid diet until the gastrointestinal tract begins to function again. Then eat a well-balanced, high-protein diet to promote healing.

CALL YOUR DOCTOR IF

- Pain, swelling, redness, drainage or bleeding increases in the surgical area.
- You develop signs of infection: headache, muscle aches, dizziness or a general ill feeling and fever.
- You experience new symptoms such as nausea, vomiting or constipation.

ANAL-FISSURE REMOVAL

GENERAL INFORMATION

DEFINITION—Removal of an anal fissure, a crack or tear in the membrane that lines the anus.

BODY PARTS INVOLVED—Anus and lining membrane; muscles around the anus.

REASONS FOR SURGERY—Relief of pain.

SURGICAL RISK INCREASES WITH
- Obesity.
- Smoking.
- Recent or chronic illness.
- Use of drugs such as: antihypertensives; muscle relaxants; tranquilizers; sleep inducers; insulin; sedatives; beta-adrenergic blockers; or cortisone.
- Use of mind-altering drugs, including: narcotics; psychedelics; hallucinogens; marijuana; sedatives; hypnotics; or cocaine.

WHAT TO EXPECT

WHO OPERATES—General surgeon or proctologist.

WHERE PERFORMED—Hospital or outpatient surgical facility.

DIAGNOSTIC TESTS—Before surgery: Blood and urine studies; anoscopy; sigmoidoscopy (see Glossary for all).

ANESTHESIA
- Local anesthesia by injection.
- Spinal anesthesia by injection.
- General anesthesia by inhalation and injection, with an airway tube placed in the windpipe.

DESCRIPTION OF OPERATION
- The sphincter is expanded with special instruments.
- The fissure is cut free from surrounding tissue and removed. Sometimes, the sphincter muscles are stretched to allow exposure.
- Bleeding vessels are tied or closed with electrocauterization.
- A drain or packing is inserted into the surgical area.
- The surgical area is left open to hasten healing. Bandages are applied.

POSSIBLE COMPLICATIONS
- Excessive bleeding or pain.
- Surgical-wound infection.

AVERAGE HOSPITAL STAY—0 to 1 day.

PROBABLE OUTCOME—Expect complete healing without complications. Allow about 3 weeks for recovery from surgery.

POSTOPERATIVE CARE

NOTE—This information is supplemental and should not replace your doctor's instructions.

GENERAL MEASURES
- Sit in a tub of warm water for 15 to 20 minutes several times a day to relieve discomfort.
- Use an electric heating pad, a heat lamp or a warm compress to relieve surgical-wound pain.
- Use soft moistened tissue to clean the anal area after bowel movements.

MEDICATION
- Your doctor may prescribe:
  Pain relievers. Don't take prescription pain medication longer than 4 to 7 days. Use *only* as much as you need.
  Stool softeners to prevent constipation.
- You may use non-prescription drugs, such as acetaminophen, for minor pain.

ACTIVITY
- Return to work and normal activity as soon as possible. This reduces postoperative depression and irritability, which are common.
- Avoid vigorous exercise for 4 weeks after surgery.
- Resume driving 1 week after returning home.

DIET—Eat a well-balanced, high-protein diet to promote healing. Increase fiber and fluid intake to prevent constipation.

CALL YOUR DOCTOR IF

- Pain, swelling, redness, drainage or bleeding increases in the surgical area.
- You experience nausea, vomiting or constipation.
- You develop signs of infection: headache, muscle aches, dizziness or a general ill feeling and fever.
- New, unexplained symptoms develop. Drugs used in treatment may produce side effects.

ANAL-FISTULA REMOVAL

GENERAL INFORMATION

DEFINITION—Removal of an anal fistula, an abnormal tract extending from inside the rectum to the skin outside of the anus.

BODY PARTS INVOLVED—Rectum; skin and underlying tissue around the rectum and anus.

REASONS FOR SURGERY
- Repeated abscesses in the anal and rectal areas.
- Chronic drainage from a fistula.

SURGICAL RISK INCREASES WITH
- Stress.
- Poor nutrition.
- Recent illness.
- Obesity.
- Smoking.
- Use of drugs such as: antihypertensives; muscle relaxants; tranquilizers; sleep inducers; insulin; sedatives; beta-adrenergic blockers; or cortisone.
- Use of mind-altering drugs, including: narcotics; psychedelics; hallucinogens; marijuana; sedatives; hypnotics; or cocaine.

WHAT TO EXPECT

WHO OPERATES—General surgeon or proctologist.

WHERE PERFORMED—Outpatient surgical facility or hospital.

DIAGNOSTIC TESTS
- Before surgery: X-rays of lower gastrointestinal tract; colonoscopy (see Glossary).
- After surgery: Blood studies.

ANESTHESIA—General anesthesia by inhalation and injection, with an airway tube placed in the windpipe.

DESCRIPTION OF OPERATION
- An incision is made in the skin around the rectum. Abscesses are drained, if necessary.
- The fistula is located with a delicate probe, cut free of connective tissue and removed.
- The space left by the removed fistula is packed with medicated gauze. A bandage is applied to control bleeding.
- The surgical wound is left open to heal from inside out.

POSSIBLE COMPLICATIONS
- Excessive bleeding.
- Surgical-wound infection.
- Slow healing or recurrence.

PROBABLE OUTCOME—Expect complete healing without complications in 4 to 5 weeks for small fistulas and up to 16 weeks for deeper ones.

POSTOPERATIVE CARE

NOTE—This information is supplemental and should not replace your doctor's instructions.

GENERAL MEASURES
- Use an electric heating pad, a heat lamp or a warm compress to relieve surgical-wound pain.
- Take warm baths as often as needed to relieve discomfort.
- Move legs often while confined to bed to decrease the likelihood of deep-vein blood clots.
- Change bandages or sanitary pads 4 to 5 times a day or as directed by your doctor.
- Clean the rectal area with soap and water after bowel movements.

MEDICATION
- Your doctor may prescribe:
  Pain relievers. Don't take prescription pain medication longer than 4 to 7 days. Use *only* as much as you need.
  Stool softeners to prevent constipation.
  Antibiotics to fight infection.
- You may use non-prescription drugs, such as acetaminophen, for minor pain.

ACTIVITY
- Resume work and normal activity as soon as possible to reduce postoperative depression and irritability, which are common.
- Avoid vigorous exercise for 6 months after surgery.
- Resume driving 1 week after returning home.
- Resume sexual relations when your doctor determines that healing is complete.

DIET—Clear liquid diet until the gastrointestinal tract functions again. Then eat a well-balanced, high-protein diet to promote healing, if your doctor does not prescribe a special diet. Increase fiber and fluid intake to prevent constipation.

CALL YOUR DOCTOR IF

- Pain, swelling, redness, drainage or bleeding increases in the surgical area.
- You develop signs of infection: headache, muscle aches, dizziness or a general ill feeling and fever.
- You experience nausea, vomiting or constipation.
- New, unexplained symptoms develop. Drugs used in treatment may produce side effects.

SURGERIES

AORTO-ILIAC BYPASS GRAFT

GENERAL INFORMATION

DEFINITION—Placement of an artificial graft to bypass a blood clot or artery closure in the arteries that supply blood to the abdomen, genital area and legs.

BODY PARTS INVOLVED—Aorta; iliac arteries.

REASONS FOR SURGERY—Restoration of normal blood circulation in the legs.

SURGICAL RISK INCREASES WITH
- Alcoholism.
- Obesity.
- Smoking.
- Diabetes mellitus; coronary artery disease; or atherosclerosis.
- Use of drugs such as: antihypertensives; muscle relaxants; tranquilizers; sleep inducers; insulin; sedatives; narcotics; beta-adrenergic blockers; or cortisone.
- Use of mind-altering drugs, including: narcotics; psychedelics; hallucinogens; marijuana; sedatives; hypnotics; or cocaine.

WHAT TO EXPECT

WHO OPERATES—General surgeon or vascular surgeon.

WHERE PERFORMED—Hospital.

DIAGNOSTIC TESTS
- Before surgery: Blood and urine studies; arteriograms (see Glossary).
- During surgery: Arteriograms.
- After surgery: Blood studies.

ANESTHESIA—General anesthesia by inhalation and injection, with an airway tube placed in the windpipe.

DESCRIPTION OF OPERATION
- An incision is made in the abdomen.
- The abdominal muscles are separated to expose the abdominal organs, which are inspected for undetected disease. Other surgeries may be performed at this time.
- The aorta and iliac arteries are located and clamped to isolate the obstruction.
- A polyester graft is fashioned and fitted in place. One end fits in the aorta and the other two ends in the iliac arteries.
- The graft is sewn in place and the clamps are released. Blood can now circulate freely.
- The muscles of the abdomen are closed in layers. The skin is closed with sutures or clips, which usually can be removed about 1 week after surgery.

POSSIBLE COMPLICATIONS
- Excessive bleeding.
- Surgical-wound infection.
- Incisional hernia.
- Inadvertent injury to the ureter.

AVERAGE HOSPITAL STAY—10 to 14 days.

PROBABLE OUTCOME—Expect complete healing without complications and restoration of normal circulation to legs. Allow about 6 weeks for recovery from surgery.

POSTOPERATIVE CARE

NOTE—This information is supplemental and should not replace your doctor's instructions.

GENERAL MEASURES
- Don't smoke.
- Keep feet clean and dry.
- A hard ridge should form along the incision. As it heals, the ridge will recede gradually.
- Use an electric heating pad, a heat lamp or a warm compress to relieve incisional pain.
- Bathe and shower as usual. You may wash the incision gently with mild unscented soap.
- Move legs often while in bed to decrease the chance of deep-vein blood clots.

MEDICATION
- Your doctor may prescribe:
  Pain relievers. Don't take prescription pain medication longer than 4 to 7 days. Use *only* as much as you need.
  Stool softeners to prevent constipation.
  Antibiotics to fight infection.
- You may use non-prescription drugs, such as acetaminophen, for minor pain.

ACTIVITY
- Resume work and normal activity as soon as possible to reduce postoperative depression, which is common.
- Avoid vigorous exercise for 6 weeks after surgery. Your doctor will prescribe an exercise program.
- Resume driving 5 weeks after returning home.
- Resume sexual relations when your doctor has determined that healing is complete.

DIET—Clear liquid diet until the gastrointestinal tract begins to function again. Then eat a well-balanced, high-protein diet to promote healing. After recovery, eat a diet low in fat and sodium (see Appendices 8 and 9).

CALL YOUR DOCTOR IF

- Pain, swelling, redness, drainage or bleeding increases in the surgical area.
- You develop signs of infection: headache, muscle aches, dizziness or a general ill feeling and fever.
- You experience new symptoms, such as nausea, vomiting, constipation or abdominal swelling.
- Your feet become cold, discolored or numb.

APPENDECTOMY

GENERAL INFORMATION

DEFINITION—Removal of the vermiform appendix, an outgrowth of tissue from the cecum, the first part of the large intestine.

BODY PARTS INVOLVED—Vermiform appendix; cecum; peritoneum.

REASONS FOR SURGERY—Treatment of an infected appendix. Signs and symptoms of infection include:
- Abdominal pain.
- Loss of appetite.
- Tenderness in the right lower abdomen.
- Low-grade fever.
- Elevated white blood-cell count.

SURGICAL RISK INCREASES WITH
- Alcoholism.
- Obesity.
- Smoking.
- Chronic heart, lung, liver or kidney disease.
- Use of drugs such as: antihypertensives; muscle relaxants; tranquilizers; sleep inducers; insulin; sedatives; beta-adrenergic blockers; cortisone; or laxatives. Caution: If you suspect you have appendicitis, do not take laxatives.
- Use of mind-altering drugs, including: narcotics; psychedelics; hallucinogens; marijuana; sedatives; hypnotics; or cocaine.

WHAT TO EXPECT

WHO OPERATES—General surgeon.

WHERE PERFORMED—Hospital.

DIAGNOSTIC TESTS
- Before surgery: Blood and urine studies, X-rays of abdomen.
- After surgery: Blood studies.

ANESTHESIA—General anesthesia by inhalation and injection, with an airway tube placed in the windpipe.

DESCRIPTION OF OPERATION
- An incision is made in the lower abdomen.
- The abdominal muscles and organs are separated and the appendix is isolated, cut free and removed. The intestine is closed, cauterized and sterilized to prevent infection.
- The area around the appendix is inspected for undetected diseases. Other surgeries may be performed at this time.
- Any fluid or pus from the infected appendix is suctioned away.
- Sometimes, a drain is placed in the area left by the removed appendix.

POSSIBLE COMPLICATIONS
- Excessive bleeding.
- Surgical-wound infection.
- Inadvertent injury to the ureter.

AVERAGE HOSPITAL STAY—3 to 5 days.

PROBABLE OUTCOME—Expect complete healing without complications. Allow about 3 weeks for recovery from surgery.

POSTOPERATIVE CARE

NOTE—This information is supplemental and should not replace your doctor's instructions.

GENERAL MEASURES
- A hard ridge should form along the incision. As it heals, the ridge will recede gradually.
- Use an electric heating pad, a heat lamp or a warm compress to relieve incisional pain.
- Bathe and shower as usual. You may wash the incision gently with mild unscented soap.
- Move legs often while resting in bed to decrease the likelihood of deep-vein blood clots.

MEDICATION
- Your doctor may prescribe:
  Pain relievers. Don't take prescription pain medication longer than 4 to 7 days. Use *only* as much as you need.
  Stool softeners to prevent constipation.
  Antibiotics to fight infection.
- You may use non-prescription drugs, such as acetaminophen, for minor pain.

ACTIVITY
- Resume work and normal activity as soon as possible to reduce postoperative depression, which is common.
- Avoid vigorous exercise for 6 weeks after surgery.
- Resume driving 9 days after returning home.

DIET—Clear liquid diet until the gastrointestinal tract begins to function again. Then eat a well-balanced, high-protein diet to promote healing.

CALL YOUR DOCTOR IF

- Pain, swelling, redness, drainage or bleeding increases in the surgical area.
- You develop signs of infection: headache, muscle aches, dizziness or a general ill feeling and fever.
- You experience new symptoms, such as nausea, vomiting, constipation or abdominal swelling.

ARTHROSCOPY

GENERAL INFORMATION

DEFINITION—Visual examination of a joint with an arthroscope, a fiber-optic instrument with a lighted tip.

BODY PARTS INVOLVED—Joint, usually in the knee.

REASONS FOR SURGERY
- Diagnosis of disease or injury inside a joint.
- Removal of bone or cartilage or repair of tendons or ligaments.

SURGICAL RISK INCREASES WITH
- Adults over 60.
- Obesity.
- Smoking.
- Poor nutrition.
- Recent illness.
- Use of drugs such as: antihypertensives; muscle relaxants; tranquilizers; sleep inducers; insulin; sedatives; beta-adrenergic blockers; or cortisone.
- Use of mind-altering drugs, including: narcotics; psychedelics; hallucinogens; marijuana; sedatives; hypnotics; or cocaine.

WHAT TO EXPECT

WHO OPERATES—Orthopedist.

WHERE PERFORMED—Hospital or outpatient surgical facility.

DIAGNOSTIC TESTS
- Before surgery: Blood and urine studies; X-rays of joint.
- After surgery: Blood studies; laboratory examination of removed fluid or tissue.

ANESTHESIA
- Local anesthesia by injection.
- Spinal anesthesia by injection.
- General anesthesia by inhalation and injection, with an airway tube placed in the windpipe.

DESCRIPTION OF OPERATION
- An incision is made at the side of the joint to be examined. The arthroscope is inserted into the joint. Diagnostic surgical procedures are then performed, depending on the problem.
- The arthroscope is removed. The skin is closed with sutures or clips, which usually can be removed about 7 to 10 days after surgery.

POSSIBLE COMPLICATIONS
- Bleeding into joint.
- Surgical-wound infection.
- Slow healing.

AVERAGE HOSPITAL STAY—0 to 1 day.

PROBABLE OUTCOME—Expect complete healing without complications. Allow about 6 weeks for recovery from surgery.

POSTOPERATIVE CARE

NOTE—This information is supplemental and should not replace your doctor's instructions.

GENERAL MEASURES
- A hard ridge should form along the incision. As it heals, the ridge will recede gradually.
- Bathe and shower as usual. You may wash the incision gently with mild unscented soap.
- Use an electric heating pad, a heat lamp or a warm compress to relieve incisional pain.
- Move legs often while resting in bed to decrease the likelihood of deep-vein blood clots.
- Use crutches or a cane to walk until your doctor determines that healing is complete.
- Physical therapy may hasten healing and restore strength. Ask your doctor.

MEDICATION
- Your doctor may prescribe:
  Pain relievers. Don't take prescription pain medication longer than 4 to 7 days. Use *only* as much as you need.
  Antibiotics to fight infection, if needed.
- You may use non-prescription drugs, such as acetaminophen, for minor pain.

ACTIVITY
- Resume work and normal activity as soon as possible to reduce postoperative depression and irritability, which are common.
- Avoid vigorous exercise for 6 weeks after surgery.
- Resume driving when your doctor determines that healing is complete.

DIET—No special diet.

CALL YOUR DOCTOR IF

- Pain, swelling, redness, drainage or bleeding increases in the surgical area.
- You develop signs of infection: headache, muscle aches, dizziness or a general ill feeling and fever.
- You experience nausea or vomiting.

BAKER'S-CYST REMOVAL

GENERAL INFORMATION

DEFINITION—Removal of Baker's cyst, a benign cystic tumor on the back of the knee joint. The cyst consists of accumulated fluid that protrudes between two groups of muscles behind the knee. Baker's cyst may result from injury or from diseases, such as arthritis, gout or inflammation of the membrane lining the knee joint.

BODY PARTS INVOLVED—Space behind the knee joint on either or both sides of the knee.

REASONS FOR SURGERY—If the cyst has resulted from disease, it usually disappears after successful treatment of the underlying disease. Otherwise, the cyst is removed when it becomes painful or unsightly. In children, the cyst is usually left to heal by itself, and is not removed unless it presses on nerves or blood vessels.

SURGICAL RISK INCREASES WITH
- Obesity.
- Smoking.
- Poor nutrition.
- Recent or chronic illness.

WHAT TO EXPECT

WHO OPERATES—General surgeon or orthopedist.

WHERE PERFORMED—Outpatient surgical facility or hospital.

DIAGNOSTIC TESTS
- Before surgery: Blood and urine studies; X-rays of both knees; arthrograms (see Glossary).
- After surgery: Blood studies.

ANESTHESIA
- Local anesthesia by injection.
- General anesthesia by inhalation and injection, with an airway tube placed in the windpipe.

DESCRIPTION OF OPERATION
- An incision is made over the cyst.
- The cyst is located, cut free from surrounding tissue and removed.
- The skin is closed with fine sutures, which usually can be removed about 2 weeks after surgery.

POSSIBLE COMPLICATIONS
- Excessive bleeding.
- Surgical-wound infection.
- Slow healing and continued pain.

AVERAGE HOSPITAL STAY—0 to 1 day.

PROBABLE OUTCOME—Expect complete healing without complications. Allow about 4 weeks for recovery from surgery.

POSTOPERATIVE CARE

NOTE—This information is supplemental and should not replace your doctor's instructions.

GENERAL MEASURES
- A hard ridge should form along the incision. As it heals, the ridge will recede gradually.
- Use an electric heating pad, a heat lamp or a warm compress to relieve incisional pain.
- Bathe and shower as usual. You may wash the incision gently with mild unscented soap.

MEDICATION
- Your doctor may prescribe:
- Pain relievers. Don't take prescription pain medication longer than 4 to 7 days. Use *only* as much as you need.
  Antibiotics to fight infection.
- You may use non-prescription drugs, such as acetaminophen, for minor pain.

ACTIVITY
- Return to work and normal activity as soon as possible. This reduces postoperative depression and irritability, which are common.
- Use crutches or a cane to walk (as directed by your doctor).
- Avoid vigorous exercise for 6 weeks after surgery.
- Resume driving 2 weeks after returning home.

DIET—Clear liquid diet until the gastrointestinal tract functions again. Then eat a well-balanced, high-protein diet to promote healing.

CALL YOUR DOCTOR IF

- Pain, swelling, redness, drainage or bleeding increases in the surgical area.
- You develop signs of infection: headache, muscle aches, dizziness or a general ill feeling and fever.
- You experience nausea or vomiting.
- New, unexplained symptoms develop. Drugs used in treatment may produce side effects.

BARTHOLIN'S-GLAND-CYST SURGERY

 ## GENERAL INFORMATION

DEFINITION—Removal or repair of a cyst in the Bartholin's glands, two small glands located in the vaginal lips.

BODY PARTS INVOLVED—Bartholin's glands; lips of vagina.

REASONS FOR SURGERY—Prevention of recurrent infection after an abscess has been drained.

SURGICAL RISK INCREASES WITH
- Obesity.
- Smoking.
- Poor nutrition.
- Recent illness.
- Alcoholism or chronic illness.
- Use of drugs such as: antihypertensives; muscle relaxants; tranquilizers; sleep inducers; insulin; sedatives; beta-adrenergic blockers; or cortisone.
- Use of mild-altering drugs, including: narcotics; psychedelics; hallucinogens; marijuana; sedatives; hypnotics; or cocaine.

 ## WHAT TO EXPECT

WHO OPERATES—Obstetrician-gynecologist, family doctor or general surgeon.

WHERE PERFORMED—Outpatient surgical facility or hospital.

DIAGNOSTIC TESTS
- Before surgery: Blood and urine studies; laboratory examination of vaginal discharge.
- After surgery: Laboratory examination of pus or secretions from opened glands.

ANESTHESIA—General anesthesia by inhalation and injection, with an airway tube placed in the windpipe.

DESCRIPTION OF OPERATION—There are two methods to treat infected Bartholin's glands. One is to remove them. The preferred method is marsupialization. In this procedure, the edges of the glands are opened and the linings are folded back and sewn shut. This forms a small pouch that drains easily. Sutures that will be absorbed by the body are used to close the pouch.

POSSIBLE COMPLICATIONS
- Excessive bleeding
- Surgical-wound infection.

AVERAGE HOSPITAL STAY—0 to 1 day.

PROBABLE OUTCOME—Expect complete healing without complications. Allow about 2 weeks for recovery from surgery.

 ## POSTOPERATIVE CARE

NOTE—This information is supplemental and should not replace your doctor's instructions.

GENERAL MEASURES
- Use an electric heating pad, a heat lamp or a warm compress to relieve surgical-wound pain.
- Wear cotton panties. Avoid panties made from nylon, polyester, silk or other non-ventilating materials. Don't wear tight clothing, such as jeans.
- Take hot baths several times a day to relieve discomfort.

MEDICATION—Your doctor may prescribe:
- Pain relievers. Don't take prescription pain medication longer than 4 to 7 days. Use *only* as much as you need.
- Stool softeners to prevent constipation.
- Antibiotics to fight infection.

ACTIVITY
- Resume work and normal activity as soon as possible. This reduces postoperative depression and irritability, which are common.
- Avoid vigorous exercise for 4 weeks after surgery.
- Resume driving 4 days after returning home.
- Resume sexual relations when your doctor determines that healing is complete.

DIET—No special diet.

 ## CALL YOUR DOCTOR IF

- Pain, swelling, redness, drainage or bleeding increases in the surgical area.
- New, unexplained symptoms develop. Drugs used in treatment may produce side effects.

BLADDER (URINARY) REMOVAL
(Cystectomy)

 GENERAL INFORMATION

DEFINITION—Removal of the urinary bladder and adjacent tissues and organs, and diversion of the urinary stream to an artificial opening, which is called an "ostomy" or "stoma."

BODY PARTS INVOLVED
- Males: Bladder; prostate; urethra; seminal vesicles; small intestine.
- Females: Urethra; ureters; cervix; vagina; small intestine.

REASONS FOR SURGERY—Cancer or suspected cancer of the bladder.

SURGICAL RISK INCREASES WITH
- Poor nutrition.
- Repeated surgeries on the bladder.

 WHAT TO EXPECT

WHO OPERATES—Urologist.

WHERE PERFORMED—Hospital.

DIAGNOSTIC TESTS
- Before surgery: Blood and urine studies; X-rays of kidneys and chest.
- During surgery: Cystoscopy (see Glossary).

ANESTHESIA—General anesthesia by inhalation and injection, with an airway tube placed in the windpipe.

DESCRIPTION OF OPERATION
- An incision is made in the abdomen. The muscles are separated and the abdominal cavity is entered.
- The blood supply and the ureters are cut and tied.
- The bladder and adjacent tissues and organs are cut free and removed.
- The ureters are diverted through an intestinal pouch to an opening made in the skin (the stoma).
- The muscles are replaced and sewn together with sutures. The skin is closed with sutures or clips, which usually can be removed about 1 week after surgery.

POSSIBLE COMPLICATIONS
- Excessive bleeding.
- Incisional hernia or infection.
- Impotence in males.

AVERAGE HOSPITAL STAY—10 to 14 days.

PROBABLE OUTCOME—Expect complete healing of surgical wounds. You will need to wear an external pouch to collect urine. The stoma will heal and shrink to its permanent size in 2 to 4 months after surgery. Allow about 6 weeks for recovery from surgery.

 POSTOPERATIVE CARE

NOTE—This information is supplemental and should not replace your doctor's instructions.

GENERAL MEASURES
- A hard ridge should form along the incision. As it heals, the ridge will recede gradually.
- Use an electric heating pad, a heat lamp or a warm compress to relieve incisional pain.
- Bathe and shower as usual. You may wash the incision gently with mild unscented soap.
- Move legs often while resting in bed to decrease the likelihood of deep-vein blood clots.
- An enterostomy specialist (see Glossary) can help you and your family learn to cope with new urination habits.
- Dry the area around the stoma by patting, not rubbing. Apply gauze soaked with 1 part vinegar to 3 parts water over the stoma to keep it clean.

MEDICATION
- Your doctor may prescribe:
  Pain relievers. Don't take prescription pain medication longer than 4 to 7 days. Use *only* as much as you need.
  Stool softeners to prevent constipation.
  Antibiotics to fight infection.
- You may use non-prescription drugs, such as acetaminophen, for minor pain.

ACTIVITY
- Return to work and normal activity as soon as possible. This reduces postoperative depression and irritability, which are common.
- Avoid vigorous exercise for 6 weeks after surgery. Avoid heavy lifting indefinitely.
- Resume driving 3 weeks after returning home.

DIET—Clear liquid diet until the gastrointestinal tract functions again. Then eat a well-balanced, high-protein diet to promote healing.

 CALL YOUR DOCTOR IF

- Pain, swelling, redness, drainage or bleeding increases in the surgical area.
- You develop signs of infection: headache, muscle aches, dizziness or a general ill feeling and fever.
- You experience nausea, vomiting, constipation or abdominal swelling.
- You have pain or difficulty with urination.
- You wish to consider penile implant surgery (if impotent).
- New, unexplained symptoms develop. Drugs used in treatment may produce side effects.

BONE GRAFT

GENERAL INFORMATION

DEFINITION—Filling space between fragments of a broken bone.

BODY PARTS INVOLVED—Bone.

REASONS FOR SURGERY
- Joining of two or more parts of a bone that have broken and not grown back together.
- Fusion of the spine after injury or surgery.

SURGICAL RISK INCREASES WITH
- Adults over 60.
- Obesity.
- Smoking.
- Poor nutrition.
- Recent illness.
- Alcoholism or chronic illness.
- Use of mind-altering drugs, including: narcotics; psychedelics; hallucinogens; marijuana; sedatives; hypnotics; or cocaine.

WHAT TO EXPECT

WHO OPERATES—Orthopedist.

WHERE PERFORMED—Hospital.

DIAGNOSTIC TESTS
- Before surgery: X-rays of area to be grafted; blood and urine studies.
- After surgery: Blood studies; X-rays of grafted area.

ANESTHESIA—General anesthesia by inhalation and injection, with an airway tube placed in the windpipe.

DESCRIPTION OF OPERATION
- If bone for the graft is to be taken from the patient, it is usually removed from the top of the hip bone or the ribs. Otherwise, bone is obtained from a bone bank (see Glossary).
- An incision is made over the affected bone. The bone is located and isolated.
- The bone to be grafted is shaped to fit the affected area. Bits and pieces of bone graft are held in place with bone wax or plastic material.
- The skin is closed with sutures or clips, which usually can be removed about 1 week after surgery.
- A splint or plaster cast keeps the affected part rigid and promotes healing (sometimes).

POSSIBLE COMPLICATIONS
- Excessive bleeding
- Surgical-wound infection.
- Rejection of transplanted bone.

AVERAGE HOSPITAL STAY—7 to 10 days.

PROBABLE OUTCOME—Expect complete healing without complications. Allow about 3 months for recovery from surgery.

POSTOPERATIVE CARE

NOTE—This information is supplemental and should not replace your doctor's instructions.

GENERAL MEASURES
- Move legs often while resting in bed to decrease the likelihood of deep-vein blood clots.
- See Appendix 17 for instructions on cast care.

MEDICATION
- Your doctor may prescribe:
  Pain relievers. Don't take prescription pain medication longer than 4 to 7 days. Use *only* as much as you need.
  Stool softeners to prevent constipation.
  Antibiotics to fight infection.
- You may use non-prescription drugs, such as acetaminophen, for minor pain.

ACTIVITY
- Resume work and normal activity as soon as possible. This reduces postoperative depression and irritability, which are common.
- Avoid vigorous exercise for 3 months after surgery.
- Resume driving when able.

DIET—No special diet.

CALL YOUR DOCTOR IF

- Pain, swelling, redness, drainage or bleeding increases in the surgical area.
- You develop signs of infection: headache, muscle aches, dizziness or a general ill feeling and fever.
- New, unexplained symptoms develop. Drugs used in treatment may produce side effects.

BONE-MARROW TRANSPLANT

GENERAL INFORMATION

DEFINITION—Removal of bone marrow from a donor for introduction into the bloodstream of a recipient.

BODY PARTS INVOLVED
- Donor: Breastbone; ilium (part of the hip joint).
- Recipient: Vein.

REASONS FOR SURGERY—Strengthening of the recipient's immune system, which has become weakened from one of the following:
- Acute leukemia.
- Severe combined immune-deficiency syndrome (see Glossary).
- Severe aplastic anemia.

SURGICAL RISK INCREASES FOR BOTH DONOR OR RECIPIENT WITH
- Obesity.
- Smoking.
- Poor nutrition.
- Recent or chronic illness.
- Use of drugs such as: antihypertensives; muscle relaxants; tranquilizers; sleep inducers; insulin; sedatives; beta-adrenergic blockers; or cortisone.
- Use of mind-altering drugs, including: narcotics; psychedelics; hallucinogens; marijuana; sedatives; hypnotics; or cocaine.

WHAT TO EXPECT

WHO OPERATES—General surgeon, hematologist or pediatrician.

WHERE PERFORMED—Hospital.

DIAGNOSTIC TESTS
- Before surgery: Blood and urine studies; studies of bone marrow of both donor and recipient.
- After surgery: Blood studies in recipient to determine success of transplant.

ANESTHESIA—Local anesthesia by injection (donor).

DESCRIPTION OF OPERATION
- Before surgery, the donor is examined for communicable diseases, and the recipient is treated with immunosuppressive drugs. Sometimes, the recipient also receives radiation treatment.
- An incision is made in the donor's chest through the breastbone or into the hip through the ilium.
- Bone marrow is removed from the breastbone with suction. The opening in the bone is closed. The skin is closed with sutures or clips.
- The bone marrow is filtered and then injected into one of the recipient's veins.

POSSIBLE COMPLICATIONS—Donor:
- Excessive bleeding.
- Surgical-wound infection.

Recipient:
- Rejection of transplanted bone marrow.
- Uncontrolled infections.

AVERAGE HOSPITAL STAY—10 to 14 days.

PROBABLE OUTCOME—This surgery is a desperate measure. A few patients—who otherwise would have died—survive as a result of it. Allow 3 weeks to determine the success of surgery.

POSTOPERATIVE CARE

NOTE—This information is supplemental and should not replace your doctor's instructions.

GENERAL MEASURES—The recipient should be isolated from attendants, family and visitors to protect the recipient from infection.

MEDICATION—For donor:
- Your doctor may prescribe:
  Pain relievers. Don't take prescription pain medication longer than 4 to 7 days. Use *only* as much as you need.
  Antibiotics to fight infection.
- You may use non-prescription drugs, such as acetaminophen, for minor pain.

For recipient:
- Immunosuppressants to prevent rejection of bone marrow.
- Antibiotics to prevent infection.

ACTIVITY—For donor and recipient:
- Return to work and normal activity as soon as possible. This reduces postoperative depression and irritability, which are common.
- Avoid vigorous exercise for 6 weeks after surgery.

DIET—Donor and recipient should have a clear liquid diet until gastrointestinal function resumes. Then a well-balanced, high-protein diet will promote healing.

CALL YOUR DOCTOR IF

Any of the following occurs in either the donor or recipient:
- Nausea or vomiting.
- Increased pain, swelling, redness, drainage or bleeding in the surgical area.
- Signs of infection: headache, muscle aches, dizziness or a general ill feeling and fever.
- New, unexplained symptoms. Drugs used in treatment may produce side effects.

BREAST-ABSCESS DRAINAGE

GENERAL INFORMATION

DEFINITION—To open and drain an abscess in the female breast.

BODY PARTS INVOLVED—Lactating breast; nipple; lactiferous ducts.

REASONS FOR SURGERY—Relief of pain and prevention of the spread of infection.

SURGICAL RISK INCREASES WITH
- Obesity.
- Smoking.
- Stress.
- Poor nutrition.
- Recent or chronic illness.
- Use of drugs such as: antihypertensives; muscle relaxants; tranquilizers; sleep inducers; insulin; sedatives; beta-adrenergic blockers; or cortisone.
- Use of mind-altering drugs, including: narcotics; psychedelics; hallucinogens; marijuana; sedatives; hypnotics; or cocaine.

WHAT TO EXPECT

WHO OPERATES—General surgeon or obstetrician-gynecologist.

WHERE PERFORMED—Hospital, emergency room or outpatient surgical facility.

DIAGNOSTIC TESTS
- Before surgery: Blood and urine studies.
- After surgery: Laboratory examination of removed pus.

ANESTHESIA
- Local anesthesia by injection.
- General anesthesia by inhalation and injection, with an airway tube placed in the windpipe.

DESCRIPTION OF OPERATION
- An incision is made in the breast extending outward from the nipple. The incision is deepened and pus is removed.
- An instrument is forced into the abscess. Pockets of pus are broken up by the surgeon's finger. The opening is enlarged and the area is irrigated with a salt solution. Gauze packing is inserted to allow drainage.
- The skin edges are brought together loosely around the drain.

POSSIBLE COMPLICATIONS
- Excessive bleeding.
- Surgical-wound infection.
- Slow healing.
- Breast engorgement, if breast is not emptied regularly of milk.

AVERAGE HOSPITAL STAY—0 to 2 days.

PROBABLE OUTCOME—Expect complete recovery without complications. Nursing can usually be resumed on the affected side in about 2 weeks. Allow about 3 weeks for complete recovery from surgery.

POSTOPERATIVE CARE

NOTE—This information is supplemental and should not replace your doctor's instructions.

GENERAL MEASURES
- A hard ridge should form along the incision. As it heals, the ridge will recede gradually.
- Use an electric heating pad, a heat lamp or a warm compress to relieve incisional pain.
- Bathe and shower as usual. After removal of the drain, you may wash the incision gently with mild unscented soap.
- Change dressings daily after bathing.
- If you continue nursing, use a breast pump on the abscessed side to prevent engorgement. Continue to nurse from the unaffected breast. The infant is unlikely to become infected.

MEDICATION
- Your doctor may prescribe:
  Pain relievers. Don't take prescription pain medication longer than 4 to 7 days. Use *only* as much as you need.
  Antibiotics to fight infection.
- You may use non-prescription drugs, such as acetaminophen, for minor pain.

ACTIVITY
- Return to work and normal activity as soon as possible. This reduces postoperative depression and irritability, which are common.
- Avoid vigorous exercise for 3 weeks after surgery.
- Resume driving 2 days after returning home.

DIET—Clear liquid diet until the gastrointestinal tract functions again. Then eat a well-balanced, high-protein diet to promote healing. Drink at least 8 glasses of water daily.

CALL YOUR DOCTOR IF

Any of the following occurs:
- Nausea or vomiting.
- Increased pain, swelling, redness, drainage or bleeding increases in the surgical area.
- Signs of infection: headache, muscle aches, dizziness or a general ill feeling and fever.
- New, unexplained symptoms. Drugs used in treatment may produce side effects.

BREAST AUGMENTATION
(Augmentation Mammoplasty)

GENERAL INFORMATION

DEFINITION—Implantation of artificial material inside the female breasts to enlarge them or give them a different shape.

BODY PARTS INVOLVED—Female breasts; underlying muscles.

REASONS FOR SURGERY
- Restoration of normal breast appearance after a mastectomy.
- Enlargement of the breasts in patients who have less breast tissue than they desire.
- Correction of asymmetry of the breasts.

SURGICAL RISK INCREASES WITH
- Smoking.
- Obesity.
- Excess alcohol consumption.
- Use of drugs such as: antihypertensives; muscle relaxants; tranquilizers; sleep inducers; insulin; sedatives; beta-adrenergic blockers; or cortisone.
- Use of mind-altering drugs, including: narcotics; psychedelics; hallucinogens; marijuana; sedatives; hypnotics; or cocaine.

WHAT TO EXPECT

WHO OPERATES—Plastic and reconstructive surgeon.

WHERE PERFORMED—Hospital; doctor's office; or outpatient surgical facility.

DIAGNOSTIC TESTS
- Before surgery: Blood studies; mammograms (see Glossary).
- After surgery: Blood studies.

ANESTHESIA—Local anesthesia by injection.

DESCRIPTION OF OPERATION
- Incisions may be made under the breast, through the nipple or in the armpit.
- The breast tissue is brought forward by raising muscles from below the breast or the muscles next to the chest wall.
- A pocket is created, and the implant (a mammary prosthesis filled with silicone or saline) is inserted. The procedures are usually repeated on the other breast.
- The skin is closed with sutures or clips, which usually can be removed about 1 week after surgery. A light bandage is applied.
- A bra or elastic bandage is fitted to give support and to reduce possible bleeding.

POSSIBLE COMPLICATIONS
- Excessive bleeding.
- Surgical-wound infection.
- Formation of a thickened band of tissue from bleeding around the breast. This will make the breast harder to the touch than usual.
- Implant may become dislodged.

AVERAGE HOSPITAL STAY—0 to 1 day.

PROBABLE OUTCOME—Expect complete healing without complications. Allow about 2 weeks for recovery from surgery. The implants do not interfere with future detection of any abnormal lumps in the breast.

POSTOPERATIVE CARE

NOTE—This information is supplemental and should not replace your doctor's instructions.

GENERAL MEASURES
- Hard ridges may form along the incision. The ridges will heal and recede gradually without treatment.
- Bathe and shower as usual. You may wash the incisions gently with mild unscented soap.
- Use ice packs to reduce swelling and to relieve incisional pain.

MEDICATION
- Your doctor may prescribe:
  Pain relievers. Don't take prescription pain medication longer than 4 to 7 days. Use *only* as much as you need.
  Antibiotics to fight infection.
- You may use non-prescription drugs, such as acetaminophen, for minor pain.

ACTIVITY
- Resume work and normal activity as soon as possible.
- Avoid vigorous exercise for 6 weeks after surgery.
- Resume driving 1 week after returning home.

DIET—No special diet.

CALL YOUR DOCTOR IF

- Pain, swelling, redness, drainage or bleeding increases in the surgical area.
- You develop signs of infection: headache, muscle aches, dizziness or a general ill feeling and fever.
- You experience new symptoms, such as nausea or vomiting.

BREAST BIOPSY BY INCISION

GENERAL INFORMATION

DEFINITION—Removal of a lump or cyst from one of the breasts.

BODY PARTS INVOLVED—Female breast; male breast (rare).

REASONS FOR SURGERY—Signs or symptoms that may indicate breast cancer. Laboratory examination of the removed tissue aids in diagnosis.

SURGICAL RISK INCREASES WITH
- Obesity.
- Stress.
- Smoking.
- Poor nutrition.
- Recent or chronic illness.
- Use of drugs such as: antihypertensives; muscle relaxants; tranquilizers; sleep inducers; insulin; sedatives; beta-adrenergic blockers; or cortisone.
- Use of mind-altering drugs, including: narcotics; psychedelics; hallucinogens; marijuana; sedatives; hypnotics; or cocaine.

WHAT TO EXPECT

WHO OPERATES—Family doctor or general surgeon.

WHERE PERFORMED—Hospital or outpatient surgical facility.

DIAGNOSTIC TESTS
- Before surgery: Blood and urine studies; X-rays of chest; mammograms (see Glossary).
- After surgery: Laboratory examination of removed tissue.

ANESTHESIA
- Local anesthesia by injection.
- General anesthesia by inhalation and injection, with an airway tube placed in the windpipe.

DESCRIPTION OF OPERATION
- An incision is made over the cyst or lump to be removed.
- The cyst or lump is cut free of surrounding tissue and removed. Bleeding is controlled with ties or electrocauterization.
- The skin is closed with sutures or clips, which usually can be removed about 1 week after surgery.

POSSIBLE COMPLICATIONS
- Excessive bleeding.
- Surgical-wound infection.
- Unsightly scar on breast (rare).

AVERAGE HOSPITAL STAY—0 to 1 day.

PROBABLE OUTCOME—Expect complete healing without complications. Allow about 2 weeks for recovery from surgery.

POSTOPERATIVE CARE

NOTE—This information is supplemental and should not replace your doctor's instructions.

GENERAL MEASURES
- A hard ridge should form along the incision. As it heals, the ridge will recede gradually.
- Use an electric heating pad, a heat lamp or a warm compress to relieve incisional pain.
- Bathe and shower as usual. You may wash the incision gently with mild unscented soap.
- Wear a supportive bra. Apply bandages to the surgical wound, and change them several times daily or as directed by your doctor.

MEDICATION
- Your doctor may prescribe pain relievers. Don't take prescription pain medication longer than 4 to 7 days. Use *only* as much as you need.
- You may use non-prescription drugs, such as acetaminophen, for minor pain.

ACTIVITY
- Return to work and normal activity as soon as possible. This reduces postoperative depression and irritability, which are common.
- Avoid vigorous exercise for 2 weeks after surgery.
- Resume driving 3 to 5 days after returning home.

DIET—Clear liquid diet until the gastrointestinal tract functions again. Then eat a well-balanced, high-protein diet to promote healing.

CALL YOUR DOCTOR IF

- Pain, swelling, redness, drainage or bleeding increases in the surgical area.
- You develop signs of infection: headache, muscle aches, dizziness or a general ill feeling and fever.

BREAST BIOPSY BY NEEDLE ASPIRATION

 GENERAL INFORMATION

DEFINITION—Removal of fluid or tissue from one of the female breasts.

BODY PARTS INVOLVED—Breast.

REASONS FOR SURGERY—Diagnosis of a thickening or lump.

SURGICAL RISK INCREASES WITH
- Obesity.
- Smoking.
- Poor nutrition.
- Recent or chronic illness.
- Use of drugs such as: antihypertensives; muscle relaxants; tranquilizers; sleep inducers; insulin; sedatives; beta-adrenergic blockers; or cortisone.
- Use of mind-altering drugs, including: narcotics; psychedelics; hallucinogens; marijuana; sedatives; hypnotics; or cocaine.

 WHAT TO EXPECT

WHO OPERATES—Family doctor or general surgeon.

WHERE PERFORMED—Hospital, doctor's office or outpatient surgical facility.

DIAGNOSTIC TESTS
- Before surgery: Medical history and physical examination; blood and urine studies; X-rays of chest; mammograms (see Glossary).
- After surgery: Laboratory examination of removed fluid or tissue.

ANESTHESIA—Local anesthesia by injection.

DESCRIPTION OF OPERATION—A small hollow needle is inserted into the thickening or lump. If the thickening or lump is a cyst, fluid usually can be removed and the cyst will shrink or disappear. The removed fluid is sent to the laboratory to be examined for abnormal cells. If a solid tumor is detected, tissue is removed through the needle for laboratory examination.

POSSIBLE COMPLICATIONS—Infection in surgical area (rare).

AVERAGE HOSPITAL STAY—0 to 1 day.

PROBABLE OUTCOME—Expect complete healing without complications. Allow about 1 week for recovery from surgery.

 POSTOPERATIVE CARE

NOTE—This information is supplemental and should not replace your doctor's instructions.

GENERAL MEASURES
- Use an electric heating pad, a heat lamp or a warm compress to relieve pain in the surgical area.
- Bathe and shower as usual. You may wash the area of needle insertion gently with mild unscented soap.
- Wear a supportive bra. Apply bandages to the surgical wound, and change them several times a day or as directed by your doctor.

MEDICATION
- Your doctor may prescribe pain relievers. Don't take prescription pain medication longer than 4 to 7 days. Use *only* as much as you need.
- You may use non-prescription drugs, such as acetaminophen, for minor pain.

ACTIVITY
- Return to work and normal activity as soon as possible. This reduces postoperative depression and irritability, which are common.
- Avoid vigorous exercise for 2 weeks after surgery.
- Resume driving 3 days after returning from the hospital.

DIET—No special diet.

 CALL YOUR DOCTOR IF

- Pain, swelling, redness, drainage or bleeding increases in the surgical area.
- You develop signs of infection: headache, muscle aches, dizziness or a general ill feeling and fever.

BREAST REDUCTION
(Reduction Mammoplasty)

GENERAL INFORMATION

DEFINITION—Removal of excess tissue and overlying skin from the female breasts. Usually, this surgery also includes reconstruction of breast shape.

BODY PARTS INVOLVED—Breasts.

REASONS FOR SURGERY
- Reduction of overly large breasts to improve appearance.
- Relief of back pain from weight of overly large breasts.
- Reconstruction of a breast to match a surgical change made in the other breast.

SURGICAL RISK INCREASES WITH
- Obesity.
- Smoking.
- Excess alcohol consumption.
- Use of drugs such as: antihypertensives; muscle relaxants; tranquilizers; sleep inducers; insulin; sedatives; beta-adrenergic blockers; or cortisone.
- Use of mind-altering drugs, including: narcotics; psychedelics; hallucinogens; marijuana; sedatives; hypnotics; or cocaine.

WHAT TO EXPECT

WHO OPERATES—Plastic and reconstructive surgeon.

WHERE PERFORMED—Hospital.

DIAGNOSTIC TESTS
- Before surgery: Blood and urine studies; mammograms (see Glossary).
- After surgery: Blood studies.

ANESTHESIA—General anesthesia by inhalation and injection, with an airway tube placed in the windpipe.

DESCRIPTION OF OPERATION
- The breast is marked where the skin will be removed and where the nipple will be after tissue is removed.
- The skin between the new nipple location and the natural nipple location is incised and removed. The nipple stays attached to underlying tissue.
- Another incision is made below the nipple. Excess tissue is removed through this incision.
- Drains are left in place to prevent fluid or blood from accumulating under the sutures.
- The skin is closed with fine sutures, which usually can be removed about 7 to 10 days after surgery.

POSSIBLE COMPLICATIONS
- Excessive bleeding.
- Surgical-wound infection.
- Discoloration of healing skin edges.

AVERAGE HOSPITAL STAY—4 to 5 days.

PROBABLE OUTCOME—Expect complete healing without complications. Allow about 4 weeks for recovery from surgery.

POSTOPERATIVE CARE

NOTE—This information is supplemental and should not replace your doctor's instructions.

GENERAL MEASURES
- A small ridge may form along the incision. The ridges will heal and recede gradually without treatment.
- Use ice packs to reduce swelling and to relieve incisional pain.
- Bathe and shower as usual. You may wash the incision gently with mild unscented soap.

MEDICATION
- Your doctor may prescribe:
  Pain relievers. Don't take prescription pain medication longer than 4 to 7 days. Use *only* as much as you need.
  Antibiotics to fight infection.
- You may use non-prescription drugs, such as acetaminophen, for minor pain.

ACTIVITY
- Resume work and normal activity as soon as possible to reduce postoperative depression, which is common.
- Avoid vigorous exercise for 6 weeks after surgery.
- Resume driving 1 month after returning home.

DIET—No special diet.

CALL YOUR DOCTOR IF

- Pain, swelling, redness, drainage or bleeding increases in the surgical area.
- You develop signs of infection: headache, muscle aches, dizziness or a general ill feeling and fever.

BRONCHOSCOPY

GENERAL INFORMATION

DEFINITION—Visual examination of the lining of the bronchial tubes and removal of tissue and secretions. Surgery is performed with a bronchoscope, an optical instrument with a lighted tip.

BODY PARTS INVOLVED—Windpipe (trachea); larynx; bronchial tree.

REASONS FOR SURGERY
- Suspected cancer in the bronchial tubes.
- Foreign matter that has been inhaled accidentally.
- Bleeding in the bronchial tubes.
- X-ray studies (bronchograms) to diagnose diseases of the lung, such as bronchiectasis or emphysema.

SURGICAL RISK INCREASES WITH
- Obesity.
- Smoking.
- Recent illness.
- Alcoholism or chronic illness.
- Use of drugs such as: antihypertensives; muscle relaxants; tranquilizers; sleep inducers; insulin; sedatives; beta-adrenergic blockers; or cortisone.
- Use of mind-altering drugs, including: narcotics; psychedelics; hallucinogens; marijuana; sedatives; hypnotics; or cocaine.

WHAT TO EXPECT

WHO OPERATES—Thoracic surgeon, general surgeon, pulmonary specialist or ear, nose and throat specialist.

WHERE PERFORMED—Hospital or outpatient surgical facility.

DIAGNOSTIC TESTS
- Before surgery: Blood and urine studies; X-rays of chest; CAT scan (see Glossary).
- During surgery: Bronchogram (see Glossary).
- After surgery: Laboratory examination of removed tissue and secretions.

ANESTHESIA—General anesthesia by inhalation and injection, with an airway tube placed in the windpipe.

DESCRIPTION OF OPERATION
- The bronchoscope is inserted in the mouth, past the back of the tongue, into the main bronchial tube and its branches.
- Foreign matter is removed, if necessary. Tissue is gathered and secretions are collected.
- The bronchoscope is removed.

POSSIBLE COMPLICATIONS
- Excessive bleeding.
- Infection in lung or bronchial tubes.
- Inadvertent injury to wall of a bronchus.

AVERAGE HOSPITAL STAY—Depends on underlying disease.

PROBABLE OUTCOME—Tissue and secretions obtained successfully without complications in virtually all cases. Allow about 1 week for recovery from surgery.

POSTOPERATIVE CARE

NOTE—This information is supplemental and should not replace your doctor's instructions.

GENERAL MEASURES—Use a vaporizer to increase moisture in the air you breathe for the first 3 to 4 nights after surgery. Don't smoke.

MEDICATION
- Your doctor may prescribe:
  Pain relievers. Don't take prescription pain medication longer than 4 to 7 days. Use *only* as much as you need.
  Antibiotics to fight infection.
- You may use non-prescription drugs, such as acetaminophen, for minor pain.

ACTIVITY
- Return to work and normal activity as soon as possible. This reduces postoperative depression and irritability, which are common.
- Avoid vigorous exercise for 7 days after surgery.
- Resume driving 4 days after returning home.

DIET—Clear liquid diet until the gastrointestinal tract functions again. Then eat a well-balanced, high-protein diet to promote healing.

CALL YOUR DOCTOR IF

- You experience excessive bleeding.
- New, unexplained symptoms develop. Drugs used in treatment may produce side effects.
- You develop signs of infection: headache, muscle aches, dizziness or a general ill feeling and fever.

SURGERIES

BUNION REMOVAL

GENERAL INFORMATION

DEFINITION—Removal of a bunion, a bony and fibrous outgrowth at the base of the big toe.

BODY PARTS INVOLVED—Foot; joint between the metatarsal bone and big toe; fluid sac that surrounds the joint.

REASONS FOR SURGERY
- Relief of pain.
- Correction of deformity.

SURGICAL RISK INCREASES WITH
- Poor nutrition.
- Recent illness.
- Alcoholism or chronic illness.

WHAT TO EXPECT

WHO OPERATES—General surgeon, orthopedist or podiatrist.

WHERE PERFORMED—Doctor's office, outpatient surgical facility or hospital.

DIAGNOSTIC TESTS
- Before surgery: X-rays of foot; blood and urine studies.
- After surgery: X-rays of foot.

ANESTHESIA
- Local anesthesia by injection.
- Spinal anesthesia by injection.
- General anesthesia by inhalation and injection, with an airway tube placed in the windpipe.

DESCRIPTION OF OPERATION
- An incision is made over the bunion.
- The capsule of the joint connecting the metatarsal bone and the big toe is opened.
- A section from the metatarsal bone is cut or filed away and removed. Another small bone (the sesamoid bone) attached to a tendon is removed also.
- Tendons attached to the base of the metatarsal and toe bones are cut. This allows the bones to straighten when healed.
- The skin is closed with sutures, which usually can be removed about 10 days after surgery.

POSSIBLE COMPLICATIONS
- Excessive bleeding.
- Surgical-wound infection.
- Slow healing.

AVERAGE HOSPITAL STAY—0 to 1 day.

PROBABLE OUTCOME—Expect complete healing without complications. Allow about 6 weeks for recovery from surgery.

POSTOPERATIVE CARE

NOTE—This information is supplemental and should not replace your doctor's instructions.

GENERAL MEASURES
- A hard ridge should form along the incision. As it heals, the ridge will recede gradually.
- Use an electric heating pad, a heat lamp or a warm compress to relieve incisional pain.
- Bathe and shower as usual. You may wash the incision gently with mild unscented soap.
- Between baths, keep the wound dry with a bandage for the first 2 or 3 days after surgery. If a bandage gets wet, change it promptly.
- Apply non-prescription antibiotic ointment to the wound before applying bandages.
- If the wound bleeds, press a clean tissue or cloth to it.

MEDICATION
- Your doctor may prescribe:
  Pain relievers. Don't take prescription pain medication longer than 4 to 7 days. Use *only* as much as you need.
  Antibiotics to prevent infection.
- You may use non-prescription drugs, such as acetaminophen, for minor pain.

ACTIVITY
- Resume work and normal activity as soon as possible to reduce postoperative depression and irritability, which are comon.
- Avoid vigorous exercise for 6 weeks after surgery. Don't put weight on the affected foot until the surgical area heals.
- Resume driving 4 days after returning home.

DIET—No special diet.

CALL YOUR DOCTOR IF

- Pain, swelling, redness, drainage or bleeding increases in the surgical area.
- You develop signs of infection: headache, muscle aches, dizziness or a general ill feeling and fever.
- New, unexplained symptoms develop. Drugs used in treatment may produce side effects.

CARDIAC CATHETERIZATION & ANGIOCARDIOGRAPHY

GENERAL INFORMATION

DEFINITION—Diagnostic procedures to examine functions of the heart.

BODY PARTS INVOLVED—Heart muscle and valves; coronary arteries; large artery in arm or leg.

REASONS FOR SURGERY
- Evaluation of chest pain.
- Diagnosis of a congenital heart defect and valvular-heart disease.
- Measurement of the heart muscle's ability to pump blood.
- Identification of narrowing or obstruction in the coronary arteries.

SURGICAL RISK INCREASES WITH
- Stress.
- Obesity.
- Smoking.
- Recent illness.
- Alcoholism or chronic illness.

WHAT TO EXPECT

WHO OPERATES—Cardiologist or general surgeon.

WHERE PERFORMED—Hospital.

DIAGNOSTIC TESTS
- Before surgery: Blood and urine studies; EKG (see Glossary).
- During surgery: Intracardiac pressures; cardiac output; cinematography; fluoroscopy; EKG (see Glossary for all).
- After surgery: EKG; blood studies.

ANESTHESIA—Local anesthesia by injection.

DESCRIPTION OF OPERATION
- The cardiac catheter is inserted into an artery in the patient's arm or leg. Fluoroscopy provides guidance for the catheter to pass through the artery to the heart.
- Blood-pressure readings are taken, and the heart's ability to pump blood is tested.
- The catheter is guided into the coronary-artery system. Fluoroscopy allows identification of any disease in the coronary arteries.
- When all examinations have been completed, the catheter is withdrawn, and the artery into which it was inserted is compressed until bleeding stops. If an arm artery was used, it may need to be repaired.
- The skin is closed with several sutures, which usually can be removed about 1 week after surgery.

POSSIBLE COMPLICATIONS
- Excessive bleeding
- Surgical-wound infection.
- Blood clot in an artery.
- Heartbeat disturbance.
- Cardiac arrest (rare).

AVERAGE HOSPITAL STAY—0 to 1 day.

PROBABLE OUTCOME—Expect complete healing without complications. Allow about 2 weeks for recovery from surgery.

POSTOPERATIVE CARE

NOTE—This information is supplemental and should not replace your doctor's instructions.

GENERAL MEASURES
- A hard ridge should form along the incision. As it heals, the ridge will recede gradually.
- Use an electric heating pad, a heat lamp or a warm compress to relieve incisional pain.
- Expect discoloration under the skin where the catheter was inserted. It should disappear in 2 weeks.
- Bathe and shower as usual. You may wash the incision gently with mild unscented soap.
- Between showers, keep the wound dry with a bandage for the first 2 or 3 days after surgery. If a bandage gets wet, change it promptly. Apply non-prescription antibiotic ointment to the wound before applying new bandages.
- If the wound bleeds during the first 24 hours after surgery, press a clean tissue or cloth to it for 10 to 15 minutes continuously.

MEDICATION
- Your doctor may prescribe pain relievers. Don't take prescription pain medication longer than 4 to 7 days. Use *only* as much as you need.
- You may use non-prescription drugs, such as acetaminophen, for minor pain.

ACTIVITY
- Avoid vigorous exercise for 2 weeks after surgery.
- Resume driving 2 days after returning home.

DIET—No special diet.

CALL YOUR DOCTOR IF

- You experience sudden or severe chest pain.
- Pain, swelling, redness, drainage or bleeding increases in the surgical area.
- You develop signs of infection: headache, muscle aches, dizziness or a general ill feeling and fever.

CAROTID-ARTERY ENDARTERECTOMY

GENERAL INFORMATION

DEFINITION—Removal of debris that has partially or totally obstructed blood supply to the brain and other parts of the head.

BODY PARTS INVOLVED—Carotid arteries.

REASONS FOR SURGERY—Prevention of stroke.

SURGICAL RISK INCREASES WITH
- Adults over 60.
- Stress.
- Obesity.
- Smoking.
- Poor nutrition.
- Excess alcohol consumption.
- Recent illness such as respiratory infection.
- Atherosclerosis; coronary artery disease; or diabetes mellitus.
- Use of drugs such as: antihypertensives; muscle relaxants; tranquilizers; sleep inducers; insulin; sedatives; beta-adrenergic blockers; or cortisone.
- Use of mind-altering drugs.

WHAT TO EXPECT

WHO OPERATES—General surgeon, cardiovascular surgeon, or peripheral vascular surgeon.

WHERE PERFORMED—Hospital.

DIAGNOSTIC TESTS
- Before surgery: Blood and urine studies; EKG; arteriograms (see Glossary).
- After surgery: Blood studies.

ANESTHESIA—General anesthesia by inhalation and injection, with an airway tube placed in the windpipe.

DESCRIPTION OF OPERATION
- An incision is made in the neck over the obstruction.
- The obstructed area is isolated. Sometimes, a tube is grafted in to circulate blood around the obstruction.
- A small incision is made over the obstruction, which is scraped away. The opened area is patched with a graft fashioned from a vein from another part of the body.
- If the bypass tube is temporary, it is removed.
- The skin is closed with sutures or clips, which usually can be removed in 2 weeks.

POSSIBLE COMPLICATIONS
- Excessive bleeding.
- Surgical-wound infection.
- Inadvertent injury to a branch of the nerves to the face.

- Breaking away of blood debris inside the artery, causing a stroke.

AVERAGE HOSPITAL STAY—7 days.

PROBABLE OUTCOME—Expect complete healing without complications and restoration of good blood flow to the brain. Allow about 2 weeks for recovery from surgery.

POSTOPERATIVE CARE

NOTE—This information is supplemental and should not replace your doctor's instructions.

GENERAL MEASURES
- A small ridge may form along the incision. As it heals, the ridge will recede gradually.
- Use an electric heating pad, a heat lamp or a warm compress to relieve incisional pain.
- Bathe and shower as usual. You may wash the incision gently with mild unscented soap.
- Move legs often while in bed to decrease the likelihood of deep-vein blood clots.

MEDICATION
- Your doctor may prescribe:
  Pain relievers. Use *only* as much as you need.
  Stool softeners to prevent constipation.
  Antibiotics to fight infection.
  Anticoagulants to prevent blood clots.
- You may use non-prescription drugs, such as acetaminophen, for minor pain.

ACTIVITY
- Resume work and normal activity as soon as possible to reduce postoperative depression, which is common.
- Avoid vigorous exercise for 6 weeks after surgery. Resume sexual relations when your doctor determines that healing is complete.
- Resume driving 3 weeks after returning home.

DIET—Clear liquid diet until the gastrointestinal tract begins to function again. Then eat a well-balanced, high-protein diet to promote healing.

CALL YOUR DOCTOR IF

Any of the following occurs:
- Pain, swelling, redness, drainage or bleeding increases in the surgical area.
- Signs of infection: headache, muscle aches, dizziness or a general ill feeling and fever.
- Nausea, vomiting or constipation.
- New, unexplained symptoms develop. Drugs used in treatment may produce side effects.

CARPAL-TUNNEL-SYNDROME REPAIR

GENERAL INFORMATION

DEFINITION—Cutting the transverse carpal ligament, the fibrous tissue extending across the wrist.

BODY PARTS INVOLVED—Transverse carpal ligament; median nerve and surrounding fibrous tissue; wrist joint.

REASONS FOR SURGERY—Relief of pain caused by carpal-tunnel syndrome.

SURGICAL RISK INCREASES WITH
- Obesity.
- Smoking.
- Poor nutrition.
- Recent illness.
- Alcoholism or chronic illness.
- Use of drugs such as: antihypertensives; muscle relaxants; tranquilizers; sleep inducers; insulin; sedatives; beta-adrenergic blockers; or cortisone.
- Use of mind-altering drugs, including: narcotics; psychedelics; hallucinogens; marijuana; sedatives; hypnotics; or cocaine.

WHAT TO EXPECT

WHO OPERATES—Hand surgeon, general surgeon, orthopedist or plastic and reconstructive surgeon.

WHERE PERFORMED—Hospital or outpatient surgical facility.

DIAGNOSTIC TESTS
- Before surgery: Blood and urine studies; X-rays of wrist; nerve-conduction tests (see Glossary).
- After surgery: Blood studies.

ANESTHESIA
- Local anesthesia by injection.
- General anesthesia by inhalation and injection, with an airway tube placed in the windpipe.

DESCRIPTION OF OPERATION
- A tourniquet is applied above the wrist to prevent bleeding in the surgical area.
- An incision is made in the underside of the wrist.
- The transverse carpal ligament is located and cut, releasing the compressed median nerve.
- The skin is closed with fine sutures, which usually can be removed about 10 days after surgery.
- A bandage is applied, and a splint is used to hold the wrist in position.

POSSIBLE COMPLICATIONS
- Excessive bleeding.
- Surgical-wound infection.
- Inadvertent injury to blood vessels or nerves.

AVERAGE HOSPITAL STAY—0 to 1 day.

PROBABLE OUTCOME—Expect complete healing without complications. Allow about 1 month for recovery from surgery.

POSTOPERATIVE CARE

NOTE—This information is supplemental and should not replace your doctor's instructions.

GENERAL MEASURES
- If the wound bleeds during the first 24 hours after surgery, press a clean tissue or cloth to it.
- A hard ridge should form along the incision. As it heals, the ridge will recede gradually.
- Use an electric heating pad, a heat lamp or a warm compress to relieve incision pain.
- Keep the wound dry with a bandage until it has healed. Protect it when bathing. If a bandage gets wet, change it promptly.
- Apply non-prescription antibiotic ointment to the wound before applying new bandages.

MEDICATION
- Your doctor may prescribe:
  Pain relievers. Don't take prescription pain medication longer than 4 to 7 days. Use *only* as much as you need.
  Antibiotics to fight infection.
- You may use non-prescription drugs, such as acetaminophen, for minor pain.

ACTIVITY
- Return to work and normal activity as soon as possible. This reduces postoperative depression and irritability, which are common.
- Resume driving 1 week after returning home.

DIET—No special diet.

CALL YOUR DOCTOR IF

- Pain, swelling, redness, drainage or bleeding increases in the surgical area.
- You develop signs of infection: headache, muscle aches, dizziness or a general ill feeling and fever.
- New, unexplained symptoms develop. Drugs used in treatment may produce side effects.

SURGERIES

CATARACT REMOVAL

GENERAL INFORMATION

DEFINITION—Removal of cataracts.

BODY PARTS INVOLVED—Eye; cornea; lens; eyelid membrane lining.

REASONS FOR SURGERY—Restoration of normal or almost-normal vision.

SURGICAL RISK INCREASES WITH
- Obesity.
- Smoking.
- Newborns and infants.
- Recent illness such as upper respiratory infection.
- Chronic illness, especially diabetes mellitus.
- Use of drugs such as: antihypertensives; muscle relaxants; tranquilizers; sleep inducers; insulin; sedatives; beta-adrenergic blockers; or cortisone.
- Use of mind-altering drugs, including: narcotics; psychedelics; hallucinogens; marijuana; sedative-hypnotics; or cocaine.

WHAT TO EXPECT

WHO OPERATES—Ophthalmologist.

WHERE PERFORMED—Hospital.

DIAGNOSTIC TESTS
- Before surgery: Blood and urine studies; eye examinations.
- After surgery: Eye examinations.

ANESTHESIA
- Local anesthesia (sometimes) by injection.
- General anesthesia by inhalation and injection, with an airway tube placed in the windpipe.

DESCRIPTION OF OPERATION
- A special instrument holds the eyelids apart, and temporary sutures hold the eye in place.
- The eye is opened around the iris, and the lens is removed. Sometimes, the lens is fragmented with ultrasound (see Glossary), and debris is suctioned away.
- Sometimes, an artificial lens is inserted to replace the diseased lens.
- The temporary sutures are removed. Pilocarpine or atropine eye-drop solutions are placed in the eye to keep the pupil open. Bandages are applied.

POSSIBLE COMPLICATIONS
- Surgical-wound infection.
- Adhesions.
- Bleeding into the eye.
- Loss of fluid from the eye.
- Retinal detachment.
- Increased pressure within the eyeball.

AVERAGE HOSPITAL STAY—2 to 3 days.

PROBABLE OUTCOME—Expect complete healing without complications. Adjusting to new glasses or contact lenses takes about 3 to 4 weeks. Allow about 2 weeks for recovery from surgery.

POSTOPERATIVE CARE

NOTE—This information is supplemental and should not replace your doctor's instructions.

GENERAL MEASURES
- Sleep with your head elevated on two pillows.
- Move legs often while resting in bed to decrease the likelihood of deep-vein blood clots.
- Avoid bending, straining or lying flat. These cause pressure inside the eye.

MEDICATION
- Your doctor may prescribe:
  Pain relievers. Don't take prescription pain medication longer than 4 to 7 days. Use *only* as much as you need.
  Stool softeners to prevent constipation.
  Antibiotic eye drops to fight infection. Keep eye drops cold, but not frozen, in the refrigerator.
- Eye drops to keep pupil dilated.
- You may use non-prescription drugs, such as acetaminophen, for minor pain.

ACTIVITY
- Return to work and normal activity as soon as possible. This reduces postoperative depression and irritability, which are common.
- Avoid vigorous exercise for 6 weeks after surgery.
- Resume driving 2 weeks after returning home.

DIET—Clear liquid diet until the gastrointestinal tract functions again. Then eat a well-balanced, high-protein diet to promote healing.

CALL YOUR DOCTOR IF

Any of the following occurs:
- Sudden loss of vision.
- Sharp pain or blood in the eye.
- Increased pain, swelling, redness or drainage in the surgical area.
- Nausea, vomiting or constipation.
- Signs of infection: headache, muscle aches, dizziness or a general ill feeling and fever.

CERVIX, BIOPSY OF

GENERAL INFORMATION

DEFINITION—Removal of tissue from the cervix, the lower third of the uterus.

BODY PARTS INVOLVED—Cervix; vagina (as route for surgery).

REASONS FOR SURGERY—Investigation of diseases of the cervix. Laboratory examination of the removed tissue aids in diagnosis.

SURGICAL RISK INCREASES WITH
- Previous bleeding disorders.
- Use of drugs such as anticoagulants or aspirin.

WHAT TO EXPECT

WHO OPERATES—Obstetrician-gynecologist, family doctor or general surgeon.

WHERE PERFORMED—Doctor's office or outpatient surgical facility.

DIAGNOSTIC TESTS
- Before surgery: Pap smear; pelvic exam; blood and urine tests.
- During surgery: Your doctor may stain the cervix before removing any sample tissue. Areas that do not hold the stain are the most important ones to examine. The staining is harmless and painless.
- After surgery: Laboratory examination of removed tissue.

ANESTHESIA—Local anesthesia by injection.

DESCRIPTION OF OPERATION
- A speculum is inserted into the vagina to hold it open and to bring the cervix into view.
- A second instrument is used to gather the tissue.
- The instruments are removed.

POSSIBLE COMPLICATIONS—Excessive bleeding or surgical-wound infection.

AVERAGE HOSPITAL STAY—Usually none.

PROBABLE OUTCOME—Tissue obtained successfully without complications in virtually all cases. Allow about 2 weeks for recovery from surgery.

POSTOPERATIVE CARE

NOTE—This information is supplemental and should not replace your doctor's instructions.

GENERAL MEASURES
- Wear cotton panties or pantyhose with a cotton crotch. Avoid panties made from nylon, polyester, silk or other non-ventilating materials.
- Use a sanitary pad to protect your clothing. Avoid tampons—they may lead to infection.
- Bathe and shower as usual. Use non-perfumed soap.
- Don't douche unless your doctor recommends it.

MEDICATION
- Your doctor may prescribe vaginal creams to relieve discomfort.
- You may use non-prescription drugs, such as acetaminophen, for minor pain.

ACTIVITY
- Resume driving 24 hours after recovering from surgery.
- Resume sexual relations in 1 week after surgery, if you wish.

DIET—No special diet.

CALL YOUR DOCTOR IF

- You develop signs of infection: headache, muscle aches, dizziness or a general ill feeling and fever.
- Vaginal discharge increases or begins to have an unpleasant odor.
- You experience discomfort that simple pain medication does not relieve quickly.
- Unusual vaginal swelling or bleeding develops.

SURGERIES

CERVIX, CONIZATION OF

GENERAL INFORMATION

DEFINITION—Removal of a cone of tissue from the cervix.

BODY PARTS INVOLVED—Cervix.

REASONS FOR SURGERY—Investigation or treatment of diseases of the cervix. Laboratory examination of the removed tissue aids in diagnosis. The surgery is also done to remove abnormal tissue after a Pap smear has revealed possible cancer of the cervix, and to treat severe inflammation or infection of the cervix (chronic cervicitis).

SURGICAL RISK INCREASES WITH
- Bleeding disorders.
- Use of drugs such as anticoagulants or aspirin.

WHAT TO EXPECT

WHO OPERATES—Obstetrician-gynecologist or general surgeon.

WHERE PERFORMED—Outpatient surgical facility or hospital.

DIAGNOSTIC TESTS
- Before surgery: Pap smear; pelvic exam; blood and urine studies; CAT scan of pelvis (see Glossary).
- After surgery: Laboratory examination of all removed tissue.

ANESTHESIA—General anesthesia by inhalation and injection, with an airway tube placed in the windpipe.

DESCRIPTION OF OPERATION
- A speculum is inserted into the vagina to hold it open and to bring the cervix into view.
- A cone of tissue at the opening of the cervix is removed either with a scalpel or a laser beam. (If the laser is used, anesthesia may not be necessary.)
- The lining membrane is closed with sutures or electrocauterization.

POSSIBLE COMPLICATIONS
- Excessive bleeding.
- Surgical-wound infection.
- Sometimes, when not enough tissue is removed, abnormal cells may develop at the edge of removed tissue.

AVERAGE HOSPITAL STAY—2 to 4 days.

PROBABLE OUTCOME—Tissue obtained successfully without complications in virtually all cases. Allow about 4 weeks for recovery from surgery.

POSTOPERATIVE CARE

NOTE—This information is supplemental and should not replace your doctor's instructions.

GENERAL MEASURES
- Wear cotton panties or pantyhose with a cotton crotch. Avoid panties made from nylon, polyester, silk or other non-ventilating materials.
- Wear a minipad to protect your clothing. Avoid tampons—they may lead to infection.
- Bathe or shower as usual. Use non-perfumed soap.
- Don't douche unless your doctor recommends it.

MEDICATION
Your doctor may prescribe:
- Pain relievers. Don't take prescription pain medication longer than 4 to 7 days. Use *only* as much as you need.
- Vaginal creams to relieve discomfort.
- Antibiotics to fight infection.

ACTIVITY
- Resume work and normal activity as soon as possible to reduce postoperative depression, which is common.
- Resume driving 1 week after returning home.
- Resume sexual relations when your doctor determines that healing is complete (about 2 to 4 weeks).

DIET—Clear liquid diet until the gastrointestinal tract begins to function again. Then eat a well-balanced, high-protein diet to promote healing.

CALL YOUR DOCTOR IF

- You develop signs of infection: headache, muscle aches, dizziness or a general ill feeling and fever.
- Vaginal discharge increases or begins to have an unpleasant odor.
- You experience discomfort that simple pain medication does not relieve quickly.
- Unusual vaginal bleeding or swelling develops.

CERVIX, CRYOSURGERY OF

GENERAL INFORMATION

DEFINITION—Destruction of abnormal (infected or damaged) cells in the cervix, the lower third of the uterus. An instrument called a cryosurgery probe is used to freeze abnormal cells with liquid nitrogen.

BODY PARTS INVOLVED—Cervix; vagina (as route for surgery).

REASONS FOR SURGERY
- Abnormal cells in the cervix.
- Inflammation or infection of the cervix (chronic cervicitis).

SURGICAL RISK INCREASES WITH—None expected.

WHAT TO EXPECT

WHO OPERATES—Obstetrician-gynecologist, family doctor or general surgeon.

WHERE PERFORMED—Doctor's office or outpatient surgical facility.

DIAGNOSTIC TESTS
- Before surgery: Pap smear; vaginal exam.
- After surgery: Pap smear in 2 to 3 months.

ANESTHESIA—Usually none.

DESCRIPTION OF OPERATION
- A speculum is inserted into the vagina to hold it open and to bring the cervix into view.
- The cryosurgery probe is held on the affected areas long enough to freeze and destroy abnormal cells.
- The instruments are removed. The procedure should be painless. Discomfort after surgery may vary from one person to the next but should not cause much distress.

POSSIBLE COMPLICATIONS—None expected.

AVERAGE HOSPITAL STAY—Usually none.

PROBABLE OUTCOME—Healing requires up to 2 months. During this time you should expect a frequent, watery vaginal discharge. Allow about 6 weeks for recovery from surgery.

POSTOPERATIVE CARE

NOTE—This information is supplemental and should not replace your doctor's instructions.

GENERAL MEASURES
- Wear cotton panties or pantyhose with a cotton crotch. Avoid panties made from nylon, polyester, silk or other non-ventilating materials.
- Use a sanitary pad to protect your clothing. Avoid tampons—they may lead to infection.
- Bathe and shower as usual. Use unscented soap.
- Don't douche unless your doctor recommends it.

MEDICATION—You may use non-prescription drugs, such as acetaminophen, to relieve minor pain.

ACTIVITY—No restrictions. Resume sexual relations when your doctor determines healing is complete.

DIET—No special diet.

CALL YOUR DOCTOR IF

- Vaginal discharge increases or develops an unpleasant odor.
- You experience pain that simple pain medication does not relieve quickly.
- You develop signs of infection: headache, muscle aches, dizziness or a general ill feeling and fever.
- Unusual vaginal swelling or bleeding develops.

CERVIX, ELECTROCAUTERIZATION OF

 GENERAL INFORMATION

DEFINITION—Destruction of abnormal (infected or damaged) cells in the cervix, in the lower third of the uterus. An instrument called an electrocautery uses electric current to destroy the abnormal tissue.

BODY PARTS INVOLVED—Cervix; vagina (as route for surgery).

REASONS FOR SURGERY
- Presence of abnormal cells in the cervix.
- Inflammation or infection of the cervix.

SURGICAL RISK INCREASES WITH—None expected.

 WHAT TO EXPECT

WHO OPERATES—Obstetrician-gynecologist, general surgeon or family doctor.

WHERE PERFORMED—Doctor's office or outpatient surgical facility.

DIAGNOSTIC TESTS
- Before surgery: Pap smear; vaginal-discharge study.
- After surgery: Vaginal-discharge study; Pap smear in about 2 months.

ANESTHESIA—Usually none.

DESCRIPTION OF OPERATION
- A speculum is inserted into the vagina to hold it open and to bring the cervix into view.
- An electrocautery is inserted into the cervix. The flow of electric current is applied to destroy abnormal cells.
- The instruments are removed. The procedure should be painless. Discomfort after surgery will vary from one person to the next, but any discomfort should be minor.

POSSIBLE COMPLICATIONS
- Surgical-wound infection.
- Inadvertent damage to normal vaginal tissue.

AVERAGE HOSPITAL STAY—None

PROBABLE OUTCOME—Healing requires up to 2 months. During this time, you will have a frequent, watery vaginal discharge. Allow about 6 weeks for recovery from surgery.

 POSTOPERATIVE CARE

NOTE—This information is supplemental and should not replace your doctor's instructions.

GENERAL MEASURES
- Wear cotton panties or pantyhose with a cotton crotch. Avoid panties made from nylon, polyester, silk or other non-ventilating materials.
- Wear a sanitary pad to protect clothing. Avoid tampons—they may lead to infection.
- Bathe or shower as usual. Use non-perfumed soap.
- Do not douche unless your doctor prescribes it.

MEDICATION
- You may use non-prescription drugs, such as acetaminophen, for minor pain.
- Your doctor may prescribe:
  Pain relievers. Don't take prescription pain medication longer than 4 to 7 days. Use *only* as much as you need.
  Vaginal creams or medicated douches.
  Antibiotics to fight infection.

ACTIVITY
- Return to work and normal activity as soon as possible. This reduces postoperative depression and irritability, which are common.
- Delay sexual relations until your doctor determines that healing is complete.

DIET—No special diet.

 CALL YOUR DOCTOR IF

- Vaginal discharge increases or begins to have an unpleasant odor.
- You experience pain that simple pain medication does not relieve quickly.
- Unusual vaginal swelling or bleeding develops.
- You develop signs of infection: headache, muscle aches, dizziness or a general ill feeling and fever.

CESAREAN SECTION

 ## GENERAL INFORMATION

DEFINITION—Delivery of a baby through an incision in the mother's lower abdominal and uterine walls.

BODY PARTS INVOLVED—Uterus; abdominal wall; placenta; placental membranes; fetus.

REASONS FOR SURGERY—Danger to the mother or baby from one or more of many causes, including:
- Baby's head too large to pass through the birth canal.
- Baby in the wrong position to pass through the birth canal.
- Insufficient contractions of the uterus.
- Abnormal attachment of placenta.
- Failure of normal labor in a patient who had a previous Cesarean section.

SURGICAL RISK INCREASES WITH
- Obesity.
- Smoking.
- Poor nutrition.
- Excess alcohol consumption.
- Placenta previa with excessive blood loss.
- Toxemia of pregnancy.
- Chronic heart or lung disease.
- Use of drugs, such as antihypertensives; cortisone; diuretics; or insulin.
- Use of mind-altering drugs.

 ## WHAT TO EXPECT

WHO OPERATES—Obstetrician-gynecologist.

WHERE PERFORMED—Hospital.

DIAGNOSTIC TESTS
- Before surgery: Blood and urine studies; sonogram (see Glossary).
- After surgery: Blood and urine studies.

ANESTHESIA—Local anesthesia by injection and spinal anesthesia by injection.

DESCRIPTION OF OPERATION
- An incision is made in the abdomen.
- Another incision is made in the uterus.
- Baby and placenta are removed.
- The uterus is closed and the abdominal contents are replaced. Connective tissue, muscles and skin are closed. The skin is closed with sutures or clips, which usually can be removed about 1 week after surgery.

POSSIBLE COMPLICATIONS—Excessive bleeding or surgical-wound infection.

AVERAGE HOSPITAL STAY—3 to 5 days.

PROBABLE OUTCOME—No complications expected. Allow about 4 weeks for recovery from surgery.

 ## POSTOPERATIVE CARE

NOTE—This information is supplemental and should not replace your doctor's instructions.

GENERAL MEASURES
- A hard ridge should form along the incision. As it heals, the ridge will recede gradually.
- Use an electric heating pad, a heat lamp or a warm compress to relieve incisional pain.
- Bathe and shower as usual. You may wash the incision gently with mild unscented soap.
- Place a heating pad or a hot-water bottle on the abdomen or back to relieve pain.
- Take hot baths to relax muscles and to relieve discomfort.
- Don't douche unless your doctor recommends it.

MEDICATION
- Your doctor may prescribe:
  Pain relievers. Use *only* as much as you need.
  Vaginal cream, if vaginal discharge develops an unpleasant odor.
  Medication to help stop lactation, if you will not be nursing your baby.
- You may use non-prescription drugs, such as acetaminophen, for minor pain.

ACTIVITY
- Resume work and normal activity as soon as possible to reduce postoperative depression, which is common.
- Resume driving 3 weeks after returning home.
- Resume sexual relations when able.

DIET—Clear liquid diet until the gastrointestinal tract begins to function again. Then eat a well-balanced, high-protein diet to promote healing.

 ## CALL YOUR DOCTOR IF

Any of the following occurs:
- Bleeding soaks more than 1 pad or tampon each hour.
- An area on the breast becomes hard, warm, tender or reddened.
- Nipples become sore or cracked.
- The urge to urinate frequently persists longer than 1 month.
- Vaginal discharge persists beyond 1 month after surgery.
- Pain, red streaks or warm areas appear on the calf of one of the legs.

SURGERIES

CHALAZION REMOVAL

 ## GENERAL INFORMATION

DEFINITION—Removal of a chalazion, a non-tender inflammation in the cartilage of the eyelid. Chalazions are caused by swelling and secretions in the meibomian glands (see Glossary).

BODY PARTS INVOLVED—Eyelids (upper or lower); meibomian glands.

REASONS FOR SURGERY—A chalazion is not cancerous or infectious. It is removed to improve appearance or to relieve pressure on an eyeball that has affected vision. Surgery is performed only after simpler treatment has failed.

SURGICAL RISK INCREASES WITH—None expected.

 ## WHAT TO EXPECT

WHO OPERATES—Ophthalmologist.

WHERE PERFORMED—Doctor's office or outpatient surgical facility.

DIAGNOSTIC TESTS—Complete eye examination before surgery.

ANESTHESIA—Local anesthesia by injection.

DESCRIPTION OF OPERATION
- The eyelid is turned inside out and held to expose its underside.
- The chalazion is identified.
- An incision is made on the surface of the chalazion.
- The chalazion is cut free and removed.
- The eye is bandaged.

POSSIBLE COMPLICATIONS
- Excessive bleeding.
- Surgical-wound infection.

AVERAGE HOSPITAL STAY—None.

PROBABLE OUTCOME—Expect complete healing without complications. Allow about 1 week for recovery from surgery. Chalazions may recur.

 ## POSTOPERATIVE CARE

NOTE—This information is supplemental and should not replace your doctor's instructions.

GENERAL MEASURES—Apply warm (not hot) compresses to the eye to relieve discomfort. Do this for 10 to 15 minutes at a time several times daily for about 2 days after surgery. Use clean cloths, and discard them after use.

MEDICATION
- Your doctor may prescribe:
  Pain relievers. Don't take prescription pain medication longer than 4 to 7 days. Use *only* as much as you need.
  Antibiotic eye drops to prevent infection. Keep eye drops cold, but not frozen, in the refrigerator.
- You may use non-prescription drugs, such as acetaminophen, to relieve minor pain.

ACTIVITY—Resume driving 2 days after returning home.

DIET—No special diet.

 ## CALL YOUR DOCTOR IF

- Pain, swelling, redness, drainage or bleeding increase in the surgical area.
- You develop signs of infection: headache, muscle aches, dizziness or a general ill feeling and fever.
- Your vision changes.

CIRCUMCISION

GENERAL INFORMATION

DEFINITION—Removal of the foreskin of the penis. This section describes circumcision performed at times other than at birth or several days after birth for religious reasons.

BODY PARTS INVOLVED—Penis; foreskin of the penis.

REASONS FOR SURGERY
- Correction of inability to retract the foreskin completely.
- Treatment of infection of the penis (balanitis).

SURGICAL RISK INCREASES WITH
- Poor nutrition.
- Recent illness.
- Alcoholism or chronic illness.

WHAT TO EXPECT

WHO OPERATES—Family doctor, general surgeon or urologist.

WHERE PERFORMED—Hospital or outpatient surgical facility.

DIAGNOSTIC TESTS
- Before surgery: Blood and urine studies.
- After surgery: Blood studies.

ANESTHESIA
- Local anesthesia by injection.
- General anesthesia (sometimes) by inhalation and injection, with an airway tube placed in the windpipe.

DESCRIPTION OF OPERATION
- The foreskin is carefully retracted from the tip of the penis.
- A clamp is placed under the foreskin.
- The clamped foreskin is slit in two places on the top and bottom of the penis.
- The foreskin between the two slits is cut free and removed.
- The mucous membrane of the foreskin is folded back on itself and sewn to the remaining skin of the penis, usually with sutures that will be absorbed by the body.
- Petroleum jelly and a bandage are applied.

POSSIBLE COMPLICATIONS
- Excessive bleeding
- Surgical-wound infection.

AVERAGE HOSPITAL STAY—0 to 1 day.

PROBABLE OUTCOME—Expect complete healing without complications. Allow about 3 weeks for recovery from surgery.

POSTOPERATIVE CARE

NOTE—This information is supplemental and should not replace your doctor's instructions.

GENERAL MEASURES
- If the wound bleeds during the first 24 hours after surgery, press a clean tissue or cloth to it for 10 minutes.
- Use ice packs to relieve pain in the surgical area for the first 24 hours after surgery.
- Use an electric heating pad, a heat lamp or a warm compress to relieve surgical-wound pain beginning 24 hours after surgery.
- Bathe and shower as usual. You may wash the surgical wound gently with mild unscented soap.
- Change the bandage daily. Between showers, keep the wound dry for the first 2 or 3 days after surgery. If a bandage gets wet, change it promptly.
- Apply non-prescription antibiotic ointment to the wound before applying new bandages.

MEDICATION
- Your doctor may prescribe:
  Pain relievers. Don't take prescription pain medication longer than 4 to 7 days. Use *only* as much as you need.
  Antibiotics to fight infection.
- You may use non-prescription drugs, such as acetaminophen, for minor pain.

ACTIVITY
- Resume work and normal activity as soon as possible to reduce postoperative depression and irritability, which are common.
- Avoid vigorous exercise for 4 weeks after surgery.
- Resume driving 5 days after returning home.
- Resume sexual relations when your doctor determines that healing is complete.

DIET—No special diet.

CALL YOUR DOCTOR IF

- Pain, swelling, redness, drainage or bleeding increases in the surgical area.
- You develop signs of infection: headache, muscle aches, dizziness or a general ill feeling and fever.
- You have difficulty urinating.
- New, unexplained symptoms develop. Drugs used in treatment may produce side effects.

CLEFT-LIP REPAIR

GENERAL INFORMATION

DEFINITION—Repair of a hereditary deformity of the upper lip called a "cleft lip" or "harelip" in which lip, nose and palate structures do not fuse correctly prior to birth. Frequently, this deformity extends to the roof of the mouth (palate) and can hamper development of normal speech.

Surgery is usually performed when the patient is about 3 months old. If a cleft palate exists, it is usually repaired in a separate surgery when the patient is 12 to 18 months old.

BODY PARTS INVOLVED—Upper lip; muscles surrounding the mouth; membrane lining the mouth; roof of the mouth (palate).

REASONS FOR SURGERY
- Prevention of nursing and feeding problems that can retard normal growth.
- Rearrangement of the distorted tissues to make the lip and palate function normally and appear as normal as possible.

SURGICAL RISK INCREASES WITH
- Other congenital abnormalities.
- Poor nutrition. This often results from inability to nurse properly because of the deformity.

WHAT TO EXPECT

WHO OPERATES—Plastic and reconstructive surgeon.

WHERE PERFORMED—Hospital.

DIAGNOSTIC TESTS
- Before surgery: Blood and urine studies.
- After surgery: Blood studies.

ANESTHESIA
- Local anesthesia by injection.
- General anesthesia by a combination of inhalation and injection, with an airway tube placed in the windpipe.

DESCRIPTION OF OPERATION
- The area where the lip, mouth and palate should be are marked.
- The skin to be relocated is cut free from its underlying tissue. Bleeding is controlled with clamps or epinephrine.
- The skin flaps are adjusted to their desired position.
- The muscles and skin edges are reconstructed with fine sutures, which usually can be removed about 7 to 10 days after surgery.

POSSIBLE COMPLICATIONS
- Excessive bleeding.
- Surgical-wound infection.

AVERAGE HOSPITAL STAY—5 to 7 days.

PROBABLE OUTCOME—Expect complete healing without complications. Allow about 4 weeks for recovery from surgery.

POSTOPERATIVE CARE

NOTE—This information is supplemental and should not replace your doctor's instructions.

GENERAL MEASURES
- A hard ridge should form along the incision. As it heals, the ridge will recede gradually.
- Bathe the child as usual. You may wash the incision gently with mild unscented soap.

MEDICATION—Your doctor may prescribe:
- Pain relievers. Don't give the child prescription pain medication longer than 4 to 7 days. Use *only* as much as the child needs.
- Antibiotics to fight infection.

ACTIVITY—No restrictions.

DIET—No special diet.

CALL YOUR DOCTOR IF

- Pain, swelling, redness, drainage or bleeding increases in the surgical area.
- You observe new symptoms, such as vomiting, constipation or abdominal swelling.

COLONOSCOPY

GENERAL INFORMATION

DEFINITION—Visual examination of the inside of the rectum and the colon (large intestine). Fecal matter, tissue or foreign matter usually are removed for laboratory examination. The procedure is performed with a colonoscope, a fiber-optic instrument that makes examination and some surgeries simple, practical and safe.

BODY PARTS INVOLVED—Anus; rectum; colon.

REASONS FOR SURGERY—Examination of the rectum and lower intestinal tract for disorders that may include: fissures; fistulas; narrowed sections of the intestine; unexplained blood in stools; benign or cancerous tumors; or pre-cancerous polyps.

SURGICAL RISK INCREASES WITH

- Adults over 60.
- Obesity.
- Smoking.
- Poor nutrition.
- Recent or chronic illness.
- Use of drugs such as: antihypertensives; muscle relaxants; tranquilizers; sleep inducers; insulin; sedatives; beta-adrenergic blockers; or cortisone.
- Use of mind-altering drugs, including: narcotics; psychedelics; hallucinogens; marijuana; sedatives; hypnotics; or cocaine.

WHAT TO EXPECT

WHO OPERATES—General surgeon, family doctor, proctologist or gastroenterologist.

WHERE PERFORMED—Hospital or outpatient surgical facility.

DIAGNOSTIC TESTS

- Before surgery: Blood and urine studies; stool examinations; X-rays of lower gastrointestinal tract.
- After surgery: Laboratory examination of removed tissue and other material.

ANESTHESIA—Local anesthesia by topical application.

DESCRIPTION OF OPERATION

- The examination is best accomplished just after a normal bowel movement. If a normal bowel movement has not occurred just before examination, it may be necessary to use a suppository or delay the test until a laxative has cleared the area to be examined.
- The colonoscope is lubricated, inserted into the rectum and passed into the colon.
- Affected areas are located, examined or treated. Fecal matter and other materials are removed for laboratory examination.
- Other minor surgical procedures may be performed. The colonoscope is removed.

POSSIBLE COMPLICATIONS

- Excessive bleeding.
- Perforation of the colon.

AVERAGE HOSPITAL STAY—Usually none.

PROBABLE OUTCOME—Expect complete healing without complications. Allow about 4 days for recovery from surgery.

POSTOPERATIVE CARE

NOTE—This information is supplemental and should not replace your doctor's instructions.

GENERAL MEASURES—No special instructions except those listed under other headings.

MEDICATION—Medicine is usually not necessary.

ACTIVITY—No restrictions.

DIET—No special diet.

CALL YOUR DOCTOR IF

Any of the following occurs:
- Increased pain, swelling, or bleeding from rectum or blood in stools.
- Signs of infection: headache, muscle aches, dizziness or a general ill feeling and fever.
- Nausea, vomiting or abdominal pain.

COLOSTOMY

GENERAL INFORMATION

DEFINITION—Creation of an artificial opening between a part of the colon (large intestine) and the surface of the body. All feces will leave the body through this opening, which is called an ostomy or stoma.

BODY PARTS INVOLVED—Large intestine.

REASONS FOR SURGERY—Creating a temporary or permanent exit for feces to leave the body above any abnormal parts of the colon.

SURGICAL RISK INCREASES WITH
- Stress.
- Obesity.
- Smoking.
- Excess alcohol consumption.
- Poor nutrition.
- Recent illness.
- Chronic illness of the heart, lungs, liver or gastrointestinal tract.
- Use of drugs such as: antihypertensives; muscle relaxants; tranquilizers; sleep inducers; insulin; sedatives; narcotics; beta-adrenergic blockers; or cortisone.
- Use of mind-altering drugs.

WHAT TO EXPECT

WHO OPERATES—General surgeon.

WHERE PERFORMED—Hospital.

DIAGNOSTIC TESTS
- Before surgery: Blood and urine studies; X-rays of kidneys, chest and gastrointestinal system; EKG (see Glossary).
- After surgery: Blood studies.

ANESTHESIA—General anesthesia by inhalation and injection, with an airway tube placed in the windpipe.

DESCRIPTION OF OPERATION
- An incision is made in the abdomen. The abdominal muscles are separated to expose the abdominal organs, which are inspected for any undetected disease. Other surgeries may be performed at this time.
- The colon section that is to be opened is isolated and clamped on both sides, then cut between the clamps. The end of the colon closer to the stomach is brought out of the abdomen and clamped outside the skin. The end farther from the stomach is closed.
- The abdominal contents are replaced, and muscles are closed around the stoma. Skin is closed with sutures or clips, which usually can be removed in about 1 week.

POSSIBLE COMPLICATIONS
- Excessive bleeding.
- Surgical-wound infection.
- Incisional hernia.
- Skin irritation around the stoma.
- Diarrhea.

AVERAGE HOSPITAL STAY—7 to 10 days.

PROBABLE OUTCOME—Expect complete healing without complications. You can look forward to a relatively normal life, except that bowel movements will now pass through the stoma instead of the rectum. Allow about 6 weeks for recovery from surgery.

POSTOPERATIVE CARE

NOTE—This information is supplemental and should not replace your doctor's instructions.

GENERAL MEASURES
- A hard ridge should form along the incision. As it heals, the ridge will recede gradually.
- Use an electric heating pad, a heat lamp or warm compress to relieve incisional pain.
- Bathe and shower as usual. You may wash the incision gently with mild unscented soap.
- An enterostomy specialist (see Glossary) can provide education and counseling for the patient and family.

MEDICATION—Your doctor may prescribe:
- Pain relievers. Don't take prescription pain medication longer than 4 to 7 days. Use *only* as much as you need.
- Antibiotics to fight infection.
- Ointment for skin around ostomy site.

ACTIVITY
- Resume work and normal activity as soon as possible to reduce postoperative depression, which is common.
- Avoid vigorous exercise for 6 weeks after surgery. Resume sexual relations when able.
- Resume driving 6 weeks after returning home.

DIET—Clear liquid diet until the gastrointestinal tract begins to function again. Then eat a well-balanced, high-protein diet to promote healing. After recovery, eat a normal diet with a high fiber content.

CALL YOUR DOCTOR IF

- You develop signs of infection: headache, muscle aches, dizziness or a general ill feeling and fever.
- Pain, swelling, redness, drainage or bleeding increases in the surgical area.
- Skin around stoma becomes irritated or infected.
- New, unexplained symptoms develop. Drugs in treatment may produce side effects.

CORNEA TRANSPLANT

 GENERAL INFORMATION

DEFINITION—Removing a diseased or injured cornea and replacing it with a healthy cornea from a donor.

BODY PARTS INVOLVED—Cornea.

REASONS FOR SURGERY—Restoration of vision or prevention of blindness.

SURGICAL RISK INCREASES WITH
- Stress.
- Obesity.
- Smoking.
- Poor nutrition.
- Recent illness.
- Alcoholism or chronic illness.
- Use of drugs such as: antihypertensives; muscle relaxants; tranquilizers; sleep inducers; insulin; sedatives; beta-adrenergic blockers; or cortisone.
- Use of mind-altering drugs, including: narcotics; psychedelics; hallucinogens; marijuana; sedatives; hypnotics; or cocaine.

 WHAT TO EXPECT

WHO OPERATES—Ophthalmologist.

WHERE PERFORMED—Hospital.

DIAGNOSTIC TESTS
- Before surgery: Blood and urine studies; eye examination.
- After surgery: Eye examination.

ANESTHESIA
- Local anesthesia by injection.
- General anesthesia by inhalation and injection, with an airway tube placed in the windpipe.

DESCRIPTION OF OPERATION
- The diseased or injured cornea is cut free with scissors and removed.
- The donor cornea (usually from an eye bank) is fastened into the area with sutures.
- The sutures holding the transplanted cornea are removed when healing has taken place, usually about 3 to 4 weeks after surgery.

POSSIBLE COMPLICATIONS
- Surgical-wound infection.
- Rejection of transplant (rare).
- Secondary glaucoma.

AVERAGE HOSPITAL STAY—2 days.

PROBABLE OUTCOME—Expect complete healing without complications. Allow 3 to 4 weeks for recovery from surgery.

 POSTOPERATIVE CARE

NOTE—This information is supplemental and should not replace your doctor's instructions.

GENERAL MEASURES—Move legs often while resting in bed to decrease the likelihood of deep-vein blood clots.

MEDICATION
- Your doctor may prescribe:
  Pain relievers. Don't take prescription pain medication longer than 4 to 7 days. Use *only* as much as you need.
  Stool softeners to prevent constipation.
  Antibiotics to fight infection.
- You may use non-prescription drugs, such as acetaminophen, for minor pain.

ACTIVITY
- Resume work and normal activity as soon as possible. This reduces postoperative depression and irritability, which are common.
- Avoid vigorous exercise for 6 weeks after surgery. Don't bend over or lift heavy objects until transplant is healed completely.
- Resume driving when your doctor determines that healing is complete.

DIET—No special diet.

 CALL YOUR DOCTOR IF

- Pain, swelling, redness, drainage or bleeding increases in the surgical area.
- You develop signs of infection: headache, muscle aches, dizziness or a general ill feeling and fever.
- You experience nausea, vomiting or constipation.
- Your vision changes.
- New, unexplained symptoms develop. Drugs used in treatment may produce side effects.

SURGERIES

CORONARY-ARTERY BYPASS GRAFT

GENERAL INFORMATION

DEFINITION—Using a section of the patient's leg vein to bypass a partial or complete blockage in the coronary-artery system.

BODY PARTS INVOLVED—Heart; coronary arteries; large veins of legs.

REASONS FOR SURGERY
- Angina pectoris.
- Restoration of blood to the heart muscle after a heart attack.
- Prevention of a possible heart attack, if coronary arteries have narrowed.

SURGICAL RISK INCREASES WITH
- Obesity.
- Smoking.
- Recent illness such as: severe heart attack; high blood pressure; thyroid disease; or diabetes mellitus.
- Chronic obstructive pulmonary disease (COPD).
- Illness that has lowered strength.
- Use of mind-altering drugs.

WHAT TO EXPECT

WHO OPERATES—Cardiovascular surgeon.

WHERE PERFORMED—Hospital.

DIAGNOSTIC TESTS
- Before surgery: Blood studies; chest X-ray; cardiac catheterization; EKG; sonogram (see Glossary for all).
- During surgery: EKG; angiograms (see Glossary).
- After surgery: EKG; chest X-ray; sonogram.

ANESTHESIA—General anesthesia by inhalation and injection, with an airway tube placed in the windpipe.

DESCRIPTION OF OPERATION
- A section of the patient's large leg vein is removed and set aside to be used as the bypass graft.
- An incision is made through the breastbone, and the chest is spread open to expose the heart.
- The heart is stopped with a mild electric shock, and the bypass graft is sewn in place. The heart-lung machine sustains life during surgery.
- The heart is given another mild electric shock that causes heartbeat to resume.
- The breastbone edges are rejoined with metal suture material, and muscles, tissue and skin are closed with lighter sutures.

POSSIBLE COMPLICATIONS
- Heart rhythm abnormalities.
- Excessive bleeding.
- Life-threatening pressure on the heart.

AVERAGE HOSPITAL STAY—7 days.

PROBABLE OUTCOME—Angina pectoris is cured in almost all cases. Probability of future heart attacks is reduced. Allow about 6 weeks for recovery from surgery.

POSTOPERATIVE CARE

NOTE—This information is supplemental and should not replace your doctor's instructions.

GENERAL MEASURES
- A hard ridge should form along the incision. As it heals, the ridge will recede gradually.
- Use an electric heating pad, a heat lamp or a warm compress to relieve incisional pain.
- Bathe and shower as usual. You may wash the incision gently with mild unscented soap.
- Move legs frequently while resting in bed to decrease the likelihood of deep-vein blood clots.

MEDICATION—Your doctor may prescribe:
- Pain relievers. Don't take prescription pain medication longer than 4 to 7 days. Use *only* as much as you need.
- Antiarrhythmics to prevent heartbeat irregularities.
- Digitalis to strengthen the heart muscle.
- Anticoagulants to decrease the likelihood of blood clots.

ACTIVITY
- Resume work and normal activity as soon as possible to reduce postoperative depression, which is common.
- Resume driving 1 month after returning home.
- Resume sexual relations when your doctor determines that healing is complete.
- Ask your doctor for advice about an exercise rehabilitation program.

DIET—Low-salt (see Appendix 9); low-fat (see Appendix 8); high-fiber.

CALL YOUR DOCTOR IF

- Pain, swelling, redness, drainage or bleeding increases in the surgical area.
- You develop signs of infection: headache, muscle aches, dizziness or a general ill feeling and fever.
- You experience new symptoms, such as a cough, heartbeat irregularities, leg pain or constipation.
- New, unexplained symptoms develop. Drugs used in treatment may produce side effects.

CRANIOTOMY

GENERAL INFORMATION

DEFINITION—Cutting through the skull (cranium) to expose and treat disorders in the brain or associated tissues.

BODY PARTS INVOLVED—Scalp; skull; brain and membrane coverings.

REASONS FOR SURGERY
- Removal of blood clots, aneurysms or tumors.
- Repair of tears in the brain's membrane coverings.
- Drainage of a brain abscess.

SURGICAL RISK INCREASES WITH
- Smoking.
- Excess alcohol consumption.
- Chronic illness.
- Recent illness, especially upper respiratory infection.
- Use of drugs such as: antihypertensives; muscle relaxants; tranquilizers; sleep inducers; insulin; sedatives; beta-adrenergic blockers; or cortisone.
- Use of mind-altering drugs, including: narcotics; psychedelics; hallucinogens; marijuana; sedatives; hypnotics; or cocaine.

WHAT TO EXPECT

WHO OPERATES—Neurosurgeon.

WHERE PERFORMED—Hospital or emergency room.

DIAGNOSTIC TESTS
- Before surgery: Blood and urine studies; X-rays of skull; angiogram; EEG; CAT scan (see Glossary for all).
- During surgery: EEG.
- After surgery: EEG; X-rays of skull; blood studies; CAT scan; angiogram (sometimes).

ANESTHESIA—General anesthesia by inhalation and injection, with an airway tube placed in the windpipe.

DESCRIPTION OF OPERATION
- The entire head is shaved. An incision is made in the scalp over the area of suspected disorder.
- A flap of bone is cut away from the skull and set aside.
- The disorder is located and treated as necessary.
- The bone flap is replaced.
- The scalp is closed with sutures or clips, which usually can be removed about 1 week after surgery.

POSSIBLE COMPLICATIONS
- Stroke.
- Excessive bleeding.
- Surgical-wound infection.
- Swelling of the brain caused by the trauma of surgery.

AVERAGE HOSPITAL STAY—10 to 14 days.

PROBABLE OUTCOME—Expect complete healing of surgical wounds. Allow about 8 weeks for recovery from surgery.

POSTOPERATIVE CARE

NOTE—This information is supplemental and should not replace your doctor's instructions.

GENERAL MEASURES
- A hard ridge should form along the incision. As it heals, the ridge will recede gradually.
- Bathe and shower as usual. You may wash the incision gently with mild unscented soap.
- Use an electric heating pad, a heat lamp or a warm compress to relieve incisional pain.
- Move legs often while resting in bed to decrease the likelihood of deep-vein blood clots.

MEDICATION
- Your doctor may prescribe:
  Pain relievers. Don't take prescription pain medication longer than 4 to 7 days. Use *only* as much as you need.
  Stool softeners to prevent constipation.
  Antibiotics to fight infection.
- You may use non-prescription drugs, such as acetaminophen, for minor pain.

ACTIVITY
- Return to work and normal activity as soon as possible. This reduces postoperative depression and irritability, which are common.
- Avoid vigorous exercise for 6 weeks after surgery.
- Resume driving about 3 weeks after returning home, depending on underlying disorder. Ask your doctor

DIET—Clear liquid diet until the gastrointestinal tract functions again. Then eat a well-balanced, high-protein diet to promote healing.

CALL YOUR DOCTOR IF

- Pain, swelling, redness, drainage or bleeding increases in the surgical area.
- You experience nausea, vomiting or constipation.
- You develop signs of infection: headache, muscle aches, dizziness or a general ill feeling and fever.
- New, unexplained symptoms develop. Drugs used in treatment may produce side effects.

CRYOSURGERY

 ## GENERAL INFORMATION

DEFINITION—Removal of abnormal or diseased tissue by freezing, usually with liquid nitrogen.

BODY PARTS INVOLVED—Any lesion on the skin; hemorrhoids; cervix; retina (rarely).

REASONS FOR SURGERY
- Removal of skin lesions.
- Treatment of cervicitis (inflammation of the cervix).
- Treatment of retinal detachment (rarely).

SURGICAL RISK INCREASES WITH—None expected.

 ## WHAT TO EXPECT

WHO OPERATES—Dermatologist or family doctor (to treat skin lesions), obstetrician-gynecologist (to treat cervicitis), or ophthalmologist (to treat retinal detachment).

WHERE PERFORMED—Hospital, outpatient surgical facility, doctor's office or emergency room.

DIAGNOSTIC TESTS
- Before surgery: Blood and urine studies.
- After surgery: None expected.

ANESTHESIA—Usually none.

DESCRIPTION OF OPERATION
- For small skin lesions, liquid nitrogen is applied to a cotton-tipped applicator. The applicator is held to the skin lesions until they are frozen and destroyed.
- Sometimes, a spray can with pressurized liquid nitrogen is used to freeze skin lesions.
- For surgery on the cervix or retina, a special instrument is used. Liquid nitrogen circulates in the tip of this instrument causing it to become almost as cold as the liquid nitrogen. The instrument tip is held on the affected areas until the abnormal tissue is frozen.

POSSIBLE COMPLICATIONS—Surgical-wound infection (rare).

AVERAGE HOSPITAL STAY—Usually none.

PROBABLE OUTCOME—For skin lesions or hemorrhoids: Initial swelling and redness become a blister in 2 or 3 days. The blister will rupture by itself about 2 weeks after surgery. It will leave a scab, but little or no scar after complete healing.
For cervical surgery: Expect complete healing without complications. Allow about 3 weeks for recovery from surgery.
For retinal detachment: Expect complete healing without complications. Allow about 1 month for recovery from surgery.

 ## POSTOPERATIVE CARE

NOTE—This information is supplemental and should not replace your doctor's instructions.

GENERAL MEASURES—Bathe and shower as usual, but keep skin wounds dry with bandages for the first 2 or 3 days after surgery. If a bandage gets wet, change it promptly.

MEDICATION—You may use non-prescription drugs, such as acetaminophen, to relieve minor pain.

ACTIVITY—No restrictions.

DIET—No special diet.

 ## CALL YOUR DOCTOR IF

- Pain, swelling, redness, drainage or bleeding increases in the surgical area.
- You develop signs of infection: headache, muscle aches, dizziness or a general ill feeling and fever.

CULDOCENTESIS

 ## GENERAL INFORMATION

DEFINITION—Piercing the "cul-de-sac," the space deep in the vagina behind and under the cervix.

BODY PARTS INVOLVED—Vagina; lowest part of pelvis behind the uterus and cervix.

REASONS FOR SURGERY—Investigation of possible ailments in the abdomen and pelvis, including: bleeding inside the lower pelvic cavity; ruptured ectopic pregnancy; ruptured ovarian cyst; ovarian cancer; or pelvic inflammatory disease. Laboratory examination of the removed fluid aids in diagnosis.

SURGICAL RISK INCREASES WITH—Recent or chronic illness.

 ## WHAT TO EXPECT

WHO OPERATES—Obstetrician-gynecologist, general surgeon or family doctor.

WHERE PERFORMED—Doctor's office; outpatient surgical facility; or hospital.

DIAGNOSTIC TESTS
- Before surgery: Pap smear; vaginal and abdominal exam; X-rays of lower abdomen.
- After surgery: Laboratory examination of removed fluid.

ANESTHESIA—Local anesthesia by injection.

DESCRIPTION OF OPERATION
- A speculum is inserted into the vagina to hold it open.
- The rear lip of the cervix is raised.
- A local anesthetic is applied to the farthest back portion of the vagina (cul-de-sac).
- The posterior wall of the vagina is penetrated with a needle and syringe.
- Fluid, if present, is aspirated. No sutures are necessary.

POSSIBLE COMPLICATIONS
- Perforation of bladder or bowel (rare).
- Excessive bleeding.
- Surgical-wound infection.

AVERAGE HOSPITAL STAY—Usually none.

PROBABLE OUTCOME—A fluid sample is obtained successfully without complications in virtually all cases. If fluid or blood confirms other findings that suggest a serious disease or condition, you may need further surgery.

If no fluid is obtained and there are no complications, but you still have your original symptoms, expect further observation or tests to diagnose your conditions. Allow about 1 week for recovery from surgery.

 ## POSTOPERATIVE CARE

NOTE—This information is supplemental and should not replace your doctor's instructions.

GENERAL MEASURES
- Resume your usual activities as soon as possible, if symptoms that caused the need for surgery disappear. If symptoms recur, see your doctor.
- Continue to use your usual birth-control methods. Your periods should not be disturbed.
- Use sanitary pads for your next menstrual period. Avoid tampons temporarily; they may lead to infection.

MEDICATION
- Your doctor may prescribe medicines according to diagnosis.
- You may use non-prescription drugs, such as acetaminophen, to relieve minor pain.

ACTIVITY—Resume normal activities gradually. Resume sexual relations when able. This will depend on various underlying causes. Ask your doctor.

DIET—No special diet.

 ## CALL YOUR DOCTOR IF

- You experience vaginal bleeding that soaks more than 1 pad or tampon each hour.
- Symptoms recur or worsen.

CYSTOSCOPY

GENERAL INFORMATION

DEFINITION—Visual examination of the lower urinary tract and collection of a urine sample from the bladder. The examination is performed with a cystoscope, a fiber-optic instrument with a lighted tip.

BODY PARTS INVOLVED—Urethra; bladder; openings into the bladder.

REASONS FOR SURGERY
- Blood in the urine (hematuria).
- Inability to control urination (incontinence).
- Urinary-tract infection.
- Congenital abnormalities of the urinary tract.
- Tumors of the bladder.
- Bladder or kidney stones.
- Tightening of the urethra or the ureters.

SURGICAL RISK INCREASES WITH
- Obesity.
- Smoking.
- Recent or chronic illness.
- Use of drugs such as: antihypertensives; muscle relaxants; tranquilizers; sleep inducers; insulin; sedatives; beta-adrenergic blockers; or cortisone.
- Use of mind-altering drugs, including: narcotics; psychedelics; hallucinogens; marijuana; sedatives; hypnotics; or cocaine.

WHAT TO EXPECT

WHO OPERATES—Urologist.

WHERE PERFORMED—Hospital, doctor's office or outpatient surgical facility.

DIAGNOSTIC TESTS
- Before surgery: Blood and urine studies; X-rays of kidneys.
- During surgery: Retrograde pyelograms (see Glossary).
- After surgery: Blood studies.

ANESTHESIA—Spinal anesthesia (sometimes) by injection.

DESCRIPTION OF OPERATION
- The patient urinates before surgery so that urine remaining in the bladder can be measured.
- The cystoscope is lubricated and inserted through the urethra into the bladder. A urine sample is collected.
- Fluid is pumped through the cystoscope to inflate the bladder, which allows visual examination of the entire bladder wall.
- Bladder or kidney stones are removed, if necessary. Tissue samples are gathered and lesions are treated, if necessary.

- Catheters are passed through the cystoscope and guided to the openings into the ureters. A harmless dye is injected through the catheters into the ureters to perform X-ray studies.
- The cystoscope is removed.

POSSIBLE COMPLICATIONS
- Excessive bleeding.
- Surgical-wound infection.
- Perforation of bladder.

AVERAGE HOSPITAL STAY—0 to 3 days.

PROBABLE OUTCOME—Examination completed and urine sample collected successfully in virtually all cases. Allow about 4 days for recovery from surgery.

POSTOPERATIVE CARE

NOTE—This information is supplemental and should not replace your doctor's instructions.

GENERAL MEASURES—Take warm baths for 10 to 15 minutes several times a day to relieve discomfort.

MEDICATION
- Your doctor may prescribe:
  Pain relievers. Don't take prescription pain medication longer than 4 to 7 days. Use *only* as much as you need.
  Antibiotics to fight infection.
- You may use non-prescription drugs, such as acetaminophen, for minor pain.

ACTIVITY
- Avoid vigorous exercise for 2 weeks after surgery.
- Resume sexual relations when your doctor determines that healing is complete.
- Resume driving 2 days after returning home.

DIET—No special diet.

CALL YOUR DOCTOR IF

- Pain, swelling, redness, drainage or bleeding increases in the surgical area.
- You develop signs of infection: headache, muscle aches, dizziness or a general ill feeling and fever.
- You experience nausea or vomiting.
- You have painful or difficult urination.
- New, unexplained symptoms develop. Drugs used in treatment may produce side effects.

DILATATION AND CURETTAGE OF THE UTERUS (D & C)

GENERAL INFORMATION

DEFINITION—Opening the cervix and scraping the inner wall of the uterus to remove tissue.

BODY PARTS INVOLVED—Uterus; cervix; vagina (as route for surgery).

REASONS FOR SURGERY
- Diagnosis of abnormal bleeding or possible cancer inside the uterus.
- Elective abortion during early pregnancy.
- Incomplete spontaneous miscarriage.
- Treatment of minor diseases of the uterus.

SURGICAL RISK INCREASES WITH
- Obesity.
- Smoking.
- Excess alcohol consumption.
- Recent or chronic illness, including anemia, diabetes mellitus, and heart or lung disease.
- Use of drugs, such as: antihypertensives; cortisone; diuretics; or insulin.
- Use of mind-altering drugs, including: narcotics; psychedelics; hallucinogens; marijuana; sedatives; hypnotics; or cocaine.

WHAT TO EXPECT

WHO OPERATES—Obstetrician-gynecologist, general surgeon or family doctor.

WHERE PERFORMED—Outpatient surgical facility or hospital.

DIAGNOSTIC TESTS
- Before surgery: Pap smear; blood and hormonal studies.
- After surgery: Blood studies; Pap smear in 2 months.

ANESTHESIA—Local anesthesia by injection, or general anesthesia by inhalation and injection, with an airway tube placed in the windpipe.

DESCRIPTION OF OPERATION
- The vagina is cleansed with an antiseptic solution.
- The cervix is carefully opened with a dilator, and a curette is inserted into the uterus.
- The curette is used to scrape away a small part of the uterine lining for laboratory analysis.
- The instruments are removed.
- Some surgeons now collect tissue by suction curettage (see Abortion in Surgery section) rather than by the procedure described here.

POSSIBLE COMPLICATIONS
- Surgical-wound infection.
- Excessive bleeding.
- Inadvertent injury to the uterus.

AVERAGE HOSPITAL STAY—0 to 1 day.

PROBABLE OUTCOME—Tissue obtained successfully without complications in virtually all cases. Allow about 4 to 6 weeks for recovery from surgery.

POSTOPERATIVE CARE

NOTE—This information is supplemental and should not replace your doctor's instructions.

GENERAL MEASURES
- Don't smoke.
- Don't douche unless your physician recommends it.
- Wear cotton panties or pantyhose with a cotton crotch. Avoid panties made from nylon, polyester, silk or other non-ventilating materials.
- Expect slight vaginal bleeding during recovery from surgery. Use a sanitary pad to protect clothing. Avoid tampons temporarily; they may lead to infection.

MEDICATION
- Your doctor may prescribe:
  Hormones to correct an imbalance.
  Pain relievers. Don't take prescription pain medication longer than 4 to 7 days. Use *only* as much as you need.
  Antibiotics to fight infection.
- You may use non-prescription drugs, such as acetaminophen, for minor pain.

ACTIVITY
- Resume driving in 1 or 2 days.
- Resume work and normal activity as soon as possible to reduce postoperative depression, which is common.
- Resume sexual relations when spotting ceases.

DIET—No special diet.

CALL YOUR DOCTOR IF

- Vaginal discharge increases or smells unpleasant.
- You experience pain that simple pain medication does not relieve quickly.
- Unusual vaginal swelling or bleeding develops.
- You develop signs of infection: headache, muscle aches, dizziness or a general ill feeling and fever.

DISK REMOVAL, RUPTURED-
(Laminectomy)

 GENERAL INFORMATION

DEFINITION—Removal of an intervertebral disk that has protruded from its normal position.

BODY PARTS INVOLVED—Spine; intervertebral disk.

REASONS FOR SURGERY—Relief of painful symptoms.

SURGICAL RISK INCREASES WITH
- Adults over 60.
- Stress.
- Obesity.
- Poor nutrition.
- Smoking.
- Chronic illness, especially back pain and alcoholism.
- Use of drugs such as: antihypertensives; muscle relaxants; tranquilizers; sleep inducers; insulin; sedatives; beta-adrenergic blockers; or cortisone.
- Use of mind-altering drugs, including: narcotics; psychedelics; hallucinogens; marijuana; sedatives; hypnotics; or cocaine.

 WHAT TO EXPECT

WHO OPERATES—Neurosurgeon, orthopedist or general surgeon (sometimes).

WHERE PERFORMED—Hospital.

DIAGNOSTIC TESTS
- Before surgery: Blood and urine studies; X-rays of back; myelogram (see Glossary).
- After surgery: Blood studies.

ANESTHESIA—General anesthesia by inhalation and injection, with an airway tube placed in the windpipe.

DESCRIPTION OF OPERATION
- An incision is made over the protruded disk.
- The arches of the spine are cut away and removed.
- The protruding disk is scooped out.
- Sometimes, the vertebral bone around the affected area is joined together with normal bone. This procedure is called fusion.
- The skin is closed with sutures or clips, which usually can be removed about 1 week after surgery.

POSSIBLE COMPLICATIONS
- Excessive bleeding.
- Surgical-wound infection.
- Injury to nerve roots, which can lead to paralysis.

AVERAGE HOSPITAL STAY—7 to 10 days.

PROBABLE OUTCOME—Expect slow healing. Some discomfort and weakness may continue. Allow about 5 weeks for recovery from surgery.

 POSTOPERATIVE CARE

NOTE—This information is supplemental and should not replace your doctor's instructions.

GENERAL MEASURES
- A hard ridge should form along the incision. As it heals, the ridge will recede gradually.
- Use an electric heating pad, a heat lamp or a warm compress to relieve incisional pain. Some patients may prefer to use ice packs instead.
- Bathe and shower as usual. You may wash the incision gently with mild unscented soap.
- Move legs often while resting in to bed to decrease the likelihood of deep-vein blood clots.

MEDICATION
- Your doctor may prescribe:
  Pain relievers. Don't take prescription pain medication longer than 4 to 7 days. Use *only* as much as you need.
  Stool softeners to prevent constipation.
  Antibiotics to fight infection.
- You may use non-prescription drugs, such as acetaminophen, for minor pain.

ACTIVITY
- Resume work and normal activity as soon as possible to reduce postoperative depression, which is common.
- Avoid vigorous exercise for 6 weeks after surgery. Then begin back exercises under medical supervision.
- Resume driving 6 weeks after returning home.
- Resume sexual relations when able.

DIET—Clear liquid diet until the gastrointestinal tract begins to function again. Then eat a well-balanced, high-protein diet to promote healing.

 CALL YOUR DOCTOR IF

Any of the following occurs:
- Increased pain, swelling, redness, drainage or bleeding in the surgical area.
- Signs of infection: headache, muscle aches, dizziness or a general ill feeling and fever.
- Nausea, vomiting, constipation or abdominal swelling.
- Return of weakness, numbness or pain in the back, buttocks or legs.
- Loss of bladder or bowel control.
- Development of new, unexplained symptoms. Drugs used in treatment may produce side effects.

DUCTUS-ARTERIOSUS CLOSURE

GENERAL INFORMATION

DEFINITION—Closure of an abnormal opening in the ductus arteriosus, a blood vessel between the heart's aorta and the pulmonary artery that usually closes at birth.

BODY PARTS INVOLVED—Ductus arteriosus.

REASONS FOR SURGERY—Performed so that normal growth and development may occur. If the abnormal opening is large, surgery is performed during the first few days after birth. Otherwise, surgery may be delayed until the child is 3 or 4 years old.

SURGICAL RISK INCREASES WITH
- Newborns and infants.
- Obesity.
- Recent or chronic illness.

WHAT TO EXPECT

WHO OPERATES—Cardiovascular surgeon.

WHERE PERFORMED—Hospital.

DIAGNOSTIC TESTS
- Before surgery: Blood and urine studies; X-rays of chest; echocardiogram; cardiac catheterization; EKG (see Glossary for all).
- During surgery: EKG monitor (see Glossary).
- After surgery: Blood studies.

ANESTHESIA—General anesthesia by inhalation and injection, with an airway tube placed in the windpipe.

DESCRIPTION OF OPERATION
- An incision is made in the chest. The muscles are divided and the chest is spread open.
- The lung is deflated to expose the ductus arteriosus.
- The ductus arteriosus is clamped in two places, cut between the clamps and tied. The ends are sewn shut to prevent bleeding from the pulmonary artery or the aorta.
- Tubes are left in place to drain fluid. A catheter is left in place to remove air from the chest so the lung can reinflate itself within 24 to 48 hours.
- The muscles are sewn together in layers with strong sutures.
- The skin is closed with sutures or clips, which usually can be removed about 1 week after surgery.

POSSIBLE COMPLICATIONS
- Excessive bleeding
- Surgical-wound infection.

AVERAGE HOSPITAL STAY—7 days.

PROBABLE OUTCOME—Expect complete healing without complications. Allow about 4 weeks for recovery from surgery.

POSTOPERATIVE CARE

NOTE—This information is supplemental and should not replace your doctor's instructions.

GENERAL MEASURES
- A hard blunt ridge should form along the incision. As it heals, the ridge will recede gradually.
- Bathe your child as usual. You may wash the incision gently with mild unscented soap.
- Use a warm compress to relieve incisional pain.
- Have the child move legs often while resting in bed to decrease the likelihood of deep-vein blood clots.

MEDICATION
- Your doctor may prescribe pain relievers. Don't give your child prescription pain medication longer than 4 to 7 days. Use *only* as much as needed.
- Antibiotics to fight infection.

ACTIVITY
- Avoid vigorous exercise for 6 weeks after surgery.
- Don't let your child ride in a car for 2 weeks after returning from the hospital.

DIET—Clear liquid diet until the gastrointestinal tract functions again. Then provide a well-balanced, high-protein diet to promote healing.

CALL YOUR DOCTOR IF

- You observe excessive bleeding.
- You observe signs of infection: headache, muscle aches, dizziness or a general ill feeling and fever.
- You observe new symptoms, such as nausea, vomiting, constipation or abdominal swelling.

DUODENAL-ULCER PERFORATION, CLOSURE OF

GENERAL INFORMATION

DEFINITION—Closure of perforated ulcer in the duodenum, the upper 12 inches of the small intestine.

BODY PARTS INVOLVED—Duodenum.

REASONS FOR SURGERY—Prevention of continuing contamination, infection and inflammation caused by leakage of digestive materials into the abdomen.

SURGICAL RISK INCREASES WITH
- Stress.
- Smoking.
- Excess alcohol consumption.
- Poor nutrition, especially vitamin deficiencies.
- Recent or chronic illness, especially: pancreatitis; hepatitis; diabetes mellitus; brain tumor; or extensive burns.

WHAT TO EXPECT

WHO OPERATES—General surgeon.

WHERE PERFORMED—Hospital.

DIAGNOSTIC TESTS
- Before surgery: Blood and urine studies; X-rays of abdomen.
- After surgery: Blood and urine studies; X-rays of abdomen.

ANESTHESIA—General anesthesia by inhalation and injection, with an airway tube placed in the windpipe.

DESCRIPTION OF OPERATION
- The patient is given a solution of antibiotics intravenously.
- An incision is made in the abdomen. Abdominal muscles are separated, and the peritoneum is opened. The perforation is located and plugged with omentum (a pad of fat inside the abdomen) or held in place with sutures.
- Sometimes, if ulcers have been chronic, a partial gastrectomy is performed, and branches of the vagus nerve to the stomach are cut to prevent stomach-acid production and further perforation of ulcers.
- Muscle layers are repaired, and the skin is closed with sutures or clips, which usually can be removed about 1 week after surgery.

POSSIBLE COMPLICATIONS
- Excessive bleeding.
- Surgical-wound infection.
- Failure to obtain complete closure of the perforated ulcer, allowing continuing leakage, causing peritonitis (infection of the peritoneum) and death.

AVERAGE HOSPITAL STAY—6 to 8 days.

PROBABLE OUTCOME—Expect complete healing without complications. Allow about 6 weeks for recovery from surgery.

POSTOPERATIVE CARE

NOTE—This information is supplemental and should not replace your doctor's instructions.

GENERAL MEASURES
- Don't smoke.
- A hard ridge should form along the incision. As it heals, the ridge will recede gradually.
- Use an electric heating pad, a heat lamp or a warm compress to relieve incisional pain.
- Bathe and shower as usual. You may wash the incision gently with mild unscented soap.

MEDICATION—Your doctor may prescribe:
- Pain relievers. Don't take prescription pain medication longer than 4 to 7 days. Use *only* as much as you need.
- Antibiotics to fight infection.
- Stool softeners to prevent constipation.

ACTIVITY
- Resume work and normal activity as soon as possible to reduce postoperative depression, which is common.
- Resume driving 12 days after returning home.

DIET—Clear liquid diet until the gastrointestinal tract begins to function again. Then eat a well-balanced, high-protein diet to promote healing. Avoid coffee, tea, cocoa, cola drinks, alcoholic beverages and any food or spice that aggravates symptoms. Bland diets apparently do not help.

CALL YOUR DOCTOR IF

Any of the following occurs:
- Pain, swelling, redness, drainage or bleeding increases in the surgical area.
- Signs of infection: headache, muscle aches, dizziness or a general ill feeling and fever.
- Increasing abdominal pain or swelling; nausea; vomiting; bleeding from rectum or black, tarry stools.
- Constipation that is not relieved with mild laxatives.
- New, unexplained symptoms develop. Drugs used in treatment may produce side effects.

EAR PIERCING

GENERAL INFORMATION

DEFINITION—Piercing small holes through the ear lobes.

BODY PARTS INVOLVED—Ear lobes.

REASONS FOR SURGERY—Creation of holes so pierced earrings can be worn.

SURGICAL RISK INCREASES WITH—None expected.

WHAT TO EXPECT

WHO OPERATES—Family doctor, general surgeon, plastic and reconstructive surgeon or trained nurse practitioner.

WHERE PERFORMED—Outpatient surgical facility or doctor's office.

DIAGNOSTIC TESTS—None, unless infection occurs. Then, blood studies are performed.

ANESTHESIA—Usually none. Sometimes a small amount of local anesthesia is applied.

DESCRIPTION OF OPERATION
- Points of holes for earrings are identified and marked. The ear lobe is sterilized with an antiseptic solution.
- A spring-loaded device is used to place the earring post quickly and painlessly through the ear lobe.
- The earring is held in place by a clip on the back of the ear lobe.
- Earrings are left in place until the holes heal and become lined with skin.

POSSIBLE COMPLICATIONS
- Surgical-wound infection. If this happens, the earrings should be removed immediately and antibiotics taken to fight infection.
- Black people sometimes develop scar tissue in the surgical area.

AVERAGE HOSPITAL STAY—Usually none.

PROBABLE OUTCOME—Expect complete healing without complications. Allow about 3 weeks for recovery from surgery.

POSTOPERATIVE CARE

NOTE—This information is supplemental and should not replace your doctor's instructions.

GENERAL MEASURES
- Clean ear lobes with a tissue or cotton ball soaked in rubbing alcohol 3 to 4 times a day for several days after surgery.
- Apply a non-prescription antibiotic ointment to help prevent infection.
- Turn earrings in their holes frequently. Don't remove earrings for 7 to 10 days after surgery.
- After healing, don't wear earrings to bed, to prevent tearing the hole.

MEDICATION
- Your doctor will prescribe local antibiotics, if infection develops.
- You may use non-prescription drugs, such as acetaminophen, for minor pain.

ACTIVITY—No restrictions.

DIET—No special diet.

CALL YOUR DOCTOR IF

- Pain, swelling, redness, drainage or bleeding increases in the surgical area.
- You develop excessive scar tissue in 4 to 6 months after surgery.

ECTROPION REPAIR

GENERAL INFORMATION

DEFINITION—Repair of an ectropion (see Illness section) by removal of excess cartilage in the edge of the eyelid.

BODY PARTS INVOLVED—Lower eyelid.

REASONS FOR SURGERY
- Improved appearance.
- Relief of redness, irritation and discomfort.
- Reduced likelihood of infection in the membrane surrounding the eye.

SURGICAL RISK INCREASES WITH
- Smoking.
- Stress.
- Poor nutrition.
- Recent illness.
- Alcoholism or chronic illness.

WHAT TO EXPECT

WHO OPERATES—Ophthalmologist.

WHERE PERFORMED—Hospital, ophthalmologist's office or outpatient surgical facility.

DIAGNOSTIC TESTS
- Before surgery: Blood and urine studies; eye examination.
- After surgery: Eye examination; laboratory examination of removed tissue.

ANESTHESIA—Local anesthesia by injection.

DESCRIPTION OF OPERATION
- An incision is made in the eyelid.
- The cartilage is cut close to the outer eyelid edge. A small wedge of cartilage is cut free and removed. The cartilage is sewn back together.
- Another wedge of cartilage is cut free and removed from the side of the eyelid close to the nose.
- The remaining cartilage is sewn together.
- The skin is closed with sutures, which usually can be removed about 10 days after surgery.

POSSIBLE COMPLICATIONS—Surgical-wound infection.

AVERAGE HOSPITAL STAY—1 to 2 days.

PROBABLE OUTCOME—Expect complete healing without complications. Allow about 2 weeks for recovery from surgery.

POSTOPERATIVE CARE

NOTE—This information is supplemental and should not replace your doctor's instructions.

GENERAL MEASURES
- Bathe and shower as usual, but keep the eye area dry for 4 to 5 days after surgery.
- Apply warm compresses to the eye to relieve discomfort.
- Sleep for several nights on 2 pillows to decrease swelling.

MEDICATION
- Your doctor may prescribe:
  Pain relievers. Don't take prescription pain medication longer than 4 to 7 days. Use *only* as much as you need.
  Antibiotic eye drops to fight infection. Keep drops cold but not frozen in the refrigerator.
- You may use non-prescription drugs, such as acetaminophen, for minor pain.

ACTIVITY
- Resume work and normal activity as soon as possible. This reduces postoperative depression and irritability, which are common.
- Avoid vigorous exercise for 2 weeks after surgery.

DIET—No special diet.

CALL YOUR DOCTOR IF

- Pain, swelling, redness, drainage or bleeding increases in the surgical area.
- You develop signs of infection: headache, muscle aches, dizziness or a general ill feeling and fever.
- You experience nausea or vomiting.
- Your vision changes.
- New, unexplained symptoms develop. Drugs used in treatment may produce side effects.

ELECTROCAUTERIZATION
(Electrocoagulation; Electrosurgery; Electrofulgeration)

 GENERAL INFORMATION

DEFINITION—Removal of abnormal or diseased tissue or control of bleeding in small blood vessels with controlled electric current.

BODY PARTS INVOLVED—Skin; blood vessels in surgical area.

REASONS FOR SURGERY
- Removal of lesions on the skin.
- Control of bleeding from small blood vessels during other surgeries.

SURGICAL RISK INCREASES WITH—None expected.

 WHAT TO EXPECT

WHO OPERATES—Family doctor, dermatologist, plastic and reconstructive surgeon or general surgeon.

WHERE PERFORMED—Hospital, outpatient surgical facility or doctor's office.

DIAGNOSTIC TESTS—Usually none.

ANESTHESIA—Local anesthesia by injection.

DESCRIPTION OF OPERATION—Usually, a lesion is numbed with local anesthesia, and removed with a curette (see Glossary). Electrocauterization with an electric instrument destroys abnormal tissue that the curette does not remove.

POSSIBLE COMPLICATIONS
- Long healing time (2 to 3 weeks).
- Tissue is destroyed, making laboratory examination impossible.

PROBABLE OUTCOME—Expect complete healing without complications. The scab will drop off spontaneously and the scar should be small. Allow 2 to 3 weeks for recovery from surgery.

 POSTOPERATIVE CARE

NOTE—This information is supplemental and should not replace your doctor's instructions.

GENERAL MEASURES
- If the wound bleeds during the first 24 hours after surgery, press a clean tissue or cloth to it for 10 minutes.
- Cover the surgical wound with a small bandage to protect it.
- Bathe and shower as usual. Between baths, keep wound dry with a bandage for the first 2 or 3 days after surgery. If a bandage gets wet, change it promptly.
- Apply non-prescription antibiotic ointment to the wound before applying new bandages.

MEDICATION—You may use non-prescription drugs, such as acetaminophen, for minor pain.

ACTIVITY—Avoid vigorous exercise for about 1 week after surgery, depending on other surgeries performed. Ask your doctor. Resume driving when able.

DIET—No special diet.

 CALL YOUR DOCTOR IF

- Pain, swelling, redness, drainage or bleeding increases in the surgical area.
- You develop signs of infection: headache, muscle aches, dizziness or a general ill feeling and fever.

SURGERIES

ENDOMETRIAL BIOPSY

 GENERAL INFORMATION

DEFINITION—Removal of tissue from the endometrium, the inner lining of the uterus.

BODY PARTS INVOLVED—Inner lining of the uterus; vagina (as route for surgery).

REASONS FOR SURGERY—Investigation of fertility in a patient who has been unable to become pregnant or investigation of bleeding between menstrual periods. Laboratory examination of the removed tissue aids in diagnosis. The surgery is performed during the last 2 weeks of the patient's menstrual cycle. This is the best time to identify possible hormonal problems and to determine if ovulation is occurring.

SURGICAL RISK INCREASES WITH—None expected.

 WHAT TO EXPECT

WHO OPERATES—Obstetrician-gynecologist, general surgeon or family doctor.

WHERE PERFORMED—Doctor's office; outpatient surgical facility; or hospital.

DIAGNOSTIC TESTS
• Before surgery: Pap smear.
• After surgery: Laboratory examination of removed tissue.

ANESTHESIA—Usually none. Your doctor may prescribe a mild tranquilizer before surgery to calm you.

DESCRIPTION OF OPERATION
• A speculum is inserted into the vagina to hold it open and to bring the cervix into view.
• A small, spoon-shaped instrument is inserted through the cervix into the uterus. It is gently scraped against the inner lining of the uterus to gather tissue.
• The instruments are removed. The surgery may cause slight pain, but it should be minor and temporary.

POSSIBLE COMPLICATIONS
• Excessive bleeding.
• Surgical-wound infection.
• Inadvertent injury to the uterus (rare).

AVERAGE HOSPITAL STAY—Usually none.

PROBABLE OUTCOME—Tissue obtained successfully without complications in virtually all cases. Allow about 1 week for recovery from surgery. During this time, you should expect vaginal discharge.

 POSTOPERATIVE CARE

NOTE—This information is supplemental and should not replace your doctor's instructions.

GENERAL MEASURES
• Bathe or shower as usual. Use non-perfumed soap.
• Wear sanitary pads for the rest of this menstrual period. Avoid tampons temporarily; they may lead to infection. Your menstrual flow may be heavier than usual.
• Wear cotton panties or pantyhose with a cotton crotch. Avoid panties made from nylon, polyester, silk or other non-ventilating materials.
• Don't douche unless your doctor recommends it.

MEDICATION
• Your doctor may prescribe hormones, if a hormonal imbalance exists.
• You may use non-prescription drugs, such as acetaminophen, for minor pain.

ACTIVITY—Resume work and normal activity as soon as possible.

DIET—No special diet.

 CALL YOUR DOCTOR IF

• Vaginal discharge increases or begins to have an unpleasant odor.
• You experience pain that simple medication does not relieve quickly.
• Unusually heavy vaginal swelling or bleeding develops.

ENTROPION REPAIR

GENERAL INFORMATION

DEFINITION—Shortening of excess tissue in the edge of the eyelid by removal of excess cartilage.

BODY PARTS INVOLVED—Skin and cartilage of the upper eyelid.

REASONS FOR SURGERY
- Improved appearance.
- Relief of redness, irritation and discomfort.

SURGICAL RISK INCREASES WITH
- Stress.
- Smoking.
- Poor nutrition.
- Recent illness.
- Alcoholism or chronic illness.

WHAT TO EXPECT

WHO OPERATES—Ophthalmologist.

WHERE PERFORMED—Hospital, ophthalmologist's office or outpatient surgical facility.

DIAGNOSTIC TESTS
- Before surgery: Blood and urine studies; eye examination.
- After surgery: Laboratory examination of removed tissue.

ANESTHESIA—Local anesthesia by injection.

DESCRIPTION OF OPERATION
- An incision is made in the eyelid.
- The cartilage is partially cut about midway between the two sides of the eyelid.
- A small amount of the cartilage is cut free of connective tissue and removed.
- The remaining cartilage is closed with silk sutures. The skin is closed over the cartilage with sutures which usually can be removed about 10 days after surgery.

POSSIBLE COMPLICATIONS—Surgical-wound infection.

AVERAGE HOSPITAL STAY—1 to 2 days.

PROBABLE OUTCOME—Expect complete healing without complications. Allow about 2 weeks for recovery from surgery.

POSTOPERATIVE CARE

NOTE—This information is supplemental and should not replace your doctor's instructions.

GENERAL MEASURES
- Bathe and shower as usual but keep the surgical area dry for 4 or 5 days after surgery.
- Apply warm compresses to the eye to relieve discomfort.
- Sleep for several nights with the head elevated on 2 pillows to decrease swelling.

MEDICATION
- Your doctor may prescribe:
  Pain relievers. Don't take prescription pain medication longer than 4 to 7 days. Use *only* as much as you need.
  Stool softeners to prevent constipation.
  Antibiotic eye drops to fight infection. Keep eye drops cold but not frozen, in the refrigerator.
- You may use non-prescription drugs, such as acetaminophen, for minor pain.

ACTIVITY
- Avoid vigorous exercise for 2 weeks following surgery.
- Resume driving 2 days after returning home.

DIET—No special diet.

CALL YOUR DOCTOR IF

- Pain, swelling, redness, drainage or bleeding increases in the surgical area.
- You develop signs of infection: headache, muscle aches, dizziness or a general ill feeling and fever.
- You experience new symptoms such as nausea or vomiting.
- Your vision changes suddenly.

EPISIOTOMY

 GENERAL INFORMATION

DEFINITION—Enlargement of the lower part of the vaginal opening.

BODY PARTS INVOLVED—Vagina; perineum.

REASONS FOR SURGERY—Usually performed during childbirth, just before the widest diameter of the baby's head passes through the outlet of the birth canal. This allows easier passage of the baby's head, decreases the likelihood of injury to the baby's head and prevents damage to the mother's vagina, bladder and rectum.

SURGICAL RISK INCREASES WITH—None expected.

 WHAT TO EXPECT

WHO OPERATES—Obstetrician-gynecologist, family doctor or midwife.

WHERE PERFORMED—Hospital or outpatient surgical facility.

DIAGNOSTIC TESTS
- Before surgery: Blood and urine studies.
- After surgery: Blood studies.

ANESTHESIA—Local anesthesia by injection.

DESCRIPTION OF OPERATION
- An incision is made in the perineum, just before the widest part of the baby's head is to be delivered. The size of the incision depends on how large an opening is required for the baby's head to pass through safely.
- The baby and placenta are delivered.
- The surgical area is repaired with sutures that will be absorbed by the body.

POSSIBLE COMPLICATIONS
- Excessive bleeding
- Surgical-wound infection.
- Inadvertent injury to sphincter or rectum.

AVERAGE HOSPITAL STAY—2 days.

PROBABLE OUTCOME—Expect complete healing without complications. Allow about 6 weeks for recovery from surgery.

 POSTOPERATIVE CARE

NOTE—This information is supplemental and should not replace your doctor's instructions.

GENERAL MEASURES
- Bathe and shower as usual. You may wash the incision gently with mild unscented soap.
- Cleanse the surgical area with warm water after urination or bowel movements.
- Take hot baths several times a day as long as you experience discomfort.
- Use ice packs made of gauze soaked in ice-cold witch hazel to relieve discomfort.

MEDICATION
- Your doctor may prescribe:
  Stool softeners to prevent constipation.
  Antibiotics to fight infection.
- You may use non-prescription drugs, such as acetaminophen, for minor pain.

ACTIVITY
- Avoid vigorous exercise for 6 weeks after surgery.
- Resume driving 10 days after returning home.
- Resume sexual relations when your doctor determines that healing is complete.

DIET—No special diet.

 CALL YOUR DOCTOR IF

- Pain, swelling, redness, drainage or bleeding increases in the surgical area.
- You develop signs of infection: headache, muscle aches, dizziness or a general ill feeling and fever.
- You experience nausea, vomiting, constipation or abdominal swelling.
- New, unexplained symptoms develop. Drugs used in treatment may produce side effects.

ESOPHAGECTOMY

GENERAL INFORMATION

DEFINITION—Removal of part of the esophagus, the tubular passage from the back of the throat to the stomach.

BODY PARTS INVOLVED—Esophagus; stomach; small intestine (sometimes).

REASONS FOR SURGERY
- Cancer of the esophagus.
- Burns and scarring of the esophagus.
- Opening a closure of the esophagus in a newborn (usually an inherited defect).

SURGICAL RISK INCREASES WITH
- Adults over 60.
- Obesity.
- Smoking.
- Excess alcohol consumption.
- Newborns and infants.
- Poor nutrition.
- Chronic or recent illness, especially pneumonia.
- Use of drugs such as: antihypertensives; muscle relaxants; tranquilizers; sleep inducers; insulin; sedatives; narcotics; beta-adrenergic blockers; or cortisone.

WHAT TO EXPECT

WHO OPERATES—General surgeon or thoracic surgeon.

WHERE PERFORMED—Hospital.

DIAGNOSTIC TESTS
- Before surgery: Blood and urine studies; X-rays of chest and upper gastrointestinal tract.
- After surgery: Blood and urine studies; X-rays of chest and upper gastrointestinal tract.

ANESTHESIA—General anesthesia by inhalation and injection, with an airway tube placed in the windpipe.

DESCRIPTION OF OPERATION
- Incisions are made in the abdomen and chest to expose the esophagus.
- The esophagus is isolated and examined.
- Abnormal tissues are removed. If the surgery is performed to treat cancer, nearby lymph glands are also removed.
- The bottom end of the remaining part of the esophagus is joined with the stomach or small intestine.
- The chest and abdomen are closed in layers. The skin is closed with sutures or clips, which usually can be removed about 1 week after surgery.

POSSIBLE COMPLICATIONS
- Excessive bleeding.
- Surgical-wound infection.
- Incisional hernia.
- Leakage of digestive material from new junction of esophagus and intestinal tract.

AVERAGE HOSPITAL STAY—18 days.

PROBABLE OUTCOME—If the surgery was performed to treat cancer in its early stages, chances of 5-year survival are good. If the surgery was performed for other reasons, expect complete healing without complications. Allow about 8 to 12 weeks for recovery from surgery.

POSTOPERATIVE CARE

NOTE—This information is supplemental and should not replace your doctor's instructions.

GENERAL MEASURES
- Don't smoke.
- A hard ridge should form along the incisions. The ridges will heal and recede gradually without treatment.
- Use an electric heating pad, a heat lamp or a warm compress to relieve incisional pain.
- Bathe and shower as usual. You may wash the incision gently with mild unscented soap.
- Move legs often while resting in bed to decrease the likelihood of deep-vein blood clots.

MEDICATION—Your doctor may prescribe:
- Pain relievers. Don't take prescription pain medication longer than 4 to 7 days. Use *only* as much as you need.
- Antibiotics to fight infection.
- Stool softeners to prevent constipation.

ACTIVITY
- Resume work and normal activity as soon as possible.
- Avoid vigorous exercise for 12 weeks after surgery.
- Resume driving 3 weeks after returning home.
- Resume sexual relations when able.

DIET—Clear liquid diet until the gastrointestinal tract begins to function again. Then eat a well-balanced, high-protein diet to promote healing. Avoid coffee, tea, cocoa, cola drinks, alcoholic beverages and any food or spice that cause indigestion.

CALL YOUR DOCTOR IF

- Pain, swelling, redness, drainage or bleeding increases in the surgical area.
- You experience vomiting, excessive weakness or black, tarry stools.
- New, unexplained symptoms develop. Drugs used in treatment may produce side effects.

SURGERIES

FACE LIFT & BLEPHAROPLASTY

GENERAL INFORMATION

DEFINITION
- Face lift: Removal of excess skin, fat and tissue from the face.
- Blepharoplasty: Removal of excess fat and skin from around the eyelids.

BODY PARTS INVOLVED—Skin and underlying tissue of the face and eyelids.

REASONS FOR SURGERY—Improved appearance of the face and improved function of the eyelids.

SURGICAL RISK INCREASES WITH
- Obesity.
- Smoking.
- Stress.
- Poor nutrition.
- Recent illness.
- Alcoholism or chronic illness.
- Use of drugs such as: antihypertensives; muscle relaxants; tranquilizers; sleep inducers; insulin; sedatives; beta-adrenergic blockers; or cortisone.
- Use of mind-altering drugs, including: narcotics; psychedelics; hallucinogens; marijuana; sedatives; hypnotics; or cocaine.

WHAT TO EXPECT

WHO OPERATES—Plastic and reconstructive surgeon.

WHERE PERFORMED—Doctor's office, outpatient surgical facility or hospital.

DIAGNOSTIC TESTS
- Before surgery: Blood and urine studies.
- After surgery: Blood studies.

ANESTHESIA
- Local anesthesia by injection.
- General anesthesia by inhalation and injection, with an airway tube placed in the windpipe.

DESCRIPTION OF OPERATION
- Incisions are made where scarring will be minimal.
- Care is taken to clamp and tie tiny bleeding vessels during the procedure to prevent collection of scar tissue under the skin.
- Flaps of skin are cut away around the eyes and face. Excess tissue is removed from underlying areas, and excess skin is trimmed away.
- The skin is closed with fine sutures, which usually can be removed about 1 week after surgery.
- Bandages and ice packs are applied to reduce swelling and bleeding.

POSSIBLE COMPLICATIONS
- Excessive bleeding.
- Surgical-wound infection.
- Collection of serum under areas where skin has been removed.

AVERAGE HOSPITAL STAY—3 to 5 days.

PROBABLE OUTCOME—Expect complete healing and improved appearance without complications. Allow about 6 weeks for recovery from surgery.

POSTOPERATIVE CARE

NOTE—This information is supplemental and should not replace your doctor's instructions.

GENERAL MEASURES
- If a wound bleeds during the first 24 hours after surgery, press a clean tissue or cloth to it for 10 minutes.
- Bathe and shower as usual. You may wash the surgical wounds gently with mild unscented soap.
- Between baths, keep the wounds dry with a bandage for the first 2 or 3 days after surgery. If a bandage gets wet, change it promptly.
- Apply non-prescription antibiotic ointment to wounds before applying new bandages.

MEDICATION
- Your doctor may prescribe:
  Pain relievers. Don't take prescription pain medication longer than 4 to 7 days. Use *only* as much as you need.
  Stool softeners to prevent constipation.
  Antibiotics to fight infection.
- You may use non-prescription drugs, such as acetaminophen, for minor pain.

ACTIVITY
- Resume work and normal activity as soon as possible. This reduces postoperative depression and irritability, which are common.
- Avoid vigorous exercise for 6 weeks after surgery.
- Resume driving 3 days after returning home.

DIET—No special diet.

CALL YOUR DOCTOR IF

- Pain, swelling, redness, drainage or bleeding increases in the surgical area.
- You develop signs of infection: headache, muscle aches, dizziness or a general ill feeling and fever.
- You experience nausea or vomiting.
- New, unexplained symptoms develop. Drugs used in treatment may produce side effects.

FASCIECTOMY

 ## GENERAL INFORMATION

DEFINITION—Removal of fascia (fibrous tissue) in the muscles of the hand that has scarred (usually called Dupuytren's contracture) as a result of an unknown cause.

BODY PARTS INVOLVED—Fascia in palm of the hand.

REASONS FOR SURGERY—Restoration of normal function of the hand.

SURGICAL RISK INCREASES WITH
- Obesity.
- Smoking.
- Poor nutrition.
- Recent illness.
- Alcoholism or chronic illness.
- Use of drugs such as: antihypertensives; muscle relaxants; tranquilizers; sleep inducers; insulin; sedatives; beta-adrenergic blockers; or cortisone.
- Use of mind-altering drugs, including: narcotics; psychedelics; hallucinogens; marijuana; sedatives; hypnotics; or cocaine.

 ## WHAT TO EXPECT

WHO OPERATES—Hand surgeon.

WHERE PERFORMED—Hospital or outpatient surgical facility.

DIAGNOSTIC TESTS
- Before surgery: Blood and urine studies.
- After surgery: Blood studies.

ANESTHESIA—Local anesthesia by injection.

DESCRIPTION OF OPERATION
- A tourniquet is applied to the patient's arm to prevent the surgical area from bleeding.
- An incision is made over the scarred fascia.
- The fascia is cut free of connective tissue and removed.
- Sometimes, a skin graft is performed to close the gap left by the removed fascia.
- The tourniquet is removed. The skin is closed with sutures, which usually can be removed about 10 days after surgery.

POSSIBLE COMPLICATIONS
- Excessive bleeding.
- Surgical-wound infection.
- Recurrent scarring of fascia.

AVERAGE HOSPITAL STAY—4 days.

PROBABLE OUTCOME—Expect complete healing without complications. Allow about 6 weeks for recovery from surgery.

 ## POSTOPERATIVE CARE

NOTE—This information is supplemental and should not replace your doctor's instructions.

GENERAL MEASURES
- A hard ridge should form along the incision. As it heals, the ridge will recede gradually.
- Use an electric heating pad, a heat lamp or a warm compress to relieve incisional pain.
- Bathe and shower as usual. You may wash the incision gently with mild unscented soap.
- Move legs often while resting in bed to decrease the likelihood of deep-vein blood clots.

MEDICATION
- Your doctor may prescribe:
  Pain relievers. Don't take prescription pain medication longer than 4 to 7 days. Use *only* as much as you need.
  Antibiotics to fight infection.
- You may use non-prescription drugs, such as acetaminophen, for minor pain.

ACTIVITY
- Resume work and normal activity as soon as possible. This reduces postoperative depression and irritability, which are common.
- Avoid vigorous exercise for 6 weeks after surgery.

DIET—Eat a well-balanced, high-protein diet to promote healing.

 ## CALL YOUR DOCTOR IF

- Pain, swelling, redness, drainage or bleeding increases in the surgical area.
- You develop signs of infection: headache, muscle aches, dizziness or a general ill feeling and fever.
- You experience nausea or vomiting.
- New, unexplained symptoms develop. Drugs used in treatment may produce side effects.

FEMORAL-POPLITEAL ARTERY, ENDARTERECTOMY OR BYPASS GRAFT

 GENERAL INFORMATION

DEFINITION—Removal or bypass of plaque or a blood clot that has blocked blood circulation in the leg.

BODY PARTS INVOLVED—Blood vessel in the leg that is called the femoral artery below the groin and the popliteal artery below the knee.

REASONS FOR SURGERY—Restoration of normal blood circulation in the leg and foot.

SURGICAL RISK INCREASES WITH
- Obesity.
- Smoking.
- Recent or chronic illness, especially atherosclerosis or diabetes mellitus.
- Use of drugs such as: antihypertensives; muscle relaxants; tranquilizers; sleep inducers; insulin; sedatives; beta-adrenergic blockers; or cortisone.
- Use of mind-altering drugs.

 WHAT TO EXPECT

WHO OPERATES—General surgeon or vascular surgeon.

WHERE PERFORMED—Hospital.

DIAGNOSTIC TESTS
- Before surgery: Blood and urine studies; arteriograms (see Glossary).
- During surgery: Arteriograms.
- After surgery: Blood studies.

ANESTHESIA—General anesthesia by inhalation and injection, with an airway tube placed in the windpipe.

DESCRIPTION OF OPERATION
- An incision is made in the thigh.
- The plaque or blood clot in the artery is located. Suction is used to remove it, if possible.
- If a bypass must be used, a large vein from the leg is selected and cut free. All large tributaries are tied off.
- The graft is sewn in place above and below the blocked artery.
- The muscles and skin are closed with sutures or clips, which usually can be removed about 1 week after surgery.

POSSIBLE COMPLICATIONS
- Excessive bleeding.
- Surgical-wound infection.
- Inadvertent injury to nerves.
- Clotting inside the damaged artery.

AVERAGE HOSPITAL STAY—10 to 14 days.

PROBABLE OUTCOME—Expect complete healing without complications. Allow about 6 weeks for recovery from surgery.

 POSTOPERATIVE CARE

NOTE—This information is supplemental and should not replace your doctor's instructions.

GENERAL MEASURES
- Don't smoke.
- Keep feet clean and dry.
- A hard ridge should form along the incision. As it heals, the ridge will recede gradually.
- Use an electric heating pad, a heat lamp or a warm compress to relieve incisional pain.
- Bathe and shower as usual. You may wash the incision gently with mild unscented soap.
- Move legs often while in to bed to decrease the likelihood of deep-vein blood clots.

MEDICATION
- Your doctor may prescribe:
  Pain relievers. Don't take prescription pain medication longer than 4 to 7 days. Use *only* as much as you need.
  Antibiotics to fight infection.
  Anticoagulants to prevent blood-clot formation.
- You may use non-prescription drugs, such as acetaminophen, for minor pain.

ACTIVITY
- Resume work and normal activity as soon as possible to reduce postoperative depression, which is common.
- Avoid vigorous exercise for 6 weeks after surgery, but start a walking exercise program as soon as your doctor recommends it.
- Resume driving 5 weeks after returning home.
- Resume sexual relations when your doctor determines that healing is complete.

DIET—Clear liquid diet until the gastro-intestinal tract begins to function again. Then eat a well-balanced, high-protein diet to promote healing. After recovery, eat a diet low in fat and salt (see Appendices 8 and 9).

 CALL YOUR DOCTOR IF

- Pain, swelling, redness, drainage or bleeding increases in the surgical area.
- You develop signs of infection: headache, muscle aches, dizziness or a general ill feeling and fever.
- You experience new symptoms, such as nausea; vomiting; constipation; or abdominal swelling.
- Your foot becomes cold, discolored or numb, or you develop pain in the calf when walking.

FIBROID-TUMOR REMOVAL
(Leiomyomectomy or Myomectomy)

 GENERAL INFORMATION

DEFINITION—Removal of fibroid tumors (leiomyoma) from the uterus through an incision in the lower abdomen.

BODY PARTS INVOLVED—Uterus.

REASONS FOR SURGERY
- Pelvic pain.
- Pressure on the bladder.
- Abnormal bleeding.
- Difficulty in becoming pregnant.
- Discomfort with sexual intercourse.

SURGICAL RISK INCREASES WITH
- Obesity.
- Smoking.
- Poor nutrition, especially inadequate iron intake that has led to anemia.
- Illness that has reduced strength.
- Use of drugs such as: cortisone; antihypertensives; beta-adrenergic blockers; or diuretics.
- Use of mind-altering drugs, including: narcotics; psychedelics; hallucinogens; marijuana; sedatives; hypnotics; or cocaine.

 WHAT TO EXPECT

WHO OPERATES—General surgeon or obstetrician-gynecologist.

WHERE PERFORMED—Hospital.

DIAGNOSTIC TESTS
- Before surgery: Blood studies; dilatation and curettage of the uterus (D & C); laparoscopy; X-rays of abdomen; barium-enema X-rays; intravenous pyelogram (see Glossary for all).
- After surgery: Blood studies.

ANESTHESIA—General anesthesia by inhalation and injection, with an airway tube placed in the windpipe.

DESCRIPTION OF OPERATION
- An incision is made in the lower abdomen.
- The muscles are separated and connective tissues are cut free to expose the uterus.
- Fibroid tumors are located on the outer uterus layers.
- Each tumor is removed separately, and each excision is repaired.
- The internal structures are closed in layers.
- The skin is closed with sutures or skin clips, which can be removed about 4 to 7 days after surgery.

POSSIBLE COMPLICATIONS
- Excessive bleeding
- Surgical-wound infection.

AVERAGE HOSPITAL STAY—2 to 3 days.

PROBABLE OUTCOME—The uterus is left intact, and you will still have menstrual periods. Your next period may be heavier than usual, but should occur at about the expected time.

Allow about 6 weeks for recovery from surgery.

 POSTOPERATIVE CARE

NOTE—This information is supplemental and should not replace your doctor's instructions.

GENERAL MEASURES
- Don't smoke.
- A hard ridge should form along the incision. As it heals, the ridge will recede gradually.
- Use an electric heating pad, a heat lamp or a warm compress to relieve incisional pain.
- Bathe and shower as usual. You may wash the incision gently with mild unscented soap.
- Wear sanitary pads—not tampons—to absorb blood.

MEDICATION
- Your doctor may prescribe:
  Pain relievers. Don't take prescription pain medication longer than 4 to 7 days. Use *only* as much as you need.
  Vaginal creams or medicated douches, if vaginal discharge develops an unpleasant odor.
- You may use non-prescription drugs, such as acetaminophen, for minor pain.

ACTIVITY
- Return to work and normal activity as soon as possible. This reduces postoperative depression, which is common.
- Resume driving about 2 weeks after returning home.
- Resume sexual relations when able.

DIET—Clear liquid diet until the gastrointestinal tract functions again. Then eat a well-balanced, high-protein diet to promote healing.

 CALL YOUR DOCTOR IF

- You experience vaginal bleeding that soaks more than 1 pad per hour.
- You develop signs of infection: headache, muscle aches, dizziness or a general feeling of ill health and fever.
- You have abdominal swelling or severe abdominal pain.
- The urge to urinate frequently persists longer than 1 month.
- Excessive vaginal discharge persists beyond 1 month after surgery.

FINGERNAIL REMOVAL

GENERAL INFORMATION

DEFINITION—Removal of a fingernail.

BODY PARTS INVOLVED—Fingernail, usually in the thumb or first finger.

REASONS FOR SURGERY
- Fingernail infection.
- Correction of abnormal fingernail growth.

SURGICAL RISK INCREASES WITH—None expected.

WHAT TO EXPECT

WHO OPERATES—General surgeon or family doctor.

WHERE PERFORMED—Hospital or outpatient surgical facility.

DIAGNOSTIC TESTS
- Before surgery: Blood and urine studies.
- After surgery: Blood studies.

ANESTHESIA—Local anesthesia by injection.

DESCRIPTION OF OPERATION
- An incision is made in the skin around the fingernail.
- The fingernail is pushed up from its bed past the cuticle with a blunt instrument.
- The nail is removed and the nail bed is scraped.
- Usually, the surgical wound is left open to heal from the bottom out.
- A special non-stick bandage is applied to prevent bleeding.

POSSIBLE COMPLICATIONS
- Excessive bleeding.
- Surgical-wound infection.

AVERAGE HOSPITAL STAY—Usually none.

PROBABLE OUTCOME—Expect complete healing without complications. Allow about 3 weeks for recovery from surgery.

POSTOPERATIVE CARE

NOTE—This information is supplemental and should not replace your doctor's instructions.

GENERAL MEASURES
- Keep the hand elevated to relieve pain and throbbing.
- Change bandages frequently. Keep bandages dry between baths. If a bandage gets wet, change it promptly.

MEDICATION
- Your doctor may prescribe:
  Pain relievers. Don't take prescription pain medication longer than 4 to 7 days. Use *only* as much as you need.
  Antibiotics to fight infection.
- You may use non-prescription drugs, such as acetaminophen, for minor pain.

ACTIVITY—No restrictions.

DIET—No special diet.

CALL YOUR DOCTOR IF

- Pain, swelling, redness, drainage or bleeding increases in the surgical area.
- You develop signs of infection: headache, muscle aches, dizziness or a general ill feeling and fever.
- New, unexplained symptoms develop. Drugs used in treatment may produce side effects.

FRACTURE REPAIR
(Fracture Reduction)

 GENERAL INFORMATION

DEFINITION—Rejoining ends of a broken bone. The term "broken bone" means the same as "fractured bone."

BODY PARTS INVOLVED—Any bone in the body.

REASONS FOR SURGERY—Restoration of normal position and function of a broken bone.

SURGICAL RISK INCREASES WITH
- Adults over 60.
- Obesity.
- Smoking.
- Poor nutrition.
- Recent illness.
- Alcoholism or chronic illness.
- Use of drugs such as: antihypertensives; muscle relaxants; tranquilizers; sleep inducers; insulin; sedatives; beta-adrenergic blockers; or cortisone.
- Use of mind-altering drugs.

 WHAT TO EXPECT

WHO OPERATES—Orthopedist, general surgeon or family doctor.

WHERE PERFORMED—Hospital, outpatient surgical facility, doctor's office or emergency room.

DIAGNOSTIC TESTS
- Before surgery: Blood and urine studies; X-ray of affected area.
- During surgery: X-rays.
- After surgery: X-rays through cast or splint to determine if rejoined pieces remain in good position for healing.

ANESTHESIA
- Local anesthesia by injection.
- General anesthesia by inhalation and injection, with an airway tube placed in the windpipe.

DESCRIPTION OF OPERATION
- The bone fragments are aligned as close as possible to their normal position without injuring the skin.
- Once the broken ends of bone are joined, the affected part is kept rigid with a plaster cast or splint.

POSSIBLE COMPLICATIONS
- Excessive bleeding.
- Improper fit of joined bone ends.
- Pressure on nearby nerves.

AVERAGE HOSPITAL STAY—0 to 6 days.

PROBABLE OUTCOME—Children's bones usually heal relatively rapidly. Fractured bones of elderly patients may never heal properly, particularly if nutrition is poor. The time required for healing depends on the type of fracture and the extent of tissue damage.

 POSTOPERATIVE CARE

NOTE—This information is supplemental and should not replace your doctor's instructions.

GENERAL MEASURES
- Do not allow pressure on any part of the cast until it is completely dry. Drying time varies, depending on the thickness of the cast, temperature and humidity.
- If the cast gets wet and a soft area appears, return to your doctor's office to have it repaired.
- Whenever possible, raise the part enclosed in the cast. This decreases the possibility of swelling. For example, prop a leg cast on a pillow when in bed and on a footstool or hassock when sitting; prop an arm cast on a pillow on the chest. For more information on care of casts, see Appendix 17.

MEDICATION
- Your doctor may prescribe:
  Pain relievers. Don't take prescription pain medication longer than 4 to 7 days. Use *only* as much as you need.
  Antibiotics to fight infection.
- You may use non-prescription drugs, such as acetaminophen, for minor pain.

ACTIVITY
- Resume work and normal activity as soon as possible to reduce postoperative depression and irritability, which are common.
- Avoid vigorous exercise for 6 weeks following surgery.
- Resume driving when your doctor determines that healing is complete.

DIET—Eat a well-balanced, high-protein diet to promote healing. Increase fiber and fluid intake if constipation occurs due to decreased activity.

 CALL YOUR DOCTOR IF

Any of the following occurs:
- Severe, persistent pain under the cast.
- Color change, coldness or numbness in tissues beyond the cast.
- Tissue swelling greater than before the cast was applied.
- New, unexplained symptoms. Drugs used in treatment may produce side effects.

FRENECTOMY

 GENERAL INFORMATION

DEFINITION—Removal of an abnormal frenum. A frenum is a band of muscle connecting the lip or cheek to the gums. In the upper jaw, an abnormal frenum may cause the two front teeth to separate, resulting in "tongue tie." Surgery is usually performed when the patient is under 2 years old. The surgery is minor and should be no more painful than other minor dental surgeries.

BODY PARTS INVOLVED—Mouth and lips; gum; frenum.

REASONS FOR SURGERY
- Prevention of separation of the front teeth during growth and development.
- Prevention of feeding and speech problems.

SURGICAL RISK INCREASES WITH—No expected risk factors in a child.

 WHAT TO EXPECT

WHO OPERATES—Dentist, oral surgeon or general surgeon.

WHERE PERFORMED—Doctor's, dentist's or oral surgeon's office.

DIAGNOSTIC TESTS—Blood and urine studies before surgery.

ANESTHESIA—Local anesthesia by injection.

DESCRIPTION OF OPERATION
- A local anesthetic is injected to numb the area around the frenum.
- The frenum is clipped with sharp scissors and removed.
- Stitches hold the incision area together during healing. They usually can be removed about 1 week after surgery.

POSSIBLE COMPLICATIONS
- Excessive bleeding.
- Surgical-wound infection.

AVERAGE HOSPITAL STAY—None.

PROBABLE OUTCOME—Expect complete recovery without complications. Allow about 2 weeks for recovery from surgery.

 POSTOPERATIVE CARE

NOTE—This information is supplemental and should not replace your doctor's instructions.

GENERAL MEASURES
- Keep a gauze bandage over the surgical area for 1 to 2 hours after surgery.
- Apply ice packs on the face over the affected area to relieve pain. Do this for 10 minutes at a time as often as needed for the first 24 hours after surgery.
- Return to the dentist about 1 week after surgery for suture removal.
- Brush the child's teeth carefully in the area of the mouth not affected by the surgery. A clean mouth heals faster.
- Do not rinse the child's mouth for at least 24 hours after surgery. After 24 hours, rinse every 1 or 2 hours with a solution of 1/2 teaspoon salt in 8 oz. warm water.

MEDICATION
- Your doctor may prescribe pain relievers. Don't give the child prescription pain medication longer than 4 to 7 days. Use *only* as much as is needed.
- You may use non-prescription drugs, such as acetaminophen, to relieve minor pain.

ACTIVITY—Avoid vigorous exercise for 1 week after surgery.

DIET—Adequate food and fluid intake after surgery will ensure more rapid healing. If your child's regular diet is too difficult, provide a high-protein liquid diet (see Appendix 7) for 2 to 3 days.

 CALL YOUR DOCTOR OR DENTIST IF

- Pain, swelling, redness, drainage or bleeding increase in the surgical area.
- You observe signs of infection: headache, muscle aches, dizziness or a general ill feeling and fever.

GALLBLADDER REMOVAL
(Cholecystectomy)

GENERAL INFORMATION

DEFINITION—Removal of the gallbladder.

BODY PARTS INVOLVED—Gallbladder; bile ducts.

REASONS FOR SURGERY
- Gallstones.
- Suspected gallbladder tumors.
- Chronic gallbladder infection.
- Sudden, severe infection of the gallbladder that does not respond rapidly to treatment.

SURGICAL RISK INCREASES WITH
- Obesity.
- Smoking.
- Recent or chronic illness, especially: alcoholism; cirrhosis of the liver; diabetes mellitus; heart disease; calcification of the gallbladder; or chronic obstructive pulmonary disease (COPD).

WHAT TO EXPECT

WHO OPERATES—General surgeon.

WHERE PERFORMED—Hospital.

DIAGNOSTIC TESTS
- Before surgery: Blood studies; X-rays of the gallbladder; ultrasonic screen (see Glossary).
- During surgery: Cholangiogram (see Glossary).
- After surgery: Blood studies.

ANESTHESIA—General anesthesia by inhalation and injection, with an airway tube placed in the windpipe.

DESCRIPTION OF OPERATION
- An incision is made under the right rib cage. Abdominal muscles are separated to expose abdominal organs, which are inspected for undetected disease. Other surgeries may be performed at this time.
- The gallbladder is cut free and removed from under the liver.
- A cholangiogram is done to determine if gallstones are lodged in the bile ducts. If necessary, the gallstones are removed.
- The incision is closed with sutures, skin clips or staples, which usually can be removed about 1 week after surgery. Frequently, 2 tubes are left in place. One connects the common bile duct to the outside, and another allows wound drainage.
- A tube running through the nose to the stomach usually remains at least 2 to 3 days after surgery until the gastrointestinal tract begins functioning again. Once normal intestinal function begins, the tube is removed and the patient can begin eating.

POSSIBLE COMPLICATIONS
- Internal bleeding.
- Peritonitis.
- Surgical-wound infection.
- Inadvertent injury to the common bile duct.

AVERAGE HOSPITAL STAY—5 to 7 days.

PROBABLE OUTCOME—Expect complete healing without complications. The surgery relieves symptoms in 90% of patients. Allow about 3 weeks for recovery from surgery.

POSTOPERATIVE CARE

NOTE—This information is supplemental and should not replace your doctor's instructions.

GENERAL MEASURES
- A hard ridge should form along the incision. As it heals, the ridge will recede gradually.
- Use an electric heating pad, a heat lamp or a warm compress to relieve incisional pain.
- Bathe and shower as usual. You may wash the incision gently with mild unscented soap.

MEDICATION—You may use non-prescription drugs, such as acetaminophen, to relieve minor pain.

ACTIVITY
- Take short walks as soon as possible.
- Resume driving 18 days after returning home.
- Resume sexual relations when able.

DIET—Your doctor will prescribe a diet.

CALL YOUR DOCTOR IF

- Pain, swelling, redness, drainage or bleeding increases in the surgical area.
- You develop signs of infection: headache, muscle aches, dizziness or a general ill feeling and fever.
- You experience new symptoms, such as hiccups, constipation or abdominal swelling.

GANGLION REMOVAL
(Ganglionectomy)

GENERAL INFORMATION

DEFINITION—Removal of ganglions, small cysts that protrude from fibrous tissue surrounding tendons. Ganglions appear near areas of repeated minor injury.

BODY PARTS INVOLVED—Fibrous tissue surrounding tendons, usually in the hand and wrist.

REASONS FOR SURGERY
- Relief of pain.
- Restored use of an affected joint.
- Improved appearance.

SURGICAL RISK INCREASES WITH
- Poor nutrition.
- Recent illness.
- Alcoholism or other chronic illness.

WHAT TO EXPECT

WHO OPERATES—General surgeon or plastic and reconstructive surgeon.

WHERE PERFORMED—Doctor's office or outpatient surgical facility.

DIAGNOSTIC TESTS
- Before surgery: Blood and urine studies.
- After surgery: Laboratory examination of removed tissue.

ANESTHESIA—Local anesthesia by injection.

DESCRIPTION OF OPERATION
- The skin is incised over the ganglion.
- The ganglion is cut free from connective tissue and removed.
- The skin is closed with sutures or clips, which usually can be removed about 10 days after surgery.
- The affected area is usually immobilized in a splint for 1 to 2 weeks.

POSSIBLE COMPLICATIONS
- Excessive bleeding.
- Surgical-wound infection.

AVERAGE HOSPITAL STAY—Usually none.

PROBABLE OUTCOME—Expect complete healing without complications. Allow about 3 weeks for recovery from surgery.

POSTOPERATIVE CARE

NOTE—This information is supplemental and should not replace your doctor's instructions.

GENERAL MEASURES
- If the wound bleeds during the first 24 hours after surgery, press a clean tissue or cloth to it for 10 minutes.
- A hard ridge should form along the incision. As it heals, the ridge will recede gradually.
- Use an electric heating pad, a heat lamp or a warm compress to relieve incisional pain.
- Bathe and shower as usual. You may wash the incision gently with mild unscented soap.
- Between baths, keep the wound dry with a bandage for the first 2 or 3 days after surgery. If a bandage gets wet, change it promptly.
- Apply non-prescription antibiotic ointment to the wound before applying new bandages.

MEDICATION
- Your doctor may prescribe pain relievers. Don't take prescription pain medication longer than 4 to 7 days. Use *only* as much as you need.
- You may use non-prescription drugs, such as acetaminophen, for minor pain.

ACTIVITY
- Return to work and normal activity as soon as possible. This reduces postoperative depression and irritability, which are common.
- Avoid vigorous exercise for 3 weeks after surgery.
- Resume driving 3 days after returning home.

DIET—No special diet.

CALL YOUR DOCTOR IF

- Pain, swelling, redness, drainage or bleeding increases in the surgical area.
- You develop signs of infection: headache, muscle aches, dizziness or a general ill feeling and fever.
- New, unexplained symptoms develop. Drugs used in treatment may produce side effects.

GASTROENTEROSTOMY FOR PYLORIC OBSTRUCTION

GENERAL INFORMATION

DEFINITION—Creation of an artificial passage between the stomach and the small intestine to bypass obstructions caused by ulcer scar tissue.

BODY PARTS INVOLVED—Stomach; duodenum; jejunum (usually).

REASONS FOR SURGERY—Restoration of normal function of the gastrointestinal tract.

SURGICAL RISK INCREASES WITH
- Adults over 60.
- Newborns and infants.
- Stress.
- Obesity.
- Smoking.
- Excess alcohol consumption.
- Poor nutrition.
- Recent or chronic illness.
- Use of drugs such as: antihypertensives; muscle relaxants; tranquilizers; sleep inducers; insulin; sedatives; narcotics; beta-adrenergic blockers; or cortisone.

WHAT TO EXPECT

WHO OPERATES—General surgeon.

WHERE PERFORMED—Hospital.

DIAGNOSTIC TESTS
- Before surgery: Blood and urine studies; gastroscopy; X-rays of upper gastrointestinal tract; serum electrolytes (see Glossary).
- After surgery: Blood and urine studies.

ANESTHESIA—General anesthesia by inhalation and injection, with an airway tube placed in the windpipe.

DESCRIPTION OF OPERATION
- An incision is made in the upper abdomen.
- The abdominal muscles are separated to expose the abdominal organs, which are inspected for any undetected disease. Other surgeries may be performed at this time.
- The stomach and jejunum are isolated. A small opening is made in each, and they are joined with sutures at the openings.
- The abdominal muscles are closed with sutures. The skin is closed with sutures or clips, which usually can be removed in about 1 week.

POSSIBLE COMPLICATIONS
- Excessive bleeding.
- Surgical-wound infection.
- Spillage of stomach contents into abdomen.
- Incisional hernia.

AVERAGE HOSPITAL STAY—7 to 10 days.

PROBABLE OUTCOME—Expect complete healing without complications. Allow about 6 weeks for recovery from surgery.

POSTOPERATIVE CARE

NOTE—This information is supplemental and should not replace your doctor's instructions.

GENERAL MEASURES
- Don't smoke.
- A hard ridge should form along the incision. As it heals, the ridge will recede gradually.
- Use an electric heating pad, a heat lamp or a warm compress to relieve incisional pain.
- Bathe and shower as usual. You may wash the incision gently with mild unscented soap.
- Move legs often while resting in bed to decrease the likelihood of deep-vein blood clots.

MEDICATION—Your doctor may prescribe:
- Pain relievers. Don't take prescription pain medication longer than 4 to 7 days. Use *only* as much as you need.
- Stool softeners to prevent constipation.
- Antibiotics to fight infection.

ACTIVITY
- Resume work and normal activity as soon as possible to reduce postoperative depression, which is common.
- Avoid vigorous exercise for 6 weeks after surgery.
- Resume driving 1 month after returning home.

DIET—Clear liquid diet until the gastrointestinal tract begins to function again. Then eat a well-balanced, high-protein diet to promote healing. Avoid coffee, tea, cocoa, cola drinks, alcoholic beverages and any food or spice that cause indigestion.

CALL YOUR DOCTOR IF

- Pain, swelling, redness, drainage or bleeding increases in the surgical area.
- You develop signs of infection: headache, muscle aches, dizziness or a general ill feeling and fever.
- You experience nausea, vomiting, constipation, abdominal swelling or black, tarry stools.
- New, unexplained symptoms develop. Drugs used in treatment may produce side effects.

HAMMERTOE CORRECTION

GENERAL INFORMATION

DEFINITION—Removal of ligaments and joining of middle joints in the toes to correct hammertoe, a deformity in which the toes bend downward. This causes the tops of the toes to become callused from rubbing against the inside of shoes. Hammertoe probably results from wearing shoes that do not fit properly, especially high-heeled shoes that place pressure on the front part of the foot and compress the smaller toes together tightly.

BODY PARTS INVOLVED—All toes except the big toes; tendons, blood vessels and nerves connected to these toes; overlying skin.

REASONS FOR SURGERY
- Relief of painful calluses.
- Prevention of permanent deformity.

SURGICAL RISK INCREASES WITH
- Obesity.
- Smoking.
- Excess alcohol consumption.
- Use of drugs such as: antihypertensives; muscle relaxants; tranquilizers; sleep inducers; insulin; sedatives; beta-adrenergic blockers; or cortisone.
- Use of mind-altering drugs, including: narcotics; psychedelics; hallucinogens; marijuana; sedatives; hypnotics; or cocaine.

WHAT TO EXPECT

WHO OPERATES—General surgeon (sometimes), podiatrist or orthopedic surgeon.

WHERE PERFORMED—Hospital or outpatient surgical facility.

DIAGNOSTIC TESTS
- Before surgery: Blood and urine studies; X-rays of feet.
- After surgery: Blood studies.

ANESTHESIA—Local anesthesia by injection.

DESCRIPTION OF OPERATION
- After local anesthesia is injected, a tourniquet is applied above the ankle to keep the surgical area from bleeding.
- An incision is made in the ball of the foot.
- The ligaments that attach to the underside of the toes are located, cut free of connective tissue to foot bones, and divided so they no longer bend downward.
- The middle joints of the affected toes are connected together permanently with fine pins and wire sutures.

- The skin is closed with fine sutures, which usually can be removed about 7 to 10 days after surgery. The tourniquet is removed.

POSSIBLE COMPLICATIONS—Excessive bleeding or surgical-wound infection.

AVERAGE HOSPITAL STAY—None.

PROBABLE OUTCOME—Expect complete healing without complications. Allow about 4 weeks for recovery from surgery.

POSTOPERATIVE CARE

NOTE—This information is supplemental and should not replace your doctor's instructions.

GENERAL MEASURES
- A hard ridge should form along the incision. As it heals, the ridge will recede gradually.
- Use an electric heating pad, a heat lamp or a warm compress to relieve incisional pain.
- Bathe and shower as usual. You may wash the incision gently with mild unscented soap.
- Wear shoes that fit well and do not cramp the toes or put undue stress on the front of the foot.
- While healing, wear flat shoes and white cotton socks.

MEDICATION
- Your doctor may prescribe pain relievers. Don't take prescription pain medication longer than 4 to 7 days. Use *only* as much as you need.
- You may use non-prescription drugs, such as acetaminophen, for minor pain.

ACTIVITY
- Avoid vigorous exercise for 6 weeks after surgery.
- Resume driving 1 week after returning home.

DIET—No special diet.

CALL YOUR DOCTOR IF

- Pain, swelling, redness, drainage or bleeding increases in the surgical area.
- You develop signs of infection: headache, muscle aches, dizziness or a general ill feeling and fever.
- You experience new symptoms such as nausea or vomiting.

HAND SURGERY

GENERAL INFORMATION

DEFINITION—Any operation performed to restore or preserve the normal function of the hand.

BODY PARTS INVOLVED—Hand.

REASONS FOR SURGERY—Preservation or restoration of normal function of the hand that has been lost or impaired by: severed nerves or blood vessels; tissue destroyed by disease or injury; severed or injured tendons; or amputated fingers.

SURGICAL RISK INCREASES WITH
- Obesity.
- Smoking.
- Poor nutrition.
- Excess alcohol consumption.
- Recent or chronic illness, especially diabetes or peripheral vascular disease.
- Use of drugs such as: antihypertensives; muscle relaxants; tranquilizers; sleep inducers; insulin; sedatives; beta-adrenergic blockers; or cortisone.
- Use of mind-altering drugs, including: narcotics; psychedelics; hallucinogens; marijuana; sedatives; hypnotics; or cocaine.

WHAT TO EXPECT

WHO OPERATES—General surgeon or hand surgeon.

WHERE PERFORMED—Doctor's office, outpatient surgical facility, hospital or emergency room.

DIAGNOSTIC TESTS
- Before surgery: Blood and urine studies; X-rays of hands.
- After surgery: Blood studies.

ANESTHESIA
- Local anesthesia (sometimes) by injection.
- General anesthesia by inhalation and injection, with an airway tube placed in the windpipe.

DESCRIPTION OF OPERATION
- The arm of the affected hand is elevated and wrapped with a blood-pressure cuff inflated to higher than normal blood pressure. This prevents the surgical area from bleeding.
- The surgery is performed carefully, but as quickly as possible. The procedures depend on the injury or disease in the hand.
- The wound is covered with gauze and padded dressings.
- After surgery, the hand and forearm are usually kept rigid with a plaster cast or splint.

POSSIBLE COMPLICATIONS
- Excessive bleeding.
- Surgical-wound infection.

AVERAGE HOSPITAL STAY—0 to 2 days.

PROBABLE OUTCOME—Expect complete healing of surgical wound. Success of surgery depends on the underlying injury. Allow about 3 weeks for recovery from surgery.

POSTOPERATIVE CARE

NOTE—This information is supplemental and should not replace your doctor's instructions.

GENERAL MEASURES
- A hard ridge should form along the incision. As it heals, the ridge will recede gradually.
- Use an electric heating pad, a heat lamp or a warm compress to relieve incisional pain.
- Bathe and shower as usual, if you don't have a cast. You may wash the incision gently with mild unscented soap.
- See Appendix 17 for complete instructions on cast care.
- Keep the affected arm above the heart to prevent or decrease swelling.

MEDICATION
- Your doctor may prescribe:
  Pain relievers. Don't take prescription pain medication longer than 4 to 7 days. Use *only* as much as you need.
  Antibiotics to fight infection.
- You may use non-prescription drugs, such as acetaminophen, for minor pain.

ACTIVITY
- Return to work and normal activity as soon as possible. This reduces postoperative depression and irritability, which are common.
- Avoid vigorous exercise for 6 weeks after surgery.
- Resume driving when the hand has healed.

DIET—Clear liquid diet until the gastrointestinal tract functions again. Then eat a well-balanced, high-protein diet to promote healing.

CALL YOUR DOCTOR IF

Any of the following occurs:
- Nausea or vomiting.
- Pain or throbbing sensation in the affected hand.
- Increased swelling, redness, drainage or bleeding in the surgical area.
- Signs of infection: headache, muscle aches, dizziness or a general ill feeling and fever.
- Nausea or vomiting.
- New, unexplained symptoms. Drugs used in treatment may produce side effects.

SURGERIES

HEART TRANSPLANT

GENERAL INFORMATION

DEFINITION—Replacement of a diseased heart with a healthy heart.

BODY PARTS INVOLVED—Diseased or abnormal heart; healthy heart from donor.

REASONS FOR SURGERY
- Coronary-artery disease.
- Cardiomyopathy.
- Valvular-heart disease with congestive heart failure.
- Severe congenital heart disease.

SURGICAL RISK INCREASES WITH
- Adults over 60.
- Stress.
- Obesity.
- Smoking.
- Poor nutrition.
- Recent illness.
- Alcoholism or other chronic illness.
- Use of drugs such as: antihypertensives; muscle relaxants; tranquilizers; sleep inducers; insulin; sedatives; beta-adrenergic blockers; or cortisone.
- Use of mind-altering drugs, including: narcotics; psychedelics; hallucinogens; marijuana; sedatives; hypnotics; or cocaine.

WHAT TO EXPECT

WHO OPERATES—Cardiovascular surgeon.

WHERE PERFORMED—Hospital.

DIAGNOSTIC TESTS
- Before surgery: Blood and urine studies; studies of the immune system; EKG; cardiac catheterization; sonograms (see Glossary for all).
- During surgery: Cardiac monitoring (see Glossary).
- After surgery: Blood studies; EKG.

ANESTHESIA—General anesthesia by inhalation and injection, with an airway tube placed in the windpipe.

DESCRIPTION OF OPERATION
- A healthy heart is obtained from a donor who has died from disease (other than heart disease) or accident.
- An incision is made in the recipient's chest to expose the heart.
- A heart-lung machine sustains life while the diseased heart is cut free and removed.
- The donor heart is sewn into place. The aorta, pulmonary artery, superior vena cava and inferior vena cava are connected to the new heart.
- The skin is closed with sutures or clips, which usually can be removed about 1 week after surgery.

POSSIBLE COMPLICATIONS
- Excessive bleeding.
- Surgical-wound infection.
- Life-threatening general infections.
- Rejection of transplanted heart.

PROBABLE OUTCOME—A successful transplant prolongs life and improves the quality of life for patients who might otherwise have died. Allow about 6 weeks for recovery from surgery. Rejection of the transplant remains a risk indefinitely. If rejection can be controlled, the patient has a life expectancy of up to 10 years.

POSTOPERATIVE CARE

NOTE—This information is supplemental and should not replace your doctor's instructions.

GENERAL MEASURES
- A hard ridge should form along the incision. As it heals, the ridge will recede gradually.
- Use an electric heating pad, a heat lamp or a warm compress to relieve incisional pain.
- Bathe and shower as usual. You may wash the incision gently with mild unscented soap.
- Move legs often while resting in bed to decrease the chance of deep-vein blood clots.

MEDICATION
- Your doctor may prescribe:
  Pain relievers. Don't take prescription pain medication longer than 4 to 7 days. Use *only* as much as you need.
  Stool softeners to prevent constipation.
  Antibiotics to fight infection.
  Immunosuppressants to decrease the likelihood of rejection.
- You may use non-prescription drugs, such as acetaminophen, for minor pain.

ACTIVITY
- Resume work and normal activity as soon as possible. This reduces postoperative depression, which is common.
- Avoid vigorous exercise for 6 weeks after surgery. Resume exercise after consulting your doctor.
- Resume sexual relations when your doctor determines that healing is complete.

DIET—Your doctor will prescribe a diet.

CALL YOUR DOCTOR IF

- Pain, swelling, redness, drainage or bleeding increases in the surgical area.
- You develop signs of infection: headache, muscle aches, dizziness or a general ill feeling and fever.
- You experience new symptoms, such as: nausea; vomiting; constipation; abdominal swelling; heartbeat irregularities; or extreme fatigue.

HEART-VALVE REPLACEMENT

GENERAL INFORMATION

DEFINITION—Replacement of one or more diseased heart valves with mechanical valves.

BODY PARTS INVOLVED—Valves that separate major sections of the heart.

REASONS FOR SURGERY—Prevention of complications resulting from valvular heart disease, especially congestive heart failure and bacterial endocarditis.

SURGICAL RISK INCREASES WITH
- Adults over 60.
- Obesity.
- Smoking.
- Poor nutrition.
- Recent illness such as acute upper respiratory infection.
- Alcoholism or chronic illness.
- Use of drugs such as: antihypertensives; muscle relaxants; tranquilizers; sleep inducers; insulin; sedatives; beta-adrenergic blockers; or cortisone.
- Use of mind-altering drugs, including: narcotics; psychedelics; hallucinogens; marijuana; sedatives; hypnotics; or cocaine.

WHAT TO EXPECT

WHO OPERATES—Cardiovascular surgeon.

WHERE PERFORMED—Hospital.

DIAGNOSTIC TESTS
- Before surgery: Blood and urine studies; X-rays of kidneys and chest; EKG (see Glossary).
- During surgery: EKG monitor.
- After surgery: Blood studies.

ANESTHESIA—General anesthesia by inhalation and injection, with an airway tube placed in the windpipe.

DESCRIPTION OF OPERATION
- An incision is made in the chest, and the breastbone is divided. The chest is opened to expose the heart.
- A heart-lung machine circulates enough blood to sustain life.
- The diseased heart valves are located through delicate incisions made in the heart.
- Diseased valves are removed and replaced with mechanical valves.
- The incisions in the heart are closed with fine sutures, and the chest cavity is reconstructed with wire sutures. The skin is closed with lighter sutures or clips, which usually can be removed about 1 week after surgery.

POSSIBLE COMPLICATIONS
- Excessive bleeding.
- Surgical-wound infection.
- Failure of the heart to resume normal heartbeat (rare).
- Complications from blood used in the heart-lung machine, including hepatitis and AIDS (rare).
- Kidney damage.
- Heart attack; congestive heart failure; cardiac arrest; deep-vein blood clots; stroke; or breathing difficulties.

AVERAGE HOSPITAL STAY—20 days.

PROBABLE OUTCOME—Expect complete healing without complications. Allow about 4 weeks for recovery from surgery.

POSTOPERATIVE CARE

NOTE—This information is supplemental and should not replace your doctor's instructions.

GENERAL MEASURES
- A hard ridge should form along the incision. As it heals, the ridge will recede gradually.
- Bathe and shower as usual. You may wash the incision gently with mild unscented soap.
- Use an electric heating pad, a heat lamp or a warm compress to relieve incisional pain.
- Move legs often while in bed to decrease the chance of deep-vein blood clots.

MEDICATION—Your doctor may prescribe:
- Pain relievers. Don't take prescription pain medication longer than 4 to 7 days. Use *only* as much as you need.
- Stool softeners to prevent constipation.
- Antibiotics to fight infection.

ACTIVITY
- Resume work and normal activity as soon as possible to reduce postoperative depression, which is common.
- Resume driving 5 weeks after returning home.
- Resume sexual relations when your doctor determines that healing is complete.

DIET—Clear liquid diet until the gastrointestinal tract begins to function again. Then eat a well-balanced, high-protein diet to promote healing. After recovery, eat a low-fat, low-salt diet (see Appendices 8 and 9).

CALL YOUR DOCTOR IF

Any of the following occurs:
- Increased pain, swelling, redness, drainage or bleeding in the surgical area.
- Signs of infection: headache, muscle aches, dizziness or a general ill feeling and fever.
- Nausea, vomiting or constipation.
- Heartbeat irregularities.
- Decreased urine output.
- Sudden chest pain.

HEEL-SPUR REMOVAL

 GENERAL INFORMATION

DEFINITION—Removal of a heel spur.

BODY PARTS INVOLVED—Bottom of the heel bone.

REASONS FOR SURGERY—Relief of pain.

SURGICAL RISK INCREASES WITH—None expected.

 WHAT TO EXPECT

WHO OPERATES—General surgeon, orthopedist or podiatrist.

WHERE PERFORMED—Outpatient surgical facility or doctor's office.

DIAGNOSTIC TESTS
- Before surgery: Blood and urine studies; X-rays of both feet.
- After surgery: Blood studies; laboratory examination of removed tissue.

ANESTHESIA
- Local anesthesia by injection.
- Spinal anesthesia by injection.

DESCRIPTION OF OPERATION
- An incision is made over the spur.
- The spur is cut free and removed with special instruments.
- The skin is closed with sutures, which usually can be removed about 10 to 14 days after surgery.

POSSIBLE COMPLICATIONS
- Excessive bleeding.
- Surgical-wound infection.

AVERAGE HOSPITAL STAY—Usually none.

PROBABLE OUTCOME—Expect complete healing without complications. Allow about 6 weeks for recovery from surgery.

 POSTOPERATIVE CARE

NOTE—This information is supplemental and should not replace your doctor's instructions.

GENERAL MEASURES
- If the wound bleeds during the first 24 hours after surgery, press a clean tissue or cloth to it for 10 minutes.
- A hard ridge should form along the incision. As it heals, the ridge will recede gradually.
- Use an electric heating pad, a heat lamp or a warm compress to relieve incisional pain.
- Bathe and shower as usual. You may wash the incision gently with mild unscented soap.
- Use crutches or a cane to walk until your doctor determines that healing is complete.
- Between baths, keep wound dry with a bandage for the first 2 or 3 days after surgery. If a bandage gets wet, change it promptly.

MEDICATION
- Your doctor may prescribe:
  Pain relievers. Don't take prescription pain medication longer than 4 to 7 days. Use *only* as much as you need.
  Antibiotics to fight infection.
- You may use non-prescription drugs, such as acetaminophen, for minor pain.

ACTIVITY
- Avoid vigorous exercise for 3 months after surgery.
- Resume driving 1 week after returning home.

DIET—No special diet.

 CALL YOUR DOCTOR IF

- Pain, swelling, redness, drainage or bleeding increases in the surgical area.
- You develop signs of infection: headache, muscle aches, dizziness or a general ill feeling and fever.
- New, unexplained symptoms develop. Drugs used in treatment may produce side effects.

HEMORRHOID REMOVAL
(Hemorrhoidectomy)

GENERAL INFORMATION

DEFINITION—Removal of hemorrhoids.

BODY PARTS INVOLVED—Dilated veins around the anus or just inside the rectum.

REASONS FOR SURGERY
- Relief of excessive itching, pain or bleeding.
- Relief of a painful thrombosed hemorrhoid (hemorrhoid containing a blood clot).

SURGICAL RISK INCREASES WITH
- Adults over 60.
- Obesity.
- Smoking.
- Poor nutrition.
- Excess alcohol consumption.
- Chronic illness.

WHAT TO EXPECT

WHO OPERATES—Proctologist, general surgeon or family physician.

WHERE PERFORMED—Doctor's office, outpatient surgical facility or hospital.

DIAGNOSTIC TESTS
- Before surgery: Blood studies.
- After surgery: Blood studies.

ANESTHESIA
- Local anesthesia by injection.
- Spinal anesthesia by injection.
- General anesthesia by inhalation and injection, with an airway tube placed in the windpipe.

DESCRIPTION OF OPERATION
- The dilated veins from around the anus and inside the rectum are cut free and removed, with care taken not to damage the sphincter muscle. Sometimes anal muscles must be dilated vigorously to expose the hemorrhoids.
- The surgical area may be sewn closed or left open, and medicated gauze is used to cover it.

POSSIBLE COMPLICATIONS
- Excessive bleeding.
- Surgical-wound infection.
- Severe pain, especially with bowel movements.

AVERAGE HOSPITAL STAY—6 days.

PROBABLE OUTCOME—Curable in most patients, no matter what age. Allow about 2 weeks for recovery from surgery.

POSTOPERATIVE CARE

NOTE—This information is supplemental and should not replace your doctor's instructions.

GENERAL MEASURES
- Warm baths every 4 hours or so relieve pain and help keep the rectal area clean. Sit in warm water for 10 to 20 minutes as often as it feels good.
- Avoid heavy lifting. If not possible, learn proper body mechanics to reduce strain contributing to recurrence.
- Don't strain with bowel movements or urination.

MEDICATION—Your doctor may prescribe:
- Pain relievers. Don't take prescription pain medication longer than 4 to 7 days. Use *only* as much as you need.
- Stool softeners or laxatives to prevent constipation.
- Analgesic ointment to relieve pain.
- Vitamins to encourage healing.

ACTIVITY
- Resume driving 1 week after returning home.
- Resume sexual relations as soon as you wish.

DIET—No special diet. Increase dietary fiber and fluid intake to prevent constipation. Straining during bowel movements can cause hemorrhoids to recur.

CALL YOUR DOCTOR IF

- Pain, swelling, redness, drainage or bleeding increase in the surgical area.
- You develop signs of infection: headache, muscle aches, dizziness or a general ill feeling and fever.

HERNIA REPAIR, FEMORAL-
(Femoral Herniorrhaphy)

 GENERAL INFORMATION

DEFINITION—Closing or repairing a femoral hernia, an internal defect or weakness in the muscles of the abdominal wall. Sometimes, an intestine protrudes through the hernia defect, causing a noticeable bulge. If the intestine becomes trapped in the hernia defect, it is called an incarcerated hernia. If the intestine's blood supply is blocked by the hernia defect, it is called a strangulated hernia.

BODY PARTS INVOLVED—Groin (muscles and ligaments inside the lower abdomen next to the genitals); abdominal muscles; the opening allowing the femoral artery to pass from the abdomen to the leg.

REASONS FOR SURGERY
- Incarcerated hernia. This is a medical emergency.
- Strangulated hernia. This is a medical emergency.
- Uncomplicated hernia. Most surgeons recommend operating on a femoral hernia even if no symptoms are present, in order to prevent the serious complications of incarceration or strangulation.

SURGICAL RISK INCREASES WITH
- Adults over 60.
- Obesity.
- Smoking.
- Excess alcohol consumption.

 WHAT TO EXPECT

WHO OPERATES—General surgeon.

WHERE PERFORMED—Hospital or outpatient surgical facility.

DIAGNOSTIC TESTS
- Before surgery: Blood and urine studies.
- After surgery: Blood studies.

ANESTHESIA
- Spinal anesthesia by injection.
- Local anesthesia by injection.
- General anesthesia by inhalation and injection, with an airway tube placed in the windpipe.

DESCRIPTION OF OPERATION
- An incision is made in the groin area. The muscles and tissue are separated, and the hernia sac is opened.
- The contents of the hernia sac are replaced in the abdominal cavity.
- The groin wall is sewn shut. The skin is closed with sutures or clips, which usually can be removed about 1 week after surgery.

POSSIBLE COMPLICATIONS
- Recurrence of hernia.
- Damage to the testicle's blood or nerve supply, if the patient is male.

AVERAGE HOSPITAL STAY—1 to 4 days.

PROBABLE OUTCOME—Expect complete healing without complications. Male virility should not be affected. Allow about 6 weeks for recovery from surgery.

 POSTOPERATIVE CARE

NOTE—This information is supplemental and should not replace your doctor's instructions.

GENERAL MEASURES
- A hard ridge should form along the incision. As it heals, the ridge will recede gradually.
- Avoid heavy lifting.
- Don't strain with urination or bowel movements.

MEDICATION
- Your doctor may prescribe:
  Pain relievers. Don't take prescription pain medication longer than 4 to 7 days. Use *only* as much as you need.
  Antibiotics to fight infection.
- You may use non-prescription drugs, such as acetaminophen, for minor pain.

ACTIVITY
- Resume work and normal activity as soon as possible. This reduces postoperative depression and irritability, which are common.
- Resume sexual relations when able.

DIET—Clear liquid diet until the gastrointestinal tract functions again. Then eat a well-balanced, high-protein diet to promote healing. Increase dietary fiber and fluid intake to prevent constipation and straining during bowel movements.

 CALL YOUR DOCTOR IF

- Pain, swelling, redness, drainage or bleeding increases in the surgical area.
- You develop signs of infection: headache, muscle aches, dizziness or a general ill feeling and fever.
- A bulge appears in the groin, the thigh, scrotum, vaginal lips or surgical area.
- You become constipated.
- New, unexplained symptoms develop. Drugs used in treatment may produce side effects.

HERNIA REPAIR, HIATAL-
(Hiatal Herniorrhaphy)

 GENERAL INFORMATION

DEFINITION—Closure of a hiatal hernia, an abnormal weakness or opening in the diaphragm.

BODY PARTS INVOLVED—Lower esophagus; diaphragm; upper part of stomach.

REASONS FOR SURGERY
- Relief of painful symptoms.
- Prevention of the stomach from shifting upward into the chest cavity.
- Prevention of the stomach from spilling digestive acid into the esophagus, causing infection and pain.

SURGICAL RISK INCREASES WITH
- Adults over 60.
- Newborns and infants.
- Obesity or poor nutrition.
- Smoking.
- Recent or chronic illness.
- Use of drugs such as: antihypertensives; muscle relaxants; tranquilizers; sleep inducers; insulin; sedatives; beta-adrenergic blockers; or cortisone.
- Alcoholism or use of mind-altering drugs.

 WHAT TO EXPECT

WHO OPERATES—General surgeon.

WHERE PERFORMED—Hospital.

DIAGNOSTIC TESTS
- Before surgery: Blood and urine studies; X-rays of chest and upper gastrointestinal tract; EKG (see Glossary).
- After surgery: Blood studies.

ANESTHESIA—General anesthesia by inhalation and injection, with an airway tube placed in the windpipe.

DESCRIPTION OF OPERATION
- An incision is made in the abdomen or the chest.
- The hernia in the diaphragm is located and closed with sutures.
- The top of the stomach is wrapped around the lower part of the esophagus and sutured in place. A prosthesis of silicone may be placed around the top of the stomach and sewn in place. This prevents the stomach from sliding into the chest cavity.
- Sometimes, the vagus nerve is removed to reduce the amount of acid the stomach produces.
- The skin is closed with sutures or clips, which usually can be removed about 1 week after surgery.

POSSIBLE COMPLICATIONS—Excessive bleeding or surgical-wound infection.

AVERAGE HOSPITAL STAY—5 to 7 days.

PROBABLE OUTCOME—Expect complete healing without complications. Allow about 6 weeks for recovery from surgery.

 POSTOPERATIVE CARE

NOTE—This information is supplemental and should not replace your doctor's instructions.

GENERAL MEASURES
- A hard ridge should form along the incision. As it heals, the ridge will recede gradually.
- Use an electric heating pad, a heat lamp or a warm compress to relieve incisional pain.
- Move legs often while resting in bed to decrease the likelihood of deep-vein blood clots.
- Bathe and shower as usual. You may wash the incision gently with mild unscented soap.

MEDICATION
- Your doctor may prescribe:
  Pain relievers. Don't take prescription pain medication longer than 4 to 7 days. Use *only* as much as you need.
  Stool softeners to prevent constipation.
  Antibiotics to fight infection.
- You may use non-prescription drugs, such as acetaminophen, for minor pain.

ACTIVITY
- Resume work and normal activity as soon as possible to reduce postoperative depression, which is common.
- Avoid heavy lifting for 6 weeks after surgery. Learn proper body mechanics to avoid strain contributing to recurrence.
- Avoid vigorous exercise for 6 weeks after surgery. Resume driving 5 weeks after returning home.
- Don't strain with urination or bowel movements.

DIET—Clear liquid diet until the gastrointestinal tract begins to function again. Then eat a well-balanced, high-protein diet to promote healing. Avoid coffee, tea, cocoa, cola drinks, alcoholic beverages and any food or spice that aggravates symptoms.

 CALL YOUR DOCTOR IF

- Pain, swelling, redness, drainage or bleeding increase in the surgical area.
- You develop signs of infection: headache, muscle aches, dizziness or a general ill feeling and fever.
- You experience nausea, vomiting, constipation or abdominal swelling.
- You vomit blood or have black, tarry stools.

HERNIA REPAIR, INCISIONAL-
(Incisional Herniorrhaphy)

 GENERAL INFORMATION

DEFINITION—Reinsertion of the intestine in the abdominal cavity. Sometimes, the intestine protrudes through a weak area in the abdomen, especially around a previously repaired hernia or abdominal incision. This protrusion causes a noticeable bulge. Surgery reinserts the intestine in its proper place.

BODY PARTS INVOLVED—Abdomen and intestines, especially where previous surgery has been performed.

REASONS FOR SURGERY
● Possible blockage of blood vessels in the gastrointestinal tract.
● Painful lump in the abdomen.

SURGICAL RISK INCREASES WITH
● Obesity.
● Smoking.
● Excess alcohol consumption.
● Use of drugs such as cortisone, diuretics or antihypertensives.
● Recent illness, especially respiratory illness or chronic cough.

 WHAT TO EXPECT

WHO OPERATES—General surgeon.

WHERE PERFORMED—Outpatient surgical facility or hospital.

DIAGNOSTIC TESTS
● Before surgery: Blood and urine studies; X-rays of the abdomen.
● After surgery: Blood studies.

ANESTHESIA—Spinal anesthesia by injection.

DESCRIPTION OF OPERATION
● An incision is made in the abdomen (at the old scar if one exists). The abdominal muscles are examined for the protruding intestine.
● The intestine is replaced in the abdominal cavity. Frequently, plastic mesh is used to strengthen the repair. The abdominal wall is reconstructed to prevent further protrusion.
● A drain is usually left in place.
● The skin is closed with sutures or clips, which usually can be removed about 1 week after surgery.

POSSIBLE COMPLICATIONS
● Surgical-wound infection.
● Inadvertent injury to intestinal tract.
● Recurrent hernia (rare).

AVERAGE HOSPITAL STAY—2 to 4 days.

PROBABLE OUTCOME—Curable in most patients, no matter what age. Allow about 2 weeks for recovery from surgery.

 POSTOPERATIVE CARE

NOTE—This information is supplemental and should not replace your doctor's instructions.

GENERAL MEASURES
● A hard ridge should form along the incision. As it heals, the ridge will recede gradually.
● Bathe and shower as usual. You may wash the incision gently with mild unscented soap.
● Use an electric heating pad, a heat lamp or a warm compress to relieve incisional pain.

MEDICATION
● Your doctor may prescribe:
Pain relievers. Don't take prescription pain medicine longer than 4 to 7 days. Use *only* as much as you need.
Antibiotics to fight infection.
● You may use non-prescription drugs, such as acetaminophen, for minor pain.

ACTIVITY
● Resume sexual relations 1 week after returning home.
● Resume driving 1 week after the surgical scar heals.
● Avoid heavy lifting for 6 weeks after surgery. Learn proper body mechanics to reduce strain contributing to recurrence after recovery.
● Don't strain with bowel movements or urination.

DIET—Clear liquid diet until the gastrointestinal tract begins to function again. Then eat a well-balanced, high-protein diet to promote healing.

 CALL YOUR DOCTOR IF

● Pain, swelling, redness, drainage or bleeding occurs in the surgical area.
● Your temperature rises to 101F (38.3C).
● You develop signs of infection: headache, muscle aches, dizziness or a general ill feeling and fever.
● You become constipated.
● New, unexplained symptoms develop. Drugs used in treatment may produce side effects.

HERNIA REPAIR, INGUINAL-
(Inguinal Herniorrhaphy)

 GENERAL INFORMATION

DEFINITION—Closing or repairing an inguinal hernia, an internal defect or weakness in the muscular layer of the abdominal wall. Sometimes an intestine protrudes through the hernia defect, causing a noticeable bulge. If the intestine becomes trapped in the hernia defect, it is called an incarcerated hernia. If the hernia defect blocks the intestine's blood supply, it is called a strangulated hernia.

BODY PARTS INVOLVED—Groin muscles and ligaments inside the lower abdomen next to the genitals; abdominal muscles.

REASONS FOR SURGERY
- Incarcerated hernia. This is a medical emergency.
- Strangulated hernia. This is a medical emergency.
- Uncomplicated hernia. Most doctors recommend operating on a hernia even if no hernia symptoms are present to prevent the serious complications of incarceration or strangulation.

SURGICAL RISK INCREASES WITH
- Adults over 60.
- Obesity.
- Smoking.
- Family history of hernias.
- Excess alcohol consumption.

 WHAT TO EXPECT

WHO OPERATES—General surgeon.

WHERE PERFORMED—Hospital or outpatient surgical facility.

DIAGNOSTIC TESTS
- Before surgery: Blood and urine studies.
- After surgery: Blood studies, if bleeding was significant during surgery.

ANESTHESIA
- Spinal anesthesia by injection.
- Local anesthesia by injection.
- General anesthesia by inhalation and injection, with an airway tube placed in the windpipe.

DESCRIPTION OF OPERATION
- An incision is made in the abdomen. The abdominal muscles are separated, and the peritoneal cavity is opened.
- The hernia is located and repaired or closed. The skin is closed with sutures or staples, which usually can be removed about 1 week after surgery.

POSSIBLE COMPLICATIONS
- Recurrent hernia.
- Surgical-wound infection.
- Damage to the testicle's blood supply or nerve supply.

AVERAGE HOSPITAL STAY
- For outpatient surgery: none (without complications).
- If hospitalized: Age 0-17, 1 to 2 days.
                    Over 17, 2 to 4 days.

PROBABLE OUTCOME—Curable in most patients, no matter what age. Male virility should not be affected. Allow about 6 weeks for recovery from surgery.

 POSTOPERATIVE CARE

NOTE: This information is supplemental and should not replace your doctor's instructions.

GENERAL MEASURES
- A hard ridge should form along the incision. As it heals, the ridge will recede gradually.
- Avoid heavy lifting for 6 weeks after surgery. Learn proper body mechanics to reduce strain contributing to recurrence after recovery.
- Don't strain with bowel movements or urination.

MEDICATION
- Your doctor may prescribe:
  Pain relievers. Don't take prescription pain medication longer than 4 to 7 days. Use *only* as much as you need.
  Stool softeners to prevent constipation.
  Antibiotics to fight infection.
- You may use non-prescription drugs, such as acetaminophen, for minor pain.

ACTIVITY
- Resume work and normal activity as soon as possible to reduce postoperative depression, which is common.
- Resume sexual relations 2 weeks after returning home.
- Resume driving 2 weeks after returning home.

DIET—Clear liquid diet until the gastrointestinal tract begins to function again. Then eat a well-balanced diet that is high in protein to promote healing and high in fiber and fluids to prevent constipation.

 CALL YOUR DOCTOR IF

- Pain, swelling, redness, drainage or bleeding increase in the surgical area.
- A bulge appears in the groin, scrotum, vaginal lips or surgical area.
- You become constipated.

SURGERIES

HERNIA REPAIR, UMBILICAL-

GENERAL INFORMATION

DEFINITION—Closure of an umbilical hernia, a weak section of muscle that allows the small intestine to protrude prominently near the navel (umbilicus). This is usually repaired in infancy, but it can be repaired into adulthood.

BODY PARTS INVOLVED—Abdominal muscular wall around the navel.

REASONS FOR SURGERY
- Improved appearance.
- Relief of pain.
- Prevention of gangrene in the intestines.

SURGICAL RISK INCREASES WITH
- Newborns and infants.
- Obesity.
- Smoking.
- Poor nutrition.
- Recent or chronic illness.
- Alcoholism.
- Use of drugs such as: antihypertensives; muscle relaxants; tranquilizers; sleep inducers; insulin; sedatives; beta-adrenergic blockers; or cortisone.

WHAT TO EXPECT

WHO OPERATES—General surgeon or pediatric surgeon.

WHERE PERFORMED—Hospital or outpatient surgical facility.

DIAGNOSTIC TESTS
- Before surgery: Blood and urine studies.
- After surgery: Blood studies.

ANESTHESIA—General anesthesia by inhalation and injection, with an airway tube placed in the windpipe.

DESCRIPTION OF OPERATION
- An incision is made slightly above or below the navel.
- An incision is made in the peritoneum to open the peritoneal cavity. The contents of the hernia sac are located and replaced in the abdominal cavity. The peritoneum is closed.
- The large abdominal muscle is pulled over the defect. The membrane covering the muscle is overlapped and tied to close the defect.
- The skin is closed with sutures or clips, which usually can be removed about 10 days after surgery.

POSSIBLE COMPLICATIONS
- Excessive bleeding.
- Surgical-wound infection.
- Incisional hernia.

AVERAGE HOSPITAL STAY—0 to 1 day.

PROBABLE OUTCOME—Expect complete healing without complications. Allow about 3 weeks for recovery from surgery.

POSTOPERATIVE CARE

NOTE—This information is supplemental and should not replace your doctor's instructions.

GENERAL MEASURES
- If the wound bleeds during the first 24 hours after surgery, press a clean tissue or cloth to it for 10 minutes.
- A hard ridge should form along the incision. As it heals, the ridge will recede gradually.
- Use a warm compress to relieve incisional pain.
- You may wash the incision gently with mild unscented soap.
- Between baths, keep the wound dry with a bandage for the first 2 or 3 days after surgery. If a bandage gets wet, change it promptly.
- Apply non-prescription antibiotic ointment to wounds before applying new bandages.

MEDICATION
- Your doctor may prescribe:
  Pain relievers. Don't use prescription pain medication longer than 4 to 7 days. Use *only* as much as you need.
  Stool softeners to prevent constipation.
  Antibiotics to fight infection.
- You may use non-prescription drugs, such as acetaminophen, for minor pain.

ACTIVITY—Vigorous exercise should be avoided for 4 weeks after surgery.

DIET—Clear liquid diet until the gastrointestinal tract functions again. Then a well-balanced, high-protein diet promotes healing.

CALL YOUR DOCTOR IF

Any of the following occur:
- Increased pain, swelling, redness, drainage or bleeding increases in the surgical area.
- Signs of infection: headache, muscle aches, dizziness or a general ill feeling and fever.
- Nausea, vomiting, constipation or abdominal swelling.
- New, unexplained symptoms. Drugs used in treatment may produce side effects.

HYDROCELECTOMY

GENERAL INFORMATION

DEFINITION—Removal of a hydrocele, fluid that has collected in a small sac usually on the testicle or in the membrane covering the testicle. Hydroceles frequently occur in infants, but may also occur in adults.

BODY PARTS INVOLVED—Scrotum; spermatic cord; membrane covering the testicle (tunica vaginalis); blood vessels and nerves connected to the scrotum.

REASONS FOR SURGERY
- In infants: completion of the repair of a congenital inguinal hernia, which frequently accompanies a congenital hydrocele.
- In adults: removal of an uncomfortable and unsightly scrotal cyst that may conceal a tumor in the testicle.

SURGICAL RISK INCREASES WITH
- Obesity.
- Chronic or recent illness.

WHAT TO EXPECT

WHO OPERATES—General surgeon or urologist.

WHERE PERFORMED—Hospital or outpatient surgical facility.

DIAGNOSTIC TESTS
- Before surgery: Blood and urine studies.
- After surgery: Usually none.

ANESTHESIA
- General anesthesia by inhalation and injection, with an airway tube placed in the windpipe in infants.
- Local anesthesia by injection.
- Spinal anesthesia by injection (sometimes) in older children and adults.

DESCRIPTION OF OPERATION
- An incision is made in the scrotum over the testicle.
- The hydrocele is located and cut free from the scrotal contents.
- The hydrocele is incised, and the fluid inside it is drained. The skin edges of the hydrocele are tucked under and sewn together to prevent refilling.
- The scrotal contents are replaced. The skin is closed with fine suture material that will be absorbed by the body.

POSSIBLE COMPLICATIONS
- Excessive bleeding.
- Surgical-wound infection.
- Damaged blood supply to the testicle.
- Twisting of the testicle.

AVERAGE HOSPITAL STAY—1 to 2 days.

PROBABLE OUTCOME—Expect complete healing without complications. Allow about 2 weeks for recovery from surgery.

POSTOPERATIVE CARE

NOTE—This information is supplemental and should not replace your doctor's instructions.

GENERAL MEASURES
- A hard ridge should form along the incision. As it heals, the ridge will recede gradually.
- Use an electric heating pad, a heat lamp or a warm compress to relieve incisional pain.
- Bathe and shower as usual. You may wash the incision gently with mild unscented soap.
- Children and adults should wear an athletic supporter for 3 to 6 weeks after surgery. Infants should wear double diapers.

MEDICATION
- Your doctor may prescribe pain relievers. Don't take prescription pain medication longer than 4 to 7 days. Use *only* as much as you need.
- You may use non-prescription drugs, such as acetaminophen, for minor pain.

ACTIVITY
- Avoid vigorous exercise for 6 weeks after surgery.
- Resume driving 1 week after returning home.
- Resume sexual relations when your doctor determines that healing is complete.

DIET—Clear liquid diet until the gastrointestinal tract begins to function again. Then eat a well-balanced, high-protein diet to promote healing.

CALL YOUR DOCTOR IF

- Pain, swelling, redness, drainage or bleeding increases in the surgical area.
- You develop signs of infection: headache, muscle aches, dizziness or a general ill feeling and fever.
- You experience nausea or vomiting.

HYMEN, OPENING OR ENLARGEMENT OF
(Hymenotomy)

 GENERAL INFORMATION

DEFINITION—Opening or enlargement of the hymen.

BODY PARTS INVOLVED—Hymen, membrane that partially or completely blocks the opening to the vagina.

REASONS FOR SURGERY
- Closed hymen that does not allow normal vaginal secretions to escape. The closed hymen may lead to swelling of the vagina, which may cause difficulty with urination and defecation.
- Hymen that does not allow menstrual blood to escape.
- Thickened hymen that causes discomfort with sexual intercourse or prevents normal insertion of the penis.

SURGICAL RISK INCREASES WITH
- Obesity.
- Smoking.
- Poor nutrition.
- Recent or chronic illness.
- Use of drugs such as: antihypertensives; muscle relaxants; tranquilizers; sleep inducers; insulin; sedatives; beta-adrenergic blockers; or cortisone.
- Use of mind-altering drugs, including: narcotics; psychedelics; hallucinogens; marijuana; sedatives; hypnotics; or cocaine.

 WHAT TO EXPECT

WHO OPERATES—Family doctor, general surgeon or obstetrician-gynecologist.

WHERE PERFORMED—Doctor's office or outpatient surgical facility.

DIAGNOSTIC TESTS—Blood and urine studies and pelvic examination before surgery.

ANESTHESIA
- Local anesthesia by topical application.
- Local anesthesia by injection.

DESCRIPTION OF OPERATION—After the anesthesia has taken effect, the hymen is cut with a scalpel quickly, simply and without discomfort.

POSSIBLE COMPLICATIONS
- Excessive bleeding.
- Surgical-wound infection.

AVERAGE HOSPITAL STAY—None.

PROBABLE OUTCOME—Expect complete healing without complications. Allow about 5 days for recovery from surgery.

 POSTOPERATIVE CARE

NOTE—This information is supplemental and should not replace your doctor's instructions.

GENERAL MEASURES
- Use an electric heating pad, a heat lamp or a warm compress to relieve pelvic pain.
- Bathe and shower as usual.
- Take 15- to 30-minute hot baths to relieve discomfort several times daily for the first 2 to 4 days after surgery.
- After bowel movements, wipe the rectal area with moist toilet paper *away* from the vagina.

MEDICATION
- Your doctor may prescribe:
  Pain relievers. Don't take prescription pain medication longer than 4 to 7 days. Use *only* as much as you need.
  Stool softeners to prevent constipation.
- You may use non-prescription drugs, such as acetaminophen, for minor pain.

ACTIVITY—No restrictions.

DIET—No special diet.

 CALL YOUR DOCTOR IF

- Pain, swelling, redness, drainage or bleeding increases in the surgical area.
- You develop signs of infection: headache, muscle aches, dizziness or a general ill feeling and fever.

HYPOSPADIAS REPAIR & URETHROPLASTY

 ## GENERAL INFORMATION

DEFINITION—Creation of a new urethra to correct hypospadias, a congenital disorder in which the urethra opening is in an abnormal location on the penis. Surgery is usually done in infancy or early childhood.

BODY PARTS INVOLVED—Urethra.

REASONS FOR SURGERY
- Prevention of urinary-tract infections.
- Establishment of sexual function.
- Correction of abnormal urination patterns.

SURGICAL RISK INCREASES WITH
- Obesity.
- Poor nutrition.
- Recent or chronic illness.

 ## WHAT TO EXPECT

WHO OPERATES—Urologist.

WHERE PERFORMED—Hospital.

DIAGNOSTIC TESTS
- Before surgery: Blood and urine studies.
- After surgery: Blood studies; laboratory examination of removed tissue.

ANESTHESIA—General anesthesia by inhalation and injection, with an airway tube placed in the windpipe.

DESCRIPTION OF OPERATION
- An incision is made over the abnormal opening of the urethra.
- An instrument is passed through the urethra and extended along its full length. Abnormal scar tissue is cut free and removed. A new urethra is fashioned from existing tissue and sewn around a catheter, which will remain in place until healing is complete.
- After healing, the catheter is removed under anesthesia.
- The skin is closed with sutures that will be absorbed by the body.

POSSIBLE COMPLICATIONS
- Excessive bleeding.
- Surgical-wound infection.
- Scarring of urethra.

AVERAGE HOSPITAL STAY—1 week.

PROBABLE OUTCOME—Expect complete healing without complications. Allow about 3 months for recovery from surgery.

 ## POSTOPERATIVE CARE

NOTE—This information is supplemental and should not replace your doctor's instructions.

GENERAL MEASURES
- A ridge should form along the incision. As it heals, the ridge will recede gradually.
- Use an electric heating pad, a heat lamp or a warm compress to relieve incisional pain.
- Bathe and shower as usual. You may wash the incision gently with mild unscented soap.

MEDICATION
- Your doctor may prescribe:
  Pain relievers. Don't take prescription pain medication longer than 4 to 7 days. Use *only* as much as you need.
  Antibiotics to fight infection.
- You may use non-prescription drugs, such as acetaminophen, for minor pain.

ACTIVITY—Vigorous exercise should be avoided for 6 weeks after surgery.

DIET—No special diet.

 ## CALL YOUR DOCTOR IF

- Pain, swelling, redness, drainage or bleeding increases in the surgical area.
- Urination is painful or difficult.
- You develop signs of infection: headache, muscle aches, dizziness or a general ill feeling and fever.
- You experience nausea or vomiting.
- New, unexplained symptoms develop. Drugs used in treatment may produce side effects.

HYSTERECTOMY (ABDOMINAL) WITH REMOVAL OF TUBES & OVARIES
(Abdominal Hysterectomy with Bilateral Salpingo-Oophorectomy)

 GENERAL INFORMATION

DEFINITION—Removal of the uterus, cervix, Fallopian tubes and ovaries through an incision in the abdomen.

BODY PARTS INVOLVED—Uterus; cervix; Fallopian tubes; ovaries; vagina.

REASONS FOR SURGERY
- Uterus:
  Cancer or suspected cancer; fibroid tumors; chronic bleeding; prolapsed (dropped) uterus; endometriosis; chronic pelvic infection; severe menstrual pain; or voluntary sterilization.
- Fallopian tubes and ovaries:
  Cancer or suspected cancer of the ovaries; precancerous or twisted ovarian cysts; ovarian pregnancy; ovarian abscess; damage to the ovaries from severe endometriosis.

SURGICAL RISK INCREASES WITH
- Obesity.
- Smoking.
- Iron-deficiency anemia; heart or lung disease; or diabetes mellitus.
- Use of drugs such as: cortisone; antihypertensives; diuretics; or beta-adrenergic blockers.
- Use of mind-altering drugs.

 WHAT TO EXPECT

WHO OPERATES—General surgeon or obstetrician-gynecologist.

WHERE PERFORMED—Hospital.

DIAGNOSTIC TESTS
- Before surgery: Blood and urine studies; X-rays of abdomen and kidneys; dilatation and curettage of the uterus (D & C.)
- After surgery: Blood studies.

ANESTHESIA—General anesthesia by inhalation and injection, with an airway tube placed in the windpipe.

DESCRIPTION OF OPERATION
- An incision is made in the abdomen.
- The abdominal organs are examined .
- The uterus, cervix, Fallopian tubes and ovaries are cut free and removed.
- The vagina is closed with sutures at its deeper end.
- The surgical wound is closed in layers.
- A catheter may remain in the bladder for several days.

POSSIBLE COMPLICATIONS
- Excessive bleeding.
- Surgical-wound Infection.
- Inadvertent injury to the bladder or ureters.

AVERAGE HOSPITAL STAY—5 to 7.

PROBABLE OUTCOME—The vagina will be shortened slightly. This should cause no lasting problem. Expect permanent sterility. Allow about 6 weeks for recovery from surgery.

 POSTOPERATIVE CARE

NOTE—This information is supplemental and should not replace your doctor's instructions.

GENERAL MEASURES
- Ignore sutures that fall out of the vagina.
- Use an electric heating pad, a heat lamp or a warm compress to relieve incisional pain.
- Bathe and shower as usual. You may wash the incision gently with mild unscented soap.
- Use sanitary napkins—not tampons—to absorb blood.

MEDICATION—Your doctor may prescribe:
- Pain relievers. Don't take prescription pain medication longer than 4 to 7 days.
- Supplemental female hormones, unless there are reasons why you should not take them. Ask your doctor.

ACTIVITY
- Resume work and normal activity as soon as possible to reduce postoperative depression, which is common.
- Resume driving 2 weeks after returning home.
- Resume sexual relations when able.

DIET—Clear liquid diet until the gastrointestinal tract functions again. Then eat a well-balanced, high-protein diet to promote healing.

 CALL YOUR DOCTOR IF

Any of the following occurs:
- Vaginal bleeding that soaks more than 1 pad per hour.
- Frequent urge to urinate or excessive vaginal discharge that persists longer than 1 month.
- Increased pain or swelling in the surgical area.
- Signs of infection: headache, muscle aches, dizziness or a general ill feeling and fever.

HYSTERECTOMY (ABDOMINAL) WITHOUT REMOVAL OF FALLOPIAN TUBES & OVARIES
(Abdominal Hysterectomy without Bilateral Salpingo-Oophorectomy)

 GENERAL INFORMATION

DEFINITION—Removal of the uterus and cervix through an incision in the abdomen. This surgery leaves the Fallopian tubes and ovaries in place.

BODY PARTS INVOLVED—Uterus; cervix; vagina.

REASONS FOR SURGERY
- Cancer or suspected cancer of the uterus.
- Fibroid tumors.
- Chronic bleeding from the uterus.
- Chronic pelvic infection.
- Endometriosis.
- Prolapsed (dropped) uterus.
- Voluntary sterilization.

SURGICAL RISK INCREASES WITH
- Obesity.
- Smoking.
- Iron-deficiency anemia; chronic heart or lung disorders; or diabetes mellitus.
- Use of drugs such as: cortisone; antihypertensives; diuretics; or beta-adrenergic blockers.
- Use of abused drugs, including: narcotics; psychedelics; hallucinogens; marijuana; sedatives; hypnotics; or cocaine.

 WHAT TO EXPECT

WHO OPERATES—General surgeon or obstetrician-gynecologist.

WHERE PERFORMED—Hospital.

DIAGNOSTIC TESTS
- Before surgery: Blood and urine studies; X-rays of abdomen and kidneys; dilatation and curettage of the uterus (D & C).
- After surgery: Blood studies.

ANESTHESIA—General anesthesia by inhalation and injection, with an airway tube placed in the windpipe.

DESCRIPTION OF OPERATION
- An incision is made in the abdomen.
- The abdominal organs are examined.
- The uterus and cervix are cut free and removed.
- The vagina is closed with sutures at its deeper end.
- The surgical wound is closed in layers.
- A catheter may remain in the bladder for several days.

POSSIBLE COMPLICATIONS
- Excessive bleeding.
- Surgical-wound infection.
- Inadvertent injury to blood supply to the ovaries.
- Inadvertent injury to the bladder or ureters.

AVERAGE HOSPITAL STAY—6 to 8 days.

PROBABLE OUTCOME—The vagina will be shortened slightly. This should cause no lasting problem. Expect permanent sterility. Allow 6 weeks for recovery from surgery.

 POSTOPERATIVE CARE

NOTE—This information is supplemental and should not replace your doctor's instructions.

GENERAL MEASURES
- Ignore sutures that fall out of the vagina.
- A hard ridge should form along the incision. As it heals, the ridge will recede gradually.
- Use an electric heating pad, a heat lamp or a warm compress to relieve incisional pain.
- Bathe and shower as usual. You may wash the incision gently with mild unscented soap.
- Use sanitary napkins—not tampons—to absorb blood.

MEDICATION—Your doctor may prescribe:
- Pain relievers. Don't take prescription pain medication longer than 4 to 7 days. Use *only* as much as you need.
- Vaginal creams or medicated douches, if vaginal discharge develops an unpleasant odor.

ACTIVITY
- Resume work and normal activity as soon as possible to reduce postoperative depression, which is common.
- Resume driving 15 days after returning home.
- Resume sexual relations when able.

DIET—Clear liquid diet until the gastrointestinal tract functions again. Then eat a well-balanced, high-protein diet to promote healing.

 CALL YOUR DOCTOR IF

Any of the following occurs:
- Vaginal bleeding that soaks more than 1 pad per hour.
- Signs of infection: headache, muscle aches, dizziness or a general ill feeling and fever.
- Excessive vaginal discharge persists beyond 1 month after surgery.
- Abdominal pain or swelling.

HYSTERECTOMY (VAGINAL) WITH BLADDER/RECTAL REPAIR
(Vaginal Hysterectomy & Anterior/Posterior Colporrhaphy)

 GENERAL INFORMATION

DEFINITION—Removal of the uterus, including cervix, through an incision made in the deepest recesses of the vagina. This surgery is frequently accompanied by plastic surgery (colporrhaphy) to repair bladder muscles and rectal muscles.

BODY PARTS INVOLVED—Uterus; cervix; bladder muscles; rectal muscles; vagina.

REASONS FOR SURGERY—Strengthening of the bladder muscles, rectal muscles and pelvic ligaments.

SURGICAL RISK INCREASES WITH
- Obesity.
- Smoking.
- Iron deficiency anemia, heart or lung disease, or diabetes mellitus.
- Use of drugs such as: antihypertensives; muscle relaxants; tranquilizers; sleep inducers; insulin; sedatives; beta-adrenergic blockers; or cortisone.
- Use of mind-altering drugs, including: narcotics; psychedelics; hallucinogens; marijuana; sedatives; hypnotics; or cocaine.

 WHAT TO EXPECT

WHO OPERATES—General surgeon or obstetrician-gynecologist.

WHERE PERFORMED—Hospital.

DIAGNOSTIC TESTS
- Before surgery: Blood and urine studies; X-rays of abdomen and kidneys; dilatation and curettage of the uterus (D & C).
- After surgery: Blood studies.

ANESTHESIA
- General anesthesia by inhalation and injection, with an airway tube placed in the windpipe.
- Spinal anesthesia by injection.

DESCRIPTION OF OPERATION
- The vaginal walls are carefully separated from the bladder and rectal muscles.
- The deepest recesses of the vagina are opened. The uterus and cervix are cut free and removed. The rear part of the vagina is closed with sutures.
- The bladder muscles and rectal muscles are sewn into their proper position.
- A small catheter is left in the bladder. The catheter will remain in for 7 to 10 days.

POSSIBLE COMPLICATIONS
- Excessive bleeding.
- Surgical-wound infection.
- Muscles supporting bladder and rectum may require a second repair.

AVERAGE HOSPITAL STAY—8 to 9 days.

PROBABLE OUTCOME—The vagina will be shortened somewhat after surgery. This should cause no lasting problem. Expect permanent sterility. Allow about 6 weeks for recovery from surgery.

 POSTOPERATIVE CARE

NOTE—This information is supplemental and should not replace your doctor's instructions.

GENERAL MEASURES
- Ignore sutures that fall out of the vagina.
- Don't use tampons for bleeding—they may cause infection. Use sanitary pads instead.

MEDICATION—Your doctor may prescribe:
- Pain relievers. Don't take prescription pain medication longer than 4 to 7 days. Use *only* as much as you need.
- Vaginal creams or medicated douches, if vaginal discharge develops a bad odor.

ACTIVITY
- Resume work and normal activity as soon as possible to reduce postoperative depression, which is common.
- Resume driving 15 days after returning home.
- Resume sexual relations when your doctor determines that healing is complete.

DIET—Clear liquid diet until the gastrointestinal tract functions again. Then eat a well-balanced, high-protein diet to promote healing.

 CALL YOUR DOCTOR IF

Any of the following occurs:
- Increased vaginal swelling, bleeding or pain (soaking more than 1 pad an hour).
- Signs of infection: headache, muscle aches, dizziness or a general ill feeling and fever.
- Frequent urination that persists longer than 1 month.
- Excessive vaginal discharge that persists longer than 1 month.
- Abdominal swelling or pain.

HYSTERECTOMY (VAGINAL) WITH REMOVAL OF TUBES & OVARIES & BLADDER/RECTAL REPAIR
(Vaginal Hysterectomy with Bilateral Salpingo-Oophorectomy & Anterior/Posterior Colporrhaphy)

 GENERAL INFORMATION

DEFINITION—Removal of the uterus, cervix, Fallopian tubes and ovaries through an incision in the deepest recesses of the vagina.

This surgery is frequently accompanied by colporrhaphy, a plastic surgery to repair weakened bladder and rectal muscles.

BODY PARTS INVOLVED—Bladder muscles; rectal muscles; uterus; cervix; Fallopian tubes; ovaries; vagina.

REASONS FOR SURGERY—Strengthening of the bladder muscles, rectal muscles and pelvic ligaments.

SURGICAL RISK INCREASES WITH
- Obesity.
- Smoking.
- Iron-deficiency anemia; heart or lung disease; or diabetes mellitus.
- Use of drugs, such as: cortisone; antihypertensives; diuretics; or beta-adrenergic blockers.
- Use of mind-altering drugs.

 WHAT TO EXPECT

WHO OPERATES—General surgeon or obstetrician-gynecologist.

WHERE PERFORMED—Hospital.

DIAGNOSTIC TESTS
- Before surgery: Blood and urine studies; X-rays of abdomen and kidneys; dilatation and curettage of the uterus (D & C).
- After surgery: Blood studies.

ANESTHESIA
- Spinal anesthesia by injection.
- General anesthesia by inhalation and injection, with an airway tube placed in the windpipe.

DESCRIPTION OF OPERATION
- The vaginal walls are separated from the bladder muscles and rectal muscles.
- The deepest recesses of the vagina are opened. The cervix, uterus, Fallopian tubes and ovaries are cut free and removed. The rear part of the vagina is closed with sutures.
- The bladder muscles and rectal muscles are sewn back in place. Supporting tissue is repaired.
- A small catheter is left in the bladder for 7 to 10 days.

POSSIBLE COMPLICATIONS
- Excessive bleeding.
- Surgical-wound infection.
- Muscles supporting bladder and rectum may require a second repair.
- Inadvertent damage to bladder, rectum or ureters.

AVERAGE HOSPITAL STAY—5 to 7 days.

PROBABLE OUTCOME—The vagina will be shortened slightly. This should cause no lasting problem. Expect permanent sterility. Allow about 6 weeks for recovery from surgery.

 POSTOPERATIVE CARE

NOTE—This information is supplemental and should not replace your doctor's instructions.

GENERAL MEASURES
- Ignore sutures that fall out of the vagina.
- Use sanitary napkins—not tampons—to absorb blood.

MEDICATION—Your doctor may prescribe:
- Pain relievers.
- Vaginal creams or medicated douches if vaginal discharge develops an unpleasant odor.

ACTIVITY
- Resume work and normal activity as soon as possible to reduce postoperative depression, which is common.
- Resume driving 2 weeks after returning home.
- Resume sexual relations as soon as able.

DIET—Clear liquid diet until the gastrointestinal tract functions again. Then eat a well-balanced, high-protein diet to promote healing.

 CALL YOUR DOCTOR IF

Any of the following occurs:
- Vaginal bleeding that soaks more than 1 pad per hour.
- Frequent urge to urinate or excessive vaginal discharge that persists longer than 1 month.
- Increased pain or swelling in the surgical area.
- Signs of infection: headache, muscle aches, dizziness or a general ill feeling and fever.
- Abdominal swelling or pain.

ILEOSTOMY

GENERAL INFORMATION

DEFINITION—Creation of an opening in the ileum, the lower part of the small intestine. After surgery, all feces leave the body through this opening, which is called an "ostomy" or "stoma."

BODY PARTS INVOLVED—Ileum; cecum.

REASONS FOR SURGERY—Ileostomy is the last step of many surgeries performed in the lower gastrointestinal tract. It provides an opening for feces to leave the body, especially after the colon has been removed.

SURGICAL RISK INCREASES WITH
- Adults over 60.
- Stress.
- Obesity.
- Smoking.
- Poor nutrition.
- Excess alcohol consumption.
- Newborns and infants.
- Recent respiratory infection.
- Chronic heart or lung disease or diabetes mellitus.
- Use of drugs such as: antihypertensives; muscle relaxants; tranquilizers; sleep inducers; insulin; sedatives; beta-adrenergic blockers; or cortisone.
- Use of mind-altering drugs, including: narcotics; psychedelics; hallucinogens; marijuana; sedatives; hypnotics; or cocaine.

WHAT TO EXPECT

WHO OPERATES—General surgeon.

WHERE PERFORMED—Hospital.

DIAGNOSTIC TESTS
- Before surgery: Blood and urine studies; EKG; sigmoidoscopy (see Glossary).
- After surgery: Blood and urine studies.

ANESTHESIA—General anesthesia by inhalation and injection, with an airway tube placed in the windpipe.

DESCRIPTION OF OPERATION
- An incision is made in the abdomen over the diseased intestinal tract.
- The muscles of the abdominal wall are separated to expose the abdominal organs, which are inspected for undetected disease. Other surgeries may be performed at this time.
- The ileum is clamped on both sides of the area to be opened, and cut between the clamps. The part closer to the stomach is brought through another small incision in the abdominal wall to accept the stoma.
- The part of the intestinal tract below the ileum, usually around the diseased part of the intestine, is closed with sutures. The abdominal contents are replaced. The muscles and skin are closed with sutures, which usually can be removed about 1 week after surgery.

POSSIBLE COMPLICATIONS
- Excessive bleeding.
- Surgical-wound infection.
- Diarrhea.
- Incisional hernia.
- Skin irritation around the stoma.

AVERAGE HOSPITAL STAY—15 days.

PROBABLE OUTCOME—Expect complete cure without complications. Allow about 6 weeks for recovery from surgery.

POSTOPERATIVE CARE

NOTE—This information is supplemental and should not replace your doctor's instructions.

GENERAL MEASURES
- A hard ridge should form along the incision. As it heals, the ridge will recede gradually.
- Bathe and shower as usual. You may wash the incision gently with mild unscented soap.
- An "enterostomy nurse" (see Glossary) can provide education and counseling for the you and your family.

MEDICATION—Your doctor may prescribe:
- Pain relievers. Don't take prescription pain medicine longer than 4 to 7 days. Use *only* as much as you need.
- Antibiotics to fight infection.

ACTIVITY
- Resume work and normal activity as soon as possible to reduce postoperative depression, which is common.
- Avoid vigorous exercise for 6 weeks after surgery.
- Resume driving about 4 weeks after returning home weeks.
- Resume sexual relations when able.

DIET—Clear liquid diet until the gastrointestinal tract begins to function again. Then eat a well-balanced, high-protein diet to promote healing. After recovery, eat a low-residue diet (see Glossary). Avoid eggs, fish and other foods that cause excess gas.

CALL YOUR DOCTOR IF

- Pain, swelling, redness, drainage or bleeding increases in the surgical area.
- You have abdominal swelling or pain.
- You develop signs of infection: headache, muscle aches, dizziness or a general ill feeling and fever.
- New, unexplained symptoms develop. Drugs used in treatment may produce side effects.

INTESTINAL OR STOMACH BYPASS

GENERAL INFORMATION

DEFINITION—Creation of a digestive passage that bypasses most of the intestinal tract.

BODY PARTS INVOLVED—Stomach; small intestine.

REASONS FOR SURGERY—Extreme obesity.

SURGICAL RISK INCREASES WITH
- Stress.
- Smoking.
- Poor nutrition.
- Recent illness.
- Alcoholism or chronic illness.
- Use of drugs such as: antihypertensives; muscle relaxants; tranquilizers; sleep inducers; insulin; sedatives; beta-adrenergic blockers; or cortisone.
- Use of mind-altering drugs.

WHAT TO EXPECT

WHO OPERATES—General surgeon.

WHERE PERFORMED—Hospital.

DIAGNOSTIC TESTS
- Before surgery: X-rays of upper gastrointestinal tract; blood and urine studies.
- After surgery: Blood studies.

ANESTHESIA—General anesthesia by inhalation and injection, with an airway tube placed in the windpipe.

DESCRIPTION OF OPERATION
- An incision is made in the abdomen.
- The abdominal muscles are divided and the peritoneum is opened. The upper jejunum is cut and joined to the ileum so that digestive flow will bypass 90% of the small intestine.
- Sometimes, the upper stomach is instead stapled across to isolate and close a section of stomach. A small opening made in the open section of stomach is joined to the lower small bowel so that digestive flow will bypass 90% of the intestinal tract.
- The peritoneum is closed and abdominal muscles are sewn together. The skin is closed with sutures or clips, which usually can be removed about 1 week after surgery.

POSSIBLE COMPLICATIONS
- Excessive bleeding.
- Surgical-wound infection.
- Diarrhea.
- Inadvertent injury to liver.
- Malnutrition.
- Infection in the bypassed segment.
- Intestinal obstruction.
- Dumping syndrome.

AVERAGE HOSPITAL STAY—7 to 10 days.

PROBABLE OUTCOME—Patients lose an average of 8 to 10 pounds per month for 6 months, then less afterwards. However, weight seldom drops below the ideal level unless severe complications develop.

POSTOPERATIVE CARE

NOTE—This information is supplemental and should not replace your doctor's instructions.

GENERAL MEASURES
- A hard ridge should form along the incision. As it heals, the ridge will recede gradually.
- Use an electric heating pad, a heat lamp or a warm compress to relieve incisional pain.
- Bathe and shower as usual. You may wash the incision gently with mild unscented soap.
- Move legs often while resting in bed to decrease the likelihood of deep-vein blood clots.

MEDICATION
- Your doctor may prescribe:
  Pain relievers. Don't take prescription pain medication longer than 4 to 7 days. Use *only* as much as you need.
  Stool softeners to prevent constipation.
  Antibiotics to fight infection.
  Vitamin B-12 injections.
- You may use non-prescription drugs, such as acetaminophen, for minor pain.

ACTIVITY
- Resume work and normal activity as soon as possible to reduce postoperative depression and irritability, which are common.
- Avoid vigorous exercise for 6 weeks after surgery. Resume sex when you feel able.
- Resume driving about 1 month after returning home.

DIET—Your doctor will prescribe:
- Supplements of vitamins and electrolytes.
- Low-fat diet (see Appendix 8).

CALL YOUR DOCTOR IF

- Pain, swelling, redness, drainage or bleeding increases in the surgical area.
- You develop signs of infection: headache, muscle aches, dizziness or a general ill feeling and fever.
- You experience nausea, vomiting, constipation or abdominal swelling.
- Symptoms of dumping syndrome (in Illness section).
- New, unexplained symptoms develop. Drugs used in treatment may produce side effects.

KIDNEY REMOVAL
(Nephrectomy)

 GENERAL INFORMATION

DEFINITION—Removal of a kidney.

BODY PARTS INVOLVED—Kidney; blood vessels connected to kidney; ureter.

REASONS FOR SURGERY
- Cancer or suspected cancer of the kidney
- Kidney transplants to treat kidney failure.

SURGICAL RISK INCREASES WITH
- Adults over 60.
- Obesity.
- Smoking.
- Newborns and infants.
- Poor nutrition.
- Recent or chronic illness.
- Alcoholism.
- Use of drugs such as: antihypertensives; muscle relaxants; tranquilizers; sleep inducers; insulin; sedatives; beta-adrenergic blockers; or cortisone.
- Use of mind-altering drugs, including: narcotics; psychedelics; hallucinogens; marijuana; sedatives; hypnotics; or cocaine.

 WHAT TO EXPECT

WHO OPERATES—General surgeon or urologist.

WHERE PERFORMED—Hospital.

DIAGNOSTIC TESTS
- Before surgery: Blood and urine studies; X-rays of kidneys, chest and lower gastrointestinal tract; EKG; sonogram or CAT scan (see Glossary for all).
- After surgery: Blood studies.

ANESTHESIA—General anesthesia by inhalation and injection, with an airway tube placed in the windpipe.

DESCRIPTION OF OPERATION
- An incision is made, usually in the left or right flank, but sometimes in the abdomen.
- The vein leading from the kidney is located, isolated and tied.
- The ureter is located, tied and cut away from the kidney.
- The artery that supplies blood to the kidney is clamped in two places and cut between the clamps.
- The kidney is freed of adhesions or adjoining connective tissue and removed.
- All disconnected blood vessels are tied, and the muscles are closed with sutures. The skin is closed with sutures or clips, which usually can be removed in about 1 week after surgery.

POSSIBLE COMPLICATIONS
- Excessive bleeding.
- Surgical-wound infection.
- Inadvertent injury to the vena cava or other organs near the kidney.

AVERAGE HOSPITAL STAY—5 to 7 days.

PROBABLE OUTCOME—Expect complete healing without complications. Allow about 4 weeks for recovery from surgery.

 POSTOPERATIVE CARE

NOTE—This information is supplemental and should not replace your doctor's instructions.

GENERAL MEASURES
- A hard ridge should form along the incision. As it heals, the ridge will recede gradually.
- Use an electric heating pad, a heat lamp or a warm compress to relieve incisional pain.
- Bathe and shower as usual. You may wash the incision gently with mild unscented soap.
- Move legs often while resting in bed to decrease the likelihood of deep-vein blood clots.

MEDICATION—Your doctor may prescribe:
- Pain relievers. Don't take prescription pain medication longer than 4 to 7 days. Use *only* as much as you need.
- Stool softeners to prevent constipation.
- Antibiotics to fight infection.

ACTIVITY
- Resume work and normal activity as soon as possible to reduce postoperative depression, which is common.
- Avoid vigorous exercise for 6 weeks after surgery.
- Resume driving 5 weeks after returning home.
- Resume sexual relations when your doctor determines that healing is complete.

DIET—Clear liquid diet until the gastrointestinal tract begins to function again. Then eat a well-balanced, high-protein diet to promote healing.

 CALL YOUR DOCTOR IF

- Pain, swelling, redness, drainage or bleeding increases in the surgical area.
- You develop signs of infection: headache, muscle aches, dizziness or a general ill feeling and fever.
- You experience nausea, vomiting, constipation or abdominal swelling.

KIDNEY-STONE REMOVAL
(Ureterolithotomy)

 GENERAL INFORMATION

DEFINITION—Removal of a kidney stone from one of the ureters.

BODY PARTS INVOLVED—Ureter; kidney.

REASONS FOR SURGERY—Restoration of normal urine flow in the ureter.

SURGICAL RISK INCREASES WITH
- Obesity.
- Smoking.
- Poor nutrition.
- Illness such as any infection.
- Alcoholism.
- Use of drugs such as: antihypertensives; muscle relaxants; tranquilizers; sleep inducers; insulin; sedatives; narcotics; beta-adrenergic blockers; or cortisone.
- Use of mind-altering drugs, including: narcotics; psychedelics; hallucinogens; marijuana; sedatives; hypnotics; or cocaine.

 WHAT TO EXPECT

WHO OPERATES—Urologist or general surgeon.

WHERE PERFORMED—Hospital.

DIAGNOSTIC TESTS
- Before surgery: Blood and urine studies; X-rays of chest; EKG; intravenous pyelogram (see Glossary).
- During surgery: Retrograde pyelogram (see Glossary).
- After surgery: Blood studies.

ANESTHESIA—General anesthesia by inhalation and injection, with an airway tube placed in the windpipe.

DESCRIPTION OF OPERATION
- An incision is made in the flank. The muscles are separated and the ureter is exposed.
- A small incision is made in the ureter. The kidney stone is pulled free and removed.
- A tube is left in the wound for drainage, and a tube is inserted in the ureter to restore urine flow. This tube is removed after healing.
- Muscle layers are closed. The skin is closed with sutures or clips, which usually can be removed about 1 week after surgery.

POSSIBLE COMPLICATIONS
- Excessive bleeding.
- Surgical-wound infection.

AVERAGE HOSPITAL STAY—4 to 5 days.

PROBABLE OUTCOME—Expect complete healing without complications. Allow about 2 weeks for recovery from surgery.

 POSTOPERATIVE CARE

NOTE—This information is supplemental and should not replace your doctor's instructions.

GENERAL MEASURES
- A hard ridge should form along the incision. As it heals, the ridge will recede gradually.
- Bathe and shower as usual. You may wash the incision gently with mild unscented soap.
- Move legs often while resting in bed to decrease the likelihood of deep-vein blood clots.

MEDICATION
- Your doctor may prescribe:
  Pain relievers. Don't take prescription pain medication longer than 4 to 7 days. Use *only* as much as you need.
  Stool softeners to prevent constipation.
  Antibiotics to fight infection.
- You may use non-prescription drugs, such as acetaminophen, for minor pain.

ACTIVITY
- Return to work and normal activity as soon as possible. This reduces postoperative depression and irritability, which are common.
- Avoid vigorous exercise for 6 weeks after surgery.
- Resume driving 2 weeks after returning home.
- Resume sexual relations when your doctor determines that healing is complete.

DIET
- Clear liquid diet until the gastrointestinal tract begins to function. Then eat a well-balanced, high-protein diet to promote healing.
- Increase daily water intake to 8 glasses or more.
- Your doctor may prescribe a special diet after examining the kidney stone.

 CALL YOUR DOCTOR IF

- Pain, swelling, redness, drainage or bleeding increases in the surgical area.
- You develop signs of infection: headache, muscle aches, dizziness or a general ill feeling and fever.
- You experience nausea, vomiting, constipation, or difficulty or pain with urination.
- New, unexplained symptoms develop. Drugs used in treatment may produce side effects.

KIDNEY TRANSPLANT

GENERAL INFORMATION

DEFINITION—Replacement of a diseased kidney with a healthy kidney obtained from a healthy donor with compatible immunological characteristics.

BODY PARTS INVOLVED—Diseased kidney; healthy donor kidney; blood vessels to and from the kidney; ureters.

REASONS FOR SURGERY—Restoration of normal kidney function.

SURGICAL RISK FOR RECIPIENT OR DONOR INCREASES WITH
- Adults over 60.
- Obesity.
- Smoking.
- Poor nutrition.
- Recent illness.
- Alcoholism or chronic illness.
- Use of drugs such as: antihypertensives; muscle relaxants; tranquilizers; sleep inducers; insulin; sedatives; beta-adrenergic blockers; or cortisone.
- Use of mind-altering drugs, including: narcotics; psychedelics; hallucinogens; marijuana; sedatives; hypnotics; or cocaine.

WHAT TO EXPECT

WHO OPERATES—General surgeon or urologist with transplant experience and training.

WHERE PERFORMED—Hospital.

DIAGNOSTIC TESTS
- Before surgery: Blood and urine studies; X-rays of kidneys.
- After surgery: Blood studies.

ANESTHESIA—General anesthesia by inhalation and injection, with an airway tube placed in the windpipe.

DESCRIPTION OF OPERATION
- The diseased kidney from the recipient may be removed several weeks in advance. During this time, dialysis (see Glossary) provides artificial kidney function.
- A kidney is removed from the donor, then chilled and preserved for up to 12 hours.
- An incision is made in the abdomen of the recipient. The abdominal cavity is examined. The new kidney is placed and sewn in position.
- The blood vessels and ureters are connected to the new kidney.
- The peritoneum and abdominal muscles are closed.
- The skin is closed with sutures or clips, which usually can be removed about 1 week after surgery.

POSSIBLE COMPLICATIONS
- Excessive bleeding.
- Surgical-wound infection.
- Rejection of transplant.

AVERAGE HOSPITAL STAY—24 to 25 days.

PROBABLE OUTCOME—A successful transplant restores almost normal life expectancy in patients who might otherwise have died. Transplants are successful in 70% to 80% of cases. Allow about 4 weeks for recovery from surgery for recipient or donor.

POSTOPERATIVE CARE

NOTE—This information is supplemental and should not replace your doctor's instructions. It applies to donor and recipient.

GENERAL MEASURES
- A hard ridge should form along the incision. As it heals, the ridge will recede gradually.
- Use an electric heating pad, a heat lamp or a warm compress to relieve incisional pain.
- Bathe and shower as usual. You may wash the incision gently with mild unscented soap.
- Move legs often while resting in bed to decrease the likelihood of deep-vein blood clots.

MEDICATION—Your doctor may prescribe:
- Pain relievers. Don't take prescription pain medication longer than 4 to 7 days. Use *only* as much as you need.
- Stool softeners to prevent constipation.
- Antibiotics to fight infection.
- Immunosuppressants to reduce the likelihood of tissue rejection.

ACTIVITY
- Resume work and normal activity as soon as possible. This reduces postoperative depression and irritability, which are common.
- Avoid vigorous exercise for 6 weeks after surgery. Resume sexual relations when you feel able.
- Resume driving 2 weeks after returning home.

DIET—Your doctor will prescribe a diet.

CALL YOUR DOCTOR IF

- Pain, swelling, redness, drainage or bleeding increases in the surgical area.
- You develop signs of infection: headache, muscle aches, dizziness or a general ill feeling and fever.
- You experience nausea, vomiting, constipation or abdominal swelling.
- New, unexplained symptoms develop. Drugs used in treatment may produce side effects.

KNEECAP REMOVAL
(Patellectomy)

 GENERAL INFORMATION

DEFINITION—Removal of the kneecap (patella).

BODY PARTS INVOLVED—Kneecap; knee joint; muscles and ligaments attached to kneecap.

REASONS FOR SURGERY
- Fracture of the kneecap.
- Recurrent dislocations of the kneecap.
- Painful degenerative arthritis in the kneecap.

SURGICAL RISK INCREASES WITH
- Obesity.
- Smoking.
- Poor nutrition.
- Recent or chronic illness.

 WHAT TO EXPECT

WHO OPERATES—Orthopedist.

WHERE PERFORMED—Hospital or outpatient surgical facility.

DIAGNOSTIC TESTS
- Before surgery: Blood and urine studies; X-rays of both knees.
- After surgery: Blood studies; X-rays of the affected knee.

ANESTHESIA
- Local anesthesia by injection.
- Spinal anesthesia by injection.
- General anesthesia by inhalation and injection, with an airway tube placed in the windpipe.

DESCRIPTION OF OPERATION
- An incision is made around the kneecap.
- The muscles and tendons attached to the kneecap are cut, and the kneecap is removed.
- The muscles are sewn back together with strong suture material.
- The skin is closed with sutures or clips, which usually can be removed about 1 week after surgery.

POSSIBLE COMPLICATIONS
- Excessive bleeding.
- Surgical-wound infection.

AVERAGE HOSPITAL STAY—6 to 8 days.

PROBABLE OUTCOME—Expect complete healing without complications. Allow about 6 weeks for recovery from surgery.

 POSTOPERATIVE CARE

NOTE—This information is supplemental and should not replace your doctor's instructions.

GENERAL MEASURES
- A hard ridge should form along the incision. As it heals, the ridge will recede gradually.
- Use an electric heating pad, a heat lamp or a warm compress to relieve incisional pain.
- Bathe and shower as usual. You may wash the incision gently with mild unscented soap.
- Move legs often while resting in bed to decrease the likelihood of deep-vein blood clots.
- While sleeping or sitting, keep the affected leg elevated with pillows under the foot or blocks under the bed.

MEDICATION
- Your doctor may prescribe:
  Pain relievers. Don't take prescription pain medication longer than 4 to 7 days. Use *only* as much as you need.
  Antibiotics to fight infection.
- You may use non-prescription drugs, such as acetaminophen, for minor pain.

ACTIVITY
- Return to work and normal activity as soon as possible. This reduces postoperative depression and irritability, which are common.
- Use crutches or a cane to walk as directed by your doctor. Don't stand for prolonged periods.
- Avoid vigorous exercise for 6 weeks after surgery. A physical therapist can teach you exercises that will restore strength to the knee.
- Resume driving 3 weeks after returning home.

DIET—Clear liquid diet until the gastrointestinal tract functions again. Then eat a well-balanced, high-protein diet to promote healing.

 CALL YOUR DOCTOR IF

- Pain, swelling, redness, drainage or bleeding increases in the surgical area.
- Toes become cold, discolored or numb.
- You develop signs of infection: headache, muscle aches, dizziness or a general ill feeling and fever.
- You experience nausea or vomiting.
- New, unexplained symptoms develop. Drugs used in treatment may produce side effects.

LACERATION REPAIR

GENERAL INFORMATION

DEFINITION—Repair of lacerations, open wounds in the skin extending to underlying tissue and sometimes muscle, blood vessels and nerves.

BODY PARTS INVOLVED—Skin; muscle; connective tissue.

REASONS FOR SURGERY
- Prevention of bleeding and infection.
- Examination to identify underlying injuries.
- Closure of the skin to hasten healing.

SURGICAL RISK INCREASES WITH
- Obesity.
- Smoking.
- Poor nutrition.
- Recent or chronic illness.
- Use of drugs such as: antihypertensives; muscle relaxants; tranquilizers; sleep inducers; insulin; sedatives; beta-adrenergic blockers; or cortisone.
- Use of mind-altering drugs, including: narcotics; psychedelics; hallucinogens; marijuana; sedatives; hypnotics; or cocaine.

OTHER—You may need an injection to prevent tetanus. Ask your doctor.

WHAT TO EXPECT

WHO OPERATES—Family doctor, general surgeon, plastic and reconstructive surgeon, orthopedist or hand surgeon.

WHERE PERFORMED—Hospital, outpatient surgical facility or emergency room.

DIAGNOSTIC TESTS
- Before surgery: Blood and urine studies.
- After surgery: Blood studies.

ANESTHESIA
- Local anesthesia by injection.
- General anesthesia by a combination of inhalation and injection, with an airway tube placed in the windpipe.

DESCRIPTION OF OPERATION
- The wound is cleansed and irrigated.
- The skin edges are examined. Shredded tissue and debris are removed. Sometimes, a ragged edge is trimmed for better cosmetic results.
- The underlying tissue is closed with sutures that will be absorbed by the body. The skin is closed with small sutures, which usually can be removed about 1 week after surgery.
- A bandage may be used to control bleeding.

POSSIBLE COMPLICATIONS
- Excessive bleeding.
- Surgical-wound infection.

AVERAGE HOSPITAL STAY—Usually none.

PROBABLE OUTCOME—Expect complete healing without complications. Allow about 3 weeks for recovery from surgery.

POSTOPERATIVE CARE

NOTE—This information is supplemental and should not replace your doctor's instructions.

GENERAL MEASURES
- If the wound bleeds during the first 24 hours after surgery, press a clean tissue or cloth to it for 10 minutes.
- Keep an arm or leg wound elevated for 24 hours after surgery to minimize swelling.
- A hard blunt ridge should form along the wound. As it heals, the ridge will recede gradually.
- Use an electric heating pad, a heat lamp or a warm compress to relieve pain in the surgical area.
- Bathe and shower as usual. You may wash the wound gently with mild unscented soap.
- Between showers, keep the wound dry with a bandage the first 2 or 3 days after surgery. If a bandage gets wet, change it promptly.
- Apply non-prescription antibiotic ointment to the wound before applying a bandage.

MEDICATION
- Your doctor may prescribe:
  Pain relievers. Don't take prescription pain medication longer than 4 to 7 days. Use *only* as much as you need.
  Antibiotics to fight infection.
- You may use non-prescription drugs, such as acetaminophen, to relieve minor pain.

ACTIVITY
- Avoid vigorous exercise for 3 to 6 weeks after surgery.
- Resume driving 2 days after returning home.

DIET—No special diet.

CALL YOUR DOCTOR IF

- Pain, swelling, redness, drainage or bleeding increases in the wound area.
- You develop signs of infection: headache, muscle aches, dizziness or a general ill feeling and fever.

LAPAROSCOPY

GENERAL INFORMATION

DEFINITION—Procedure that allows visual examination and some treatments of the pelvic and abdominal organs. Surgery is performed with a laparoscope, a fiber-optic instrument.

BODY PARTS INVOLVED—Abdomen and all its contents.

REASONS FOR SURGERY
- Diagnosis of reasons for infertility in women.
- Minimal endometriosis.
- Complications from pelvic disease.
- Masses or cysts in the pelvis.
- Undiagnosed pelvic pain.
- Fibroid tumors of the uterus.
- Voluntary sterilization.

SURGICAL RISK INCREASES WITH
- Obesity.
- Smoking.
- Heart or lung disease.
- Advanced pregnancy.
- Previous abdominal surgery, especially hernias.
- Use of drugs such as: antihypertensives; antiarrhythmics; diuretics; or beta-adrenergic blockers.
- Use of mind-altering drugs.

WHAT TO EXPECT

WHO OPERATES—General surgeon or obstetrician-gynecologist.

WHERE PERFORMED—Outpatient surgical facility or hospital.

DIAGNOSTIC TESTS
- Before surgery: Blood studies.
- During surgery. Dye passed through Fallopian tubes.

ANESTHESIA—General anesthesia by inhalation and injection, with an airway tube placed in the windpipe.

DESCRIPTION OF OPERATION
- A small incision is made in or below the patient's navel. A needle is inserted to inflate the abdomen with carbon dioxide.
- The operating table is tilted to allow the bowel and carbon dioxide to float up toward the chest. The laparoscope is used to examine the abdomen visually.
- The laparoscope is used to perform surgeries, if necessary.
- The laporoscope is removed, and the carbon dioxide is allowed to escape from the abdomen.
- Small sutures under the skin and an adhesive bandage are used to close the wound.

POSSIBLE COMPLICATIONS—Perforation of the bowel or liver (rare).

AVERAGE HOSPITAL STAY—0 to 2 days.

PROBABLE OUTCOME—Expect full recovery without complications. You may experience slight discomfort for 24 to 48 hours. You may have aches in your shoulders and chest from the carbon dioxide that was used to inflate your abdomen. No treatment is necessary. Allow 6 days for full recovery from surgery.

POSTOPERATIVE CARE

NOTE—This information is supplemental and should not replace your doctor's instructions.

GENERAL MEASURES
- Change the adhesive bandage daily.
- Bathe and shower as usual. You may wash the incision gently with mild soap.
- Ask your doctor about contraception methods. If surgery was for sterilization and you were taking birth-control pills, finish your present package; then you no longer need birth-control methods.
- Use sanitary pad (not tampons) to stop slight vaginal bleeding, which may occur after surgery.
- Sit in a hot tub of water for 10 to 15 minutes at a time to relieve discomfort.

MEDICATION—Your doctor may prescribe pain relievers. Don't take prescription pain medication longer than 4 to 7 days. Use *only* as much as you need.

ACTIVITY
- Return to work and normal activity as soon as possible. This reduces postoperative depression and irritability, which are common.
- Resume driving 24 hours after recovery from surgery.
- Resume sexual relations in 2 or 3 days after recovery from surgery.

DIET
- Avoid carbonated beverages for 48 hours after surgery.
- Eat a clear liquid diet until the gastrointestinal tract functions again. Then eat a well-balanced, high-protein diet to promote healing.

CALL YOUR DOCTOR IF

- You develop signs of infection: headache, muscle aches, dizziness or a general ill feeling and fever.
- You have excessive bleeding or discharge from either the surgical area or the vagina.
- You experience abdominal swelling or pain.

SURGERIES

LAPAROTOMY

GENERAL INFORMATION

DEFINITION—Any opening made into the abdomen.

BODY PARTS INVOLVED—Skin; abdominal muscles; peritoneum; abdominal organs.

REASONS FOR SURGERY
- Repair or removal of abnormal tissue.
- Removal of diseased organs.
- Diagnostic examination of the abdominal organs.
- Collection of tissue samples for diagnosis.
- Closure of hernias in the abdominal wall.
- Correction of unsightly or disfiguring abnormalities.

SURGICAL RISK INCREASES WITH
- Stress.
- Obesity.
- Smoking.
- Excess alcohol consumption.
- Poor nutrition.
- Recent acute infection.
- Chronic illness.
- Use of drugs such as: antihypertensives; muscle relaxants; tranquilizers; sleep inducers; insulin; sedatives; beta-adrenergic blockers; or cortisone.
- Use of mind-altering drugs, including: narcotics; psychedelics; hallucinogens; marijuana; sedatives; hypnotics; or cocaine.

WHAT TO EXPECT

WHO OPERATES—General surgeon.

WHERE PERFORMED—Hospital.

DIAGNOSTIC TESTS
- Before surgery: Blood and urine studies; X-rays of kidneys and chest; EKG (see Glossary).
- After surgery: Blood studies.

ANESTHESIA—General anesthesia by inhalation and injection, with an airway tube placed in the windpipe.

DESCRIPTION OF OPERATION
- An incision is made in the abdomen. The abdominal muscles are separated, and the peritoneum is opened.
- Blood vessels cut during the surgery are clamped and tied.
- Wound edges are retracted with a special instrument.
- Fluid in the abdominal cavity is often removed for laboratory examination.
- The abdominal organs are examined. Other surgeries may be performed at this time.
- Samples of suspicious tissue are gathered or diseased areas are treated.
- The peritoneum is closed, and the muscles are reconstructed with heavy sutures.

- The skin is closed with sutures or clips, which usually can be removed about 1 week after surgery.

POSSIBLE COMPLICATIONS
- Excessive bleeding.
- Surgical-wound infection.
- Incisional hernia.

AVERAGE HOSPITAL STAY—5 to 7 days.

PROBABLE OUTCOME—Expect complete healing without complications. Allow about 4 weeks for recovery from surgery.

POSTOPERATIVE CARE

NOTE—This information is supplemental and should not replace your doctor's instructions.

GENERAL MEASURES
- A hard ridge should form along the incision. As it heals, the ridge will recede gradually.
- Use an electric heating pad, a heat lamp or a warm compress to relieve incisional pain.
- Bathe and shower as usual. You may wash the incision gently with mild unscented soap.
- Move legs often while resting in bed to decrease the chance of deep-vein blood clots.

MEDICATION
- Your doctor may prescribe:
  Pain relievers. Don't take prescription pain medication longer than 4 to 7 days. Use *only* as much as you need.
  Stool softeners to prevent constipation.
  Antibiotics to fight infection.
- You may use non-prescription drugs, such as acetaminophen, for minor pain.

ACTIVITY
- Return to work and normal activity as soon as possible. This reduces postoperative depression, which is common.
- Avoid vigorous exercise for 6 weeks after surgery. Resume sexual relations when doctor's exam reveals complete healing.
- Resume driving about 3 weeks after returning home.

DIET—Clear liquid diet until the gastrointestinal tract functions again. Then eat a well-balanced, high-protein diet to promote healing. Your doctor may prescribe another diet, depending on your condition.

CALL YOUR DOCTOR IF

- Pain, swelling, redness, drainage or bleeding increases in the surgical area.
- You develop signs of infection: headache, muscle aches, dizziness or a general ill feeling and fever.
- You experience new symptoms, such as nausea, vomiting, constipation, abdominal swelling or severe pain.

LARYNX REMOVAL
(Laryngectomy)

 GENERAL INFORMATION

DEFINITION—Removal of the larynx.

BODY PARTS INVOLVED—Larynx (voice box), organ at the top of the windpipe that controls the voice.

REASONS FOR SURGERY—Cancer of the larynx.

SURGICAL RISK INCREASES WITH
- Adults over 60.
- Obesity.
- Smoking.
- Stress.
- Poor nutrition.
- Recent illness.
- Chronic illness, especially alcoholism.
- Use of drugs such as: antihypertensives; muscle relaxants; tranquilizers; sleep inducers; insulin; sedatives; beta-adrenergic blockers; or cortisone.
- Use of mind-altering drugs, including: narcotics; psychedelics; hallucinogens; marijuana; sedatives; hypnotics; or cocaine.

 WHAT TO EXPECT

WHO OPERATES—Ear, nose and throat specialist.

WHERE PERFORMED—Hospital.

DIAGNOSTIC TESTS
- Before surgery: Blood and urine studies.
- After surgery: Blood studies.

ANESTHESIA—General anesthesia by inhalation and injection, with an airway tube placed in the windpipe.

DESCRIPTION OF OPERATION
- An incision is made in the neck. The muscles that attach the larynx to the windpipe are divided.
- The blood vessels and nerves that supply the larynx are located and cut.
- The larynx is cut free and removed.
- A tracheostomy tube (device to prevent obstruction of air passage) is fitted and positioned.
- The muscles and skin edges are closed around the tube with sutures or clips, which usually can be removed about 1 week after surgery.

POSSIBLE COMPLICATIONS
- Excessive bleeding.
- Surgical-wound infection.
- Inadvertent injury to the esophagus or trachea.

AVERAGE HOSPITAL STAY—5 to 7 days.

PROBABLE OUTCOME—Expect complete healing of the surgical wound. Allow about 4 weeks for recovery from surgery.

 POSTOPERATIVE CARE

NOTE—This information is supplemental and should not replace your doctor's instructions.

GENERAL MEASURES
- Keep the surgical area dry.
- Keep your head elevated.
- Don't try to talk. Communicate by writing messages.
- Consult a speech therapist as soon as possible.
- Move legs often while resting in bed to decrease the likelihood of deep-vein blood clots.
- Treat crusting and secretions around the surgical wound with petroleum jelly, antibiotic ointment and gauze.
- A hard ridge should form along the incision. As it heals, the ridge will recede gradually.
- Use an electric heating pad, a heat lamp or a warm compress to relieve incisional pain.

MEDICATION
- Your doctor may prescribe:
  Pain relievers. Don't take prescription pain medication longer than 4 to 7 days. Use *only* as much as you need.
  Stool softeners to prevent constipation.
  Antibiotics to fight infection.
- You may use non-prescription drugs, such as acetaminophen, for minor pain.

ACTIVITY
- Return to work and normal activity as soon as possible. This reduces postoperative depression and irritability, which are common.
- Avoid vigorous exercise for 6 weeks after surgery.
- Resume driving 2 weeks after returning home.

DIET—Tube or intravenous feedings for first 2 days after surgery. Then resume your normal diet gradually.

 CALL YOUR DOCTOR IF

- Pain, swelling, redness, drainage or bleeding increases in the surgical area.
- You develop signs of infection: headache, muscle aches, dizziness or a general ill feeling and fever.
- New, unexplained symptoms develop. Drugs used in treatment may produce side effects.

SURGERIES

LIPOMA REMOVAL

GENERAL INFORMATION

DEFINITION—Removal of a lipoma (benign, fatty tumor).

BODY PARTS INVOLVED—Skin and underlying tissue, usually on the back, arms and legs.

REASONS FOR SURGERY
- Improved appearance.
- Prevention of cancer.

SURGICAL RISK INCREASES WITH—Recent illness.

WHAT TO EXPECT

WHO OPERATES—Family doctor, general surgeon, dermatologist or plastic and reconstructive surgeon.

WHERE PERFORMED—Doctor's office or outpatient surgical facility.

DIAGNOSTIC TESTS
- Before surgery: Blood and urine studies.
- After surgery: Laboratory examination of removed tissue.

ANESTHESIA—Local anesthesia by injection.

DESCRIPTION OF OPERATION
- An incision is made over the lipoma.
- The lipoma is opened, cut free from connective tissue and removed.
- The skin is closed with sutures or clips, which usually can be removed about 1 week after surgery.

POSSIBLE COMPLICATIONS
- Excessive bleeding.
- Surgical-wound infection.

AVERAGE HOSPITAL STAY—None.

PROBABLE OUTCOME—Expect complete healing without complications. Allow about 3 weeks for recovery from surgery.

POSTOPERATIVE CARE

NOTE—This information is supplemental and should not replace your doctor's instructions.

GENERAL MEASURES
- If the wound bleeds during the first 24 hours after surgery, press a clean tissue or cloth to it for 10 minutes.
- A hard ridge should form along the incision. As it heals, the ridge will recede gradually.
- Use an electric heating pad, a heat lamp or a warm compress to relieve incisional pain.
- Bathe and shower as usual. You may wash the incision gently with mild unscented soap.
- Between showers, keep the wound dry with a bandage for the first 2 or 3 days after surgery. If a bandage gets wet, change it promptly.
- Apply non-prescription antibiotic ointment to the wound before applying new bandages.

MEDICATION
- Your doctor may prescribe pain relievers. Don't take prescription pain medication longer than 4 to 7 days. Use *only* as much as you need.
- You may use non-prescription drugs, such as acetaminophen, for minor pain.

ACTIVITY
- Avoid vigorous exercise for 4 weeks after surgery.
- Resume driving 2 days after returning home.

DIET—No special diet.

CALL YOUR DOCTOR IF

- Pain, swelling, redness, drainage or bleeding increases in the surgical area.
- You develop signs of infection: headache, muscle aches, dizziness or a general ill feeling and fever.

LIVER TRANSPLANT

GENERAL INFORMATION

DEFINITION—Replacement of a diseased liver with a healthy liver obtained immediately after death from a donor with compatible immunological characteristics.

BODY PARTS INVOLVED—Diseased or abnormal liver; healthy donor liver; blood vessels and bile ducts connected to liver.

REASONS FOR SURGERY—End-stage liver failure from liver cancer or other chronic liver disease.

SURGICAL RISK INCREASES WITH
- Infants.
- Obesity.
- Smoking.
- Excess alcohol consumption.
- Stress.
- Poor nutrition.
- Recent or chronic illness.
- Use of drugs such as: antihypertensives; muscle relaxants; tranquilizers; sleep inducers; insulin; sedatives; beta-adrenergic blockers; or cortisone.
- Use of mind-altering drugs, including: narcotics; psychedelics; hallucinogens; marijuana; sedatives; hypnotics; or cocaine.

WHAT TO EXPECT

WHO OPERATES—General surgeon with transplant experience and training.

WHERE PERFORMED—Hospital.

DIAGNOSTIC TESTS
- Before surgery: Immune-system and liver-matching procedures; studies of body systems.
- After surgery: Blood studies.

ANESTHESIA—General anesthesia by inhalation and injection, with an airway tube placed in the windpipe.

DESCRIPTION OF OPERATION
- Liver is removed from donor, then chilled and preserved up to 12 hours until surgery.
- An incision is made under the recipient's ribs. The abdominal muscles are separated or split, and the peritoneal cavity is opened.
- The liver and its bile ducts are isolated.
- The liver is cut free and removed. The donor liver is positioned and sewn in place. Blood vessels and bile ducts are connected.
- The peritoneum and abdominal muscles are closed. The skin is closed with sutures or clips, which usually can be removed about 1 week after surgery.

POSSIBLE COMPLICATIONS
- Excessive bleeding.
- Surgical-wound infection.
- Rejection of transplant.
- Bile-duct obstruction.
- Recurrence of cancerous growth.

AVERAGE HOSPITAL STAY—3 weeks.

PROBABLE OUTCOME—A successful transplant prolongs life and improves the quality of life for a few months to a few years in patients who might otherwise have died. Allow about 6 months for recovery from surgery.

POSTOPERATIVE CARE

NOTE—This information is supplemental and should not replace your doctor's instructions.

GENERAL MEASURES
- A hard ridge should form along the incision. As it heals, the ridge will recede gradually.
- Bathe and shower as usual. You may wash the incision gently with mild unscented soap.
- Use an electric heating pad, a heat lamp or a warm compress to relieve incisional pain.
- Move legs often while resting in bed to decrease the likelihood of deep-vein blood clots.

MEDICATION—Your doctor may prescribe:
- Pain relievers. Don't take prescription pain medication longer than 4 to 7 days. Use *only* as much as you need.
- Stool softeners to prevent constipation.
- Antibiotics to fight infection.
- Immunosuppressants to decrease the likelihood of rejection.

ACTIVITY
- Resume work and normal activity as soon as possible to reduce postoperative depression, which is common.
- Avoid vigorous exercise for 6 weeks after surgery.
- Resume driving when your doctor determines that healing is complete.

DIET—Your doctor will prescribe a diet.

CALL YOUR DOCTOR IF

- Pain, swelling, redness, drainage or bleeding increases in the surgical area.
- You develop signs of infection: headache, muscle aches, dizziness or a general ill feeling and fever.
- You experience new symptoms such as: nausea; vomiting; constipation; abdominal swelling; back pain; jaundice; or fluid retention in abdomen, eyes or ankles.

SURGERIES

LUNG RESECTION

GENERAL INFORMATION

DEFINITION—Removal of tissue from the lungs. If part of a lung (usually called a lobe) is removed, the surgery is called lobectomy. If the entire lung is removed, the surgery is called pneumonectomy.

BODY PARTS INVOLVED—Lung; bronchial tubes; blood vessels in chest; ribs.

REASONS FOR SURGERY
● Cancer or suspected cancer of the lung.
● Diseased lobes of the lung caused by several chronic conditions, especially bronchiectasis.

SURGICAL RISK INCREASES WITH
● Adults over 60.
● Obesity.
● Smoking.
● Excess alcohol consumption.
● Poor nutrition.
● Alcoholism or chronic illness.
● Recent illness, especially upper-respiratory infection.
● Use of drugs such as: antihypertensives; muscle relaxants; tranquilizers; sleep inducers; insulin; sedatives; narcotics; beta-adrenergic blockers; or cortisone.
● Use of mind-altering drugs, including: narcotics; psychedelics; hallucinogens; marijuana; or cocaine.

WHAT TO EXPECT

WHO OPERATES—Thoracic surgeon.

WHERE PERFORMED—Hospital.

DIAGNOSTIC TESTS
● Before surgery: Blood and urine studies; X-rays of chest; EKG (see Glossary).
● During surgery: EKG monitor.
● After surgery: Blood studies.

ANESTHESIA—General anesthesia by inhalation and injection, with an airway tube placed in the windpipe.

DESCRIPTION OF OPERATION
● An incision is made in the chest. Sometimes, a rib is removed for better exposure to the lungs.
● The blood supply to the diseased area is isolated and tied off.
● The diseased area is located and examined. The growth, the lobe in which it appears or the entire lung is cut free and removed.
● A tube is inserted to drain fluid and air from the surgical area.
● The muscles are reconstructed with strong sutures. The skin is closed with sutures or clips, which usually can be removed about 1 week after surgery.

POSSIBLE COMPLICATIONS—Excessive bleeding; surgical-wound infection; or pneumonia.

AVERAGE HOSPITAL STAY—10 to 14 days.

PROBABLE OUTCOME—In some cases, underlying lung disease may be cured. In other cases, quality of life may be improved. Allow about 6 weeks for recovery from surgery.

POSTOPERATIVE CARE

NOTE—This information is supplemental and should not replace your doctor's instructions.

GENERAL MEASURES
● A hard ridge should form along the incision. As it heals, the ridge will recede gradually.
● Bathe and shower as usual. You may wash the incision gently with mild unscented soap.
● Use an electric heating pad, a heat lamp or a warm compress to relieve incisional pain.
● Move legs often while in bed to decrease the likelihood of deep-vein blood clots.
● Breathe deeply and cough often to keep secretions from pooling inside the lungs. Respiratory therapists can help you learn to keep bronchial tubes clear. Ask your doctor.

MEDICATION
● Your doctor may prescribe:
  Pain relievers. Don't take prescription pain medication longer than 4 to 7 days. Use *only* as much as you need.
  Antibiotics to fight infection.
● A vaccine to prevent pneumonia.
● You may use non-prescription drugs, such as acetaminophen, for minor pain.

ACTIVITY
● Resume work and normal activity as soon as possible to reduce postoperative depression, which is common.
● Avoid vigorous exercise for 6 weeks after surgery. Resume sexual relations when able.
● Resume driving 5 weeks after returning home.

DIET—Clear liquid diet until the gastrointestinal tract begins to function again. Then eat a well-balanced, high-protein diet to promote healing.

CALL YOUR DOCTOR IF

● Pain, swelling, redness, drainage or bleeding increases in the surgical area.
● You develop signs of infection: headache, muscle aches, dizziness or a general ill feeling and fever.
● You experience nausea, vomiting or shortness of breath.
● You develop a "bubbly" feeling under skin of your chest.

LUNG TRANSPLANT

GENERAL INFORMATION

DEFINITION—Replacement of diseased lungs with healthy lungs obtained immediately after death from a donor with compatible immunological characteristics.

BODY PARTS INVOLVED—Diseased or abnormal lungs; healthy donor lungs; blood vessels and bronchial tubes to the lungs.

REASONS FOR SURGERY—Pulmonary hypertension (see Glossary) or respiratory failure.

SURGICAL RISK INCREASES WITH
- Adults over 60.
- Obesity.
- Smoking.
- Stress.
- Poor nutrition.
- Recent or chronic illness.
- Alcoholism.
- Use of drugs such as: antihypertensives; muscle relaxants; tranquilizers; sleep inducers; insulin; sedatives; beta-adrenergic blockers; or cortisone.
- Use of mind-altering drugs.

WHAT TO EXPECT

WHO OPERATES—Thoracic surgeon or cardiovascular surgeon with transplant experience and training.

WHERE PERFORMED—Hospital.

DIAGNOSTIC TESTS
- Before surgery: Evaluation of body systems, especially the respiratory system; immune-system and lung-matching procedures.
- During surgery: Cardiac monitor.
- After surgery: Blood studies.

ANESTHESIA—General anesthesia by inhalation and injection, with an airway tube placed in the windpipe.

DESCRIPTION OF OPERATION
- Healthy lungs are removed from the donor, chilled and preserved up to 12 hours.
- An incision is made in the recipient's chest and the chest is spread apart.
- The heart-lung machine (see Glossary) sustains life during surgery.
- The lungs are cut free of the connecting bronchial tubes and blood vessels and removed.
- The donor lungs are positioned and sewn in place. Blood vessels and bronchial tubes are connected. Chest tubes remain for drainage.
- The chest muscles are closed. The skin is closed with sutures or clips, which usually can be removed about 1 week after surgery.

POSSIBLE COMPLICATIONS
- Excessive bleeding.
- Surgical-wound infection.
- Pneumonia.
- Rejection of transplanted lung.

AVERAGE HOSPITAL STAY—3 weeks.

PROBABLE OUTCOME—A few transplants are successful. When successful, a lung transplant prolongs life up to a few years and improves the quality of life in patients who might otherwise have died. Allow about 6 months for recovery from surgery.

POSTOPERATIVE CARE

NOTE—This information is supplemental and should not replace your doctor's instructions.

GENERAL MEASURES
- Oxygen will be necessary for 1 to 7 days.
- A hard ridge should form along the incision. As it heals, the ridge will recede gradually.
- Use an electric heating pad, a heat lamp or a warm compress to relieve incisional pain.
- Bathe and shower as usual. You may wash the incision gently with mild unscented soap.
- Move legs often while resting in bed to decrease the likelihood of deep-vein blood clots.

MEDICATION—Your doctor may prescribe:
- Pain relievers. Don't take prescription pain medication longer than 4 to 7 days. Use *only* as much as you need.
- Stool softeners to prevent constipation.
- Antibiotics to fight infection.
- Immunosuppressants to decrease the likelihood of rejection.

ACTIVITY
- Resume work and normal activity as soon as possible. This reduces postoperative depression, which is common.
- Avoid vigorous exercise for 6 weeks after surgery.
- Resume sexual relations when your doctor determines that healing is complete.

DIET—Your doctor will prescribe a special diet.

CALL YOUR DOCTOR IF

Any of the following occur:
- Increased pain, swelling, redness, drainage or bleeding in the surgical area.
- Signs of infection: headache, muscle aches, dizziness or a general ill feeling and fever.
- Nausea or vomiting.
- Fatigue, coughing, shortness of breath or blood in the sputum.
- New, unexplained symptoms. Drugs used in treatment may produce side effects.

MALIGNANT-MELANOMA REMOVAL

 GENERAL INFORMATION

DEFINITION—Removal of any lesion on the skin that might be malignant melanoma, the most dangerous form of skin cancer.

BODY PARTS INVOLVED—Skin.

REASONS FOR SURGERY—Treatment of malignant melanoma.

SURGICAL RISK INCREASES WITH
- Obesity.
- Smoking.
- Poor nutrition.
- Recent or chronic illness.
- Use of drugs such as: antihypertensives; muscle relaxants; tranquilizers; sleep inducers; insulin; sedatives; beta-adrenergic blockers; or cortisone.
- Use of mind-altering drugs, including: narcotics; psychedelics; hallucinogens; marijuana; sedatives; hypnotics; or cocaine.

 WHAT TO EXPECT

WHO OPERATES—General surgeon, dermatologist or plastic and reconstructive surgeon.

WHERE PERFORMED—Hospital or outpatient surgical facility.

DIAGNOSTIC TESTS
- Before surgery: Blood and urine studies.
- During surgery: Microscopic examination of skin margins to determine how much skin to remove.
- After surgery: Laboratory examination of removed tissue.

ANESTHESIA—Local anesthesia by injection.

DESCRIPTION OF OPERATION
- Surgery is directed primarily toward cure and secondarily toward preservation of normal appearance.
- Cancerous cells are cut free and removed with a scalpel.
- The depth of the incision depends on findings during surgery. All skin and tissue that appears abnormal is removed. Bordering skin and tissue are removed to improve the likelihood of removing all cancerous cells.
- The skin is closed with fine suture material or clips, which usually can be removed about 10 days after surgery.

POSSIBLE COMPLICATIONS
- Surgical-wound infection.
- Residual cancer due to not removing enough diseased skin.

AVERAGE HOSPITAL STAY—1 to 2 days.

PROBABLE OUTCOME—Expect complete healing of the surgical wounds. Examination of removed skin and tissue may reveal that additional treatment will be necessary. Further treatment such as radiation, laser surgery or anticancer drugs depends on each patient's case. Allow about 2 weeks for recovery from surgery.

 POSTOPERATIVE CARE

NOTE—This information is supplemental and should not replace your doctor's instructions.

GENERAL MEASURES
- If the wound bleeds during the first 24 hours after surgery, press a clean tissue or cloth to it for 10 minutes.
- A hard blunt ridge should form along the incisions. As it heals, the ridge will recede gradually.
- Use an electric heating pad, a heat lamp or a warm compress, to relieve incisional pain.
- Bathe and shower as usual. You may wash the incisions gently with mild unscented soap.
- Between baths, keep the wound dry with a bandage for the first 2 or 3 days after surgery. If a bandage gets wet, change it promptly.
- Apply non-prescription antibiotic ointment to wounds before applying bandages.

MEDICATION
- Your doctor may prescribe:
  Pain relievers. Don't take prescription pain medication longer than 4 to 7 days. Use *only* as much as you need.
  Antibiotics to ward off infection.
- You may use non-prescription drugs, such as acetaminophen to relieve minor pain.

ACTIVITY
- Return to work and normal activity as soon as possible. This reduces postoperative depression and irritability, which are common.
- Avoid vigorous exercise for 2 weeks after surgery.
- Resume driving 3 days after returning home.

DIET—No special diet.

 CALL YOUR DOCTOR IF

- Pain, swelling, redness, drainage or bleeding increases in the surgical area.
- You develop signs of infection: headache, muscle aches, dizziness or a general ill feeling and fever.

MASTECTOMY, MODIFIED RADICAL
(Total Mastectomy)

GENERAL INFORMATION

DEFINITION—Removal of the breast.

BODY PARTS INVOLVED—Breast; lymph glands (sometimes).

REASONS FOR SURGERY—Cancer of the breast.

SURGICAL RISK INCREASES WITH
- Obesity or poor nutrition.
- Smoking.
- Stress.
- Recent or chronic illness.
- Use of drugs such as: antihypertensives; muscle relaxants; tranquilizers; sleep inducers; insulin; sedatives; beta-adrenergic blockers; or cortisone.
- Use of mind-altering drugs.

WHAT TO EXPECT

WHO OPERATES—General surgeon or oncological surgeon.

WHERE PERFORMED—Hospital.

DIAGNOSTIC TESTS
- Before surgery: Blood and urine studies; mammogram; needle biopsy (see Glossary for all).
- During surgery: Laboratory examination of removed tissue by frozen section.
- After surgery: Blood studies; laboratory examination of removed tissue.

ANESTHESIA—General anesthesia by inhalation and injection, with an airway tube placed in the windpipe.

DESCRIPTION OF OPERATION
- An incision is made encompassing the entire breast.
- The underlying tissue is cut free and removed in one piece with the lymph glands from the armpit. Bleeding is controlled with ties and electrocauterization. A tube is inserted for drainage.
- The skin is closed with sutures or clips, which usually can be removed about 1 week after surgery.

POSSIBLE COMPLICATIONS
- Excessive bleeding.
- Surgical-wound infection.
- Depression.
- Accumulation of blood under the skin in the surgical area.
- Limited shoulder motion.

AVERAGE HOSPITAL STAY—6 to 8 days.

PROBABLE OUTCOME—Expect complete healing of the surgical wound. Allow about 6 weeks for recovery from surgery.

POSTOPERATIVE CARE

NOTE—This information is supplemental and should not replace your doctor's instructions.

GENERAL MEASURES
- Support groups can help you learn to cope with the loss of a breast.
- A hard ridge should form along the incision. As it heals, the ridge will recede gradually.
- Use an electric heating pad, a heat lamp or a warm compress to relieve incisional pain.
- Bathe and shower as usual. You may wash the incision gently with mild unscented soap.
- Move legs often while resting in bed to decrease the likelihood of deep-vein clots.
- Wear long sleeves to protect the arm and hand. Avoid injuries to the arm and hand, such as injections or blood drawing, in the affected arm and hand.

MEDICATION
- Your doctor may prescribe:
  Pain relievers. Don't take prescription pain medication longer than 4 to 7 days. Use *only* as much as you need.
  Stool softeners to prevent constipation.
  Antibiotics to fight infection.
- You may use non-prescription drugs, such as acetaminophen, for minor pain.

ACTIVITY
- Return to work and normal activity as soon as possible. This reduces postoperative depression and irritability, which are common.
- Avoid vigorous exercise for 6 weeks after surgery. After recovery, exercise your arm as directed by your doctor.
- Resume driving 2 weeks after returning home.
- Resume sexual relations when able.

DIET—Clear liquid diet until the gastrointestinal tract functions again. Then eat a well-balanced, high-protein diet to promote healing.

CALL YOUR DOCTOR IF

Any of the following occurs:
- Increased pain, swelling, redness, drainage or bleeding in the surgical area.
- Nausea, vomiting or constipation.
- Signs of infection: headache, muscle aches, dizziness or a general ill feeling and fever.
- Redness, warmth, swelling, stiffness or hardness in the affected arm or hand.
- New, unexplained symptoms. Drugs used in treatment may produce side effects.

SURGERIES

MASTECTOMY, PARTIAL
(Lumpectomy)

 GENERAL INFORMATION

DEFINITION—Removal of a lump from the female breast that is known or suspected to be cancerous.

BODY PARTS INVOLVED—Breast.

REASONS FOR SURGERY—Cancer or suspected cancer of the breast. Surgeries to treat breast cancer are controversial and vary considerably. Consult with your doctor before deciding to undergo any surgery.

SURGICAL RISK INCREASES WITH
- Obesity.
- Smoking.
- Stress.
- Poor nutrition.
- Recent or chronic illness.
- Use of drugs such as: antihypertensives; muscle relaxants; tranquilizers; sleep inducers; insulin; sedatives; beta-adrenergic blockers; or cortisone.
- Use of mind-altering drugs, including: narcotics; psychedelics; hallucinogens; marijuana; sedatives; hypnotics; or cocaine.

 WHAT TO EXPECT

WHO OPERATES—General surgeon or oncological surgeon.

WHERE PERFORMED—Hospital.

DIAGNOSTIC TESTS
- Before surgery: Blood and urine studies; X-rays of chest; mammograms (see Glossary).
- During surgery: Laboratory examination of the removed lump by frozen section.
- After surgery: Blood studies; laboratory examination of removed tissue.

ANESTHESIA—General anesthesia by inhalation and injection, with an airway tube placed in the windpipe.

DESCRIPTION OF OPERATION
- An incision is made over the lump to be removed.
- The lump and a small surrounding area of normal tissue are cut free and removed. Bleeding is controlled with ties and electrocauterization.
- The skin is closed with sutures or clips, which usually can be removed about 1 week after surgery.

POSSIBLE COMPLICATIONS
- Excessive bleeding.
- Surgical-wound infection.
- Need for additional surgery (sometimes).

AVERAGE HOSPITAL STAY—1 to 2 days.

PROBABLE OUTCOME—Expect complete healing of the surgical wound. Allow about 2 weeks for recovery from surgery.

 POSTOPERATIVE CARE

NOTE—This information is supplemental and should not replace your doctor's instructions.

GENERAL MEASURES
- A hard ridge should form along the incision. As it heals, the ridge will recede gradually.
- Use an electric heating pad, a heat lamp or a warm compress to relieve incisional pain.
- Bathe and shower as usual. You may wash the incision gently with mild unscented soap.

MEDICATION
- Your doctor may prescribe:
  Pain relievers. Don't take prescription pain medication longer than 4 to 7 days. Use *only* as much as you need.
  Stool softeners to prevent constipation.
  Antibiotics to fight infection.
- You may use non-prescription drugs, such as acetaminophen, for minor pain.

ACTIVITY
- Return to work and normal activity as soon as possible. This reduces postoperative depression and irritability, which are common.
- Avoid vigorous exercise for 4 weeks after surgery.
- Resume driving 1 week after returning home.

DIET—Clear liquid diet until the gastrointestinal tract functions again. Then eat a well-balanced, high-protein diet to promote healing.

 CALL YOUR DOCTOR IF

- Pain, swelling, redness, drainage or bleeding increases in the surgical area.
- You develop signs of infection: headache, muscle aches, dizziness or a general ill feeling and fever.
- You experience nausea or vomiting.
- New, unexplained symptoms develop. Drugs used in treatment may produce side effects.

MENISCECTOMY

 GENERAL INFORMATION

DEFINITION—Removal of injured cartilage in the knee. Usually, injury has resulted from a torn ligament.

BODY PARTS INVOLVED—Knee and all its parts.

REASONS FOR SURGERY—Prevention of permanent damage to the knee joint.

SURGICAL RISK INCREASES WITH
- Obesity.
- Smoking.
- Recent or chronic illness.
- Use of drugs such as: antihypertensives; muscle relaxants; tranquilizers; sleep inducers; insulin; sedatives; beta-adrenergic blockers; or cortisone.
- Use of mind-altering drugs, including: narcotics; psychedelics; hallucinogens; marijuana; sedatives; hypnotics; or cocaine.

 WHAT TO EXPECT

WHO OPERATES—Orthopedist.

WHERE PERFORMED—Hospital or outpatient surgical facility.

DIAGNOSTIC TESTS
- Before surgery: Blood and urine studies; X-rays of both knees.
- After surgery: X-rays of affected knee; blood studies.

ANESTHESIA
- Spinal anesthesia by injection.
- General anesthesia by inhalation and injection, with an airway tube placed in the windpipe.

DESCRIPTION OF OPERATION
- The affected area can be approached by arthroscopy (see Glossary) or by incision into the knee joint. Either approach exposes the injured cartilage.
- The cartilage is removed with forceps or suction. Any injured ligaments are sewn together.
- The skin is closed with sutures or clips, which usually can be removed about 1 week after surgery.

POSSIBLE COMPLICATIONS
- Excessive bleeding.
- Surgical-wound infection.
- Weakened knee joint.

AVERAGE HOSPITAL STAY—6 to 8 days.

PROBABLE OUTCOME—Expect complete recovery without complications. Allow about 6 weeks for recovery from surgery.

 POSTOPERATIVE CARE

NOTE—This information is supplemental and should not replace your doctor's instructions.

GENERAL MEASURES
- A hard ridge should form along the incision. As it heals, the ridge will recede gradually.
- Use an electric heating pad, a heat lamp or a warm compress to relieve incisional pain.
- Bathe and shower as usual. You may wash the incision gently with mild unscented soap.
- Move legs often while resting in bed to decrease the likelihood of deep-vein blood clots.
- When sleeping or sitting, keep the affected leg elevated with pillows under the foot or blocks under the bed.

MEDICATION
- Your doctor may prescribe:
  Pain relievers. Don't take prescription pain medication longer than 4 to 7 days. Use *only* as much as you need.
  Antibiotics to fight infection.
- You may use non-prescription drugs, such as acetaminophen, for minor pain.

ACTIVITY
- Return to work and normal activity as soon as possible. This reduces postoperative depression and irritability, which are common.
- Use crutches or a cane to walk as directed by your doctor. Don't stand for prolonged periods.
- Avoid vigorous exercise for 4 weeks after surgery. A physical therapist can teach you exercises that will restore strength to the knee.
- Resume driving 3 weeks after returning home.

DIET—Clear liquid diet until the gastrointestinal tract functions again. Then eat a well-balanced, high-protein diet to promote healing.

 CALL YOUR DOCTOR IF

- Pain, swelling, redness, drainage or bleeding increases in the surgical area.
- Toes become cold, discolored or numb.
- You develop signs of infection: headache, muscle aches, dizziness or a general ill feeling and fever.
- You experience nausea or vomiting.
- New, unexplained symptoms develop. Drugs used in treatment may produce side effects.

MORTON'S-NEUROMA REMOVAL

GENERAL INFORMATION

DEFINITION—Removal of Morton's neuroma, a small benign tumor in the nerve that serves the toes. Its cause is unknown, and it produces severe pain.

BODY PARTS INVOLVED—A small tumor between the 2nd and 3rd toes or the 3rd and 4th toes. It may occur in either or both feet.

REASONS FOR SURGERY—Relief of pain caused by the neuroma.

SURGICAL RISK INCREASES WITH
- Obesity.
- Smoking.
- Poor nutrition.
- Recent or chronic illness.
- Use of drugs such as: antihypertensives; muscle relaxants; tranquilizers; sleep inducers; insulin; sedatives; beta-adrenergic blockers; or cortisone.
- Use of mind-altering drugs, including: narcotics; psychedelics; hallucinogens; marijuana; sedatives; hypnotics; or cocaine.

WHAT TO EXPECT

WHO OPERATES—General surgeon or podiatrist.

WHERE PERFORMED—Hospital, outpatient surgical facility, doctor's office or emergency room.

DIAGNOSTIC TESTS
- Before surgery: Blood and urine studies; X-rays of the foot.
- After surgery: Laboratory examination of removed tissue.

ANESTHESIA—Local anesthesia by injection.

DESCRIPTION OF OPERATION
- A tourniquet is wrapped around the leg to prevent the surgical area from bleeding.
- The neuroma is located, cut free from surrounding tissue and removed.
- The skin is closed with sutures, which usually can be removed about 10 to 14 days after surgery. The tourniquet is removed.

POSSIBLE COMPLICATIONS
- Excessive bleeding.
- Surgical-wound infection.

AVERAGE HOSPITAL STAY—1 day.

PROBABLE OUTCOME—Expect complete healing without complications. Allow about 3 weeks for recovery from surgery.

POSTOPERATIVE CARE

NOTE—This information is supplemental and should not replace your doctor's instructions.

GENERAL MEASURES
- If the wound bleeds during the first 24 hours after surgery, press a clean tissue or cloth to it for 10 minutes.
- A hard ridge should form along the incision. As it heals, the ridge will recede gradually.
- Use an electric heating pad, a heat lamp or a warm compress to relieve incisional pain.
- Bathe and shower as usual. You may wash the incision gently with mild unscented soap.
- Between baths, keep the wound dry with a bandage for the first 2 or 3 days after surgery. If a bandage gets wet, change it promptly. Apply non-prescription antibiotic ointment to the wound before applying new bandages.
- Keep the foot elevated as much as possible during recovery.

MEDICATION
- Your doctor may prescribe:
  Pain relievers. Don't take prescription pain medication longer than 4 to 7 days. Use *only* as much as you need.
  Antibiotics to fight infection.
- You may use non-prescription drugs, such as acetaminophen, for minor pain.

ACTIVITY
- Return to work and normal activity as soon as possible. This reduces postoperative depression and irritability, which are common.
- Avoid vigorous exercise for 6 weeks after surgery.
- Resume driving 1 week after returning home.

DIET—No special diet.

CALL YOUR DOCTOR IF

- Pain, swelling, redness, drainage or bleeding increases in the surgical area.
- You develop signs of infection: headache, muscle aches, dizziness or a general ill feeling and fever.
- New, unexplained symptoms develop. Drugs used in treatment may produce side effects.

MYRINGOTOMY

GENERAL INFORMATION

DEFINITION—Opening the eardrum (tympanic membrane) to remove fluid in the middle ear. This fluid consists of blood, pus, water and debris, and usually collects because of infection or allergy. Frequently small tubes are inserted in the middle ear to maintain drainage.

BODY PARTS INVOLVED—Eardrum; middle ear; external ear canal (route for surgery).

REASONS FOR SURGERY
- Relief of pain caused by pressure.
- Prevention of temporary or permanent hearing loss.

SURGICAL RISK INCREASES WITH
- Smoking.
- Recent illness, especially upper-respiratory infection.
- Chronic illness.
- Previous perforation of the eardrum.

WHAT TO EXPECT

WHO OPERATES—Ear, nose and throat specialist.

WHERE PERFORMED—Hospital or outpatient surgical facility.

DIAGNOSTIC TESTS
- Before surgery: Blood and urine studies; hearing tests.
- After surgery: Blood studies; hearing tests.

ANESTHESIA—Local anesthesia by topical application.

DESCRIPTION OF OPERATION
- An instrument called an ear speculum is placed in the external ear canal, and the operative microscope is positioned.
- An incision is made around the eardrum, with care taken not to injure the small bones in the middle ear.
- The fluid is drained, and small tubes are usually left in place to continue drainage.
- No sutures are placed in the eardrum. It will heal by itself, if infection is minimal or absent.
- The tubes will prevent premature closure of the eardrum and allow the middle ear to heal. Usually, the tubes can be removed 1 to 3 weeks after surgery.

POSSIBLE COMPLICATIONS
- Excessive bleeding.
- Surgical-wound infection.
- Hearing loss.

AVERAGE HOSPITAL STAY—0 to 1 day.

PROBABLE OUTCOME—Expect complete healing without complications. Hearing should improve noticeably. Allow about 4 weeks for recovery from surgery.

POSTOPERATIVE CARE

NOTE—This information is supplemental and should not replace your doctor's instructions.

GENERAL MEASURES
- Keep the ear dry.
- Apply warm compresses or a heating pad to relieve discomfort.

MEDICATION
- Your doctor may prescribe:
  Pain relievers. Don't take prescription pain medication longer than 4 to 7 days. Use *only* as much as you need.
  Antibiotics to fight infection.
- You may use non-prescription drugs, such as acetaminophen, for minor pain.

ACTIVITY
- Return to work and normal activity as soon as possible. This reduces postoperative depression, which is common.
- Resume driving about 1 week after returning home.

DIET—Liquid diet the first day after surgery, then no special diet.

CALL YOUR DOCTOR IF

- Pain, swelling, redness, drainage or bleeding increases in the surgical area.
- You develop signs of infection: headache, muscle aches, dizziness or a general ill feeling and fever.
- You experience new symptoms, such as nausea or vomiting.

NASAL-POLYPS REMOVAL
(Nasal Polypectomy)

 GENERAL INFORMATION

DEFINITION—Removal of nasal polyps, accumulations of fluid under the membrane lining inside the nose.

BODY PARTS INVOLVED—Nose and its membrane lining.

REASONS FOR SURGERY—Restoration of normal breathing.

SURGICAL RISK INCREASES WITH—None expected.

 WHAT TO EXPECT

WHO OPERATES—Ear, nose and throat specialist or general surgeon.

WHERE PERFORMED—Doctor's office, hospital or outpatient surgical facility.

DIAGNOSTIC TESTS—Blood and urine studies before surgery.

ANESTHESIA
- Local anesthesia by topical application.
- Local anesthesia by injection.

DESCRIPTION OF OPERATION
- The nose is held open with a speculum.
- The polyps are located, clamped and removed with a wire loop.
- Bleeding is controlled with electrocautery.
- Petroleum jelly and gauze may be applied to the surgical area to prevent bleeding. Your doctor will remove this dressing, usually 3 to 4 days after surgery.

POSSIBLE COMPLICATIONS
- Excessive bleeding.
- Surgical-wound infection.

AVERAGE HOSPITAL STAY—0 to 1 day.

PROBABLE OUTCOME—Expect complete healing without complications. Allow about 2 weeks for recovery from surgery.

 POSTOPERATIVE CARE

NOTE—This information is supplemental and should not replace your doctor's instructions.

GENERAL MEASURES
- Don't blow your nose for the first 3 days after surgery.
- Beginning 24 hours after surgery, apply warm compresses to the nose to relieve discomfort. Do this for 15 to 20 minutes several times daily, for as long as needed.

MEDICATION
- Your doctor may prescribe:
  Pain relievers. Don't take prescription pain medication longer than 4 to 7 days. Use *only* as much as you need.
  Antibiotics to fight infection.
- You may use non-prescription drugs, such as acetaminophen, to relieve minor pain.

ACTIVITY—Resume driving 3 days after returning home.

DIET—Eat a well-balanced, high-protein diet to promote healing.

 CALL YOUR DOCTOR IF

- Pain, swelling, redness, drainage or bleeding increase in the surgical area.
- You develop signs of infection: headache, muscle aches, dizziness or a general ill feeling and fever.
- You experience new symptoms, such as nausea or vomiting.

NECK, RADICAL DISSECTION OF

GENERAL INFORMATION

DEFINITION—Removal of cancerous growths in the tissues in the neck.

BODY PARTS INVOLVED—Neck muscles; lymph glands; windpipe.

REASONS FOR SURGERY—Cancer in the oral cavity or neck, which will spread to other parts of the body, if not removed.

SURGICAL RISK INCREASES WITH
- Adults over 60.
- Obesity.
- Smoking.
- Poor nutrition.
- Recent or chronic illness, especially respiratory illness.
- Alcoholism or chronic illness.
- Use of drugs such as: antihypertensives; muscle relaxants; tranquilizers; sleep inducers; insulin; sedatives; beta-adrenergic blockers; or cortisone.
- Use of mind-altering drugs, including: narcotics; psychedelics; hallucinogens; marijuana; sedatives; hypnotics; or cocaine.

WHAT TO EXPECT

WHO OPERATES—Ear, nose and throat specialist or general surgeon.

WHERE PERFORMED—Hospital.

DIAGNOSTIC TESTS
- Before surgery: Blood and urine studies; X-rays of chest; EKG (see Glossary).
- After surgery: Blood studies.

ANESTHESIA—General anesthesia by inhalation and injection, with an airway tube placed in the windpipe.

DESCRIPTION OF OPERATION
- An incision shaped like an "H" is made in the neck. Skin flaps are separated from the underlying tissue.
- The lymph glands, muscles and connective tissue are cut free and removed.
- Sometimes, a tracheostomy is performed.
- Tubes are left in the surgical area to drain secretions.
- The connective tissue is closed, and the skin is closed with sutures or clips, which usually can be removed about 1 week after surgery.

POSSIBLE COMPLICATIONS
- Excessive bleeding.
- Surgical-wound infection.
- Restricted breathing.
- Inadvertent injury to the large blood vessels and nerves in the neck, tip of the lung, thoracic duct or laryngeal nerve.

AVERAGE HOSPITAL STAY—13 to 15 days.

PROBABLE OUTCOME—Expect complete healing. Removing tissue in the neck may cause some unavoidable disfigurement. However, some cancers can be cured completely with this surgery. Allow about 4 weeks for recovery from surgery.

POSTOPERATIVE CARE

NOTE—This information is supplemental and should not replace your doctor's instructions.

GENERAL MEASURES
- A hard ridge should form along the incision. As it heals, the ridge will recede gradually.
- Use an electric heating pad, a heat lamp or a warm compress to relieve incisional pain.
- Bathe and shower as usual. You may wash the incision gently with mild unscented soap.
- Move legs often while resting in bed to decrease the likelihood of deep-vein blood clots.

MEDICATION—Your doctor may prescribe:
- Pain relievers. Don't take prescription pain medication longer than 4 to 7 days. Use *only* as much as you need.
- Stool softeners to prevent constipation.
- Antibiotics to fight infection.

ACTIVITY
- Resume work and normal activity as soon as possible to reduce postoperative depression, which is common.
- Avoid vigorous exercise for 6 weeks after surgery.
- Resume driving 5 weeks after returning home.

DIET—Clear liquid diet until the gastrointestinal tract begins to function again. Then eat a well-balanced, high-protein diet to promote healing.

CALL YOUR DOCTOR IF

- Pain, swelling, redness, drainage or bleeding increases in the surgical area.
- You develop signs of infection: headache, muscle aches, dizziness or a general ill feeling and fever.
- You experience new symptoms such as: nausea; vomiting; constipation; abdominal swelling; hoarseness; or difficulty with breathing.

OVARIAN-CYST OR TUMOR REMOVAL

 GENERAL INFORMATION

DEFINITION—Removal of cysts on an ovary.

BODY PARTS INVOLVED—Ovary.

REASONS FOR SURGERY
- Cancer or suspected cancer in the ovaries.
- Rupture or twisting of an ovarian cyst.

SURGICAL RISK INCREASES WITH
- Adults over 60.
- Stress.
- Obesity.
- Smoking.
- Poor nutrition.
- Recent or chronic illness.
- Alcoholism.
- Use of drugs such as: antihypertensives; muscle relaxants; tranquilizers; sleep inducers; insulin; sedatives; beta-adrenergic blockers; or cortisone.
- Use of mind-altering drugs.

 WHAT TO EXPECT

WHO OPERATES—Obstetrician-gynecologist or general surgeon.

WHERE PERFORMED—Hospital.

DIAGNOSTIC TESTS
- Before surgery: Blood and urine studies; CAT scan of pelvic organs; laparoscopy or culdoscopy; ultrasound; X-rays of chest, lower abdomen and lower intestinal tract; culdocentesis (see Glossary for all).
- During surgery: Laboratory examination of removed tissue by frozen section (see Glossary).
- After surgery: Blood studies.

ANESTHESIA—General anesthesia by inhalation and injection, with an airway tube placed in the windpipe.

DESCRIPTION OF OPERATION
- An incision is made in the abdomen. The abdominal muscles are separated and the peritoneum is opened.
- Blood vessels supplying the ovaries are located, clamped and tied.
- The tumor or cyst in the ovary is located, cut free and removed. If examination reveals signs of cancer, the ovary is removed.
- The peritoneum is closed, and the abdominal muscles are sewn together with heavy sutures.
- The skin is closed with sutures or clips, which usually can be removed about 10 days after surgery.

POSSIBLE COMPLICATIONS
- Excessive bleeding.
- Surgical-wound infection.

AVERAGE HOSPITAL STAY—5 to 7 days.

PROBABLE OUTCOME—Expect complete healing of surgical wound. If cancer is detected, your doctor will prescribe treatment with radiation or anticancer drugs. Allow about 4 weeks for recovery from surgery.

 POSTOPERATIVE CARE

NOTE—This information is supplemental and should not replace your doctor's instructions.

GENERAL MEASURES
- A hard ridge should form along the incision. As it heals, the ridge will recede gradually.
- Use an electric heating pad, a heat lamp or a warm compress to relieve incisional pain.
- Bathe and shower as usual. You may wash the incision gently with mild unscented soap.
- Move legs often while resting in bed to decrease the likelihood of deep-vein blood clots.

MEDICATION
- Your doctor may prescribe:
  Pain relievers. Don't take prescription pain medication longer than 4 to 7 days. Use *only* as much as you need.
  Stool softeners to prevent constipation.
  Hormone supplements.
  Antibiotics to fight infection.
- You may use non-prescription drugs, such as acetaminophen, for minor pain.

ACTIVITY
- Resume work and normal activity as soon as possible. This reduces postoperative depression and irritability, which are common.
- Avoid vigorous exercise for 6 weeks after surgery.
- Resume sexual relations when your doctor determines that healing is complete.

DIET—Clear liquid diet until the gastrointestinal tract functions again. Then eat a well-balanced, high-protein diet to promote healing.

 CALL YOUR DOCTOR IF

- Pain, swelling, redness, drainage or bleeding increases in the surgical area.
- You develop signs of infection: headache, muscle aches, dizziness or a general ill feeling and fever.
- You experience nausea, vomiting, constipation, abdominal swelling or hot flashes.
- New, unexplained symptoms develop. Drugs used in treatment may produce side effects.

PACEMAKER INSERTION

 GENERAL INFORMATION

DEFINITION—Insertion of a pacemaker into the chest. A pacemaker is an electronic device consisting of an electrode connected to the heart muscle and a regulatory device and power source implanted in the skin. It provides regular, mild electric shocks that stimulate the heart muscle and maintain normal heartbeat.

BODY PARTS INVOLVED—Veins in neck; tissue under the skin below the collarbone; heart.

REASONS FOR SURGERY
- Regulation of heartbeat that has slowed due to heart disease.
- Prevention of heart block.

SURGICAL RISK INCREASES WITH
- Adults over 60.
- Stress.
- Obesity.
- Smoking.
- Excess alcohol consumption.
- Use of drugs such as: antihypertensives; muscle relaxants; tranquilizers; sleep inducers; insulin; sedatives; beta-adrenergic blockers; or cortisone.
- Use of mind-altering drugs, including: narcotics; psychedelics; hallucinogens; marijuana; sedatives; hypnotics; or cocaine.

 WHAT TO EXPECT

WHO OPERATES—Cardiovascular surgeon.

WHERE PERFORMED—Outpatient surgical facility or hospital.

DIAGNOSTIC TESTS
- Before surgery: Blood and urine studies; X-rays of chest; EKG (see Glossary for all).
- During surgery: EKG monitor; fluoroscopy (see Glossary for both).
- After surgery: EKG.

ANESTHESIA—Local anesthesia by injection.

DESCRIPTION OF OPERATION
- Small incisions are made below the collarbone and in the vein under the collarbone. An electrode is passed through the vein into the heart. The implantation site is confirmed.
- The electrode is attached to the power and regulating units. The entire device is inserted under the skin in a pouch created from tissue under the collarbone.
- The skin is closed with suture material, which usually can be removed about 1 week after surgery.

POSSIBLE COMPLICATIONS
- Excessive bleeding.
- Surgical-wound infection.
- Rupture in the heart muscle (rare).
- Some pacemakers may be affected by radiation from microwave ovens. Ask your doctor.

AVERAGE HOSPITAL STAY—0 to 2 days.

PROBABLE OUTCOME—Expect complete healing without complications. Allow about 2 weeks for recovery from surgery.

 POSTOPERATIVE CARE

NOTE—This information is supplemental and should not replace your doctor's instructions.

GENERAL MEASURES
- A hard ridge should form along the incision. As it heals, the ridge will recede gradually.
- Use an electric heating pad, a heat lamp or a warm compress to relieve incisional pain.
- Bathe or shower as usual. You may wash the incision gently with mild unscented soap.

MEDICATION
- Your doctor may prescribe pain relievers. Don't take prescription pain medication longer than 4 to 7 days. Use *only* as much as you need.
- You may use non-prescription drugs, such as acetaminophen, for minor pain.

ACTIVITY
- Return to work and normal activity as soon as possible. This reduces postoperative depression, which is common.
- Avoid vigorous exercise for 2 weeks after surgery.
- Resume driving about 1 week after returning home.
- Resume sexual relations when able.

DIET—No special diet.

 CALL YOUR DOCTOR IF

- Pain, swelling, redness, drainage or bleeding increases in the surgical area.
- You develop signs of infection: headache, muscle aches, dizziness or a general ill feeling and fever.

PANCREAS TRANSPLANT

GENERAL INFORMATION

DEFINITION—Replacement of a diseased pancreas with a healthy pancreas obtained immediately after death from a donor with compatible immunological characteristics. The duodenum is also replaced to allow drainage of pancreatic secretions into the gastrointestinal tract.

BODY PARTS INVOLVED—Diseased or abnormal pancreas and duodenum; healthy donor pancreas and duodenum.

REASONS FOR SURGERY—Prevention of complications of severe diabetes mellitus, such as kidney failure and damage to the retinas.

SURGICAL RISK INCREASES WITH
- Adults over 60.
- Obesity.
- Smoking.
- Stress.
- Poor nutrition.
- Excess alcohol consumption.
- Recent or chronic illness.
- Alcoholism.
- Use of drugs such as: antihypertensives; muscle relaxants; tranquilizers; sleep inducers; insulin; sedatives; beta-adrenergic blockers; or cortisone.
- Use of mind-altering drugs.

WHAT TO EXPECT

WHO OPERATES—General surgeon.

WHERE PERFORMED—Hospital.

DIAGNOSTIC TESTS
- Before surgery: Evaluation of all body systems; immune-system and pancreas matching procedures.
- After surgery: Blood studies.

ANESTHESIA—General anesthesia by inhalation and injection, with an airway tube placed in the windpipe.

DESCRIPTION OF OPERATION
- The pancreas is removed from the donor, chilled and preserved up to 12 hours until surgery.
- An incision is made under the ribs.
- The abdominal muscles are divided and the peritoneal cavity is entered.
- The pancreas and duodenum are cut free and removed.
- The donor pancreas and duodenum are positioned and connected to blood vessels.
- Sometimes, only the cells of the pancreas that produce insulin (islet cells) are transplanted. In some patients, this is all that is necessary to re-establish normal function.

- The peritoneum and muscles are closed. The skin is closed with sutures or clips, which usually can be removed in 1 week.

POSSIBLE COMPLICATIONS
- Excessive bleeding.
- Surgical-wound infection.
- Rejection of transplant.

AVERAGE HOSPITAL STAY—3 weeks.

PROBABLE OUTCOME—Islet-cell transplants are usually successful in giving young diabetics near-normal life expectancy. In adults, a successful transplant prolongs life and improves the quality of life for patients who might otherwise have died, but life expectancy is currently unknown. Allow about 6 months for recovery from surgery.

POSTOPERATIVE CARE

NOTE—This information is supplemental and should not replace your doctor's instructions.

GENERAL MEASURES
- A hard ridge should form along the incision. As it heals, the ridge will recede gradually.
- Bathe and shower as usual. You may wash the incision gently with mild unscented soap.
- Use an electric heating pad, a heat lamp or a warm compress to relieve incisional pain.
- Move legs often while resting in bed to decrease the chance of deep-vein blood clots.

MEDICATION—Your doctor may prescribe:
- Pain relievers. Don't take prescription pain medication longer than 4 to 7 days. Use *only* as much as you need.
- Stool softeners to prevent constipation.
- Antibiotics to fight infection.
- Immunosuppressants to decrease the likelihood of rejection.

ACTIVITY
- Resume work and normal activity as soon as possible. This reduces postoperative depression and irritability, which are common.
- Avoid vigorous exercise for 6 months.

DIET—You doctor will prescribe a diet.

CALL YOUR DOCTOR IF

Any of the following occur:
- Increased pain, swelling, redness, drainage or bleeding in the surgical area.
- Headache, muscle aches, dizziness or a general ill feeling and fever.
- Nausea, vomiting, constipation or abdominal swelling.
- Increased frequency of urination or increased thirst.
- New, unexplained symptoms. Drugs used in treatment may produce side effects.

PARATHYROIDECTOMY

GENERAL INFORMATION

DEFINITION—Removal of parathyroid tumors or the parathyroid glands.

BODY PARTS INVOLVED—Parathyroid glands (at least 4 glands, sometimes up to 7).

REASONS FOR SURGERY
- Hyperparathyroidism.
- Cancer or suspected cancer.

SURGICAL RISK INCREASES WITH
- Obesity.
- Smoking.
- Stress.
- Poor nutrition.
- Recent or chronic illness.
- Alcoholism.
- Use of drugs such as: antihypertensives; muscle relaxants; tranquilizers; sleep inducers; insulin; sedatives; beta-adrenergic blockers; or cortisone.
- Use of mind-altering drugs, including: narcotics; psychedelics; hallucinogens; marijuana; sedatives; hypnotics; or cocaine.

WHAT TO EXPECT

WHO OPERATES—General surgeon.

WHERE PERFORMED—Hospital.

DIAGNOSTIC TESTS
- Before surgery: Blood and urine studies; X-rays of upper gastrointestinal tract.
- During surgery: Laboratory examination of removed tissue by frozen section (see Glossary).
- After surgery: Blood studies; laboratory examination of removed tissue.

ANESTHESIA—General anesthesia by inhalation and injection, with an airway tube placed in the windpipe.

DESCRIPTION OF OPERATION
- An incision is made in the neck just under the Adam's apple.
- The parathyroid glands are located. A section of one is cut free, removed, frozen and examined.
- If a benign tumor is detected, it is removed. If the tissue is an enlarged, overactive gland rather than a tumor, all except one of the other parathyroid glands are cut free and removed. One of the glands is left in place to help prevent hypoparathyroidism.

POSSIBLE COMPLICATIONS
- Excessive bleeding.
- Surgical-wound infection.
- Hypoparathyroidism.
- Inadvertent injury to thyroid gland or vocal-cord nerves.
- Kidney stones.

AVERAGE HOSPITAL STAY—7 to 10 days.

PROBABLE OUTCOME—Expect complete healing without complications. Allow about 4 weeks for recovery from surgery.

POSTOPERATIVE CARE

NOTE—This information is supplemental and should not replace your doctor's instructions.

GENERAL MEASURES
- A hard ridge should form along the incision. As it heals, the ridge will recede gradually.
- Use an electric heating pad, a heat lamp or a warm compress to relieve incisional pain.
- Bathe and shower as usual. You may wash the incision gently with mild unscented soap.
- Move legs often while resting in bed to decrease the likelihood of deep-vein blood clots.

MEDICATION
- Your doctor may prescribe:
  Pain relievers. Don't take prescription pain medication longer than 4 to 7 days. Use *only* as much as you need.
  Stool softeners to prevent constipation.
  Antibiotics to fight infection.
- You may use non-prescription drugs, such as acetaminophen, for minor pain.
- Don't take thiazide diuretics or antacids that contain calcium. These may cause calcium, potassium or sodium imbalance.

ACTIVITY
- Resume work and normal activity as soon as possible. This reduces postoperative depression and irritability, which are common.
- Avoid vigorous activity for 6 weeks after surgery.
- Resume driving 2 weeks after returning home.

DIET—Your doctor will prescribe a diet. Drink at least 3 quarts of liquids daily from now on. Include 1 or 2 glasses of cranberry juice daily to prevent kidney stones from forming.

CALL YOUR DOCTOR IF

- Pain, swelling, redness, drainage or bleeding increases in the surgical area.
- You develop signs of infection: headache, muscle aches, dizziness or a general ill feeling and fever.
- You experience nausea, vomiting, constipation or abdominal swelling.
- You have numbness or tingling around the mouth or hands.
- New, unexplained symptoms develop. Drugs used in treatment may produce side effects.

PAROTID-GLAND TUMOR, REMOVAL OF

 ## GENERAL INFORMATION

DEFINITION—Removal of benign or cancerous tumors in the parotid glands.

BODY PARTS INVOLVED—Parotid glands, one of three paired sets of salivary glands, located inside the cheeks.

REASONS FOR SURGERY—Cancer or suspected cancer of the parotid glands.

SURGICAL RISK INCREASES WITH
- Adults over 60.
- Smoking.
- Poor nutrition.
- Recent illness, especially upper-respiratory illness.
- Alcoholism or chronic disease.
- Use of drugs such as: antihypertensives; muscle relaxants; tranquilizers; sleep inducers; insulin; sedatives; beta-adrenergic blockers; or cortisone.
- Use of mind-altering drugs, including: narcotics; psychedelics; hallucinogens; marijuana; sedatives; hypnotics; or cocaine.

 ## WHAT TO EXPECT

WHO OPERATES—Ear, nose and throat specialist, general surgeon or oral surgeon.

WHERE PERFORMED—Hospital.

DIAGNOSTIC TESTS
- Before surgery: Blood and urine studies.
- After surgery: Laboratory examination of removed tissue; blood studies.

ANESTHESIA—General anesthesia by inhalation and injection, with an airway tube placed in the windpipe.

DESCRIPTION OF OPERATION
- An incision shaped like a "Y" is made behind and in front of the ear, just below the jaw.
- The facial nerve is located and protected while the parotid gland is removed.
- Abnormal tissue is removed. If laboratory analysis of the tissue reveals the tumor to be cancerous, surgery to remove lymph glands in the neck must be anticipated. If cancer is detected, the facial nerve may have to be cut to remove all suspicious tissue.
- The skin is closed with sutures or clips, which usually can be removed about 1 week after surgery.

POSSIBLE COMPLICATIONS
- Excessive bleeding.
- Surgical-wound infection.
- Inadvertent or unavoidable injury to the facial nerve, causing facial distortion.
- Flushing of the skin and increased sweating at mealtime in the area of the removed parotid gland. The cause of this complication is unknown. It may not appear for up to a year after surgery.

AVERAGE HOSPITAL STAY—4 to 5 days.

PROBABLE OUTCOME—Expect complete healing without complications. Allow about 3 weeks for recovery from surgery.

 ## POSTOPERATIVE CARE

NOTE—This information is supplemental and should not replace your doctor's instructions.

GENERAL MEASURES
- A hard ridge should form along the incision. As it heals, the ridge will recede gradually.
- Use an electric heating pad, a heat lamp or a warm compress to relieve incisional pain.
- Bathe and shower as usual. You may wash the incision gently with mild unscented soap.

MEDICATION
- Your doctor may prescribe:
  Pain relievers. Don't take prescription pain medication longer than 4 to 7 days. Use *only* as much as you need.
  Stool softeners to prevent constipation.
  Antibiotics to fight infection.
- You may use non-prescription drugs, such as acetaminophen, for minor pain.

ACTIVITY
- Resume work and normal activity as soon as possible to reduce postoperative depression, which is common.
- Avoid vigorous exercise for 6 weeks after surgery.
- Resume driving about 1 week after returning home.

DIET—Clear liquid diet until the gastrointestinal tract begins to function again. Then eat a well-balanced, high-protein diet to promote healing.

 ## CALL YOUR DOCTOR IF

- Pain, swelling, redness, drainage or bleeding increases in the surgical area.
- You develop signs of infection: headache, muscle aches, dizziness or a general ill feeling and fever.
- You experience new symptoms such as nausea or vomiting.
- You experience difficulty in smiling or closing the eyelid on the side of the face where surgery was performed.

PENILE IMPLANT

GENERAL INFORMATION

DEFINITION—Insertion of semiflexible plastic bars or an inflatable prosthesis in the penis. The former produces a permanent, partial erection. The latter can be inflated at will.

BODY PARTS INVOLVED—Penis.

REASONS FOR SURGERY—Impotence.

SURGICAL RISK INCREASES WITH
- Obesity.
- Smoking.
- Stress.
- Poor nutrition.
- Recent or chronic illness.
- Alcoholism.
- Use of drugs such as: antihypertensives; muscle relaxants; tranquilizers; sleep inducers; insulin; sedatives; beta-adrenergic blockers; or cortisone.
- Use of mind-altering drugs, including: narcotics; psychedelics; hallucinogens; marijuana; sedatives; hypnotics; or cocaine.

WHAT TO EXPECT

WHO OPERATES—Urologist.

WHERE PERFORMED—Hospital.

DIAGNOSTIC TESTS
- Before surgery: Blood and urine studies.
- After surgery: Blood studies.

ANESTHESIA
- Spinal anesthesia by injection.
- General anesthesia by inhalation and injection, with an airway tube placed in the windpipe.

DESCRIPTION OF OPERATION
Plastic Implant:
- An incision is made in the underside of the penis.
- The tissues on both sides of the urethra are expanded to allow placement of the implants.
- An implant is placed on each side of the urethra.
- The skin is closed with sutures that will be absorbed by the body.
Inflatable Prosthesis:
- An incision is made in the top side of the penis.
- The penile tissue is stretched to allow placement of the prosthesis. The fluid reservoir for the prosthesis is implanted under the skin above the bladder at the base of the pelvis. The prosthesis can be inflated by applying pressure on the reservoir.
- The skin is closed with sutures that will be absorbed by the body.

POSSIBLE COMPLICATIONS—Surgical-wound infection.

AVERAGE HOSPITAL STAY—3 to 7 days.

PROBABLE OUTCOME—Expect complete recovery without complications. Allow about 4 weeks for recovery from surgery. Penile sensations and sexual arousal should be near normal.

POSTOPERATIVE CARE

NOTE—This information is supplemental and should not replace your doctor's instructions.

GENERAL MEASURES
- A hard ridge should form along the incision. As it heals, the ridge will recede gradually. After healing, the prosthesis should cause no discomfort.
- Use an electric heating pad, a heat lamp or a warm compress to relieve incisional pain.
- Bathe and shower as usual. You may wash the incision gently with mild unscented soap.

MEDICATION
- Your doctor may prescribe:
  Pain relievers. Don't take prescription pain medication longer than 4 to 7 days. Use *only* as much as you need.
  Antibiotics to fight infection.
- You may use non-prescription drugs, such as acetaminophen, for minor pain.

ACTIVITY
- Avoid vigorous exercise for 6 weeks after surgery.
- Resume sexual relations when your doctor determines that healing is complete.
- Resume driving 1 week after returning home.

DIET—No special diet.

CALL YOUR DOCTOR IF

- Pain, swelling, redness, drainage or bleeding increases in the surgical area.
- You develop signs of infection: headache, muscle aches, dizziness or a general ill feeling and fever.
- You experience new symptoms such as nausea, vomiting, constipation or abdominal swelling.
- You have pain or difficulty with urination.
- New, unexplained symptoms develop. Drugs used in treatment may produce side effects.

PEPTIC-ULCER SURGERY

GENERAL INFORMATION

DEFINITION—Surgery to treat the complications of peptic ulcer disease, especially destruction of the protective lining of the gastrointestinal tract that leads to ulcer craters.

BODY PARTS INVOLVED—Esophagus; stomach; duodenum; jejunum.

REASONS FOR SURGERY—Treatment of complications of peptic ulcers:
- Bleeding.
- Intolerable pain.
- Blockage of stomach contents from emptying.
- Perforation. If an ulcer perforates, the contents of the gastrointestinal tract are dumped into the abdominal cavity, causing peritonitis. This is a medical emergency requiring immediate surgery.

SURGICAL RISK INCREASES WITH
- Adults over 60.
- Stress.
- Alcoholism.
- Poor nutrition, especially vitamin and mineral deficiencies.
- Use of any drugs that irritate the stomach.
- Pancreatitis; hepatitis; diabetes mellitus; brain tumor; or extensive burns.

WHAT TO EXPECT

WHO OPERATES—General surgeon.

WHERE PERFORMED—Hospital.

DIAGNOSTIC TESTS
- Before surgery: Blood and urine studies; X-rays of abdomen.
- After surgery: Blood and urine studies; X-rays of abdomen.

ANESTHESIA—General anesthesia by inhalation and injection, with an airway tube placed in the windpipe.

DESCRIPTION OF OPERATION—Any of the following procedures is used to perform this surgery:
- Vagotomy and pyloroplasty: The nerve that stimulates stomach-acid production is severed, and the outlet of the stomach that leads to the duodenum is enlarged.
- Gastric resection: The part of the stomach that produces acid is removed, and the remaining stomach is attached with sutures to the duodenum or the jejunum.
- Closure of perforated ulcer: The perforated ulcer is closed by various methods. Incisions that are made are closed with sutures or clips, which usually can be removed about 1 week after surgery.

POSSIBLE COMPLICATIONS
- Excessive bleeding.
- Surgical-wound infection.
- Incisional hernia.

AVERAGE HOSPITAL STAY—6 to 8 days.

PROBABLE OUTCOME—Expect complete healing without complications. Allow about 4 to 6 weeks for recovery from surgery.

POSTOPERATIVE CARE

NOTE—This information is supplemental and should not replace your doctor's instructions.

GENERAL MEASURES
- Don't smoke.
- A hard ridge should form along the incision. As it heals, the ridge will recede gradually.
- Bathe and shower as usual. You may wash the incision gently with mild unscented soap.
- Use an electric heating pad, a heat lamp or a warm compress to relieve incisional pain.

MEDICATION—Your doctor may prescribe pain relievers. Don't take prescription pain medication longer than 4 to 7 days. Use *only* as much as you need. Don't take aspirin.

ACTIVITY
- Return to work and normal activity as soon as possible. This reduces postoperative depression, which is common.
- Resume driving about 2 weeks after returning home.

DIET—Clear liquid diet until the gastrointestinal tract functions again. Then eat a well-balanced, high-protein diet to promote healing. Avoid coffee, tea, cocoa, cola drinks, alcoholic beverages and any food or spice that aggravates symptoms.

CALL YOUR DOCTOR IF

Any of the following occurs:
- Increased pain, swelling, redness, drainage or bleeding in the surgical area.
- Headache, muscle aches, dizziness or a general ill feeling and fever.
- Increasing abdominal pain or swelling; constipation; nausea; vomiting; bleeding from the rectum or black, tarry stools.
- New, unexplained symptoms develop. Drugs used in treatment may produce side effects.

PERIODONTAL SURGERY

GENERAL INFORMATION

DEFINITION—Removal of infected tissue from the gums and reshaping of the bone underlying the gums.

BODY PARTS INVOLVED—Gums; surrounding bone.

REASONS FOR SURGERY—Prevention of the spread of gum infection.

SURGICAL RISK INCREASES WITH
- Adults over 60.
- Smoking.
- Excess alcohol consumption.
- Poor nutrition.
- Chronic illness.
- Recent illness such as upper respiratory infection.
- Use of drugs such as: antihypertensives; muscle relaxants; tranquilizers; sleep inducers; insulin; sedatives; beta-adrenergic blockers; or cortisone.
- Use of mind-altering drugs, including: narcotics; psychedelics; hallucinogens; marijuana; sedatives; hypnotics; or cocaine.

WHAT TO EXPECT

WHO OPERATES—Dentist or periodontist.

WHERE PERFORMED—Hospital, outpatient surgical facility or dentist's or periodontist's office.

DIAGNOSTIC TESTS
- Before surgery: Blood and urine studies; X-rays of the mouth.
- After surgery: Blood studies.

ANESTHESIA
- Local anesthesia by injection.
- General anesthesia (sometimes) by inhalation and injection, with an airway tube placed in the windpipe.

DESCRIPTION OF OPERATION
- The diseased periodontal tissue is carefully cut free and removed.
- The bone under the gum is reshaped, if necessary.
- Special dressings are applied that control bleeding and hasten healing. Your dentist will remove or replace dressings 5 to 10 days after surgery.

POSSIBLE COMPLICATIONS
- Excessive bleeding
- Surgical-wound infection.

AVERAGE HOSPITAL STAY—0 to 1 day.

PROBABLE OUTCOME—Expect complete healing without complications. The affected gum tissue should heal and return to its normal pink color again in 2 to 3 weeks.

POSTOPERATIVE CARE

NOTE—This information is supplemental and should not replace your doctor's instructions.

GENERAL MEASURES
- Do not disturb the dressing.
- Apply ice packs to relieve pain. Do this for 10 minutes at a time as often as needed for the first 24 hours after surgery.
- Keep your teeth free of plaque (germs, food debris and saliva). Brush your teeth and use dental floss as directed by your dentist. Mouth irrigations also help to prevent plaque.

MEDICATION
- Your doctor may prescribe:
  Pain relievers. Don't take prescription pain medication longer than 4 to 7 days. Use *only* as much as you need.
  Antibiotics to fight infection.
- You may use non-prescription drugs, such as acetaminophen, for minor pain.

ACTIVITY
- Return to work and normal activity as soon as possible. This reduces postoperative depression and irritability, which are common.
- Avoid vigorous exercise for 3 weeks after surgery.
- Resume driving 2 days after returning home.

DIET—Clear liquid diet until healing occurs. Then eat a well-balanced, high-protein diet to promote healing.

CALL YOUR DOCTOR IF

- The dressing becomes loose.
- You experience new symptoms, such as nausea or vomiting.
- Pain, swelling, redness, drainage or bleeding increases in the surgical area.
- Bleeding recurs 48 hours or longer after surgery.
- You develop signs of infection: headache, muscle aches, dizziness or a general ill feeling and fever.

PILONIDAL-CYST REMOVAL

 GENERAL INFORMATION

DEFINITION—Removal of a pilonidal cyst, a cyst that contains elements found in the skin, including hair, sweat and glands.

BODY PARTS INVOLVED—Area over the tailbone.

REASONS FOR SURGERY—Relief of pain and prevention of the spread of infection.

SURGICAL RISK INCREASES WITH
- Obesity.
- Smoking.
- Recent or chronic illness.
- Use of drugs such as: antihypertensives; muscle relaxants; tranquilizers; sleeping pills; insulin; sedatives; beta-adrenergic blockers; or cortisone.
- Use of mind-altering drugs, including: narcotics; psychedelics; hallucinogens; marijuana; sedatives; hypnotics; or cocaine.

 WHAT TO EXPECT

WHO OPERATES—General surgeon or proctologist.

WHERE PERFORMED—Hospital or outpatient surgical facility.

DIAGNOSTIC TESTS
- Before surgery: Blood and urine studies; sigmoidoscopy (see Glossary).
- After surgery: Blood tests.

ANESTHESIA
- Local anesthesia by injection.
- General anesthesia by inhalation and injection, with an airway tube placed in the windpipe.

DESCRIPTION OF OPERATION
- The cyst and its cavities (also called sinuses) over the tailbone are identified with probes. An incision is made in the cyst.
- The cyst and all affected sinuses are removed.
- Bleeding is controlled with sutures or electrocauterization.
- The skin is usually left open to heal from the bottom out.

POSSIBLE COMPLICATIONS
- Excessive bleeding.
- Surgical-wound infection.
- Slow healing.
- Recurrence of cyst.

AVERAGE HOSPITAL STAY—0 to 4 days.

PROBABLE OUTCOME—Expect complete healing without complications. Allow about 2 months for recovery from surgery.

 POSTOPERATIVE CARE

NOTE—This information is supplemental and should not replace your doctor's instructions.

GENERAL MEASURES
- Take warm baths to relieve discomfort. Do this for 15 to 20 minutes several times daily for the first week after surgery.
- Don't dry the surgical area with a towel. Drip dry or use a blow dryer after bathing.
- Sit on a rubber ring (available in drugstores) to relieve discomfort, if necessary.

MEDICATION
- Your doctor may prescribe:
  Pain relievers. Don't take prescription pain medication longer than 4 to 7 days. Use *only* as much as you need.
  Stool softeners to prevent constipation.
  Antibiotics to fight infection.
- You may use non-prescription drugs, such as acetaminophen, for minor pain.

ACTIVITY
- Return to work and normal activity as soon as possible. This reduces postoperative depression and irritability, which are common.
- Avoid vigorous exercise for 6 weeks after surgery.
- Resume driving 1 week after returning home.
- Resume sexual relations when your doctor determines that healing is complete.

DIET—Clear liquid diet until the gastrointestinal tract functions again. Then eat a well-balanced, high-protein diet to promote healing.

 CALL YOUR DOCTOR IF

- Pain, swelling, redness, drainage or bleeding increases in the surgical area.
- You develop signs of infection: headache, muscle aches, dizziness or a general ill feeling and fever.
- New, unexplained symptoms develop. Drugs used in treatment may produce side effects.

POPLITEAL-ARTERY EMBOLECTOMY

 ## GENERAL INFORMATION

DEFINITION—Removal of a blood clot that has blocked blood supply to the leg and foot.

BODY PARTS INVOLVED—Blood vessel in the leg that is called the femoral artery below the groin and the popliteal artery below the knee.

REASONS FOR SURGERY—Restoration of normal blood circulation in the legs. Re-establishing blood flow can restore muscular function, prevent gangrene and enable patients to return to normal or almost normal activities.

SURGICAL RISK INCREASES WITH
- Obesity.
- Smoking.
- Rheumatic heart disease or coronary-artery disease.
- Use of drugs such as: antihypertensives; muscle relaxants; tranquilizers; sleep inducers; insulin; sedatives; narcotics; beta-adrenergic blockers; or cortisone.

 ## WHAT TO EXPECT

WHO OPERATES—General surgeon or vascular surgeon.

WHERE PERFORMED—Outpatient surgical facility or hospital.

DIAGNOSTIC TESTS
- Before surgery: Blood and urine studies; arteriogram (see Glossary).
- During surgery: Arteriogram after blood clot is removed.
- After surgery: Blood studies.

ANESTHESIA—Spinal anesthesia by injection.

DESCRIPTION OF OPERATION
- An incision is made over the artery where the clot is lodged.
- The artery is clamped above and below the blood clot.
- The artery is opened above the blood clot.
- A special catheter is passed into the artery beyond the blood clot. The catheter is expanded with air beyond the clot and then withdrawn, forcing the clots out of the artery.
- An anticoagulant is injected into the artery, and normal blood circulation is restored.
- The clamps are removed from the arteries. Muscles and connective tissue are sewn together in layers. The skin is closed with sutures or clamps, which usually can be removed about 1 week after surgery.

POSSIBLE COMPLICATIONS
- Excessive bleeding.
- Surgical-wound infection.
- Inadvertent injury to the large nerves.

AVERAGE HOSPITAL STAY—0 to 3 days.

PROBABLE OUTCOME—Expect complete healing without complications. Allow about 3 weeks for recovery from surgery.

 ## POSTOPERATIVE CARE

NOTE—This information is supplemental and should not replace your doctor's instructions.

GENERAL MEASURES
- Don't smoke.
- Keep feet clean and dry.
- A hard ridge should form along the incision. As it heals, the ridge will recede gradually.
- Use an electric heating pad, a heat lamp or a warm compress to relieve incisional pain.
- Bathe and shower as usual. You may wash the incision gently with mild unscented soap.
- Move legs often while resting in bed to decrease the likelihood of deep-vein blood clots.

MEDICATION
- You may use non-prescription drugs, such as acetaminophen, for minor pain.
- Your doctor may prescribe pain relievers. Don't take prescription pain medication longer than 4 to 7 days. Use *only* as much as you need.

ACTIVITY
- Resume work and normal activity as soon as possible to reduce postoperative depression, which is common.
- Avoid vigorous exercise for 3 weeks after surgery, but start a walking exercise program as soon as your doctor recommends.
- Resume driving about 1 week after returning home.

DIET—No special diet.

 ## CALL YOUR DOCTOR IF

- Pain, swelling, redness, drainage or bleeding increases in the surgical area.
- You develop signs of infection: headache, muscle aches, dizziness or a general ill feeling and fever.
- Your foot becomes cold, discolored or numb.
- Preoperative symptoms don't improve.

PORTACAVAL SHUNT

GENERAL INFORMATION

DEFINITION—Connection of the portal vein with the vena cava to release backed-up pressure in the venous system (veins) that drains the intestinal tract.

BODY PARTS INVOLVED—Portal vein (the large vein that drains the liver); vena cava (the largest vein in the body that drains all the blood from the intestines and the lower part of the body).

REASONS FOR SURGERY—Treatment or prevention of bleeding from esophageal varices (large veins in the lower esophagus).

SURGICAL RISK INCREASES WITH
- Adults over 60.
- Obesity.
- Smoking.
- Poor nutrition.
- Recent or chronic illness.
- Alcoholism.
- Use of drugs such as: antihypertensives; muscle relaxants; tranquilizers; sleep inducers; insulin; sedatives; beta-adrenergic blockers; or cortisone.
- Use of mind-altering drugs.

WHAT TO EXPECT

WHO OPERATES—General surgeon or vascular surgeon.

WHERE PERFORMED—Hospital.

DIAGNOSTIC TESTS
- Before surgery: Blood and urine studies; X-rays of chest and upper gastrointestinal tract; EKG; esophagoscopy (see Glossary).
- After surgery: Blood studies.

ANESTHESIA—General anesthesia by inhalation and injection, with an airway tube placed in the windpipe.

DESCRIPTION OF OPERATION
- An incision is made in the abdomen.
- The portal vein and vena cava are located and isolated.
- The portal vein is clamped in two places and divided between the clamps. A "window" is cut into the vena cava. One end of the severed portal vein is tied and the other end is sewn into the window in the vena cava. This allows blood from the portal vein to drain directly into the vena cava.
- The abdominal cavity is closed, and the muscle layers are reconstructed with sutures.
- The skin is closed with sutures or clips, which usually can be removed about 1 week after surgery.

POSSIBLE COMPLICATIONS—Excessive bleeding; surgical-wound infection; incisional hernia or inadvertent injury to parts of the body near the surgical area, including the arteries, nerves and common bile duct.

AVERAGE HOSPITAL STAY—12 to 14 days.

PROBABLE OUTCOME—Expect complete healing without complications. Allow about 2 months for recovery from surgery.

POSTOPERATIVE CARE

NOTE—This information is supplemental and should not replace your doctor's instructions.

GENERAL MEASURES
- A hard ridge should form along the incision. As it heals, the ridge will recede gradually.
- Use an electric heating pad, a heat lamp or a warm compress to relieve incisional pain.
- Bathe and shower as usual. You may wash the incision gently with mild unscented soap.
- Move legs often while resting in bed to decrease the likelihood of deep-vein blood clots.

MEDICATION
- Your doctor may prescribe:
  Pain relievers. Don't take prescription pain medication longer than 4 to 7 days. Use *only* as much as you need.
  Stool softeners to prevent constipation.
  Antibiotics to fight infection.
- You may use non-prescription drugs, such as acetaminophen, for minor pain.

ACTIVITY
- Resume work and normal activity as soon as possible to reduce postoperative depression, which is common.
- Avoid vigorous exercise for 6 weeks after surgery.
- Resume driving 4 weeks after returning home.

DIET—Clear liquid diet until the gastrointestinal tract begins to function again. Then eat a well-balanced, high-protein diet to promote healing. Avoid coffee, tea, cocoa, cola drinks, alcoholic beverages and any food or spice that causes indigestion.

CALL YOUR DOCTOR IF

- Pain, swelling, redness, drainage or bleeding increases in the surgical area.
- You develop signs of infection: headache, muscle aches, dizziness or a general ill feeling and fever.
- You experience nausea, vomiting, constipation or abdominal swelling.
- You vomit blood or have black, tarry stools.

PROSTATE-GLAND REMOVAL, SUPRAPUBIC

 ## GENERAL INFORMATION

DEFINITION—Removal of part or all of an enlarged prostate gland through an opening above the pubic bone.

BODY PARTS INVOLVED—Prostate gland; bladder; rectum; urethra.

REASONS FOR SURGERY—Restoration of normal passage of urine.

SURGICAL RISK INCREASES WITH
- Adults over 60.
- Stress.
- Smoking.
- Obesity.
- Poor nutrition.
- Recent illness, especially upper-respiratory infection.
- Alcoholism or chronic illness.
- Use of drugs such as: antihypertensives; muscle relaxants; tranquilizers; sleep inducers; insulin; sedatives; beta-adrenergic blockers; or cortisone.
- Use of mind-altering drugs, including: narcotics; psychedelics; hallucinogens; marijuana; sedatives; hypnotics; or cocaine.

 ## WHAT TO EXPECT

WHO OPERATES—Urologist.

WHERE PERFORMED—Hospital.

DIAGNOSTIC TESTS
- Before surgery: Blood and urine studies; kidney function studies; X-rays of lower tract, kidneys and chest; EKG (see Glossary).
- After surgery: Blood studies.

ANESTHESIA
- Spinal anesthesia by injection.
- General anesthesia by inhalation and injection, with an airway tube placed in the windpipe.

DESCRIPTION OF OPERATION
- An incision is made in the lower abdomen.
- The bladder and urethra are opened, and the enlarged parts of the prostate gland cut free and removed.
- Two catheters are placed in the bladder, and a tube to drain secretions is placed next to the bladder. The urethra and bladder are closed with sutures. One of the catheters will pass through the penis, and the other will be brought out through the incision along with the drain.
- The muscles are repositioned and sewn in place. The skin is closed with sutures or clips, which usually can be removed about 1 week after surgery.

POSSIBLE COMPLICATIONS
- Excessive bleeding.
- Surgical-wound infection.
- Inability to control urinary stream.
- Impotence (usually) and sterility.

AVERAGE HOSPITAL STAY—7 to 10 days.

PROBABLE OUTCOME—Expect complete healing without complications. Allow about 6 weeks for recovery from surgery.

 ## POSTOPERATIVE CARE

NOTE—This information is supplemental and should not replace your doctor's instructions.

GENERAL MEASURES
- A hard ridge should form along the incision. As it heals the ridge will recede gradually.
- Use an electric heating pad, a heat lamp or a warm compress to relieve incisional pain.
- Bathe and shower as usual. You may wash the incision gently with mild unscented soap.
- Move legs often while resting in bed to decrease the likelihood of deep-vein blood clots.

MEDICATION
- Your doctor may prescribe:
  Pain relievers. Don't take prescription pain medication longer than 4 to 7 days. Use *only* as much as you need.
  Stool softeners to prevent constipation.
  Antibiotics to fight infection.
- You may use non-prescription drugs, such as acetaminophen, for minor pain.

ACTIVITY
- Resume work and normal activity as soon as possible to reduce postoperative depression, which is common.
- Resume driving 5 weeks after returning home.
- Resume sexual relations when able.

DIET—Clear liquid diet until the gastrointestinal tract begins to function again. Then eat a well-balanced, high-protein diet to promote healing. Avoid coffee, tea, cocoa, cola drinks, alcoholic beverages and any food or spice that aggravates symptoms.

 ## CALL YOUR DOCTOR IF

- Pain, swelling, redness or drainage increases in the surgical area.
- You experience excessive bleeding.
- You develop signs of infection: headache, muscle aches, dizziness or a general ill feeling and fever.
- You experience new symptoms, such as: nausea; vomiting; constipation; abdominal swelling or pain; or difficulty with urination.

PROSTATE-GLAND REMOVAL, TRANSURETHRAL

 GENERAL INFORMATION

DEFINITION—Removal of part or all of an enlarged prostate gland with a cystoscope, an instrument that is passed up through the urethra.

BODY PARTS INVOLVED—Penis; prostate gland; urethra; bladder.

REASONS FOR SURGERY—Restoration of normal passage of urine.

SURGICAL RISK INCREASES WITH
- Stress.
- Obesity.
- Poor nutrition.
- Smoking.
- Recent illness.
- Alcoholism or chronic illness.
- Use of drugs such as: antihypertensives; muscle relaxants; tranquilizers; sleep inducers; insulin; sedatives; beta-adrenergic blockers; or cortisone.
- Use of mind-altering drugs, including: narcotics; psychedelics; hallucinogens; marijuana; sedatives; hypnotics; or cocaine.

 WHAT TO EXPECT

WHO OPERATES—Urologist.

WHERE PERFORMED—Hospital.

DIAGNOSTIC TESTS
- Before surgery: Blood and urine studies; kidney-function studies; X-rays of kidneys and chest; EKG (see Glossary).
- After surgery: Blood studies.

ANESTHESIA
- Spinal anesthesia by injection.
- General anesthesia by inhalation and injection, with an airway tube placed in the windpipe.

DESCRIPTION OF OPERATION
- A cystoscope is passed up through the urethra to the prostate gland.
- A miniature telescope and light inside the cystoscope make the prostate gland visible.
- An electrical current in the cystoscope tip is used to cauterize and remove the enlarged or diseased parts of the prostate gland.

POSSIBLE COMPLICATIONS
- Excessive bleeding.
- Surgical-wound infection.
- Impotence (sometimes) and sterility.
- Epididymitis.

AVERAGE HOSPITAL STAY—11 to 12 days.

PROBABLE OUTCOME—Expect complete healing without complications. Allow about 3 weeks for recovery from surgery.

 POSTOPERATIVE CARE

NOTE—This information is supplemental and should not replace your doctor's instructions.

GENERAL MEASURES—Move legs often while resting in bed to decrease the likelihood of deep-vein blood clots.

MEDICATION
- Your doctor may prescribe:
  Pain relievers. Don't take prescription pain medication longer than 4 to 7 days. Use *only* as much as you need.
  Stool softeners to prevent constipation.
  Antibiotics to fight infection.
- You may use non-prescription drugs, such as acetaminophen, for minor pain.

ACTIVITY
- Resume work and normal activity as soon as possible to reduce postoperative depression, which is common.
- Avoid vigorous exercise for 6 weeks after surgery.
- Resume driving 1 month after returning home.
- Try to resume sexual relations when your doctor determines that healing is complete.

DIET—Clear liquid diet until the gastrointestinal tract begins to function again. Then eat a well-balanced, high-protein diet to promote healing. Avoid coffee, tea, cocoa, cola drinks, alcoholic beverages and any food or spice that aggravates symptoms.

 CALL YOUR DOCTOR IF

- Pain, swelling, redness, drainage or bleeding increases in the surgical area.
- You develop signs of infection: headache, muscle aches, dizziness or a general ill feeling and fever.
- You experience new symptoms such as nausea, vomiting, constipation, pain or difficulty with urination.
- You remain impotent longer than 3 months after surgery.

PTERYGIUM REMOVAL

GENERAL INFORMATION

DEFINITION—Removal of a pterygium, an abnormal tissue that grows from the edge of the eye and extends to attach to the cornea.

BODY PARTS INVOLVED—Eye; cornea; membrane lining eyelid (conjunctiva).

REASONS FOR SURGERY
- Restoration of normal vision.
- Improved appearance.

SURGICAL RISK INCREASES WITH—None expected.

WHAT TO EXPECT

WHO OPERATES—Ophthalmologist.

WHERE PERFORMED—Hospital or outpatient surgical facility.

DIAGNOSTIC TESTS
- Before surgery: Blood and urine studies; complete eye examination.
- After surgery: Complete eye examination.

ANESTHESIA
- Local anesthesia by topical application.
- Local anesthesia by injection.

DESCRIPTION OF OPERATION
- An incision is made in the cornea around the pterygium.
- The pterygium is cut and brought upward, clear of the cornea.
- The lower edge of the pterygium is cut free and the entire pterygium is removed.
- Open areas in the membrane covering the eye are closed with fine sutures, which usually can be removed about 1 week after surgery.

POSSIBLE COMPLICATIONS—Surgical-wound infection.

AVERAGE HOSPITAL STAY—0 to 1 day.

PROBABLE OUTCOME—Expect complete healing without complications. Allow about 3 weeks for recovery from surgery.

POSTOPERATIVE CARE

NOTE—This information is supplemental and should not replace your doctor's instructions.

GENERAL MEASURES—Beginning 24 hours after surgery, apply warm compresses to the eye to relieve discomfort. Do this for 10 to 15 minutes each hour as long as discomfort continues.

MEDICATION
- Your doctor may prescribe:
  Pain relievers. Don't take prescription pain medication longer than 4 to 7 days. Use *only* as much as you need.
  Antibiotic eye drops to fight infection. Keep eye drops cold in the refrigerator, but not frozen.
- You may use non-prescription drugs, such as acetaminophen, to relieve minor pain.

ACTIVITY
- Return to work and normal activity as soon as possible. This reduces postoperative depression and irritability, which are common.
- Avoid vigorous exercise for 3 weeks after surgery.
- Resume driving about 1 week after returning home.

DIET—No special diet.

CALL YOUR DOCTOR IF

- Pain, swelling, redness, drainage or bleeding increase in the surgical area.
- Vision changes.
- You develop signs of infection: headache, muscle aches, dizziness or a general ill feeling and fever.
- New, unexplained symptoms develop. Drugs used in treatment may produce side effects.

RECTAL- OR COLON-POLYP REMOVAL
(Polypectomy)

GENERAL INFORMATION

DEFINITION—Removal of a polyp from the membrane lining inside the rectum or colon.

BODY PARTS INVOLVED—Membrane lining of the rectum and colon.

REASONS FOR SURGERY—Removal of a possible source of cancer.

SURGICAL RISK INCREASES WITH
- Obesity.
- Smoking.
- Poor nutrition.
- Recent or chronic illness.
- Use of drugs such as: antihypertensives; muscle relaxants; tranquilizers; sleep inducers; insulin; sedatives; beta-adrenergic blockers; or cortisone.
- Use of mind-altering drugs, including: narcotics; psychedelics; hallucinogens; marijuana; sedatives; hypnotics; or cocaine.

WHAT TO EXPECT

WHO OPERATES—General surgeon or proctologist.

WHERE PERFORMED—Hospital or outpatient surgical facility.

DIAGNOSTIC TESTS
- Before surgery: Blood and urine studies; X-rays of lower gastrointestinal tract; colonoscopy (see Glossary).
- After surgery: Blood studies; laboratory examination of removed tissue.

ANESTHESIA—Intravenous sedative and narcotic pain killer.

DESCRIPTION OF OPERATION
- Surgery is preceded by medicated enemas.
- A colonoscope or sigmoidoscope is inserted through the rectum into the sigmoid colon. The polyp is located and removed with a wire snare, ultrasound or a laser beam.
- Bleeding is controlled with electric current or pressure applied with gauze soaked in epinephrine (see Glossary).

POSSIBLE COMPLICATIONS
- Excessive bleeding.
- Surgical-wound infection.
- Inadvertent injury to the colon.

AVERAGE HOSPITAL STAY—0 to 1 day.

PROBABLE OUTCOME—Expect complete healing without complications. Allow about 12 days for recovery from surgery.

POSTOPERATIVE CARE

NOTE—This information is supplemental and should not replace your doctor's instructions.

GENERAL MEASURES—Watch for signs of excessive bleeding, such as bloody or black, tarry stools.

MEDICATION
- Your doctor may prescribe:
  Pain relievers. Don't take prescription pain medication longer than 4 to 7 days. Use *only* as much as you need.
  Stool softeners to prevent constipation.
- You may use non-prescription drugs, such as acetaminophen, to relieve minor pain.

ACTIVITY
- Return to work and normal activity as soon as possible. This reduces postoperative depression and irritability, which are common.
- Avoid vigorous exercise for 4 weeks after surgery.
- Resume driving 3 days after returning home.

DIET—Clear liquid diet until the gastrointestinal tract functions again. Then eat a well-balanced, high-protein diet to promote healing. Increase intake of dietary fiber and fluids to prevent constipation. Avoid coffee, tea, cocoa, cola drinks, alcoholic beverages and any food or spice that causes painful or irritating digestive symptoms.

CALL YOUR DOCTOR IF

Any of the following occurs:
- Increased pain, swelling, redness, drainage or bleeding in the surgical area.
- Signs of infection: headache, muscle aches, dizziness or a general ill feeling and fever.
- Nausea, vomiting, constipation, abdominal swelling or pain.
- Bloody or black, tarry stools.
- New, unexplained symptoms. Drugs used in treatment may produce side effects.

RECTO-VAGINAL-FISTULA REPAIR

GENERAL INFORMATION

DEFINITION—Repair of a fistula (an abnormal tract) between the rectum and vagina that usually results from tearing during childbirth.

BODY PARTS INVOLVED—Vagina; rectum; connective tissue; blood vessels and nerves in the perineum.

REASONS FOR SURGERY—Prevention of fecal matter from contaminating the vagina or urinary tract.

SURGICAL RISK INCREASES WITH
- Obesity.
- Smoking.
- Poor nutrition.
- Recent or chronic illness.
- Alcoholism.
- Use of drugs such as: antihypertensives; muscle relaxants; tranquilizers; sleep inducers; insulin; sedatives; beta-adrenergic blockers; or cortisone.
- Use of mind-altering drugs, including: narcotics; psychedelics; hallucinogens; marijuana; sedatives; hypnotics; or cocaine.

WHAT TO EXPECT

WHO OPERATES—Urologist, proctologist or general surgeon.

WHERE PERFORMED—Hospital.

DIAGNOSTIC TESTS
- Before surgery: Blood and urine studies; X-rays of lower gastrointestinal tract and kidneys.
- After surgery: Blood studies.

ANESTHESIA—General anesthesia by inhalation and injection, with an airway tube placed in the windpipe.

DESCRIPTION OF OPERATION
- An incision is made in the perineum.
- Scar tissue and the fistula between the vagina and rectum are cut free and removed.
- The openings into the rectum and vagina are closed with sutures that will be absorbed by the body.
- The skin is closed with sutures, which usually may be removed about 1 week after surgery.

POSSIBLE COMPLICATIONS
- Excessive bleeding.
- Surgical-wound infection.
- Failure to heal completely.

AVERAGE HOSPITAL STAY—8 to 10 days.

PROBABLE OUTCOME—Expect complete healing without complications. Allow about 6 weeks for recovery from surgery.

POSTOPERATIVE CARE

NOTE—This information is supplemental and should not replace your doctor's instructions.

GENERAL MEASURES
- Take hot baths several times a day to relieve discomfort.
- Bathe after bowel movements to prevent infection.
- Use sanitary pads instead of tampons during menstrual periods for 6 months.

MEDICATION
- Your doctor may prescribe:
  Pain relievers. Don't take prescription pain medication longer than 4 to 7 days. Use *only* as much as you need.
  Stool softeners to prevent constipation.
  Antibiotics to fight infection.
- You may use non-prescription drugs, such as acetaminophen, for minor pain.

ACTIVITY
- Resume work and normal activity as soon as possible. This reduces postoperative depression and irritability, which are common.
- Avoid vigorous exercise for 6 weeks after surgery. Resume sexual relations when your doctor determines that healing is complete.
- Resume driving 1 week after returning home.

DIET—Clear liquid diet until the gastrointestinal tract functions again. Then eat a well-balanced, high-protein diet to promote healing.

CALL YOUR DOCTOR IF

- Pain, swelling, redness, drainage or bleeding increases in the surgical area.
- You develop signs of infection: headache, muscle aches, dizziness or a general ill feeling and fever.
- You experience nausea, vomiting, constipation or diarrhea.
- New, unexplained symptoms develop. Drugs used in treatment may produce side effects.

RETINAL-DETACHMENT REPAIR

 GENERAL INFORMATION

DEFINITION—Reattachment of a retina that has become separated from the rest of the eye.

BODY PARTS INVOLVED—The eye and all its parts.

REASONS FOR SURGERY—Prevention of vision loss.

SURGICAL RISK INCREASES WITH
- Obesity.
- Smoking.
- Poor nutrition.
- Recent or chronic illness.
- Alcoholism.
- Use of drugs such as: antihypertensives; muscle relaxants; tranquilizers; sleep inducers; insulin; sedatives; beta-adrenergic blockers; or cortisone.
- Use of mind-altering drugs, including: narcotics; psychedelics; hallucinogens; marijuana; sedatives; hypnotics; or cocaine.

 WHAT TO EXPECT

WHO OPERATES—Ophthalmologist.

WHERE PERFORMED—Hospital or outpatient surgical facility.

DIAGNOSTIC TESTS
- Before surgery: Complete eye examination; blood and urine studies.
- After surgery: Complete eye examination.

ANESTHESIA
- Local anesthesia by injection or topical application.
- General anesthesia by inhalation and injection, with an airway tube placed in the windpipe.

DESCRIPTION OF OPERATION
- Sometimes, tears or holes in the retina are repaired with laser beams that coagulate the eye tissue and cause it to readjust to its normal position.
- Otherwise, the membrane lining the eye is cut. A cryosurgical probe is placed around the detached retina. The probe applies extreme cold, causing eye tissue to coagulate and to adhere to its normal position.
- If a cornea transplant is required, it is performed.
- The membrane around the eye is closed with fine sutures, which usually can be removed about 1 week after surgery.

POSSIBLE COMPLICATIONS
- Surgical-wound infection.
- Partial or total vision loss in the affected eye from recurrence of retinal detachment.

AVERAGE HOSPITAL STAY—3 to 4 days.

PROBABLE OUTCOME—Surgery is successful in preserving eyesight in over 90% of patients. About 10% will require another operation, which is usually successful. Allow about 2 weeks for recovery from surgery.

 POSTOPERATIVE CARE

NOTE—This information is supplemental and should not replace your doctor's instructions.

GENERAL MEASURES
- Rest with your head elevated on two pillows. You may move your head in any direction.
- Use dark glasses in bright light until you no longer need to keep the pupils dilated with eye drops. Don't rub the eyes.
- Don't bend over or strain with lifting, bowel movements or urination for at least 6 months after surgery.

MEDICATION—Your doctor may prescribe:
- Pain relievers. Don't take prescription pain medication longer than 4 to 7 days. Use *only* as much as you need.
- Stool softeners to prevent constipation.
- Antibiotics to fight infection.
- Eye drops to keep the pupil dilated during healing.

ACTIVITY
- Return to work and normal activity as soon as possible. This reduces postoperative depression and irritability, which are common.
- Avoid vigorous exercise for 6 weeks after surgery.
- Resume driving 4 weeks after returning home.

DIET—No special diet.

 CALL YOUR DOCTOR IF

Any of the following occur:
- Loss of vision.
- Constipation.
- Increased pain, swelling, redness, drainage or bleeding in the surgical area.
- Signs of infection: headache, muscle aches, dizziness or a general ill feeling and fever.
- New, unexplained symptoms. Drugs used in treatment may produce side effects.

RHINOPLASTY & SUBMUCOUS RESECTION

 ## GENERAL INFORMATION

DEFINITION—Reconstruction of the tip of nose and removal of deformities of the septum.

BODY PARTS INVOLVED—Nose, including nasal cartilage and bone and mucous membrane of the septum.

REASONS FOR SURGERY
- Opening of blocked nasal passages.
- Improved appearance.

SURGICAL RISK INCREASES WITH
- Obesity.
- Smoking.
- Poor nutrition.
- Excess alcohol consumption.
- Recent or chronic illness.
- Use of drugs such as: antihypertensives; muscle relaxants; tranquilizers; sleeping pills; insulin; sedatives; beta-adrenergic blockers; or cortisone.
- Use of mind-altering drugs, including: narcotics; psychedelics; hallucinogens; marijuana; sedatives; hypnotics; or cocaine.

 ## WHAT TO EXPECT

WHO OPERATES—Plastic and reconstructive surgeon or ear, nose and throat specialist.

WHERE PERFORMED—Hospital or outpatient surgical facility.

DIAGNOSTIC TESTS
- Before surgery: Blood and urine studies; X-rays of facial bones.
- After surgery: Blood studies.

ANESTHESIA—General anesthesia by inhalation and injection, with an airway tube placed in the windpipe.

DESCRIPTION OF OPERATION
- The nostril is held open with a speculum.
- An incision is made in the nose. The bone or cartilage is fractured, trimmed and molded into the desired shape.
- The mucous membrane is closed with fine sutures, which usually can be removed about 10 days after surgery. Bandages are applied.

POSSIBLE COMPLICATIONS
- Excessive bleeding.
- Surgical-wound infection.

AVERAGE HOSPITAL STAY—0 to 1 day.

PROBABLE OUTCOME—Expect complete healing without complications. Allow about 3 weeks for recovery from surgery.

 ## POSTOPERATIVE CARE

NOTE—This information is supplemental and should not replace your doctor's instructions.

GENERAL MEASURES
- Apply ice packs to the nose to relieve discomfort. Do this for 10 to 20 minutes at a time 4 to 8 times a day during the first 2 days after surgery.
- Beginning 2 days after surgery, use an electric heating pad, a heat lamp or a warm compress to relieve incisional pain.
- Don't blow the nose forcefully for 1 month. Don't blow it at all in the first week.

MEDICATION
- Your doctor may prescribe:
  Pain relievers. Don't take prescription pain medication longer than 4 to 7 days. Use *only* as much as you need.
  Antibiotics to fight infection.
- You may use non-prescription drugs, such as acetaminophen, for minor pain.

ACTIVITY
- Return to work and normal activity as soon as possible. This reduces postoperative depression and irritability, which are common.
- Avoid vigorous exercise for 3 weeks after surgery.
- Resume driving 1 week after returning home.

DIET—Eat a well-balanced, high-protein diet to promote healing.

 ## CALL YOUR DOCTOR IF

Any of the following occurs:
- Nausea or vomiting.
- Increased pain, swelling, redness, drainage or bleeding in the surgical area.
- Signs of infection: headache, muscle aches, dizziness or a general ill feeling and fever.
- New, unexplained symptoms. Drugs used in treatment may produce side effects.

SALIVARY-GLAND-TUMOR REMOVAL

GENERAL INFORMATION

DEFINITION—Removal of a cancerous tumor of the salivary glands.

BODY PARTS INVOLVED—Salivary glands under the tongue (sublingual) or under the jawbone (submaxillary).

REASONS FOR SURGERY—Cancer or suspected cancer of the sublingual or submaxillary salivary glands.

SURGICAL RISK INCREASES WITH
- Adults over 60.
- Obesity.
- Smoking.
- Excess alcohol consumption.
- Stress.
- Poor nutrition.
- Recent or chronic illness.
- Alcoholism.
- Use of drugs such as: antihypertensives; muscle relaxants; tranquilizers; sleep inducers; insulin; sedatives; beta-adrenergic blockers; or cortisone.
- Use of mind-altering drugs, including: narcotics; psychedelics; hallucinogens; marijuana; sedatives; hypnotics; or cocaine.

WHAT TO EXPECT

WHO OPERATES—Ear, nose and throat specialist or general surgeon.

WHERE PERFORMED—Hospital.

DIAGNOSTIC TESTS
- Before surgery: Blood and urine studies; X-rays of the head, neck, upper gastrointestinal tract and chest.
- After surgery: Blood studies.

ANESTHESIA—General anesthesia by inhalation and injection, with an airway tube placed in the windpipe.

DESCRIPTION OF OPERATION
- Incisions are made in the mucous membrane over the tumor.
- The tumor is isolated, cut free and removed.
- The tissue is examined to determine if the tumor is benign or cancerous.
- If the tumor is benign, the mucous membrane over the tumor is closed with fine silk sutures.
- If the tumor is cancerous, a radical neck dissection (in Surgery section) is usually performed.

POSSIBLE COMPLICATIONS
- Excessive bleeding.
- Surgical-wound infection.
- Spread of cancer to nearby or distant tissues.

AVERAGE HOSPITAL STAY—4 to 7 days.

PROBABLE OUTCOME—Expect complete healing without complications. Your doctor may prescribe further treatment with radiation and anticancer drugs depending on findings from surgery. Allow about 3 months for recovery from surgery.

POSTOPERATIVE CARE

NOTE—This information is supplemental and should not replace your doctor's instructions.

GENERAL MEASURES
- Move legs often while resting in bed to decrease the likelihood of deep-vein blood clots.
- Rinse your mouth every 2 to 3 hours with a solution of 1 teaspoon salt in 8 oz. warm water. A clean mouth heals faster.

MEDICATION
- Your doctor may prescribe:
  Pain relievers. Don't take prescription pain medication longer than 4 to 7 days. Use *only* as much as you need.
  Stool softeners to prevent constipation.
  Antibiotics to fight infection.
- You may use non-prescription drugs, such as acetaminophen, for minor pain.

ACTIVITY
- Resume work and normal activity as soon as possible. This reduces postoperative depression and irritability, which are common.
- Avoid vigorous exercise for 6 weeks after surgery.

DIET—Clear liquid diet until the gastrointestinal tract functions again. Then eat a well-balanced, high-protein diet to promote healing.

CALL YOUR DOCTOR IF

- Pain, swelling, redness, drainage or bleeding increases in the surgical area.
- You develop signs of infection: headache, muscle aches, dizziness or a general ill feeling and fever.
- You experience nausea, vomiting or constipation.
- New, unexplained symptoms develop. Drugs used in treatment may produce side effects.

SEBACEOUS-CYST REMOVAL
(Epidermoid-Cyst Removal)

 GENERAL INFORMATION

DEFINITION—Removal of sebaceous cysts, sometimes called epidermoid cysts.

BODY PARTS INVOLVED—Sebaceous cysts, usually occurring on the skin of the trunk, face, scalp and neck. They often appear behind the ear.

REASONS FOR SURGERY
- Prevention of infections.
- Improved appearance.

SURGICAL RISK INCREASES WITH—Any bleeding disorder.

 WHAT TO EXPECT

WHO OPERATES—Family doctor, general surgeon or dermatologist.

WHERE PERFORMED—Doctor's office or outpatient surgical facility.

DIAGNOSTIC TESTS
- Before surgery: Blood and urine studies.
- After surgery: Laboratory examination of removed tissue.

ANESTHESIA—Local anesthesia by injection.

DESCRIPTION OF OPERATION
- An incision is made over the cyst, with care taken not to rupture its confining wall. Leakage from the cyst can cause inflammation and delay healing.
- The cyst and its contents are removed intact.
- The skin is closed with sutures or clips, which usually can be removed about 1 week after surgery.

POSSIBLE COMPLICATIONS
- Excessive bleeding.
- Surgical-wound infection.

AVERAGE HOSPITAL STAY—Usually none.

PROBABLE OUTCOME—Expect complete healing without complications. Allow about 2 weeks for recovery from surgery.

 POSTOPERATIVE CARE

NOTE—This information is supplemental and should not replace your doctor's instructions.

GENERAL MEASURES
- If the wound bleeds during the first 24 hours after surgery, press a clean tissue or cloth to it for 10 minutes.
- A hard ridge should form along the incision. As it heals, the ridge will recede gradually.
- Use an electric heating pad, a heat lamp or a warm compress to relieve incisional pain.
- Bathe and shower as usual. You may wash the incision gently with mild unscented soap.
- Between baths, keep the wound dry with a bandage for the first 2 days after surgery. If a bandage gets wet, change it promptly.
- Apply non-prescription antibiotic ointment to the wound before applying bandages.

MEDICATION
- Your doctor may prescribe antibiotics to prevent infection.
- You may use non-prescription drugs, such as acetaminophen, to relieve minor pain.

ACTIVITY
- Avoid vigorous exercise for 2 weeks after surgery.
- Resume driving 2 days after returning home.

DIET—No special diet.

 CALL YOUR DOCTOR IF

- Pain, swelling, redness, drainage or bleeding increases in the surgical area.
- You develop signs of infection, headache, muscle aches, dizziness or a general ill feeling and fever.
- New, unexplained symptoms develop. Drugs used in treatment may produce side effects.

SIGMOID-COLON REMOVAL
(Sigmoid Colectomy)

 GENERAL INFORMATION

DEFINITION—Removal of the sigmoid colon.

BODY PARTS INVOLVED—Sigmoid colon, the part of the large intestine (colon) that extends from the descending colon to the rectum.

REASONS FOR SURGERY
- Diverticulitis with bleeding and infection.
- Diverticulitis with ruptured diverticula and peritonitis from infection caused by perforations.
- Cancer or precancerous polyps.

SURGICAL RISK INCREASES WITH
- Adults over 60 years.
- Obesity.
- Smoking.
- Stress.
- Poor nutrition.
- Newborns and infants.
- Excess alcohol consumption.
- Chronic illness.
- Recent illness such as acute diverticulitis.
- Family history of diverticulitis disease.
- Use of drugs such as: antihypertensives; muscle relaxants; tranquilizers; sleep inducers; insulin; sedatives; beta-adrenergic blockers; or cortisone.
- Use of mind-altering drugs, including: narcotics; psychedelics; hallucinogens; marijuana; sedatives; hypnotics; or cocaine.

 WHAT TO EXPECT

WHO OPERATES—General surgeon.

WHERE PERFORMED—Hospital.

DIAGNOSTIC TESTS
- Before surgery: Blood and urine studies; X-rays of upper and lower gastrointestinal tract; EKG (see Glossary).
- After surgery: Blood studies.

ANESTHESIA—General anesthesia by inhalation and injection, with an airway tube placed in the windpipe (trachea).

DESCRIPTION OF OPERATION
- An incision is made in the abdomen, and the abdominal muscles are opened.
- The sigmoid colon is isolated and clamps are placed at each end.
- All of the diseased sigmoid colon is cut free and removed. The two healthy ends are brought back together and joined.
- The abdominal contents are replaced into the abdomen, and the muscles are closed. The skin is closed with sutures or skin clips, which usually can be removed about 1 week after surgery.

POSSIBLE COMPLICATIONS
- Excessive bleeding.
- Surgical-wound infection.
- Deep-vein blood clots.
- Leaking from the repair area that can result in peritonitis or incisional hernia. If surgery is performed to treat infection or tumor, a temporary colostomy may be necessary.

AVERAGE HOSPITAL STAY—7 to 10 days.

PROBABLE OUTCOME—Expect complete healing without complications. Allow 6 weeks for recovery from surgery.

 POSTOPERATIVE CARE

NOTE—This information is supplemental and should not replace your doctor's instructions.

GENERAL MEASURES
- A hard ridge should form along the incision. As it heals, the ridge will recede gradually.
- Use an electric heating pad, a heat lamp or a warm compress to relieve incisional pain.

MEDICATION—Your doctor may prescribe:
- Pain relievers. Don't take prescription pain medication longer than 4 to 7 days. Use *only* as much as you need.
- Stool softeners to prevent constipation.
- Antibiotics to fight infection.

ACTIVITY
- Return to work and normal activity as soon as possible. This reduces postoperative depression, which is common.
- Resume driving about 3 weeks after returning home.
- Resume sexual relations when able.

DIET—Clear liquid diet until the gastrointestinal tract functions again. Then eat a well-balanced, high-protein diet to promote healing. After recovery, eat a normal diet with adequate bulk.

 CALL YOUR DOCTOR IF

- You develop signs of leaking in the surgical area: fever, fast pulse or abdominal swelling.
- Pain, swelling, redness, drainage or bleeding increase in the surgical area.
- New, unexplained symptoms develop. Drugs used in treatment may produce side effects.

SKIN GRAFT

GENERAL INFORMATION

DEFINITION—Taking skin from one area of the body and attaching it to another area where no skin exists.

BODY PARTS INVOLVED—Skin (donor sites and recipient sites).

REASONS FOR SURGERY—Extensive wounds, burns or certain surgeries may require skin grafts for healing to occur.

SURGICAL RISK INCREASES WITH
- Adults over 60.
- Newborns and infants.
- Obesity.
- Smoking.
- Poor nutrition.
- Anemia.
- Recent or chronic illness.
- Use of drugs such as: antihypertensives; muscle relaxants; tranquilizers; sleep inducers; insulin; sedatives; beta-adrenergic blockers; or cortisone.
- Use of mind-altering drugs, including: narcotics; psychedelics; hallucinogens; marijuana; sedatives; hypnotics; or cocaine.

WHAT TO EXPECT

WHO OPERATES—General surgeon or plastic and reconstructive surgeon.

WHERE PERFORMED—Hospital, outpatient surgical facility or emergency room (rarely).

DIAGNOSTIC TESTS
- Before surgery: Blood and urine studies.
- After surgery: Blood studies.

ANESTHESIA
- Local anesthesia by injection.
- General anesthesia by inhalation and injection, with an airway tube placed in the windpipe.

DESCRIPTION OF OPERATION
- Skin is removed from a donor site. The donor site is covered with gauze.
- Debris is cleared from the recipient site.
- The skin from the donor site is placed on the recipient site and fastened at each corner with sutures. Bandages are applied. New blood vessels begin growing from the recipient area into the transplanted skin within 36 hours.

POSSIBLE COMPLICATIONS
- Excessive bleeding.
- Surgical-wound infection.
- Collection of serum under recipient site that prevents growth of new blood vessels.
- Loss of grafted skin.

AVERAGE HOSPITAL STAY—2 to 12 days, depending on extent of surgery.

PROBABLE OUTCOME—Allow about 6 weeks for recovery from surgery. Most skin grafts are successful, but in some cases they don't "take" and must be done again. This often occurs if skin edges are injured from stitches. Skillful postoperative nursing care is critical to the graft's success.

POSTOPERATIVE CARE

NOTE—This information is supplemental and should not replace your doctor's instructions.

GENERAL MEASURES
- Apply non-prescription antibiotic ointment to new bandages, if instructed by your doctor. Keep bandages dry while bathing. If a bandage gets wet, change it promptly.
- If the wound bleeds, press a clean tissue or cloth to it for 10 minutes.

MEDICATION
- Your doctor may prescribe:
  Pain relievers. Don't take prescription pain medication longer than 4 to 7 days. Use *only* as much as you need.
  Antibiotics to fight infection.
- You may use non-prescription drugs, such as acetaminophen, for minor pain.

ACTIVITY
- Return to work and normal activity as soon as possible. This reduces postoperative depression and irritability, which are common.
- Avoid vigorous exercise for 6 weeks following surgery.
- Resume driving 1 week after returning home.

DIET—No special diet.

CALL YOUR DOCTOR IF

Any of the following occur:
- Pain, swelling, redness, drainage, bleeding or odor in the surgical area.
- Signs of infection: headache, muscle aches, dizziness or a general ill feeling and fever.
- New, unexplained symptoms. Drugs used in treatment may produce side effects.

SURGERIES

SKIN-LESION REMOVAL

 GENERAL INFORMATION

DEFINITION—Removal of any benign or cancerous lesion on the skin.

BODY PARTS INVOLVED—Abnormal growth on the skin. The most common are warts, moles, skin cancers, molluscum contagiosum or senile keratoses.

REASONS FOR SURGERY
- Diagnosis of the abnormal growth.
- Removal of any abnormality suspected to be cancerous.

SURGICAL RISK INCREASES WITH—None expected.

 WHAT TO EXPECT

WHO OPERATES—Family doctor, dermatologist, general surgeon or plastic and reconstructive surgeon.

WHERE PERFORMED—Hospital, emergency room, doctor's office or outpatient surgical facility.

DIAGNOSTIC TESTS
- Before surgery: Blood and urine studies.
- After surgery: Laboratory examination of removed tissue.

ANESTHESIA—Local anesthesia by injection.

DESCRIPTION OF OPERATION—Techniques to remove abnormal growths from the skin include:
- Scraping the abnormality away (curettement).
- Cutting, removing and sewing.
- Cutting with scissors, especially if the lesion is on a stalk.
- Removing a plug of skin for diagnosis.
- Freezing warts and benign superficial keratoses (cryotherapy).
- Using heat (electrosurgery).
- Incising the skin with a cold scalpel, removing the lesion and sewing the skin edges together.

The technique chosen depends on the nature of the lesion and the condition of the patient. If sutures or clips are used to close the wound, they usually can be removed about 1 week after surgery.

POSSIBLE COMPLICATIONS
- Excessive bleeding.
- Surgical-wound infection.

AVERAGE HOSPITAL STAY—None.

PROBABLE OUTCOME—Expect complete healing without complications. Allow about 2 weeks for recovery from surgery.

 POSTOPERATIVE CARE

NOTE—This information is supplemental and should not replace your doctor's instructions.

GENERAL MEASURES
- If the wound bleeds during the first 24 hours after surgery, press a clean tissue or cloth to it for 10 minutes.
- If an incision was made, a hard blunt ridge should form along it in 4 to 5 days after surgery. As it heals, the ridge will recede gradually.
- Use an electric heating pad, a heat lamp or a warm compress to relieve incisional pain.
- Bathe and shower as usual. You may wash the incision gently with mild unscented soap.
- Between showers, keep the wound dry with a bandage for the first 2 or 3 days after surgery. If the bandage gets wet, change it promptly.
- Apply a non-prescription antibiotic ointment to the wound before applying bandages.

MEDICATION—You may use non-prescription drugs, such as acetaminophen, to relieve minor pain.

ACTIVITY
- Avoid vigorous exercise for 2 weeks after surgery.
- Resume driving 2 days after returning home.

DIET—No special diet.

 CALL YOUR DOCTOR IF

Any of the following occurs:
- Nausea or vomiting.
- Increased pain, swelling, redness, drainage or bleeding in the surgical area.
- Signs of infection: headache, muscle aches, dizziness or a general ill feeling and fever.

SMALL-BOWEL RESECTION

GENERAL INFORMATION

DEFINITION—Removal of diseased section of the small bowel (small intestine).

BODY PARTS INVOLVED—Small intestine, including muscles and peritoneum layer around it.

REASONS FOR SURGERY—Tumor, gangrene, narrowing or obstruction in the small intestine.

SURGICAL RISK INCREASES WITH
- Adults over 60.
- Obesity.
- Smoking.
- Poor nutrition.
- Previous abdominal surgery.
- Recent or chronic illness.
- Use of drugs such as: antihypertensives; muscle relaxants; tranquilizers; sleep inducers; insulin; sedatives; beta-adrenergic blockers; or cortisone.
- Use of mind-altering drugs, including: narcotics; psychedelics; hallucinogens; marijuana; sedatives; hypnotics; or cocaine.

WHAT TO EXPECT

WHO OPERATES—General surgeon.

WHERE PERFORMED—Hospital.

DIAGNOSTIC TESTS
- Before surgery: Blood and urine studies; X-rays of chest and gastrointestinal tract.
- After surgery: Blood studies.

ANESTHESIA—General anesthesia by inhalation and injection, with an airway tube placed in the windpipe.

DESCRIPTION OF OPERATION
- An incision is made in the abdomen.
- The muscles are separated or cut, and the abdominal cavity is entered.
- The intestine is examined for disease.
- The small intestine is clamped above and below the diseased section. The diseased section between the clamps is cut free and removed.
- The two open ends of the remaining small bowel are fastened together with sutures or staples.
- The peritoneum and muscles are closed with sutures. The skin is closed with sutures or clips, which usually can be removed about 1 week after surgery.

POSSIBLE COMPLICATIONS
- Excessive bleeding.
- Surgical-wound infection.
- Recurrence of intestinal obstructions caused by adhesions.

AVERAGE HOSPITAL STAY—7 to 10 days.

PROBABLE OUTCOME—Expect complete healing of surgical wound. Allow about 4 weeks for recovery from surgery.

POSTOPERATIVE CARE

NOTE—This information is supplemental and should not replace your doctor's instructions.

GENERAL MEASURES
- A hard ridge should form along the incision. As it heals, the ridge will recede gradually.
- Use an electric heating pad, a heat lamp or a warm compress to relieve incisional pain.
- Bathe and shower as usual. You may wash the incision gently with mild unscented soap.
- Move legs often while resting in bed to decrease the likelihood of deep-vein blood clots.

MEDICATION
- Your doctor may prescribe:
  Pain relievers. Don't take prescription pain medication longer than 4 to 7 days. Use *only* as much as you need.
  Stool softeners to prevent constipation.
  Antibiotics to fight infection.
- You may use non-prescription drugs, such as acetaminophen, for minor pain.

ACTIVITY
- Return to work and normal activity as soon as possible. This reduces postoperative depression and irritability, which are common.
- Avoid vigorous exercise for 6 weeks after surgery.
- Resume driving 3 weeks after returning home.

DIET—Intravenous feeding for several days, then return slowly to a diet your doctor will prescribe.

CALL YOUR DOCTOR IF

- Pain, swelling, redness, drainage or bleeding increases in the surgical area.
- You develop signs of infection: headache, muscle aches, dizziness or a general ill feeling and fever.
- You experience nausea, vomiting, constipation, abdominal swelling, or bloody or tarry stools.
- New, unexplained symptoms develop. Drugs used in treatment may produce side effects.

SURGERIES

SPINAL TAP
(Lumbar Puncture)

GENERAL INFORMATION

DEFINITION—Removal of spinal fluid from the spinal canal, either for laboratory analysis or prior to surgery with spinal anesthesia.

BODY PARTS INVOLVED—Skin; muscles; covering of spinal cord (meninges).

REASONS FOR SURGERY
- Diagnosis of disorders of the central nervous system that may involve the brain, spinal cord or their coverings.
- Injection of spinal anesthesia.

SURGICAL RISK INCREASES WITH
- Recent or chronic illness.
- Alcoholism.

WHAT TO EXPECT

WHO OPERATES—General surgeon, family doctor, neurologist, neurosurgeon, anesthesiologist or internist.

WHERE PERFORMED—Hospital, outpatient surgical facility or emergency room

DIAGNOSTIC TESTS
- Before surgery: Blood and urine studies.
- During surgery: Pressure of spinal fluid measured with a manometer (see Glossary).
- After surgery: Laboratory examination of removed fluid.

ANESTHESIA—Local anesthesia by injection.

DESCRIPTION OF OPERATION
- The patient is positioned on his side with the knees drawn as close to the chest as possible.
- A hollow needle is inserted in the back between the 4th and 5th lumbar vertebrae.
- The spinal canal is penetrated with the needle. Fluid pressure is measured and then fluid is removed.
- The surgical wound will heal by itself.

POSSIBLE COMPLICATIONS
- Surgical-wound infection.
- Headaches (common during the first 24 hours after surgery).

AVERAGE HOSPITAL STAY—Usually 6 to 24 hours in the surgical facility.

PROBABLE OUTCOME—Expect complete healing without complications. Allow about 3 days for recovery from surgery.

POSTOPERATIVE CARE

NOTE—This information is supplemental and should not replace your doctor's instructions.

GENERAL MEASURES—Moving the head and neck as little as possible for 12 hours after surgery helps prevent headache. Resume activity slowly.

MEDICATION
- Your doctor may prescribe pain relievers. Don't take prescription pain medication longer than 4 to 7 days. Use *only* as much as you need.
- You may use non-prescription drugs, such as acetaminophen, for minor pain.

ACTIVITY
- Avoid vigorous exercise for 2 weeks after surgery.
- Resume driving in 3 days after returning home.

DIET—No special diet. Increase fluid intake. This may prevent post-spinal-tap headaches.

CALL YOUR DOCTOR IF

- Pain, swelling, redness, drainage or bleeding increases in the surgical area.
- You develop signs of infection: headache, muscle aches, dizziness or a general ill feeling and fever.
- You experience nausea or vomiting.

SPLEEN REMOVAL
(Splenectomy)

GENERAL INFORMATION

DEFINITION—Removal of the spleen.

BODY PARTS INVOLVED—The spleen, a large organ on the left side of the upper abdominal cavity next to the stomach.

REASONS FOR SURGERY
- Injury to the spleen causing rupture and bleeding.
- Various blood diseases, including spherocytosis, thrombocytopenia or lymphatic leukemia (see Glossary for all).
- Splenic-vein thrombosis caused by esophageal varices (see Glossary).
- Benign or cancerous tumors.

SURGICAL RISK INCREASES WITH
- Adults over 60.
- Newborns and infants.
- Obesity.
- Smoking.
- Excess alcohol consumption.
- Poor nutrition.
- Chronic weakening illness.
- Use of drugs such as: antihypertensives; muscle relaxants; tranquilizers; sleep inducers; insulin; sedatives; beta-adrenergic blockers; or cortisone.
- Use of mind-altering drugs.

WHAT TO EXPECT

WHO OPERATES—General surgeon.

WHERE PERFORMED—Hospital.

DIAGNOSTIC TESTS
- Before surgery: Blood and urine studies; X-rays of abdomen.
- After surgery: Blood studies.

ANESTHESIA—General anesthesia by inhalation and injection, with an airway tube placed in the windpipe.

DESCRIPTION OF OPERATION
- An incision is made in the abdomen.
- The spleen is located and isolated.
- Blood vessels to the spleen are cut and tied off.
- The spleen is rotated and removed from its bed where it is attached to the coverings of the stomach, kidney and diaphragm (see Glossary).
- If the spleen has been ruptured, the abdomen is explored to identify any other injured organs or blood vessels. Other surgeries may be performed at this time.
- The muscles are closed in layers. The skin is closed with sutures or skin clips, which usually can be removed in about 1 week.

POSSIBLE COMPLICATIONS
- Excessive bleeding.
- Infection, especially in young children.
- Incisional hernia.
- Atelectasis.
- Pancreatitis.
- Deep-vein blood clots.
- Pneumonia.

AVERAGE HOSPITAL STAY—5 to 7 days.

PROBABLE OUTCOME—Expect complete healing without complications. Allow about 4 weeks for recovery from surgery.

POSTOPERATIVE CARE

NOTE—This information is supplemental and should not replace your doctor's instructions.

GENERAL MEASURES
- A hard ridge should form along the incision. As it heals, the ridge will recede gradually.
- Use an electric heating pad, a heat lamp or a warm compress to relieve incisional pain.
- Bathe and shower as usual. You may wash the incision gently with mild unscented soap.

MEDICATION
- Your doctor may prescribe:
  Pain relievers. Don't take prescription pain medication longer than 4 to 7 days. Use *only* as much as you need.
  Antibiotics to fight infection.
  Stool softeners to prevent constipation.
  Pneumonia vaccinations.
- You may use non-prescription drugs, such as acetaminophen, for minor pain.

ACTIVITY
- Return to work and normal activity as soon as possible. This reduces postoperative depression, which is common.
- Avoid vigorous exercise for 6 weeks after surgery. Resume sexual relations when your doctor determines that healing is complete.
- Resume driving 4 weeks after returning home.

DIET—Clear liquid diet until the gastrointestinal tract functions again. Then eat a well-balanced, high-protein diet to promote healing.

CALL YOUR DOCTOR IF

- You develop signs of infection: headache, muscle aches, dizziness or a general ill feeling and fever.
- Pain, swelling, redness, drainage or bleeding increases in the surgical area.
- New, unexplained symptoms develop. Drugs used in treatment may produce side effects.

STAPES REMOVAL
(Stapedectomy)

GENERAL INFORMATION

DEFINITION—Removal of the stapes, one of the bones in the middle ear that transmit sound waves to the inner ear. The stapes is also called the stirrup.

BODY PARTS INVOLVED—External ear canal; eardrum; middle ear; stapes.

REASONS FOR SURGERY—Improvement of hearing ability or prevention of continued hearing loss, usually due to otosclerosis.

SURGICAL RISK INCREASES WITH
- Obesity.
- Smoking.
- Poor nutrition.
- Recent or chronic illness.
- Use of drugs such as: antihypertensives; muscle relaxants; tranquilizers; sleeping pills; insulin; sedatives; beta-adrenergic blockers; or cortisone.
- Use of mind-altering drugs, including: narcotics; psychedelics; hallucinogens; marijuana; sedatives; hypnotics; or cocaine.

WHAT TO EXPECT

WHO OPERATES—Ear, nose and throat specialist.

WHERE PERFORMED—Hospital or outpatient surgical facility.

DIAGNOSTIC TESTS
- Before surgery: Blood and urine studies; hearing tests.
- After surgery: Hearing tests.

ANESTHESIA—General anesthesia by inhalation and injection, with an airway tube placed in the windpipe.

DESCRIPTION OF OPERATION
- The operating microscope is positioned, and an incision is made in the middle ear.
- The small bones in the ear are identified, and the stapes is isolated and removed.
- Sometimes, a prosthesis made of stainless steel wire and cellulose sponge is inserted to replace it.
- Blood and fluid are suctioned gently from the ear.
- The wound is closed with fine sutures, which usually can be removed about 1 week after surgery.

POSSIBLE COMPLICATIONS
- Excessive bleeding.
- Surgical-wound infection.

AVERAGE HOSPITAL STAY—5 to 6 days.

PROBABLE OUTCOME—Expect complete healing of the surgical wound without complications. Hearing should improve immediately. Allow about 3 weeks for recovery from surgery.

POSTOPERATIVE CARE

NOTE—This information is supplemental and should not replace your doctor's instructions.

GENERAL MEASURES
- Lie flat during the first 24 to 48 hours after surgery.
- Don't blow your nose for at least 1 week after surgery.
- Protect ears from moisture or cold. Take tub baths instead of showers for 2 weeks after surgery.
- Don't strain, bend or lift for 3 weeks after surgery.
- Avoid people with upper-respiratory infections until your healing is complete.
- Avoid loud noises and sudden pressure changes, such as those caused by flying in non-pressurized aircraft or scuba diving, for the rest of your life.

MEDICATION
- Your doctor may prescribe:
  Pain relievers. Don't take prescription pain medication longer than 4 to 7 days. Use *only* as much as you need.
  Stool softeners to prevent constipation.
  Antibiotics to fight infection.
- You may use non-prescription drugs, such as acetaminophen, for minor pain.

ACTIVITY
- Return to work and normal activity as soon as possible. This reduces postoperative depression and irritability, which are common.
- Avoid vigorous exercise for 6 weeks after surgery.
- Resume driving 3 weeks after returning home.

DIET—Clear liquid diet until the gastrointestinal tract functions again. Then eat a well-balanced, high-protein diet to promote healing.

CALL YOUR DOCTOR IF

- Hearing does not improve within 2 days after surgery.
- Pain, swelling, redness, drainage or bleeding increases in the surgical area.
- You develop signs of infection: headache, muscle aches, dizziness or a general ill feeling and fever.
- You experience new symptoms, such as nausea, vomiting or constipation.

STOMACH-CANCER SURGERY

GENERAL INFORMATION

DEFINITION—Removal of cancerous tissue (gastric carcinoma) in the stomach.

BODY PARTS INVOLVED—Stomach; small intestine.

REASONS FOR SURGERY—Cancer of the stomach.

SURGICAL RISK INCREASES WITH
- Adults over 60.
- Obesity.
- Smoking.
- Stress.
- Poor nutrition.
- Recent illness.
- Alcoholism or other chronic illness.
- Use of drugs such as: antihypertensives; muscle relaxants; tranquilizers; sleep inducers; insulin; sedatives; beta-adrenergic blockers; or cortisone.
- Use of mind-altering drugs, including: narcotics; psychedelics; hallucinogens; marijuana; sedatives; hypnotics; or cocaine.

WHAT TO EXPECT

WHO OPERATES—General surgeon.

WHERE PERFORMED—Hospital.

DIAGNOSTIC TESTS
- Before surgery: X-rays of gastrointestinal tract; blood and urine studies.
- During surgery: Laboratory examination of removed tissue by frozen section (see Glossary).
- After surgery: Blood studies; laboratory examination of removed tissue.

ANESTHESIA—General anesthesia by inhalation and injection, with an airway tube placed in the windpipe.

DESCRIPTION OF OPERATION
- A tube is passed from the nose into the stomach to keep the stomach decompressed.
- An incision is made below the ribs.
- Abdominal muscles are cut or retracted, the peritoneum is opened and the stomach is isolated.
- The cancerous part of the stomach is cut free and removed.
- The remaining stump of stomach is joined to a loop of small intestine (usually the jejunum) to allow normal digestive flow.
- The peritoneum is closed and the muscles are sewn together. The skin is closed with sutures or clips, which usually can be removed about 10 days after surgery.

POSSIBLE COMPLICATIONS
- Excessive bleeding.
- Surgical-wound infection.
- Incisional hernia.

AVERAGE HOSPITAL STAY—10 to 14 days.

PROBABLE OUTCOME—Expect complete healing of the surgical wound. Your doctor may recommend further treatment with radiation and anticancer drugs. Allow about 6 weeks for recovery from surgery.

POSTOPERATIVE CARE

NOTE—This information is supplemental and should not replace your doctor's instructions.

GENERAL MEASURES
- A hard ridge should form along the incision. As it heals, the ridge will recede gradually.
- Use an electric heating pad, a heat lamp or a warm compress to relieve incisional pain.
- Bathe and shower as usual. You may wash the incision gently with mild unscented soap.
- Move legs often while resting in bed to decrease the likelihood of deep-vein blood clots.

MEDICATION
- Your doctor may prescribe:
  Pain relievers. Don't take prescription pain medication longer than 4 to 7 days. Use *only* as much as you need.
  Stool softeners to prevent constipation.
  Antibiotics to fight infection.
- You may use non-prescription drugs, such as acetaminophen, for minor pain.

ACTIVITY
- Resume work and normal activity as soon as possible to reduce postoperative depression and irritability, which are common.
- Resume driving 2 weeks after returning home.
- Avoid vigorous exercise for 6 weeks after surgery.

DIET—Your doctor will prescribe a diet.

CALL YOUR DOCTOR IF

- Pain, swelling, redness, drainage or bleeding increases in the surgical area.
- You develop signs of infection: headache, muscle aches, dizziness or a general ill feeling and fever.
- You experience nausea, vomiting, constipation or abdominal swelling.
- New, unexplained symptoms develop. Drugs used in treatment may produce side effects.

SYMPATHECTOMY, CERVICODORSAL

GENERAL INFORMATION

DEFINITION—Removing a section of the sympathetic nerves located near the spinal cord in the upper back.

BODY PARTS INVOLVED—Cervicodorsal sympathetic nerves (part of the autonomic nervous system) that control contraction and expansion of small arteries in the arms; lungs; ribs.

REASONS FOR SURGERY—Restoration of normal blood supply to the arms. Removing part of the sympathetic nervous system stops spasms in the blood vessels that can cause or aggravate partial obstruction.

SURGICAL RISK INCREASES WITH
- Obesity.
- Smoking.
- Excess alcohol consumption.
- Atherosclerosis or diabetes mellitus.
- Chronic illness.
- Use of drugs such as: antihypertensives; muscle relaxants; tranquilizers; sleep inducers; insulin; sedatives; beta-adrenergic blockers; or cortisone.
- Use of mind-altering drugs, including: narcotics; psychedelics; hallucinogens; marijuana; sedatives; hypnotics; or cocaine.

WHAT TO EXPECT

WHO OPERATES—General surgeon, neurosurgeon or vascular surgeon.

WHERE PERFORMED—Hospital.

DIAGNOSTIC TESTS
- Before surgery: Blood and urine studies; X-rays of chest; EKG (see Glossary).
- After surgery: Blood studies.

ANESTHESIA—General anesthesia by inhalation and injection, with an airway tube placed in the windpipe.

DESCRIPTION OF OPERATION
- An incision is made in the armpit.
- The muscles are divided, and part of the 3rd rib is removed.
- One lung is allowed to collapse temporarily to allow easier entry into the chest cavity.
- The cervical and dorsal sympathetic nerve chains are identified and divided.
- The ribs are reconstructed and held in place with heavy sutures. The lung is re-expanded. The muscles and skin edges are closed with sutures or clips, which usually can be removed about 1 week after surgery.

POSSIBLE COMPLICATIONS
- Excessive bleeding.
- Surgical-wound infection.
- Inadvertent injury to lung tissue.

AVERAGE HOSPITAL STAY—7 days.

PROBABLE OUTCOME—Expect complete healing without complications. Circulation will improve in 3 to 4 days. Allow about 4 weeks for recovery from surgery.

POSTOPERATIVE CARE

NOTE—This information is supplemental and should not replace your doctor's instructions.

GENERAL MEASURES
- Don't smoke.
- A hard ridge should form along the incision. As it heals, the ridge will recede gradually.
- Use an electric heating pad, a heat lamp or a warm compress to relieve incisional pain.
- Bathe and shower as usual. You may wash the incision gently with mild unscented soap.
- Move legs often while resting in bed to decrease the likelihood of deep-vein blood clots.

MEDICATION
- Your doctor may prescribe:
  Pain relievers. Don't take prescription pain medication longer than 4 to 7 days. Use *only* as much as you need.
  Stool softeners to prevent constipation.
  Antibiotics to fight infection.
- You may use non-prescription drugs, such as acetaminophen, for minor pain.

ACTIVITY
- Return to work and normal activity as soon as possible. This reduces postoperative depression, which is common.
- Avoid vigorous exercise for 6 weeks after surgery.
- Resume driving 18 days after returning home.

DIET—Clear liquid diet until the gastrointestinal tract functions again. Then eat a well-balanced, high-protein diet to promote healing. After recovery, eat a low-fat, low-salt diet (see Appendices 8 and 9).

CALL YOUR DOCTOR IF

Any of the following occurs:
- Increased pain, swelling, redness, drainage or bleeding in the surgical area.
- Signs of infection: headache, muscle aches, dizziness or a general ill feeling and fever.
- Nausea, vomiting, constipation or abdominal swelling.
- Coldness, discoloration or numbness in the hand.
- Cough, shortness of breath or chest pain.

SYMPATHECTOMY, LUMBAR

GENERAL INFORMATION

DEFINITION—Removing a section of the sympathetic nerves located near the spinal cord in the lower back.

BODY PARTS INVOLVED—The lumbar sympathetic nerves (part of the autonomic nervous system) that control contraction and expansion of small arteries in the legs.

REASONS FOR SURGERY—Restoration of normal blood supply to the legs. Removing part of the sympathetic nervous system stops spasms in the blood vessels that can cause or aggravate partial obstruction.

SURGICAL RISK INCREASES WITH
- Obesity.
- Smoking.
- Atherosclerosis or diabetes mellitus.
- Chronic illness.
- Use of drugs such as: antihypertensives; muscle relaxants; tranquilizers; sleep inducers; insulin; sedatives; beta-adrenergic blockers; or cortisone.
- Use of mind-altering drugs, including: narcotics; psychedelics; hallucinogens; marijuana; sedatives; hypnotics; or cocaine.

WHAT TO EXPECT

WHO OPERATES—General surgeon, neurosurgeon or vascular surgeon.

WHERE PERFORMED—Hospital.

DIAGNOSTIC TESTS
- Before surgery: Blood and urine studies.
- After surgery: Blood studies.

ANESTHESIA—General anesthesia by inhalation and injection, with an airway tube placed in the windpipe.

DESCRIPTION OF OPERATION
- A large incision is made, extending from the abdomen around the flank, almost to the backbone. The muscles are separated.
- The lumbar sympathetic chain of nerves is located, cut free and removed.
- The muscles are sewn together with large sutures.
- The skin is closed with sutures or clips, which usually can be removed about 1 week after surgery.

POSSIBLE COMPLICATIONS
- Excessive bleeding.
- Surgical-wound infection.
- Incisional hernia.
- Inadvertent injury to the ureter.

AVERAGE HOSPITAL STAY—7 days.

PROBABLE OUTCOME—Expect complete healing without complications. Circulation will improve in 3 to 4 days. Allow about 4 weeks for recovery from surgery.

POSTOPERATIVE CARE

NOTE—This information is supplemental and should not replace your doctor's instructions.

GENERAL MEASURES
- Don't smoke.
- A hard ridge should form along the incision. As it heals, the ridge will recede gradually.
- Use an electric heating pad, a heat lamp or a warm compress to relieve incisional pain.
- Bathe and shower as usual. You may wash the incision gently with mild unscented soap.
- Move legs often while resting in bed to decrease the likelihood of deep-vein blood clots.

MEDICATION
- Your doctor may prescribe:
  Pain relievers. Don't take prescription pain medication longer than 4 to 7 days. Use *only* as much as you need.
  Stool softeners to prevent constipation.
  Antibiotics to fight infection.
- You may use non-prescription drugs, such as acetaminophen, for minor pain.

ACTIVITY
- Return to work and normal activity as soon as possible. This reduces postoperative depression, which is common.
- Avoid vigorous exercise for 6 weeks after surgery. Start a walking exercise program when your doctor prescribes it.
- Resume driving 18 days after returning home.
- Resume sexual relations when your doctor determines that healing is complete.

DIET—Clear liquid diet until the gastrointestinal tract functions again. Then eat a well-balanced, high-protein diet to promote healing. After recovery, eat a low-fat, low-salt diet (see Appendices 8 and 9).

CALL YOUR DOCTOR IF

- Pain, swelling, redness, drainage or bleeding increases in the surgical area.
- You develop signs of infection: headache, muscle aches, dizziness or a general ill feeling and fever.
- You experience new symptoms, such as nausea, vomiting, constipation or abdominal swelling.
- Your foot becomes cold, discolored or numb.

SURGERIES

TEAR DUCT, OPENING OF

GENERAL INFORMATION

DEFINITION—Opening of tear ducts (also called lacrimal ducts) in the corners of the eyes closer to the nose. They may be blocked by infection or foreign material, or may be incompletely open in newborns.

BODY PARTS INVOLVED—Tear glands and tear ducts, usually in newborns, infants or young children.

REASONS FOR SURGERY—Infection or complete blockage that does not respond to simple treatment.

SURGICAL RISK INCREASES WITH
- Obesity.
- Poor nutrition.
- Recent or chronic illness.

WHAT TO EXPECT

WHO OPERATES—Ophthalmologist, pediatric surgeon, general surgeon or ear, nose and throat specialist.

WHERE PERFORMED—Hospital or outpatient surgical facility.

DIAGNOSTIC TESTS
- Before surgery: Blood and urine studies.
- After surgery: Blood studies.

ANESTHESIA
- Local anesthesia by injection or topical application (sometimes).
- General anesthesia by inhalation and injection, with an airway tube placed in the windpipe.

DESCRIPTION OF OPERATION
- The tear duct is expanded, probed and irrigated until fluid flows freely through it. The procedure is repeated on the other tear duct.
- Sutures are not needed. Bleeding should not be a problem.

POSSIBLE COMPLICATIONS—Surgical-wound infection.

AVERAGE HOSPITAL STAY—0 to 1 day.

PROBABLE OUTCOME—Expect complete healing without complications. Allow about 10 days for recovery from surgery.

POSTOPERATIVE CARE

NOTE—This information is supplemental and should not replace your doctor's instructions.

GENERAL MEASURES
- Bathe your child as usual.
- Use a warm compress to relieve pain in the surgical area.

MEDICATION
- Your doctor may prescribe antibiotic eye drops to fight infection. Keep eye drops cold, but not frozen, in the refrigerator.
- You may give your child non-prescription drugs, such as acetaminophen, for minor pain.

ACTIVITY—Avoid vigorous exercise for 1 week after surgery.

DIET—No special diet.

CALL YOUR DOCTOR IF

Any of the following occurs:
- Nausea or vomiting.
- Pain, swelling, redness or drainage in the surgical area.
- Signs of infection: headache, muscle aches, dizziness or a general ill feeling and fever.

TENDON REPAIR

GENERAL INFORMATION

DEFINITION—Reattaching tendons to their connective tissue or sewing sections of broken tendons together.

BODY PARTS INVOLVED—Injured tendons, most frequently in the hand, foot, ankle, wrist, shoulder, hip, knee and elbow.

REASONS FOR SURGERY—Restoration of normal function of joints or tissue surrounding tendons.

SURGICAL RISK INCREASES WITH
- Adults over 60.
- Obesity.
- Smoking.
- Poor nutrition.
- Recent or chronic illness.
- Alcoholism.
- Use of drugs such as: antihypertensives; muscle relaxants; tranquilizers; sleep inducers; insulin; sedatives; beta-adrenergic blockers; or cortisone.
- Use of mind-altering drugs, including: narcotics; psychedelics; hallucinogens; marijuana; sedatives; hypnotics; or cocaine.

WHAT TO EXPECT

WHO OPERATES—Hand surgeon or general surgeon.

WHERE PERFORMED—Hospital, outpatient surgical facility or emergency room.

DIAGNOSTIC TESTS
- Before surgery: Blood and urine studies; X-rays of the injured part.
- After surgery: Blood studies.

ANESTHESIA
- Local anesthesia by injection.
- Spinal anesthesia by injection.

DESCRIPTION OF OPERATION
- An incision is made over the injured tendon.
- The severed ends of the tendon are located and sewn together. If the tendon has been injured severely, a tendon graft may be required.
- If necessary, tendons are reattacted to surrounding connective tissue.
- The surgical area is examined for injuries to nerves and blood vessels.
- The skin is closed with sutures, which usually can be removed about 10 days after surgery.
- Usually, the injured part is kept rigid with a splint or plaster cast.

POSSIBLE COMPLICATIONS
- Excessive bleeding.
- Surgical-wound infection.
- Partial loss of function in joint served by the injured tendon(s).

AVERAGE HOSPITAL STAY—0 to 1 day.

PROBABLE OUTCOME—Expect complete healing without complications. Allow about 1 month for recovery from surgery.

POSTOPERATIVE CARE

NOTE—This information is supplemental and should not replace your doctor's instructions.

GENERAL MEASURES
- If the wound bleeds during the first 24 hours after surgery, press a clean tissue or cloth to it for 10 minutes.
- A hard ridge should form along the incision. As it heals, the ridge will recede gradually.
- Use an electric heating pad, a heat lamp or a warm compress to relieve incisional pain.
- Bathe or shower as usual after the splint is removed.
- Between bathings, keep the wound dry with a bandage for the first 2 or 3 days after the splint is removed. If a bandage gets wet, change it promptly.
- See Appendix 17 for complete instructions on care of casts.

MEDICATION
- Your doctor may prescribe:
  Pain relievers. Don't take prescription pain medication longer than 4 to 7 days. Use *only* as much as you need.
  Antibiotics to fight infection.
- You may use non-prescription drugs, such as acetaminophen, for minor pain.

ACTIVITY
- Resume work and normal activity as soon as possible. This reduces postoperative depression and irritability, which are common.
- Avoid vigorous exercise for 6 weeks after surgery.
- Resume driving 4 weeks after returning home.

DIET—No special diet.

CALL YOUR DOCTOR IF

- Pain, swelling, redness, drainage or bleeding increases in the surgical area.
- Skin below the cast becomes cold, discolored or numb.
- You develop signs of infection: headache, muscle aches, dizziness or a general ill feeling and fever.
- You experience nausea or vomiting.
- New, unexplained symptoms develop. Drugs used in treatment may produce side effects.

TESTICLE FIXATION
(Orchiopexy)

 GENERAL INFORMATION

DEFINITION—Fastening an undescended or twisted testicle in its normal position.

BODY PARTS INVOLVED—Scrotum; testicle; vas deferens; blood vessels and nerves in the scrotum.

REASONS FOR SURGERY—Placement of an undescended testicle in its normal position, or correction of a twisted testicle.

SURGICAL RISK INCREASES WITH
- Chronic illness.
- Use of drugs such as: antihypertensives; muscle relaxants; tranquilizers; insulin; or cortisone.
- Use of mind-altering drugs, including: narcotics; psychedelics; hallucinogens; marijuana; sedatives; hypnotics; or cocaine.

 WHAT TO EXPECT

WHO OPERATES—Urologist or general surgeon.

WHERE PERFORMED—Hospital.

DIAGNOSTIC TESTS
- Before surgery: Blood and urine studies.
- After surgery: Blood studies.

ANESTHESIA
- Spinal anesthesia by injection.
- Local anesthesia by injection.

DESCRIPTION OF OPERATION
- An incision is made in the scrotum.
- The blood supply and nerves leading to the testicle are located and carefully preserved.
- If the testicle has not descended from the abdomen, the surgeon reaches into the inguinal canal with special instruments and gently pulls it down.
- The testicle and its blood supply and nerves are pulled to the bottom of the scrotum and sewn in place.
- The skin is closed with sutures that will be absorbed by the body.

POSSIBLE COMPLICATIONS
- Excessive bleeding.
- Surgical-wound infection.

AVERAGE HOSPITAL STAY—3 to 6 days.

PROBABLE OUTCOME—Expect complete healing without complications. Allow about 3 weeks for recovery from surgery.

 POSTOPERATIVE CARE

NOTE—This information is supplemental and should not replace your doctor's instructions.

GENERAL MEASURES
- Apply an ice pack to the surgical area as needed for the first 24 hours after surgery to prevent excessive swelling.
- Use an electric heating pad, a heat lamp or a warm compress to relieve incisional pain beginning 24 hours after surgery.
- The incision may be washed gently with mild unscented soap.
- 2 pairs of jockey shorts should be worn for 4 to 6 weeks.

MEDICATION
- Your doctor may prescribe:
  Pain relievers. Pain medication should not be used longer than 4 to 7 days. Use *only* as much as you need.
  Stool softeners to prevent constipation.
  Antibiotics to fight infection.
- You may use non-prescription drugs, such as acetaminophen, for minor pain.

ACTIVITY—Normal activity may be resumed as soon as possible. This reduces postoperative depression and irritability, which are common.

DIET—A well-balanced, high-protein diet promotes healing.

 CALL YOUR DOCTOR IF

Any of the following occur:
- Nausea or vomiting.
- Discomfort or difficulty in urination.
- Increased pain, swelling, redness, drainage or bleeding in the surgical area.
- Signs of infection: headache, muscle aches, dizziness or a general ill feeling and fever.

TESTICLE REMOVAL
(Orchiectomy)

GENERAL INFORMATION

DEFINITION—Removal of one of the testicles (orchiectomy).

BODY PARTS INVOLVED—Scrotum; testicle; vas deferens; blood vessels and nerves in the scrotum.

REASONS FOR SURGERY—Cancer or gangrene of the testicle.

SURGICAL RISK INCREASES WITH
- Adults over 60.
- Smoking.
- Chronic illness.
- Use of drugs such as: antihypertensives; muscle relaxants; tranquilizers; sleep inducers; insulin; sedatives; beta-adrenergic blockers; or cortisone.
- Use of mind-altering drugs, including: narcotics; psychedelics; hallucinogens; marijuana; sedatives; hypnotics; or cocaine.

WHAT TO EXPECT

WHO OPERATES—Urologist or general surgeon.

WHERE PERFORMED—Hospital.

DIAGNOSTIC TESTS
- Before surgery: Blood and urine studies.
- After surgery: Blood studies.

ANESTHESIA
- Spinal anesthesia by injection.
- Local anesthesia by injection.

DESCRIPTION OF OPERATION
- An incision is made in the scrotum. The blood supply and nerves leading to the testicle are located and cut free.
- The testicle is cut free from surrounding tissue and removed.
- The skin is closed with sutures that will be absorbed by the body.

POSSIBLE COMPLICATIONS
- Excessive bleeding.
- Surgical-wound infection.

AVERAGE HOSPITAL STAY—3 to 6 days.

PROBABLE OUTCOME—Expect complete healing without complications. Allow about 3 weeks for recovery from surgery.
   Removal of one testicle should not interfere with normal sexual function or the ability to have children.

POSTOPERATIVE CARE

NOTE—This information is supplemental and should not replace your doctor's instructions.

GENERAL MEASURES
- Apply an ice pack to the surgical area as needed for the first 24 hours after surgery to prevent excessive swelling.
- Use an electric heating pad, a heat lamp or a warm compress to relieve incisional pain beginning 24 hours after surgery.
- Bathe and shower as usual. You may wash the incision gently with mild unscented soap.
- Wear an athletic supporter for 4 to 6 weeks.

MEDICATION
- Your doctor may prescribe:
   Pain relievers. Don't take prescription pain medication longer than 4 to 7 days. Use *only* as much as you need.
   Stool softeners to prevent constipation.
   Antibiotics to fight infection.
- You may use non-prescription drugs, such as acetaminophen, for minor pain.

ACTIVITY
- Return to work and normal activity as soon as possible. This reduces postoperative depression and irritability, which are common.
- Avoid vigorous exercise for 6 weeks after surgery.
- Resume driving 2 weeks after returning home.
- Resume sexual relations when your doctor determines that healing is complete.

DIET—Clear liquid diet until the gastrointestinal tract functions again. Then eat a well-balanced, high-protein diet to promote healing.

CALL YOUR DOCTOR IF

- You experience nausea, vomiting, or discomfort or difficulty in urination.
- Pain, swelling, redness, drainage or bleeding increases in the surgical area.
- You develop signs of infection: headache, muscle aches, dizziness or a general ill feeling and fever.
- New, unexplained symptoms develop. Drugs used in treatment may produce side effects.

THYROGLOSSAL-DUCT & CYST REMOVAL

GENERAL INFORMATION

DEFINITION—Removal of a thyroglossal duct that has a cyst. The cyst results from remnants of the thyroid gland that do not descend normally during early fetal development. The cyst usually appears during childhood, attached to the hyoid bone by the duct. The duct then passes upward to its origin at the base of the tongue. Surgery is usually performed when the patient is between 6 and 10 years old.

BODY PARTS INVOLVED—Thyroglossal cyst; remnants of the thyroglossal duct; hyoid bone.

REASONS FOR SURGERY
- Prevention of infections.
- Relief of pressure on the airway that causes difficulty in breathing or swallowing.

SURGICAL RISK INCREASES WITH
- Obesity.
- Poor nutrition.
- Recent or chronic illness.
- Other congenital disorders.

WHAT TO EXPECT

WHO OPERATES—General surgeon or ear, nose and throat specialist.

WHERE PERFORMED—Hospital.

DIAGNOSTIC TESTS
- Before surgery: Blood and urine studies.
- After surgery: Blood studies.

ANESTHESIA—General anesthesia by inhalation and injection, with an airway tube placed in the windpipe.

DESCRIPTION OF OPERATION
- An incision is made in the neck over the thyroglossal cyst.
- The cyst is cut free of muscle and connective tissue. The part of the hyoid bone to which the cyst is attached is cut, and the cyst and bone are removed.
- The thyroglossal duct is located, tied, cut and removed.
- The neck muscles are closed with fine sutures.
- The skin is closed with either sutures or clips, which usually can be be removed about 4 to 7 days after surgery.

POSSIBLE COMPLICATIONS
- Excessive bleeding.
- Surgical-wound infection.
- Inadvertent injury to larynx.

AVERAGE HOSPITAL STAY—2 to 4 days.

PROBABLE OUTCOME—Expect complete healing without complications. Allow about 6 weeks for recovery from surgery.

POSTOPERATIVE CARE

NOTE—This information is supplemental and should not replace your doctor's instructions.

GENERAL MEASURES
- A hard, blunt ridge should form along the incision. As it heals, the ridge will recede gradually.
- Use an electric heating pad, a heat lamp or a warm compress to relieve incisional pain.
- The child should bathe and shower as usual, and wash the incision gently with mild unscented soap.

MEDICATION
- Your doctor may prescribe:
  Pain relievers. Don't give your child prescription pain medication longer than 4 to 7 days. Use *only* as much as needed. Antibiotics to fight infection.
- You may use non-prescription drugs, such as acetaminophen, for minor pain.

ACTIVITY
- Return to normal activity as soon as possible. This reduces postoperative depression and irritability, which are common.
- Avoid vigorous exercise for 6 weeks after surgery.

DIET—Clear liquid diet until the gastrointestinal tract functions again. Then provide a well-balanced, high-protein diet to promote healing.

CALL YOUR DOCTOR IF

Any of the following occurs:
- Increased pain, swelling, redness, drainage or bleeding in the surgical area.
- Nausea or vomiting.
- Signs of infection, such as headache, muscle aches, dizziness or a general ill feeling and fever.
- Hoarseness that doesn't go away within 2 weeks after surgery.

THYROID-GLAND REMOVAL
(Thyroidectomy)

GENERAL INFORMATION

DEFINITION—Removal of part or all of the thyroid gland.

BODY PARTS INVOLVED—Thyroid gland, the organ in the neck below the Adam's apple that controls the body's metabolism.

REASONS FOR SURGERY
- Hyperthyroidism in pregnant women and children.
- Benign or cancerous tumors of the thyroid.
- Thyroglossal cysts (see Glossary).

SURGICAL RISK INCREASES WITH
- Adults over 60.
- Obesity.
- Smoking.
- Poor nutrition.
- Untreated hyperthyroidism.
- Use of antithyroid medication and iodides before surgery decreases risk. Ask your doctor.

WHAT TO EXPECT

WHO OPERATES—General surgeon.

WHERE PERFORMED—Hospital.

DIAGNOSTIC TESTS
- Before surgery: Blood studies; sonograms; CAT scan; needle biopsy; or radioactive-iodine uptake and scan (see Glossary).
- After surgery: Blood studies.

ANESTHESIA—General anesthesia by inhalation and injection, with an airway tube placed in the windpipe.

DESCRIPTION OF OPERATION
- An incision is made in the neck following natural skin lines.
- Blood supply to the thyroid gland is clamped.
- All or part of the thyroid gland is cut free and removed, and a drain is left in place. In certain cases, some normal thyroid gland tissue is left intact.
- The skin is closed with sutures or clips, which can usually be removed in 2 to 10 days after surgery.

POSSIBLE COMPLICATIONS
- Hoarseness, if vocal-cord nerves are damaged during surgery.
- Hypothyroidism.
- Hypoparathyroidism.
- Excessive bleeding.
- Surgical-wound infection.

AVERAGE HOSPITAL STAY—3 to 7 days.

PROBABLE OUTCOME—Underlying problem cured in most patients. Cancer that is present but has not spread may require radiation treatment. Allow about 6 weeks for recovery from surgery.

POSTOPERATIVE CARE

NOTE—This information is supplemental and should not replace your doctor's instructions.

GENERAL MEASURES
- A hard ridge should form along the incision. As it heals, the ridge will recede gradually.
- Use an electric heating pad, a heat lamp or a warm compress to relieve incisional pain.
- Bathe and shower as usual. You may wash the incision gently with mild unscented soap.

MEDICATION—Your doctor may prescribe:
- Pain relievers. Don't take prescription pain medication longer than 4 to 7 days. Use *only* as much as you need.
- Thyroid hormones.

ACTIVITY
- Return to work and normal activity as soon as possible. This reduces postoperative depression and irritability, which are common.
- Resume driving 2 weeks after you return home.
- Resume sexual relations when able.

DIET—No special diet.

CALL YOUR DOCTOR IF

- Pain, swelling, redness, drainage or bleeding increases in the surgical area.
- You develop signs of infection: headache, muscle aches, dizziness or a general ill feeling and fever.
- You develop symptoms of hypothyroidism: excessive weakness, fatigue, intolerance to cold, menstrual irregularities, constipation, or dry and coarse skin and hair.

TOENAIL REMOVAL

 GENERAL INFORMATION

DEFINITION—Removal of part or all of a toenail.

BODY PARTS INVOLVED—Toenail, usually in the big toe.

REASONS FOR SURGERY
● Relief of painful symptoms of an ingrown toenail, with or without an infection.
● Toenails may be removed for reasons other than ingrown toenail, including: injury with part of the toenail torn away; splinters that cannot be removed without removing the toenail; or warts under the nail.

SURGICAL RISK INCREASES WITH
● Illnesses such as: diabetes mellitus; arterial occlusive disease with poor circulation to the feet; other infections of the foot; alcoholism.
● Use of drugs such as: antihypertensives; muscle relaxants; tranquilizers; sleep inducers; insulin; sedatives; beta-adrenergic blockers; or cortisone.
● Use of mind-altering drugs, including: narcotics; psychedelics; hallucinogens; marijuana; sedatives; hypnotics; or cocaine.

 WHAT TO EXPECT

WHO OPERATES—General surgeon, family doctor, dermatologist or podiatrist.

WHERE PERFORMED—Doctor's office or outpatient surgical facility.

DIAGNOSTIC TESTS—None required.

ANESTHESIA—Local anesthesia by injection.

DESCRIPTION OF OPERATION
● A section of skin is cut on the affected side of the toe.
● Part or all of the nail is pulled up along its bed and cut free of its underlying tissue.
● The nail bed along the affected side is scraped.
● A special non-stick bandage is applied tightly to prevent bleeding. Usually, no sutures are needed.

POSSIBLE COMPLICATIONS
● Excessive bleeding.
● Surgical-wound infection.

AVERAGE HOSPITAL STAY—None.

PROBABLE OUTCOME—Expect complete healing without complications. Allow about 3 weeks for recovery from surgery. The toenail should eventually grown back.

 POSTOPERATIVE CARE

NOTE—This information is supplemental and should not replace your doctor's instructions.

GENERAL MEASURES
● Keep the surgical area dry until after the dressing is changed for the first time. Change dressings as needed.
● After the dressing is changed the first time, soak the affected area in plain or salt water at 101 to 104F (38.3 to 40C) for 10 to 20 minutes several times a day to reduce pain and swelling.
● Avoid shoes that fit tightly, especially those with narrow toes. Wear white cotton socks.
● To prevent a recurrence when the toenail grows back, cut it straight across instead of rounding off at the corners.

MEDICATION
● Your doctor may prescribe:
   Pain relievers. Don't take prescription pain medication longer than 4 to 7 days. Use *only* as much as you need.
   Antibiotics or antifungal medication to fight infection.
● You may use non-prescription drugs, such as acetaminophen, for minor pain.

ACTIVITY—Avoid vigorous exercise until the nail heals. Don't put any weight on the affected foot for 24 hours, then resume walking gradually.

DIET—No special diet.

 CALL YOUR DOCTOR IF

● Pain, swelling, redness, drainage or bleeding increases in the surgical area.
● You develop signs of infection: headache, muscle aches, dizziness or a general ill feeling and fever.
● New, unexplained symptoms develop. Drugs used in treatment may produce side effects.

TONGUE, CHEEK OR GUM BIOPSY

GENERAL INFORMATION

DEFINITION—Removal of tissue from the oral cavity.

BODY PARTS INVOLVED—Tongue; cheek; gums; roof of mouth; salivary glands under the tongue.

REASONS FOR SURGERY—Usually performed to determine if any unusual lesion in the mouth is cancerous. Laboratory examination of the removed tissue aids in diagnosis.

SURGICAL RISK INCREASES WITH
● Adults over 60.
● Smoking.
● Excess alcohol consumption.
● Use of drugs such as: antihypertensives; muscle relaxants; tranquilizers; sleep inducers; insulin; sedatives; beta-adrenergic blockers; or cortisone.
● Use of mind-altering drugs, including: narcotics; psychedelics; hallucinogens; marijuana; sedatives; hypnotics; or cocaine.

WHAT TO EXPECT

WHO OPERATES—Dentist, oral surgeon, general surgeon or ear, nose and throat specialist.

WHERE PERFORMED—Hospital, outpatient surgical facility or doctor's, dentist's or oral surgeon's office.

DIAGNOSTIC TESTS
● Before surgery: Blood and urine studies.
● After surgery: Laboratory examination of removed tissue.

ANESTHESIA
● Local anesthesia by injection.
● General anesthesia (sometimes) by inhalation and injection, with an airway tube placed in the windpipe.

DESCRIPTION OF OPERATION
● The area where the tissue is to be gathered is numbed with a local anesthetic.
● Abnormal tissue and a small amount of healthy surrounding tissue is removed.
● Small stitches may be needed to close the incision. These usually can be removed in 3 to 5 days after surgery.

POSSIBLE COMPLICATIONS
● Excessive bleeding.
● Surgical-wound infection.

AVERAGE HOSPITAL STAY—None.

PROBABLE OUTCOME—Tissue obtained successfully without complications in virtually all cases. Allow about 2 weeks for recovery from surgery.

POSTOPERATIVE CARE

NOTE—This information is supplemental and should not replace your doctor's instructions.

GENERAL MEASURES
● Beginning 24 hours after surgery, rinse your mouth every 1 or 2 hours with a solution of 1/2 teaspoon salt in 8 oz. warm water.
● Brush your teeth with a soft toothbrush. A clean mouth heals faster.

MEDICATION
● Your doctor may prescribe pain relievers. Don't take prescription pain medication longer than 4 to 7 days. Use *only* as much as you need.
● You may use non-prescription drugs, such as acetaminophen, for minor pain.

ACTIVITY—No restrictions.

DIET—Resuming normal food and fluid intake after surgery will ensure rapid healing. If your regular diet is too difficult, try a high-protein liquid diet (see Appendix 7) for 2 or 3 days.

CALL YOUR DOCTOR IF

● Pain, swelling, redness, drainage or bleeding increases in the surgical area.
● You develop signs of infection: headache, muscle aches, dizziness or a general ill feeling and fever.

SURGERIES

TONSIL & ADENOID REMOVAL
(Tonsillectomy & Adenoidectomy)

 GENERAL INFORMATION

DEFINITION—Removal of the tonsils and adenoids.

BODY PARTS INVOLVED—Tonsils; adenoids; opening from the nose into the throat; back of the throat.

REASONS FOR SURGERY—In tonsils:
- More than 5 attacks of tonsillitis in 1 year.
- Peritonsillar abscess (see Glossary).

In adenoids:
- Obstruction of air through the nose.
- Infections in the middle ear.

SURGICAL RISK INCREASES WITH
- Obesity.
- Smoking.
- Poor nutrition.
- Recent or chronic illness.
- Use of drugs such as: antihypertensives; muscle relaxants; tranquilizers; sleep inducers; insulin; sedatives; beta-adrenergic blockers; or cortisone.
- Use of mind-altering drugs, including: narcotics; psychedelics; hallucinogens; marijuana; sedatives; hypnotics; or cocaine.

 WHAT TO EXPECT

WHO OPERATES—Ear, nose and throat specialist or general surgeon.

WHERE PERFORMED—Hospital or outpatient surgical facility.

DIAGNOSTIC TESTS
- Before surgery: Blood and urine studies.
- After surgery: Laboratory examination of removed tissue; blood studies.

ANESTHESIA—General anesthesia by inhalation and injection, with an airway tube placed in the windpipe.

DESCRIPTION OF OPERATION
- The mouth is held open to expose the tonsils.
- The tonsils are grasped with clamps and pulled toward the middle of the mouth. The tonsils are cut free of surrounding membrane and removed.
- Bleeding is controlled by pressure, sutures or clamps and ties.
- The adenoids are located and removed with a special instrument.

POSSIBLE COMPLICATIONS
- Excessive bleeding.
- Surgical-wound infection.
- Adenoid-tissue regrowth.
- Inadvertent injury to the uvula, soft palate or eustachian tubes.

AVERAGE HOSPITAL STAY—1 to 2 days.

PROBABLE OUTCOME—Expect complete healing without complications. You will experience moderate nasal congestion and drainage, a sore throat and earaches for a few days after surgery. Allow about 3 weeks for recovery from surgery. During this time, avoid becoming hot, tired or excited.

 POSTOPERATIVE CARE

NOTE—This information is supplemental and should not replace your doctor's instructions.

GENERAL MEASURES
- Bathe and shower as usual.
- Apply ice packs to relieve pain.
- Try not to talk, swallow, cough, clear the throat, cry or sing for 1 week after surgery.

MEDICATION
- Your doctor may prescribe:
  Pain relievers. Don't take prescription pain medication longer than 4 to 7 days. Use *only* as much as you need.
  Stool softeners to prevent constipation.
  Antibiotics to fight infection.
- You may use non-prescription drugs, such as acetaminophen, to relieve minor pain.

ACTIVITY
- Rest in bed for 2 to 3 days, then resume normal activities slowly. This reduces postoperative depression and irritability, which are common.
- Avoid vigorous exercise for 6 weeks after surgery.

DIET—Avoid spicy and hard-to-digest foods. Eat soft foods, such as gelatin and custard, for 3 to 4 days after surgery. Gradually return to a normal diet.

 CALL YOUR DOCTOR IF

Any of the following occur:
- Nausea or vomiting.
- Coughing, spitting or vomiting blood.
- Increased pain, swelling, redness, drainage or bleeding in the surgical area.
- Signs of infection: headache, muscle aches, dizziness or a general ill feeling and fever.
- New, unexplained symptoms. Drugs used in treatment may produce side effects.

TOOTH EXTRACTION

 ## GENERAL INFORMATION

DEFINITION—Removal (extraction) of a tooth.

BODY PARTS INVOLVED—Teeth; gums; bones in jaw.

REASONS FOR SURGERY—Routine removals:
- Loss of supporting tissue, bone or gums.
- Infection of the nerve in the tooth.
- Fractured teeth that cannot be restored.

Impacted-tooth removals:
- Infection and pain around the lower wisdom teeth.
- Pain upon closing the jaws.
- Destruction or erosion of nearby teeth and bone due to growth of surrounding tissue.
- Lack of space for normal tooth growth.

SURGICAL RISK INCREASES WITH
- Smoking.
- Poor nutrition.
- Chronic disease, especially: rheumatic fever with rheumatic heart disease; heart or blood disease; hypertension; or alcoholism.
- Use of drugs such as: antihypertensives; muscle relaxants; tranquilizers; sleep inducers; insulin; sedatives; beta-adrenergic blockers; or cortisone.
- Use of mind-altering drugs, including: narcotics; psychedelics; hallucinogens; marijuana; sedatives; hypnotics; or cocaine.

 ## WHAT TO EXPECT

WHO OPERATES—Dentist or oral surgeon.

WHERE PERFORMED—Hospital, outpatient surgical facility or dentist's or oral surgeon's office.

DIAGNOSTIC TESTS
- Before surgery: Blood and urine studies; X-rays of mouth.
- After surgery: Blood studies.

ANESTHESIA
- Local anesthesia by injection.
- General anesthesia (sometimes) by inhalation and injection, with an airway tube placed in the windpipe.

DESCRIPTION OF OPERATION
- For impacted teeth, the gum is incised over the tooth to be removed.
- For all extractions, the tooth is grasped with special instruments, rotated and pulled from the surrounding gum and bone.
- A gauze sponge is packed into the space left by the extracted tooth.
- Sometimes, sutures are used to close the gum edges. They usually come out by themselves, but may need removal in 3 or 4 days after surgery.

POSSIBLE COMPLICATIONS—Excessive bleeding or surgical-wound infection.

AVERAGE HOSPITAL STAY—0 to 1 day.

PROBABLE OUTCOME—Expect complete healing without complications. Allow about 3 weeks for recovery from surgery.

 ## POSTOPERATIVE CARE

NOTE—This information is supplemental and should not replace your doctor's instructions.

GENERAL MEASURES
- Do not smoke or use drinking straws for the next 24 hours.
- Keep your mouth closed firmly on the gauze sponge. Don't spit.
- Change the gauze sponge about every 30 minutes if it becomes soaked with blood. If not, leave it in place for about 3 to 4 hours after surgery.
- Use ice to relieve pain. Apply an ice pack for 10 minutes at a time every hour for 12 hours after surgery.
- Beginning 24 hours after surgery, rinse your mouth gently as needed with a solution of 1/2 teaspoon of salt in 8 oz. lukewarm water.

MEDICATION
- Your doctor or dentist may prescribe: Pain relievers. Don't take prescription pain medication longer than 4 to 7 days. Use *only* as much as you need. Antibiotics to fight infection.
- You may use non-prescription drugs, such as acetaminophen, for minor pain.

ACTIVITY—Rest quietly at home for 24 hours after surgery, then resume limited activity for 1 or 2 days. Then, no restrictions.

DIET—Soft or liquid diet (See Appendix 7) for 24 hours after surgery. Do not drink alcoholic beverages during this time.

 ## CALL YOUR DOCTOR OR DENTIST IF

- Nausea or vomiting begins.
- Medication does not relieve pain.
- Sutures drop out during the first 48 hours after surgery.
- Excessive bleeding (one gauze sponge becoming deep red in 10 to 15 minutes) continues for more than 4 hours after surgery.
- Pain, swelling, redness, drainage or bleeding increases in the surgical area.
- Signs of infection begin: headache, muscle aches, dizziness or a general ill feeling and fever.

SURGERIES

TOOTH REPLANTATION

GENERAL INFORMATION

DEFINITION—Replanting a tooth that has been knocked out of its normal position. Best results are obtained when the tooth is replanted within 2 hours after injury.

BODY PARTS INVOLVED—Mouth; teeth; gums.

REASONS FOR SURGERY—Prevention of permanent loss of a tooth.

SURGICAL RISK INCREASES WITH
- Smoking.
- Poor nutrition.
- Recent or chronic illness.
- Poor dental hygiene or gum disease.
- Use of drugs such as: antihypertensives; muscle relaxants; tranquilizers; sleep inducers; insulin; sedatives; beta-adrenergic blockers; or cortisone.
- Use of mind-altering drugs, including: narcotics; psychedelics; hallucinogens; marijuana; sedatives; hypnotics; or cocaine.

WHAT TO EXPECT

WHO OPERATES—Oral surgeon or dentist.

WHERE PERFORMED—Hospital, oral surgeon's or dentist's office, outpatient surgical facility, doctor's office or emergency room.

DIAGNOSTIC TESTS
- Before surgery: Usually none, because of the need for immediate surgery.
- After surgery: Blood studies.

ANESTHESIA
- Local anesthesia by injection.
- General anesthesia (if time allows) by inhalation and injection, with an airway tube placed in the windpipe.

DESCRIPTION OF OPERATION—If you or your child has a tooth knocked out, try to find the tooth, wash it and replace it in the socket as quickly as possible. Go to your dentist as soon as possible.

If you cannot replace the tooth in its socket, wash it and keep it wet. Go to your dentist immediately.

Usually the root-canal nerve of the tooth is removed and filled with plastic material before the tooth is reinserted. Some dentists simply place the tooth back into the socket immediately.

The replanted tooth is anchored to neighboring teeth with wire or plastic.

POSSIBLE COMPLICATIONS
- Excessive bleeding.
- Surgical-wound infection.
- Rejection of tooth (rare).

AVERAGE HOSPITAL STAY—0 to 1 day.

PROBABLE OUTCOME—Expect complete healing without complications. Allow about 4 weeks for recovery from surgery. The tooth often appears normal. If it darkens, a plastic dental veneer can be applied to make it cosmetically acceptable.

POSTOPERATIVE CARE

NOTE—This information is supplemental and should not replace your doctor's instructions.

GENERAL MEASURES
- Do not rinse your mouth, spit, smoke or use drinking straws for 24 hours after surgery.
- Beginning 24 hours after surgery, rinse your mouth with a solution of 1/2 teaspoon salt in 8 oz. lukewarm water every 1 or 2 hours.
- Brush your teeth with a soft toothbrush in the area not affected by surgery. A clean mouth heals faster.
- Do not bite down on the affected tooth until healing is complete.

MEDICATION
- Your doctor or dentist may prescribe: Pain relievers. Don't take prescription pain medication longer than 4 to 7 days. Use *only* as much as you need. Antibiotics to fight infection.
- You may use non-prescription drugs, such as acetaminophen, for minor pain.

ACTIVITY—Avoid vigorous exercise for 6 weeks after surgery.

DIET—Resuming your normal food and fluid intake will promote more rapid healing. If your regular diet is too difficult, try a high-protein liquid diet (see Appendix 7) for 2 or 3 days. Avoid alcoholic beverages until healing is complete.

CALL YOUR DOCTOR OR DENTIST IF

- Pain, swelling, redness, drainage or bleeding increases in the surgical area.
- You develop signs of infection: headache, muscle aches, dizziness or a general ill feeling and fever.
- You experience nausea or vomiting.
- New, unexplained symptoms develop. Drugs used in treatment may produce side effects.

TOOTH TRANSPLANT

GENERAL INFORMATION

DEFINITION—Replacement of an injured or diseased first or second molar with a third molar (wisdom tooth).

BODY PARTS INVOLVED—Mouth; teeth; gums.

REASONS FOR SURGERY—Restoration of normal tooth function.

SURGICAL RISK INCREASES WITH
- Recent or chronic illness.
- Smoking.

WHAT TO EXPECT

WHO OPERATES—Dentist or oral surgeon.

WHERE PERFORMED—Dentist's or oral surgeon's office, outpatient surgical facility or hospital.

DIAGNOSTIC TESTS
- Before surgery: Blood and urine studies.
- After surgery: Blood studies.

ANESTHESIA
- Local anesthesia by injection.
- General anesthesia (sometimes) by inhalation and injection, with an airway tube placed in the windpipe.

DESCRIPTION OF OPERATION
- A wisdom tooth is pulled.
- Sometimes, the root of the pulled tooth may be shortened for better fit.
- The socket where the tooth will be transplanted is enlarged.
- The wisdom tooth is inserted in the socket and secured to a neighboring tooth. This provides support during healing.

POSSIBLE COMPLICATIONS
- Excessive bleeding.
- Surgical-wound infection.
- Rejection of transplanted tooth (rare).

AVERAGE HOSPITAL STAY—0 to 1 day.

PROBABLE OUTCOME—Expect complete healing without complications. Allow about 1 month for recovery from surgery.

POSTOPERATIVE CARE

NOTE—This information is supplemental and should not replace your doctor's instructions.

GENERAL MEASURES
- Do not rinse your mouth, spit, smoke or use drinking straws for 24 hours after surgery.
- Beginning 24 hours after surgery, rinse your mouth with a solution of 1/2 teaspoon salt in 8 oz. lukewarm water every 1 or 2 hours.
- Brush your teeth with a soft toothbrush in the area of the mouth not affected by surgery. A clean mouth heals faster.
- Do not bite down on the affected tooth until healing is complete.

MEDICATION
- Your doctor or dentist may prescribe:
  Pain relievers. Don't take prescription pain medication longer than 4 to 7 days. Use *only* as much as you need.
  Antibiotics to fight infection.
- You may use non-prescription drugs, such as acetaminophen, for minor pain.

ACTIVITY—Avoid vigorous exercise for 3 weeks after surgery.

DIET—Resuming your normal food and fluid intake will promote more rapid healing. If you find that your regular diet is too difficult, try a high-protein liquid diet (see Appendix 7) for 2 or 3 days. Avoid alcoholic beverages until healing is complete.

CALL YOUR DOCTOR OR DENTIST IF

- Pain, swelling, redness, drainage or bleeding increases in the surgical area.
- You develop signs of infection: headache, muscle aches, dizziness or a general ill feeling and fever.
- You experience nausea and vomiting.
- New, unexplained symptoms develop. Drugs used in treatment may produce side effects.

TRACHEOSTOMY

GENERAL INFORMATION

DEFINITION—Creation of an opening in the windpipe (trachea) that will function as an airway either temporarily or permanently. The opening bypasses obstructions that prevent air from being inhaled.

BODY PARTS INVOLVED—Windpipe; muscles, blood vessels and nerves in the neck.

REASONS FOR SURGERY
- Restoration of normal breathing.
- Control of secretions from the nose and throat, particularly in patients who are unconscious.
- Creation of an open airway in patients who require prolonged breathing assistance.

SURGICAL RISK INCREASES WITH
- Newborns and infants.
- Adults over 60.
- Obesity.
- Smoking.
- Poor nutrition.
- Recent illness, especially upper-respiratory infection.
- Alcoholism or chronic illness.
- Use of drugs such as: antihypertensives; muscle relaxants; tranquilizers; sleep inducers; insulin; sedatives; beta-adrenergic blockers; or cortisone.

WHAT TO EXPECT

WHO OPERATES—Ear, nose and throat specialist or general surgeon.

WHERE PERFORMED—Hospital, outpatient surgical facility or emergency room.

DIAGNOSTIC TESTS—Blood and urine studies and X-rays of chest before and after (if necessary) surgery.

ANESTHESIA
- Local anesthesia (in emergencies) by injection.
- General anesthesia (when time allows) by inhalation and injection, with an airway tube placed in the windpipe.

DESCRIPTION OF OPERATION
- An incision is made in the neck. The muscles and connective tissue around the windpipe are divided.
- A section at the front of the windpipe is cut free and removed.
- A tracheostomy tube is fitted into the opening in the windpipe to function as an airway. The patient will breathe through this tube as long as it is in place.
- The skin is closed around the tube with sutures or clips, which usually can be removed about 1 week after surgery.

POSSIBLE COMPLICATIONS
- Excessive bleeding.
- Surgical-wound infection.
- Inadvertent damage to the vocal cords, vocal-cord nerves or esophagus.

AVERAGE HOSPITAL STAY—3 to 5 days.

PROBABLE OUTCOME—Expect complete healing without complications. Allow about 2 weeks for recovery from surgery.

POSTOPERATIVE CARE

NOTE—Follow your doctor's instructions. These instructions are supplemental.

GENERAL MEASURES
- A hard ridge should form along the incision. As it heals, the ridge will recede gradually.
- Use a heat lamp or a warm compress to relieve incisional pain.
- Keep the surgical area dry.
- Consult a speech therapist as soon as possible.

MEDICATION
- Your doctor may prescribe:
  Pain relievers. Don't take prescription pain medication longer than 4 to 7 days. Use *only* as much as you need.
  Antibiotics to fight infection.
- You may use non-prescription drugs, such as acetaminophen, for minor pain.

ACTIVITY
- Return to work and normal activity as soon as possible. This reduces postoperative depression and irritability, which are common.
- Avoid vigorous exercise for 6 weeks after surgery.

DIET—Clear liquid diet until the gastrointestinal tract functions again. Then eat a well-balanced, high-protein diet to promote healing.

CALL YOUR DOCTOR IF

- Pain, swelling, redness, drainage or bleeding increases in the surgical area.
- You develop signs of infection: headache, muscle aches, dizziness or a general ill feeling and fever.
- You experience new symptoms, such as nausea or vomiting.
- Speech difficulties persist after a temporary tracheostomy tube has been removed.

TUBAL LIGATION

GENERAL INFORMATION

DEFINITION—Tying the Fallopian tubes to accomplish sterilization in a woman.

BODY PARTS INVOLVED—Fallopian tubes.

REASONS FOR SURGERY—Prevention of unwanted pregnancy. It is important to receive professional counseling before deciding to undergo this surgery. Sterilization is usually irreversible.

SURGICAL RISK INCREASES WITH
- Obesity.
- Smoking.
- Poor nutrition.
- Recent or chronic illness.
- Use of drugs such as: antihypertensives; muscle relaxants; tranquilizers; sleeping pills; insulin; sedatives; beta-adrenergic blockers; or cortisone.
- Use of mind-altering drugs, including: narcotics; psychedelics; hallucinogens; marijuana; sedatives; hypnotics; or cocaine.

WHAT TO EXPECT

WHO OPERATES—Obstetrician-gynecologist or general surgeon.

WHERE PERFORMED—Hospital or outpatient surgical facility.

DIAGNOSTIC TESTS
- Before surgery: Blood and urine studies.
- After surgery: Blood studies.

ANESTHESIA
- Local anesthesia by injection.
- Spinal anesthesia by injection.
- General anesthesia by inhalation and injection, with an airway tube placed in the windpipe.

DESCRIPTION OF OPERATION—Several techniques are used to expose the Fallopian tubes for surgery. The most common are laparoscopy, posterior colpotomy (approach through the rear of the vagina) and minilaparotomy (approach through an incision just above the pubic-hair line).

Once the Fallopian tubes are exposed, a small section of each tube is cut free and removed. The severed ends are tied.

If an incision was made, the skin is closed with sutures or clips, which usually can be removed about 1 week after surgery.

POSSIBLE COMPLICATIONS
- Excessive bleeding.
- Surgical-wound infection.
- Inadvertent injury to bowel.
- Shoulder pain (after laparoscopy).

AVERAGE HOSPITAL STAY—0 to 1 day.

PROBABLE OUTCOME—Expect complete healing without complications with sterility for life. Your menstrual periods will continue as usual. Allow about 2 weeks for recovery from surgery.

POSTOPERATIVE CARE

NOTE—This information is supplemental and should not replace your doctor's instructions.

GENERAL MEASURES
- Use an electric heating pad, a heat lamp or a warm compress to relieve surgical-wound pain.
- Bathe and shower as usual. You may wash the incision gently with mild unscented soap.

MEDICATION
- Your doctor may prescribe:
  Pain relievers. Don't take prescription pain medication longer than 4 to 7 days. Use *only* as much as you need.
  Stool softeners to prevent constipation.
  Antibiotics to fight infection.
- You may use non-prescription drugs, such as acetaminophen, for minor pain.

ACTIVITY
- Return to work and normal activity as soon as possible. This reduces postoperative depression and irritability, which are common.
- Avoid vigorous exercise for 2 weeks after surgery.
- Resume driving 3 days after returning home.
- Resume sexual relations when your doctor has determined that healing is complete.

DIET—Clear liquid diet until the gastrointestinal tract functions again. Then eat a well-balanced, high-protein diet to promote healing.

CALL YOUR DOCTOR IF

- Pain, swelling, redness, drainage or bleeding increases in the surgical area.
- You develop signs of infection: headache, muscle aches, dizziness or a general ill feeling and fever.
- You experience nausea, vomiting, constipation or abdominal swelling.
- New, unexplained symptoms develop. Drugs used in treatment may produce side effects.

TUMMY TUCK
(Abdominoplasty)

GENERAL INFORMATION

DEFINITION—Removal of excess skin and fat from the abdomen.

BODY PARTS INVOLVED—Fat between skin and muscles in abdomen; skin.

REASONS FOR SURGERY—Improved appearance.

SURGICAL RISK INCREASES WITH
- Stress.
- Smoking.
- Poor nutrition.
- Previous abdominal surgery.
- Recent or chronic illness.
- Alcoholism.
- Use of drugs such as: antihypertensives; muscle relaxants; tranquilizers; sleep inducers; insulin; sedatives; beta-adrenergic blockers; or cortisone.
- Use of mind-altering drugs, including: narcotics; psychedelics; hallucinogens; marijuana; sedatives; hypnotics; or cocaine.

WHAT TO EXPECT

WHO OPERATES—Plastic and reconstructive surgeon.

WHERE PERFORMED—Hospital.

DIAGNOSTIC TESTS
- Before surgery: Blood and urine studies.
- After surgery: Blood studies.

ANESTHESIA—General anesthesia by inhalation and injection, with an airway tube placed in the windpipe.

DESCRIPTION OF OPERATION
- A large, elliptical incision is made in the abdomen.
- Excessive skin and the underlying apron of excess fat are cut free and removed.
- Drains are left under the operative site to prevent accumulation of blood and fluid from tissue drainage.
- Both edges of the skin are gently stretched and carefully sewn together with sutures.
- Sutures can usually be removed in 10 to 14 days.

POSSIBLE COMPLICATIONS
- Wide scars.
- Excessive bleeding.
- Surgical-wound infection.
- Blood or serum collection beneath the flap where fat was removed.

AVERAGE HOSPITAL STAY—6 days.

PROBABLE OUTCOME—Expect complete healing without complications and improved appearance. Allow about 10 weeks for recovery from surgery.

Excess abdominal fat will return if caloric intake is not controlled.

POSTOPERATIVE CARE

NOTE—This information is supplemental and should not replace your doctor's instructions.

GENERAL MEASURES
- A hard ridge should form along the incision. As it heals, the ridge will recede gradually.
- Use an electric heating pad, a heat lamp or a warm compress to relieve incisional pain.
- Bathe and shower as usual. You may wash the incision gently with mild unscented soap.
- Between showers, keep the wound dry with a bandage for the first 2 or 3 days after surgery. If a bandage gets wet, change it promptly.
- Apply non-prescription antibiotic ointment to the wound before applying new bandages.

MEDICATION
- Your doctor may prescribe:
  Pain relievers. Don't take prescription pain medication longer than 4 to 7 days. Use *only* as much as you need.
  Stool softeners to prevent constipation.
  Antibiotics to fight infection.
- You may use non-prescription drugs, such as acetaminophen, for minor pain.

ACTIVITY
- Resume work and normal activity as soon as possible. This reduces postoperative depression and irritability, which are common.
- Resume sexual relations when able.
- Exercise will help maintain improved appearance. Consult your doctor about an exercise program after recovery.

DIET—No special diet, but diet must be controlled to maintain improved appearance.

CALL YOUR DOCTOR IF

- Pain, swelling, redness, drainage or bleeding increases in the surgical area.
- You develop signs of infection: headache, muscle aches, dizziness or a general ill feeling and fever.
- You experience nausea, vomiting, constipation or abdominal swelling.

TYMPANOPLASTY

GENERAL INFORMATION

DEFINITION—Repair, removal or bypass of an obstruction or defect in the middle ear that prevents sound waves from reaching the inner ear. This is called conductive hearing loss, which can be total or partial. Usually, it is caused by chronic infection in the middle ear.

BODY PARTS INVOLVED—Eardrum (tympanic membrane); middle ear cavity; skin separating middle ear from inner ear; inner ear.

REASONS FOR SURGERY—Restoration of or improvement in hearing ability.

SURGICAL RISK INCREASES WITH
- Obesity.
- Smoking.
- Chronic illness.
- Use of drugs such as: antihypertensives; muscle relaxants; tranquilizers; sleep inducers; insulin; sedatives; beta-adrenergic blockers; or cortisone.
- Use of mind-altering drugs, including: narcotics; psychedelics; hallucinogens; marijuana; sedatives; hypnotics; or cocaine.

WHAT TO EXPECT

WHO OPERATES—Ear, nose and throat specialist.

WHERE PERFORMED—Hospital.

DIAGNOSTIC TESTS
- Before surgery: Blood and urine studies; hearing tests.
- After surgery: Blood studies; hearing tests.

ANESTHESIA—General anesthesia by inhalation and injection, with an airway tube placed in the windpipe.

DESCRIPTION OF OPERATION
- An instrument called an ear speculum is placed in the external ear canal, and the operating microscope is positioned.
- The middle ear is entered through an incision in the eardrum.
- Depending on the defect, one of the following methods is used:
  Repair of a defect in the eardrum.
  Closure of a defect in the eardrum with a skin graft.
  Fenestration, the creation of a new opening into a part of the inner ear. This method is used to treat otosclerosis.

POSSIBLE COMPLICATIONS
- Excessive bleeding.
- Surgical-wound infection.

AVERAGE HOSPITAL STAY—3 to 5 days.

PROBABLE OUTCOME—Expect complete healing without complications. Hearing should improve noticeably. Allow about 4 weeks for recovery from surgery.

POSTOPERATIVE CARE

NOTE—This information is supplemental and should not replace your doctor's instructions.

GENERAL MEASURES
- Keep the ear dry.
- Use warm compresses or heat lamps to relieve discomfort beginning 24 hours after surgery.

MEDICATION
- Your doctor may prescribe:
  Pain relievers. Don't take prescription pain medication longer than 4 to 7 days. Use *only* as much as you need.
  Antibiotics to fight infection.
- You may use non-prescription drugs, such as acetaminophen, for minor pain.

ACTIVITY
- Return to work and normal activity as soon as possible. This reduces postoperative depression, which is common.
- Avoid vigorous exercise for 4 weeks after surgery.
- Resume driving about 2 weeks after returning home.

DIET—Liquid diet the first day after surgery, then no special diet.

CALL YOUR DOCTOR IF

- Pain, swelling, redness, drainage or bleeding increases in the surgical area.
- You develop signs of infection: headache, muscle aches, dizziness or a general ill feeling and fever.

URETHRAL-CARUNCLE REMOVAL

GENERAL INFORMATION

DEFINITION—Removal of a urethral caruncle, a small benign tumor that develops at the opening of the female urethra.

BODY PARTS INVOLVED—Urethra; vagina (route for surgery).

REASONS FOR SURGERY—Treatment of excessive bleeding or discomfort.

SURGICAL RISK INCREASES WITH
- Adults over 60.
- Obesity.
- Smoking.
- Poor nutrition.
- Recent or chronic illness.
- Alcoholism.
- Use of drugs such as: antihypertensives; muscle relaxants; tranquilizers; sleep inducers; insulin; sedatives; beta-adrenergic blockers; or cortisone.
- Use of mind-altering drugs, including: narcotics; psychedelics; hallucinogens; marijuana; sedatives; hypnotics; or cocaine.

WHAT TO EXPECT

WHO OPERATES—Urologist or obstetrician-gynecologist.

WHERE PERFORMED—Hospital, outpatient surgical facility or doctor's office.

DIAGNOSTIC TESTS
- Before surgery: Pap smear; pelvic examination; blood and urine studies.
- After surgery: Pelvic examination.

ANESTHESIA—Local anesthesia by injection and topical application.

DESCRIPTION OF OPERATION
- The vagina is held open with a speculum. The caruncle is located, cleansed and anesthetized with local anesthesia.
- The caruncle is then removed with electrocauterization or a scalpel.
- Bleeding is controlled with pressure or electrocauterization.

POSSIBLE COMPLICATIONS
- Excessive bleeding.
- Surgical-wound infection.

AVERAGE HOSPITAL STAY—Usually none.

PROBABLE OUTCOME—Expect complete healing without complications. Allow about 2 weeks for recovery from surgery.

POSTOPERATIVE CARE

NOTE—This information is supplemental and should not replace your doctor's instructions.

GENERAL MEASURES
- Bathe and shower as usual. Wash the vaginal area gently with mild unscented soap and water after urination.
- Use an electric heating pad, a heat lamp or a warm compress in the genital area to relieve surgical-wound pain.

MEDICATION
- Your doctor may prescribe:
  Pain relievers. Don't take prescription pain medication longer than 4 to 7 days. Use *only* as much as you need.
  Antibiotics to fight infection.
- You may use non-prescription drugs, such as acetaminophen, for minor pain.

ACTIVITY
- Resume work and normal activity as soon as possible. This reduces postoperative depression and irritability, which are common.
- Avoid vigorous exercise for 2 weeks after surgery.
- Resume driving 3 days after returning home.
- Sexual relations may be resumed when your doctor determines that healing is complete.

DIET—No special diet.

CALL YOUR DOCTOR IF

- Pain, swelling, redness, drainage or bleeding increases in the surgical area.
- Urination is painful or difficult.
- You develop signs of infection: headache, muscle aches, dizziness or a general ill feeling and fever.
- New, unexplained symptoms develop. Drugs used in treatment may produce side effects.

VAGOTOMY

 GENERAL INFORMATION

DEFINITION—Disconnecting branches of the vagus nerve to slow acid production in the stomach. Usually, this surgery is performed before other surgeries such as gastroenterostomy.

BODY PARTS INVOLVED—Stomach; branches of the vagus nerve.

REASONS FOR SURGERY—Treatment of the complications of peptic ulcers such as: obstruction of digestive flow; ulcer perforation; bleeding of an ulcer; or intolerable pain.

SURGICAL RISK INCREASES WITH
- Obesity.
- Smoking.
- Stress.
- Poor nutrition.
- Recent or chronic illness.
- Use of drugs such as: antihypertensives; muscle relaxants; tranquilizers; sleeping pills; insulin; sedatives; beta-adrenergic blockers; or cortisone.
- Use of mind-altering drugs, including: narcotics; psychedelics; hallucinogens; marijuana; sedatives; hypnotics; or cocaine.

 WHAT TO EXPECT

WHO OPERATES—General surgeon.

WHERE PERFORMED—Hospital.

DIAGNOSTIC TESTS
- Before surgery: Blood and urine studies; X-rays of gastrointestinal tract; gastroscopy (see Glossary).
- After surgery: Blood studies.

ANESTHESIA—General anesthesia by inhalation and injection, with an airway tube placed in the windpipe.

DESCRIPTION OF OPERATION
- An incision is made in the abdomen, and the abdominal muscles are separated.
- The vagus nerve is identified, and the branches that control stomach-acid production are isolated, divided and clipped.
- The abdominal muscles are sewn together in layers. The skin is closed with sutures or clips, which usually can be removed about 7 to 10 days after surgery.

POSSIBLE COMPLICATIONS
- Excessive bleeding.
- Surgical-wound infection.
- Incisional hernia.
- Dumping syndrome.
- Diarrhea.

AVERAGE HOSPITAL STAY—7 days.

PROBABLE OUTCOME—Expect complete healing without complications. Allow about 6 weeks for recovery from surgery.

 POSTOPERATIVE CARE

NOTE—This information is supplemental and should not replace your doctor's instructions.

GENERAL MEASURES
- A hard ridge should form along the incision. As it heals, the ridge will recede gradually.
- Bathe and shower as usual. You may wash the incision gently with mild unscented soap.
- Use an electric heating pad, a heat lamp or a warm compress to relieve incisional pain.
- Move legs often while resting in bed to decrease the likelihood of deep-vein blood clots.

MEDICATION
- Your doctor may prescribe:
  Pain relievers. Don't take prescription pain medication longer than 4 to 7 days. Use only as much as you need.
  Stool softeners to prevent constipation.
  Antibiotics to fight infection.
- You may use non-prescription drugs, such as acetaminophen and antacids, for minor pain. Avoid aspirin and other non-steroidal anti-inflammatory drugs because they can irritate the lining of the stomach.

ACTIVITY
- Return to work and normal activity as soon as possible. This reduces postoperative depression and irritability, which are common.
- Avoid vigorous exercise for 6 weeks after surgery.
- Resume driving 2 weeks after returning home.

DIET—Clear liquid diet until the gastrointestinal tract functions again. Then eat a well-balanced, high-protein diet to promote healing. Avoid coffee, tea, cocoa, cola drinks, alcoholic beverages and any food or spice that aggravates ulcer symptoms.

 CALL YOUR DOCTOR IF

- Pain, swelling, redness, drainage or bleeding increases in the surgical area.
- You develop signs of infection: headache, muscle aches, dizziness or a general ill feeling and fever.
- You experience nausea, vomiting, constipation, diarrhea, black tarry stools or abdominal swelling.
- New, unexplained symptoms develop. Drugs used in treatment may produce side effects.

SURGERIES

VARICOCELE REMOVAL
(Varicocelectomy)

 GENERAL INFORMATION

DEFINITION—Removal of a varicocele, a swelling in the scrotum caused by veins that have dilated and filled with blood.

BODY PARTS INVOLVED—Scrotum and its contents; varicocele.

REASONS FOR SURGERY
- Relief of discomfort in the scrotum.
- Reduced congestion of the venous system around the testicles.
- Improved quality and quantity of sperm production (sometimes).

SURGICAL RISK INCREASES WITH—Risk factors are unknown.

 WHAT TO EXPECT

WHO OPERATES—General surgeon or urologist.

WHERE PERFORMED—Hospital or outpatient surgical facility.

DIAGNOSTIC TESTS
- Before surgery: Blood and urine studies.
- After surgery: Blood studies.

ANESTHESIA
- Local anesthesia by injection.
- Spinal anesthesia by injection.

DESCRIPTION OF OPERATION
- An incision is made in the scrotum.
- The spermatic cord is identified, and the blood vessels are cut.
- Abnormal veins are cut and tied. The tortuous, dilated vein or veins that form the varicocele are cut free and removed.
- The skin is closed with sutures that will be absorbed by the body.

POSSIBLE COMPLICATIONS
- Excessive bleeding.
- Surgical-wound infection.
- Inadvertent injury to the spermatic cord.

AVERAGE HOSPITAL STAY—0 to 1 day.

PROBABLE OUTCOME—Expect complete healing without complications. Allow about 1 week for recovery from surgery.

 POSTOPERATIVE CARE

NOTE—Follow your doctor's instructions. These instructions are supplemental.

GENERAL MEASURES
- A hard ridge should form along the incision. As it heals, the ridge will recede gradually.
- Apply ice packs to the surgical area to relieve discomfort immediately after surgery. Beginning 24 hours later use an electric heating pad, a heat lamp or a warm compress to relieve pain.
- Bathe and shower as usual. You may wash the incision gently with mild unscented soap.
- Wear an athletic supporter or two jockey shorts for support for 2 months after surgery.

MEDICATION
- Your doctor may prescribe pain relievers. Don't take prescription pain medication longer than 4 to 7 days. Use *only* as much as you need.
- You may use non-prescription drugs, such as acetaminophen, for minor pain.

ACTIVITY
- Return to work and normal activity as soon as possible. This reduces postoperative depression and irritability, which are common.
- Avoid vigorous exercise for 6 weeks after surgery.
- Resume driving 3 days after returning home.

DIET—Clear liquid diet until the gastrointestinal tract functions again. Then eat a well-balanced, high-protein diet to promote healing.

 CALL YOUR DOCTOR IF

Any of the following occurs:
- Excessive bleeding.
- Discomfort with urination.
- Nausea or vomiting.
- Increased pain, swelling, redness or drainage from the surgical area.
- Signs of infection: headache, muscle aches, dizziness or a general ill feeling and fever.

VARICOSE-VEIN REMOVAL

GENERAL INFORMATION

DEFINITION—Removal of varicose veins.

BODY PARTS INVOLVED—Diseased veins in the legs, usually in the greater and lesser saphenous veins, the largest veins in the lower body.

REASONS FOR SURGERY
- Improvement of blood circulation in the legs and feet.
- Relief of painful symptoms.

SURGICAL RISK INCREASES WITH
- Family history of varicose veins.
- Stress.
- Obesity.
- Smoking.
- Excess alcohol consumption.
- Adults over 60.
- Poor nutrition.

WHAT TO EXPECT

WHO OPERATES—General surgeon.

WHERE PERFORMED—Outpatient surgical facility or hospital.

DIAGNOSTIC TESTS
- Before surgery: Blood and urine studies.
- After surgery: Blood studies.

ANESTHESIA—General anesthesia by inhalation and injection, with an airway tube placed in the windpipe.

DESCRIPTION OF OPERATION
- An incision is made over the top of the saphenous-femoral vein system (see Glossary).
- The large, diseased veins are identified. The upper and lower ends of each diseased vein are cut and tied. An instrument is passed through the inside of the entire vein and tied to the bottom end. The entire vein is stripped out from bottom to top.
- After the main veins have been removed, smaller veins are identified, incisions are made and the smaller veins are tied individually and removed.
- The skin is closed with sutures, which usually can be removed about 1 week after surgery.
- The legs are wrapped snugly in elastic bandages.

POSSIBLE COMPLICATIONS
- Excessive bleeding.
- Surgical-wound infection.
- Inadvertent injury to nearby arteries or nerves.
- Deep-vein blood clots (rare).

AVERAGE HOSPITAL STAY—3 to 5 days.

PROBABLE OUTCOME—Expect complete healing without complications. Allow about 11 weeks for recovery from surgery.

POSTOPERATIVE CARE

NOTE—This information is supplemental and should not replace your doctor's instructions.

GENERAL MEASURES
- A hard ridge should form along the incision. As it heals, the ridge will recede gradually.
- Use an electric heating pad, a heat lamp or a warm compress to relieve incisional pain.
- Bathe and shower as usual. You may wash the incision gently with mild unscented soap.
- Keep your legs elevated whenever possible. Raise the foot of your bed, and use foot rests when sitting.
- Move legs often while resting in bed to decrease the likelihood of deep-vein blood clots.

MEDICATION
- Your doctor may prescribe:
  Pain relievers. Don't take prescription pain medication longer than 4 to 7 days. Use *only* as much as you need.
  Antibiotics to fight infection.
- You may use non-prescription drugs, such as acetaminophen, for minor pain.

ACTIVITY
- Return to work and normal activity as soon as possible. This reduces postoperative depression, which is common.
- Avoid vigorous exercise for 6 weeks after surgery.
- Resume driving 2-1/2 to 3 weeks after returning home.
- Resume sexual relations when able.

DIET—Clear liquid diet until the gastrointestinal tract functions again. Then eat a well-balanced, high-protein diet to promote healing.

CALL YOUR DOCTOR IF

- Pain, swelling, redness, drainage or bleeding increases in the surgical area.
- Your foot becomes cold, numb or discolored.
- You develop signs of infection: headache, muscle aches, dizziness or a general ill feeling and fever.

VASECTOMY

 GENERAL INFORMATION

DEFINITION—Cutting and tying the vas deferens (sperm channels inside the scrotum). The surgery stops the flow of sperm, and provides a safe, effective form of birth control without affecting sexual desire or ability.

BODY PARTS INVOLVED—Scrotum; vas deferens.

REASONS FOR SURGERY
- Voluntary sterilization.
- Recurrent epididymitis when caused by chronic prostate infection.

SURGICAL RISK INCREASES WITH
- Emotional instability.
- Recent illness, especially one with fever.

 WHAT TO EXPECT

WHO OPERATES—General surgeon, family doctor, urologist or plastic and reconstructive surgeon.

WHERE PERFORMED—Doctor's office, outpatient surgical facility or hospital.

DIAGNOSTIC TESTS
- Before surgery: Sperm studies.
- After surgery: Sperm studies, at least twice during 10 weeks after surgery.

ANESTHESIA—Local anesthesia by injection.

DESCRIPTION OF OPERATION
- The scrotum is shaved at home before surgery.
- Incisions are made on both sides of the scrotum. The vas deferens is identified, tied in two places and cut between the ties.
- The divided vas deferens is returned to the scrotum.
- The edges of incised skin are reconstructed with fine sutures, which usually fall out in about 7 days.

POSSIBLE COMPLICATIONS
- Collection of blood in scrotum.
- Excessive bleeding.
- Surgical-wound infection.
- Epididymitis .
- Sperm granuloma (benign lump in the surgical area).
- Small possibility of re-establishing fertility.

AVERAGE HOSPITAL STAY—Usually none.

PROBABLE OUTCOME—Expect sterility without complications. You may have up to 30 ejaculations before sperm completely disappears from semen. Allow 6 days for full recovery from surgery.

 POSTOPERATIVE CARE

NOTE—This information is supplemental and should not replace your doctor's instructions.

GENERAL MEASURES
- Return home immediately. Rest in bed to for 24 hours. Apply ice bags to both sides of the scrotum for 20 minutes out of each hour for the first 6 to 8 hours.
- Hard blunt ridges should form along the incisions. While healing, the ridges will recede gradually.
- Use an electric heating pad, a heat lamp or a warm compress to relieve incisional pain (beginning 24 hours after surgery).
- Bathe and shower as usual. You may wash the incisions gently with mild unscented soap.
- Wear scrotal support or two pairs of jockey shorts for 4 to 6 weeks after surgery.

MEDICATION
- Your doctor may prescribe:
  Pain relievers. Don't take prescription pain medication longer than 4 to 7 days. Use *only* as much as you need.
  Antibiotics to fight infection.
- You may use non-prescription drugs, such as acetaminophen, for minor pain.

ACTIVITY
- Return to work and normal activity as soon as possible (usually 24 hours after surgery).
- Resume sexual relations when able, as soon as 1 week after surgery. Use birth-control measures until laboratory studies confirm sterility.

DIET—No special diet.

 CALL YOUR DOCTOR IF

- Pain, swelling, redness, drainage or bleeding increases in the surgical area.
- You develop signs of infection: headache, muscle aches, dizziness or a general ill feeling and fever.

VENA-CAVA (INFERIOR) PLICATION

GENERAL INFORMATION

DEFINITION—Creation of a partial blockage in the vena cava, the body's largest vein.

BODY PARTS INVOLVED—Vena cava.

REASONS FOR SURGERY—Protection of the lungs from dangers caused by blood clots that have broken away from veins in the legs or pelvis.

SURGICAL RISK INCREASES WITH
- Adults over 60.
- Stress.
- Obesity.
- Smoking.
- Excess alcohol consumption.
- Poor nutrition.
- Illness, surgery or injury that has required prolonged bed rest.
- Use of drugs such as: antihypertensives; muscle relaxants; tranquilizers; sleep inducers; insulin; sedatives; beta-adrenergic blockers; or cortisone.
- Use of mind-altering drugs, including: narcotics; psychedelics; hallucinogens; marijuana; sedatives; hypnotics; or cocaine.

WHAT TO EXPECT

WHO OPERATES—General surgeon or vascular surgeon.

WHERE PERFORMED—Hospital.

DIAGNOSTIC TESTS
- Before surgery: Blood and urine studies; X-rays of upper and lower gastrointestinal tract; EKG (see Glossary).
- After surgery: Blood studies.

ANESTHESIA—General anesthesia by inhalation and injection, with an airway tube placed in the windpipe.

DESCRIPTION OF OPERATION
- A slanting incision is made from the top of the hip bone to just below the navel.
- The muscles of the flank are separated and the vena cava is located and exposed.
- The vena cava is permanently tied or clamped. Blood from the veins below the partial closure now reaches the heart through other blood channels where clots are less likely to cause harm.
- The vena cava is returned to its normal position. The muscles are joined with sutures. The skin is closed with sutures or clips, which usually can be removed about 1 week after surgery.

POSSIBLE COMPLICATIONS
- Excessive bleeding.
- Surgical-wound infection.
- Inadvertent injury to the ureter.

- Dislodged blood clot that passes on into the lungs.
- Adhesions.

AVERAGE HOSPITAL STAY—7 to 10 days.

PROBABLE OUTCOME—Expect complete healing without complications. Allow about 2 weeks for recovery from surgery.

POSTOPERATIVE CARE

NOTE—This information is supplemental and should not replace your doctor's instructions.

GENERAL MEASURES
- A hard ridge should form along the incision. As it heals, the ridge will recede gradually.
- Use an electric heating pad, a heat lamp or a warm compress to relieve incisional pain.
- Bathe and shower as usual. You may wash the incision gently with mild unscented soap.
- Move legs often while resting in to bed to decrease the likelihood of deep-vein blood clots.

MEDICATION
- Your doctor may prescribe:
  Pain relievers. Don't take prescription pain medication longer than 4 to 7 days. Use *only* as much as you need.
  Anticoagulants to prevent blood-clot formation.
  Stool softeners to prevent constipation.
  Antibiotics to fight infection.
- You may use non-prescription drugs, such as acetaminophen, for minor pain.

ACTIVITY
- Resume work and normal activity as soon as possible to reduce postoperative depression, which is common.
- Resume driving about 4 weeks after returning home.
- Resume sexual relations when your doctor determines that healing is complete.

DIET—Clear liquid diet until the gastrointestinal tract begins to function again. Then eat a well-balanced, high-protein diet to promote healing.

CALL YOUR DOCTOR IF

- Pain, swelling, redness, drainage or bleeding increases in the surgical area.
- You develop signs of infection: headache, muscle aches, dizziness or a general ill feeling and fever.
- You experience nausea, vomiting, constipation or abdominal swelling.
- New, unexplained symptoms develop. Drugs used in treatment may produce side effects.

SURGERIES

VESICO-VAGINAL-FISTULA REPAIR

GENERAL INFORMATION

DEFINITION—Repair of a vesico-vaginal fistula, an abnormal tract between the bladder and the vagina that usually results from tearing in childbirth.

BODY PARTS INVOLVED—Vagina and bladder.

REASONS FOR SURGERY
- Control of urine flow from the bladder.
- Prevention of vaginal and urinary-tract infections.

SURGICAL RISK INCREASES WITH
- Adults over 60.
- Obesity.
- Smoking.
- Stress.
- Poor nutrition.
- Recent or chronic illness.
- Alcoholism.
- Previous pelvic surgery.
- Use of drugs such as: antihypertensives; muscle relaxants; tranquilizers; sleep inducers; insulin; sedatives; beta-adrenergic blockers; or cortisone.
- Use of mind-altering drugs, including: narcotics; psychedelics; hallucinogens; marijuana; sedatives; hypnotics; or cocaine.

WHAT TO EXPECT

WHO OPERATES—Obstetrician-gynecologist, urologist or general surgeon.

WHERE PERFORMED—Hospital.

DIAGNOSTIC TESTS
- Before surgery: Blood and urine studies.
- After surgery: Blood studies; laboratory examination of removed tissue.

ANESTHESIA
- Spinal anesthesia by injection.
- General anesthesia by inhalation and injection, with an airway tube placed in the windpipe.

DESCRIPTION OF OPERATION
- A speculum is used to hold the vagina open.
- Scar tissue around the fistula is cut free and removed.
- The bladder wall and vaginal wall are closed with sutures that will be absorbed by the body.
- The bladder is filled with sterile water to search for leaks. If leaks exist, further repairs are made. If no leaks are found, a catheter is placed in the bladder.
- The catheter usually can be removed about 5 to 7 days after surgery.

POSSIBLE COMPLICATIONS
- Excessive bleeding.
- Surgical-wound infection.
- Urinary-tract infection.
- Continued urine leakage through fistula.

AVERAGE HOSPITAL STAY—6 days.

PROBABLE OUTCOME—Expect complete healing without complications. Allow about 6 weeks for recovery from surgery.

POSTOPERATIVE CARE

NOTE—This information is supplemental and should not replace your doctor's instructions.

GENERAL MEASURES
- Use an electric heating pad, a heat lamp or a warm compress to relieve surgical-wound pain.
- Take warm baths several times a day to relieve discomfort.
- Move legs often while resting in bed to decrease the likelihood of deep-vein blood clots.

MEDICATION
- Your doctor may prescribe:
  Pain relievers. Don't take prescription pain medication longer than 4 to 7 days. Use *only* as much as you need.
  Stool softeners to prevent constipation.
  Antibiotics to fight infection.
- You may use non-prescription drugs, such as acetaminophen, for minor pain.

ACTIVITY
- Resume work and normal activity as soon as possible. This reduces postoperative depression and irritability, which are common.
- Avoid vigorous exercise for 6 weeks after surgery.
- Resume driving 3 weeks after returning home.
- Resume sexual relations when your doctor determines that healing is complete.

DIET—Your doctor will prescribe a diet.

CALL YOUR DOCTOR IF

- Pain, swelling, redness, drainage or bleeding increases in the surgical area.
- You develop signs of infection: headache, muscle aches, dizziness or a general ill feeling and fever.
- You experience nausea, vomiting or constipation.
- You develop urinary frequency and stinging or burning on urination.
- New, unexplained symptoms develop. Drugs used in treatment may produce side effects.

VITRECTOMY

GENERAL INFORMATION

DEFINITION—Removal of fluid from the eyeball that has clouded and blocked light from reaching the retina, causing loss of vision. A chemical solution is injected to replace the removed fluid.

BODY PARTS INVOLVED—Eye and all its parts.

REASONS FOR SURGERY—Restoration of normal vision or prevention of continued vision loss resulting from disease that blocks light from reaching the retina. These include: bleeding, injury or infection inside the eyeball; diabetes mellitus; sickle-cell disease; complications of cataract surgery; or glaucoma.

SURGICAL RISK INCREASES WITH
- Adults over 60.
- Obesity.
- Smoking.
- Stress.
- Poor nutrition.
- Recent or chronic illness.
- Alcoholism.
- Use of drugs such as: antihypertensives; muscle relaxants; tranquilizers; sleep inducers; insulin; sedatives; beta-adrenergic blockers; or cortisone.
- Use of mind-altering drugs, including: narcotics; psychedelics; hallucinogens; marijuana; sedatives; hypnotics; or cocaine.

WHAT TO EXPECT

WHO OPERATES—Ophthalmologist.

WHERE PERFORMED—Hospital.

DIAGNOSTIC TESTS
- Before surgery: Eye examination; blood and urine studies.
- After surgery: Eye examination.

ANESTHESIA
- Local anesthesia by injection.
- General anesthesia by inhalation and injection, with an airway tube placed in the windpipe.

DESCRIPTION OF OPERATION
- A small instrument is inserted behind the cornea. The instrument is used to cut free and remove the clouded vitreous fluid and scar tissue.
- This surgery often causes a retinal detachment. Usually, this is corrected by injecting gas into the vitreous cavity.
- A chemical solution that promotes healing and stimulates normal vitreous fluid production is injected.
- If sutures are needed to close the surgical wound, they will be absorbed by the body.

POSSIBLE COMPLICATIONS
- Surgical-wound infection in the eye.
- Recurrent retinal detachment.

AVERAGE HOSPITAL STAY—1 to 4 days.

PROBABLE OUTCOME—Expect complete healing without complications. Allow about 6 weeks for recovery from surgery. Vision will greatly improve by then.

POSTOPERATIVE CARE

NOTE—This information is supplemental and should not replace your doctor's instructions.

GENERAL MEASURES
- Move legs often while resting in bed to decrease the likelihood of deep-vein blood clots.
- Use warm compresses over the eyes to relieve discomfort.
- Don't lift heavy objects, bend over or strain with bowel movements until your doctor determines that healing is complete.

MEDICATION—Your doctor may prescribe:
- Pain relievers. Don't take prescription pain medication longer than 4 to 7 days. Use *only* as much as you need.
- Stool softeners to prevent constipation.
- Antibiotic eye drops to fight infection.

ACTIVITY
- Resume work and normal activity as soon as possible. This reduces postoperative depression and irritability, which are common.
- Avoid vigorous exercise for 6 weeks after surgery.

DIET—Clear liquid diet until the gastrointestinal tract functions again. Then eat a well-balanced, high-protein diet to promote healing.

CALL YOUR DOCTOR IF

- Pain, swelling, redness, drainage or bleeding increases in the surgical area.
- You develop signs of infection: headache, muscle aches, dizziness or a general ill feeling and fever.
- You experience nausea, vomiting or constipation.
- New, unexplained symptoms develop. Drugs used in treatment may produce side effects.

APPENDIX 1

Well-Balanced Diet

The well-balanced diet is for all patients whose condition does not require dietary treatment. There are no restrictions in types of foods that may be consumed as part of this diet.

This diet provides the Recommended Dietary Allowances (RDA) established by the Food and Nutrition Board of the National Research Council, if foods are eaten daily from the Basic Four Food Groups.

BASIC FOUR FOOD GROUPS

1. **Milk and Milk Products Group**—Skim or low-fat milk, cheese, yogurt, ice cream. 2 or more cups a day.

2. **Meat Group**—Lean meats, poultry, fish, eggs, beans. 2 or more servings a day.

3. **Vegetable and Fruit Group**—4 or more servings a day.

4. **Bread and Cereals Group**—Unrefined, unsweetened, whole-grain cereals and breads. 4 or more servings a day.

Most dietetic experts recommend a regular diet with increased fiber (roughage) to promote normal bowel function. Increased roughage also protects against diverticulosis, some forms of intestinal cancer and perhaps even atherosclerosis—thus protecting against heart attack and stroke.

Daily fat intake should not exceed 30% of total calories in the regular diet. A low-fat diet (see Appendix 8) will help control obesity and decrease the likelihood of atherosclerosis.

For optimal health, reduce intake of refined sugars, such as those in candy, in the regular diet. Eat unrefined sugars such as those found in fresh fruits, vegetables, potatoes and whole-grain breads and cereals.

Reduce salt intake (except during pregnancy) to 3 to 4 grams (usually in the form of table salt) a day. See Appendix 9 for suggestions.

A healthy, well-balanced diet should include minimum salt; reduced fat; lots of complex carbohydrates and fiber; more fish, seafood and poultry; less red meat; and less fatty, salty, prepared meats and snacks.

APPENDIX 2

Diet Suggestions for Persons Over 50

A well-balanced diet is just as essential for this age group as it is for all age groups. Since metabolism is decreased in persons over 50, you probably will not require as many calories per day as younger people. Eat every 5 hours or so. Do not let more than 14 hours pass between an evening meal and breakfast.

The recommended daily caloric intake for persons of normal weight, capable of normal activity, who are 51 or over, is 2,400 calories for men, and 1,800 calories for women.

SAMPLE GENERAL DIET

Suggested Meal Plan	Sample Menu
BREAKFAST	
Citrus fruit or juice	Orange juice
Cereal	Oatmeal
Meat or meat substitute	Soft-cooked eggs
Bread, butter or margarine	Toast, butter or margarine, jelly
Milk	Milk
Beverage	Decaffeinated coffee or tea
LUNCH (CAN BE NOON OR EVENING MEAL)	
Meat or meat substitute	Baked meat loaf with gravy
Potato or potato substitute	Whipped potatoes
Vegetable and/or	Buttered green beans
salad	Tossed green salad with oil and vinegar dressing
Dessert	Lemon sponge cake
Bread, butter or margarine	Bread with butter or margarine
Beverage	Decaffeinated coffee or tea
DINNER (CAN BE EVENING OR NOON MEAL)	
Soup or juice	Consomme
Meat or meat substitute	Creamed chicken on toast
Vegetable and/or	Buttered peas
salad	Sliced tomato on lettuce with mayonnaise
Dessert	Baked apple with cinnamon
Bread, butter or margarine	Bread with butter or margarine
Milk	Milk
Beverage	Decaffeinated coffee or tea

(Adapted from The Arizona Diet Manual, by the Diet Therapy Section of The Arizona Dietetic Association, Inc.)

APPENDIX 3

Pregnancy and Breast-Feeding Diet

General guidelines:
- Increase your normal caloric intake about 10% above what you should normally consume if you were not pregnant.
- Except under unusual circumstances, don't try to *lose* weight during pregnancy. The average weight gain in an uncomplicated pregnancy is 22 to 27 pounds.
- Make sure your diet contains adequate protein during pregnancy and during breast-feeding. Protein is the "building block" of body tissue.
- Iron, vitamins, minerals and calcium supplements are helpful to maintain proper nutrition. Follow your doctor's recommendations. Remember that calcium tablets are not a substitute for milk.
- Use iodized salt.
- Caffeine should be avoided during pregnancy. Either eliminate coffee, cola, cocoa, tea and other caffeine-containing substances from your diet, or reduce the amount you consume drastically.

DAILY DIET FOR PREGNANCY AND BREAST-FEEDING

Foods	During First Half of Pregnancy	During Second Half of Pregnancy	During Breast-Feeding
MILK GROUP Pasteurized milk includes: whole, skim, evaporated, reliquified dry or buttermilk. (1-1/2 ounces cheddar cheese may be substituted for each cup of milk.)	2 cups (to drink or use in cooking)	4 to 6 cups (to drink or use in cooking)	4 to 6 cups (to drink or use in cooking)

The diet as directed during pregnancy and breast-feeding supplies adequate nutrients as recommended by the National Research Council, with the possible exception of vitamin D. The daily need of 400 International Units of vitamin D may be met by consuming 1 quart of vitamin-D milk or a prescribed supplement.

Foods	During First Half of Pregnancy	During Second Half of Pregnancy	During Breast-Feeding
MEAT GROUP Lean cooked meat, fish, poultry (include liver frequently.)	1 serving (2 to 3 ounces)	1 to 2 servings (5 ounces)	1 to 2 servings (5 ounces)
Meat alternate: 1 serving of any variety cheese; mature shelled beans or peas (dried or fresh); nuts; or peanut butter. Egg	1	1	1

APPENDIX 3 (continued)

**VEGETABLE AND
FRUIT GROUP**

Vitamin A—Dark green vegetables and fruits	1 serving	1 serving	1 to 2 servings
Other vegetables or fruits	1 serving	2 servings	2 servings
Vitamin-C-rich foods:			
Good Sources—citrus fruit or juice (fresh, frozen or canned); cantaloupe; strawberries; broccoli; green pepper; sweet red pepper.	1 good source or 2 fair sources	1 good source and 2 fair sources or 2 good sources	1 good source and 2 fair sources or 2 good sources

Fair Sources—honeydew melon; tangerines; watermelon; asparagus; Brussels sprouts; raw cabbage; greens; potatoes and sweet potatoes cooked in their skins; spinach; strawberries; tomatoes or tomato juice; watercress.

**BREAD AND
CEREALS GROUP**

Whole-grain or enriched cereal	1 serving	1 serving	1 serving
Whole-grain or enriched bread	2 to 3 slices	2 to 3 slices	3 slices

**BUTTER OR
FORTIFIED MARGARINE**

	As caloric intake permits	As caloric intake permits	As caloric intake permits.

(Adapted from The Arizona Diet Manual, by the Diet Therapy Section of The Arizona Dietetic Association, Inc.)

Milk-Restricted Diet

This diet is used for treatment of lactose intolerance and milk allergy.

Lactose Intolerance—Lactose intolerance is caused by a deficiency of the enzyme lactase, which breaks down lactose, the form of sugar found in milk. This intolerance is commonly found in several ethnic groups, including blacks, American Indians, Mexican-Americans and Orientals.

For infants, the substitution of formulas that do not contain lactose, such as soybean formula, will relieve symptoms of lactose intolerance.

Some adults with lactase-enzyme deficiency can tolerate small amounts of milk products, especially when they are consumed with a meal or other foods. This contributes valuable calcium to the diet. The diet should be individualized, depending on what the person can tolerate.

Pregnant women and children should take a calcium supplement, if they consume only small amounts of milk products.

Milk Allergy—A milk allergy is a reaction caused by hypersensitivity to the protein found in milk. This allergy may occur more frequently in infants than in adults, and can frequently cause an allergic reaction.

Milk allergy is treated with a diet using soybean or meat-based formulas that contain no milk. Commercially available soybean formulas vary considerably in mineral content, and deficiencies of both vitamin A and thiamine have been reported in infants consuming these formulas. Ask your doctor about vitamin supplements.

Some people who are allergic to milk in one form may be able to use milk that has been boiled, evaporated or dried, because these processes change the protein. Milk is an important source of calcium, protein, vitamins A and D and riboflavin. Foods rich in these nutrients should be selected when milk has been excluded from the diet. When milk products are excluded from the diet, high-calcium foods from the list below should be substituted.

More than 1,000 mg. per serving size
3/4 cup dry barley, oatmeal or rice cereal

More than 100 mg. per serving size

1/2 cup collard greens
3/4 cup kale
1/2 cup mustard greens
12 oysters
3-1/2 oz. salmon (if bones are eaten)

12 shrimp
1 cup cooked instant creamed wheat
  (no milk added)
1/2 cup cooked barley cereal (no
  milk added)

More than 50 mg. per serving size
1/2 cup broccoli
1 cup Brussels sprouts

(Adapted from The Arizona Diet Manual, by the Diet Therapy Section of The Arizona Dietetic Association, Inc.)

Gluten-Restricted Diet

This diet is used to eliminate the consumption of gluten (a protein substance found in grain), usually because of gastrointestinal disease.

FOODS	ALLOWED	OMITTED
Beverage	Coffee; tea; decaffeinated coffee; pure instant coffee*; carbonated beverages; artificially flavored fruit drinks.	Cereal beverages; coffee beverages containing cereal grains; root beer+.
Meat	Pure meat, fish, poultry and eggs; guaranteed pure-meat cold cuts,* frankfurters* and sausage*; aged cheese; cottage cheese, cream cheese; peanut butter; soybeans; peanuts.	Commercially prepared meat and egg products;+ breaded meats, meatloaf and meat patties; processed cheese+; cheese foods+ and dips+; products that contain texturized or hydrolized vegetable protein.
Fat	Butter; margarine; cream; vegetable oil; shortening; nuts; olives; mayonnaise; gravies and sauces made with allowed thickening agents (below).	Non-dairy cream substitutes+; commercially prepared salad dressings, gravies and sauces.
Milk	Milk; yogurt.	Commercial chocolate milk; malted milk; instant milk drinks+; hot cocoa mixes+.
Starch	Specially prepared bread and other baked products made with the following flours: corn, rice, potato, soybean, wheat starch.	Any homemade or commercially prepared baked goods or mixes containing wheat (except wheat starch), oats, rye, graham, barley, buckwheat pancakes+, bran, or wheat germ; commercially prepared corn muffins+; gluten bread.
	Corn and rice cereals++.	Cereals containing wheat, oats, rye, barley, bran, wheat germ, graham, bulgur, or millet.
	Potatoes; rice; hominy grits; low-protein wheat-starch pastas.	Commercial rice mixes; pasta, noodles, spaghetti, and macaroni products.
	Snack foods, chips, and wafers made only of rice, corn, or potatoes; corn tortillas; popcorn.	Crackers, chips+, and other snack foods+.
	Thickening agents: corn flour, corn starch, cornmeal, potato flour, potato starch, wheat starch, soybean starch, arrowroot starch, tapioca, gelatin.	All others.
Vegetable	All except those in omitted column.	Any commercially prepared with cheese sauce+ or cream sauce; canned baked beans.
Fruit	All except those in omitted column.	Commercially prepared pie fillings+; thickened fruit+.

FOODS	ALLOWED	OMITTED
Soup	Homemade broth, vegetable, or cream soups thickened with allowed flours or starches.	Commercially prepared soup+; soup mixes+; bouillon+; and broth+; any containing barley, pasta, or noodles.
Dessert	Gelatin; meringues; custard; corn-starch, rice, and tapioca puddings; specially prepared desserts made of allowed flours and cereal-free baking powder; junket.	Commercially prepared desserts and mixes: cookies, cakes, pie, piecrust, pastries, pudding; ice cream+; sherbet+; ice cream cones.
Sweets	Sugar; honey; jelly; jam; molasses; corn syrup; pure maple syrup; pure baking chocolate; pure cocoa; coconut.	Flavored syrups+; chocolate and other commercial candies+.
Miscellaneous	Salt; pepper; other spices and herbs; dry yeast; food coloring and extracts.	Prepared catsup+, mustard+, and horseradish+; bottled meat sauces+; soy sauce+; pickles+; seasoning mixes+; cake yeast+; chewing gum+; baking powder+.
	Wine; rum; brandy; vermouth; cognac.	Beer; ale; alcoholic beverages distilled from cereal grains.

Read product labels carefully and avoid sources of gluten: wheat, oats, rye, barley, bran, wheat germ, bulgur, millet, graham, durham, and malt. Possible sources of gluten in processed foods include stabilizers, emulsifiers, cereal additives, and vegetable protein. If there is any doubt, the product should be avoided until absence of gluten is verified by the manufacturer or by a brand name list prepared by the research unit of a hospital or university.

*Check label carefully to be sure gluten is not an ingredient.
+Avoid unless absence of gluten is verified by the manufacturer or by a special brand name products lists.
++Ready-to-eat corn and rice cereals may contain a small amount of malt as flavoring, but the amount usually is well tolerated.

(Adapted from Mayo Clinic Diet Manual, Fifth Edition, Philadephia, W. B. Saunders Company, 1981.)

APPENDIX 6

Allergy Diet

Many people suffer allergic reactions after eating certain foods. This diet is used to prevent or reduce those reactions by eliminating the offending foods.

FOODS	ALLOWED	OMITTED
Highly Seasoned Foods		Highly seasoned foods.
Beverages	Tea; carbonated beverages; cereal beverages.	Coffee; cola beverages; chocolate-flavored beverages.
Meats	Any except those in omitted column; cottage cheese.	Highly seasoned meats (such as cold cuts); fresh pork; fish; shellfish; eggs*; other cheeses; peanut butter; corned beef; cheese spreads.
Fats	Any except those in omitted column.	Cream cheese; nuts; salad dressings made with eggs or cheese.
Milk	Milk; milk drinks.	Chocolate milk; eggnog; hot cocoa.
Bread	Any except those in omitted column.	Commercially prepared mixes; any bread made with eggs or nuts; cornbread.
Vegetables	Any except those in omitted column.	Tomatoes; tomato products (puree, sauce, catsup, etc.).
Fruits	Any except those in omitted column.	Fresh or frozen: apples; cherries; berries+. Fresh, frozen, dried or cooked: bananas; grapes; mangoes; papayas; pineapple; rhubarb; raisins.
Soups	Any except those in omitted column.	Any made with corn, tomatoes or shellfish.
Desserts	Any except those in omitted column.	Any made with chocolate, cocoa, eggs, nuts or omitted fruits; commercially prepared mixes.
Sweets	Any except those in omitted column.	Jelly, jam or marmalade made with omitted fruits; candy with chocolate, eggs, nuts or omitted fruits.
Miscellaneous	Salt, spices, herbs except those omitted; vinegar; pickles; gravy; white sauce.	Garlic; strong spices; chocolate; cocoa.

*Eggs in all forms should be avoided when the diet is used for children. Adults, however, may have small amounts of cooked eggs, such as those found in most desserts. The allergic protein in eggs is denatured by cooking.
+Cooking denatures some allergens. Therefore, *cooked* apples, cherries and berries may be consumed. Other fruits may be extremely allergenic in some patients, and cooking does not denature the allergens.

(Adapted from The Mayo Clinic Diet Manual, Fourth and Fifth Editions. Philadelphia, W. B. Saunders Company, 1981.)

APPENDIX 7

Liquid Diet

This diet is for patients who cannot chew or swallow solid foods. It is a modified form of the normal diet with changes in consistency or texture. The diet as outlined will satisfy the daily nutrient needs (except for iron and thiamine) recommended by the National Research Council, which is part of the National Academy of Sciences.

Food Groups	Foods Allowed

MILK GROUP
4 or more 8-ounce
cups milk
	Milk: whole; skim; buttermilk.
	Milk drinks such as eggnog, milkshakes and malted milk.
	
	Substitutes for 1 cup milk:
	  3 to 4 tablespoons dry milk.
	  4 ounces evaporated milk.
	  1 pint ice cream without fruit or nuts.
	  Milk may be used in other foods, such
	  as puddings, custards and strained cream soups.

MEAT GROUP
2 or more servings
or substitute
	Finely strained meats (about 2 tbsp. per serving) added to strained soups or broths.
	
	Substitute for 1 serving of meat:
	  2 eggs (in eggnog or soft custard).
	  Commercially prepared strained meats and egg yolks.

VEGETABLE-FRUIT GROUP 4 or more servings	**Sources of Vitamin C (1 Daily):** Strained grapefruit, orange, tangerine, or tomato juices. **Sources of Vitamin A (1 Every Other Day):** Strained apricots; carrots; spinach; or winter squash. **Other Fruits and Vegetables:** All other strained fruits and fruit juices. Other mild-flavored strained vegetables (fresh or canned) added to strained soups.
BREAD-CEREAL GROUP 4 or more servings	Strained cooked cereals. Cereal may be thinned with extra milk.
FATS	Cream; butter; margarine; oils.
SWEETS AND DESSERTS	Sugar; honey; molasses; corn syrup; ice cream; sherbet, ices; fruit whips or gelatin without nuts, seeds and whole fruits; soft-custard or rennet desserts.
SOUPS AND SAUCES	Strained soups.
BEVERAGES	Any beverages such as coffee, tea, cocoa, carbonated drinks.
MISCELLANEOUS	Salt and seasonings as tolerated.

(Adapted from The Arizona Diet Manual, by the Diet Therapy Section of The Arizona Dietetic Association, Inc.)

Low-Fat Diet

Most diet experts agree that Americans eat too much fat. A low-fat diet can help prevent obesity and the dangers it causes to health. Use the diet suggestions below for general good health or for dietary treatment of your condition as recommended by your doctor.

FOODS	ALLOWED	OMITTED
Beverages	Coffee, tea, carbonated beverages.	No restrictions.
Breads and Cereals	4 servings or more a day of whole-grain or enriched cereals; white, whole wheat, rye or French bread; plain rolls; saltines; graham crackers; wheat crackers; corn or flour tortillas.	Biscuits, cornbread, pancakes and waffles, unless made with allowed vegetable oils, egg white and skim milk or buttermilk; doughnuts; commercial coffee cakes; cheese crackers; pretzels; rusks.
Desserts	Angel food cake; cakes and cookies made with skim milk, oil and egg whites; fruit (preferred); fruit pie and cobblers (of pastry made with allowed oils); fruit whips; fruit meringues; gelatin desserts; puddings and custards made with skim milk; sherbet; fruit ices.	Desserts containing butter or margarine, chocolate, cream, egg yolk (unless from day's allowance), shortening or whole milk (such as ice cream and regular puddings); commercial cakes, cookies and pastries.
Eggs	Egg whites as desired, but limit egg yolks to not more than 3 per week, including those used in cooking; low-cholesterol egg substitute.	
Fats (Use sparingly)	Corn oil; cottonseed oil; safflower oil; soybean oil; non-hydrogenated vegetable-oil margarine; sunflower seed oil; commercial mayonnaise and salad dressings; peanut oil; olive oil.	All visible fat on meats; butter; chocolate; coconut oil; cream; lard; hydrogenated (hardened) fats; margarine (except non-hydrogenated vegetable oil); bacon drippings.
Fruits	2 servings or more a day.	Avocado.
Meats and Meat Substitutes	5 ounces daily total of lean meat, fish or poultry (trim all visible fat from meat before cooking); low-fat cottage cheese; sapsago cheese; mozzarella cheese; specially prepared low-cholesterol cheeses; mature shelled beans and peas; peanut butter (for second entree when possible); barbecue (using only sauce without fat), broil, boil or roast on a rack so that fat will drip out; nuts (particularly peanuts and walnuts if caloric allowance permits); tripe; beef or veal liver once a month.	Liver; duck; goose; bacon; salt pork; sausage; lunch meat; frankfurters; brisket; shortribs; club, porterhouse and T-bone steaks; prime rib roasts; cheese (except those allowed); any fish prepared with fats other than allowed oils; cashew nuts.

APPENDIX 8 (continued)

FOODS	ALLOWED	OMITTED
Milk	1-1/2 pints a day of skim milk or buttermilk; cocoa prepared with skim milk.	Whole milk; evaporated milk; Bulgarian buttermilk; beverages containing chocolate (note: cocoa is allowed); ice cream; ice milk; eggs; cream.
Miscellaneous	Herbs; catsup; mustard; pickles; spices; gravies made from pan drippings skimmed free of fat (let stand in refrigerator until fat forms); popcorn cooked in oil or non-hydrogenated vegetable-oil margarine; olives (use sparingly).	Coconut; buttered popcorn.
Potato or Substitute	White or sweet potato; brown or restored rice; corn; hominy; enriched grits; macaroni or noodles; dried beans and peas.	Fried potatoes and potato chips (unless cooked in oil).
Soups	Meat and chicken soups (soups should be cooled and fat removed from the top before reheating and serving); fat-free broth and bouillon; soups made with skim milk and allowed vegetable-oil margarine.	Any soup made with butter, ordinary margarine or whole milk; most canned soups.
Sweets	Gumdrops; hard candy; homemade candies made without cream, whole milk, chocolate, or butter; honey; jam; jelly; jelly beans; marshmallows; mints made with allowed ingredients; molasses; syrup; sugar.	Candies containing fats such as butter, chocolate, cocoa butter, coconut or cream.
Vegetables	2 servings or more of any vegetable. Do not cook vegetables with meat; season with non-hydrogenated vegetable-oil margarine.	Any vegetables prepared with butter, ordinary margarine, cream, salt pork or bacon grease.

(Adapted from The Arizona Diet Manual, by the Diet Therapy Section of The Arizona Dietetic Association, Inc.)

APPENDIX 9

Low-Salt Diet

This is a normal diet, restricted only in certain foods that have excessive salt or sodium. Avoid canned and prepared frozen foods. Read all labels carefully.

FOODS	ALLOWED	OMITTED
Beverages	All tea, coffee, milk.	No restrictions.
Bread and Cereals	Regular bread and cereals.	Crackers with salted tops; pretzels; salted popcorn.
Desserts	All, in moderation.	No restrictions.
Fats	All except those in omitted column.	Bacon and bacon fat; salt pork; olives; prepared meats.
Fruits	All.	No restrictions.
Meat and Meat Substitutes	Meat; fish; poultry; eggs; cottage cheese; dried beans and peas; all cheeses except those omitted; cured meats and fish may be consumed once a week.	Any meat, fish or poultry that is smoked, brine-cured or salted, including: bacon; bologna; chipped beef; corned beef; frankfurters; luncheon meats; ham; kosher meats; salt pork; sausages; salted or smoked fish such as herring, sardines, anchovies or salted codfish; processed cheese; cheese spreads; or cheese such as Roquefort or Camembert.
Potatoes and Substitutes	All except potato chips.	Potato chips.
Seasonings and Flavorings	A small amount of salt or other seasoning may be used in cooking.	Salt at the table; catsup; pickles; relishes; soy sauce.
Soups	Cream soups; canned soups.	Bouillon cubes, prepared soup bases and canned soups containing smoked or salty meats.
Vegetables	All except those in omitted column.	Sauerkraut and other vegetables prepared in brine.

(Adapted from The Arizona Diet Manual, by the Diet Therapy Section of The Arizona Dietetic Association, Inc.)

Weight-Reduction Diet

This is a simple "exchange list" diet for individuals who want to lose weight. The diet provides 1,000 to 1,200 calories per day. If meals are chosen from a variety of foods, this diet will meet the adult Recommended Dietary Allowances (RDA). A diet of less than 1,000 calories per day may not meet requirements for vitamins and minerals.

Plan your meals by selecting items from the Breakfast, Lunch and Dinner columns (Portions from Food Lists). For example, breakfast allows you two different fruit portions (or two portions of the same fruit). Select two portions from the Fruit List. You may also have one portion from the Starch List for breakfast, and so on. Amounts of each portion are indicated in each food list.

Portions can be interchanged among breakfast, lunch and dinner as long as the total for the day doesn't exceed those indicated. For example, you can eat all your fruits for breakfast if desired, but don't exceed 4 portions for the day.

Before starting any diet, ask your doctor for specific recommendations.

PORTIONS FROM FOOD LISTS
(See lists below)

BREAKFAST	LUNCH	DINNER
2 Fruits	2 Meats	3 Meats
1 Starch	1 Vegetable	1 Fat
1/2 Milk	1 Fat	1 Bread
1 Fat	2 Breads	2 Vegetables
	1/2 Milk	1 Fruit
	1 Fruit	

FREE ITEMS: You may have these as desired.

Beverages: coffee, tea, sugar-free beverages.
Pickles, except sweet pickles.
Boullion and consommes.
All spices, herbs, flavorings and artificial sweeteners.
Catsup, mustard, soy sauce, vinegars and Worcestershire sauce.

FRUIT LIST: A portion is 1 small piece or 1/2 cup unless listed.

Apples: Juice or Sauce	Fruit Cocktail	Plums (2)
Apricots (2)	Grapefruit or Juice	Prunes (2)
Apricots, dried (2)	Grapes (12)	Prune Juice (1/4 cup)
Banana	Grape Juice	Raspberries
Blackberries	Lemon	Raisins (2 Tbsp.)
Blueberries	Orange or	Rhubarb
Cantaloupe	Orange Juice	Strawberries (10)
Cherries	Peach	Tangerine
Dates (2)	Pear	Watermelon (1 cup)
	Pineapple	

VEGETABLE LIST: A portion is 1 cup raw or 1/2 cup cooked.

Artichoke	Celery	Parsley
Asparagus	Cucumber	Peppers
Beans, sprouts, green or wax	Eggplant	Peas
Beets	Endive	Pumpkin
Broccoli	Greens	Radish
Brussels Sprouts	Lettuce	Rutabaga
Cabbage or Sauerkraut	Mixed Vegetables	Spinach
Cauliflower	Mushrooms	Squash
Carrot	Okra	Tomato
	Onions	Turnips

Some vegetables are shown in the Starch List.

APPENDIX 10 (continued)

STARCH LIST

Angel Food Cake (1 oz.)
Bagel (1/2)
Beans, canned (1/2 cup)
Biscuit (1)
Bread (1 slice)
Bun (1/2)
Cereal (1/2 cup)
Corn (1/3 cup)
Cookies (1 or 2 small)
Cornbread (1 in. cube)
Cornstarch (2 Tbsp.)
English Muffin (1/2)
Flour (2-1/2 Tbsp.)
Graham Crackers (2)
Jello (1/2 cup)
Pancakes (1)
Pastas (1/2 cup)
Popcorn, fat free (3 cups)
Potato, white (1/2 cup)
Potato, sweet (1/3 cup)
Pretzels (5 small)
Rice (1/2 cup)
Saltines (5)
Taco Shell (1)
Tortilla (one 6-inch)

MEAT OR MEAT SUBSTITUTE
(A portion is 1 ounce or 1/4 cup or as listed.)

Beef (lean cuts)
Eggs (3 per week)
Cheese (skim milk types)
Cold Cuts or Frankfurters
Cottage Cheese (1/3 cup)
Fish (all types)
Shellfish
Lamb (leg, roasted)
Pork (chops, ham or roast)
Peanut Butter (1 Tbsp.)
Poultry or Game Hen
Soybeans, cooked (1/3 cup)
Veal

FAT LIST

Bacon, crisp (1 slice)
Cheese, cream (1 Tbsp.)
Coconut (1 Tbsp.)
Cream, light (2 Tbsp.)
Gravy (2 Tbsp.)
Margarine (1 teaspoon)
Mayonnaise (1 teaspoon)
Nuts (6 to 10)
Oils (1 teaspoon)
Olives (5 small)
Salad Dressings (1 Tbsp.)
Seeds (1 Tbsp.)

MILK

Skim milk (1 cup)
Buttermilk (1 cup)
Yogurt (2/3 cup)

- Purchase fruits fresh, fresh-frozen or canned unsweetened, or in natural juices. All juices should be unsweetened.
- Vegetable and fruit portions are for the edible amounts of the item.
- Allowed amounts of meats are *after* cooking; amounts shown are for edible parts only (excluding bones). Be sure to trim all extra fat away from meat prior to cooking. Remove skin from all poultry. Roasting or broiling of meats is preferred.

Soft Diet

This diet is used frequently as a transition between a liquid diet and a regular diet. Usually, this diet is used during recovery from surgery, especially dental surgeries.

FOODS	ALLOWED	OMITTED
Beverages	Milk; cocoa; tea; coffee; fruit juices; carbonated beverages; decaffeinated coffee; cereal beverages.	No restrictions.
Cereals and Breads	Eat 4 or more servings daily of the following: dry or cooked refined cereals such as creamed wheat, farina, oatmeal, hominy grits, rice, cornmeal; cornflakes; puffed rice, puffed wheat; plain or toasted white or wheat-blend breads; saltines; flour tortillas.	All whole-grain breads; all hot breads including cornbread, pancakes, fried breads and sweet rolls; all whole-grain cereals except oatmeal.
Condiments	Salt and pepper in moderation; cinnamon; nutmeg; paprika; flavoring extracts.	All others, including chili and garlic.
Desserts	Simple desserts such as custard, gelatin, plain ice cream and sherbets; simple cakes and cookies; allowed fruits.	Rich pastries; any dessert containing dates, nuts, raisins or coconut.
Fats	Butter, cream, margarine and crisp bacon in moderation; mayonnaise.	Lard; pork fat; highly spiced salad dressings.
Fruits	Drink 1 serving of citrus juice daily; eat 2 or more servings of other fruits such as ripe avocado or banana, sectioned citrus fruit without membrane; fruit juices; cooked or canned apples; pears, peaches, white cherries, apricots, fruit cocktail or pineapple.	All fruits containing seeds and skins; all raw fruits except those allowed.

APPENDIX 11 (continued)

FOODS	ALLOWED	OMITTED
Meat, Fish Poultry, Eggs	Eat 2 or more 3-ounce servings daily of broiled, roasted, baked or stewed tender lean beef, mutton, lamb, veal, chicken, turkey, liver, pork, ham, bacon or whitefish; canned tuna, salmon or oysters; cottage cheese or other mild cheese used in cooking; poached, soft-cooked, hard-cooked, creamed or scrambled eggs.	All fried meat, fish or fowl; fried eggs; all strong-flavored cheese.
Milk	2 or more cups daily for adults; 3 to 4 cups daily for children.	
Potatoes or Substitute	White or sweet potatoes; rice; noodles; spaghetti; macaroni.	Fried potatoes; potato chips or corn chips.
Soups	Broths or creamed soups made with allowed vegetables, strained tomatoes or creamed corn.	All soups not made with allowed vegetables; highly seasoned soups.
Sweets	Sugar; syrup; jelly; honey; plain hard candies; molasses.	Rich candies; jam with seeds.
Vegetables	Vegetable juices; cooked vegetables with low-fiber content such as: young peas, asparagus tips, carrots, beets, green beans, spinach, squash, cooked tomatoes or wax beans.	All gas-forming vegetables such as: corn; radishes; Brussels sprouts; onions; dried beans and peas; broccoli; cabbage; parsnips; turnips; chili peppers; or hominy.

(Adapted from The Arizona Diet Manual, by the Diet Therapy Section of The Arizona Dietetic Association, Inc.)

APPENDIX 12

Suggestions to Help You Live Longer

The following list represents the conclusions of a group of researchers headed by Drs. Belloc and Breslow of the University of California at Los Angeles. They studied the physical health status and health practices of thousands of adults.

The conclusions scientifically validate what we have known all along. Simple as they seem, they require accepting and reviewing and following—if you desire to maintain optimum health and stay at your highest level of physical fitness, mental alertness and creativity.

Here are some suggestions for healthy living based on results of the study:

GET ENOUGH SLEEP

Get the right amount of sleep (average 8 hours for men, 7 for women) each night. The right amount must also be coupled with the right *quality* of sleep. Consider some of these suggestions for good sleep:

- **Use the bedroom for sleep and intimacy only.** Avoid taking business or private worries to bed with you. Avoid getting caught up in suspenseful reading or television while relaxing in bed. If you toss and turn on occasion and can't get to sleep, go to another room and do something productive.

- **Learn relaxation techniques.** Try meditation or breathing exercises, or alternate tensing and relaxing muscles. Use one or more of these techniques, followed by a warm bath, before going to bed at night.

EAT A GOOD BREAKFAST

Don't skip breakfast! Failing to eat because "you don't have time" or ill-advised reduction of calories per day can lead to poor health. The scientific evidence for this recommendation is convincing.

EAT THREE MEALS A DAY AT REGULAR TIMES

Regular meals keep the metabolic and digestive systems functioning at their most efficient levels. If you get hungry between meals, don't resort to fatty, salty or refined-sugar snacks. Instead, eat fruit, raw vegetables or whole grain snacks.

EXERCISE REGULARLY

Exercise that you enjoy is most likely to be successful and continued. See Appendix 20 for recommendations.

CONTROL YOUR WEIGHT

Even small amounts of excessive weight can shorten your life! Extreme obesity is associated with many physical and mental disorders. If you need to reduce, do so. If your weight is ideal, work to keep it that way.

DRINK ALCOHOL MODERATELY—OR NOT AT ALL!

Alcohol abuse can cause serious diseases, reduce your lifespan and make your life miserable. Moderate consumption can be defined as drinking no more than 3 ounces of alcohol in any form on any day.

DON'T SMOKE

There is overwhelming evidence that smoking damages the human body and shortens life. Cigarette smoking is a risk factor for many illnesses, particularly lung cancer, chronic lung disease, hardening of the arteries, heart attack, and damage to unborn children of pregnant women who smoke. Anyone who smokes is at greater risk of problems with anesthesia during surgery.

DON'T ABUSE DRUGS

Evidence is mounting about the cumulative ill effects of drug abuse. Common sense dictates avoiding them if you want to stay mentally and physically healthy.

How to Cope with Stress and Psychosomatic Illness

Changes in lifestyle and disruptions in your normal routine can bring about stress. Some of the common causes of stress are:

- Recent death of a loved one—spouse, child, friend.
- Loss of anything valuable to you.
- Injuries or severe illnesses.
- Getting fired or changing jobs.
- Recent move to a new home.
- Sexual difficulties between you and your partner.
- Business or financial reverses, or taking on a large debt, such as purchasing a new home.
- Regular conflict between you and a family member, close friend or business associate.
- Constant fatigue brought about by inadequate rest, sleep or recreation.

STRESS-RELATED DISORDERS

A certain amount of stress is not always bad. It varies from person to person how much stress one can handle easily. Sometimes, stress can push us on to greater achievement. But excessive stress can be self-defeating. Too much stress can also lead to any of the following disorders:

- Mental and emotional upheavals.
- Skin eruptions, such as eczema and neurodermatitis.
- Digestive system problems, including peptic ulcers, colitis and irritable colon.
- Endocrine disorders, including overactive thyroid, adrenal- or pituitary-gland overactivity or underactivity, changes in menstrual patterns, impotence and premature ejaculation in men, or orgasmic dysfunction in women.
- Lung disorders associated with spasm of the bronchial tubes, such as in asthma.
- Pain syndromes, such as chronic or recurrent disabling headaches or back pain.

Many doctors believe that stress has a role in almost any disorder. Practically no one doubts that stress can complicate an illness by preventing normal recovery, prolonging pain and sustaining disability.

SELF-HELP TIPS FOR COPING

Here are some tips that may help you reduce stress:

- Learn a meditation technique and practice it regularly—daily if possible. There are many methods available. Most of them include "tuning in to" and giving complete attention to a word, sound, sentence or concept that you silently repeat to yourself. Don't try to banish other thoughts that enter your mind during your period of concentration, but don't focus on them enough to stop you from meditating. The purpose of meditation is to empty your mind of all disturbing thoughts for a given period of time to encourage mental relaxation. Mental relaxation, in turn, will help reduce stress.

- Take a short period of time away from any stressful situation you encounter during a day. Practice a muscle-tensing and muscle-relaxing technique. Close your eyes. Take a series of deep breaths. Then start with the muscle groups in your face. Consciously tense them and hold the contraction for a few seconds. Then consciously relax them. Continue through all major muscle groups in the body: neck, shoulders, hands, abdomen, back and legs. When you become skillful, you can use this technique to produce relaxation quickly any time you need to and in almost any environment.

- Adopt an exercise program (see Appendix 20). People in good physical condition are less likely to suffer the negative effects of stress, anxiety or depression.

- Avoid taking your problems to bed with you. At the end of the day, spend a few minutes reviewing your entire day's experiences, event by event, as if you're replaying a tape. Release all negative emotions you have harbored (anger, feelings of insecurity or anxiety). Relish all good energy or emotion (loving thoughts, praise, feeling good about your work or yourself). Reach a decision about unfinished events, and release mental or muscular tension. Now you're ready for a relaxing and emotionally healing sleep.

APPENDIX 13 (continued)

PSYCHOSOMATIC ILLNESS

We can't separate our bodies from our minds or our spirits. Most departures from good health have some connection with these elements.

Psychosomatic illness is a term used to describe an illness in which factors other than physical ones are dominant. They may also play an important part in complications. Such illnesses are real—not imagined—as many people think. The links between mind, spirit and body may be poorly defined at times, but they are provable by accepted scientific methods.

Although medical researchers are beginning to understand the basic mechanisms, we still have much to learn about psychosomatic illness. One group of researchers believes that mental, emotional or spiritual stress can trigger almost any illness in a person genetically predisposed to that illness. Such illnesses include asthma, cancer, digestive disturbances, heart disease—all these and others are more common in certain families.

Yet, all members of the same genetic makeup do not succumb to the same illnesses.

SUGGESTIONS

Here are some simple suggestions to help you improve, prevent or cope with psychosomatic illness:

- Define and resolve all personal conflicts. Define and confront areas of personal conflict in spiritual, emotional, occupational, civic or recreational involvements. If you can't resolve these conflicts alone, seek help from family, friends or competent counselors.
- Be moderate in all your activities.
- Seek a balanced life of work, intellectual and physical challenges, recreation, intimacy, reflection and rest.
- Be of good humor whenever possible.
- Be a friend.
- Give and receive love.
- Keep a positive outlook on life. Considerate, respectful and loving attitudes toward yourself and others are powerful allies.

APPENDIX 14

Breast Self-Exam

WHY SHOULD YOU EXAMINE YOUR BREASTS MONTHLY?

Most breast cancer is first discovered by women themselves. Since breast cancer found early and treated promptly has an excellent chance for cure, learning how to examine your breasts properly can help save your life. Use the simple 3-step breast self-examination (BSE) procedure described below.

WHEN TO EXAMINE YOUR BREASTS

Follow the same procedure once a month about 1 week after your period, when your breasts are usually not tender or swollen.

After menopause, check your breasts on the first day of each month. After a hysterectomy, consult with your doctor or clinic for an appropriate time of the month.

Doing a monthly self-exam will give you peace of mind, and seeing your doctor once a year will reassure you there is nothing wrong.

3-Step Breast Self-Exam

1. IN THE SHOWER

Examine your breasts during a bath or shower—hands glide easier over wet skin. With the fingers flat, move the hand gently over every part of each breast. Use your right hand to examine the left breast, left hand for the right breast. Check for any lump, hard knot or thickening.

2. IN FRONT OF A MIRROR

Inspect your breasts with arms at your sides. Next, raise your arms high overhead. Look for any changes in contour of each breast, such as a swelling, dimpling of skin or changes in the nipple.

3. LYING DOWN ON YOUR BACK

To examine your right breast, put a pillow or folded towel under your right shoulder. Place your right hand under your head—this distributes breast tissue more evenly on the chest.

With the left hand, fingers flat, press gently in small circular motions around an imaginary clock face. Begin at the outermost top of your right breast for 12 o'clock, then move to 1 o'clock, and so on around the circle back to 12. A ridge of firm tissue in the lower curve of each breast is normal. Then move in an inch, toward the nipple, and keep circling to examine every part of your breast, including the nipple. This requires at least three more circles.

Now slowly repeat the procedure on your left breast with a pillow under your left shoulder and the left hand under your head. Notice how your breast structure feels.

Finally, squeeze the nipple of each breast gently between thumb and index finger. Any discharge, clear or bloody, should be reported to your doctor immediately.

WHAT TO DO IF YOU FIND A LUMP OR THICKENING

If a lump, dimple or discharge is discovered during a self-exam, it is important to see your doctor as soon as possible. Don't be frightened. Most breast lumps or changes are not cancer, but only your doctor can make the diagnosis.

(Courtesy of the American Cancer Society)

APPENDIX 15

Back Care

EXERCISES WHILE BACK PAIN IS PRESENT

While lying on your back:

- Bring one knee up to the chest. Lower it slowly, but do not straighten leg. Relax. Repeat with each leg 10 times.
- Bring both knees slowly up to the chest. Tighten the abdominal muscles and press the back flat against bed. Hold knees to chest 20 seconds, then lower slowly. Relax. Repeat 5 times. This exercise gently stretches shortened muscles of the lower back, while strengthening abdominal muscles. Clasp knees, bring them up to chest, at the same time coming to a sitting position. Rock back and forth.

EXERCISES AFTER BACK PAIN SUBSIDES

Use these inconspicuous exercises whenever you have a spare moment during the day, both to reduce tension and improve the tone of important muscle groups.

- Rotate shoulders, forward and backward.
- Turn head slowly side to side.
- Turn your head down and to the right as if stretching to see your right armpit. Stretch your neck slowly up, around and down, switching to a gaze at your left armpit. Repeat, starting on the left side.
- Slowly, touch left ear to left shoulder, then right ear to right shoulder. Raise both shoulders to touch ears, drop them as far down as possible.
- At any pause in the day (such as waiting for an elevator or traffic light), pull in the abdominal muscles, tighten and hold for the count of 8 without breathing. Relax slowly. Increase the count gradually after the first week, and practice breathing normally with the abdomen flat and contracted. Do this while sitting, standing and walking.

RULES TO PREVENT RECURRENT BACK PAIN

- Never bend from the waist only. Bend both hips and knees.
- Never lift a heavy object higher than your waist.
- Always turn and face the object you wish to lift.
- Avoid carrying unbalanced loads. Hold heavy objects close to your body.
- Never carry anything heavier than you can easily manage.
- Never lift or move heavy furniture alone. Get help from someone who knows the principles of leverage.
- Avoid sudden movements that "overload" muscles. Learn to move deliberately, swinging the legs from the hips.
- Train yourself to use your abdominal muscles to flatten your lower abdomen. In time, this muscle contraction will become a habit.
- For good posture, concentrate on strengthening "nature's corset," the abdominal and buttock muscles.
- For proper bed posture, a firm mattress is essential. If you have a soft mattress, put a 3/4-inch piece of plywood under it. Lie and sleep on your side with the knees flexed.
- Learn to keep the head in line with the spine when standing, sitting and lying in bed.
- Don't sit in soft chairs and deep couches. During prolonged sitting, cross your legs to rest your back.
- Use a rocking chair. Rocking rests the back.
- Avoid exercise that arches or overstrains the lower back, such as backward bends, forward bends or touching the toes with the knees straight.

APPENDIX 16

Immunizations

Immunizations protect children and adults from serious diseases that can be fatal. The schedule below is the current recommendation of the Center for Disease Control, an agency of the U.S. Public Health Service.

Don't consider the recommended ages as absolute. For example, "2 months" can mean a range of 6 to 10 weeks. Immunizations may not be a good idea at the recommended time if your child is ill or taking immunosuppressants or cortisone. Rely on the judgment of informed professionals.

SCHEDULE OF IMMUNIZATIONS

Age Recommended	Vaccines
2 months	DPT 1 [Diphtheria, Pertussis (whooping cough), Tetanus] OPV 1 (Oral Polio Vaccine)
4 months	DPT 2, OPV 2
6 months	DPT 3
15 months	MMR [Measles, Mumps, Rubella (German Measles)]
18 months	DPT 4, OPV 3
4 to 6 years	DPT 5, OPV 4
14 to 16 years	TD (Adult Tetanus and Diphtheria toxoid combined)
Every 10 years thereafter	TD

Vaccines are also available to protect against pneumococcal pneumonia, influenza, hepatitis, rabies, typhoid fever and other diseases. These vaccines are given only under special circumstances.

Ask your doctor, health department or travel agent about vaccinations required or recommended before travel in another country. Inquire several months before your expected departure.

APPENDIX 17

Care of Casts

Casts are used to help immobilize an injured part of the body after fractures or other injuries.

Casts are usually applied by placing a splint along the injured part and then wrapping it with gauze saturated with plaster of Paris. Before the injury heals, it may be necessary to change the cast one or more times. The time that the cast remains in place depends on how much time is needed for healing. Some casts are needed for only two weeks. Others remain in place for several months.

X-rays through the cast will determine that there is satisfactory alignment of the bones involved, and later check for signs of healing.

CARE OF THE CAST

● Do not allow pressure on any part of the cast until it is completely dry. The time required for drying varies, depending on the thickness of the cast, temperature and humidity. Drying can require 24 hours or longer.

● If the cast accidentally gets wet and a soft area appears, return to the doctor's office, emergency room or outpatient surgical facility for repairs.

CARE OF THE PATIENT IN A CAST

● Whenever possible, raise the part enclosed in the cast. This decreases the likelihood of swelling of the tissues underneath the cast. Prop a leg cast on a pillow when in bed and on a footstool or chair when sitting. Prop an arm cast on a pillow placed on the chest.

● No matter how carefully the injured tissues are handled and no matter how expertly the cast is applied, it is still possible for swelling to occur under the cast. If this happens, one or more of the following symptoms will probably become noticeable:

1. Severe and persistent pain.
2. Change in color of the tissues beyond the cast, such as a change to blue or gray under the nails of the fingers or toes.
3. Coldness of the tissues beyond the cast when the remaining part of the body is warm.
4. Numbness or complete loss of feeling in the skin beyond the cast.
5. Swelling of the tissue to a greater extent than was present before the cast was applied.

If any of the above signs or symptoms occur, contact your doctor or an emergency room as soon as possible for treatment.

APPENDIX 18

Soaks

Soaks are used to treat symptoms and diseases of the skin. They are used to:
1. Surround a scraped, injured or denuded part of the skin with fluid. Fluid frequently calms nerve endings that transmit pain and itching sensations.
2. Soften and dissolve crusts (such as scabs) and remove material that may invite secondary bacterial infection or cause fluid to collect and damage the skin.

WRAPPED SOAKS

Moisten and wring out strips of cotton cloth just enough so they are not dripping wet. Wrap the strips around the affected area. Keep the strips moist, and keep them applied for at least 30 minutes at a time. Repeat soaks several times a day.

IMMERSION SOAKS

Use a bathtub, sitz bath or foot pan with enough lukewarm or cool water to cover the affected area. Use soaks 30 to 40 minutes at a time, repeated several times a day. Use swirling water, such as a whirlpool bath or spa, if possible.

Water temperature for any kind of soak is not critical, but in general, cool water relieves itching and warm water relieves pain.

Chronic skin ulcers may require several weeks of soaks. Patients with other skin problems should use soaks for only 2 or 3 days. Otherwise, the skin may become dehydrated and the underlying problem will worsen.

APPENDIX 19

How to Reduce Fever

Fever is the body's reaction to infection or inflammation. It is not a disease in itself, but rather a sign of a problem.

The normal temperature in children varies with activity, eating and the time of day, ranging from 99F (37.2C) to 100F (37.8C) *rectally* in healthy children. Rectal thermometers are the most accurate and are the preferred method of taking temperature in children under 10 years old.

The thermometer has its line at 98.6F (37C), which is *not* the normal rectal temperature.

FLUIDS

Fluids are the only important requirement in the diet of the child with fever. Provide water, weak tea, ginger ale, broth, nectar or liquid jello. Some of the best-tolerated foods are saltines, cereal, applesauce, bananas, carrots and lean meat. Offer food, but don't force it. Fluids in small, frequent doses are all that is important for the first few days.

HOW TO REDUCE FEVER

If temperature in a child rises to 103F (39.4C) or above, your doctor may recommend sponging the child's body with warm water to reduce the fever temporarily. This is one common technique:

- Remove all clothing and lay the child down on a towel.
- Fill a basin with warm water.
- Dip a washcloth (preferably a new one that is still a little bit rough) into the warm water. Wring it out until it is damp but not soggy.
- Using the washcloth, begin massaging all over the body, covering as much surface as you can. The child should not be dripping wet, but should feel moist all over.
- Continue constant gentle massaging. This increases the flow of warm blood to the skin.
- When the washcloth begins to cool off, dip it into the warm water and wring it out again.
- Repeat massages. In 5 to 15 minutes, the child's temperature will probably be on its way down.
- Don't use a fan, alcohol, ice or cold water, and don't use cold baths or leave your child covered with wet towels!

DOSAGE SCHEDULE FOR FEVER-REDUCING MEDICINES

Age	Average Weight	Acetaminophen Drops	Acetaminophen Syrup
3 mos. or less	13 lbs. or less	0.3 cc	1/4 teaspoon
3 mos. to 1 yr.	13 to 21 lbs.	0.6 cc	1/2 teaspoon
1 to 2 years	21 to 28 lbs.	0.9 cc	3/4 teaspoon
2 to 3 years	28 to 32 lbs.	1.2 cc	1 teaspoon
3 to 4 years	32 to 36 lbs.	2.4 cc	1-1/2 teaspoon
4 to 5 years	36 to 41 lbs.	2.4 cc	2 teaspoons

APPENDIX 20

Benefits of Exercise and Physical Fitness

Regular exercise can play a key role in staying healthy or getting healthier. Exercise can be an important part of treating many medical problems, such as hypertension, sleep disorders, depression, anxiety, diabetes and high blood-fat levels (especially high levels of low-density cholesterol).

Regular exercise also can help improve your body image and increase your energy level. It can help control weight, reduce stress and protect from heart and blood-vessel disease.

EXERCISE PRESCRIPTION

After obtaining a medical history and performing a physical examination, your doctor may address four components of your exercise "prescription."

Type of Exercise—Popular ones include brisk walking, swimming, bike riding, jogging.

Frequency of Exercise—It's best to start at about three exercise sessions per week, then increase gradually to four, five or more.

Duration of Exercise—The ideal duration is 30 minutes of continuous activity. It's best to begin with 10 or 15 minutes and increase as your tolerance for exercise improves.

Intensity of Exercise—This component varies greatly depending on your age, sex and medical condition. If your doctor prescribes an exercise program, he or she will give specific instructions that uniquely apply to you after your physical checkup.

KEYS TO SUCCESS OF AN EXERCISE PROGRAM

- Fit exercise into your normal daily schedule and lifestyle.
- Exercise regularly—increase your pace gradually.
- Recruit a spouse or a friend to make exercise fun.
- Vary your activity. Alternate forms of exercise to avoid boredom.
- Increase exercise in easy, day-by-day activities. For example, park your car far enough away from a destination to allow a good walk, walk up a flight of stairs, use manual rather than power tools.

AEROBIC EXERCISE

An exercise is aerobic if it provides:
1. Sustained physical activity that uses major muscle groups of the body.
2. Regulated intensity, long-duration exercise for 20 minutes or more.

Medical experts recommend aerobic exercise as a good program for achieving and maintaining cardio-pulmonary-vascular fitness—strong and healthy heart, lungs and blood vessels.

Proper aerobic benefit is based on sufficient exercise to accelerate the heart rate to a prescribed level and keep it there a certain length of time. Most exercise routines call for aerobic sessions three to five times per week for maximum benefit.

Best forms of aerobic exercise include brisk walking, swimming, bike riding, jogging, rope jumping and rowing. Sports such as tennis and golf have good recreational effects, but they do not require enough effort to reach sustained aerobic levels.

Good sources for additional reading about aerobics include *The New Aerobics,* by Dr. Kenneth Cooper, a recognized international authority on the subject.

MuscleAerobics: The Ultimate Workout For Body Shaping, by Patricia Patano and Linette Savage, published by The Body Press, is a new approach that combines aerobics with the use of body-shaping hand weights.

APPENDIX 21

Safe Use of Medicine

Some suggestions for wise, safe use of medicine apply to all medicines. Your doctor and dentist must have complete information to prescribe drugs wisely for you. Always give the following information to your physician, dentist or other health-care professional:

YOUR COMPLETE MEDICAL HISTORY

Tell the important facts of your medical history dealing with medicines. Include allergic reactions, side effects or adverse reactions you have experienced in the past. Describe the allergic problems you have, such as hay fever, asthma, eye watering and itching, throat irritation and reactions to food. People who have allergies to common substances are more likely to develop side effects or adverse reactions to drugs.

MEDICINES YOU ARE TAKING NOW

List all prescription and non-prescription drugs. Don't forget common ones such as laxatives; vitamin or mineral supplements; skin, rectal or vaginal medicines; antacids; antihistamines; cold and cough remedies; aspirin and aspirin-containing pain pills; motion sickness remedies; weight-loss aids; salt and sugar substitutes; caffeine (in coffee, tea, cola drinks and cocoa); oral contraceptives; sleeping pills; or "tonics."

KNOW THIS INFORMATION BEFORE TAKING ANY MEDICINE

- Generic names and brand names of all the medicines you take. Write them down to help you remember. If a drug is a mixture of two or more generic ingredients, learn the names of each.
- Uses for each medicine you take.
- How to take each medicine—for example, with or without water, or with food.
- When to take.
- What to do if you forget a dose.
- How each drug works in your body.
- Time lapse before drug works.
- Symptoms and treatment of overdose.
- Possible adverse reactions and side effects and what to do if they occur.
- Interactions with other drugs and other substances such as alcohol, food, beverages, cocaine, marijuana and tobacco. When mixed with some medicines, these substances can sometimes cause life-threatening interactions.
- Know all warnings and precautions that apply to special circumstances, such as:
  1. Reasons not to take the drug in the presence of some medical conditions. These reasons are called *contraindications*.
  2. Special considerations for elderly patients; pregnant or breast-feeding women; infants and children.
  3. Implications for prolonged use; exposure to sun and sunlight; driving; piloting aircraft; hazardous work; flying in airplanes.
  4. Instructions before discontinuing the drug.

OTHER SAFETY TIPS

- Before taking any prescribed medicine, discuss plans with your doctor that you may have for elective surgery, pregnancy, and breast-feeding.
- Don't hesitate to ask questions about a drug. Your doctor, nurse and pharmacist will be able to provide more information if they are familiar with you and your past medical history, especially regarding medicines.
- Never take medicine in the dark! It is always possible to take the wrong one. Recheck the label before each drug use.
- Tell your doctor about any new or unexpected symptoms you develop while taking medicine. You may need to change medicines or have a dose adjustment.
- Store all medicines out of children's reach. Keep drugs in a cool, dry place, such as a kitchen cabinet or bedroom. Avoid medicine cabinets in bathrooms—they get too moist and warm at times. Keep medicine in its original container, tightly closed. Don't remove the label! If directions call for refrigeration, keep cool but don't freeze.
- Don't save leftover oral or injectable medicine to use later. Discard it before or on the expiration date shown on the container. Dispose of it safely to protect children and pets.
- Study any information you can find about the specific drugs you take. An excellent reference is *Complete Guide to Prescription and Non-Prescription Drugs,* published by HPBooks.
- Don't take any drug prescribed for someone else.
- Prior to any surgery (including oral surgery or simple dental procedures), tell your doctor or dentist about all medicines you take or have taken in the past few weeks.

Glossary

A

Abdominal Aorta—Section of the aorta that passes through the abdomen to supply blood to the lower part of the body.

Abscess—Swollen, inflamed, tender area of infection containing pus.

Accident Proneness—Tendency of some persons to have more accidents than normal. It may be due to a risk factor such as poor vision, but unconscious factors are often the cause.

Acetaminophen—Non-prescription medication used to relieve minor pain and to reduce fever. Its analgesic effects are similar to aspirin, but it does not reduce inflammation or swelling. It is less irritating to the stomach than aspirin.

Achylasia—Condition of the esophagus that disrupts normal swallowing.

Acupuncture—Method of anesthesia and treatment of pain developed by the Chinese. Needles are inserted through the skin to stimulate precise areas.

Acute—Beginning suddenly; also severe, but of short duration.

Addiction—Intense craving for substances such as alcohol, tobacco or narcotics, or a compulsive behavior such as gambling.

Adenoids—Infection-fighting tissue (part of the lymphatic system) in the upper throat, near the tonsils.

Adenoids, Enlarged—Adenoids that have swollen and impaired speech.

Adenovirus—Group of viruses that cause certain respiratory and eye infections.

Adhesions—Small strands of fibrous tissue that cause organs in the abdomen and pelvis to cling together abnormally, creating a risk of intestinal obstruction.

Adolescence—Time of life from the beginning of puberty until maturity.

Adrenal Glands—Two glands attached to the kidneys. Each has an outer layer (cortex) that produces steroid hormones and an inner layer (medulla) that produces adrenalin.

Adrenalin—Hormone produced by the adrenal glands that increases heart rate and prepares the body for crisis. Also called epinephrine.

Aging—The normal process of gradual physical and mental decline.

Airways—Tubular passages that air passes through to the lungs: the trachea (windpipe), bronchi and bronchioles.

Alveoli—Lung cells at ends of the airways where oxygen enters the blood and waste gases leave the blood.

Ambulatory Medical Center—A health-care facility for patients who do not require prolonged bed rest or hospitalization.

Amniotic Sac—The thin, transparent membrane filled with fluid in which the fetus lives until born.

Amphetamine Drugs—Habit-forming drugs that stimulate the brain and central nervous system, increase blood pressure, reduce nasal stuffiness or suppress appetite.

Amyloid Deposits—Abnormal protein material deposited in tissues, usually caused by diseases. These deposits cause impairment of certain organs.

Analgesics—Medications that relieve pain.

Anemia—Condition in which red blood cells or hemoglobin (oxygen-carrying substance in blood) is inadequate.

Anesthesia, General—Causing temporary loss of consciousness and inability to feel pain by use of inhaled gases or injected anesthetics.

Anesthesia, Local—Temporary prevention of pain by injecting medication (local anesthetic).

Anesthesia, Local (Nerve Block)—Injection of the local anesthetic near the nerves of the surgical area.

Aneurysm—Abnormal swelling or ballooning of a blood vessel.

Angina—Pain or pressure beneath the breastbone caused by inadequate blood supply to the heart.

GLOSSARY

Angiogram, Angiography—Study of arteries and veins by injecting material into them that X-rays can outline.

Anoscopy—Visual examination of the anus by means of a short tube called an anoscope, an optical instrument with lenses and a lighted tip.

Antacid—Medicine taken orally that reduces or neutralizes stomach acid.

Antiarrhythmics—Medications used to treat heartbeat irregularities (arrhythmias).

Antibiotics—Medications that attack germs and fight infection.

Antibiotics, Cephalosporin—Class of antibiotics related to penicillin, capable of destroying more kinds of germs than penicillin.

Antibiotics, Erythromycin—Class of antibiotics that destroys germs similar to those destroyed by penicillin. Often used to treat infections in patients who are allergic to penicillin.

Antibodies—Proteins created in blood and body tissue by the immune system to neutralize or destroy sources of disease.

Anticancer Drugs—Medications that weaken or destroy cancerous tissues without harming healthy tissues.

Anticholinergic Drugs—Medications that reduce nerve impulses in the parasympathetic nervous system. They control some activities of the gastrointestinal system, heart, bladder and other organs.

Anticoagulants—Medications that slow or delay blood clotting.

Anticonvulsants—Medications that control seizures (convulsions), pain or conditions in which the brain or nerves are overly sensitive.

Antidepressants—Medications that help control depression.

Antiemetic Drugs—Medications that prevent or stop nausea and vomiting.

Antifungal Drugs—Medications used to treat fungus diseases.

Antigens—Germs or other sources of disease that antibodies (produced by the immune system) neutralize or destroy.

Antihelminthic Drugs—Medications used to treat worms in the intestines.

Antihistamines—Medications used to treat allergies.

Antihyperlipidemic Drugs—Medications that reduce fat (cholesterol) in the blood. They help prevent blood-vessel disease.

Antihypertensives—Medications used to reduce blood pressure.

Anti-Inflammatory Drugs—Medications used to control inflammation not caused by infection.

Antimalarial Drugs—Medications used to prevent or treat malaria.

Antimetabolite Drugs—Medications that are used to treat some cancers and autoimmune diseases.

Antimicrobial Drugs—Same as *Antibiotics*.

Antinuclear Antibody—Substance that appears in the blood, indicating presence of an autoimmune disease.

Antiparkinsonism Drugs—Medications used to treat Parkinson's disease.

Antiprotozoal Drugs—Medications used in treatment of single-celled parasites (protozoa).

Antipruritic Drugs—Medications that reduce itching.

Antispasmodic Drugs—Medications that improve digestion and relieve intestinal cramps.

Antistreptococcal Titer—Blood test that measures body's response to infection by streptococcal bacteria.

Antithyroid Drugs—Medications used to counter the effects of an overactive thyroid gland.

Antiviral Drugs—Medications used to treat infections caused by viruses.

Anus—A muscular band at the end of the rectum that opens and expands to allow passage of feces.

Anus, Imperforate—Congenital abnormality of newborn infants in which the anus cannot pass feces.

Anxiety—Uncomfortable feeling that something unpleasant or dangerous will happen.

Aorta—Body's largest blood vessel, arising from the top of the heart. It carries blood from the heart to all parts of the body.

Aphrodisiac—Substance claimed to increase sexual arousal or pleasure.

Appendage—Body part that has a minor role (or no role at all) in normal body function. For example, the appendix is an appendage to the colon that seems to have no function.

GLOSSARY

Arteriogram, Arteriography—Studying arteries by injecting material into them that X-rays can outline.

Artery—Blood vessels that carry blood from the heart to the body.

Arthrograms—X-rays of the joints taken with an arthroscope.

Arthroscope—Slender optical instrument with a lighted tip that allows direct visual examination of some joints. It can also be used to correct some defects in joints.

Artificial Limbs—Mechanical substitutions for amputated arms or legs.

Ascending Colon—First part of the large colon (intestine) extending from the lower end of the small intestine.

Aspiration—1) Removal of accumulated pus or fluid with a needle. 2) Accidental inhalation of objects or fluids into the lungs.

Astigmatism—Visual impairment caused by abnormal eye shape.

Asymmetrical—Uneven in size, shape or position.

Atriums—Small chambers in the heart that pump blood into the ventricles. Also called auricles.

Atropine—Medication used to treat diseases of the eye, heart, gastrointestinal system and nervous system.

Audiogram, Audiometry—Test of hearing ability.

Autism—Mental illness of children in which they seem unaware of their surroundings.

Autoimmune, Autoimmunity—Disease in which a person's immune system attacks its own tissues.

Autoimmune Assays (ANA Tests)—Blood tests to identify autoimmune disease.

Autoimmune Disorder—Disease in which the immune system produces antibodies that attack the body's own tissues.

Autonomic Nervous System—Part of the nervous system that controls organs that function involuntarily, such as the heart, lungs, digestive system and blood vessels.

B

Bacteria—One-celled micro-organisms that can sometimes cause disease.

Balloon Angioplasty—Treatment for obstructed arteries, especially those supplying blood to the heart and brain. A small uninflated balloon is passed up the artery to the obstruction, and then expanded to release the obstruction.

Barium Enema X-Rays—Examining the colon by filling it with a barium solution that is detected by X-rays.

Bartholin's Glands—Small glands in the lips of the vagina that secrete a lubricating fluid, especially during sexual arousal.

Belladonna—Medication derived from a plant used to treat some diseases of the gastrointestinal system. It is similar to atropine.

Benign—1) Tumor or growth that is neither cancerous nor located where it might impair normal function. 2) Harmless.

Beta-Adrenergic Blockers (Beta-Blockers)—Medications that reduce heart or blood-vessel overactivity to improve blood circulation. Also used to prevent migraine headaches, high blood pressure and angina.

Bile—A digestive juice produced in the liver and stored in the gallbladder. Bile empties into the small intestine for digestive processes.

Bile Duct—A small tube that allows bile to pass from the gallbladder into the intestines.

Bilirubin—A yellowish, red-blood-cell waste product in bile that the blood carries to the liver. It contributes to urine's yellowish color and can cause jaundice if it builds up in the blood.

Biopsy—Removal of a small amount of tissue or fluid for laboratory examination that aids in diagnosis.

Biopsy Needle—Instrument often used to perform a biopsy.

Birth Canal—Passageway through the cervix and the vagina through which the baby passes during childbirth.

Bladder—An organ that holds fluids such as urine (urinary bladder) or bile (gallbladder).

Blood Cells, Red—Microscopic cells in the blood that carry oxygen to tissues of the body. One drop of blood contains about 200 million red cells.

Blood Cells, White—Microscopic cells in the blood that help fight infection by destroying germs. One drop of blood contains about 400,000 white cells.

GLOSSARY

Blood Chemistries—Tests that measure chemicals in the blood.

Blood Count—Counting red and white blood cells to aid in diagnosis of many diseases.

Blood Platelets—See *Platelet Count.*

Blood Studies—Examination of a blood sample to measure white blood cells, red blood cells, hemoglobin, hematocrit and chemical substances. See *Blood Chemistries.*

Blood Vessels—Arteries, veins and capillaries; the tubes in which blood circulates through the body.

Bone Bank—Facility where human bone is stored and made available for transplantation.

Bone Spurs—Abnormal and sometimes painful protrusions of bone with sharp points near joints or tendons.

Bronchial Tubes (Bronchi)—Hollow air passageways that branch from the windpipe (trachea) into the lungs. They carry oxygen into the lungs and pass waste gases (mostly carbon dioxide) out of the body.

Bronchioles—Small air passageways that serve the same purpose as bronchial tubes. Bronchioles are the smallest parts of the respiratory system.

Bronchodilator Drugs—Medications used to treat diseases of the bronchi that cause shortness of breath, such as asthma. The medicines help constricted tubes to relax.

Bronchogram—Diagnosing lung diseases by placing a material in the lung that X-rays can outline.

Bronchoscope—An optical instrument with a lighted tip that is passed into the windpipe, then into the bronchi.

Bruising—Discoloration under the skin caused by injury or bleeding.

C

Calcification—A process in which calcium from the blood is deposited abnormally into tissues due to injury, infection or aging. Often it is part of healing and not a sign of active disease.

Calcium-Channel Blocker Drugs—Medication used to treat angina, hypertension and heartbeat irregularities.

Cancerous Growths—Extensions of cancerous tissues that invade nearby healthy tissues.

Cancers—Destructive tumors that can arise in almost all parts of the body. Cancer can destroy nearby healthy tissue and may spread to distant organs.

Capillaries—Microscopic vessels that supply all body cells and tissues with blood.

Carbohydrates, Complex—Starches, sugars, cellulose and gums. Complex carbohydrates are those contained in whole grains, fresh fruits and fresh vegetables. These are considered more nutritious than simple carbohydrates.

Carbohydrates, Simple—Refined carbohydrates (sugars) that have lower molecular weights than complex carbohydrates. They produce a quick rise in blood-sugar levels. Most nutrition counselors recommend that daily diets contain minimal amounts of refined sugars. So-called "junk foods" are frequently very high in simple carbohydrates.

Cardiac Catheter—A slender tube that is inserted into an artery or vein and then passed into the heart. It is used to examine the heart and nearby blood vessels by injecting material into the heart that X-rays can detect.

Cardiac Catheterization—Studying heart function with a cardiac catheter.

Cardiopulmonary Resuscitation (CPR)—Emergency treatment for a patient whose heart has stopped (cardiac arrest).

Cardiovascular—Relating to the heart and blood vessels.

Cardiovascular Surgeon—Doctor specially trained to operate on the heart and blood vessels.

Cardiovascular System—System that supplies the body with blood. It consists of the heart and blood vessels (arteries, capillaries, veins).

Carotid Arteries—Large arteries that supply much of the blood to the brain.

Cartilage—Rubbery, dense connective tissue that permits smooth movement of joints. It also helps shape flexible parts of the nose and external ear.

Caruncle—Small, red protrusion of tissue near a body opening. The most common caruncles arise from the urethra or cervix.

GLOSSARY

CAT (or CT) Scan (Computerized Axial Tomography) — A computerized X-ray procedure that provides exceptionally clear images of parts of the body. It aids in diagnosis of diseases that cannot be diagnosed by ordinary X-ray methods.

Catheter — A hollow tube used to introduce fluids into the body or to drain fluids away.

Caudal Anesthesia — Form of local (low-spinal) anesthesia used to reduce pain during childbirth and surgery on pelvic areas.

Cauterant — Chemical used to destroy abnormal or diseased cells on the skin.

Cautery — Destroying small areas of diseased tissue by burning with an electric needle or laser beam, freezing with low-temperature instruments or using a chemical that destroys tissue.

Cecum — The part of the intestinal tract at the beginning of the large colon (intestine).

Central Nervous System — System that controls the body's voluntary acts. It consists of the brain and spinal cord.

Cervical Spine — Bones in the neck at the top of the spinal column.

Cervix — Lower third of the uterus, which protrudes into the vagina.

Cesarean Section — Delivery of a baby through incisions in the mother's abdomen and uterus. It is performed when normal vaginal delivery would be dangerous for the mother or baby.

Chancre — Hard, slightly ulcerated, painless lesion that forms where syphilis enters the body, usually on the genital lips.

Chemocautery — Destruction of abnormal tissue by means of acids, caustics or poisons.

Chemotherapy — Treatment of cancer by injecting medications that kill cancer cells without harming healthy tissue. It is used to treat cancers that cannot be completely cured or treated with surgery or radiation.

Chiggers — Small red biting insects. Also called "red bugs."

Child — Person in the first 10 years of life.

Chiropractor — Practitioner of chiropractic treatment of disease, which involves massage and manipulations that chiropractors claim restore normal body functions.

Chokes — Severe breathing difficulty experienced by scuba divers and others who go from high to normal air pressure too rapidly. Bubbles of nitrogen develop in the blood stream and obstruct blood supply to vital organs, sometimes resulting in severe injury or death.

Cholangiogram, Cholangiography — X-ray procedures to diagnose diseases of the bile system (liver, gallbladder, bile ducts). Special medications are used to make the bile system visible on X-rays.

Cholera — Acute, severe, infectious disease causing extreme diarrhea and dehydration.

Choroiditis — Inflammation of the part of the eye that supports the retina and supplies blood to it.

Chromosome — Structures inside the nucleus of living cells which contain hereditary information. Defects in chromosomes cause many birth defects and inherited diseases.

Chronic — Long-term, continuing. Chronic illnesses are usually not curable, but they can often be prevented from worsening. Symptoms usually can be controlled.

Cinematography — Form of motion-picture photography used to record a fast-moving series of X-ray images.

Circulatory System — The system that provides blood to the body, consisting of the heart, arteries, veins and lymphatic system.

Clinician — Health-care professional who has direct contact with patients. The word literally means "someone who is at the patient's bedside."

Clips — See *Skin Clips*.

Clot Retraction Test — Measurement of the time necessary for a tube of blood to form a clot. Abnormal results often indicate a defect in blood platelets, cells important in blood coagulation.

Clotting — Activity of the blood and blood vessels that cause blood to form a jellylike clot, usually near an injury. Clotting helps stop bleeding. The body's clotting mechanism is slowed or reduced ("thinning the blood") with anticoagulants to treat certain diseases.

Coagulation — Same as *Clotting*.

Cocaine—Medication applied directly to mucous membranes to control pain in the nose and throat. Used illegally as a mind-altering drug, it is addicting and dangerous.

Colic, Colicky—A pain that recurs in a regular pattern every few seconds or minutes.

Collagen—A gelatinous protein from which body tissues are formed.

Colon—The last major portion of the gastrointestinal tract, where waste material is formed into feces and held for elimination. It is also known as the large intestine.

Colonoscopy—Method of diagnosing diseases of the colon by visual examination of the inside of the colon through a *flexible colonoscope,* a fiber-optic instrument with a lighted tip.

Color-Blindness—Inability to recognize red and green, which appear to be gray. It is usually hereditary.

Colposcopy—Visual examination of the cervix by means of a colposcope, a slender optical instrument with a lighted tip.

Combined Immunodeficiency Disease—Serious inherited disease in which the immune system of infants is unable to defend against disease.

Complication—Undesirable event during disease or treatment that causes further symptoms and delay in recovery.

Compress—Cloth, sometimes soaked in warm water or coated with medication. It is applied to the skin to relieve discomfort.

Compression—Applying pressure to the surface of the body, usually to stop bleeding.

Compulsion, Compulsive—Intense, irrational urge to perform some action.

Condom—A thin sheath, usually of rubber, applied to the penis before sexual intercourse. It is used to prevent disease of the genitals and as a contraceptive.

Congenital—Abnormality of the body, present at birth, usually meaning a defect. Congenital defects may be inherited or caused by conditions occurring while the fetus grows in the uterus.

Congenital Hypoplastic Anemia—See *Hypoplastic Anemia.*

Conization of the Cervix—Removal of a cone of tissue from the cervix. Laboratory examination of the removed tissue identifies possible cancer.

Conjunctiva—The mucous membrane lining the outermost surface of the eye ("white of the eye").

Connective Tissue—Body's supporting framework of tissue consisting of strands of collagen, elastic fibers and simple cells.

Contact Lenses—Small plastic lenses worn on the eyes to correct nearsightedness, farsightedness or astigmatism.

Contagious—Disease or condition that spreads from one person to another.

Convalescence—Recovery from an illness or surgery.

COPD (Chronic Obstructive Pulmonary Disease)—Several usually incurable lung diseases associated with gradually increasing breathing difficulty.

Copious—Large in amount.

Cornea—Clear thickened surface of the eye through which light passes. It has no blood supply and can be transplanted without danger of rejection.

Coronary—Referring to the blood vessels supplying the heart. Sometimes, it refers to a heart attack resulting from coronary-artery obstruction.

Coronary-Care Unit (CCU)—Area of a hospital equipped to care for patients who have suffered a heart attack or other life-threatening heart conditions.

Cortisone Drugs—Medications similar to natural hormones produced by the central core of the adrenal glands.

Cosmetic Surgery—Surgery to improve appearance.

Coxsackie Viruses—Group of viruses causing infections such as poliomyelitis, aseptic meningitis, herpangina and myocarditis.

CPR—See *Cardiopulmonary Resuscitation.*

Cranium—Bones that make up the skull.

Cryosurgery—Destruction of abnormal tissue by applying freezing temperatures, usually with liquid nitrogen.

Cryotherapy—The use of cold (below -200F) temperatures in treatment.

CT Scan—See *CAT Scan.*

GLOSSARY

Culdocentesis—Piercing of the space deep in the vagina under the cervix, to obtain fluid. Laboratory examination of the removed fluid aids in diagnosis of ectopic pregnancy and other disorders.

Culdoscopy—Visual examination of the female pelvic organs by means of a slender instrument brought into the pelvic cavity by penetrating through the space deep in the vagina under the cervix.

Culture—Identification of bacteria, fungi and viruses. Material (pus, blood or urine) from an area infected is collected, placed on nutrient material, and kept warm (usually in an incubator) until the infecting agent has grown. The resulting growth is examined with a microscope.

Curettage—Scraping process frequently used to obtain tissue from the lining of the uterus for laboratory examination. Laboratory examination of the removed tissue aids in diagnosis.

Curette—Instrument with a sharp end used to scrape tissue from the inner lining of the uterus and to scrape away skin lesions.

Cyst—Sac or cavity filled with fluid or diseased matter.

Cyst Aspiration—Removal of cyst contents for examination, or drainage for relief of symptoms.

Cystoscopy—Visual examination of the inside of the urinary bladder by means of a cystoscope, a slender optical instrument with a lighted tip.

Cytotoxic Drugs—Medications used to destroy cancerous cells with minimal harm to healthy cells.

D

Debilitating—Causing a general weakening or deterioration in health.

Defibrillation, Cardiac—Applying an electric current to the chest over the heart to interrupt fibrillation, a disturbance of heartbeat.

Dehydration—Loss of essential fluids from the tissues and blood of the body.

Dependence—Condition in which a person requires substances such as narcotics or alcohol to remain comfortable. If the substances are not used, withdrawal symptoms develop.

Dermatome—Area of the skin to which feeling (sensation) is provided by a nerve to the spinal cord.

Descending Colon—The part of the colon in the left side of the abdomen that stores feces until they are passed from the body.

Diabetic Retinopathy—Degeneration of the retina that develops in patients with diabetes mellitus. It may cause vision impairment or blindness.

Diagnosis—Identifying disease. A complete diagnosis names the part of the body affected, the disease process (such as inflammation, cancer or allergy) and the cause of disease.

Dialysis—Removal of natural wastes from the bloodstream. It is used to treat patients with kidney failure.

Diaphragm—Thin, broad sheet of muscle separating the chest cavity from the abdominal cavity.

Diathermy—Treatment in which mild heat is generated within the body by high-frequency radio waves.

Digestive System—Organs in which food is processed for absorption into the blood stream. The major digestive organs are the mouth, esophagus, stomach, duodenum, small bowel (small intestine), colon (large intestine), and rectum. The liver, gallbladder and pancreas are also considered parts of the digestive system.

Digitalis—A drug used to treat congestive heart failure and some other heart diseases.

Dilate, Dilation—To widen, expand or open up.

Dilator—Instrument used to widen organs that have narrowed because of disease.

Discolored Teeth—A yellowish-brown discoloration of the teeth frequently occurring in infants whose mothers took tetracycline while pregnant. Children may also be affected if they take tetracycline before they have their permanent teeth.

Discomfort—Unpleasant physical or mental sensation.

Disease—Adverse change in health; sickness or ailment. A disease can be defined by the body part involved (for example, the heart or liver), by the abnormality present (cancer, infection, allergy, degeneration, etc.) or by its cause (bacteria, poisons, injury, etc.).

Disk—Same as *Intervertebral Disk*.

GLOSSARY

Disorder—Same as *Disease*.

Diuretics—Medications that force the kidneys to excrete more urine, sodium and potassium than normal, which helps eliminate excessive body fluid.

Diverticulum—Small pouch or sac that develops in the wall of tubular organs such as the esophagus or colon.

Dizziness—Sensation of faintness, lightheadedness or spinning (vertigo).

Donor—Person who gives to someone else. In transplantation surgery, the donor gives up an organ (such as a kidney) to be transplanted into the recipient.

Doppler Sonography—See *Sonogram;* this is one of several methods of sonography.

Dormant—Sleeping or inactive state of living things. Also, an inactive state of a disease.

Drainage—Passage of fluids out of the body through an opening or incision.

Ductus Arteriosus—Small blood vessel connecting the aorta and the pulmonary artery, which is the main artery to the lung. The vessel is open during the time the fetus is in the uterus, but normally closes at birth.

Duodenum—First 12 inches of the small intestine.

Dupuytren's Contracture—Chronic condition in which scar tissue forms in the palms. In severe cases, it can impair use of the fingers.

Dwarfism—Condition of being undersized for one's age. It may be due to endocrine disorders, malnutrition or an inherited defect.

E

Ear Canal—Passageway extending from the outer ear inward to the eardrum.

Ear, Nose and Throat (ENT) Specialist—A physician specially trained to treat diseases of the ears, nose and throat.

Echocardiogram, Echocardiography—Studying the heart by examining sound waves created by an instrument placed on the chest. The waves reflected from the heart form an image (echocardiogram) on a monitor, aiding in diagnosis of heart diseases.

Edema—Accumulation of fluid under the skin, in the lungs or elsewhere.

EEG (Electroencephalography)—Studying the brain by measuring electric activity ("brain waves") with an electroencephalograph. The record produced is the electroencephalogram.

EKG (Electrocardiography)—Method of diagnosing heart diseases by measuring electrical activity of the heart with an electrocardiograph. The record produced is called an electrocardiogram.

Electrocardiography—See *EKG*.

Electrocautery—Destruction of tissue by heat applied with a controlled electric current.

Electroencephalography—See *EEG*.

Electrolyte—A chemical that is dissolved in the blood and all other body fluids. Electrolytes play an essential role in all body functions. The major electrolytes are: sodium, potassium, chloride, calcium, phosphorus, magnesium and carbon dioxide. Electrolytes come from food. They are regulated mostly by the kidneys and lungs.

Electrolyte Measurement—Laboratory test on blood or urine to identify and measure the electrolytes present.

Electrolyte Supplements—Electrolytes taken to correct or to prevent body-fluid or electrolyte imbalance.

Electromyography—Studying nerve and muscle disorders by recording electrical activity of muscles with an electromyograph. The record produced is the electromyogram.

Endemic—Disease that is constantly present in a community or group of people. Endemic disease may affect only a few people at any one time.

Endocrine System—System of organs that secrete hormones into the blood to regulate basic functions of cells and tissues. The endocrine organs are the anterior and posterior pituitary glands, thyroid and parathyroid glands, pancreas, adrenal glands, ovaries (in women) and testicles (in men).

Endocrinologist—Doctor specially trained in diagnosis and treatment of endocrine disorders.

GLOSSARY

Endoscopy—Method of diagnosing diseases in hollow organs. An endoscope (an optical instrument with a lighted tip) is inserted into the organ, which allows visual examination of the cavity. Used in the abdomen, pelvis, lumen of the bronchial tubes, or intestines.

Endotracheal Tube—Tube temporarily placed in the trachea (windpipe) of patients who are unable to breathe normally because of disease or surgery.

Enteric—Relating to the small intestine. Enteric-coated medicine is coated with a hard shell that dissolves when it reaches the small intestine.

Enterostomy—Surgically created artificial opening for elimination of feces. An enterostomy nurse or enterostomy specialist is a professional who teaches patients how to care for the artificial opening.

Enzymes—Proteins manufactured by the body that regulate the rate of essential life processes (metabolism).

Epinephrine—Same as *Adrenalin*.

Episcleritis—Inflammation of tissues on the sclera (the 'white of the eye').

Epithelial Horn—Thick, rough lesion protruding from the skin. It may become cancerous if not removed.

Equine Virus—Virus that causes a serious form of encephalitis in horses and man.

Ergot—Medication derived from a fungus that grows on rye plant. It is used to treat migraine headache and to increase strength of uterine contractions during and immediately after childbirth.

Esophageal Varices—Enlarged veins on the lining of the esophagus. They are subject to severe bleeding and often appear in patients with severe liver disease.

Esophagoscopy—Method of diagnosing diseases of the esophagus by means of an esophagoscope, an optical instrument with lenses and a lighted tip.

Esophagus—Muscular tube connecting the throat and stomach.

Estrogen—Female sex hormone, primarily secreted by the ovaries. It can also be produced synthetically for use in estrogen replacement therapy.

Estrogen Receptor Value—Used in the study of breast-cancer cells to determine the best treatment.

Etiology—Cause or causes of a disease.

Eustachian Tubes—Slender passages between the throat and the middle ear that maintain normal air pressure in the middle ear.

Excise—To remove by cutting out.

Exploratory Laparotomy—Diagnosing abdominal disease by surgically opening the abdomen and examining its contents.

Extremities—Arms and legs.

Eye Bank—Facility where living corneas are stored and made available for transplantation.

Eyes, Crossed—Condition in which muscles controlling the eyes are unbalanced. The eyes point in different directions. Also called squint or strabismus.

F

Fallopian Tubes—Organs of the female reproductive tract through which an egg (ovum) passes from the ovary to the uterus. Tying these tubes (tubal ligation) accomplishes sterility.

Familial Polyposis—Inherited condition in which the lining of the intestines contains many polyps, some of which may become cancerous.

Family History—Information about illnesses that tend to occur within a family. This information is used to determine the likelihood of diseases occurring in other members of the family.

Farsightedness—Same as *Hypermetropia*.

Fascia—Sheet or band of tough, fibrous tissue that covers muscles and other body organs.

Fecal—Relating to feces, waste products eliminated through the lower intestinal tract.

Fecal-Oral—Pathway by which some fecal germs gain entry into the bloodstream. Sewage in drinking water, hand-to-mouth transmission after bowel movements or sexual contact can cause infection.

Feces—Body waste formed of undigested food that has passed through the gastrointestinal system to the colon. Feces are produced and stored in the colon until eliminated.

Fetal Monitoring—Measuring the heart rate of the fetus during labor.

GLOSSARY

Fetal-Scalp Electrodes—Fine wires attached to the scalp of a fetus to measure heart rate and rhythm during labor.

Fetal-Scalp Monitoring—Measuring the well-being of the fetus during labor by obtaining blood from the scalp or by measuring the heart rate of the fetus or contraction strength of the uterus.

Fever—Above-normal body temperature. Normal mouth temperature is 98.6F (37C). Normal rectal temperature is 99.6F (37.6C).

Fiber—A non-nutritious ingredient of many complex carbohydrates. Fiber increases bulk in the diet. Many nutritionists recommend including ample fiber in the diet. Experimental studies and clinical studies show that people who eat high-fiber diets are less likely to develop colon cancer, diverticulitis, atherosclerosis and gallbladder disease.

Fiber Optics—System of transmitting light and images through thread-like strands of glass. Fiber-optic instruments make some examinations and surgical procedures simple, safe and effective.

Fibrin—Protein formed by the action of blood clotting on fibrogen.

Fibrinogen—Protein in the blood needed for blood clotting.

Fibrositis—Inflammatory conditions affecting connective tissue of muscles, joints, ligaments and tendons.

First Molars—First permanent flat teeth, used for grinding food, which appear at about age 6 to 7.

Fissure—Break in the skin or inner lining of organs.

Fistula—Abnormal passage between two organs or between the body and the outside.

Flank—Area on the side of the body below the ribs and above the hip.

Fleas—Tiny biting insects. Most cause minor skin irritation; some carry and transmit serious diseases such as plague and typhus.

Fluorescein-Dye Test—Method of diagnosis using fluorescein, a dye, to study tissues and germs. When these dyed tissues are exposed to ultraviolet light, they glow. Substances to which the dye does not cling do not glow.

Fluorescent Antibody Studies—Tests used to study some allergic and infectious conditions. When antibodies created by these conditions are present in the blood, they can be made to glow by using a dye and a microscope with ultraviolet light.

Fluoroscopy—Method of X-ray diagnosis in which moving organs (such as the heart or intestinal tract) can be studied in action.

Foley Catheter—Slender, flexible tube used to drain urine from the bladder of patients who are unable to urinate normally.

Forceps—Instrument with two blades and handles. It is used to grasp tissue, body parts or sterile materials. Also used to deliver babies when progress of labor is slow.

Fracture—Break; usually used to refer to a bone or tooth.

Frei Test—Test used to make a precise diagnosis of lymphogranuloma, a sexually transmitted disease.

Friedreich's Ataxia—Rare, inherited nervous-system disease that causes loss of balance and coordination, awkward walking, speech difficulty and tremors.

Frozen Section—A study in a pathology laboratory of fresh tissue that was removed during surgery. The purpose is to determine if a suspicious area is or is not cancerous.

Fungus—Mold or yeast that may infect skin, internal surfaces (mouth, vagina) or tissues.

Fungus Infection—Infection caused by fungus.

Fusiform Bacteria—Bacteria shaped like slender rods.

G

Galactorrhea—1) Continued breast-milk flow after weaning. 2) Excess breast-milk flow during nursing.

Galactosemia—Inherited disease of infants in which milk cannot be digested. Milk should be eliminated from the infant's diet to prevent malnutrition, liver and kidney disease, and mental retardation.

Gallbladder—Small organ under the liver that stores bile. For digestion, the gallbladder contracts to empty bile into the intestines.

GLOSSARY

Gamma Globulin—Protein in the blood manufactured by the immune system to help destroy or neutralize infection-causing germs. Gamma globulin derived and concentrated from blood of other humans is used to help create temporary immunity to some diseases.

Gammaglobulinemia—Extremely low levels in the blood of gamma globulin brought about by a disease of the immune system. The deficiency causes increased susceptibility to many infections by bacteria, viruses and fungi. Also called hypogammaglobulinemia.

Gangrene—Death of tissue, usually due to . partial or total loss of blood supply.

Gastrectomy—Removal of part or all of the stomach.

Gastroenterologist—Doctor who specializes in the diagnosis and treatment of diseases of the gastrointestinal system.

Gastrointestinal Series (Upper GI Series)—X-rays of the upper digestive system (esophagus, stomach and duodenum).

Gastrointestinal Tract—See *Digestive System.*

Gastroscopy—Visual examination of the inside of the stomach by means of a gastroscope, an optical instrument with a lighted tip.

Gene—Basic unit of protein molecules in chromosomes of cells. Genes transmit inherited characteristics such as eye color, blood type, gender or body shape. Defective genes cause many kinds of birth defects and inborn diseases.

Gene, Dominant or Recessive—Dominant gene, if present in either the mother's egg or father's sperm, will transmit its characteristics to the newborn child. Recessive genes must be present in both parents before its characteristic will be transmitted.

General Surgeon—A doctor specially trained to perform operations.

Genetic Counseling—Counseling to help couples decide whether to have children or not when there is a risk of genetic disease being transmitted to the child.

Genetics—Science of determining inherited factors that result in the unique make-up of every human being; also, science that traces the appearance patterns to genetic (inherited) disease.

Genitourinary Tract—Body system that forms, stores and eliminates urine. Also has a role in male and female reproductive functions. Organs include the kidneys, ureters, bladder, urethra, uterus, Fallopian tubes, ovaries, vagina, cervix, penis, scrotum and testicles.

Germs—Organisms that cause infection such as bacteria, viruses or fungi.

Gestation—Time spent in the mother's uterus by the fetus. Average gestation time for the human infant, from conception to delivery, is approximately 39 weeks.

Gigantism—Condition in which the body or a body part grows excessively, sometimes due to an overactive pituitary gland.

Glucagon—Hormone secreted by the pancreas that increases blood sugar. A synthetic form is sometimes used as emergency treatment for patients with diabetes who have temporarily low blood sugar.

Glucose—Major form of sugar in the blood, stored primarily in the liver. It provides energy to most tissues, organs and systems.

Glucose-Tolerance Test—Method of diagnosing diabetes mellitus or functional hypoglycemia. The patient drinks a measured amount of glucose (sugar). The blood and urine are tested at measured intervals for glucose content.

Gluten—Protein found in wheat and other foods that cannot be digested by some persons because of genetic disease. A gluten-free diet allows persons with the disorder to digest food and grow normally.

Gonads—Parts of the reproductive system that produce and release female eggs (ovaries) or male sperm (testes).

Growth Disorders—Conditions in children that result in underdevelopment or overdevelopment of the body. Diseases of the endocrine glands, nutritional problems or genetic abnormalities are frequently the causes.

Gynecologist—Doctor specially trained to treat diseases of the female reproductive system.

GLOSSARY

H

H-2 Blocker Drugs—Class of antihistamines that reduce the production of stomach acid for treatment of peptic ulcers.

Hallucinogens—Substances that produce hallucinations, apparent sights, sounds or other experiences that do not actually exist.

Hand Surgeon—Surgeon specially trained to treat hand diseases, injuries, infections and arthritic conditions.

Hangover—Unpleasant aftereffects of excessive consumption of alcoholic beverages. Symptoms include irritability, headache and nausea. Sometimes, the same feelings result from using certain medications.

Hashimoto's Thyroiditis—One of several kinds of inflammation of the thyroid gland.

Heart Catheterization—Same as *Cardiac Catheterization*.

Heart Murmur—Same as *Murmur*.

Heart Tumors—Rare tumors that grow in the heart wall or in the heart chambers, interfering with normal heart function.

Heart-Lung Machine—Complex mechanical device that provides artificial function of a patient's heart and lungs for a short time during open-heart surgery and heart or lung transplantation.

Hematocrit—Blood test used to detect anemia and other blood disorders. It is expressed as the percentage of blood made up of red blood cells (remainder of the blood is made up of serum or plasma). Normal hematocrit range is approximately 35 to 45%, but it varies with age and sex.

Hematologist—Doctor specially trained to diagnose and treat diseases of the blood and blood-forming organs.

Hemochromatosis—Disease in which excessive iron accumulates in the liver, pancreas and skin, resulting in liver disease, diabetes mellitus and a bronzed skin color.

Hemoglobin, Hemoglobin Range—
1) Component that carries oxygen to body tissues. 2) Blood test used to detect anemia and other blood disorders, expressed in grams per 100 cubic centimeters. The normal hemoglobin range is approximately 12 to 18 grams per 100 cubic centimeters and varies according to age and sex.

Hirschsprung's Disease—Congenital defect of infants in which the colon cannot eliminate feces, resulting in severe constipation.

Histamine—Chemical in body tissues that dilates the smallest blood vessels, constricts the muscle around the bronchial tubes, stimulates stomach secretions and produces an allergic response.

Holter Monitor—Instrument that detects heartbeat-rhythm abnormalities 24 hours or longer. The device is portable for patients to carry wherever they go.

Hormones—Powerful substances manufactured by the endocrine glands and carried by the blood to body tissues and organs. Hormones determine growth and structure of many organs (such as during growth and maturation) and also control many vital body functions.

Host—Person or animal with an infection that has been received from another person, animal or plant, or the environment.

Hyaline-Membrane Disease—Serious condition of premature infants in which the lungs can't expand normally. Cause is unknown.

Hydatidiform Mole—Disease occurring during early pregnancy resulting in death of the fetus and an overgrowth of tissue within the uterus.

Hydraminos and Polyhydraminos—Condition in which amniotic fluid (fluid in the uterus that surrounds the fetus until birth) becomes excessive.

Hygiene—Personal self-care and cleanliness that reduces the risk of infections and diseases.

Hyoid Bone—V-shaped bone located just above the larynx.

Hyperalimentation—Method of supplying total nutritional needs of patients unable to eat normally. The method (usually intravenous or by tube through the nose into the stomach) provides nutrients containing essential proteins, fats, carbohydrates and vitamins.

Hyperbaric Chamber—Large, sealed room in which air pressure can be raised above normal levels. It is used primarily to treat patients with either decompression sickness or severe burns (sometimes).

GLOSSARY

Hypercalcemia—Presence of excessive calcium in the blood, occasionally a sign of malignancy.

Hyperlipoproteinemia—Condition in which excessive lipoproteins (cholesterol and other fatty materials) accumulate in the blood.

Hypermetropia—Seeing distant objects clearly while nearby objects appear blurred; also called farsightedness.

Hypersensitivity—Extreme sensitivity to any agent (drugs, pollens, chemicals, etc.) that causes allergic reactions. Some reactions can be life-threatening, but most are less serious.

Hypnotics—Medications that produce sleep.

Hypochondriasis—Mental illness in which a person is convinced that serious disease is present, despite examination that proves otherwise. The symptoms of the imagined disease seem real to the patient (often called a hypochondriac).

Hypoplastic Anemia (Aplastic Anemia)—Group of anemias that decrease blood-producing bone marrow. This can be life-threatening.

Hypothalamus—Part of the brain that regulates body functions such as temperature, blood pressure, appetite and thirst.

Hysteria—1) Condition in which a person becomes anxious and excitable and experiences impaired sensory and motor abilities. Sometimes, hysterical persons simulate conditions of diseases such as deafness or blindness. 2) Outbreak of uncontrolled emotions, such as fits of laughing or crying.

Hysterosalpingography—Studying the uterus and Fallopian tubes by injecting material into the uterus that X-rays can detect. It is used primarily to determine if the passageway for the ovum (egg) is open all the way to the uterus. The X-ray image is the hysterosalpingogram.

Hysteroscope—An instrument with lens system and lighted tip used in direct visual examination of the cervix and cavity of the uterus.

Hysterostomy—Incision of the uterus to prepare for Cesarean-section delivery of a baby.

I

I-131 Uptake—Measuring thyroid activity with radioactive iodine and radiation emission counters.

Idiopathic—Condition caused by unknown factors.

Ileum—Part of the small intestine just above the large intestine (colon).

Ileus—Condition of the small intestine in which either an obstruction or paralysis prevents material from passing through the intestine.

Iliac Arteries—Large arteries in the inner pelvis that supply blood to the legs.

Immune, Immunity—Resistance or protection against infection by the body's natural defenses. A person may be immune to one kind of infection but not immune to another. Some infections, such as measles, chickenpox or mumps, cause the body to become immune permanently to that infection.

Immune System—Body's system of defense against infection.

Immunization—Producing immunity by giving a vaccine (orally or by injection) of germs that have been altered so they cannot produce significant disease. The vaccine causes the body's immune system to produce antibodies that create immunity.

Immunosuppressants—Drugs used in immunosuppression treatment to weaken the immune system and to inhibit immune response.

Immunosuppression—Prevention of the body from forming a normal immune response. It is used to treat diseases (especially when organs must be transplanted) where certain antibodies must be inactivated.

Impotence—Male's inability to achieve or to sustain an erection or to ejaculate sperm during sexual intercourse.

Incise, Incision—To cut open or cut into.

Incomplete Spontaneous Miscarriage—Naturally occurring miscarriage in which the fetus is expelled, but part of the placenta remains in the uterus. Excessive bleeding and infection can result unless the uterus is emptied, usually by dilatation and curettage of the uterus (D & C) or suction curettage.

GLOSSARY

Incubation Period—The time between exposure to an infecting germ and the appearance of symptoms indicating an infection. Also describes the period of bacterial growth in laboratory cultures.

Infant—Child between the ages of 2 weeks and 1 year.

Infection, Infectious—Disease caused by germs (bacteria, viruses, fungi) that enter the body and cause inflammation or other processes that have an adverse effect on health.

Inflammation, Inflammatory Process—Process by which the body attempts to overcome illness-producing causes such as germs, injuries such as burns, or diseases such as arthritis. The process causes increased body heat (fever or local warmth), swelling, pain and tenderness. If the inflammation is near the skin, redness results.

Inhalation—Breathing air into the lungs.

Inherited—Body characteristic that is transmitted from one generation to the next by chromosomes in the mother's egg and father's sperm. Some inherited characteristics such as brown eyes are normal; others such as Down's syndrome are disorders.

Inoculation—Injection of infected material such as pus into a nutrient medium where the germs will grow, or incubate. They are then stained and analyzed through a microscope. Also describes any kind of immunization.

Insufflation Test—See *Rubin's Insufflation Test.*

Insulin—Hormone produced by the pancreas that helps regulate sugar in the blood and helps produce energy.

Intensive Care Unit (ICU)—Area of a hospital where patients who are seriously ill or recovering from serious surgery are given more care than is available in other hospital units. As soon as the condition improves, the patient is transferred from the ICU to a regular hospital unit.

Intermittent—Happening only occasionally or under certain conditions.

Internist—Doctor specially trained in non-surgical diagnosis and treatment of diseases in adults.

Intervertebral Disk—Cartilage that connects adjacent vertebrae in the spinal column.

Intestinal Tract—All parts of the gastrointestinal tract except the mouth, esophagus and stomach. The intestinal tract organs are: duodenum, small bowel, ileum, cecum, appendix, ascending colon, transverse colon, descending colon, sigmoid colon, rectum and anus.

Intestine, Large—Last major portion of the gastrointestinal tract located just under the small intestine. It is also called the colon or large bowel. It processes waste material into feces, which are stored until eliminated from the body.

Intestine, Small—Longest section of the gastrointestinal tract, located just under the stomach and duodenum. It absorbs digested food into the bloodstream and passes waste material into the large intestine.

Intrauterine Death—Death of a fetus while inside the mother's uterus.

Intrauterine Device (IUD)—Birth-control method in which a small device placed permanently in the uterus prevents growth of fertilized eggs.

Intravenous—Within the vein. Fluids, medications and nutrients that cannot be taken orally are given intravenously by a needle placed in a large vein near the surface of the skin.

Intravenous Pyelogram (IVP)—See *Pyelogram, Intravenous.*

IQ (Intelligence Quotient)—Supposedly a measure of a person's intelligence, rather than what one has learned. Recent research on intelligence raises questions about the accuracy and meaning of the I.Q. test.

Iridectomy—Surgery performed to treat some kinds of glaucoma.

Irrigation—Flooding with water or other liquid. It is used frequently to clean wounds or areas of the body that will undergo surgery.

GLOSSARY

Isolation, Reverse Isolation—Procedures to prevent spread of infection in a hospital. Isolation protects hospital staff and visitors from contracting a contagious disease from a patient. Reverse isolation protects a patient susceptible to infection because of immunosuppression from contracting infection from hospital staff or visitors.

IUD—See *Intrauterine Device.*

J

Jaundice—Yellow skin and whites of the eyes, dark urine and light stools, symptoms of diseases of the liver and blood.

Joint—Structure that enables two or more bones to move easily in relation to each other. A joint consists of ligaments and cartilage that hold bones together.

Joint Capsule—Tough, fibrous tissue that surrounds a joint.

Joint Replacement—Replacement of diseased joints with mechanical joints. The wrist, hip and knee joints are among the most common joints replaced.

K

Ketoacidosis—Serious complication of diabetes mellitus in which the body produces acids that cause fluid and electrolyte disorders, dehydration and sometimes coma.

Klinefelter's Syndrome—Inherited disease of young males in which secondary sex characteristics are underdeveloped. The condition does not become evident until puberty. Mental deficiency and some female characteristics are present.

L

Laceration—Wound with jagged edges.

Lactiferous Ducts—Network of tubes in the female breast that collects milk and delivers it to the nipple.

Laparoscopy—Exploratory examination of the organs inside the abdominal cavity with a laparoscope, an optical instrument with a lighted tip. The laparoscope is inserted into the abdomen through a small incision. Visual examination can then be made of many abdominal organs.

Laparotomy—Exploratory surgery in the abdomen performed to diagnose and sometimes treat abdominal disease.

Laryngeal Nerve—Nerve located in the neck that controls the vocal cords and enables a person to speak.

Larynx—Structure of muscle and cartilage in the upper neck. It contains the vocal cords. Air passes through the larynx into the windpipe and then into the lungs. The "Adam's apple" is part of the larynx.

Laser Therapy—Using a laser beam to treat many diseases. Sharply focused laser light creates intense heat and is valuable in cutting tissue, destroying unwanted tissue and joining tissue together. It is most often used to treat retinal detachment, endometriosis or atherosclerosis.

Latent—Present but inactive; something that exists in an undeveloped form.

Laxatives—Medications used to treat constipation.

Lesion—General term for injury or damage to an organ or tissue.

Lethargy—Fatigue or lack of usual physical or mental energy.

Libido—Sexual desire.

Life Cycle—Growth and development from birth to death.

Ligaments—Strong, flexible cords of tissue near joints that hold bones together and permit bone motion.

Lipoproteins (High Density and Low Density)—Components of the fluid in blood that are measured to help predict the likelihood of atherosclerosis (hardening of the arteries).

Liquid Nitrogen—Nitrogen that has been cooled until it becomes a liquid. It is used most often in cryosurgery.

Local Anesthesia—See *Anesthesia, Local.*

Low-Residue Diet—Diet consisting of foods that are digested almost entirely, leaving minimal material to form feces.

GLOSSARY

Low-Spinal Anesthesia—Also called "saddle-block" anesthesia. An injection into the lower spinal canal provides anesthesia to the lower body.

Lower GI Series—Same as *Barium-Enema X-rays.*

Lumbar Puncture (Spinal Tap)—A diagnostic procedure in which a needle is inserted between 2 bones (vertebra) of the lower spine to collect spinal fluid for laboratory examination.

Lumbar Spine—Lower part of the spine, from the lowest ribs to the bottom of the spine.

Lymph (or Lymphatic) System—Lymph channels and lymph glands considered as a single body system.

Lymph Channels—Tubes of tissue that carry lymph fluid away from tissues and back to the bloodstream. Lymph fluid is composed of proteins and water, varying in composition in different parts of the body.

Lymph Glands—Small collections of tissue (nodes) located along lymph channels in areas such as the elbow, armpit or groin. When infection is present, nearby lymph glands enlarge, become tender and destroy germs that enter lymph channels. Lymph glands also manufacture antibodies to help fight infection.

Lymphangiogram, Lymphangiography—Diagnostic method of studying the lymphatic system by infecting a material into the lymph channels that X-rays can detect. The image on X-ray film is the lymphangiogram.

Lymphatic Leukemia—Class of leukemias, involving primarily lymphatic cells, affecting children and adults.

Lymphocytes—One of several types of white blood cells that help fight infection.

Lymphosarcoma—Class of cancers of the lymphatic system.

M

Macular Degeneration of the Eye—Condition of the macula (area on the retina that provides detailed vision) in which impaired blood supply causes gradual vision loss.

Macule—General term for any discolored spot or patch on the skin, such as a freckle.

Malignant—Capable of causing great harm, including death. It usually refers to cancerous growth.

Mammogram, Mammography—Diagnostic method of studying the female breast by an X-ray technique that detects cancerous growths while they are still treatable. The image on X-ray film is the mammogram.

Manic-Depressive Illness—Mental illness in which behavior alternates between unrealistic enthusiasm and deep depression.

MAO Inhibitors—See *Monamine Oxidase Inhibitors.*

Marijuana—Mood-altering substance that is usually taken into the body by smoking. It is derived from Indian hemp or Cannabis leaves, stems and seed pods.

Marrow—Core of many bones, where most of the body's blood cells are produced.

Mastoiditis—Infection of the mastoid (bony area just behind the ear).

Mediators—Substances that: 1) help nerve impulses travel from one cell to the next; 2) participate in the allergic process.

Medic Alert—Non-profit agency that maintains a medical-record system. Subscribers receive a bracelet or pendant that states their medical condition and provides a toll-free number for more information. The service can save the life of a person with a major medical condition who may not be able to provide medical history. For information write: Medic Alert Foundation, P.O. Box 1009, Tulock, CA 95381.

Medical History—Essential facts about past and present medical conditions. Knowing your medical history enables your doctor to plan the best possible health care. Carry a card stating essential health details in your purse or wallet, and consider joining the Medic-Alert program (see above).

Meibomian Glands—Small glands on the inner eyelid. They secrete a fluid that helps the eyelids move easily over the surface of the eye.

Membrane—Thin tissue lining a body cavity, covering an internal organ or dividing a space.

Meninges—Three-layered membrane covering the brain.

Mental System (Mind)—Functions of the brain that provide the abilities to perceive surroundings, to have emotions, imagination, memory, will, and to process information.

Metastases—Cancerous cells or infectious germs that spread from their original location to other parts of the body.

Metatarsal Bones—Bones in the middle of the foot.

Midwife—Nurse with special training and experience in childbirth.

Mole—Skin lesion, often dark-brown or black.

Monamine Oxidase (MAO) Inhibitors—Medications used to treat some forms of depression.

Motor Nerve—Nerve that transmits the stimulus that causes muscles to contract.

Mucous Membrane—Thin tissue lining internal cavities (nose, mouth, vagina) and tubular systems (respiratory and gastrointestinal) that produce mucus.

Mucus—Slippery liquid produced by the lining of internal cavities and tubular systems to protect tissue.

Murmur—Sound of blood rushing through the heart and blood vessels, detected by a stethoscope. Some murmurs are innocent, meaning they are not caused by disease. Other murmurs arise from heart disease or partial obstruction in the arteries.

Muscle—Tissue that contracts, often with considerable force, when stimulated by the motor-nerve impulses.

Muscle Relaxants—Medications that relieve muscle spasms. They also can have significant side effects.

Muscle Tumors—Benign or cancerous tumors arising from muscle tissue.

Musculo-Skeletal System—The system of bones, muscles, ligaments and tendons that enable the body to move.

Myelogram—Special X-ray of the spinal canal and spinal cord, requiring a spinal tap and injection of dye that is visible on X-ray film. Myelograms frequently are used to identify the location of ruptured disks.

Myoma—Tumor of the muscle.

Myopia—Disease of the eye in which close objects are clearly visible while distant objects are blurred. Also called nearsightedness.

N

Narcotics—Medications used to control severe pain. Narcotics should be used only when necessary because of their serious side effects: addiction; reduced breathing; nausea and vomiting; low blood pressure; reduced cough reflex; and constipation.

Naso-Gastric Tube—Slender tube passed through the nose into the stomach. It is used to drain away stomach secretions or to feed patients unable to eat normally.

Naturopathy—Health-care system relying on diet, sunshine, exercises, herbs and other non-medicinal treatment.

Nausea—Unpleasant sensation of being about to vomit.

Nearsightedness—Same as *Myopia*.

Nebulizer—Device for administering medications used to treat asthma and similar conditions. It converts medication into a fine mist that is inhaled deeply into the lungs.

Nerve-Block Local Anesthesia—See *Anesthesia, Nerve Block or Local.*

Nerve-Conduction Test—Diagnostic test that measures the rate at which an electrical impulse moves along a nerve. It is used to diagnose disorders of the peripheral nerves and muscle.

Nervous Breakdown—Non-technical term for mental illness serious enough to interfere with daily activities.

Neuritis—Inflammation of a nerve.

Neurological—Relating to the body's nervous system.

Neurologist—Doctor specially trained to diagnose and treat diseases of the nervous system.

Neuroma—Tumor arising from nerve tissue.

Neuro-Muscular System—Nerves and muscles acting together as a system to control body movements.

Neurosis—Mental illness in which anxiety is controlled by avoidance, blaming others, developing bodily complaints or other mechanisms.

Neurosurgeon—Doctor specially trained to diagnose and treat surgically diseases of the brain, spinal cord and nerves.

Nodes—See *Lymph Glands.*

Nodule—Small, rounded lump or firm swelling underneath the skin.

Non-Steroidal Anti-Inflammatory Drugs—Medications that control inflammation other than that caused by infection. Usually used to treat conditions of the joints and muscles and pain such as menstrual cramps or headache. "Non-steroidal" means they are not steroid hormones such as cortisone, prednisone, dextramethasone and others.

Nurse Practitioner (NP)—Registered nurse with additional medical training who can diagnose and treat common illness. Nurse practitioners usually work closely with a doctor, although in some states the practitioner can prescribe medicine and work independently of a physician.

Nutrient—Food or material containing elements needed to promote growth and development or to support life.

O

Obsessions—Unpleasant, frightening, senseless thoughts that won't go away despite reasoning.

Obstetrician-Gynecologist—Doctor specially trained to treat diseases of the female reproductive system and provide health care for pregnant mothers.

Obstructive Pulmonary Disease—See *COPD (Chronic Obstructive Pulmonary Disease)*.

Occlusion—Closing or obstruction. Usually used to describe blockage in blood vessels. In dentistry, it means the way the teeth come together when the mouth is closed.

Oncologist—Doctor specially trained to diagnose and treat cancer.

Operative Death Rate—Percentage of patients who die as a result of a certain surgery. It provides general measure of the risk of a surgery.

Ophthalmologist—Doctor specially trained to diagnose and treat diseases of the eyes.

Optic Neuritis—Inflammation of the nerve that conducts vision impulses from the eye to the brain.

Oral—Relating to the mouth.

Oral-Fecal—See *Fecal-Oral*.

Organic—Conditions or diseases resulting from change in body organs that can be measured or seen. Organic diseases are distinct from functional diseases in which no change can be observed in an organ that is not functioning normally.

Organic Psychosis—Mental illness that results from disease in the brain.

Orthodontia—Straightening teeth by applying temporary braces.

Orthopedic Surgeon (Orthopedist)—Doctor specially trained to diagnose and treat diseases of the muscles, bones and joints using surgical or mechanical means. A *rheumatologist* is an internist who diagnoses and treats similar conditions primarily with medications and other non-surgical means.

Osteogenesis Imperfecta—Inherited condition in which the bones are brittle and easily broken.

Otorhinolaryngologist or Otolaryngologist—See *Ear, Nose and Throat Specialist*.

Ovary—Female sexual gland where eggs mature and ripen for fertilization.

Ovulation—Monthly process in which an egg leaves the ovary for possible fertilization by a sperm cell.

Ovum—Egg produced by the ovary.

P

Pain—Unpleasant sensation arising from stimulation of sensory nerves located in almost every part of the body. Disease, injury and strenuous activity can all cause pain.

Palate—Roof of the mouth, consisting of a bony front portion (hard palate), and a soft back portion (soft palate).

Palpitations—Irregular rapid heartbeat, noticeable to the patient.

Pancreas—Organ located on the back abdominal wall that produces and secretes digestive juices into the small intestine. It also produces and secretes insulin into the bloodstream to regulate the level of sugar and other nutrients.

Pap Smear—Test done to detect cancer of the cervix in an early and treatable stage.

GLOSSARY

Papule—Small, raised skin lesion. Papules may be red, brown, yellow, white or skin-colored. They may be flat-topped, pointed or dome-shaped.

Paranoia—Mental illness in which a person believes that he or she is being talked about or plotted against.

Parasite—Organism that lives within, upon or at the expense of another living organism. Human parasites include disease-causing agents such as amoebas or worms that infect the digestive system, or fungi that live on the skin.

Parasympathetic Nervous System—System of nerves that controls digestion, heartbeat, and relaxation or contraction of small muscles.

Parathyroid Glands—Small glands that control calcium levels in the blood and bones. They are located within or next to the thyroid glands at the base of the neck.

Passive Exercises—Exercises in which a therapist moves the arms and legs of a patient while the patient relaxes. These exercises keep the joints limber until the patient is able to move without assistance.

Patency—Blood vessels or any hollow organs that clog or become blocked are said to lose their patency.

Pathological—Relating to an abnormal condition.

Pathological Examination—Laboratory study of abnormal tissue to establish or confirm a diagnosis.

Pediatrician—Doctor specially trained to care for children and adolescents, especially to foster normal growth and development.

Pediculicide—Medication that cures body lice (pediculosis). Usually applied to the skin.

Pelvic Examination—Examination of a woman's reproductive organs to diagnose pregnancy or detect diseases.

Pelvic Ultrasonography—Examination of a woman's reproductive organs that uses high-frequency sound waves to create an image. It is used to determine the age, size and position of a fetus in the uterus or to diagnose disease of the pelvic organs.

Pelvis—Lower part of the trunk of the body.

Penis—Male organ used for urination and sexual intercourse.

Perforation—Abnormal hole or opening.

Perforation, Intestinal—Complication of conditions such as ulcers, cancers, or injury to the digestive system. When this occurs, intestinal contents enter the abdominal cavity, causing severe inflammation.

Perfusionist—Medical technician who controls the heart-lung machine to sustain a patient's life during open-heart and lung-transplant surgery.

Perineum—Area between the vulva and anus in females, and between the scrotum and anus in males.

Peripheral Nervous System—Nerves that connect to all parts of the body and carry information via electrical impulses to and from the brain and spinal cord.

Peripheral Vascular System—Network of arteries, veins and lymphatic channels supplying the head, arms and legs.

Perirectal—Skin and underlying tissue around the rectum.

Peristalsis—Rhythmic movements of hollow muscular organs (such as the intestines) that move contents (such as digestive material) in one direction.

Peritoneal Cavity—Space enclosed by the peritoneum.

Peritoneum—Very thin, two-layered tissue. One layer lines the outer surface of all the abdominal organs. The other layer lines the abdominal wall.

Peritonsillar Abscess—Abscess forming in the back of the throat near the tonsils.

Pessary—Small ring-shaped device that is inserted into the vagina to help maintain the uterus in a normal position.

pH Balance—Measure of blood's acidity or alkalinity. The pH is controlled by body fluids and electrolytes. Body tissues cannot function normally if the pH varies from a limited range.

Phenothiazine Drugs—Medications used to slow and regulate mental-system activity. Usually used to treat anxiety and other mental conditions; also useful in producing sleep.

Phlebotomy—Removing blood from the blood vessels. This was once believed to cure many diseases; today, it is done to remove blood for diagnostic testing.

Phobia—Fear that cannot be overcome by reason.

GLOSSARY

Physical Therapy—Treatment of diseases of the bone, muscular and nervous systems to help restore normal function after disease or injury.

Physician's Assistant (PA)—Someone trained to do some of the simpler tasks ordinarily performed by a doctor. The PA works under the direction of the doctor.

Pilocarpine—Medication used principally in eye drops to treat glaucoma.

Pituitary Gland—Small endocrine gland at the base of the brain that controls growth and regulates other endocrine glands.

Placenta—Disk-shaped organ that attaches and grows inside the uterus during pregnancy. It enables the fetus to receive nutrients from and transfer natural wastes to the mother's bloodstream. The umbilical cord connects the placenta to the fetus.

Plaque—1) Small raised area of abnormal material on a surface such as the skin or lining of a blood vessel. 2) Mixture of bacteria and calcium deposited on the teeth that can cause cavities and gum diseases.

Plasma—Liquid part of blood that remains when blood cells are removed.

Plastic and Reconstructive Surgeon (Plastic Surgeon)—Doctor specially trained to perform plastic and reconstructive surgery.

Plastic and Reconstructive Surgery—Special surgery to repair and change body parts to improve function or appearance. The face, hands, breasts and skin are areas most frequently treated.

Platelet Count—Platelets are blood cells (much smaller than red or white blood cells) that assist in the blood-clotting process. A drop of blood contains about 12.5 million platelets. A platelet count determines if the number of platelets is normal.

Pleura—Thin tissue lining the lungs and chest cavity. Inflammation of the pleura (pleurisy) is a painful condition caused by lung diseases.

Pleural Effusion (Pleural Fluid Effusion)—Fluid that collects around the lungs, usually caused by inflammation of the lungs and pleura or congestive-heart failure.

Podiatrist—Health-care professional trained in the medical and surgical treatment of foot diseases.

Polyp—A growth, often on a stalk arising from dry mucous membranes, such as in the nose, cervix or colon.

Portal-Vein System—Veins that drain blood from the gastrointestinal system. The smaller veins empty into the portal vein, which transports blood into the liver.

Postmature Infant—Infant that spends 3 weeks or more beyond the normal 39 weeks of pregnancy in the womb.

Postoperative—Period of recuperation and return to normal health after surgery.

Postural Drainage—Exercises and body positions that promote drainage of fluid and secretions that collect in the lungs and airways.

Potassium—Electrolyte present in all body cells, blood and body fluids. Potassium is important in maintaining normal heart contractions and the strength and contractions of all muscles. Foods high in potassium include: dried apricots and peaches; whole-grain cereals; plain cocoa; dried lentils and peas; bananas; and molasses.

Precancerous—Characteristic of a growth that has the potential to become cancerous.

Predisposition—Tendency. For example, a person who gets many infections has a predisposition to infection.

Premature Labor—Labor beginning before the usual 39 weeks of pregnancy.

Presbyopia—Form of nearsightedness that normally accompanies aging.

Primary Disorder—Basic disease that may result in complications. Diabetes mellitus, for example, is a primary disorder that often causes secondary complications involving the kidneys, blood vessels and eyes.

Proctoscope, Proctoscopy—Method of examining the rectum and lower part of the colon with a proctoscope, an optical instrument with a lighted tip.

Prolapse—Pushing or falling out of a part or an organ from its normal position.

Prolapsed (Dropped) Uterus—Uterus that has moved from its normal position because of loose pelvic muscles and ligaments. In severe cases, it can protrude completely outside the vagina.

Prophylaxis—Measures taken to prevent an illness.

GLOSSARY

Prophylaxis, Dental—Regular care (including cleaning) of the teeth and gums that helps prevent tooth decay and gum inflammation.

Prostaglandins—Natural substances found in semen, menstrual fluid and many body tissues. They are involved in basic body functions such as inflammation, immune response and activities of the lungs, heart, kidneys, uterus and digestive system.

Prostate (Prostate Gland)—Male sex gland located at the base of the urinary bladder. It produces a fluid that is added to sperm to produce semen.

Prosthesis—Artificial device used as a substitute for a missing or badly functioning part of the body.

Prothrombin Time—Test to measure one of the components of the body's blood-clotting mechanism. It is used to diagnose clotting diseases and to control blood-thinning (anticoagulation) in treatment of some diseases of the heart and blood vessels.

Psychiatrist—Doctor specially trained to diagnose and treat mental illnesses.

Psychoanalysis—Treatment of some mental illness that involves a detailed understanding of how past events in a person's life may have resulted in mental disturbances.

Psychologist—Health-care professional specially trained to diagnose and treat some kinds of mental illness.

Psychopathy—Psychological or mental illness.

Psychosis—Mental illness characterized by deranged personality, loss of contact with reality, and possible delusions, hallucinations or illusions.

Psychosocial—Influences of society on growth and development.

Psychosomatic Illness—Illness in which thoughts and emotions play an important role.

Psychotherapist—Professional specially trained to diagnose and treat some mental illnesses.

Puberty—Period in early adolescence when hormonal changes bring about full sexual maturity and capacity to reproduce.

Pubic Bone—One of the bones of the pelvis located above the genitals in both sexes.

Pulmonary—Relating to the lungs and breathing.

Pulmonary Hypertension—Increased pressure in the blood vessels of the lungs.

Pulse—Heartbeat (contraction of the heart) as felt in an artery. Heart rate is often measured by counting the pulse felt in the artery in the wrist.

Pus—Thick fluid, usually green or yellow, that forms to fight local infection. Pus often collects in an enclosed sac, an abscess, at the site of an infection.

Pyelogram, Intravenous—Method of studying the kidneys and urinary tract by injecting into the bloodstream a medication that X-rays can detect.

Pyelogram, Retrograde—Method of studying the kidneys, similar to an intravenous pyelogram, but in which the medication detected by X-rays is placed in the urinary system by a catheter inserted through the bladder into the ureters.

R

Radiation Therapy or Treatment—Use of high-energy waves (generated by special X-ray machines, cobalt machines and other devices) to treat some forms of cancer. Radiation destroys cancerous tissue but does little harm to healthy tissue.

Radioactive Chromium Studies—Diagnostic method used to measure total blood in the body.

Radioactive Iodine Uptake and Scan—Same as *Thyroid Scan*.

Radioactive Studies—Same as *Radioisotope Studies*.

Radioactive Technetium 99 Scan—Radioisotope scan method used to diagnose some disorders of the heart, liver, spleen and other organs.

Radioisotope—Radioactive form of chemicals normally present in the body.

Radioisotope Scan—Scan of radioisotopes given orally or intravenously to a patient that become concentrated in organs such as the heart, lungs or brain. Instruments measure the radiation given off by the radioisotopes and create a photographic image of the organ being studied.

GLOSSARY

Radioisotope Studies—Radioisotopes are chemical elements that give off radiation. A radioisotope of a chemical element normally present in the body (such as carbon), if injected into the body, will mix with the non-isotopes. The body doesn't know the difference, but radiation from the isotopes can be detected with special instruments. Determining where radioisotopes go in the body allows diagnosis of diseases that cannot be detected otherwise.

Radioisotope Therapy—Treatment of some cancers with radioisotopes.

Radiologist—Doctor specially trained to use X-rays and other kinds of radiation in diagnosis and treatment.

Recovery Room—Specially equipped and staffed area of a hospital for observing and caring for patients who have just undergone surgery. Postoperative patients usually remain in the recovery room until they are awake and their vital signs (blood pressure, pulse and respiration) are satisfactory.

Rectum—End of the large intestine, located in the pelvis below the sigmoid colon and above the anus.

Regenerate—Ability of some parts of the body to grow back to normal after being damaged.

Regurgitate—To vomit.

Relapse—Stage of illness in which the patient gets worse after having improved.

Remission—Stage of a chronic illness when the patient's condition improves.

Renal Dialysis—Mechanical and chemical method of removing normal wastes from the body of a patient whose kidneys cannot function adequately. It is also used to remove harmful poison or a drug overdose from the bloodstream.

Reproductive Organs, Female—Organs of a woman's body that enable her to become pregnant and deliver a baby. The major organs are the vagina, uterus, Fallopian tubes and ovaries.

Reproductive Organs, Male—Organs of a man's body that enable him to produce sperm and impregnate the woman. The major organs are the penis, testicles, seminal vesicles and prostate gland.

Reproductive System—Body system enabling impregnation and delivery of a baby. It also provides characteristic male or female appearance.

Resect—Surgical removal of a part of the body.

Respiratory-Distress Syndrome—A condition of newborn infants (often born prematurely) in which the lungs cannot supply adequate oxygen to the body.

Retained Placenta—Condition occurring immediately after childbirth in which part of the placenta remains attached to the uterus, creating a risk of serious bleeding or infection.

Retina—Light-sensitive part of the eye at the back of the eyeball on which the lens focuses images. The retina converts the image to impulses that go to the brain.

Retinal-Vein Occlusion—Condition in which a clot forms in the vein supplying the retina with blood.

Retinoblastoma—Cancerous tumor that forms in the eye of an infant.

Retrovirus—Group of viruses that cause AIDS (Acquired Immunodeficiency Syndrome) and some types of lymphoma and leukemia.

Rh Negative Blood—A subtype of red blood cells. Blood subtypes are inherited. The major subtypes are types A, B, O and Rh negative.

Rheumatologist—A specialist in internal medicine who subspecializes in medical diagnosis and treatment of rheumatic and arthritic disorders..

Rinne Test—Test using a tuning fork to diagnose hearing disorders.

Rubin's Insufflation Test—Test used in diagnosing fertility problems in women. A harmless gas is introduced into the uterus to determine if there is a blockage in the Fallopian tubes.

S

Sacroiliac Region—Area of the lower back where the spine meets the pelvic bone.

Saline—Salt-containing solution similar to normal body fluid that is given intravenously to help correct fluid and electrolyte imbalances.

GLOSSARY

Salivary Glands—Glands located inside the mouth around the jaw that secrete saliva into the mouth.

Saphenous-Femoral Vein System—Network of large veins in the legs that helps return blood from the leg to the inferior vena cava, then to the heart.

Scale, Scaling—Flakes of dried skin which form as whitish skin lesions.

Schizophrenia—Mental illness characterized by a distorted sense of reality, bizarre behavior and fragmentation of the personality.

Sciatic Nerve—Large nerve that begins at the base of the spine and passes through the buttocks down the back side of the thigh and down the leg.

Sciatica—Painful condition resulting from irritation of the sciatic nerve.

Scleritis—Inflammation of the sclera (the white of the eye).

Scoliosis—Curvature of the spine.

Scopolamine—Medication used to treat hyperactive or spastic conditions of the digestive system and to prevent motion sickness.

Scrotum—Organ of the male reproductive system that contains the testicles, blood vessels and the vas deferens.

Scurvy—Disease of bones, gums and blood vessels caused by a deficiency of vitamin C.

Second Molars—Permanent grinding teeth that appear at about age 11 to 13.

Secondary Infection—Infection that results from some other problem. It may occur after surgery or develop during antibiotic treatment of another infection.

Sedative—Medication used to produce relaxation or sleep.

Sedative-Hypnotics—Class of medications that help relieve anxiety and promote sleep.

Sedimentation Rate—Blood test measuring the rate that blood settles in a test tube. It identifies infection, inflammation or tissue damage.

Self-Care—Treatment that patients can administer for themselves.

Seminal Vesicles—Small sacs next to the prostate that help make and store seminal fluid, and contract to eject semen.

Senile Dementia—Permanent loss of mental functions of older persons, resulting from conditions such as Alzheimer's disease and atherosclerosis (hardening of the arteries).

Senile Keratosis—Same as *Seborrheic Keratoses*. (See Illness section.)

Sensitivity Studies (Antibiotics)—Laboratory method of determining which antibiotic will most likely be successful in treating infections caused by bacteria.

Sensory—Ability to feel or experience sensations such as sound, light or pain.

Septic—Infected.

Serological Tests—Tests of serum (blood without cells) used to diagnose a variety of diseases, especially infections and autoimmune conditions.

Serum—Liquid portion of blood that remains after blood cells and blood clots have been removed.

Serum Alkaline Phosphatase—Material present in excessive amounts in the blood of patients with some bone and liver diseases.

Serum Electrolytes—Same as *Electrolytes*.

Sesamoid Bones—Small oval-shaped bones in the tendons of the hands and feet.

Sever's Disease—Painful condition of the heel bone of growing children.

Sexual Dysfunction—Inability to participate in sexual relations that are satisfactory for both partners.

Shave Biopsy—Procedure to diagnose skin disorders in which a thin layer of tissue from under a skin lesion is shaved away for laboratory examination.

Shock—Condition in which the blood pressure falls below the level needed to supply blood to the body. Signs and symptoms include weakness, paleness, rapid heartbeat, dry mouth, cold sweat and feelings of doom.

Sick-Sinus Syndrome—Form of heart-rhythm disorder (arrhythmia).

Sigmoid Colon—Lower part of the large colon (intestine) located in the pelvis just above the rectum.

Sigmoidoscope, Sigmoidoscopy—Same as *Proctoscope, Proctoscopy*.

GLOSSARY

Signs—Evidence of disease that can be observed and measured, in contrast to *symptoms,* which only patients can experience. For example, blood-pressure measurement or red tonsils are *signs;* headache or nausea are *symptoms.*

Silicone—Artificial compound used by plastic and reconstructive surgeons to reshape parts of the body, such as the breast.

Silver Nitrate—Chemical used for cautery.

Sims-Huhner Test—Test used in diagnosis of reasons for infertility in women in which the mucus from the cervix is examined, especially for presence of sperm after sexual intercourse.

Skin Clips—Small U-shaped metal strips used instead of stitches to close skin that has been incised during surgery.

Skin Tests for Allergy—Diagnostic method used to determine whether a particular substance is causing allergic reactions. The test is carried out by introducing a small amount of the suspected material, such as pollen or dust, under the skin or on the skin. If inflammation results, the patient is allergic to the material.

Sleep Inducers—Medications used to produce sleep.

Sleep-Study Laboratory—Laboratory where persons are studied with sensitive instruments while asleep. Information from sleep study aids in diagnosis of sleep disorders.

Slow Viruses—Group of viruses that infect the brain but do not cause disease until many years afterward.

Soaks—Applying moisture—either plain water or water with dissolved medicines—to an inflamed area of the skin.

Soft Palate—Fleshy part of the roof of the mouth close to the throat.

Sonogram, Sonography—Diagnostic method in which high-frequency (ultrasound) sound waves are transmitted into the body. Their reflections create images of body organs.

Spasmodic—Sudden intermittent symptom, or intermittent muscle spasm.

Spastic, Spasticity—A description of muscles that are continuously contracting and in a state of excessive tension.

Speculum—Instrument used to examine the interior of openings such as the vagina, nose, ear or rectum.

Sperm—Male reproductive cells manufactured in testicles and ejaculated in semen.

Spherocytosis—Abnormally shaped red blood cells caused by some anemias. These cells are sphere-shaped, in contrast to the doughnut shape of normal red blood cells.

Spikes, Temperature—High but brief episodes of fever.

Spina Bifida—Congenital (inherited) disorder in which the base of the spine remains open, sometimes exposing the spinal cord and nerves.

Spinal Anesthesia—Method to provide anesthesia to the lower body by injecting an anesthetic into the fluid in the space that surrounds the lower spinal cord.

Spirometry—Test of lung (pulmonary) function.

Spleen—A large organ in the upper abdomen on the left side, located close to the left side of the stomach. It is the largest structure of the lymph system. The spleen causes disintegration of old red blood cells in adults, manufactures red blood cells in the fetus and newborn, and serves as an important reservoir of blood.

Splenic-Vein Thrombosis—Clot in the major vein that carries blood away from the spleen.

Splints—Rigid supports, made of metal, plastic or plaster, used to immobilize an injured or inflamed part of the body. Splints are used temporarily in the case of injury, following some surgical procedures on joints or ligaments, or occasionally in the case of arthritis.

Spore—Microscopic seed form of fungi. Spores are extremely hardy, and survive extremes of temperature. If they enter the body of a susceptible person, they can cause fungal disease.

Sputum—Secretion of the lungs, coughed up in large amounts in some lung diseases.

Staphylococcus—Bacteria which frequently cause boils, abscesses, pneumonias, bone infections and infections in other tissues or organs.

GLOSSARY

Staples—Small U-shaped metal wires used in place of stitches to close incised skin after some surgeries, especially in the digestive system. Also used to close off some portions of the stomach during operations for extreme obesity.

Sterilized—1) Made completely free of all germs, usually by steam heat, toxic gas or chemicals. All instruments used in surgeries are sterilized, as is most other medical equipment. 2) Made unable to conceive children.

Steroids—Medications which resemble hormones produced by the cortex of the adrenal glands, ovaries and testicles.

Stethoscope—Instrument used to listen to the sounds produced by the heart, lungs, blood vessels and pregnant uterus.

Still's Disease—Form of arthritis in children similar to rheumatoid arthritis in adults.

Stimulant Drugs—Medications that increase the activity of the brain and nervous system.

Stomatitis—Inflammation of the mouth.

Stool—Feces.

Streptococcus—Bacteria that cause illnesses such as laryngitis, cellulitis of the skin, pneumonia, meningitis and others. If not treated, streptococcal infections may also cause serious heart and kidney diseases as complications that appear after the original infection has cleared.

Sublingual Salivary Glands—Small glands near the base of the tongue that secrete saliva into the mouth.

Submaxillary Salivary Glands—Small glands near the jaw that secrete saliva into the mouth.

Sulfonamides (Sulfa Drugs)—Class of drugs used to fight infections.

Sulfonurea Drugs—Medications taken orally to treat some forms of diabetes mellitus.

Surgery—Treatment in which the body is restored to a healthy condition by physical methods (or operations) such as cutting, removing, replacing, straightening, repairing or joining.

Surgical Suite—Group of rooms used to perform surgery. In addition to operating rooms, where surgery takes place, there are supply areas, a recovery room, administrative rooms and a lounge for the staff to rest between surgeries.

Suture—Thread-like material used to hold tissues or skin edges together.

Symmetry, Symmetrical—Refers to the arrangement of the body in pairs, such as two arms, legs, kidneys, lungs, etc.

Sympathomimetics—Medications similar to adrenalin in their actions.

Symptoms—Effects of disease that only the patient can experience, such as pain, nausea, dizziness, anxiety, depression and others.

Synovial Membranes—Delicate tissue that lines the inside of joints.

Systemic—Conditions that affect most or all of the body, in contrast to conditions that affect only a limited area. For example, diabetes mellitus is a systemic condition; an abscess is a local condition.

T

Tartar—Hard deposit that forms on the teeth and causes inflammation of the gums.

Temperature Spike—See *Spikes, Temperature.*

Temporo-Mandibular Joint—Joint that joins the jaw to the other head bones.

Tenderness—Condition that causes pain when pressure is applied.

Tendon—Tough cord of tissue at the end of muscles that attach to bone. Tendons transmit the force of muscle contraction to cause movement.

Testes or Testicles—Male sex glands that produce sex hormones and sperm.

Therapeutic Trial—Form of diagnosis and treatment where medication is used even though the diagnosis is not firmly established. If the patient improves after treatment with a medication known to be useful in treating a specific condition, the improvement suggests that the specific disease was present. Therapeutic trials are somewhat risky and are used only when other forms of diagnosis and treatment have failed.

GLOSSARY

Therapist—Health-care professional specially trained to provide therapy.

Thermogram, Thermography—Method of diagnosis that measures body heat. The area being studied is scanned by a heat-sensitive instrument capable of producing an image (thermogram) of areas of increased heat. They are useful in studying female breast tumors and some blood-vessel conditions.

Thiazide Diuretics—Class of medications that promote excretion of excess fluids by the kidneys.

Third Molars—Permanent grinding teeth that appear at about age 17 to 25.

Thoracic Duct—The largest channel of the lymphatic system through which lymph fluid enters the vena cava.

Thoracic Spine—That part of the spinal column below the neck and above the back. Ribs attach to the thoracic spine.

Thoracic Surgeon—A surgeon who specializes in surgical treatment of disorders of the organs in the thorax (chest), including lungs, pericardium, heart, pleura (covering of lungs), bronchial tubes and large blood vessels.

Thyroglossal Duct—Small passageway, normally closed, located in the upper neck. It extends from the back of the tongue to just above the larynx. If an abnormally open duct becomes filled with fluid, a *thyroglossal cyst* results.

Thyroid Cartilage—Larynx (also called the voice box, or Adam's apple), made of semihard cartilage.

Thyroid Gland—Endocrine gland located in the lower neck next to the trachea that produces hormones that regulate the rate at which all body cells function. Thyroid hormones are also essential for normal growth and development.

Thyroid Scan—Method of examination of the thyroid gland in which a small amount of radioactive iodine introduced into the body collects in the thyroid gland. An instrument passed over the thyroid produces an image of the gland based on the concentration of the radioactive iodine.

Ticks—Small biting insects that may cause inflammation of the skin or serious infections such as Rocky Mountain Spotted Fever.

Tics—Brief, uncontrollable muscle spasms.

Tissue—Building blocks of body organs; living cells all of one type.

Tonsils—Lymphatic tissues that help fight infection located at the entrance of the throat. They frequently become infected, especially in children.

Topical—Medications applied to the skin, conjunctiva, or mucous membrane of the mouth, nose, vagina or rectum.

Tourniquet—Cord or band wrapped around an arm or leg tightly enough to stop blood circulation temporarily.

Toxic, Toxicity—Harmful; capable of causing body damage.

Toxin—Poison. Usually refers to the chemicals produced by some living organisms that harm the human body.

Traction—Method of treating some conditions of bones, muscles, and ligaments by exerting a steady pull on the affected parts. Some bone fractures and back pain due to a ruptured disk are treated this way.

Tranquilizer—Medication used to help diminish anxiety and to produce calmness.

Tranquilizers, Benzodiazepine—Class of tranquilizers commonly used to treat anxiety, nervousness or tension.

Transfuse—To give a patient blood, necessary in treatment of some conditions.

Transfusion—Process of introducing blood through a needle placed in the patient's vein.

Transfusion Reaction—Undesirable symptom or condition resulting from a blood transfusion.

Transmission, Transmit—Passing a disease to another person.

Transplant—Living organ (such as kidney, cornea, heart, bone marrow or skin), removed from one person (donor), and placed in the body of another (recipient).

Transverse Colon—Middle part of the colon (intestine), lying horizontally in the middle or upper abdomen.

Trauma—Force that injures or damages any part of the body.

Tricyclic Antidepressant Drugs (Tricyclics)—Class of medications used to treat depression.

Trophoblastic Tumors—See *Hydatidiform Mole.*

GLOSSARY

Tube Feeding—Providing nutrients through a small tube placed in the stomach of patients who are unable to eat. The tube may pass through the nose to the stomach or be inserted through an incision in the stomach.

Tuberous Sclerosis—Rare inherited condition of the skin, nervous system and other organs of the body.

Tumor—Literally, a swelling; usually used to refer to a benign or cancerous growth.

U

Ulceration—Wearing away of the surface or lining of an organ, exposing underlying tissue. Ulceration of the lining of the stomach exposes blood vessels, which may bleed. Ulceration may erode through the wall of an organ (perforation). Ulceration frequently affects the skin, if rubbed excessively or if diseased.

Ultrasonography—See *Sonography*.

Ultrasound Treatment—Method of treatment in which high-energy sound waves are focused on the affected area, producing mild heat that helps relieve inflammation. It is especially useful in treatment of muscular symptoms.

Underlying—Beneath, below or more basic. Thus, losing weight may result from an underlying condition such as diabetes mellitus or cancer.

Upper Gastrointestinal Series—X-ray examination of the esophagus, stomach and duodenum accomplished by having the patient swallow barium solution that X-rays can detect.

Upper Respiratory System—Upper part of the breathing system, consisting of the nose, throat, larynx, trachea and bronchial tubes.

Uremia—A serious condition associated with kidney failure in which body wastes build up in the blood and body tissues.

Ureters—Slender muscular tubes that carry urine from the kidneys to the urinary bladder, where it is stored until eliminated from the body.

Urethra—Tubular passageway extending from the urinary bladder to the outside of the body.

Uric Acid—Chemical normally produced in the body from metabolism or breakdown of protein and eliminated in the urine. If the level of uric acid rises in the body as a result of disease, gout or kidney stones may result.

Urinalysis—Laboratory test performed on a urine sample that helps diagnose diseases of the kidney and other parts of the body.

Urinary Bladder—Muscular sac in the lower abdomen that stores urine brought to it from the kidneys by the ureters. The bladder stores urine until it can be eliminated through the urethra by contractions of the bladder muscles.

Urinary Studies—Laboratory or X-ray tests of the urinary tract.

Urinary Tract—Organs that produce, store and eliminate urine. The organs are the kidneys, ureters, urinary bladder and urethra.

Uterus—Organ of the female reproductive system on the wall of which the fertilized egg (ovum) attaches and develops to form a fetus.

Uveitis—Inflammation of the parts of the eyes that make up the iris (the colored tissue encircling the clear center—the pupil).

Uvula—Soft tissue hanging down from the soft palate at the back of the throat.

V

Vaccination—Method of providing protection against disease (immunity) by giving a patient a small amount of the disease-causing germ that is weakened, killed or otherwise modified so that it cannot itself cause disease. Same as *Immunization*.

Vaccine—Medication used to provide immunity by vaccination. Vaccines are given mostly by injection or by mouth.

Vagus Nerve—Long cranial nerve, arising in the base of the brain and passing to the chest and abdomen. It helps regulate heart rate, breathing, swallowing, digestion and many other body functions.

Varicose—Swollen and twisting, usually used to describe varicose veins.

Vas Deferens—Tube that carries sperm manufactured by the testicles toward the prostate gland and seminal vesicles.

Vasculitis—Inflammation of blood vessels, the basis of many illnesses.

GLOSSARY

Vasoconstrictor Drugs—Medications that cause blood vessels to contract, tighten or become smaller.

Vasodilator Drugs—Medications that cause small arteries to widen, providing more blood to an area of the body where the blood vessels are constricted by spasm, narrowed or obstructed.

Vector—1) An imaginary line that represents both direction and quantity used to study electrocardiograms (EKG's).
2) An agent that transmits infectious germs from one organism to another.

Veins—Blood vessels that return blood from body organs to the heart and lungs. Veins are much thinner than arteries. Veins carry blood at a much lower pressure than do arteries.

Vena Cava—Largest vein in the body. It collects blood from the venous system and carries it to the heart.

Venereal—Related to sexual intercourse or sexual contact. Venereal diseases such as genital herpes, gonorrhea, or syphilis are now usually referred to as "sexually transmitted diseases."

Venous System—Network of veins that extend from all body organs and transport blood back to the heart.

Ventricles—Chambers containing fluid. The ventricles of the heart pump blood; ventricles of the brain contain cerebrospinal fluid.

Ventricular Aneurysm—Ballooning of the wall of the heart resulting from a weakening of the heart muscle, a complication of scarring from a previous heart attack.

Vertebrae—Bones of the spine that form the vertebral column (backbone).

Vertebral Column—The spine; the bones of the back.

Virulent—Extremely dangerous or harmful. Virulent bacteria are ones capable of causing diseases.

Viruses—Small germs responsible for a variety of infectious illnesses. Viruses are not alive until they enter cells of the body, where they grow and reproduce, causing viral illnesses.

Visual Acuity—Clarity with which objects are seen.

Vitamins—Chemical substances found in food that are necessary for healthy body growth, function and tissue repair.

Vitreous—Clear fluid that fills much of the eye.

Vocal Cords—Two narrow bands of fibrous and muscular tissue in the larynx that vibrate to create the sounds of the voice.

Volvulus—Twisting of loops of intestines, which become closed off (obstructed) and may lose their blood supply.

W

Warts—Small, often hard and rough skin growths caused by viruses that infect the skin.

Wasting of Body or Muscles—Severe loss of body tissues (other than surplus fat), especially muscles and vital organs, resulting in weakness, susceptibility to infection, bone fractures and sometimes death.

Weber Test—Hearing test performed with a tuning fork.

Wheezes—High-pitched sounds and whistles produced in the lungs where secretions have partially blocked air passages.

Whirlpool Treatment—Method of treating minor blood-vessel and musculo-skeletal diseases by immersion in a pool where jets of warm water enter and swirl under high pressure.

Wisdom Teeth—Same as *Third Molars*.

X

Xeroradiogram—Method of X-ray diagnosis, usually of the female breast, which uses a process similar to that used to produce photocopies.

X-Rays—High energy, invisible waves capable of penetrating the body and creating shadows on photographic film. The shadows provide images of the body tissues through which the X-rays pass.

Z

Zoster—"Girdle," used to describe a form of virus infection (herpes zoster, shingles) that often produces bands of inflammation across the chest or abdomen.

RESOURCES FOR ADDITIONAL INFORMATION

Abortion

Alternatives to Abortion International
Hillcrest Hotel, Suite 511
16th and Madison Sts.
Toledo, OH 43699
(419) 248-4471

National Abortion Rights Action League
825 15th St. N. W.
Washington, DC 20005
(202) 347-7774

Aging

National Center on Arts and the Aging
National Council on the Aging
600 Maryland Ave. S. W.
Washington, DC 20024
(202) 479-1200

Alcoholism

Al-Anon Family Group Headquarters
1 Park Ave.
New York, NY 10016
(212) 481-6565

Alateen World Service Headquarters
1 Park Ave.
New York, NY 10016
(212) 481-6565

Alcoholics Anonymous World Services
P. O. Box 459
Grand Central Station
New York, NY 10163
(212) 686-1100

General Service Board of
  Alcoholics Anonymous (AA)
468 Park Ave. S.
New York, NY 10016
(212) 686-1100

Amputation

National Amputation Foundation, Inc.
12-45 150th St.
Whitestone, NY 11357
(212) 767-8400

Amyotrophic Lateral Sclerosis

Amyotrophic Lateral Sclerosis
  Society of America
15300 Ventura Blvd., Suite 315
P. O. Box 5951
Sherman Oaks, CA 91403
(213) 990-2151

National ALS Foundation, Inc.
185 Madison Ave.
New York, NY 10016
(212) 679-4016

Anorexia Nervosa

American Anorexia Nervosa Association
133 Cedar La.
Teaneck, NJ 07666
(201) 836-1800

The National Association of Anorexia
  Nervosa & Associated Disorders
Box 271
Highland Park, IL 60035
(312) 831-3438

Arthritis

Arthritis Foundation (AF)
3400 Peachtree Rd. N. E.
Atlanta, GA 30326
(404) 266-0795

American Rheumatism Association (ARA)
c/o Arthritis Foundation

National Institute of Arthritis
  & Metabolic Diseases
Bldg. 31
9000 Rockville Pike
Bethesda, MD 20205

Asthma & Allergy

Asthma & Allergy Foundation of America
9604 Wisconsin Ave., Suite 100
Bethesda, MD 20814
(301) 493-6552

Autism

National Society for Children and Adults
  with Autism
1234 Massachusetts Ave. N. W.
Suite 1017
Washington, DC 20005
(202) 783-0125

Biofeedback

Biofeedback Society of America
c/o Francine Butler, Ph. D.
4301 Owens St.
Wheat Ridge, CO 80033
(303) 420-2889

Birth Control & Family Planning

Association for Voluntary Sterilization
122 E. 42nd St.
New York, NY 10168
(212) 986-3880

Planned Parenthood Federation of America
810 Seventh Ave.
New York, NY 10019
(212) 541-7800

Birth Defects

National Foundation March of Dimes
1275 Mamaroneck Ave.
White Plains, NY 10605
(914) 428-7100

Blindness

American Foundation for the Blind (AFB)
15 W. 16th St.
New York, NY 10011
(212) 620-2000

Eye Bank Association of America
6560 Fannin, Level 9
Houston, TX 77030
(713) 790-5949

New Eyes for the Needy
549 Milburn Ave.
Short Hills, NJ 07078
(201) 376-4903

Breast-Feeding

La Leche League International, Inc.
9619 Minneapolis Ave.
Franklin Park, IL 60131
(312) 455-7730

Burns

National Institute of Burn Medicine
909 E. Ann St.
Ann Arbor, MI 48104
(313) 769-9000

Cancer

American Cancer Society (ACS)
777 3rd Ave.
New York, NY 10017
(212) 371-2900

Breast Cancer Advisory Center
P. O. Box 224
Kensington, MD 20895
(301) 984-1020

International Association of
Laryngectomees (IAL)
c/o American Cancer Society

Reach to Recovery Foundation
c/o American Cancer Society

United Ostomy Association
1111 Wilshire Blvd.
Los Angeles, CA 90017
(213) 481-2811

Cerebral Palsy

United Cerebral Palsy Association (ACPA)
66 E. 34th St.
New York, NY 10016
(212) 481-6300

Cleft Palate

American Cleft Palate Association
331 Salk Hall
University of Pittsburgh
Pittsburgh, PA 15261
(412) 681-9620

Cystic Fibrosis

Cystic Fibrosis Foundation
6000 Executive Blvd.
Suite 309
Rockville, MD 20852
(301) 881-9130

Dental Problems

American Dental Association
211 E. Chicago Ave.
Chicago, IL 60611
(312) 440-2500

Diabetes

American Association of Diabetes
  Educators (AADE)
Box 56, N. Woodbury Rd.
Pitman, NJ 08071
(609) 589-4831

American Diabetes Association (ADA)
2 Park Ave.
New York, NY 10016
(212) 683-7444

Juvenile Diabetes Foundation (JDF)
23 E. 26th St.
New York, NY 10010
(212) 889-7575

Drugs

Food & Drug Administration
5600 Fisher's Lane
Rockville, MD 20857

Endocrine Disorders
  **(Thyroid, Parathyroid, Pituitary,
  Sex Glands, Adrenals)**

National Institute of Metabolic Disease
9650 Rockville Pike
Bethesda, MD 20205

Epilepsy

Epilepsy Foundation of America (EFA)
4351 Garden City, Suite 406
Landover, MD 20785
(301) 459-3700

Foot Disorders

American Podiatry Association
20 Chevy Chase Circle N. W.
Washington, DC 20015

Genetics

National Genetics Foundation
555 W. 57th St.
New York, NY 10019
(212) 586-5800

Handicapped

Disabled American Veterans
P. O. Box 14301
Cincinnati, OH 45214

Goodwill Industries of America
9200 Wisconsin Ave.
Bethesda, MD 20814-3896
(301) 530-6500

Information Center for Individuals
  with Disabilities, Inc.
20 Park Plaza, Suite 330
Boston, MA 02116
(617) 727-5540

Institute for the Crippled & Disabled
400 First Ave.
New York, NY 10010

National Easter Seal Society
2023 W. Ogden Ave.
Chicago, IL 60612
(312) 243-8400

National Society for Crippled
  Children & Adults
2023 W. Ogden Ave.
Chicago, IL 60612

Hearing or Speech Impairment

Alexander Graham Bell Association
  for the Deaf
3417 Volta Place N. W.
Washington, DC 20007
(202) 337-5220

American Hearing Society
919 18th St. N. W.
Washington, DC 20006

American Speech-Language-Hearing
  Association
10801 Rockville Pike
Rockville, MD 20852
(301) 897-5700

National Association of the Deaf
814 Thayer Ave.
Silver Spring, MD 20910
(301) 587-1788

Self Help for Hard of Hearing People, Inc.
P. O. Box 34889
Bethesda, MD 20817
(301) 469-7222

Heart Disease

American Heart Association
7320 Greenville Ave.
Dallas, TX 75231
(214) 750-5300

Hemophilia

National Hemophilia Foundation (NHF)
19 W. 34th St., Room 1204
New York, NY 10001
(212) 563-0211

Herpes, Genital

Herpes Resource Center
Box 100
Palo Alto, CA 94302

Hypertension

Citizens for the Treatment of
   High Blood Pressure, Inc.
1140 Connecticut Ave. N. W., Suite 604
Washington, DC 20036
(202) 296-7747

National High Blood Pressure
   Information Center
NIH 120/80
Bethesda, MD 20014

Hypoglycemia

Adrenal Metabolic Research Society
   of the Hypoglycemia Foundation, Inc.
153 Pawling Ave.
Troy, NY 12180
(518) 272-7154

Infectious Diseases

Centers for Disease Control (CDC)
1600 Clifton Rd. N. E.
Atlanta, GA 30333
(404) 329-3311

Kidney Disease

National Kidney Foundation
2 Park Ave.
New York, NY 10016

Leukemia

Leukemia Society of America, Inc.
800 Second Ave.
New York, NY 10017
(212) 573-8484

Lung Disease

National Heart, Lung & Blood Institute
Information Center
Bethesda, MD 20014

Lupus Erythematosus

American Lupus Society
23751 Madison St.
Torrance, CA 90505
(213) 373-1335

National Lupus Erythematosus Foundation
   (NLEF)
5430 Van Nuys Blvd., Suite 206
Van Nuys, CA 91401
(213) 885-8787

Mental Health

Community Guidance Service
120 W. 58th St.
New York, NY 10019

Institute for the Development
   of Emotional and Life Skills
P. O. Box 391
State College, PA 16801
(814) 237-4805

National Mental Health Association
1800 N. Kent St.
Arlington, VA 22209
(703) 528-6405

Recovery, Inc.
116 S. Michigan Ave.
Chicago, IL 60603

Mental Retardation

Association for Children with
   Retarded Mental Development, Inc.
   (A/CRMD)
817 Broadway
New York, NY 10003
(212) 470-7200

President's Committee on Mental
   Retardation
Regional Office, Bldg. 3
7th & D Sts. S. W.
Washington, DC 20201
(202) 245-7634

Migraine

National Migraine Foundation
5252 N. Western Ave.
Chicago, IL 60625
(312) 878-7715

Miscellaneous

American Red Cross (ARC)
17th and D Sts. N. W.
Washington, DC 20006
(202) 737-8300

Medic Alert Foundation
Box K-7
Turlock, CA 95380

U. S. Committee for the World Health
  Organization (USA-WHO)
777 United Nations Plaza, 9A
New York, NY 10017
(212) 986-8451

Multiple Sclerosis

National Multiple Sclerosis Society (NMSS)
205 E. 42nd St.
New York, NY 10017
(212) 986-3240

Muscular Dystrophy

Muscular Dystrophy Association, Inc.
810 7th Ave.
New York, NY 10019
(212) 586-0808

Myasthenia Gravis

Myasthenia Gravis Foundation
15 E. 26th St.
New York, NY 10010
(212) 889-8157

Ostomy

International Association for
  Enterostomal Therapy
505 N. Tustin Ave., Suite 282
Santa Ana, CA 92705
(714) 972-1720

United Ostomy Association, Inc.
2001 W. Beverly Blvd.
Los Angeles, CA 90057
(213) 413-5510

Parkinson's Disease

American Parkinson Disease Association
116 John St. , Suite 417
New York, NY 10038
(212) 732-9550

National Parkinson Foundation (NPF)
1501 N. W. 9th Ave.
Miami, FL 33136
(305) 324-0156

United Parkinson Foundation (UPF)
220 S. State St.
Chicago, IL 60604
(312) 922-9734

Plastic Surgery

Society for the Rehabilitation
  of the Facially Disfigured, Inc.
550 First Ave.
New York, NY 10016

Psoriasis

National Psoriasis Foundation
6415 S. W. Canyon Court, Suite 200
Portland, OR 97221
(503) 297-1545

Rape Crisis

Women Organized Against Rape
P. O. Box 64
Harrisburg, PA 17108
(800) 692-7445

Reye's Syndrome

National Reye's Syndrome Foundation, Inc.
426 N. Lewis
P. O. Box 829
Bryan, OH 43506
(419) 636-2679

Scleroderma

United Scleroderma Foundation
305 W. Beach St.
P. O. Box 350
Watsonville, CA 95077-0350
(408) 728-2202

Scoliosis

Scoliosis Association, Inc.
One Penn Plaza
New York, NY 10119
(212) 845-1760

Sexuality

American Association of Sex Educators,
Counselors and Therapists (AASECT)
11 Dupont Circle, N. W.
Suite 220
Washington, DC 20036

American Social Health Association
260 Sheridan Ave.
Palo Alto, CA 94306

Sex Information and Education
Council of the U. S. (SIECUS)
80 Fifth Ave., Suite 801
New York, NY 10011
(212) 929-2300

Sickle-Cell Anemia

National Association for Sickle Cell Disease
3460 Wilshire Blvd., Suite 1012
Los Angeles, CA 90010
(213) 731-1166

Smoking

Smokenders
37 N. 3rd St.
Easton, PA 18042

Spinal Injury

American Spinal Injury Association
250 E. Superior, Room 619
Chicago, IL 60611
(312) 649-3425

Sudden Infant Death Syndrome

National Sudden Infant Death
Syndrome Foundation (NSIDSF)
310 S. Michigan Ave., Suite 1904
Chicago, IL 60604
(312) 663-0650

Tay-Sachs Disease

National Tay-Sachs &
Allied Diseases Association, Inc.
(NTSAD)
92 Washington Ave.
Cedarhurst, NY 11516
(516) 569-4300

Weight Control

TOPS Club, Inc.
4575 S. Fifth St.
P. O. Box 07489
Milwaukee, WI 53207
(414) 482-4620

SUGGESTED READING FOR ADDITIONAL INFORMATION

AIDS

Fettner, Ann Giudici. *The Truth About A. I. D. S.: Evolution of an Epidemic.* New York: Rinehart & Winston, 1984.

Kassler, Jeanne. *Gay Men's Health: A Guide to the AID Syndrome and Other Sexually Transmitted Diseases.* New York: Harper Row, 1983.

Alcoholism

Elkin, Michael. *Families Under the Influence: Changing Alcoholic Patterns.* New York: Norton, 1984.

Mumey, Jack. *The Joy of Being Sober: A Book For Recovering Alcoholics—and Those Who Love Them.* Chicago: Contemporary Books, 1984.

O'Brien, Robert, ed. *Encyclopedia of Alcoholism.* New York: Facts on File, 1982.

Alzheimer's Disease

Heston, Leonaro L. *Dementia: A Practical Guide to Alzheimer's Disease and Related Illnesses.* New York: W. H. Freeman, 1983.

Arthritis

Fries, James F. *Arthritis: A Comprehensive Guide.* Reading, Ma.: Addison-Wesley, 1979.

Hart, F. Dudley. *Overcoming Arthritis.* New York: Arco, 1981.

*McCarty, Daniel J., ed. *Arthritis and Allied Conditions: A Textbook of Rheumatology,* 10th ed. Philadelphia: Lea & Febiger, 1984.

Asthma

Berland, Theodore. *Living With Your Allergies and Asthma.* New York: St. Martin, 1983.

Lane, Donald J., and Anthony Storr. *Asthma: The Facts.* New York: Oxford University Press, 1979.

Back Pain

Stoddard, Alan. *The Back—Relief From Pain. Patterns of Back Pain—How to Deal With and Avoid Them.* New York: Arco, 1979.

*Textbook or medical reference containing technical language.

Blood Disorders

*Beck, William S., ed. *Hematology,* 3rd ed. Cambridge, Ma.: MIT Press, 1981.

Cancer

Burns, Sheila. *Cancer: Understanding and Fighting It.* New York: Messner, 1982.

*Del Ragato, Juan, and Harlan Spjut. *Ackerman and Del Ragato's Cancer: Diagnosis, Treatment, and Prognosis,* 5th ed. St. Louis, Mo.: Mosby, 1977.

Hausman, Patricia. *Foods that Fight Cancer: A Diet & Vitamin Program That Protects the Entire Family.* New York: Rawson Assoc., 1984.

Levitt, Paul. *The Cancer Reference Book: Direct and Clear Answers to Everyone's Questions,* rev. ed. New York: Facts on File, 1983.

McKhann, Charles F. *The Facts About Cancer: A Guide for Patients, Family and Friends.* New York: Prentice-Hall, 1981.

Margie, Joyce Daly. *Nutrition and the Cancer Patient.* Huntington Beach, Ca.: Chilton, 1983.

National Research Council on Diet, Nutrition and Cancer. *Diet, Nutrition, and Cancer.* Washington, DC: National Academy Press, 1982.

Rosenbaum, Ernest H., and Isadora Rosenbaum. *A Comprehensive Guide for Patients and Their Families.* Palo Alto, Ca.: Bull Publishing Co., 1980.

White, Kristin. *Diet and Cancer.* New York: Bantam, 1984.

Children's Health

Boston Children's Medical Center. *Child Health Encyclopedia.* New York: Dell, 1978.

Boston Women's Health Book Collective. *Ourselves and Our Children: A Book By and For Parents.* New York: Random, 1978.

Diagram Group. *Child's Body: A Parent's Manual.* New York: Paddington, 1977.

Haessler, Herbert. *How to Make Sure Your Baby is Well and Stays that Way: The First Guide to over 400 Medical Tests and Treatments You Can Do at Home to Check Your Baby's Daily Health and Growth.* New York: Rawson Assoc., 1984.

Hart, Terril H. *The Parent's Guide to Baby and Child Medical Care.* Deephaven, Mn.: Meadowbrook, 1982.

Pomeranz, Virginia E. *The Mother's and Father's Medical Encyclopedia,* rev. ed. New York: New American Library, 1984.

*Silver, Henry K. *Handbook of Pediatrics,* 14th ed. Los Altos, Ca.: Lange, 1983.

*Textbook or medical reference containing technical language.

Cold, Common

Murphy, Wendy B. *Coping With the Common Cold.* Alexandria, Va.: Time-Life, 1981.

Dental Care

Wood, Norman. *The Complete Book of Dental Care.* New York: Hart, 1979.

Diabetes

Court, John M. *Helping Your Diabetic Child.* New York: Taplinger, 1974.

Jorgenson, Carol Dow. *The ABC's of Diabetes.* New York: Crown, 1978.

Down's Syndrome

Pueschel, Siegfried M. *The Young Child With Down Syndrome.* New York: Human Sciences Press, 1984.

Drug Abuse

Ausubel, David P. *What Every Well-Informed Person Should Know About Drug Addiction.* Chicago: Nelson-Hall, 1980.

Baron, Jason D. *Kids and Drugs: A Parent's Handbook of Drug Abuse Treatment and Prevention.* New York: Putnam Pub. Group, 1983.

O'Brien, Robert, ed. *Encyclopedia of Drug Abuse.* New York: Facts on File, 1984.

Rolling Stone, eds. *How to Get Off Drugs.* New York: Simon & Schuster, 1984.

Drugs

*Goodman, L. S., and A. Gilman, eds. *The Pharmacological Basis of Therapeutics,* 6th ed. New York: MacMillan, 1980.

Griffith, H. Winter. *Complete Guide to Prescription & Non-Prescription Drugs,* rev. ed. Tucson, Az.: HPBooks, 1985.

Long, James W. *Essential Guide to Prescription Drugs: What You Need to Know for Safe Drug Use,* 4th ed. New York: Harper Row, 1985.

Physician's Desk Reference, 39th ed. Oradell, N. J.: Medical Economics, 1985.

*Textbook or medical reference containing technical language.

Eating Disorders

Arenson, Gloria. *Binge Eating: How to Stop It Forever.* New York: Rawson Associates, 1984.

Kinoy, Barbara P. *When Will We Laugh Again? Living and Dealing With Anorexia Nervosa and Bulimia.* New York: Columbia University Press, 1984.

Levenkron, Steven. *Treating and Overcoming Anorexia Nervosa.* New York: Scribner, 1982.

Elderly, Health Care for

Blacker, M. M., and D. R. Wekstein. *Your Health After 60.* New York: Dutton, 1979.

*Reichel, William, ed. *Clinical Aspects of Aging: A Comprehensive Text,* 2nd ed. Prepared under the direction of the American Geriatric Society. Baltimore, Md.: Williams & Wilkins, 1983.

Emergency Care

American Medical Association. *The American Medical Association's Handbook of First Aid and Emergency Care.* New York: Random, 1980.

Green, Martin I. *Lifesavers: The Complete Home Medical & Emergency Handbook.* New York: Ballantine, 1982.

Hocutt, John E. *Emergency Medicine: A Quick Reference for Primary Care.* East Norwalk, Ct.: Appleton-Century-Crofts, 1982.

Emphysema

Shayevitz, Myra and Berton Shayevitz. *Living Well With Emphysema & Bronchitis: A Handbook for Everyone With Chronic Obstructive Pulmonary Disease.* New York: Doubleday, 1985.

Endocrinology

*Williams, Robert H. *Textbook of Endocrinology,* 6th ed. Philadelphia: Saunders, 1981.

Epilepsy

Sands, Harry, ed. *Epilepsy: The Mental Health Professional Guide.* New York: Brunner-Mazel, 1981.

*Textbook or medical reference containing technical language.

Eye

Eden, John. *The Eye Book.* New York: Viking, 1978.

*Newell, Frank W. *Ophthalmology: Principles and Concepts,* 5th ed. St. Louis, Mo.: Mosby, 1982.

Vaughan, Daniel. *General Ophthalmology,* 10th ed. Los Altos, Ca.: Lange, 1983.

Fertility

Stangel, John J. *Fertility and Conception: An Essential Guide For Childless Couples.* New York: Facts on File, 1979.

Foot Care

Feigel, William, and Dennis Zamzow. *Foot Care Book.* Mountain View, Ca.: Anderson World, 1982.

Gastrointestinal Disorders

*Sleinsenger, Marvin H., and John S. Fordtran. *Gastrointestinal Disease: Pathophysiology, Diagnosis, Management,* 3rd ed. Philadelphia: Saunders, 1983. 2 vols.

General

The American Medical Association. *Family Medical Guide.* New York: Random, 1982.

Consumer Guide, eds. *Family Medical Guide: The Illustrated Medical and Health Advisor.* New York: Morrow, 1983.

* *Dorland's Medical Dictionary.* New York: Harper and Row, 1982.

Good Housekeeping Concise Medical Encyclopedia. New York: Hearst, 1981.

Gottlieb, Bill, ed. *Prevention's New Encyclopedia of Common Diseases.* Emmaus, Pa.: Rodale Press, 1984.

Horton, Edward, and Felicity Smart, eds. *The Illustrated Encyclopedia of Family Health.* London: Marshall Cavendish Ltd.: 1984. 24 vols.

*Isselbacher, K. J., ed. *Harrison's Principles of Internal Medicine,* 10th ed. New York: McGraw-Hill, 1983. 2 vols.

Johnson, G. Timothy. *Doctor! What You Should Know About Health Care Before You Call a Physician.* New York: McGraw-Hill, 1975.

*Krupp, Marcus A., and Milton J. Chatton. *Current Medical Diagnosis and Treatment.* Los Altos, Ca.: Lange, 1984.

Landers, Ann. *Ann Landers' Encyclopedia A to Z.* New York: Ballantine, 1979.

*Textbook or medical reference containing technical language.

Merck Manual of Diagnosis and Therapy, 14th ed. Rahway, N. J.: Merck, 1982.

Mosby's Medical and Nursing Dictionary. St. Louis, Mo.: Mosby, 1983.

Moskowitz, Mark A., and Michael E. Osband. *Complete Book of Medical Tests.* New York: Norton, 1984.

The Physicians' Manual For Patients. New York: Times Books, 1984.

Professional Guide to Diseases. Springhouse, Pa: Intermed Communications, 1982.

*Rakel, Robert E., ed. *Conn's Current Therapy,* 1985. Philadelphia: W. B. Saunders Co., 1985.

*Rakel, Robert, and Howard F. Conn. *Textbook of Family Practice,* 3rd ed. Philadelphia: Saunders, 1984.

Headache

Murphy, Wendy B. *Dealing With Headaches.* Alexandria, Va.: Time-Life, 1982.

Saper, Joel R., and Kenneth R. Magee. *Freedom From Headaches: A Personal Guide For Understanding and Treating Headache, Face and Neck Pain.* New York: Simon & Schuster, 1980.

Wilkinson, Marcia. *Migraine & Headaches: Understanding, Controlling, and Avoiding the Pain.* New York: Arco, 1982.

Heart Disease

American Heart Association. *The American Heart Association Cookbook.* New York: Ballantine, 1980.

American Heart Association. *Heartbook: A Guide to Prevention and Treatment of Cardiovascular Diseases.* New York: Dutton, 1980.

Amsterdam, Ezra A. *Take Care of Your Heart.* New York: Facts on File, 1984.

Gasner, Douglas. *The American Medical Association's Book of Heart Care.* New York: Random, 1982.

Hochman, Gloria. *Heart Bypass: What Every Patient Must Know.* New York: St. Martin, 1982.

*Hurst, John Willis. *The Heart: Arteries and Veins,* 5th ed. New York: McGraw-Hill, 1982. 2 vols.

Phibbs, Brendan. *The Human Heart: A Consumer's Guide to Cardiac Care.* St. Louis, Mo: Mosby, 1982.

Yalof, Ina L. *Open Heart Surgery: A Guidebook For Patients and Families,* 1st ed. New York: Random, 1983.

*Textbook or medical reference containing technical language.

Hypertension

Freis, Edward D., and Gina Bari Kolata. *The High Blood Pressure Book: A Guide for Patients and Their Families.* New York: Dutton, 1979.

O'Brien, Eoin T. *High Blood Pressure: What it Means for You, and How to Control It.* New York: Arco, 1981.

Infectious Diseases

*Top, F. H., and P. F. Wehrle, eds. *Communicable and Infectious Diseases,* 9th ed. St. Louis, Mo: Mosby, 1981.

Kidney Disease

*Brenner, B. M., and F. C. Rector. *The Kidney,* 2nd ed. Philadelphia: Saunders, 1981. 2 vols.

Cameron, Stewart. *Kidney Disease: The Facts.* New York: Oxford University Press, 1981.

Lung Disorders

Better Living and Breathing: A Manual for Patients, 2nd ed. St. Louis, Mo.: Mosby, 1980.

Lupus Erythematosus, Systemic

Blau, Sheldon Paul. *Lupus: The Body Against Itself,* rev. ed. New York: Doubleday, 1984.

Mental Health

Benson, Herbert. *Beyond the Relaxation Response: How to Harness the Healing Power of Your Personal Beliefs.* New York: Times Books, 1984.

*Freeman, Alfred M. *Comprehensive Textbook of Psychiatry,* 3rd ed. Baltimore, Md.: Williams & Wilkins, 1980. 2 vols.

Mishara, Brian, and Robert Patterson. *The Consumer's Guide to Mental Health: How to Find, Select, and Use Help.* New York: Times Books, 1977.

Rubin, Theodore Isaac. *Not to Worry: The American Family Book of Mental Health.* New York: Viking, 1984.

Wender, Paul H. *Mind, Mood, and Medicine: A Guide to the New Biopsychiatry.* New York: New American Library, 1982.

*Textbook or medical reference containing technical language.

Multiple Sclerosis

Scheinberg, Labe C., ed. *Multiple Sclerosis: A Guide For Patients and Their Families.* New York: Raven, 1983.

Nutrition

*Goodhart, Robert S., and Maurice E. Shils, eds. *Modern Nutrition in Health and Disease: Dietotherapy,* 6th ed. Philadelphia: Lea & Febiger, 1980.

Stare, Frederick. *Nutrition for Good Health.* Philadelphia: G. F. Stickley, 1982.

Obesity

Mirkin, Gabe. *Getting Thin: All About Fat—How You Get It, How You Lose It, How You Keep It Off For Good.* Boston, Ma.: Little, Brown & Co., 1983.

Orthopedics

*Brashear, Robert H., and Richard Beverly Raney. *Shand's Handbook of Orthopedic Surgery,* 9th ed. St. Louis, Mo.: Mosby, 1978.

Ostomy

Vukovich, Virginia. *Care of the Ostomy Patient.* St. Louis, Mo.: Mosby, 1982.

Parkinson's Disease

Duvoisin, Roger C. *Parkinson's Disease: A Guide for Patient and Family,* 2nd ed. Mahonoy City, Pa.: Raven, 1984.

Plastic Surgery

Cirillo, Dennis P. *The Complete Book of Cosmetic Facial Surgery: A Step-by-Step Guide to the Physical and Psychological Process, by a Plastic Surgeon and a Psychiatrist.* New York: Simon & Schuster, 1984.

Heidi, Gloria. *New Beginnings: Cosmetic Surgery for Men and Women.* New York: Putnam, 1982.

Poisoning

*Dreisbach, Robert M. *Handbook of Poisoning: Prevention, Diagnosis and Treatment,* 11th ed. Los Altos, Ca.: Lange, 1983.

*Textbook or medical reference containing technical language.

Pregnancy

Cherry, Sheldon H. *Rovinsky & Guttmacher's Medical, Surgical & Gynecological*

Russell, Keith P. *Eastman's Expectant Motherhood.* Boston: Little, Brown & Co., 1983.

Freeman, Roger K. *Safe Delivery: Protecting Your Baby During High Risk Pregnancy.* New York: Facts on File, 1982.

Sexual Dysfunction

*Kaplan, Helen S. *The Evaluation of Sexual Disorders: Psychological & Medical Aspects.* New York: Brunner-Mazel, 1983.

Sexually Transmitted Diseases

Lumiere, Richard. *Healthy Sex—and Keeping it That Way: A Complete Guide to Sexual Infections.* New York: Simon & Schuster, 1983.

Skin Disorders

*Fitzpatrick, Thomas B., ed. *Dermatology in General Medicine,* 2nd ed. New York: McGraw Hill, 1979.

Goldstein, Norman. *The Skin You Live In: How to Recognize and Prevent Skin Problems and Keep Your Skin Youthful and Attractive.* New York: Hart, 1978.

Sterilization

Wylie, Evan M. *All About Voluntary Sterilization.* New York: Berkley, 1977.

Stroke

Sarno, John E., and Martha Taylor Sarno. *Stroke: A Guide for Patients and Their Families.* New York: McGraw-Hill, 1979.

Sudden Infant Death Syndrome (SIDS)

Bergman, Abraham B. *Why Did My Baby Die? The Phenomenon of Sudden Infant Death Syndrome & How to Cope With It.* New York: Okpaku Communications, 1975.

*Textbook or medical reference containing technical language.

Surgery, General

Crile, George, Jr. *Surgery: Your Choices, Your Alternatives.* New York: Delacorte, 1978.

*Sabiston, David G., ed. *David-Christopher Textbook of Surgery,* 12th ed. Philadelphia: Saunders, 1981. 2 vols.

Schneider, Robert G. *When to Say No to Surgery: How to Evaluate the Most Often Performed Operations.* New York: Prentice-Hall, 1982.

*Way, Lawrence W., ed. *Current Surgical Diagnosis and Treatment,* 6th ed. Los Altos, Ca.: Lange, 1983.

Urology

*Smith, Donald R. *General Urology,* 11th ed. Los Altos, Ca.: Lange, 1984.

Women's Health

Boston Women's Health Book Collective. *The New Our Bodies, Ourselves.* New York: Simon & Schuster, 1985.

Cherry, Sheldon H. *For Women of All Ages: A Gynecological Guide to Modern Female Health Care.* New York: MacMillan, 1979.

*Danforth, David N., ed. *Obstetrics and Gynecology,* 4th ed. New York: Harper, 1982.

Diagram Group. *Woman's Body: An Owner's Manual.* New York: Paddington, 1977.

Gifford-Jones, W. *What Every Woman Should Know About Hysterectomy.* New York: Funk & Wagnalls, 1977.

Holt, Linda Hughey. *The American Medical Association Guide to Womancare,* rev. ed. New York: Random, 1984.

Scott, Joseph W. *Woman, Know Thyself.* Thorofare, N. J.: Charles B. Slack, 1976.

Stewart, Felicia Hance. *My Body, My Health: The Concerned Women's Guide to Gynecology.* New York: Bantam, 1981.

*Textbook or medical reference containing technical language.

Index

INDEX

INDEX

INDEX

INDEX

INDEX

EMERGENCY FIRST AID

ANAPHYLAXIS (Severe allergic reaction)

Symptoms

Itching, rash, hives, runny nose, wheezing, paleness, cold sweats, low blood pressure, coma, cardiac arrest.

Treatment

If Victim is Unconscious, Not Breathing:

1. Yell for help. Don't leave victim.
2. Begin mouth-to-mouth breathing immediately.
3. If there is no heartbeat, give external cardiac massage.
4. Have someone call 0 (operator) or 911 (emergency) for an ambulance or medical help.
5. Don't stop cardiopulmonary resuscitation (CPR) until help arrives.

If Victim is Unconscious and Breathing:

1. Dial 0 (operator) or 911 (emergency) for an ambulance or emergency medical help.
2. If you can't get help immediately, take patient to nearest emergency room or other facility with adequate equipment and personnel to care for medical emergencies.

BLEEDING

Symptoms

Bleeding caused by any serious injury should be treated in an emergency facility. There is usually a lot of bright-red blood pumping from an injured artery, or darker blood if a large vein has been injured.

Treatment

1. Call for ambulance or take to emergency room. In the meantime, render first aid yourself.
2. Cover entire injured area with cloth or bare hands if no cloth is available.
3. Apply strong pressure directly on injured area for 10 minutes while awaiting ambulance or transporting to emergency room.
4. If direct pressure doesn't control brisk bleeding and emergency assistance will not be available within 5 minutes, use a tourniquet *as a last resort* to prevent death from bleeding. Make a tourniquet from a length of cloth or similar material. Wrap and tie the tourniquet around extremity above the wound. Place a stick or other rigid object between the cloth and the extremity. Twist the rigid object several times until tight pressure has been applied and bleeding stops. Note how long the tourniquet is in place so emergency medical personnel will know.

BURNS

Symptoms

First- and second-degree burns are not usually life-threatening.
First-degree burns cause only red skin and mild swelling.
Second-degree burns cause blisters, pain and oozing.
Third-degree burns can be life-threatening if extensive. Skin turns white or appears charred.

Treatment

For first- and second-degree burns:

1. Apply lotion to cool first-degree burns. However, if marked swelling develops, seek emergency care.
2. Immerse small second- or third-degree burn areas (as from hot-grease splatters) in cold water for 10 minutes to reduce pain and swelling.
3. Keep the burn area clean. Soak in a tub or use warm compresses once a day. You may add 2 tablespoons of powdered detergent to the tub to help soak off crusting areas. Use plain water for compresse..
4. Prop the burn area higher than the rest of the body, if possible.
5. Use dressings on the burned area, if you wish.

For third-degree burns:

1. Don't use ice to "relieve" pain!
2. Keep patient lying flat and lightly covered to prevent shock.
3. Remove clothes and jewelry unless they are sticking to burned skin.
4. Take to emergency room.

Special instructions:

Electrical Burns — Turn off the source of electricity, if possible. If not, use a non-conductive material, such as a board or wooden chair, to pull the victim away from the electrical source. Don't use your bare hands. If the victim is not breathing, begin mouth-to-mouth breathing.

Chemical Burns of the Eye or Skin — Hold the victim's head or other burned area beneath a faucet. Turn on cool water at medium pressure. Rinse for at least 15 minutes, directing the water away from the unaffected area.

For Burns of Large Areas — Prepare a solution for the victim to drink on the way to the emergency room. Mix 1 quart of water with 1/3 teaspoon of salt and 1/3 teaspoon of baking soda. This may help prevent kidney failure.

CHOKING

Symptoms

Clutching at throat. Gagging or gasping for air. Sudden collapse without previous illness. Unable to speak. Breathing labored and wheezing if breathing is possible at all.

Treatment

1. Stand behind person, bend patient forward and give 3 or 4 sharp blows to back between shoulder blades.
2. If this doesn't dislodge obstruction, perform the Heimlich Maneuver as follows:

Heimlich Maneuver

1. Stand behind person, place both arms around his upper abdomen and grasp your wrists halfway between bottom of ribs and waistline, just above navel.
2. Give 3 or 4 quick forceful squeezes, pushing in and up.

Note: If you are alone and are choking, lean forward on your abdomen against back of a chair and push forcefully.

FRACTURES OR DISLOCATIONS

Symptoms

Extreme pain and tenderness in any injured area; change in appearance of injured part, such as swelling, protruding bone or blood under skin. Extremity, such as finger, arm or leg, may be bent out of normal alignment.

Treatment

1. Immobilize any injured area and keep movement to minimum. For obvious fractures of fingers, wrists, arms, legs, ankles or feet, improvise a splint from stiff rolled-up paper, scrap wood or metal.
2. Attach splint firmly to injured extremity with strips of cloth, twine or similar material to prevent movement.
3. If leg, back or neck is severely injured and possibly fractured or dislocated, keep patient warm and still until ambulance arrives. Don't move the victim.

HEART ATTACK

Symptoms

Chest pain lasting more than 2 minutes that radiates into jaw or arm. Heavy sweating without obvious other cause. Weakness, nausea, pale skin. Irregular pulse.

Treatment

If Victim is Unconscious, Not Breathing:

1. Yell for help. Don't leave victim.
2. Begin mouth-to-mouth breathing immediately.
3. If there is no heartbeat, give external cardiac massage.
4. Have someone call 0 (operator) or 911 (emergency) for an ambulance or medical help.
5. Don't stop cardiopulmonary resuscitation (CPR) until help arrives.

If Victim is Unconscious and Breathing:

1. Dial 0 (operator) or 911 (emergency) for an ambulance or emergency medical help.
2. If you can't get help immediately, take patient to nearest emergency room or other facility with adequate equipment and personnel to care for medical emergencies.

Conversion to Metric Measure

When You Know	Symbol	Multiply By	To Find	Symbol
VOLUME				
teaspoons	tsp.	4.93	milliliters	ml
tablespoons	tbsp.	14.79	milliliters	ml
fluid ounces	fl. oz.	29.57	milliliters	ml
cups	c.	0.24	liters	l
pints	pt.	0.47	liters	l
quarts	qt.	0.95	liters	l
gallons	gal.	3.79	liters	l
LENGTH				
inches	in	25.4	millimeters	mm
inches	in.	2.54	centimeters	cm
feet	ft.	30.48	centimeters	cm
yards	yd.	0.91	meters	m
TEMPERATURE				
Fahrenheit	F	0.56 (after subtracting 32)	Celsius	C